Essentials of Psychiatry

Third Edition

Essentials of Psychiatry

Third Edition

Edited by

Robert E. Hales, M.D., M.B.A.
Stuart C. Yudofsky, M.D.
Glen O. Gabbard, M.D.

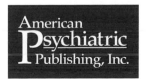

American Psychiatric Publishing, Inc.

Washington, DC
London, England

Copyright © 2011 American Psychiatric Publishing, Inc.
ALL RIGHTS RESERVED

Manufactured in the United States of America on acid-free paper
14 13 12 11 10   5 4 3 2 1
Third Edition

Typeset in Adobe's AvantGarde and Palatino.

American Psychiatric Publishing, Inc.
1000 Wilson Boulevard
Arlington, VA 22209-3901
www.appi.org

Library of Congress Cataloging-in-Publication Data
Essentials of psychiatry / edited by Robert E. Hales, Stuart C. Yudofsky, Glen O. Gabbard. — 3rd ed.
        p. ; cm.
    Rev. ed. of: Essentials of clinical psychiatry / edited by Robert E. Hales, Stuart C. Yudofsky. 2nd ed. c2004.
    Includes bibliographical references and index.
    ISBN 978-1-58562-933-6 (pbk. : alk. paper) 1. Psychiatry. I. Hales, Robert E. II. Yudofsky, Stuart C. III. Gabbard, Glen O. IV. American Psychiatric Publishing. V. Essentials of clinical psychiatry.
    [DNLM: 1. Mental Disorders. 2. Psychiatry. WM 140]
    RC454.E823 2010
    616.89—dc22
                                                                                2010030415

British Library Cataloguing in Publication Data
A CIP record is available from the British Library.

CONTENTS

Robert E. Hales, M.D., M.B.A.
Stuart C. Yudofsky, M.D.
Glen O. Gabbard, M.D.

1

Linda B. Andrews, M.D.

2

H. Florence Kim, M.D.
Paul E. Schulz, M.D.
Elisabeth A. Wilde, Ph.D.
Stuart C. Yudofsky, M.D.

3

James A. Bourgeois, O.D., M.D., F.A.P.M.
Jeffrey S. Seaman, M.S., M.D.
Mark E. Servis, M.D.

4

Martin H. Leamon, M.D.
Tara M. Wright, M.D.
Hugh Myrick, M.D.

5

Michael J. Minzenberg, M.D.
Jong H. Yoon, M.D.
Cameron S. Carter, M.D.

6

John A. Joska, M.D., M.Med.(Psych.), F.C.Psych.(S.A.)
Dan J. Stein, M.D., Ph.D.

CONTRIBUTORS

Linda B. Andrews, M.D.
Associate Dean for Graduate Medical Education, Director of Residency Education, Psychiatry, Baylor College of Medicine, Houston, Texas

L. Jarrett Barnhill, M.D.
Professor of Psychiatry and Director of the Developmental Neuropharmacology Clinic, Department of Psychiatry, Division of Child and Adolescent Psychiatry, University of North Carolina, Chapel Hill, North Carolina

Aaron T. Beck, M.D.
Professor of Psychiatry, University of Pennsylvania School of Medicine, Philadelphia, Pennsylvania

Heather A. Berlin, Ph.D., M.P.H.
Assistant Professor, Department of Psychiatry, Mount Sinai School of Medicine, New York, New York

Jed E. Black, M.D.
Associate Professor, Sleep Medicine Division, Stanford University; Medical Director, Stanford Sleep Medicine Clinic, Stanford, California

Dan G. Blazer, M.D., Ph.D.
J.P. Gibbons Professor of Psychiatry and Behavioral Sciences, Duke University School of Medicine, Durham, North Carolina

James A. Bourgeois, O.D., M.D., F.A.P.M.
Professor and Vice Chair, Education, Department of Psychiatry and Behavioural Neurosciences, Faculty of Health Sciences, Michael G. DeGroote School of Medicine, McMaster University, Hamilton, Ontario, Canada

Daniel J. Buysse, M.D.
Professor of Psychiatry, University of Pittsburgh School of Medicine; Director, Neuroscience Clinical and Translational Research Center, Department of Psychiatry, Western Psychiatric Institute and Clinic, Pittsburgh, Pennsylvania

Cameron S. Carter, M.D.
Professor of Psychiatry and Psychology; and Director, Imaging Research Center, University of California, Davis, School of Medicine, Sacramento, California

Stephen J. Cozza, M.D.
Associate Professor, Department of Psychiatry, and Associate Director, Center for the Study of Traumatic Stress, F. Edward Hébert School of Medicine, Uniformed Services University of the Health Sciences, Bethesda, Maryland

Glen C. Crawford, M.D.
Director of Medical Services and Clinical Support Services, Staff Child and Adolescent Forensic Psychiatrist, U.S. Naval Hospital, Naples, Italy; Assistant Professor of Psychiatry, F. Edward Hébert School of Medicine, Uniformed Services University of the Health Sciences, Bethesda, Maryland

Mantosh J. Dewan, M.D.
SUNY Distinguished Service Professor and Chair, Department of Psychiatry and Behavioral Sciences, SUNY Upstate Medical University, Syracuse, New York

Mina K. Dulcan, M.D.
Margaret C. Osterman Professor of Child Psychiatry and Psychiatrist-in-Chief, Children's Memorial Hospital; Head, Warren Wright Adolescent Center, Northwestern Memorial Hospital; Head, Child and Adolescent Psychiatry and Professor of Psychiatry and Behavioral Sciences and Pediatrics, Feinberg School of Medicine, Northwestern University, Chicago, Illinois

Glen O. Gabbard, M.D.
Brown Foundation Chair of Psychoanalysis and Professor of Psychiatry, Baylor College of Medicine, Houston, Texas

Roger P. Greenberg, Ph.D.
SUNY Distinguished Teaching Professor and Head, Psychology Division, Department of Psychiatry and Behavioral Sciences, SUNY Upstate Medical University

John G. Gunderson, M.D.
Professor of Psychiatry, Harvard Medical School, Boston; and Director, Psychosocial and Personality Research, McLean Hospital, Belmont, Massachusetts

Robert E. Hales, M.D., M.B.A.
Joe P. Tupin Endowed Chair, and Professor and Chair, Department of Psychiatry and Behavioral Sciences, University of California-Davis School of Medicine, Sacramento, California

Katherine A. Halmi, M.D.
Professor of Psychiatry, Eating Disorder Program, New York Presbyterian Hospital—Westchester Division, White Plains, New York

Eric Hollander, M.D.
Esther and Joseph Klingenstein Professor, Chair of Psychiatry; Director, Seaver and NY Autism Center of Excellence; Director of Clinical Psychopharmacology; Director, Compulsive, Impulsive, and Anxiety Dis-

orders Program; Mount Sinai School of Medicine, New York, New York

John A. Joska, M.D., M.Med.(Psych.), F.C.Psych.(S.A.)
Senior Specialist and Lecturer, Department of Psychiatry and Mental Health, University of Cape Town, South Africa

Paul H. Kartheiser, M.D.
Attending Child and Adolescent Psychiatrist, Dorothea Dix Hospital, Raleigh, North Carolina; Assistant Professor of Psychiatry, Department of Psychiatry, Division of Child and Adolescent Psychiatry, University of North Carolina, Chapel Hill, North Carolina

H. Florence Kim, M.D.
Assistant Professor, Medical Director, Neuropsychiatry Programs, Department of Psychiatry and Behavioral Sciences, Baylor College of Medicine, Houston, Texas

Kimberly G. Klipstein, M.D.
Director, Behavioral Medicine and Consultation Psychiatry, Department of Psychiatry, and Assistant Professor of Psychiatry, Mount Sinai School of Medicine, New York, New York

Susan G. Lazar, M.D.
Adjunct Professor, Department of Psychiatry, George Washington University School of Medicine, Washington, D.C.; Adjunct Professor, Department of Psychiatry, Uniformed Services University of the Health Sciences, F. Edward Hébert School of Medicine, Bethesda, Maryland; Training and Supervising Analyst, Washington Psychoanalytic Institute, Washington, D.C.

Martin H. Leamon, M.D.
Associate Professor of Clinical Psychiatry, Department of Psychiatry and Behavioral Sciences, University of California, Davis; Medical Director, Sacramento County Mental Health Treatment Center, Sacramento, California

Lauren B. Marangell, M.D.
Brown Foundation Chair, Psychopharmacology of Mood Disorders; Associate Professor of Psychiatry; and Director, Mood Disorders Research, Menninger Department of Psychiatry, Baylor College of Medicine; Associate Director of Research, South Central MIRECC, Department of Veterans Affairs, Houston, Texas

James M. Martinez, M.D.
Clinical Research Physician, Eli Lilly and Company, Indianapolis, Indiana; Assistant Professor of Psychiatry, and Associate Director, Mood Disorders Center, Menninger Department of Psychiatry, Baylor College of Medicine, South Central MIRECC, Department of Veterans Affairs, Houston, Texas

Melissa Martinez, M.D.
Assistant Professor of Psychiatry, Menninger Department of Psychiatry, Baylor College of Medicine, Houston, Texas

Michael J. Minzenberg, M.D.
Associate Professor, Imaging Research Center, University of California, Davis, School of Medicine, Sacramento, California

Hugh Myrick, M.D.
Associate Professor of Psychiatry, Medical University of South Carolina, Ralph H. Johnson VAMC, Charleston, South Carolina

Jeffrey H. Newcorn, M.D.
Associate Professor of Psychiatry and Pediatrics and Director, Division of Child and Adolescent Psychiatry, Mount Sinai Medical Center, New York, New York

Brooke S. Parish, M.D.
Assistant Professor of Psychiatry, Department of Psychiatry, University of New Mexico, Albuquerque, New Mexico

Paul E. Schulz, M.D.
Associate Professor, Department of Neurology, Baylor College of Medicine, Houston, Texas

Jeffrey S. Seaman, M.S., M.D.
Residency Training Director, Associate Professor of Psychiatry, Department of Psychiatry and Behavioral Sciences, University of Oklahoma Health Sciences Center, Oklahoma City, Oklahoma

Mark E. Servis, M.D.
Roy T. Brophy Professor and Vice Chair for Education, Department of Psychiatry and Behavioral Sciences, University of California Davis, School of Medicine, Sacramento, California

Daniel W. Shuman, J.D.
Professor of Law, Southern Methodist University, Dedman School of Law, Dallas, Texas

Daphne Simeon, M.D.
Associate Professor, Co-Director, Compulsive Impulsive Disorders Program; Director, Depersonalization and Dissociation Program, Mount Sinai School of Medicine, New York, New York

Robert I. Simon, M.D.
Clinical Professor of Psychiatry; Director, Program in Psychiatry and Law, Georgetown University School of Medicine, Washington, D.C.; Chair, Department of Psychiatry, Suburban Hospital/Johns Hopkins Medicine, Bethesda, Maryland

Andrew E. Skodol, M.D.
President, Institute for Mental Health Research, Phoenix, Arizona; and Research Professor of Psychiatry, University of Arizona College of Medicine, Tucson, Arizona

Stephen M. Sonnenberg, M.D.
Clinical Professor, Department of Psychiatry, Baylor College of Medicine, Houston, Texas; Adjunct Professor, Department of Psychiatry, Uniformed Services University of the Health Sciences, F. Edward Hébert School of Medicine, Bethesda, Maryland; Training and Supervising Analyst, Hous-

ton–Galveston Psychoanalytic Institute, Austin, Texas

Brett N. Steenbarger, Ph.D.
Clinical Associate Professor, Department of Psychiatry and Behavioral Sciences, SUNY Upstate Medical University, Syracuse, New York

Dan J. Stein, M.D., Ph.D.
Professor and Chair, Department of Psychiatry, University of Cape Town, South Africa; Visiting Professor, Department of Psychiatry, Mount Sinai School of Medicine, New York, New York

James J. Strain, M.D.
Professor of Psychiatry, Mount Sinai School of Medicine, New York, New York

Patrick J. Strollo Jr., M.D.
Associate Professor of Medicine, University of Pittsburgh School of Medicine; Medical Director, Sleep Medicine Center, University of Pittsburgh Medical Center, Pittsburgh, Pennsylvania

Michael E. Thase, M.D.
Professor of Psychiatry, University of Pittsburgh Medical Center, Pittsburgh, Pennsylvania

Amy M. Ursano, M.D.
Assistant Professor of Psychiatry, Department of Psychiatry, Division of Child and Adolescent Psychiatry, University of North Carolina, Chapel Hill, North Carolina

Robert J. Ursano, M.D.
Professor and Chairman, Department of Psychiatry, Uniformed Services University of the Health Sciences, F. Edward Hébert School of Medicine, Bethesda, Maryland; teaching faculty, Washington Psychoanalytic Institute, Washington, D.C.

Elisabeth A. Wilde, Ph.D.
Assistant Professor, Departments of Physical Medicine and Rehabilitation and of Neurology and Radiology, Baylor College of Medicine, Houston, Texas

John W. Winkelman, M.D., Ph.D.
Associate Professor of Psychiatry, Harvard Medical School, Boston, Massachusetts; Medical Director, Sleep Health Center, Brigham and Women's Hospital, Brighton, Massachusetts

Jesse H. Wright, M.D., Ph.D.
Professor and Vice Chair for Academic Affairs and Director, Depression Center, Department of Psychiatry and Behavioral Sciences, University of Louisville, Louisville, Kentucky

Tara M. Wright, M.D.
Assistant Professor of Psychiatry, Medical University of South Carolina, Ralph H. Johnson VAMC, Charleston, South Carolina

Jong H. Yoon, M.D.
Assistant Professor, Imaging Research Center, University of California, Davis, School of Medicine, Sacramento, California

Stuart C. Yudofsky, M.D.
D.C. and Irene Ellwood Professor and Chairman, Menninger Department of Psychiatry and Behavioral Sciences, Baylor College of Medicine; Chairman, Department of Psychiatry, The Methodist Hospital, Houston, Texas

Sean H. Yutzy, M.D.
Associate Professor of Psychiatry, Department of Psychiatry, University of New Mexico, Albuquerque, New Mexico

Phyllis G. Zee, M.D., Ph.D.
Professor of Neurology, Northwestern University, Chicago, Illinois

Disclosure of Interests

The contributors have declared all forms of support received within the 12 months prior to manuscript submittal that may represent a competing interest in relation to their work published in this volume, as follows:

Aaron T. Beck, M.D. The author may receive a portion of profits from sale of software "Good Days Ahead" for computer-assisted CBT discussed in this text. The publisher of the software is Mindstreet, LLC, Louisville, KY.

Jed E. Black, M.D. *Consultant/Grant Support:* Takeda, Boehringer-Ingelheim, Jazz Pharmaceuticals, GlaxoSmithKline, Cephalon.

Daniel J. Buysse, M.D. *Consultant:* Actelion, Arena, Cephalon, Eli Lilly, GlaxoSmithKline, Merck, Neurocrine, Neurogen, Pfizer, Respironics, sanofi-aventis, Sepracor, Servier, Somnus, Stress Eraser, Takeda, Transcept.

Mina K. Dulcan, M.D. *ADHD Advisory Board:* Eli Lilly; *Consultant/Editorial Board:* Care Management Technologies (develops medication guidelines).

Eric Hollander, M.D. *Consultant:* Transcept.

Lauren B. Marangell, M.D. *Grant Support:* Bristol-Myers Squibb, Eli Lilly, Cyberonics, Neuronetics, National Institute of Mental Health, Stanley Foundation; *Consultant/ Honoraria:* Eli Lilly, GlaxoSmithKline, Cyberonics, Pfizer, Medtronic, Forest, Aspect Medical Systems, Novartis.

James M. Martinez, M.D. *Research Support:* Aspect Medical Systems, AstraZeneca, Bristol-Myers Squibb, Cyberonics, Eli Lilly, Forest Pharmaceuticals, Neuronetics, sanofi-aventis, National Institute of Mental Health, Stanley Foundation; *Speakers' Bureau:* Astra-Zeneca, Bristol-Myers Squibb, Cyberonics, Eli Lilly, Forest Pharmaceuticals, Glaxo-SmithKline, Janssen, Pfizer, Wyeth Ayerst; *Consultant:* Cyberonics.

Melissa Martinez, M.D. *Research Support:* Cyberonics.

Jeffrey H. Newcorn, M.D. *Advisory Board/ Consultant:* Abbott, McNeil, Eli Lilly, Shire, Novartis, Cortex, Pfizer, Lupin; *Research Support:* McNeil, Eli Lilly, Shire, Novartis; *Speakers' Bureau:* Novartis, Shire

Paul E. Schulz, M.D. *Speakers' Bureau:* Pfizer, Forest Pharmaceuticals.

Jeffrey S. Seaman, M.S., M.D. *Clinical Trials:* Bristol-Myers Squibb, Cephalon.

Dan J. Stein, M.D., Ph.D. *Grant Support/Consultant Honoraria:* AstraZeneca, Eli Lilly, GlaxoSmithKline, Johnson & Johnson, Lundbeck, Orion, Pfizer, Pharmacia, Rocher, Servier, Solvay, Sumitomo, Tikvah, Wyeth.

Patrick J. Strollo Jr., M.D. *Grant Support:* ResMed, Respironics.

Michael E. Thase, M.D. *Scientific Consultation:* AstraZeneca, Bristol-Myers Squibb, Eli Lilly, Forest, Gerson Lehman Group, GlaxoSmithKline, Guidepoint Global, H. Lundbeck A/S, MedAvante, Neuronetics, Novartis, Otsuka, Ortho-McNeil, PamLab, Pfizer, Schering-Plough, Shire US, Supernus, Takeda (Lundbeck), Transcept; *Speakers' Bureau:* AstraZeneca, Bristol-Myers Squibb, Eli Lilly, Pfizer; *Grant Funding:* Eli Lilly, GlaxoSmithKline, Sepracor. Equity Holdings: MedAvante. *Royalty Income:* American Psychiatric Publishing, Guilford, Herald House, Oxford University Press, W.W. Norton. Dr. Thase's wife is employed as the Group Scientific Director for Embryon (formerly Advogent, which does business with BMS and Pfizer/Wyeth).

Robert J. Ursano, M.D. *Consultant:* Abbott, GlaxoSmithKline; *Speakers' Bureau:* McNeil.

John W. Winkelman, M.D., Ph.D. *Consultant/ Advisory Board:* GlaxoSmithKline, Impax, Luitpold, Pfizer, UCB, Zeo; *Research Support:* GlaxoSmithKline.

Jesse H. Wright, M.D., Ph.D. *Royalties/Stock Ownership:* Mindstreet (from sale of "Good Days Ahead" software for computer-assisted CBT); *Consultant:* Wyeth.

Phyllis G. Zee, M.D. *Consultant/Advisory Board:* Boehringer-Ingelheim, GlaxoSmithKline, Jazz, sanofi-aventis, Takeda.

The following contributors stated that they had no competing interests during the year preceding manuscript submission: Linda B. Andrews, M.D.; L. Jarrett Barnhill, M.D.; Heather A. Berlin, Ph.D., M.P.H.; Dan G. Blazer, M.D., Ph.D.; James A. Bourgeois, O.D., M.D., F.A.P.M.; Cameron S. Carter, M.D.; Stephen J. Cozza, M.D.; Glen C. Crawford, M.D.; Mantosh J. Dewan, M.D.; Glen O. Gabbard, M.D.; Roger P. Greenberg, Ph.D.; John G. Gunderson, M.D.; Robert E. Hales, M.D., M.B.A.; Katherine A. Halmi, M.D.; John A. Joska, M.D., M.Med.(Psych.), F.C.Psych.(S.A.); Paul H. Kartheiser, M.D.; H. Florence Kim, M.D.; Kimberly G. Klipstein, M.D.; Susan G. Lazar, M.D.; Martin H. Leamon, M.D.; Michael J. Minzenberg, M.D.; Hugh Myrick, M.D.; Brooke S. Parish, M.D.; Mark E. Servis, M.D.; Daniel W. Shuman, J.D.; Daphne Simeon, M.D.; Robert I. Simon, M.D.; Andrew E. Skodol, M.D.; Stephen M. Sonnenberg, M.D.; Brett N. Steenbarger, Ph.D.; James J. Strain, M.D.; Amy M. Ursano, M.D.; Elisabeth A. Wilde, Ph.D.; Tara M. Wright, M.D.; Jong H. Yoon, M.D.; Stuart C. Yudofsky, M.D.; Sean H. Yutzy, M.D.; Phyllis G. Zee, M.D., Ph.D.

PREFACE

The Third Edition of *Essentials of Psychiatry* provides a synopsis of the most important material included within the fifth edition of *The American Psychiatric Publishing Textbook of Psychiatry* and was developed specifically for those needing a concise reference of clinical psychiatry. Although this work will provide psychiatry residents, fourth-year medical students on psychiatry electives, and practicing psychiatrists a complete, yet abridged, overview of clinical psychiatry, it will also serve anyone seeking a clear and direct reference on this subject. As such, it will prove useful to both physicians in other fields as well as laypersons who are interested in clinical psychiatry.

With its more concise structure, this book intends to provide core knowledge to the busy trainee or practitioner on psychiatric assessment and treatment of children, adolescents, adults, and seniors. It takes a biopsychosocial approach to patient treatment, including both psychotherapy and psychopharmacology.

The Third Edition has fewer pages (790 vs. 1008) and two less chapters than the prior edition. It was felt that readers wanted more condensed and clinically relevant material. Of the 55 authors of chapters in this edition, 34 (or 61%) are new, making this edition the most extensively revised version yet.

To develop the subject matter of this work, we carefully reviewed the 44 chapters contained within *The American Psychiatric Publishing Textbook of Psychiatry* and selected the 22 that we felt were most important and relevant for clinical practice in a variety of settings: inpatient, partial hospitalization, outpatient, and rehabilitation programs. Our goal was create an economical paperback version of the *Textbook* that remained focused on key clinical information concerning selected psychiatric disorders. At the same time, we endeavored to present this essential knowledge base and the methods of psychiatric treatment in a manner that was both exciting and accessible.

One important feature that gives *Essentials of Psychiatry* its particular effectiveness is the combined effort of senior and junior authors in certain chapters. The addition of junior authors has infused the chapters with new research insights and fresh and expanded perspectives on the subject matter. The senior authors have complemented these new ideas with their considerable wisdom and vast research and clinical experience. We believe that these collaborations both increase the appeal of the chapters to readers at all levels of educational and clinical experience and enrich the diversity and quality of the material presented. We hope that you will enjoy this edition!

Acknowledgments

The challenging task of condensing the 1,786-page Textbook of Psychiatry into an abbreviated volume required outstanding editorial skills from the APPI team. We are fortunate that Rebecca Richters assumed the role of Project Editor and performed in her usual outstanding fashion. A number of other people at American Psychiatric Publishing, Inc. (APPI) also helped us a great deal with this project. First, we would like to thank CEO Ron McMillen for his support and encouragement in developing the work. In addition, John McDuffie, Editorial Director, and Greg Kuny, Managing Editor of Books, provided a number of helpful suggestions concerning its structure and formatting. Bob Pursell, Director of Marketing, designed an effective marketing strategy to "spread the word" on the book and its approach to its subjects.

The editorial headquarters for this work was located at the University of California, Davis. Susan Mortensen handled all of the complex interactions with our 55 authors and APPI editorial staff with her usual efficiency, skill, and good humor. The project would not have been accomplished on time without her invaluable help.

Last and most importantly, we would like to thank our outstanding authors for carefully reviewing their chapters and skillfully sculpting them into well-edited summaries of their topics. Because of their efforts, readers of this work will find the information it contains is easily accessible, concise, and clinically relevant to psychiatric practice. As a result, we believe that *Essentials of Psychiatry* will prove to be a useful companion volume to the fourth edition of *The American Psychiatric Publishing Textbook of Psychiatry* and will establish itself as a vital source for clinical information.

Robert E. Hales, M.D., M.B.A.
Sacramento, California

Stuart C. Yudofsky, M.D.
Houston, Texas

Glen O. Gabbard, M.D.
Houston, Texas

THE PSYCHIATRIC INTERVIEW AND MENTAL STATUS EXAMINATION

Linda B. Andrews, M.D.

Requisite Physician Preparation

An effective psychiatric interview allows the clinician both to connect with a patient and to gather pertinent data. Although medical technology has advanced tremendously in recent years and has increased the amount of laboratory and neuroimaging information available to assist psychiatrists in making more accurate diagnoses and developing more specific treatment plans for patients, these tests cannot supplant the importance of gathering critical data via the traditional psychiatric interview. The psychiatric interview is the single most important method of arriving at an understanding of a patient who exhibits the signs and symptoms of a psychiatric illness (Scheiber 2003). The psychiatric interview is similar to the general medical interview in that both include the patient's chief complaint, history of present illness, past history, social and family history, and review of systems. However, the psychiatric interview differs from the traditional medical interview because the psychiatric interview also includes a more thorough examination of the patient's developmental history, including the patient's feelings about important life events and exploration of the patient's significant interpersonal relationships, patterns of adaptation, and character traits (MacKinnon et al. 2006; Scheiber 2003). The psychiatric interview includes a formal examination of the patient's mental status as well.

Connecting with a patient and gathering pertinent data via the psychiatric interview requires considerable preparation and practice. Psychiatric interviewing is a skill founded on extensive knowledge of normal and abnormal human behavior (MacKinnon et al. 2006).

Conduct of the Psychiatric Interview

Goals and Purpose

If the psychiatric interviewer and the patient wish to complete a successful interview, it is very helpful, and probably necessary, for the psychiatric interviewer and the patient to agree on the purpose of the interview. Relevant questions to establish the goals and purpose of the interview include the following:

- Is this interview being conducted for diagnostic or therapeutic purposes?
- Will the psychiatrist see this patient for this interview alone with the expressed goal to establish a psychiatric diagnosis, or does this interview represent the first of many appointments with this patient within a newly developed therapeutic or treatment relationship?
- Under what circumstances is the psychiatric interview occurring?
- Who requested and who made arrangements for the psychiatric interview to take place?
- Will the results of the psychiatric interview be confidential?
- Is the patient participating voluntarily in the interview?
- How much time does the psychiatrist have to conduct the psychiatric interview?
- Does the psychiatric evaluation consist of one or more than one actual meetings with the patient?
- Where will the psychiatric interview occur?
- Does the psychiatrist or patient expect other persons to be interviewed as part of the psychiatric evaluation?
- Is the patient expected to pay for the psychiatric interview? If so, how will the fee be determined and how will the billing be handled?

Different answers to each of these questions will significantly influence how the psychiatrist conducts the psychiatric interview, what results the psychiatrist obtains from the psychiatric interview, and what the psychiatrist does with the obtained results.

Pre-Interview Contact

The psychiatrist must decide whether he or she should have telephone or e-mail contact with the patient before, during, and after the formal psychiatric evaluation. In the current age of electronic communication, patients may expect to communicate with their physicians via e-mail. As with most guidelines for conducting the psychiatric interview and mental status examination, no absolute rule exists about communications with patients outside of the actual psychiatric interview. Patients should be clearly instructed about how they should handle medical or psychiatric emergencies that might occur before or after the formal evaluation or between appointments if the psychiatrist and patient plan to meet more than once. Most commonly, this involves the psychiatrist either giving the patient an after-hours contact number or instructing the patient to go to a particular hospital emergency department in the case of a true medical or psychiatric emergency. For patient questions other than emergencies, each psychiatrist must decide for him- or herself how to manage phone calls and e-mails.

Process of the Psychiatric Interview

Once all of the questions on the goals and purposes of the interview have been answered, the psychiatrist is ready to begin the actual psychiatric interview and mental status examination. The next—and perhaps most important—task is to establish rapport with the patient being interviewed (Table 1–1). Establishing an effective working relationship will be necessary to accomplish all of the other tasks discussed throughout this chapter. Developing this working alliance

---

Table 1–1. Tasks for the therapist conducting a psychiatric interview

---

1. Establish goals.
2. Establish rapport.
3. Develop a collaborative doctor–patient relationship.
4. Communicate empathically.
5. Maintain appropriate boundaries.
6. Communicate in a language that the patient understands, and avoid psychiatric jargon.
7. Monitor the emotional intensity of the interview and adjust as necessary.
8. Gather pertinent psychiatric history data.
9. Perform a mental status examination.
10. Assess patient reliability.
11. Assess patient safety.
12. Develop a plan for possible emergencies.
13. Review previous records and other available data.
14. Interview others as appropriate.
15. Document accurately.
16. Manage time.

---

with the patient is generally accomplished by communicating respect and empathy to the patient. Communicating respect includes an appropriate introduction of one's self to the patient and respectfully asking the patient how he or she wishes to be addressed during the interview. Respectful and empathic communication involves making appropriate eye contact, observing nonverbal cues, and limiting interruptions. Empathic communications show the patient that the psychiatrist is trying to listen and observe from the patient's perspective.

Based on an empathic connection with the patient, the psychiatrist should be able to adjust his or her interview style to match the needs of a particular patient at any particular point in the interview. This empathic connection should also allow the psychiatrist to follow a patient's cues or leads as appropriate.

Empathic attunement also allows the psychiatrist to focus on more emotionally relevant topics. Open-ended questions generally assist in this effort and allow a patient to give more detailed and emotionally meaningful responses to such questions.

Empathic communication may also allow the psychiatric interviewer to recognize when a patient is becoming overwhelmed with the emotional load of the interview and to reduce the intensity of the interview by using more focused, close-ended questions. This type of question more often generates a brief, even "yes" or "no" response from the patient. Such questions generally focus on gathering factual data from the patient rather than on understanding emotional meaning for the patient. Close-ended questions are also useful when interviewing patients with disturbances of thought content or production, perceptual disturbances, or cognitive deficits. Empathic attunement also allows the psychiatrist to recognize when an interview should be stopped before completion because a patient has become acutely agitated, dangerous, or medically compromised. Gathering data should never supersede keeping a patient safe during an interview.

Empathic and respectful communication should allow the patient to understand the psychiatrist's questions or comments. The psychiatrist should adjust his or her use of words to match the patient's intellectual abilities, perceived educational level, and language and cultural needs. The psychiatrist should avoid the use of medical jargon. The psychiatrist should enlist the assistance of a translator when necessary. The psychiatrist can demonstrate that he or she is actively listening to the patient by verifying that he or she has heard the patient correctly. Doing so allows the patient to correct any errors in the psychiatrist's understanding of the patient, which should lead to improved overall patient care.

As the psychiatrist gathers information throughout the interview, he or she should remain cognizant of assessing the patient's reliability. Information obtained during the psychiatric interview is only as valid as the information's source. Confirming information given by the patient with information that can be verified by medical records or other valid sources should help the psychiatrist determine the patient's overall reliability.

Although the interviewer cannot ever anticipate or control every possible exchange that might take place with a new patient, the psychiatric interviewer should begin each relationship with a new patient by having some personally and professionally established guidelines about self-disclosure. For most first interviews, the psychiatrist will remain focused on gathering information about the patient and would rarely intend to be self-disclosing at this juncture in the physician–patient relationship. If the relationship with the patient were to develop into a therapeutic relationship, then the psychiatrist would need to judge whether, and when, self-disclosure might be beneficial in deepening the collaborative therapeutic relationship with the patient.

If, during a psychiatric interview, a patient becomes agitated or threatening toward the psychiatrist, the psychiatrist must rather abruptly adjust his or her interview focus to manage this acute situation. Flexible interviewing strategies, such as rearranging the chairs in the examination room, opening the door, letting a patient stand during the interview, or inviting a professionally trained colleague or comforting family member to join the interview, may allow the patient to continue the interview and provide additional safety for both the patient and the interviewer.

Documentation is an important and necessary responsibility for the physician caring for patients. When conducting a psychiatric interview, the psychiatrist should determine ahead of time if and how records of the interview will be kept. Patients must give informed consent to be audiotaped or videotaped. In a clinical setting, the psychiatrist should explain to the patient that he or she will take notes that will become part of the patient's medical record, but that the content of these notes are covered by the Health Insurance Portability and Accountability Act of 1996 and will be privacy protected to the fullest extent allowed by law. During the psychiatric interview itself, the psychiatrist should take notes to ensure that an accurate recording of the dialogue is kept but should not take such voluminous notes so as to interfere with establishing and maintaining rapport or remaining empathically connected to the patient. In most settings, the patient will have the right to view his or her medical record.

Ideally, the psychiatrist will review all of the available patient data prior to conducting the psychiatric interview of the patient. If this is not possible, the psychiatrist should at least review these records before developing a final diagnosis and treatment plan. This review would include reading any available medical records or psychiatric records as well as the results of all laboratory tests, neuropsychological testing, or neuroimaging scans that have been performed.

A thorough psychiatric interview could also include interviewing other individuals who have firsthand knowledge of the patient. This could include, but is not limited to, family members, teachers, colleagues, other physicians, or other health care providers. Whenever possible, the psychiatric interviewer should inform and obtain consent from the patient to interview these other individuals.

Throughout the interview, the psychiatrist must remain cognizant of time constraints. The psychiatric interviewer should have decided before beginning the interview whether he or she plans to make diagnostic and treatment recommendations during the first interview or if these issues will be presented to and discussed with the patient at a subsequent visit. If the psychiatric interviewer plans to discuss diagnosis and treatment during the first appointment, then the interviewer should manage the interview to leave adequate time toward the end for patient questions and to discuss significant diagnostic and treatment issues. If the psychiatrist has decided to have this discussion at the next appointment, then he or she should leave a few minutes at the end of this first appointment to allow the patient to ask questions and to schedule the next appointment together.

Content of the Psychiatric Interview

Once the introductions, instructions, and consents have been completed, the psychiatrist may focus on obtaining information from the patient. If time allows, the interviewer should cover all key elements of the psychiatric history and mental status examination. For the psychiatric history, these key elements include the chief complaint or primary reason for the evaluation, history of the present illness, past psychiatric history, family psychiatric history, past medical history, family medical history, social history, developmental history, and a review of systems. For the mental status examination, these key elements include general appearance, orientation, speech, motor, affect, mood, thought production, thought content, perceptions, suicidal/homicidal ideation, memory/cognition, insight, and judgment.

Chief Complaint and History of Present Illness

It is usually best to begin the interview with a relatively open-ended, unstructured question to elicit the patient's chief complaint or primary concern. Examples of this type of question include the following: "How are you doing today?" "What brings you to the clinic today?" or "Are you having any troubles today?" These types of questions allow the patient to direct the conversation initially and to decide what is discussed first between the patient and the doctor. The psychiatric interviewer should then slowly direct the questions to obtain more details about the chief complaint and allow the chief complaint to be expanded to include a more thorough discussion of the history of present illness. It is extremely important to spend adequate time and effort to flesh out considerable details about the history of the present illness. Questions about the history of present illness should include a review of current psychiatric symptoms: their onset, frequency, intensity, duration, precipitating factors, relieving or aggravating factors, and associated symptoms.

Past Psychiatric History

Expanding the history of present illness to inquire whether such symptoms have ever occurred before will lead to questions about the patient's past psychiatric history. This discussion should include past symptom frequency, intensity, and duration; precipitating, relieving, or aggravating factors; and associated symptoms. The review of the patient's past psychiatric history should include questions about past treatment with medications, therapy, or electroconvulsive therapy; previous hospitalizations; previous treatment for alcohol or substance abuse or dependence; and previous suicidal or homicidal ideation or attempts. With respect to previous medications, the psychiatrist should ask the patient to list all previously taken medications, including their dosages, side effects, length of treatment, compliance with treatment, and, if relevant, reason(s) for stopping treatment. With respect to psychotherapy, the psychiatrist should ask the patient to describe all previous experiences in psychotherapy, including therapy type, format, frequency, duration, and adherence. With respect to treatment for substance abuse, the psychiatrist should ask the patient to describe his or her substance use history, including quantity; frequency; route of administration; pattern of use; functional, interpersonal, or legal consequences of use; tolerance or withdrawal phenomena; and experience in any previous addiction treatment programs, including type and duration of the program and the patient's compliance with or completion of any such addiction treatment program (Vergare et al. 2006). The psychiatric interviewer should try to understand the patient's opinion about the efficacy of all previous treatments. The psychiatrist should avoid recommending a treatment deemed by the patient to have been previously unsuccessful. The psychiatrist should pay particular attention to treatments that have been successful in the past, because the patient is more likely to respond to such treatments again in the future. Family members' positive responses to a particular treatment may also predict a good response for the patient being evaluated.

Family Psychiatric History

The interviewer should gather detailed information about the patient's family psychiatric history, including the presence or absence of psychiatric illnesses in parents, grandparents, siblings, aunts, uncles, cousins, and children. The psychiatric interviewer may need to use less medical jargon when inquiring about the patient's family psychiatric history, because family stories and lore about family members' previous experiences with mental illness vary widely.

Medical History

The interviewer must inquire about the patient's past and current medical problems. Specifically, the psychiatrist needs to know what medications the patient takes regularly and if the patient is allergic to any medications or other things. Inquiry about medications should also include over-the-counter medications, herbal or energy supplements, vitamins, and complementary or alternative medical treatments (Vergare et al. 2006). The patient should be asked about any history of side effects to medications taken. Even if the patient denies any medical problems, it is important for the psychiatrist to ask specific questions about several medical illnesses, such as diabetes mellitus, seizure disorder, hypo- or hyperthyroidism, and cardiac disease, because a patient having any of these

illnesses may alter the psychiatrist's diagnostic impressions or treatment plans. The psychiatrist should also inquire about a family history of medical problems.

Social History

Gathering information about the patient's social history is an extremely important part of the psychiatric interview because stability or instability in the patient's surroundings may dramatically affect the status of the patient's psychiatric illness. The psychiatric interviewer should inquire about the patient's living situation:

- Does the patient have a stable place of residence that is safe and affordable?
- Has anything about the patient's living situation changed recently?
- Are any changes expected in the near future?
- Does the patient have a reliable source of income?
- Is the patient working?
- Does the patient rely on some sort of subsidy, such as Medicare, Medicaid, or Social Security disability, for financial resources?
- Does the patient have an adequate support system, including family, friends, neighbors, and so on?
- Is the patient's support system reliable and available in times of need?
- Is the patient married, single, divorced, separated?
- Does the patient have children?
- Does the patient have family nearby and available to help?
- What is the nature of the patient's relationship with his or her family—that is, is the family supportive and helpful or intrusive and difficult?

Understanding the family system and dynamics is particularly important. Even if a patient wishes to change his or her problematic behaviors, the family's willingness to support such change will be critical. The family's resistance to such change may severely undermine the patient's efforts for change.

The psychiatrist should ask about the patient's level of education. The interviewer should gather some information about the patient's ethnic and cultural beliefs, because symptoms considered to be problematic and indicative of serious psychiatric illness in Western cultures are often believed to be normal behaviors in other cultures. The psychiatrist should ask the patient if he or she has strong connections to or receives support from a particular faith or spiritual group.

The interviewer should ask the patient if he or she has any habits that could negatively affect the efficacy of any psychiatric treatments prescribed, such as tobacco use, alcohol or drug use, or sexual promiscuity. When inquiring about these types of habits, the interviewer must ask specific questions to elicit meaningful answers. Patients do not generally easily or openly discuss behaviors about which they have some concern, embarrassment, or shame.

The interviewer should also ask the patient about any current or pending legal problems. The interviewer should also ask whether the patient is now serving or has ever served in the U.S. military. If yes, the interviewer should ask the patient to describe his or her experiences in the military. Patients who serve or did serve in the military may be eligible for specialized medical and psychological services through the federal government. Questions about domestic violence should be covered at some time during the interview, and for many psychiatrists, doing so concurrent with discussions about the patient's social history seems most appropriate.

Developmental History

Gathering information about the patient's developmental history is another critical aspect of the psychiatric interview. Understanding a patient's development will greatly improve the likelihood that the psychiatrist will be able accurately to contextualize the patient's current psychiatric symptoms. A truly thorough developmental history will include questioning along a number of developmental continua, including motor, language, physical, sexual, emotional, and moral. The psychiatrist should ask about any unusual perinatal events and whether the patient achieved most developmental milestones, such as talking, walking, reading, and so on, in a normal fashion. Sometimes, a patient will not remember this information, but family members, especially parents or siblings, can be particularly helpful in obtaining a thorough and accurate developmental history.

Also, the psychiatrist will try to ascertain the quality of the patient's attachments to parental figures, the patient's experiences of various separations in childhood, and the quality of the patient's peer relationships, considering issues of attachment, trust, and intimacy to be of critical importance. Many adult manifestations of personality health or disorder relate significantly to the presence or absence of and the quality of these early childhood relationships. The psychiatric interviewer should ask if the patient experienced any verbal, emotional, physical, or sexual abuse as a child or teenager.

Because development extends beyond the childhood years, the psychiatric interviewer should assess the patient's ongoing development through adolescence and early, middle, and late adulthood, as appropriate, including an assessment of patterns of response to normal life transitions and major life events as well as the quality of ongoing interpersonal relationships. Some important areas to consider include how the patient handled the following events: moving away from home for the first time, going to college, getting married, having children, losing a job, losing a parent, and so on. Most psychiatrists include questions about sexual orientation in the social history portion of the interview as well.

Review of Systems

The psychiatric interviewer should complete this portion of the evaluation by reviewing any general medical systems or psychiatric illness categories that have not previously been discussed. The psychiatric interviewer should ask every patient about his or her sleep and appetite patterns, weight regulation, and sexual functioning (MacKinnon et al. 2006). The psychiatric interviewer should also ask every patient at least one or two questions about thought, mood, anxiety, substance use, and cognitive disorders, if these have not already been covered elsewhere.

The Mental Status Examination

The psychiatric interviewer completes the mental status examination by combining a series of observations with a series of formal questions (Table 1–2). The purpose of the mental status examination is to provide as clear a picture as possible of the patient's actual mental state at the time of the psychiatric interview or evaluation. It is truly a "state" rather than "trait" examination, meaning that it describes the patient's mental function at a given moment in time and does not necessarily represent a historical perspective of the patient's mental illness. It is, therefore, quite common, and probably expected, that the patient's mental status examination will differ from interview to interview. For this reason, the psychiatrist can use changes in a patient's mental status examination across multiple appointments to help clarify diagnostic questions and/or to update treatment decisions. Careful documentation and appropriate use of standard terminology of the mental status examination may allow these diagnostic and therapeutic decisions to be made even when different practitioners see the patient over time.

General Appearance

The psychiatric interviewer should observe the patient's general appearance throughout

Table 1–2. Outline of the mental status examination

1. General appearance
2. Orientation
3. Speech
4. Motor activity
5. Affect and mood
6. Thought production
7. Thought content
8. Perceptual disturbances
9. Suicidal and homicidal ideation
10. Attention, concentration, and memory
11. Abstract thinking
12. Insight/judgment

the interview. The interviewer's report should include some comment on the patient's posture, grooming, clothing, and body habitus. If the psychiatrist has been treating a patient over time, he or she should mention any changes in the patient's general appearance.

Orientation

When a psychiatrist interviews a patient for the first time, he or she should complete some formal assessment of orientation, asking the patient his or her full name, the full date (number, month, and year), and the place where the interview is occurring (city, state, building, floor, clinic name). In subsequent appointments with the same patient, the interviewer may decide to only ask these very specific orientation questions again if the patient's attention or focus seems to have changed from previous meetings.

Speech

The psychiatrist should include commentary about the patient's speech as part of the formal mental status examination. For example, the psychiatrist should describe the patient's rate, volume, articulation, coherence, and spontaneity of speech as observed throughout the psychiatric interview.

Motor Activity

The mental status examination should include specific mention of the patient's motor behavior. This should include comment on the patient's gait and station, gestures, abnormal movements, tics, and overall general body movements as witnessed throughout the entire interview. Monitoring changes in motor activity over time may help the clinician track the patient's illness progression over time, including compliance with and response to psychiatric medications.

Affect

The psychiatrist should observe and then comment on the patient's affect. *Affect* describes the patient's expressed emotional state that the psychiatrist observes throughout the interview. Words such as *sad, sullen, bubbly,* or *agitated* could be used. The interviewer should note whether the patient's affect changes throughout the interview, and if so, whether the affect changes occur gradually or abruptly and whether the changes are congruent with the interview content and appropriate for the interview setting.

Mood

Reporting the patient's *mood* is the only element of the mental status examination that actually is historical and not observed. The interviewer should ask the patient to report his or her mood for the past few days and weeks. Whenever possible, the psychiatric interviewer should use words directly reported by the patient, such as "The patient states that her mood has been gloomy over the past few weeks."

Thought Production

Thought process or *production* describes how the patient's thoughts are expressed during the psychiatric interview. The psychiatric interviewer should comment on the patient's thought production rate and flow, including comments about whether the patient's thinking is logical, goal-directed, circumstantial, or tangential, or shows loosening of associations or flight of ideas (i.e., ideas are not connected one to the next). A patient's flow of thought can usually be described somewhere on the continuum between goal-directed and disconnected.

Thought Content

A description of the patient's thought content should include mention of important themes and the presence or absence of delusional or obsessional thinking and suicidal or homicidal thoughts. *Delusional thinking* includes fixed false beliefs that are persecutory, erotomanic, grandiose, somatic, or jealous in content. Patients with delusions believe that their fixed false beliefs are reality. *Obsessions* are defined as recurrent, persistent thoughts that intrude involuntarily into a person's thinking. Obsessions appear to be senseless and are not based in reality. Patients with obsessions recognize that their intrusive thoughts are not normal. A patient's awareness that these thoughts are senseless, as opposed to believing them to be reality, distinguishes obsessions from delusions.

Perceptual Disturbances

The psychiatric interviewer must inquire about the patient's perceptual abilities. The interviewer must ask if the patient sees, hears, smells, or feels anything that is not based on an actual sensory stimulus. Of course, the interviewer probably should word the question more clearly to a patient, such as "Do you ever see things that other people don't see?" or "Do you ever hear voices talking to you and then realize that no one is actually in the room with you?" Perceptual disturbances such as hearing, seeing, smelling, or feeling things in the absence of an actual sensory stimulus are called *hallucinations*. During a psychiatric interview, the interviewer may be able to observe a patient who is responding to internal stimuli because the patient is answering a question even though a question has not been asked or is turning to talk to someone in a different part of the room when another person is not actually present. A patient may or may not acknowledge or admit to having such perceptual disturbances. Patients often will only admit to these hallucinations after establishing some sort of therapeutic relationship with the doctor, after several appointments together.

Suicidal and Homicidal Ideation

A competent psychiatric interview should always include an assessment of suicidality and homicidality. The suicide assessment is particularly critical for patients with a personal or family history of suicide attempts or a family history of completed suicide and should include exploring for the presence or absence of current suicidal ideation, intent, and plan. The homicide assessment is particularly critical for patients with a prior history of violence or trouble with the law. If, during a psychiatric interview, the psychiatrist learns that a patient is actively suicidal or homicidal, the psychiatrist must redirect his or her interviewing efforts to manage this acute situation. Such management might be to organize admission to a psychiatric hospital for an acutely suicidal patient or to call the police to get assistance with an acutely agitated or homicidal patient. The interviewer should be knowledgeable about state laws regarding the duty to warn, should a patient threaten to harm another person.

Attention, Concentration, and Memory

As part of the mental status examination, the psychiatric interviewer should assess the patient's attention, concentration, and memory. Most clinicians will ask at least a few testing questions before concluding that the patient's attention, concentration, and memory are within normal limits. Some tests include the following:

- "Please spell the word 'world' forward for me. Now spell the word 'world' backward."
- "Start with the number 100, subtract 7, and continue to count backward by 7s until I tell you to stop."
- "Who is the current president of the United States? Who was president before him? Who were the previous four presidents of the United States before him?"

The psychiatric interviewer must carefully choose the questions to assess attention, concentration, and memory to ensure that the questions match the patient's educational level and cultural background. For patients who appear to have cognitive deficits, it is recommended that the psychiatric interview include a formal Mini-Mental State Exam (MMSE), which includes a specific set of questions whose answers are scored and compared with a 30-point maximum score. Patients with cognitive disorders as well as cognitive impairment secondary to other psychiatric disorders usually have lower MMSE scores (Folstein et al. 1975). For patients who have lower MMSE scores, the psychiatrist should repeat the MMSE at each subsequent appointment and track the patient's performance over time to monitor for cognitive changes.

Abstract Thinking

As part of the mental status examination, most psychiatrists perform some assessment of abstraction abilities. Most often, the psychiatric interviewer will ask the patient to interpret a proverb by saying something similar to the following: "Please tell me what this saying might mean, as if you were trying to explain its meaning to a small child. 'Don't cry over spilled milk' or 'People who live in glass houses shouldn't throw stones.'" Patients with less than an eighth-grade education or patients who have not yet fully acculturated into the Western culture may struggle with this type of question, regardless of any superimposed psychiatric illness. The psychiatrist should incorporate data from the entire interview when determining whether a patient's thinking is more concrete than would otherwise be expected for the patient's level of education or acculturation.

Insight/Judgment

Toward the end of the psychiatric interview and mental status examination, the interviewer should consider the degree to which the patient understands and appreciates the impact of his or her psychiatric illness on the rest of the patient's life. Psychiatrists refer to this capacity to understand one's illness as *insight*. Patients with greater insight into their illnesses generally demonstrate greater compliance with treatment recommendations. Compliance can serve as a measure of judgment. Psychiatrists assume that patients with better judgment will be more compliant with treatment recommendations.

Some interviewers ask questions to assess judgment more formally. Suggested questions include "What would you do if you ran out of your medications 1 week before your next scheduled doctor's appointment?" and "What would you do if you developed severe diarrhea 2 days after starting a new medication for your depression?" These questions allow the physician to test the patient's judgment and also introduce an effective way to discuss such important treatment issues as compliance and medication side effects.

Diagnostic Formulation and Treatment Planning

In beginning to consolidate an understanding of the patient, the psychiatrist may decide to complete various rating scales to help document the presence or absence of symptoms or to quantify the severity of specific illnesses identified. A wide variety of such rating scales exists and should be chosen carefully and specifically for each patient (MacKinnon et al. 2006).

The biopsychosocial formulation allows the interviewer to assimilate the primary bio-

logical, psychological, and social factors into a brief but integrated understanding of the patient. The primary function of the biopsychosocial formulation is to provide a succinct conceptualization of the patient and thereby guide a treatment plan. The biopsychosocial formulation is a hypothesis or set of hypotheses that attempt to explain the patient's symptoms. If the psychiatric interviewer sees the patient over time, the biopsychosocial formulation should be revised regularly as new data appear (Kassaw and Gabbard 2002; Perry et al. 1987). Particularly for the psychological portion of the formulation, the psychiatrist should not try to make the formulation all-inclusive but should focus on one or two key themes at the core of the patient's problems, identify key developmental experiences and relevant stressors, and use the here-and-now transference and countertransference data from the interview to link the patient's past and present problems (Kassaw and Gabbard 2002).

Using the biopsychosocial formulation as a guide, the psychiatrist should next develop a working diagnosis using the five-axis classification system delineated in DSM-IV-TR (Table 1–3; American Psychiatric Association 2000).

In developing a treatment plan, the psychiatrist should include relevant biological, psychological, and social treatment recommendations. The first treatment decision involves determining the appropriate setting in which treatment should occur. Specifically, can the patient and his or her illness be managed in the outpatient setting? If not, the psychiatric interviewer must make the necessary arrangements to hospitalize the patient. Once the setting has been determined, the psychiatrist can proceed in creating a biopsychosocial treatment plan.

The biological portion of the treatment plan may include performing or arranging for a physical examination to be performed. Next, the psychiatrist should determine any laboratory tests as well as any neuroimaging studies that should be completed. The biolog-

Table 1–3. DSM-IV-TR multiaxial assessment and differential diagnosis

Axis I	All primary psychiatric disorders of thought, mood, anxiety, cognition, and substance abuse and other conditions that might be a focus of clinical attention
Axis II	Personality disorders and disorders first diagnosed in childhood, including mental retardation
Axis III	Concurrent general medical conditions
Axis IV	Psychosocial and environmental problems
Axis V	Global assessment of functioning based on a standard scoring system from 1 to 100, with 1 being severe impairment of function and 100 being no impairment of function

Source. Adapted from American Psychiatric Association 2000, pp. 27–33.

ical portion of the biopsychosocial treatment plan should also include the list of any psychiatric medications that the patient is currently taking with explicit instructions about whether those medications will be continued and, if so, how they should be taken. It should include instructions for any medication blood levels or other laboratory tests that the patient will need to obtain following the first appointment. The biological portion of the treatment plan should also include a discussion about any medical illness management issues that need to be addressed, such as referral to an internist to improve hypertension or diabetes mellitus control or referral to a dietitian for weight loss management.

The psychological portion of the treatment plan should include recommendations for indicated neuropsychological testing as well as a discussion of all possible psychotherapeutic interventions. Psychotherapy treatment options should include individual psychotherapy, group psychotherapy, couples therapy, or family therapy as indicated by the patient's particular treatment needs. Individual psychotherapy recommendations could include long- or short-term psychodynamic psychotherapy; brief focused therapies, such as cognitive-behavioral therapy, interpersonal psychotherapy, or dialectical behavior therapy; and long- or short-term supportive psychotherapy. The psychotherapeutic treatment plan must be specifically tailored to each patient. The treatment recommendations may include more than one form of psychotherapy.

The key to successful psychotherapy depends on carefully selecting patients suited to the particular psychotherapy chosen. Two principal assessments must be made when recommending psychotherapy: 1) Are the patient's clinical symptoms likely to respond to the particular therapy being recommended? and 2) If considering psychodynamic therapy, does the patient have the psychological characteristics suitable for the psychodynamic approach (Gabbard 2004)?

The patient's ability to afford the recommended psychotherapy, both from a financial and a time perspective, must be considered when developing a final treatment plan. If the patient's financial resources are limited, the psychiatrist should familiarize him- or herself with any lower-fee psychotherapy services available within the area.

The social portion of the treatment plan may include recommendations to improve the patient's living, work, financial, or support network situations, as relevant to the particular patient.

Each portion of the treatment plan must be carefully tailored to meet an individual patient's needs. Implementation of each treatment recommendation should be plausible and feasible. The patient's potential resistance for any element of the treatment plan should be addressed as directly as possible, to minimize opportunities for the patient to sabotage the treatment plan. The psychiatrist should ensure that the patient fully understands each aspect of the treatment plan. The patient should be given ample opportunity to ask questions and to consider alternative options, if acceptable treatment substitutes exist.

The psychiatrist should document if the patient refuses any portion of the treatment plan. If the psychiatrist believes that the patient's treatment refusal will cause serious harm to the patient or others or that the patient's psychiatric illness will deteriorate significantly without treatment, the psychiatrist might need to pursue mandated treatment, including possibly appointing another person to serve as the patient's guardian to force treatment adherence.

Finally, the psychiatrist and patient should discuss and agree on a follow-up plan. Whenever possible, the date and time of the next appointment should be determined before the patient leaves the psychia-

trist's office. Last, as discussed previously, the psychiatrist should give the patient specific contact information for his or her office and instructions about how to handle any urgent or emergent situations regarding the patient's mental health that might arise before the next appointment.

Conclusion

The psychiatric interview, including the mental status examination, continues to be one of the most important tools for patient assessment, even with recent advances in medical technology. As is the case with all critical medical skills, psychiatrists must maintain their expertise through continued education and regular practice.

Key Points

- Establish rapport and communicate respect. Introduce yourself, use patient's name, make eye contact, and limit interruptions.

- Use empathic connection to guide and adjust interview to match the particular patient and situation. Follow the patient's leads or cues whenever possible and use open ended questions to increase depth of understanding and information gathered (fewer topics covered, greater depth). Use focused questions to increase breadth of understanding and information gathered (more topics covered, less depth). Increase focus of questions for patients with disturbances of thought content or production, perceptual disturbances, or cognitive deficits. Abbreviate the interview for acutely agitated, dangerous, or medically compromised patients. Use words that the patient can understand—avoid medical jargon; assess the patient's education, language, and cultural needs; and use a translator when necessary. Clarify and verify that the patient understands you and that you understand the patient.

- Assess the patient's safety, including assessment of suicide risk in every patient. Assess dangerousness early and often during an interview with a potentially dangerous patient.

- Take notes to record necessary data, but do not let note taking interfere with your ability to establish and maintain rapport with the patient. Review available medical records and test results before completing your assessment and developing your treatment plan. Interview other relevant persons in the patient's life.

- Cover all key elements of the psychiatric history and mental status examination. Psychiatric history includes chief complaint, history of present illness, past psychiatric history, past medical history, social history, developmental history, family psychiatric and medical history, and review of systems. For the mental status examination, observe or assess the following aspects of behavior and thought: general appearance; orientation; speech; motor activity; affect and mood; thought production; thought content; perceptual disturbances; suicidal or homicidal ideation; attention, concentration, and memory; abstract thinking; and insight/judgment.

- Formulate the data gathered during psychiatric interview and develop a biopsychosocial formulation and a thorough differential diagnosis, including information for all five DSM-IV-TR axes. Develop a treatment plan that includes appropriate biological, psychological, and social interventions and considers the patient's overall prognosis. Ensure that the patient understands the treatment goals and plan, and verify that the patient can afford the treatment recommendations. Document if the patient refuses treatment. Establish follow-up plans (e.g., next appointment, tests to complete).

Suggested Readings

MacKinnon RA, Yudofsky SC: Principles of the Psychiatric Evaluation, 2nd Edition. Philadelphia, PA, JB Lippincott, 1991

MacKinnon RA, Michels R, Buckley PJ: The Psychiatric Interview in Clinical Practice, 2nd Edition. Washington, DC, American Psychiatric Publishing, 2006

References

American Psychiatric Association: Diagnostic and Statistical Manual of Mental Disorders, 4th Edition, Text Revision. Washington, DC, American Psychiatric Association, 2000

Folstein MF, Folstein SE, McHugh PR: "Mini-Mental State": a practical method for grading the cognitive state of patients for the clinician. J Psychiatr Res 12:189–198, 1975

Gabbard GO: Long-Term Psychodynamic Psychotherapy. Washington, DC, American Psychiatric Publishing, 2004

Kassaw K, Gabbard GO: Creating a psychodynamic formulation from a clinical evaluation. Am J Psychiatry 159:721–726, 2002

MacKinnon RA, Michels R, Buckley PJ: The Psychiatric Interview in Clinical Practice, 2nd Edition. Washington, DC, American Psychiatric Publishing, 2006

Perry S, Cooper AM, Michels R: The psychodynamic formulation: its purpose, structure and clinical application. Am J Psychiatry 144:543–551, 1987

Scheiber SC: The psychiatric interview, psychiatric history, and mental status examination, in The American Psychiatric Publishing Textbook of Clinical Psychiatry, 4th Edition. Edited by Hales RE, Yudofsky SC. Washington, DC, American Psychiatric Publishing, 2003, pp 155–188

Vergare MJ, Binder RL, Cook IA, et al: Practice guideline for the psychiatric evaluation of adults, 2nd edition. Am J Psychiatry 163:1–36, 2006

LABORATORY TESTING AND IMAGING STUDIES IN PSYCHIATRY

H. Florence Kim, M.D.
Paul E. Schulz, M.D.
Elisabeth A. Wilde, Ph.D.
Stuart C. Yudofsky, M.D.

Laboratory and diagnostic testing traditionally have not held a central role in the diagnosis and treatment of patients with psychiatric disorders. This contrasts with the other specialties of modern medicine, which have come to rely heavily on laboratory and imaging modalities to provide the necessary information to diagnose and treat patients with disorders such as cancer, heart disease, and pulmonary problems.

Psychiatric diagnoses, on the other hand, continue to be made primarily on clinical grounds, with laboratory and diagnostic testing being relegated to informing clinicians about medical causes of psychiatric symptoms that might be excluded from the differential diagnoses or used to monitor psychotropic drug levels during treatment. Yet clinical laboratory and diagnostic imaging is on the threshold of a new era.

New methods such as pharmacogenetic and pharmacogenomic testing are becoming widespread and more widely available for clinical use. Research into structural and functional neuroimaging abnormalities in psychiatric disorders is providing valuable information about the possible pathophysiology underlying these disease states, and neuroimaging studies hold promise for eventual use as routine diagnostic modalities. Research into the use of combined laboratory and imaging modalities is leading us to our eventual goal of early identification, treatment, and ultimately prevention of psychiatric illnesses. In this chapter, we present what is currently available for clinical diagnostic testing and imaging of psychiatric patients and what the future holds for these modalities as the arsenal of diagnostic modalities grows ever larger for the clinical psychiatrist.

Approach to Screening Laboratory and Diagnostic Testing of Psychiatric Patients

Laboratory assessment is essential to the workup of the psychiatric patient because any number of neurological and medical illnesses can give rise to psychiatric symptomatology. A careful neuropsychiatric history and physical examination and judicious clinical laboratory testing are still the first and very important steps in the workup. They can focus or even obviate neuroimaging or electrophysiological testing, which can be expensive, invasive, and physically and emotionally uncomfortable to the patient.

Moreover, psychiatric symptoms that on the surface may appear to be similar may, in fact, have dissimilar etiologies. For example, hallucinations can occur in the context of schizophrenia as well as in Alzheimer's disease, Parkinson's disease, frontotemporal dementia, delirium from other chronic medical illnesses, and alcohol withdrawal. Table 2–1 lists some of the many medical and neurological illnesses that may present with prominent neuropsychiatric symptoms. Clinical laboratory assessment and diagnostic testing can help determine which of these many causes is responsible for a patient's hallucinations. Importantly, a number of these etiologies may have potentially curative remediations, and hence accurate diagnosis is critical.

A complete psychiatric assessment, including a medical and psychiatric history, physical examination, and mental status examination, must be conducted before the initiation of any clinical and diagnostic testing. Such initial assessments will guide the clinician in his or her choices for relevant, cost-effective laboratory testing. Laboratory costs accounted for 10%–12% of total health care costs in 1990, and unnecessary tests should be avoided if they are unlikely to alter the patient's treatment and outcome (Sheline and Kehr 1990). At present, there are no consensus guidelines for the initial laboratory screening of psychiatric patients without known medical illnesses. Clinicians are generally guided by the history, physical examination, and mental status examination and by their own clinical judgment to decide what tests are appropriate to obtain.

Screening Chest Radiographs

In several studies, investigators have retrospectively reviewed the utility of the screening chest radiograph in the evaluation of psychiatric patients. Data from several studies suggest that there is little evidence that a routine chest radiograph will yield beneficial information for a patient without respiratory or neurological symptoms (Brown and Gaar 1995; Gomez-Gil et al. 2002; Harms and Hermans 1994; Hughes and Barraclough 1980; Liston et al. 1979; Mookhoek and Sterrenburg-vdNieuwegiessen 1998). These data, in addition to the absence of current screening guidelines for chest radiographs in the general population, indicate that the *routine* screening chest radiograph is not indicated for a person being evaluated for the presence of a psychiatric disorder. However, chest radiographs are clearly indicated for specific clinical situations. For example, for an elderly patient with sudden onset of fever, shortness of breath, chest pain, or delirium, a chest radiograph should be ordered on an emergency basis.

Table 2–1. Selected medical conditions with psychiatric manifestations

Neurological
  Cerebrovascular disease
  Multiple sclerosis
  Multiple systems atrophy
  Parkinson's disease
  Progressive supranuclear palsy
  Alzheimer's disease
  Frontotemporal dementias
  Dementia associated with Lewy bodies
  Seizure disorder
  Huntington's disease
  Traumatic brain injury
  Anoxic brain injury
  Migraine headache
  Sleep disorders (narcolepsy, sleep apnea)
  Normal pressure hydrocephalus

Neoplastic
  Central nervous system tumors, primary
    and metastatic
  Pancreatic carcinoma
  Paraneoplastic syndromes
  Endocrine tumors
  Pheochromocytoma

Infectious
  HIV
  Neurosyphilis
  Creutzfeldt-Jakob disease
  Systemic viral and bacterial infections
  Viral and bacterial meningitis and
    encephalitis
  Tuberculosis
  Infectious mononucleosis
  Pediatric autoimmune neuropsychiatric
    disorder associated with streptococcal
    infections (PANDAS)

Nutritional
  Vitamin deficiencies
    B_{12}: pernicious anemia
    Folate: megaloblastic anemia
    Nicotinic acid deficiency: pellagra
  Thiamine deficiency: Wernicke-Korsakoff
    syndrome
  Trace mineral deficiency (zinc, magnesium)

Table 2–1. Selected medical conditions with psychiatric manifestations *(continued)*

Autoimmune
  Systemic lupus erythematosus
  Sarcoidosis
  Sjögren syndrome
  Behçet syndrome

Endocrine/metabolic
  Wilson's disease
  Fluid and electrolyte disturbances
    (syndrome of inappropriate
    antidiuretic hormone secretion
    [SIADH], central pontine myelinolysis)
  Porphyrias
  Uremias
  Hypercapnia
  Hepatic encephalopathy
  Hyper-/hypocalcemia
  Hyper-/hypoglycemia
  Thyroid and parathyroid disease
  Diabetes mellitus
  Pheochromocytoma
  Pregnancy
  Gonadotropic hormonal disturbances
  Panhypopituitarism

Drugs and toxins
  Environmental toxins: organophosphates,
    heavy metals, carbon monoxide
  Drug or alcohol intoxication/withdrawal
  Adverse effects of prescription and over-
    the-counter medications

Source. Adapted from Ringholz 2001; Sadock and Sadock 2007; Wallach 2000.

Screening Electrocardiograms

Several studies have shown that the routine performance of screening electrocardiograms on young, medically healthy psychiatric patients who do not have cardiovascular symptoms is unnecessary (Hollister 1995). However, studies differ regarding the importance of electrocardiography in the elderly, with some finding an increased prevalence of electrocardiographic abnormalities in people over age 50. Furthermore, the conclusions of these studies differ with regard to the clinical importance or outcome that these abnormalities might have for the patient's health (Hall et al. 1980; Harms and Hermans 1994; Hollister 1995; Mookhoek and Sterrenburg-vdNieuwegiessen 1998). However, all agree that, regardless of age, an electrocardiogram is indicated when the history, review of systems, or findings from the physical examination suggest cardiovascular disease, or if a patient is initiating treatment with a psychotropic drug, such as a tricyclic antidepressant (TCA) or an antipsychotic, that is known to alter cardiac function or increase cardiac conduction times.

Screening Electroencephalograms

The electroencephalogram (EEG) can be very useful when a patient has altered mental status, such as delirium or encephalopathy. It can be useful for distinguishing between possible diagnoses. For example, it can diagnose complex partial status epilepticus. It can also be useful for diagnosing metabolic encephalopathy, which is generally due to a systemic illness that is having an effect on the nervous system, such as a urinary tract infection, endocrine disorder, toxin(s), or metabolic derangement(s). The EEG is also useful for distinguishing some specific etiologies of encephalopathy. For example, it might show the di- and triphasic waves characteristic of renal failure, hepatic failure, or anoxia. In the patient who is frankly comatose, the EEG can be very valuable for identifying the level of nervous system impairment. For example, it can show an alpha coma pattern or a theta coma pattern characteristic of brain stem lesions producing coma or may show a delta coma pattern characteristic of bihemispheric disease. In the patient who appears to be obtunded, the EEG can be useful for demonstrating whether a patient is catatonic, and hence has a normal awake-looking EEG, versus encephalopathic, where there might be diffuse slowing or triphasic waves (metabolic encephalopathy).

Although the acute computed tomography (CT) scan has generally superseded the EEG for diagnosing strokes, strokes may not be demonstrable in the first 24 hours after they occur. In that setting, an EEG may be useful for diagnosing a focal deficit before it is visible on a CT scan. Thus, it might be useful, for example, to distinguish a functional right hemiparesis and aphasia due to a stroke that is not yet visible on a head CT. When these symptoms are due to a large middle cerebral artery stroke, there will be focal slowing on the EEG. The EEG will be normal, in contrast, in a functional hemiparesis and aphasia.

Screening Structural Neuroimaging Examinations

A screening head CT scan is very easy to perform, takes only a few minutes, produces little discomfort, and has a fairly high resolution and sensitivity. It can thus be easily performed in any psychiatric patient admitted with clinical features that do not appear to be classic for the disorder diagnosed. For example, if a patient has late-onset depression or mood disorder, then a head CT scan can be useful for screening for vascular disease, demyelinating disease, subdural hematoma, subarachnoid hemorrhage, and so on.

Magnetic resonance imaging (MRI) of the brain has the advantage over the head CT of being more sensitive. It is much more likely to detect vascular disease and demyelinating disease. It is also useful for detecting mild neurodegenerative changes that might point to degenerative dementias. However, MRI does take longer (about 45 minutes) than CT scans, and it is at least twice as expensive. In most places, MRI is also not available at night and hence is not useful for rapid screening.

Overall Role of Screening Laboratory and Diagnostic Testing

The consensus of studies evaluating the role and value of laboratory testing is that patients who have psychiatric signs and symptoms but who do not exhibit other physical complaints or symptoms will benefit from a small screening battery that includes serum glucose concentration, blood urea nitrogen (BUN) concentration, creatinine clearance, and urinalysis. Female patients older than 50 years will also benefit from a screening thyroid-stimulating hormone (TSH) test regardless of the presence or absence of mood symptoms. Broader screening panels are costly and are generally unnecessary. However, for psychiatric patients who have concomitant physical complaints or findings on physical examination, more extensive laboratory workup may become necessary. Likewise, more extensive laboratory workup is warranted for patients who are of higher risk, such as elderly or institutionalized patients or those with low socioeconomic status, self-neglect, alcohol or drug dependence, or cognitive impairment. Imaging may also be helpful when atypical features are present, such as an older age at onset of psychiatric illness, or when cognitive impairment is present.

Laboratory Approach to Specific Clinical Situations in Psychiatry

In this section, we discuss the specific clinical situations that may arise with the psychiatric patient that would warrant more extensive laboratory and diagnostic workup. These situations include, but are not limited to, new-onset psychosis, new-onset mood symptoms, anxiety symptoms, altered mental status, cognitive decline, and substance abuse.

New-Onset Psychosis

A careful evaluation is important for a patient with a first episode of psychosis in order to rule out the many possible medical and neurological causes of psychosis. Routine screening tests often include serum chemistries for sodium, potassium, chloride, carbon dioxide, BUN, and creatinine; liver function tests such as total protein, total and direct bilirubin, se-

rum aspartate transaminase/serum glutamic-oxaloacetic transaminase (AST/SGOT), and alanine aminotransferase/serum glutamic pyruvic transaminase (AAT/SGPT); complete blood count (CBC) with platelets and differential; TSH; a rapid plasma reagin for syphilis; HIV serology; serum alcohol level; urinalysis; and urine toxicology screen for drugs of abuse. Other tests to consider during the initial workup include structural neuroimaging (head CT or brain MRI) and electroencephalography. If appropriate, the clinician should also consider ordering a urine pregnancy test and baseline electrocardiogram, especially if he or she is planning to initiate or change antipsychotic medication. If these initial tests do not immediately yield an etiology, the clinician may also consider a lumbar puncture to analyze cerebrospinal fluid (CSF) for the presence of red and white blood cells, protein, and glucose; opening pressure; and bacterial culture, cryptococcal antigen, and viral serologies. Antinuclear antibodies, rheumatoid factor, erythrocyte sedimentation rate, urine porphyrins, blood cultures, and assays for heavy metals (manganese and mercury) and bromides are other tests to consider. There are many causes of psychosis that need to be considered, including central nervous system (CNS) or systemic infections, temporal lobe epilepsy, substance intoxication and withdrawal, metabolic or endocrine disorders, CNS tumors, and heavy metal poisoning. Table 2–2 summarizes some of the recommended tests in the diagnostic approach to a patient with new-onset psychosis.

Mood Disturbance: Depressive or Manic Symptoms

A thorough laboratory screening is also recommended for the evaluation of adult patients with new-onset mood symptoms such as depression or mania. Tests might include TSH, serum chemistries, CBC, urinalysis, and urine toxicology screen for drugs of abuse. If appropriate, the clinician should also consider

---

Table 2–2.   Recommended diagnostic workup for a patient with new-onset psychosis

---

Routine screening

Complete blood count with differential and platelets

Serum chemistries, including liver and renal function tests

Thyroid-stimulating hormone

Rapid plasma reagin

HIV serology

Erythrocyte sedimentation rate

Serum alcohol level

Urine toxicology screen

Head computed tomography or brain magnetic resonance imaging scan

Electroencephalogram

Urine pregnancy test

Baseline electrocardiogram

Therapeutic drug levels

Consider per clinical suspicion

Antinuclear antibody

Rheumatoid factor

Blood cultures

Serum B_{12} and folate levels

Metal assays: serum and urine copper, serum ceruloplasmin; lead; mercury; manganese

Cerebrospinal fluid analysis: red blood cell count; white blood cell count; protein; glucose; opening pressure; bacterial cultures; cryptococcal antigen; viral serologies

Urine porphyrins

---

ordering a urine pregnancy test and electrocardiogram, especially if he or she is considering starting a mood-stabilizing medication. Measuring levels of therapeutic drugs can be helpful to confirm the presence of a drug if noncompliance is suspected or if therapeutic effect is not obtained, to determine whether toxicity may be contributing to the patient's clinical presentation, or to determine whether drug interactions have altered the desired therapeutic levels (Wallach 1992). Serum trough levels of mood stabilizers such as lith-

ium, valproate, or carbamazepine and TCAs can be obtained to monitor therapeutic response in accordance with therapeutic levels. (For additional information, see the sections "Medication Monitoring and Maintenance" and "Pharmacogenetics and Pharmacogenomics" later in this chapter.)

Neuroimaging and electroencephalography are often helpful as well in understanding the etiology of a patient's mood symptoms. Multiple neurological and medical disorders have mood manifestations that may often be the presenting complaint. For example, stroke, seizure disorders, Parkinson's disease, Huntington's disease, frontotemporal dementia, and thyroid and other endocrine abnormalities may all present with depression, mania/hypomania, or psychosis as the primary complaint, with only subtle physical and cognitive manifestations that may be missed by cursory clinical examination. Further workup with laboratory tests, structural and sometimes functional imaging, and electroencephalography can uncover medical or neurological etiologies, thus providing the patient with effective treatment or prophylaxis against further episodes. The diagnostic approach to a patient with new-onset depressive or manic symptoms is summarized in Table 2–3.

Anxiety

The initial workup for anxiety symptoms should include serum chemistries, serum glucose, and TSH and other endocrine measures (Table 2–4). Many different medical diseases can also manifest with anxiety, including angina and myocardial infarction, mitral valve prolapse, substance intoxication and withdrawal, and metabolic and endocrine disorders such as thyroid abnormalities, pheochromocytoma, and hypoglycemia. Neurological disorders, such as many forms of dementia, can also present with anxiety. A cardiac workup is important because cardiac symptoms may masquerade as panic attacks and are often misdiagnosed as such, especially in female patients. Therefore, electrocardiography, Holter monitoring, stress test, and/or

Table 2–3. Recommended diagnostic workup for a patient with new-onset depressive or manic symptoms

Routine screening

Complete blood count with differential and platelets

Serum chemistries, including liver and renal function tests

Thyroid-stimulating hormone

Rapid plasma reagin

HIV serology

Urinalysis

Urine toxicology screen

Serum alcohol level (if suspected)

Urine pregnancy test

Electrocardiogram

Therapeutic drug levels (if patient is already on psychiatric medications)

Consider per clinical suspicion

Structural neuroimaging (brain magnetic resonance imaging)

Electroencephalogram

Table 2–4. Recommended diagnostic workup for a patient with new-onset anxiety symptoms

Routine screening

Serum chemistries, including liver and renal function tests

Serum glucose

Thyroid-stimulating hormone

Referral for cardiac evaluation: electrocardiogram, Holter monitoring, stress test and/or echocardiogram

Consider per clinical suspicion

Referral for respiratory evaluation: chest radiograph; pulmonary function tests

Electroencephalogram

Urine porphyrins and vanillylmandelic acid levels

Urine metanephrines

Blood gas

echocardiography may be necessary. Respiratory function should also be evaluated with a chest radiograph or pulmonary function tests to rule out chronic obstructive pulmonary disease as a contributory factor. Other tests to consider if one has clinical suspicion include electroencephalography, urine porphyrins, and urine vanillylmandelic acid.

Altered Mental Status

Patients with a fluctuating mental status of acute onset most likely will have one or more underlying medical or neurological causes for their impaired consciousness. This often constitutes a medical emergency, and comprehensive laboratory and diagnostic testing are indicated on an emergency basis, as summarized in Table 2–5. In addition to a complete physical examination and as much history as can be obtained from the patient and ancillary sources, the clinician should order serum chemistries, CBC, erythrocyte sedi-

mentation rate, HIV serology, urinalysis and urine toxicology, electrocardiogram, and chest radiograph. A CT scan, blood cultures, lumbar puncture with CSF analysis, and EEG can be helpful as well, if clinically indicated. Many medical and neurological disorders can cause impairment in mental status, including seizures, CNS and systemic infection, kidney or liver failure, cardiac arrhythmias, stroke, myocardial infarction, and substance intoxication and withdrawal.

As noted previously, the EEG can be very helpful in the workup of patients with encephalopathy. It can diagnose seizures. It can also suggest that an encephalopathy is due to a nonneurological etiology. For example, it can show a metabolic etiology (metabolic encephalopathy), which often suggests that systemic issues are at the root of encephalopathy. Such etiologies include electrolyte disturbances, infections, and toxins.

The head CT scan can also be helpful in the workup of the patient with altered mental status. It can detect subdural hematomas or subarachnoid hemorrhage, and a CT with contrast can suggest infections such as meningitis or an abscess. Strokes do not typically

Table 2–5. Recommended diagnostic workup for a patient with altered mental status

Routine screening

Serum chemistries, including liver and renal function tests

Complete blood count

Erythrocyte sedimentation rate

HIV serology

Antinuclear antibody

Rheumatoid factor

B_{12}

Folate

Rapid plasma reagin

Urinalysis

Urine toxicology

Serum alcohol level

Therapeutic drug levels

Electrocardiogram

Chest radiograph

Head computed tomography scan

Electroencephalogram

Consider per clinical suspicion

Cerebrospinal fluid analysis: red blood cell count; white blood cell count; protein; glucose; opening pressure; bacterial cultures; cryptococcal antigen; viral serologies

Urine porphyrins

Serum ammonia level

Brain magnetic resonance imaging

Arterial blood gases

Blood cultures

present as altered mental status. However, a right middle cerebral artery stroke or a thalamic stroke can occasionally present with altered mental status, and the head CT scan can be very useful for detecting these etiologies.

Cognitive Decline

Dementias

Laboratory testing is a major component of the comprehensive evaluation of cognitive decline. The current American Academy of Neurology (2007) practice recommendations for evaluation of reversible causes of dementia include testing for vitamin B_{12} deficiency and hypothyroidism. These laboratory tests are recommended in addition to structural imaging (noncontrast head CT or MRI studies) and evaluation of depression to rule out so-called pseudodementia, or dementia-like symptoms that stem from depression. Syphilis serology screening is necessary only in patients with dementia who are at risk for neurosyphilis. Neuropsychological testing is also recommended. It can be very useful for differentiating between dementia and pseudodementia, for distinguishing among the many types of dementia, and for determining whether a patient is responding to treatment.

Other imaging modalities—such as linear and volumetric imaging, single photon emission computed tomography (SPECT), and positron emission tomography (PET)—are not recommended routinely at this time because there are insufficient data on the validity of these tests to diagnose illnesses that lead to cognitive disorders and dementia. However, PET and SPECT are approved to distinguish between Alzheimer's dementia and frontotemporal dementia.

Likewise, there are no serum or CSF biomarkers or genetic tests currently recommended for routine use in the diagnosis of dementia, although the clinical utility of several tests is being investigated. One exception is the immunoassay for CSF 14–3–3 protein, which is useful for the confirmation of Creutzfeldt-Jakob disease in a patient with rapidly progressive dementia and pathognomonic neurological symptoms (e.g., myoclonic jerks). False-positive results can occur with some other neurological conditions such as viral encephalitis, stroke, and paraneoplastic neurological disorders. Table 2–6 lists the laboratory and diagnostic tests that would be included in the workup of a patient with cognitive impairment.

Mild Cognitive Impairment

There are no current clinical recommendations for the laboratory assessment of pa-

Table 2–6. Recommended diagnostic workup for a patient with cognitive decline

Routine screening

Complete blood count with differential and platelets

Serum chemistries including liver and renal function tests

Erythrocyte sedimentation rate

Antinuclear antibody

Rheumatoid factor

B_{12} and folate levels

Thyroid-stimulating hormone

Structural neuroimaging studies (head computed tomography or brain magnetic resonance imaging scan)

Consider per clinical suspicion

Rapid plasma reagin

HIV serology

C-reactive protein

Cerebrospinal fluid (CSF) analysis: red blood cell count; white blood cell count; protein; glucose; opening pressure; bacterial cultures; cryptococcal antigen; viral serologies; CSF 14–3–3 protein immunoassay (if Creutzfeldt-Jakob disease is suspected); CSF tau and A beta 1–42 levels for frontotemporal dementia vs. Alzheimer's disease

Urine porphyrins

Functional neuroimaging studies (single photon emission computed tomography or positron emission tomography)

Electroencephalogram

Apolipoprotein E genotyping

Neuropsychological testing

Fasting lipids, triglycerides, and blood sugar when a vascular etiology is suspected

tients who have mild cognitive impairment. By definition, such patients do not yet meet criteria for dementia. However, patients with mild cognitive impairment are at very high risk for developing dementia or Alzheimer's disease (Petersen et al. 2005). However, the utility of a diagnostic workup, aside from cognitive screening, is as yet unknown. Patients who have symptoms of mild cognitive impairment will likely benefit from a thyroid screen. Other laboratory tests typically ordered for the evaluation of dementia may be of use should signs and symptoms be elicited from the history, review of systems, or physical examination. For example, it may be useful to measure folate and vitamin B_{12} levels in a patient with mild cognitive impairment who has a long history of alcohol abuse or who is discovered to have peripheral neuropathy on the neurological examination. Because one-third of patients with mild cognitive impairment progress to Alzheimer's disease over 3 years (Petersen et al. 2005), many clinicians feel it prudent to order the same tests they would to rule out reversible causes of dementia. However, as of yet, there are no studies that have proven the clinical utility of this strategy.

Substance Abuse

In a study of 345 consecutive patients who presented to the emergency department of an urban teaching hospital with primary psychiatric complaints, 141 of these patients (41%) had positive urine toxicology screens for substances of abuse, and 90 (26%) had positive ethanol screens (Olshaker et al. 1997). Clearly, laboratory testing is essential to the evaluation, monitoring, and subsequent treatment of patients who abuse alcohol, prescribed addictive medications, or illicit drugs.

Laboratory detection of drugs of abuse, as well as test results indicative of end-organ damage related to the abuse, can provide valuable hard evidence for the treating clinician, which can be used to inform and monitor his or her patient's progress. These data are also frequently useful in confronting the denial of substance abuse by the patient or his or her family. Laboratory testing can be conducted with blood and urine specimens or with saliva and hair samples. Urine specimens are typically preferred, because the detectable length of time that a particular drug of abuse and its metabolites are present is

Table 2–7. Toxic levels and urine detection times of commonly abused substances

Agent	Toxic level	Urine detection time
Alcohol	300 mg/dL at any time or >100 g ingested	7–12 hours
Amphetamines		48 hours
Barbiturates	>6 μg/mL	24 hours (short-acting) 3 weeks (long-acting)
Benzodiazepines	Varies with medication Lorazepam: >25–100 mg Diazepam: >250 mg	3 days
Cannabis	50–200 μg/kg	4–6 weeks
Cocaine	>1.2 g	6–8 hours 2–4 days (metabolites)
Opiates	Varies with medication Heroin: >100–250 mg Codeine: >500–1,000 mg Morphine: >50–100 μg/kg	2–3 days
Phencyclidine	>10–20 mg	1–2 weeks

Source.   Adapted from Wallach 2000.

longer in urine than in blood. However, some substances, such as alcohol or barbiturates, are best detected in blood specimens.

The length of time that a drug of abuse is detectable in the urine varies based on the amount and duration of substance consumed, kidney and liver function, and the specific drug itself. Laboratory methodologies vary. If the screening tests yield a positive result, follow-up with more specific tests, including quantitative analyses, can be ordered for confirmation. Table 2–7 reviews common drugs of abuse and the toxic level and urine detection time of each.

Medication Monitoring and Maintenance

Measuring levels of therapeutic drugs to evaluate for toxicity and effective levels can be extremely helpful in the workup and treatment of the psychiatric patient. Therapeutic drug monitoring should be used to confirm the presence and level of the drug if noncompliance is suspected, if the desired therapeutic effect is not obtained, or if signs or symptoms of toxicity occur; to determine whether toxicity may be contributing to the patient's clinical presentation; or to determine whether drug interactions have altered desired levels of therapeutic drugs (Wallach 1992). Serum trough levels of mood stabilizers (such as lithium, valproate, or carbamazepine) and TCAs can be obtained to monitor therapeutic response in accordance with therapeutic levels for acute exacerbation and maintenance treatment of bipolar disorder.

Mood Stabilizers

Blood tests are important for screening for end-organ damage before the initiation of treatment with these mood stabilizers. Follow-up testing during maintenance treatment is recommended at regular intervals, although the utility of these routine screens in detecting asymptomatic end-organ damage—such as an increase in liver function with valproate or renal impairment with lithium—is unclear. No clear consensus exists as to the appropriate interval for routine monitoring during the use of mood stabilizers.

Most experts recommend screening every 3–6 months; however, some experts recommend that clinical monitoring of signs of toxicity may be more effective than periodic screening. That may especially be the case for drugs like valproate for which the routine monitoring of liver function tests may have little predictive value in terms of hepatotoxicity (Marangell et al. 2002; Pellock and Willmore 1991; Willmore et al. 1991). Although there is a lack of consensus regarding the recommended screening tests, a potential set of guidelines, which most authors appear to support, is listed in Table 2–8. The table shows the psychotropic medications for which therapeutic drug monitoring may be useful as well as therapeutic and toxic drug levels and ancillary tests that are recommended to monitor for the prevention of end-organ damage.

Tricyclic Antidepressants

Drug levels of TCAs may also be obtained, although it is unclear whether blood levels of antidepressants correlate with therapeutic response. Four TCAs—imipramine, desipramine, amitriptyline, and nortriptyline—have been well studied, and generalizations can be made about the relationship of drug levels to therapeutic response. For imipramine, optimal response rates occur as blood levels reach 200–250 ng/mL, and levels greater than 250 ng/mL often produce more side effects but no change in antidepressant response (American Psychiatric Association Task Force on the Use of Laboratory Tests in Psychiatry 1985). Nortriptyline, in contrast, appears to have a specific therapeutic window between 50 and 150 ng/mL, and poor clinical response occurs both above and below that window. Desipramine also appears to have a linear relationship between drug concentration and clinical outcome, with plasma concentrations greater than 125 ng/mL being significantly more effective. Amitriptyline has been fairly well studied; however, some studies have found a linear relationship similar to that of imipramine, others have found a curvilinear relationship, and

others have found no relationship between blood levels and clinical outcomes (American Psychiatric Association Task Force on the Use of Laboratory Tests in Psychiatry 1985). For the other TCAs that have been less well studied, drug levels can still be useful to confirm the presence of the drug or to confirm extremely high serum levels (Hyman et al. 1995).

Neuroleptics

The monitoring of blood levels for neuroleptics is not routinely used in clinical practice. Different methods for monitoring neuroleptic drugs have been developed, but a reliable therapeutic range has not been established because there does not appear to be a consistent relationship between blood levels of neuroleptics and clinical response (Curry 1985). However, there are several clinical situations in which it may be useful to obtain blood levels of neuroleptics.

Blood level monitoring may be useful to confirm the presence of the neuroleptic when adherence is a concern. It may be used to ascertain the presence of drug interactions in a patient who has relapsed or experienced an exacerbation of symptoms after a period of stabilization and who has been taking drugs that may interact with neuroleptics, such as carbamazepine or fluoxetine. It may also be helpful to obtain drug levels in patients who develop excessive side effects to moderate dosages of neuroleptics (Bernardo et al. 1993).

Diagnostic and laboratory monitoring are important components of care for patients receiving neuroleptic medications. In patients who are over the age of 50, or who have pre-existing cardiac disease, a screening electrocardiogram should be ordered before institution of antipsychotic medications, such as thioridazine or ziprasidone, that may cause prolongation of the QT_c interval (a marker for potentially life-threatening cardiac arrhythmias such as torsades de pointes). Follow-up electrocardiograms should be ordered for any patient receiving treatment with antipsychotic medications in whom symptoms indic-

Table 2–8. Medication monitoring

Medication type	Medication	Therapeutic range	Toxic level	Recommended screening
Mood stabilizer	Lithium	0.8–1.2 mEq/L	>1.5 mEq/L	Initiation: sodium, potassium, calcium, phosphate, BUN, creatinine, TSH, T$_4$, CBC, urinalysis, beta-HCG if appropriate; ECG in patient older than 50 years or with preexisting cardiac disease
				Maintenance: TSH, BUN/creatinine recommended every 6 months; ECGs as needed in patient older than 40 years or with preexisting cardiac disease
	Valproate	50–150 µg/mL	>150 µg/mL	Initiation: CBC with platelets, LFTs; beta-HCG if appropriate
				Maintenance: LFTs, CBC recommended every 6 months
	Carbamazepine	8–12 µg/mL	>12 µg/mL	Initiation: CBC with platelets, LFTs, BUN/creatinine
				Maintenance: CBC with platelets, LFTs, BUN/creatinine
Tricyclic antidepressant (TCA)	Imipramine + desipramine	125–250 ng/mL	>500 ng/mL or >1 g ingested	Desipramine is metabolite of imipramine
				Initiation: ECG in patient older than 40 years or with preexisting cardiac disease for all TCAs
	Doxepin + (metabolite) desmethyldoxepin	100–275 ng/mL	>500 ng/mL	Initiation: ECG in patient older than 40 years or with preexisting cardiac disease for all TCAs
	Amitriptyline + nortriptyline	75–225 ng/mL	>500 ng/mL	Initiation: ECG in patient older than 40 years or with preexisting cardiac disease for all TCAs
	Nortriptyline only	50–150 ng/mL	>50 ng/mL	Initiation: ECG in patient older than 40 years or with preexisting cardiac disease for all TCAs
Antipsychotic	Olanzapine, quetiapine, risperidone, ziprasidone			Fasting serum glucose, triglycerides every 6 months ECG in patient older than 50 years or with preexisting cardiac disease for agents that can cause prolongation of the QTc interval

Note. BUN=blood urea nitrogen; CBC=complete blood count; ECG=electrocardiogram; HCG=human chorionic gonadotropin; LFT=liver function test; T$_4$=thyroxine; TSH=thyroid-stimulating hormone.

Source. Adapted from Wallach 2000; Hyman et al. 1995.

ative of cardiac compromise appear. It is also recommended that screening laboratory studies be performed at regular intervals (every 6 months) to test for glucose and metabolic dysregulation (hyperlipidemias, diabetes, hypothyroidism), which are often associated with atypical antipsychotic medications.

Pharmacogenetics and Pharmacogenomics

Recent progress in drug metabolism research has resulted in newly available tests that may have significant clinical utility for psychopharmacology. Human drug metabolism is highly variable, making it difficult to predict therapeutic dosage levels and ranges, and can lead to unanticipated adverse outcomes, toxicity, and therapeutic failure. Clearly, adverse drug reactions are a serious problem, as estimated by a meta-analysis of serious adverse drug reactions (Lazarou et al. 1998). It was estimated that in 1994, more than 2 million hospitalized patients had serious adverse drug reactions, with more than 100,000 resulting in death in the United States alone.

Most psychiatric drugs are metabolized by microsomal enzymes called the cytochrome P450 (CYP) enzyme system. The CYP enzymes are a superfamily of more than 20 related enzymes, although only six metabolize more than 90% of all medications (Streetman 2000). These six enzymes that are important to human drug metabolism are CYP1A2, CYP2C9, CYP2C19, CYP2D6, CYP2E1, and CYP3A. Enzymes are identified by numbers and letters that identify the family and subfamily grouping. For example, CYP2D6 is in family 2 and subfamily 2D and is structurally related to CYP2C19 in the same family, but it is not similar to CYP3A, which is in a different family (Streetman 2000).

The majority of CYP enzyme metabolism occurs in the liver, although metabolism can occur elsewhere in the body, such as the small intestine (CYP3A4), the brain (CYP2D6), and the lung (CYP1A1). The CYP enzyme system, in addition to metabolizing drugs, also metabolizes exogenous substances, such as environmental toxins and dietary nutrients, and endogenous substances, such as steroids and prostaglandins. Through drug metabolism, a medication is made more hydrophilic or water soluble in order to be excreted by the kidneys. Table 2–9 lists many of the psychiatric drugs that are metabolized by selected CYP enzymes (substrates) as well as those that may decrease enzyme activity (inhibitors). CYP drug metabolism is highly variable due to several factors, including genetic polymorphisms, effects of concomitant medications (inhibition or induction of enzymes), physiological or disease status, and environmental or exogenous factors such as toxins and diet (Ingelman-Sundberg et al. 1999).

Pharmacogenetics is the study of genetic variation as it relates to drug response and metabolism. Research in pharmacogenetics to date has focused largely on genes that encode receptors targeted by drugs such as the serotonin and dopamine receptor subtypes or those that encode CYP enzymes. Research on the latter has been significantly more helpful to our understanding of the genetic basis of variability in medication response than research on the former.

The pharmacokinetic effects of the CYP enzyme system, specifically CYP2D6 and CYP2C19 polymorphisms, on psychiatric medications have been studied extensively. The allele sequence that produces a normally functioning enzyme is coded by the wild-type gene (given the suffix "*1"). Thereafter, differing genetic sequence polymorphisms are numbered sequentially (e.g.,*2, *3). Thus, multiple copies of a functional CYP enzyme gene can occur, resulting in enzyme overactivity. Conversely, polymorphisms may be inactivating, resulting in decreased CYP enzyme activity or even a complete loss of activity.

Four general phenotypes have been used to describe the outcomes of these CYP genetic polymorphisms (Table 2–10): ultrarapid metabolizers, extensive metabolizers, intermediate metabolizers, and poor metabolizers. Ex-

Table 2–9.　Psychiatric drug metabolism by specific P450 enzymes

Enzyme	CYP2D6	CYP2C19
Substrates (drugs metabolized by specific enzyme)	Antidepressants 　Amitriptyline 　Desipramine 　Duloxetine 　Fluoxetine 　Fluvoxamine 　Imipramine 　Nortriptyline 　Paroxetine 　Sertraline 　Trazodone 　Venlafaxine Antipsychotics 　Aripiprazole 　Clozapine 　Fluphenazine 　Haloperidol 　Olanzapine 　Perphenazine 　Risperidone 　Thioridazine Other drugs 　Donepezil 　Methadone	Antidepressants 　Amitriptyline 　Citalopram 　Clomipramine 　Escitalopram ' 　Imipramine Other drugs 　Diazepam
Inhibitors	Antidepressants 　Amitriptyline 　Bupropion 　Desipramine 　Fluoxetine 　Paroxetine 　Sertraline Antipsychotics 　Clomipramine 　Clozapine 　Thioridazine	Amitriptyline Citalopram Clomipramine Fluoxetine Fluvoxamine

Source.　Data adapted from Kirchheiner et al. 2001; Streetman 2000.

tensive metabolizers have the normal two copies of fully active CYP enzyme alleles for a particular microsomal enzyme. Poor metabolizers do not have the active enzyme gene allele, resulting in increased concentrations of medications due to reduced metabolism, and may have more adverse effects at usual, recommended dosages. In contrast, ultrarapid metabolizers will have multiple copies of the functional enzyme allele, resulting in an increased rate of drug metabolism, and may not reach therapeutic concentrations at the recommended dosage.

There is significant ethnic variability in allele frequencies, with 4%–10% of Caucasians completely lacking the CYP2D6 enzyme compared with only 1%–3% of African Americans and Chinese. Similarly, discrepancy in allele

Table 2–10. Drug metabolizer phenotype classification

Type	Number of active enzyme gene alleles	Expected response to substrate drug
Poor metabolizer	None	Reduced metabolism of drug may result in increased concentrations and more adverse effects
Intermediate metabolizer	One active and one inactive allele, or two gene alleles with reduced activity	Lesser degree of adverse effects related to reduced metabolism
Extensive metabolizer (normal)	2	Expected response to standard medication dosage
Ultrarapid metabolizer	>2	Rapid clearance of medications, so may not reach therapeutic concentrations at recommended dosages

Source. Adapted from Ingelman-Sundberg et al. 1999; Mrazek 2006.

frequencies occur for the CYP2C19 enzyme, with up to 20% of Asians lacking the active enzyme gene allele compared with only 2%–5% of Caucasians (de Leon et al. 2006).

Cerebrospinal Fluid Studies

Laboratory examination of CSF can be helpful in the diagnosis of some neuropsychiatric disorders. CSF studies are often employed in the secondary evaluation of a psychiatric patient when a neurological and possibly reversible cause is suspected, including infections, such as encephalitis or meningitis, which may be caused by bacteria; acid-fast bacilli (e.g., tuberculosis); spirochetes (e.g., syphilis, Lyme disease); viruses (e.g., herpes simplex, cytomegalovirus, Epstein-Barr virus, West Nile virus); prions (e.g., Creutzfeldt-Jakob disease); or fungi (e.g., *Cryptococcus*). CSF analysis can also reveal subarachnoid hemorrhage, which can present with altered mental status, headache, coma, and/or focal findings.

Spinal fluid analysis can also be useful for investigating inflammatory etiologies for neuropsychiatric complaints. These include autoimmune demyelinating disorders (e.g., multiple sclerosis or acute demyelinating encephalomyelitis) and autoimmune neuronal disorders (systemic lupus erythematosus). CSF analysis can also reveal disorders of CSF production that produce elevated (e.g., pseudotumor cerebri) or low pressure. Finally, CSF analysis can be very useful for identifying neoplastic processes within the nervous system, including direct tumor invasion (e.g., lymphoma), carcinomatous meningitis (e.g., prostate cancer), or a paraneoplastic syndrome.

The utility of spinal fluid analysis is being investigated for the diagnosis or differentiation between various neurodegenerative dementias. CSF tau and A beta 1–42 levels can sometimes distinguish between Alzheimer's disease and frontotemporal dementia. Spinal fluid analysis is not sensitive or specific enough to be a diagnostic test, but it can be a useful adjuvant. Other spinal fluid markers are the subject of intense investigation, with the goal of identifying one capable of diagnosing neurological and psychiatric disorders.

CSF is obtained through lumbar puncture and should always be accompanied by a blood sample drawn simultaneously and sent for protein, glucose, and serum protein electrophoresis. Except under emergency conditions, lumbar puncture should not be performed until a head CT scan has been obtained to rule out increased intracranial pressure or a mass lesion in a position that could produce herniation after a lumbar puncture. A lumbar puncture can be obtained fluoroscopically if it cannot be readily obtained due to the large size of the patient or lumbar spinal abnormalities.

Electrophysiological Testing

Standard Electroencephalogram

The standard EEG is a noninvasive recording of electrical activity of the brain. Electrodes placed on the scalp record extracellular current flow of neurons. The EEG is used in the evaluation of the psychiatric patient to exclude the contribution of a general medical condition, such as epilepsy or delirium, to a patient's clinical presentation. In general, an abnormal EEG will consist of one or more of the following: 1) paroxysmal activity indicative of transient, episodic neuronal discharges as seen in epilepsy; 2) nonparoxysmal slowing of activity, as seen in delirium; 3) asymmetric activity as observed with mass lesions or infarction; or 4) sleep abnormalities consistent with sleep apnea, rapid eye movement sleep behavior disorder, or narcolepsy.

No clear guidelines exist for the use of electroencephalographic evaluation in routine screening of the psychiatric patient. An EEG would be prudent to obtain in a patient with new-onset psychosis, episodic behavioral disturbance, or altered mental status. In a patient with altered mental status, the EEG can be diagnostically useful because it can differentiate between a diffuse encephalopathy, nonmotoric status epilepticus, or focal lesion (Boutros and Struve 2004). A normal EEG does not exclude seizure disorder from the differential diagnosis, because 20% of patients with epilepsy will have normal EEGs, and 2% of patients without epilepsy will have spike and wave formations (Engel 1992).

Polysomnography

Polysomnography entails the recording of multiple physiological variables during sleep to determine the presence of sleep disorders. It is a useful technique to implement in the psychiatric patient if a sleep disorder is suspected to be responsible for or exacerbating psychiatric symptoms. Hypnagogic hallucinations, which occur at the interface between sleep and wakefulness, can often be mistaken for symptoms of a primary psychotic disorder. Furthermore, there is considerable overlap in symptoms of depression and sleep disorders, such as insomnia, daytime fatigue, or excessive daytime sleepiness. A typical polysomnogram will consist of an EEG, electrocardiogram, electro-oculogram, and electromyogram and measurement of respiratory airflow and oxygenation, blood pressure, and body temperature. Again, no definitive guidelines exist as to the usefulness of polysomnography in the clinical workup of the psychiatric patient. Although psychiatric disorders often go hand in hand with disturbed sleep, sleep studies are not ordered for the routine evaluation of the psychiatric patient. Instead, a polysomnogram is ordered when there is clinical suspicion of parasomnia or hypersomnia (narcolepsy), a breathing disorder such as sleep apnea, or limb movements during sleep.

Evoked Potentials

Auditory, visual, somatosensory, or cognitive stimuli can be used to evoke electrical potentials that can be recorded. Repetitive stimuli result in small-magnitude electrical changes that are mathematically manipulated or "averaged," resulting in the evoked potential. Evoked potential testing provides clinically useful information about processing of sensory stimuli, which is helpful in discerning medical versus psychogenic causes of some symptoms. For example, visual evoked potentials can be useful to differentiate psychogenic blindness from true blindness, and auditory evoked potentials can be used to differentiate psychogenic deafness from catatonia in a mute, unresponsive patient.

Quantitative EEG

Quantitative EEG uses 1–2 minutes of a resting EEG that is analyzed using fast Fourier transform to quantify the power at each frequency of the EEG averaged across the entire sample (Hughes and John 1999). For each of the four frequency bands (delta [1.5–3.5 Hz], theta [3.5–7.5 Hz], alpha [7.5–12.5 Hz], and beta [12.5–20 Hz]), results obtained include absolute power (total microV2), relative power (percentage of total power for each band), coherence (synchronization between bands), and symmetry between bands. Thus, quantification allows comparison of these variables between patient groups. Despite numerous studies of quantitative EEG in dementias, cerebrovascular disease, schizophrenia, mood and anxiety disorders, learning disorders, and substance abuse disorders, there are few data available to support its use in the clinical evaluation of psychiatric patients. However, this analytical tool holds great promise for the future.

Neuroimaging Studies in Psychiatry

Brain imaging research in psychiatry has exploded in the past two decades, spurred on by increasingly sophisticated neuroimaging modalities. Although neuroimaging does not yet play a diagnostic role for any of the primary psychiatric disorders, it is still an integral part of the clinical workup for psychiatric patients to rule out underlying medical causes of psychiatric symptoms. In this section, we discuss current clinical and research neuroimaging modalities as they relate to psychiatric disorders.

Current neuroimaging methods provide both structural and functional data about the brain. Structural imaging techniques such as CT and MRI provide a fixed image of the brain's anatomy and spatial distribution. Newer functional neuroimaging techniques such as PET and SPECT provide information about brain metabolism, blood flow, the presynaptic uptake of transmitter precursors, neurotransmitter transporter activity, and postsynaptic receptor activity. Functional scans should always be interpreted in the context of the underlying structural images. With these techniques, one can find a grossly normal brain, structurally speaking, with abnormal function. Alternately, one can have abnormal brain structures that can lead to reduced or increased metabolic function (e.g., a brain tumor).

Structural Neuroimaging Modalities

Computed Tomography

CT scanning enlists a focused beam of X rays that passes through the brain at many angles. The many images evoked are then joined together to provide a cross-sectional view of the brain. The X rays are attenuated as they pass through tissue, which absorbs their energy. The degree of energy absorbed varies, based on the radiodensity of the tissue. This differential X-ray attenuation is transformed into a two-dimensional grayscale map of the brain by computers, with bone appearing most radiopaque, or white, and air the least radiopaque, or black. Brain tissue, CSF, and water have varying degrees of radiopacity (Figure 2–1).

CT has many advantages. It is widely available, less expensive than MRI, has a quick scanning time, and is relatively more comfortable and convenient than other structural imaging modalities. Thus, CT is quick and efficient and is used to rule out life-threatening conditions such as skull fracture, hemorrhage, or brain tumor.

CT also has limitations. A brain CT scan involves some radiation exposure. Deep brain structures, including those of the posterior fossa such as brain stem and cerebellum, are poorly visualized with CT because of the surrounding bony structures. Furthermore, discrimination between gray and white matter in the brain is limited due to their similar radiodensities.

Tissue	Relative attenuation values (in Hounsfield units)	Appearance on CT
Metal	1,000	White
Bone/calcium	100–1,000	
Blood		
Acute	80–85	
Subacute	25–50	
Chronic	0–25	
Gray matter	35–40	
White matter	25–30	
Water	0	
Fat	–100	
Air	–1,000	Black

Figure 2–1. Computed tomography (CT) tissue attenuation values and appearance.

Source. Adapted from J. Levine lecture "Structural Neuroimaging in Psychiatry," given as part of the Neuroimaging in Psychiatry lecture series, Department of Psychiatry, Baylor College of Medicine, March 2006.

Magnetic Resonance Imaging

MRI relies upon nuclear magnetic resonance. Hydrogen nuclei in the body have paramagnetic properties, and their spins align when placed in a static magnetic field. The magnetic field is pulsed, causing the hydrogen protons to align. When the magnetic pulses are terminated, the protons relax toward their original positions and release energy at a detectable radiofrequency. The collective magnetic behavior of the realigning hydrogen atoms within the magnetic field constitutes T1, or longitudinal relaxation, and T2, or transverse relaxation. The bulk of the MRI signaling comes from hydrogen atoms in water. MRI can distinguish between hydrogen nuclei in free water and those in blood, fat, or muscle based on differential relaxation rates in different tissues. These resonant frequencies are nonionizing and not harmful. The quality of the images produced is determined by the strength of the static magnet. Most clinical MRI scanners use a superconducting magnet of 1.5 tesla strength, although MRI scanners for research use often use 3.0 tesla or more.

In clinical practice, T2-weighted images can be very useful for visualizing lesions because they show edema as an increase in signal intensity. T1-weighted images are useful for demonstrating structural anatomy. Gradient echo images can reveal past hemorrhages. Fluid-attenuated inversion recovery images are useful for removing fluids like CSF, but retaining fluid changes as observed with the gliosis of past infarcts. One can thus observe, for example, the extent of past small-vessel ischemic changes. Figure 2–2 illustrates axial MRI images of a patient with bipolar disorder compared with an age-matched control patient.

Comparison of CT and MRI

MRI has many advantages over CT. First and foremost, it has superior visualization of brain tissue, providing enhanced gray/white matter discrimination versus CT and allowing quantitative or volumetric measurement of brain regions. Deep brain structures such as the cerebellum and brain stem are better visualized with MRI. Furthermore, axial, coronal, and sagittal images may be acquired. MRI image acquisition is complex, and depending on parameters, can produce T1-, T2-, or proton density–weighted images, spin-echo sequence, and inversion-recovery images. Table 2–11 provides a summary comparison of CT

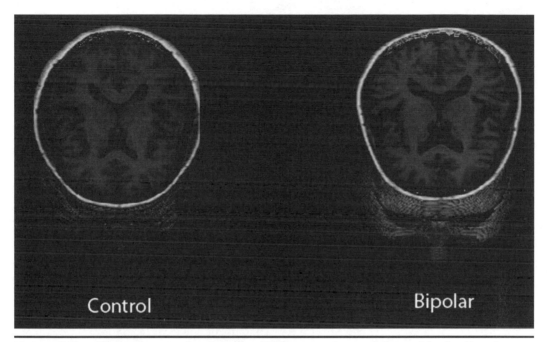

Figure 2–2. Magnetic resonance imaging (MRI) comparison axial cuts, bipolar disorder patient versus matched control subject.

MRI (T1-weighted) images of a 58-year-old healthy control patient *(left)* as compared with a patient of comparable age with bipolar disorder *(right)* but without any significant medical or substance abuse history. Although not diagnostic, common findings in neuroimaging research studies with bipolar disorder patients include diffuse gray matter loss, enlargement of the ventricles, and mild prefrontal volume loss. *Source.* Images courtesy of Elisabeth A. Wilde, Ph.D., Department of Physical Medicine and Rehabilitation, Baylor College of Medicine, Houston, Texas.

and MRI imaging. Figure 2–3 is a comparison of images available with CT versus MRI.

Clinical Use of CT and MRI in Psychiatry

For the primary psychiatric disorders, the clinical use of structural neuroimaging such as CT and MRI is largely limited to the identification of medical causes of psychiatric symptomatology. Structural imaging is ordered to evaluate for evidence of tangible abnormalities such as stroke, brain tumor, trauma, or developmental abnormalities that might underlie psychiatric symptoms. The clinical utility of structural imaging modalities has been evaluated in several retrospective studies (Agzarian et al. 2006; Hollister and Shah 1996; McClellan et al. 1988; Moles et al. 1998). There appears to be little justification

for routine screening of psychiatric patients (Agzarian et al. 2006; McClellan et al. 1988).

In the study by Agzarian et al. (2006), 397 consecutive psychiatric patients without focal neurological signs were screened with CT scans over a 2-year period, and 95% (377) of these scans were normal. The authors found that an abnormal cognitive examination (Folstein Mini-Mental State Exam was used in this study), an abnormal neurological examination, and age were the most sensitive predictors of abnormal CT findings that would influence treatment.

The clinical utility of MRI in the evaluation of adult psychiatric patients has been addressed in a few studies (Erhart et al. 2005; Hollister and Shah 1996). In a retrospective chart review of psychiatric patients referred for brain MRI evaluation (excluding those referred for evaluation of dementia) over a

Table 2–11. Comparison of computed tomography (CT) and magnetic resonance imaging (MRI)

	CT	MRI
Mechanism	X-ray attenuation	Proton magnetic resonance
Imaging planes	Axial (transverse) only	Axial, coronal, sagittal
Image acquisition time	Short (5–10 minutes)	Longer (45 minutes)
Slice thickness	2–5 mm	1–3 mm
Spatial resolution	1–2 mm	<1 mm
Cost	$300–$500	$800–$1,000
Advantages	Widely available Rapid acquisition Useful in evaluating for acute, life-threatening conditions such as hemorrhage or trauma	No radiation exposure Gray–white contrast excellent Excellent visualization of posterior fossa
Disadvantages	Radiation exposure Limited visualization of posterior fossa	Unable to use if metal or pacemakers present Slow acquisition

6-year period, 15% (38 of 253) had MRI findings that modified treatment recommendations. For 6 patients (2%), MRI identified a new medical condition requiring treatment. Thus, the authors concluded that MRI evaluation can be valuable in patients with suspected underlying medical problems causing psychiatric manifestations (Erhart et al. 2005). In a study of CT and MRI scans ordered in a psychiatric hospital over a 2-year period, 18% (12 of 68) of scans were abnormal. The authors concluded that brain imaging scans are indicated for psychiatric patients with cognitive impairment (to evaluate for dementia), a first psychotic break, personality change in a patient older than 50 years, or new or unexplained focal neurological signs (Hollister and Shah 1996).

Although evidence is limited, structural neuroimaging appears to be indicated for psychiatric patients in the following clinical situations: new or unexplained focal neurological signs, cognitive changes or impairment, new-onset psychosis, or prior to the initiation of electroconvulsive therapy. For psychiatric patients older than 50 years, any change in mental status, mood, personality, or behavior may warrant an MRI (Rauch and Renshaw 1995). A CT is valuable when evaluating for suspected hemorrhage or skull fracture or when MRI is contraindicated (e.g., presence of metal implants) (Table 2–12).

Neuroimaging of Psychiatric Disorders

Structural and functional neuroimaging of psychiatric disorders has exploded in recent decades, given the many new and powerful imaging techniques that are now available. Yet these marked advances have led to few conclusive findings about the pathophysiology and workings of the mysterious human brain. A comprehensive discussion of the research findings to date from neuroimaging studies of the major psychiatric disorders is beyond the scope of this chapter. However, Table 2–13 summarizes the structural and functional neuroimaging findings in selected psychiatric disorders that may be of interest to the psychiatric clinician.

Conclusion

Laboratory assessment and imaging studies are particularly important to the evaluation of the psychiatric patient. Their influence and scope, although of limited clinical use in the past, have the potential to increase tremendously, as promising new modalities

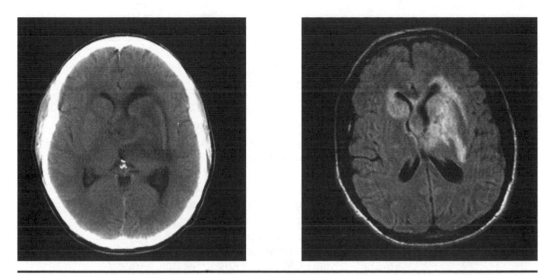

Figure 2–3. Side-by-side comparison of structural imaging modalities: computed tomography (CT) and magnetic resonance imaging (MRI).

The sensitivity of head CT versus MRI of the brain in the same patient is demonstrated here in a patient who presented with memory loss. Head CT scan at *left* shows a large area of decreased density consistent with edema. It is difficult to ascertain whether there is an underlying mass or what its shape might be. The image on the *right* is from a brain MRI (T2 image) and also demonstrates an area of increased intensity of about the same shape as the CT abnormality. The patient was found to be HIV positive, and a subsequent brain biopsy demonstrated that the mass was a B-cell lymphoma.
Source. Images courtesy of Paul E. Schulz, M.D., Department of Neurology, Baylor College of Medicine, Houston, Texas.

Table 2–12. Indications for computed tomography (CT), prior to or instead of magnetic resonance imaging (MRI)

Noncontrast CT

Evaluation of new-onset or acute neurological abnormality

Acute stroke

Subarachnoid hemorrhage

Trauma

Mass with edema, hydrocephalus, mass effect

Evaluation of ventricular size

Sinus disease

CT with or without contrast

Bone pathology (with or without contrast)

Source. Adapted from J. Levine lecture "Structural Neuroimaging in Psychiatry," given as part of the Neuroimaging in Psychiatry lecture series, Department of Psychiatry, Baylor College of Medicine, March 2006.

become more widely available and demonstrate ever-increasing clinical possibilities.

Judicious choice of laboratory testing, guided by a complete psychiatric assessment—including a thorough medical and psychiatric history, review of systems, and physical examination—may often uncover an unsuspected medical or neurological etiology underlying primarily psychiatric symptomatology. Likewise, structural and functional neuroimaging are powerful tools that can provide evidence of tangible abnormalities that might underlie psychiatric symptoms. One hopes that through advances in neuroimaging and laboratory testing, promising genetic and biological markers will be discovered and will attain a level of clinical utility so that a new and important dimension may be added to the uses of laboratory testing: the identification, biological treatment, and ultimately prevention of psychiatric illnesses.

Table 2–13. Summary of neuroimaging findings in selected psychiatric disorders

Disorder/imaging modality	Findings
Schizophrenia and primary psychotic disorders	
Structural imaging studies	Ventricular enlargement; abnormalities in medial temporal lobe structures and superior temporal gyrus (Shenton et al. 2001).
	Majority of studies report frontal lobe abnormalities (prefrontal gray matter and orbitofrontal regions) (Shenton et al. 2001).
	Subcortical abnormalities involving cavum septum pellucidum, basal ganglia, corpus callosum, and thalamus (Shenton et al. 2001).
	Ventricular enlargement and decreased gray matter volumes in first-episode schizophrenic patients (Lim et al. 1996).
Functional imaging studies	Positron emission tomography shows relative hypometabolism in the prefrontal cortex (Buchsbaum et al. 1982; Tamminga et al. 1992).
	Metabolic abnormalities of limbic areas (temporal lobe, anterior cingulum) (Nordahl et al. 2001; Tamminga et al. 1992).
Magnetic resonance spectroscopy	Decreased N-acetylaspartate levels in frontal, temporal, and thalamic regions (Bertolino et al. 1998; Deicken et al. 1998; Nasrallah et al. 1994; Yurgelun-Todd et al. 1996).
	Antipsychotic medications associated with selective increase in N-acetylaspartate in dorsolateral prefrontal cortex (Bertolino et al. 2001).
Mood disorders	
Structural imaging studies	Abnormal signal hyperintensities in frontal cortex and basal ganglia (Videbech 1997).
	Ventricular enlargement and increased sulcal prominence in patients with bipolar disorder and unipolar depression (Elkis et al. 1995).
Functional imaging studies	Depression: hypometabolism in limbic and dorsolateral prefrontal cortical regions, but hypermetabolism of ventrolateral frontal cortex (Brody et al. 2001; Ketter et al. 1996).
Magnetic resonance spectroscopy	Major depression: increased choline levels in basal ganglia and anterior cingulate (Renshaw et al. 2001; Soares et al. 1999).
Anxiety disorders/obsessive-compulsive disorder (OCD)	
Structural imaging studies	OCD: unclear findings; no volume differences in striatal or ventricular regions (Aylward et al. 1996)
Functional imaging studies	Hypermetabolism in the orbitofrontal cortex and anterior cingulum (Nordahl et al. 1989; Swedo et al. 1989).
	Successful treatment of OCD associated with decreased metabolism in orbitofrontal cortex, anterior cingulum, and caudate nucleus (Baxter et al. 1992; Benkelfat et al. 1990; Swedo et al. 1992).

Key Points

- Laboratory testing of the psychiatric patient in the past has been utilized mainly to uncover medical or neurological causes of psychiatric symptoms.

- The consensus of studies evaluating the role and value of laboratory testing is that patients who have psychiatric signs and symptoms but who do not exhibit other physical complaints or symptoms will benefit from a small screening battery that includes serum glucose concentration, BUN concentration, creatinine clearance, and urinalysis. Female patients older than 50 years will also benefit from a screening TSH test regardless of the presence or absence of mood symptoms.

- More extensive laboratory screening may be necessary for psychiatric patients who do have concomitant physical complaints or findings on physical examination or for patients who are of higher risk, such as elderly or institutionalized patients or those with low socioeconomic status, self-neglect, alcohol or drug dependence, or cognitive impairment.

- Newer laboratory testing methods such as pharmacogenetic testing and testing for investigational genetic and biological markers have the potential to transform and dramatically increase the importance of laboratory testing in the workup of the psychiatric patient.

- Imaging may also be helpful when atypical features are present, such as an older age at onset of psychiatric illness, or when cognitive impairment is present.

- Neuroimaging does not yet play a diagnostic role for any of the primary psychiatric disorders, but it is still an integral part of the clinical workup for psychiatric patients to rule out underlying medical causes of psychiatric symptoms.

- Current neuroimaging methods provide both structural and functional data about the brain. Structural imaging techniques such as CT and MRI provide a fixed image of the brain's anatomy and spatial distribution. Newer functional neuroimaging techniques such as PET and SPECT provide information about brain metabolism, blood flow, the presynaptic uptake of transmitter precursors, neurotransmitter transporter activity, and postsynaptic receptor activity.

- Functional scans should always be interpreted in the context of the underlying structural images.

Suggested Readings

Baumann P, Hiemke C, Ulrich S, et al: The AGNP-TDM Expert Group consensus guidelines: therapeutic drug monitoring in psychiatry. Pharmacopsychiatry 37:243–265, 2004

Cabeza R, Nyberg L: Imaging cognition II: an empirical review of 275 PET and fMRI studies. J Cogn Neurosci 12:1–47, 2000

de Leon J, Armstrong SC, Cozza KL: Clinical guidelines for psychiatrists for the use of pharmacogenetic testing for CYP450 2D6 and CYP450 2C19. Psychosomatics 47:75–85, 2006

Yudofsky SC, Kim HF (eds): Neuropsychiatric Assessment (Review of Psychiatry Series, Vol 23; Oldham JM and Riba MB, series eds). Washington, DC, American Psychiatric Publishing, 2004

References

Agzarian MJ, Chryssidis S, Davies RP, et al: Use of routine computed tomography brain scanning of psychiatry patients. Australas Radiol 50:27–28, 2006

American Academy of Neurology: American Academy of Neurology practice guidelines for dementia. Continuum 13(2):Appendix A, 2007

American Psychiatric Association Task Force on the Use of Laboratory Tests in Psychiatry: Tricyclic antidepressants: blood level measurements and clinical outcome. An APA Task Force report. Am J Psychiatry 142:155–162, 1985

Aylward EH, Harris GL, Hoehn-Saric R, et al: Normal caudate nucleus in obsessive-compulsive disorder assessed by quantitative neuroimaging. Arch Gen Psychiatry 53:577–584, 1996

Baxter LR Jr, Schwartz JM, Bergman KS, et al: Caudate glucose metabolic rate changes with both drug and behavior therapy for obsessive-compulsive disorder. Arch Gen Psychiatry 49:681–689, 1992

Benkelfat C, Nordahl TE, Semple WE, et al: Local cerebral glucose metabolic rates in obsessive-compulsive disorder patients treated with clomipramine. Arch Gen Psychiatry 47:840–848, 1990

Bernardo M, Palao DJ, Arauxo A, et al: Monitoring plasma level of haloperidol in schizophrenia. Hosp Community Psychiatry 44:115, 118, 1993

Bertolino A, Callicott JH, Elman I, et al: Regionally specific neuronal pathology in untreated patients with schizophrenia: a proton magnetic resonance spectroscopic imaging study. Biol Psychiatry 43:641–648, 1998

Bertolino A, Callicott JH, Mattay VS, et al: The effect of treatment with antipsychotic drugs on brain N-acetylaspartate measures in patients with schizophrenia. Biol Psychiatry 49:39–46, 2001

Boutros N, Struve F: Electrophysiological testing, in Neuropsychiatric Assessment. Edited by Yudofsky SC, Kim HF (Review of Psychiatry Series, Vol 23; Oldham JM and Riba MB, series eds). Washington, DC, American Psychiatric Publishing, 2004, pp 69–104

Brody AL, Barsom MW, Bota RG, et al: Prefrontal-subcortical and limbic circuit mediation of major depressive disorder. Semin Clin Neuropsychiatry 6:102–112, 2001

Brown D, Gaar SJ: Alaska services for children and youth with dual sensory impairments final performance report, October 1, 1992 to September 30, 1995. Washington, DC, U.S. Department of Education, Office of Educational Research and Improvement, Educational Resources Information Center, 1995

Buchsbaum MS, Ingvar DH, Kessler R, et al: Cerebral glucography with positron tomography: use in normal subjects and in patients with schizophrenia. Arch Gen Psychiatry 39:251–259, 1982

Curry S: The strategy and value of neuroleptic drug monitoring. J Clin Psychopharmacol 5:263–271, 1985

Deicken RF, Zhou L, Schuff N, et al: Hippocampal neuronal dysfunction in schizophrenia as measured by proton magnetic resonance spectroscopy. Biol Psychiatry 43:483–488, 1998

de Leon J, Armstrong S, Cozza KL: Clinical guidelines for psychiatrists for the use of pharmacogenetic testing for CYP450 2D6 and CYP450 2C19. Psychosomatics 47:75–85, 2006

Elkis H, Friedman L, Wise A, et al: Meta-analyses of studies of ventricular enlargement and cortical sulcal prominence in mood disorders: comparisons with controls or patients with schizophrenia. Arch Gen Psychiatry 52:735–746, 1995

Engel J Jr: The epilepsies, in Cecil Textbook of Medicine, 19th Edition, Vol 2. Edited by Wyngaarden JB, Smith LH, Bennett JC. Philadelphia, PA, WB Saunders, 1992, pp 2202–2213

Erhart SM, Young AS, Marder SR, et al: Clinical utility of magnetic resonance imaging radiographs for suspected organic syndromes in adult psychiatry. J Clin Psychiatry 66:968–973, 2005

Gomez-Gil E, Trilla A, Corbella B, et al: Lack of clinical relevance of routine chest radiography in acute psychiatric admissions. Gen Hosp Psychiatry 24:110–113, 2002

Hall RC, Gardner ER, Stickney SK, et al: Physical illness manifesting as psychiatric disease, II: analysis of a state hospital inpatient population. Arch Gen Psychiatry 37:989–995, 1980

Harms H, Hermans P: Admission laboratory testing in elderly psychiatric patients without organic mental syndromes: should it be routine? Int J Geriatr Psychiatry 9:133–140, 1994

Hollister LE: Electrocardiographic screening in psychiatric patients. J Clin Psychiatry 56:26–29, 1995

Hollister LE, Shah NN: Structural brain scanning in psychiatric patients: a further look. J Clin Psychiatry 57:241–244, 1996

Hughes J, Barraclough BM: Value of routine chest radiography of psychiatric patients. Br Med J 281:1461–1462, 1980

Hughes JR, John ER: Conventional and quantitative electroencephalography in psychiatry. J Neuropsychiatry Clin Neurosci 11:190–208, 1999

Hyman SE, Arana GW, Rosenbaum JF: Handbook of Psychiatric Drug Therapy, 3rd Edition. Boston, MA, Little, Brown, 1995

Ingelman-Sundberg M, Oscarson M, McLellan RA: Polymorphic human cytochrome P450 enzymes: an opportunity for individualized drug treatment. Trends Pharmacol Sci 20: 342–349, 1999

Ketter TA, George MS, Kimbrell TA, et al: Functional brain imaging, limbic function, and affective disorders. The Neuroscientist 2:55–65, 1996

Kirchheiner J, Brosen K, Dahl ML, et al: CYP2D6 and CYP2C19 genotype-based dose recommendations for antidepressants: a first step towards subpopulation-specific dosages. Acta Psychiatr Scand 104:173–192, 2001

Lazarou J, Pomeranz BH, Corey PN: Incidence of adverse drug reactions in hospitalized patients: a meta-analysis of prospective studies. JAMA 279:1200–1205, 1998

Lim KO, Tew W, Kushner M, et al: Cortical gray matter volume deficit in patients with first-episode schizophrenia. Am J Psychiatry 153:1548–1553, 1996

Liston EH, Gerner RH, Robertson AG, et al: Routine thoracic radiography for psychiatric inpatients. Hosp Community Psychiatry 30:474–476, 1979

Marangell LB, Martinez JM, Silver JM, et al: Concise Guide to Psychopharmacology. Washington, DC, American Psychiatric Publishing, 2002

McClellan RL, Eisenberg RL, Giyanani VL, et al: Routine CT screening of psychiatry inpatients. Radiology 169:99–100, 1988

Moles JK, Franchina JJ, Sforza PP: Increasing the clinical yield of computerized tomography for psychiatric patients. Gen Hosp Psychiatry 20:282–291, 1998

Mookhoek EJ, Sterrenburg-vdNieuwegiessen IM: Screening for somatic disease in elderly psychiatric patients. Gen Hosp Psychiatry 20:102–107, 1998

Mrazek DA: The context of genetic testing in clinical psychiatric practice. CNS Spectr 11:3–4, 2006

Nasrallah HA, Skinner TE, Schmalbrock P, et al: Proton magnetic resonance spectroscopy (1H MRS) of the hippocampal formation in schizophrenia: a pilot study. Br J Psychiatry 165:481–485, 1994

Nordahl TE, Benkelfat C, Semple WE, et al: Cerebral glucose metabolic rates in obsessive compulsive disorder. Neuropsychopharmacology 2:23–28, 1989

Nordahl TE, Carter CS, Salo RE, et al: Anterior cingulate metabolism correlates with Stroop errors in paranoid schizophrenia patients. Neuropsychopharmacology 25:139–148, 2001

Olshaker JS, Browne B, Jerrard DA, et al: Medical clearance and screening of psychiatric patients in the emergency department. Acad Emerg Med 4:124–128, 1997

Pellock JM, Willmore LJ: A rational guide to routine blood monitoring in patients receiving antiepileptic drugs. Neurology 41:961–964, 1991

Petersen RC, Thomas RG, Grundman M, et al: Vitamin E and donepezil for the treatment of mild cognitive impairment. N Engl J Med 352:2379–2388, 2005

Rauch SL, Renshaw PF: Clinical neuroimaging in psychiatry. Harv Rev Psychiatry 2:297–312, 1995

Renshaw PF, Parow AM, Hirashima F, et al: Multinuclear magnetic resonance spectroscopy studies of brain purines in major depression. Am J Psychiatry 158:2048–2055, 2001

Ringholz GR: Differential Diagnosis. Lecture presented at Current Neurology conference, Houston, Texas, November 2001

Sadock BJ, Sadock VA: Laboratory tests in psychiatry, in Kaplan and Sadock's Synopsis of Psychiatry, 10th Edition. Baltimore, MD, Lippincott Williams & Wilkins, 2007, pp 255–267

Sheline Y, Kehr C: Cost and utility of routine admission laboratory testing for psychiatric inpatients. Gen Hosp Psychiatry 12:329–334, 1990

Shenton ME, Dickey CC, Frumin M, et al: A review of MRI findings in schizophrenia. Schizophr Res 49:1–52, 2001

Soares JC, Boada F, Spencer S, et al: NAA and choline measures in the anterior cingulate of bipolar disorder patients (abstract). Biol Psychiatry 45 (8 suppl):119S, 1999

Streetman DS: Metabolic basis of drug interactions in the intensive care unit. Crit Care Nurs Q 22:1–13, 2000

Swedo SE, Schapiro MB, Grady CL, et al: Cerebral glucose metabolism in childhood-onset obsessive-compulsive disorder. Arch Gen Psychiatry 46:518–523, 1989

Swedo SE, Pietrini P, Leonard HL, et al: Cerebral glucose metabolism in childhood-onset obsessive-compulsive disorder: revisualization during pharmacotherapy. Arch Gen Psychiatry 49:690–694, 1992

Tamminga CA, Thaker GK, Buchanan R, et al: Limbic system abnormalities identified in schizophrenia using positron emission tomography with fluorodeoxyglucose and neocortical alterations with deficit syndrome. Arch Gen Psychiatry 49:522–530, 1992

Videbech P: MRI findings in patients with affective disorder: a meta-analysis. Acta Psychiatr Scand 96:157–168, 1997

Wallach J: Interpretation of Diagnostic Tests. Boston, MA, Little, Brown, 1992

Wallach J: Interpretation of Diagnostic Tests, 7th Edition. Philadelphia, PA, Lippincott Williams & Wilkins, 2000

Willmore LJ, Triggs WJ, Pellock JM: Valproate toxicity: risk-screening strategies. J Child Neurol 6:3–6, 1991

Yurgelun-Todd DA, Renshaw PF, Gruber SA, et al: Proton magnetic resonance spectroscopy of the temporal lobes in schizophrenics and normal controls. Schizophr Res 19:55–59, 1996

3

DELIRIUM, DEMENTIA, AND AMNESTIC AND OTHER COGNITIVE DISORDERS

James A. Bourgeois, O.D., M.D., F.A.P.M.

Jeffrey S. Seaman, M.S., M.D.

Mark E. Servis, M.D.

Delirium, dementia, and amnestic and other cognitive disorders are classified as cognitive disorders in DSM-IV-TR (American Psychiatric Association 2000). As a group, they represent psychiatric disturbances formerly described as exclusively due to "organic" as opposed to "functional" etiological factors. As research into the etiology and treatment of other psychiatric disorders has progressed, the artificial distinction between *organic* (an anachronistic term in current clinical practice) and *functional* psychiatric illness has blurred substantially. Nonetheless, these cognitive disorders generally have clear structural and functional disturbances in brain function as their primary causes. Psychological factors are still very relevant in the pa-

tient's experience of symptoms and his or her behavioral and emotional response to illness. Delirium, dementia, and the other cognitive disorders make clear the need for psychiatric evaluation based on the biopsychosocial model of psychiatric illness.

Delirium

Definition

Delirium is an acute brain disorder manifested by a syndromal array of neuropsychiatric symptoms. Engel and Romano (1959) portrayed delirium as a "syndrome of cerebral insufficiency," analogous to heart failure or renal insufficiency. They were the first to assert delirium not only complicated the treatment of concurrent systemic illnesses but also carried "the serious possibility of permanent irreversible brain damage" in its own right. In other words, Engel and Romano proposed delirium is *brain failure*—a "new" conceptualization fundamental to an updated understanding of delirium.

The DSM-IV-TR model describes delirium as an acute, *reversible* neuropsychiatric syndrome *caused* by general medical conditions and/or exogenous substances. A survey by Ely et al. (2004b) confirmed that many clinicians believe delirium to be transient and lacking in long-term consequences on the brain. This belief system is in direct conflict, however, with current scientific evidence on several fronts. For one, delirium has been shown to markedly and *independently* affect patient outcomes such as length of stay, subsequent institutionalization, and death, among others (e.g., Edelstein et al. 2004; Marcantonio et al. 2005; Thomason et al. 2005). Equally striking are studies (McCusker et al. 2001; Rockwood et al. 1999; Serrano-Duenas and Bleda 2005) demonstrating new and permanent cognitive deficits *postrecovery* that may be linked to hypothesized pathological processes occurring within the delirious brain (Gaudreau and Gagnon 2005; Munford and Tracey 2002; Pratico et al. 2005).

Clinical Features

The DSM-IV-TR diagnostic criteria for delirium require a disturbance in *consciousness/attention* and a change in *cognition* that develop *acutely* and *tend* to fluctuate (Table 3–1). Lipowski (1983, 1987) characterized delirium as a disorder of attention, wakefulness, cognition, and motor behavior. The disruption of attention is often considered the core symptom. Patients struggle to sustain attentional focus, are easily distracted, and often vary in their level of alertness. Delirium is not always a "fortunate complication" of being hospitalized and seriously ill. The 50% of patients who recall their delirious episode rate the experience as highly distressing (Breitbart et al. 2002). The families and staff caring for the delirious patient rate their experiences as quite miserable as well (Morita et al. 2004).

Delirium Subtypes

Consistent with the ancient descriptions of phrenitis and lethargus, hyperactive and hypoactive subtypes of delirium have been reported. Liptzin and Levkoff (1992) first

---

Table 3–1. DSM-IV-TR diagnostic criteria for delirium due to...[indicate the general medical condition]

A. Disturbance of consciousness (i.e., reduced clarity of awareness of the environment) with reduced ability to focus, sustain, or shift attention.

B. A change in cognition (such as memory deficit, disorientation, language disturbance) or the development of a perceptual disturbance that is not better accounted for by a preexisting, established, or evolving dementia.

C. The disturbance develops over a short period of time (usually hours to days) and tends to fluctuate during the course of the day.

D. There is evidence from the history, physical examination, or laboratory findings that the disturbance is caused by the direct physiological consequences of a general medical condition.

Coding note: If delirium is superimposed on a preexisting vascular dementia, indicate the delirium by coding 290.41 vascular dementia, with delirium.

Coding note: Include the name of the general medical condition on Axis I, e.g., 293.0 delirium due to hepatic encephalopathy; also code the general medical condition on Axis III (see DSM-IV-TR Appendix G for codes).

characterized delirious patients with rest-lessness, hypervigilance, rapid speech, irrita-bility, and combativeness as *hyperactive*, whereas those showing slowed speech and kinetics, apathy, and reduced alertness were designated *hypoactive*. The mixed type vacil-lated or included elements of the two other subtypes. Hypoactive patients tend to be older (McCusker et al. 2001; Peterson et al. 2006), to have more severe cognitive distur-bances (Koponen et al. 1989b), to be less likely to be diagnosed (Inouye et al. 2001), and to have a poorer prognosis (Andrew et al. 2005; Liptzin and Levkoff 1992).

Etiopathogenesis

One key to sustained progress in understand-ing delirium is a *refutation* of the misleading model wherein delirium is believed to be *caused* by the comorbid systemic disease. We suggest instead that comorbid disease states, environmental stressors, and certain medica-tions may *precipitate* delirium in vulnerable patients. The vast number and disparate na-ture of the identified precipitants (Elie et al. 1998) innately argue against most of them having *direct* causality for delirium. Further-more, it is recognized clinically that delirium often persists *well after* the precipitants have been successfully addressed and removed. This occurs most typically in patients clini-cally estimated to have less cerebral reserve.

Precipitants can initiate a cascade of neu-rochemical and metabolic events in the brain. More robust patients can resist this cascade and not become delirious or, if they do be-come delirious, recover rapidly and without sequelae. Variations on this theme may exist where selected precipitants have partial causal links, such as medications with hefty anticholinergic or prodopaminergic activity. Investigations into the etiology of delirium have looked at neuronal integrity, the role of oxygen, cardiovascular and respiratory re-serves, oxygen demand and anemia, anoxia, neurotransmitter roles, melatonin, and neu-roanatomic loci.

Epidemiology

Delirium is epidemic among hospitalized pa-tients, especially in the elderly. Inouye (2006) estimated that delirium annually complicates the hospitalizations of 2.5 million elderly Americans, is present for about 17 million in-patient days, and accounts for $7 billion in Medicare costs alone, *excluding* the substan-tial postdischarge morbidity costs. Delirium was also shown to *directly* increase hospital costs by 40% (Milbrandt et al. 2004). In a 2005 paper, Pandharipande et al. calculated that delirium may directly increase intensive care unit (ICU) costs by up to $20 billion per year. Inpatient studies have reported a delirium prevalence of 12%–40% among geriatric pa-tients (Francis and Kapoor 1992; Inouye and Charpentier 1996; Inouye et al. 1998; O'Keeffe and Lavan 1997), 10%–15% across patients of all ages (Cameron et al. 1987), and 37% among postoperative patients (Dyer et al. 1995).

Clinical Evaluation
History

A thorough history provides the majority of the diagnostic information (Table 3–2).

Central to the history gathering is estab-lishing what the patient's premorbid base-line was, whether a recent change occurred, and when. Not only is this information key in distinguishing delirium from dementia, but it may also serve to identify precipitants. Prime sources of information are those who have known the patient for some time, such as family and treatment team members. Re-view of the patient's current medical or sur-gical illness is also essential. Assessment of the treatment environment with a focus on variables that could confuse, disorient, and disrupt circadian cycles is standard. These variables may include visual or hearing aids; light, dark, and noise cycles; communication efforts and assistive devices; familiar versus unfamiliar caretakers, objects, and routines; and depersonalization factors.

Table 3–2. Evaluation of delirium

Standard

Vital signs

Complete history

Medication review: recent past and current

Neurological examination

Bedside testing: months of the year
  backward, verbal Trails B, clock
  drawing, "A" test for vigilance

As clinically warranted

Laboratory work: complete blood count,
  electrolytes, blood urea nitrogen,
  creatinine, glucose, calcium, pulse
  oximetry or arterial blood gas,
  urinalysis, drug screen, liver function
  test with serum albumin, cultures, HIV
  screening, cerebrospinal fluid
  examination

Tests: chest X ray, electrocardiogram,
  brain imaging, electroencephalogram

Medication Review

Every delirium evaluation warrants a medication review inclusive of current and recently discontinued drugs, whether prescription, over-the-counter, herbal, or illicit. Medications with anticholinergic properties should be avoided if possible. The potential for drug–drug interactions should be reviewed.

Interview and Observation

The interview itself should focus on establishing a global image of the patient's cognitive functioning. It is helpful to observe the patient for decreased attention capacity, psychosis, short-term memory deficits, disorientation, executive dysfunction, and changes in mood or kinetics. Bedside examinations (e.g., the "A" test for vigilance) and tests sensitive to frontal lobe dysfunction (Royall et al. 1998) are quick and easy to administer. These tests have not been validated as delirium screens but can function to rapidly illuminate key cognitive domains.

In regard to the Mini-Mental State Exam (MMSE; Folstein et al. 1975), one study (C.A. Ross et al. 1991) reported the mean MMSE score to be 14.3 for delirious patients, versus 29.6 for control subjects. A single MMSE is not sensitive (33%) for identifying delirium, however, and is incapable of discriminating delirium from dementia (Trzepacz et al. 1986). Serial MMSEs, on the other hand, can help identify improvement or worsening of delirium (O'Keeffe et al. 2005; Tune and Folstein 1986) and assist in delirium screening when baseline MMSEs are clearly known (Fayers et al. 2005).

Rating Scales

Diagnostic and rating tools are critical for objectifying and unifying diagnostic and research efforts in delirium. The most-cited and -validated instruments are the Delirium Rating Scale (DRS) and the Delirium Rating Scale—Revised–98 (DRS-R-98; Trzepacz et al. 1988a, 2001), the Confusion Assessment Method (CAM; Inouye et al. 1990), and the Memorial Delirium Assessment Scale (MDAS; Breitbart et al. 1997).

Neurological Examination

Unexplained or new focal neurological signs beyond cognitive disturbances are atypical in delirium and warrant discussion with a neurologist. Neuroimaging should be considered for patients with head injuries, focal findings, cancer, stroke risk, AIDS, and atypical presentations (e.g., young, healthy, lack of identifiable precipitants).

Laboratory Tests

Laboratory tests are important but are not the foundation of a delirium evaluation. Tests are thus warranted on an individually tailored basis. Not only is such a practice fiscally responsible, but it also avoids the error of pursuing clinically irrelevant and/or false-positive results. Evaluations may include a complete blood count, electrolytes, blood urea nitrogen, creatinine, glucose, calcium, pulse oximetry or arterial blood gas, and urinalysis. Other tests commonly obtained are urine drug screens, liver function tests with serum albumin, cultures, chest X ray, and electrocardiogram. Cerebrospinal fluid examination should also be considered for cases in which meningitis or encephalitis is suspected as well as for atypical cases of delirium.

Electroencephalography

Utilizing electroencephalography, Romano and Engel (1944) first demonstrated delirious patients had progressive disorganization of rhythms and generalized slowing (Figure 3–1). Delirious patients specifically have slowing of the peak and average frequencies in addition to increased theta and delta but decreased alpha rhythms (Koponen et al. 1989a). It is also important to realize that there are instances when the electroencephalogram (EEG) may be read as

"normal" in a delirious patient but is actually *abnormal* for the individual when compared with the baseline EEG—particularly for those patients whose usual electroencephalographic frequencies reside in the fast range (Engel and Romano 1959).

The EEG is useful in the uncommon situation where one is trying to distinguish delirium from other psychiatric states, for example, catatonia, depression, conversion disorder, and malingering. EEG changes normalize before cognitive dysfunction clears (Trzepacz et al. 1992), whereas cognitive testing remains sensitive throughout the course of the delirium (Trzepacz et al. 1988b). Nondelirious elderly patients can additionally exhibit electroencephalographic slowing, particularly if they have dementia (Obrist 1979).

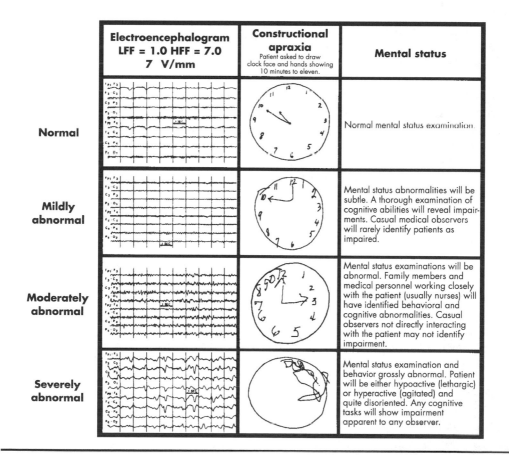

Figure 3–1. Comparison of electroencephalogram, constructional apraxia, and mental status in delirium.

HFF=high-frequency filter; LFF=low-frequency filter.

Table 3–3. Delirium versus dementia

Feature	Delirium	Dementia
Onset	Acute	Insidious
Cognitive dysfunction	Acute/acutely worse	Chronic
Attention	Disrupted	Intact (except Lewy body dementia and end-stage disease)
Fluctuation	Common	No (except Lewy body dementia)
Speech	Disorganized/confused	Impoverished

Differential Diagnosis

Delirium needs to be distinguished most frequently from dementia (Table 3–3). Dementia has an insidious rather than an acute onset, features chronic memory and executive disturbances, and—unless it is Lewy body dementia (LBD) or there is a superimposed delirium—tends to not fluctuate. A nondelirious dementia patient typically has intact attention and alertness. Dementia is also characterized by impoverished speech and thinking, as opposed to the confused or disorganized pattern seen in delirium. "Beclouded dementia" describes delirium that develops in a patient who already has dementia. Beclouded dementia should be approached like any other case of delirium (Trzepacz et al. 1998), albeit with the understanding such patients are highly sensitive to precipitants and medications.

Other possibilities to consider in the differential diagnosis include drug intoxication and withdrawal, schizophrenia, catatonia, and Bell's mania (Table 3–4). A thorough history, physical examination, and toxicology screen should identify most intoxication cases. Stimulants, hallucinogens, and dissociative drugs are commonly abused agents capable of mimicking or precipitating delirium. It is worth noting that agents such as mescaline and lysergic acid diethylamide (LSD) do not cause diffuse electroencephalographic slowing like that seen in delirium (Engel and Romano 1959). The *first episode* of a psychotic disorder can also be difficult to differentiate from delirium, particularly if the mental status change developed acutely without a prolonged prodrome. Attentional difficulties, disorganization, and diffuse cognitive dysfunction can occur in both illnesses. A trial of antipsychotics and observation may suffice if no localizing neurological abnormalities or identifiable deliriogenic precipitants are present in an otherwise healthy young person. If the cause was delirium, it typically clears rapidly in this population. On the other hand, it is likely the first episode of a primary psychotic disorder if the negative signs of schizophrenia persist with residual delusions or hallucinations, but attention and cognitive function improve. Catatonia can be difficult to differentiate at times, particularly if there are no motor findings (Seaman 2005). Serial examinations, a trial of intravenous lorazepam, and an EEG are often most helpful.

Risk Factors: Precipitants and Baseline Vulnerability

The term *precipitant* has been used to subsume risk factors that are generally transient or acute (e.g., a urinary tract infection). Similarly, *baseline vulnerability* describes those risk factors that are, by definition, chronic and innate to the patient (e.g., cerebral atrophy). We advocate that there are numerous and widely varying precipitants that can activate delirium in susceptible (high-baseline-vulnerability) patients.

One of the most common precipitants of delirium is medication. Numerous medications across many classes have been noted to precipitate delirium (Brown and Stoudemire 1998). The commonly used benzodiazepine lorazepam has been shown to independently

Table 3–4. Delirium differential beyond dementia

Diagnosis	Similarities	Differences
Depression	Withdrawn, hypoactive	Intact attention, insidious, EEG
Catatonia	Hypo- or hyperactive, odd behavior, limited or no speech	Motor findings, resolves with lorazepam/ECT, EEG
Bell's mania	Hyperactive, confused	Responsive to ECT, other manic symptoms and history, EEG
First-break schizophrenia	Disorganized, poor attention, diffuse cognitive dysfunction	Young age, no precipitants, persistent psychotic symptoms after confusion cleared, EEG
Drug/alcohol intoxication or withdrawal	Hypo- or hyperactive, hallucinations, poor attention	Positive drug screen or history, EEG

Note.   ECT = electroconvulsive therapy; EEG = electroencephalogram.

increase delirium development in ICU patients (Pandharipande et al. 2006). Importantly, the capacity of a medication to exert anticholinergic activity has been shown to correlate with its propensity to trigger delirium (L. Han et al. 2001). A 1992 study found that 14 of the 25 drugs most commonly prescribed for elderly patients (i.e., furosemide, digoxin, Dyazide, Lanoxin, dipyridamole, theophylline, warfarin, prednisone, nifedipine, isosorbide dinitrate, codeine, cimetidine, captopril, and ranitidine) had detectable anticholinergic effects (Tune et al. 1992). It is important to note although that a single medication may have a low serum level of anticholinergic activity (SAA) by itself, the combined effect of several such medications (Tune et al. 1992) may precipitate delirium in a susceptible individual. Last, some general anesthetic agents such as isoflurane and ketamine are potent inhibitors of nicotinic acetylcholine receptors and thus may be pertinent for examining postoperative delirium risk (Fodale and Santamaria 2003).

Prospective studies have identified many other precipitants and baseline risks for delirium. Two of the most frequently reported are preexisting cognitive decline and advanced age. In a cohort of patients with an average age of 86 years, Voyer et al. (2006) illustrated a dose–response relationship between the degree of prior cognitive impairment and subsequent likelihood of developing delirium.

Prognosis

Mortality

Lipowski (1983) described delirium as a "grave prognostic sign," and a wealth of published data support this view. Many dozens of studies have reported elevated death rates for delirious inpatients, and a few studies of delirious patients discharged to postacute facilities (i.e., Bellelli and Trabucchi 2006) are now available. When the most robust studies were combined in a meta-analysis (Cole and Primeau 1993), patients with delirium were reported to have an average 1-month mortality of 14.2% (vs. 4.8% in control

subjects) and a 6-month mortality of 22.2% (vs. 10.6% in control subjects).

Morbidity

Delirium also often portends poor clinical outcomes. The length of hospital stay is longer (Ely et al. 2004a; Thomason et al. 2005), the readmission rate higher (Marcantonio et al. 2005), and the loss of independent living more common (Adamis et al. 2006; Bourdel-Marchasson et al. 2004; Francis and Kapoor 1992; Pitkala et al. 2005) among patients who had been delirious. These differences persist even after control for variables such as illness severity, preexisting chronic cognitive impairment, and activities of daily living status. Delirium also independently predicted increased nursing home placements and decreased ability to perform activities of daily living (Inouye et al. 1998; Marcantonio et al. 2000; O'Keeffe and Lavan 1997). Overall, a meta-analysis (Cole and Primeau 1993) found that patients with delirium had a mean length of hospital stay of 20.7 days (vs. 8.9 days for control subjects) and a reduced rate of independent living 6 months after admission of 56.8% (vs. 91.7% in control subjects).

Duration

Average delirium episodes of 3–13 days are typically reported, although 20 days was the mean in a sample of patients with beclouded dementia (Koponen et al. 1989b). Persistence beyond 30 days has been described to occur in as many as 13%–50% of delirious elderly (Marcantonio et al. 2000). Patients with hypoactive delirium have been shown to have longer episodes than those with the mixed or hyperactive subtypes (Kelly et al. 2001). Studies have also noted some delirium symptoms persist at time of discharge in as many as 60%–96% of elderly patients who experienced delirium during their stay (Kelly et al. 2001). One investigation (Kiely et al. 2004) found that half of the 15% patients in skilled-nursing facilities with delirium at the time of admission remained delirious 1 month into their stay. Independent predictors of the delirium persistence included age older than 85 years, preexisting cognitive impairment, and severe delirium (MDAS score >5).

Treatment and Prevention

The precipitant–vulnerability brain-failure model presented earlier can serve to guide modern delirium management. Once the delirium diagnosis is made, the first task of the psychiatrist is to *not* recommend that the primary team "search for an underlying cause of delirium" and to recommend antipsychotics if the patient is agitated. Our first task in delirium treatment is to be a *diligent observer* and an *active learner.* Active data collection enables the physician to more selectively seek to address modifiable precipitants and to choose when and which pharmacological agents would best serve the patient.

Modifiable precipitants may be an undetected urinary tract infection, pneumonia, organ failure, sepsis, select medications, or a host of other variables. Anticholinergics, benzodiazepines, corticosteroids, powerful dopamine agonists, and some opioids are best limited when feasible (Morita et al. 2005), although uncertainty remains in this arena (Gaudreau et al. 2005). The goal of treating delirium is not solely to control agitation or hallucinations; rather, the preeminent objective is *to prevent and reverse the delirium and thus mitigate associated morbidity and mortality risks.*

Nonpharmacological Interventions

Several comprehensive, primarily nonpharmacological intervention protocols have been published. One large, well-designed study was Inouye et al.'s (1999) Elder Life Program. This prevention program selected 426 nondelirious patients at risk for delirium and sought to address baseline cognitive impairment, sleep, mobility, vision, hearing, and dehydration. The authors reported a decline in delirium incidence in the intervention group compared with a usual-care group (10% vs.

15%). The cost of the program was $327 per patient; it saved an average of $6,341 for each patient who did not develop delirium. One year after discharge, the intervention group demonstrated a 15% reduction in costs and lengths of stay at nursing homes compared with the control group (Leslie et al. 2005).

Pharmacotherapy

Although tailored environmental manipulations and supportive care are crucial, medications offer further advantages. First, interventions directed at delirium precipitants should be instituted. Unless the delirium clears very rapidly or is mild, the concurrent use of delirium-specific treatments is recommended. Elevated dopamine levels are known to occur in delirium; thus, the judicious use of dopamine-receptor antagonists is rational. Although further study is needed, patients with the nonagitated, hypoactive subtype of delirium may be among the *most important to treat* with delirium-specific medication (Platt et al. 1994), considering their poor prognosis.

Haloperidol has been the most studied treatment for delirium. The American Psychiatric Association (1999) practice guideline supported haloperidol as a first-line agent for delirium because of its minimal anticholinergic effects, minimal orthostasis, limited sedation, and flexibility in dosing and administration with oral, intramuscular, and intravenous routes. Both oral and intravenous forms have been used for more than 40 years and have an extensive track record of safety and efficacy in even the most severely ill medical and surgical patients (Cassem and Sos 1978). Haloperidol has also been proven clearly superior to benzodiazepines given alone in delirium (Breitbart et al. 1996). The recommended dosage of haloperidol (American Psychiatric Association 1999) is 1–2 mg every 2–4 hours as needed, with further titration until desired effects are seen. In severe delirium refractory to boluses, continuous haloperidol infusions of 3–25 mg/hour have been used safely (Riker et al. 1994), although the practice guideline suggested a ceiling of 5–10 mg/hour. Electrocardiographic monitoring is recommended with continuous infusion because of concerns about torsades de pointes, although no specific dosage threshold has been designated (American Psychiatric Association 1999; Sharma et al. 1998). Awareness and management of risk factors for QTc prolongation (hypokalemia, hypomagnesemia, bradycardia, congenital long-QT syndrome, preexisting cardiac disease, and drug–drug interactions) are advised (Gury et al. 2000). Prolonged QTc intervals beyond 450 msec or 25% above baseline should prompt a cardiology consultation, a dosage reduction, or discontinuation of the antipsychotic agent (American Psychiatric Association 1999).

Other, more rarely utilized agents for delirium include propofol (Mirenda and Broyles 1995), other typical antipsychotics, intravenous ondansetron (a 5-HT$_3$ antagonist; Bayindir et al. 2000), and valproic acid (Bourgeois et al. 2005; Ichikawa et al. 2005).

There are numerous reports regarding the use of atypical antipsychotics for delirium in recent years, but few double-blind randomized trials (C.S. Han and Kim 2004; Hu et al. 2004; Lonergan et al 2007). Specialists in psychosomatic medicine have been successfully using these agents in clinical practice for the past decade despite scanty literature support. The advantages are the lowered risk of extrapyramidal symptoms or electrocardiographic abnormalities (Titier et al. 2004), mood-modulating effects, and possibly enhanced efficacy in select patients. These agents also may exert their effectiveness via blockade at 5-HT$_{2A}$, D$_4$, and α_1 receptors and agonism at 5-HT$_{1A}$ (Meltzer 2002). Interestingly, olanzapine, risperidone, and ziprasidone may also enhance net cholinergic activity in the prefrontal cortex (Ichikawa et al. 2002; Parada et al. 1997) via several serotonin–acetylcholine receptor interactions (Kennedy et al. 2001).

Prevention

An absolute duty in the management of delirium is prevention (Lipowski 1983). Ideally, patients could be quickly screened for delirium at intake (Monette et al. 2001) and scored with a predictive model. Patients would be eligible for prophylactic interventions if judged to be at high risk for developing delirium. Such screening practices would be much like what is currently done to reduce the risks of other illnesses (e.g., subcutaneous heparin for pulmonary-embolus prophylaxis). Candidates for preventive interventions could include both pharmacological and nonpharmacological measures (Siddiqi et al. 2007).

Additional hypothesized mechanisms are emerging and may become targets of future biological therapies for delirium. One group (J.R. Maldonado et al. 2003) used dexmedetomidine in a postoperative sedation protocol. They reported a stunning 5% 3-day incidence of delirium in the group receiving the α_2 agonist versus a 51% incidence for those who received standard sedation protocols. A second group also found dexmedetomidine to be effective in preventing postoperative agitation or delirium in a rare study in children, reporting a delirium incidence of 26% with dexmedetomidine versus 61% with placebo (Shukry et al. 2005). The mechanisms underlying the potential effectiveness of this α_2 agonist remain elusive but may be associated with sleep regulation pathways. Additional hypotheses point to reduced intraoperative anesthetic requirements with dexmedetomidine use and its role in modulating autonomic reactivity to surgery (Stumita et al. 2007).

Delirium: Summary

The era of contentment with our understanding of delirium has thankfully expired. Aggressive examination of this pervasive and destructive disorder is under way as we question delirium's etiopathogenesis and neurotoxicity, which in turn will inform data-driven prevention and treatment strategies. Continued cultivation of an objectively defined paradigm for delirium may lead us to the day when we can routinely prevent delirium and offer better protection for our patients against spiraling functional and cognitive decline.

Dementia

The dementias are a heterogeneous group of psychiatric disorders characterized by loss of previous levels of cognitive, executive, and memory (anterograde and/or retrograde) function in a state of full alertness. The loss of socioeconomic productivity and burdens to family caregivers are profound. With the increasing age of the population, the prevalence of dementia is expected to double by 2030 (Doraiswamy et al. 1998). Dementia directly increases health care expenditures and complicates the management of comorbid medical conditions. Patients with dementia have increased rates of institutionalization and mortality. The average duration from diagnosis to death is 3–10 years (Doraiswamy et al. 1998).

Although the typical course of most dementias is progressive cognitive and functional decline until death, physicians are now urged to view the dementias as treatable illnesses. Contemporary advances in psychopharmacology equip the physician with a greater range of medications to maximize function, delay disease progression, and minimize disruption to patients and caregivers. Early identification of cases is now imperative, given that prompt evaluation and diagnosis facilitate early use of cognition-enhancing and neuroprotective therapies and supportive care to the patient and family. Thorough evaluation and management of comorbid systemic and neuropsychiatric illness are essential to foster the best clinical outcomes.

Clinical Features of the Dementias

DSM-IV-TR Classification of Dementias

According to DSM-IV-TR, core features of the dementias include multiple cognitive deficits (anterograde and/or retrograde memory impairment and aphasia, apraxia, agnosia, or disturbance in executive functioning) that cause impairment in role functioning and represent a significant decline (American Psychiatric Association 2000). Dementia subtypes specified in DSM-IV-TR are shown in Table 3–5. Although the dementias share core features, specific dementia syndromes differ in terms of the sequence of presentation of these and additional associated clinical features.

Cortical Versus Subcortical Dementias

A distinction is made between dementias with primarily cortical and those with primarily subcortical pathology (Table 3–6). Whereas all dementias exhibit the same core clinical features, cortical and subcortical dementias often differ in their specific clinical presentation. Cortical dementia is characterized by prominent memory impairment (recall *and* recognition), language deficits, apraxia, agnosia, and visuospatial deficits (Doody et al. 1998; Paulsen et al. 1995). Subcortical dementia features greater impairment in recall memory, decreased verbal fluency without anomia, bradyphrenia (slowed thinking), depressed mood, affective lability, apathy, and decreased attention/concentration (Doody et al. 1998; Paulsen et al. 1995). Cortical dementias generally lack prominent motor signs, whereas subcortical dementias typically feature such signs (Geldmacher and Whitehouse 1997).

Cortical Dementias

Dementia of the Alzheimer's type (DAT), the most common dementia, is estimated to affect nearly 2 million white Americans (Hy and Keller 2000). There is an important conceptual and semantic distinction between the DSM-IV-TR diagnoses of DAT and Alzheimer's disease (AD) (Rabins et al. 1997). DAT is a clinical diagnosis, based on the findings of insidious onset and gradual, steady progression of cognitive deficits. Because symptoms

---

Table 3–5. Diagnostic features of the dementias

Features common to all dementias:

Multiple cognitive deficits that do not occur exclusively during the course of delirium, including memory impairment and aphasia, apraxia, agnosia, or disturbed executive functioning that represent a decline from previous level of functioning and impair role functioning

Dementia of the Alzheimer's type, additional features:

Gradual onset and continuing cognitive decline, deficits are not due to other central nervous system, systemic, or substance-induced conditions and not better attributed to another Axis I disorder

Vascular dementia, additional features:

Focal neurological signs and symptoms or laboratory/radiological evidence indicative of cerebrovascular disease etiologically related to deficits

Dementia due to other general medical conditions, additional feature:

Clinical evidence that cognitive disturbance is direct physiological consequence of one of the following: HIV, head trauma, Parkinson's disease, Huntington's disease, Pick's disease, Creutzfeldt-Jakob disease, or another general medical condition (includes Lewy body dementia)

Substance-induced persisting dementia, additional features:

Deficits persist beyond usual duration of substance intoxication or withdrawal with clinical evidence that deficits are etiologically related to the persisting effects of substance use

Dementia due to multiple etiologies, additional feature:

Clinical evidence that the disturbance has more than one etiology

Dementia not otherwise specified, additional feature:

Dementia that does not meet criteria for one of the specified types above

---

Source.   Adapted from American Psychiatric Association 2000.

and signs consistent with DAT may be present with other types of neuropathology, a clinical diagnosis of AD should be made only after medical evaluation fails to reveal other causes for the dementia symptoms (Rabins et al. 1997). Even so, the clinical diagnosis of AD can be *definitively* validated only by microscopic examination of neural tissue, typically at autopsy, for characteristic neuropathology (Rabins et al. 1997). A *clinical* diagnosis of AD (after ruling out other dementia causes) is pathologically validated in 70%–90% of cases (Rabins et al. 1997). Established and proposed risk factors for DAT are shown in Table 3–7 (Blennow et al. 2006; Moceri et al. 2000).

Amnesia and other cognitive symptoms may be present early in the disease, although poor insight regarding memory loss is common. Decreased visual attention may be a key factor in cognitive impairment (Rizzo et al. 2000). The patient may become spatially disoriented and wander aimlessly. Apraxias for self-care behaviors may be evident. Deficits in memory, concentration, attention, and executive functions eventually render the patient unable to maintain employment or safely operate a motor vehicle.

The noncognitive symptoms in dementia are also referred to as the behavioral and psychological symptoms of dementia (Lawlor 2004). These include psychiatric symptoms and behavioral manifestations that cross the boundaries of DSM-IV-TR categories of psychiatric disorders. Over the course of a case of

Table 3–6. Cortical and subcortical dementia types

Cortical dementias

Dementia of the Alzheimer's type (DAT)
Frontotemporal dementia, including
   dementia due to Pick's disease
Dementia due to Creutzfeldt–Jakob disease
Dementia due to chronic subdural
   hematoma

Subcortical dementias

Dementia due to HIV
Dementia due to Parkinson's disease
Dementia due to Huntington's disease
Dementia due to multiple sclerosis

Dementias with cortical and subcortical features

Vascular dementia (formerly multi-infarct
   dementia)*
Vascular dementia (poststroke dementia)*
Mixed dementia (DAT + vascular
   dementia)
Lewy body variant of Alzheimer's disease*
Lewy body dementia*
Dementia due to fragile X–associated
   tremor/ataxia syndrome
Dementia due to normal pressure
   hydrocephalus

*Relative amount of cortical and subcortical features is dependent on location of neuropathology.

Table 3–7. Established and proposed risk factors for dementia of the Alzheimer's type

Increased age
Female gender
Head trauma
Small head size
Family history
Low childhood intelligence
Limited education
Childhood rural residence
Large sibships
Smoking
Never having married
Depression
Diabetes mellitus
Increased total cholesterol
Vascular disease
Hypertension
Increased platelet membrane fluidity
Apolipoprotein E (APOE) ε4 allele on
   chromosome 19
Abnormalities on chromosomes 1, 6, 12, 14,
   and 21
Trisomy 21

dementia, the symptoms tend to fluctuate as the patient's cognitive status changes. Mood symptoms that occur before cognitive deficits may represent a prodromal state (Berger et al. 1999). Depressive disorders have been reported in up to 86% of patients with DAT, with a median estimate of 19% (Aalten et al. 2003; Zubenko et al. 2003). Depression is more common in mild DAT, whereas psychosis is more common in moderate to severe DAT (Rabins et al. 1997; Rao and Lyketsos 1998). Apathy is common and may occur in the absence of full-syndrome depression; apathy, agitation, dysphoria, and aberrant motor behavior all increase with illness progression and increasing cognitive impairment (Aalten et al. 2003; Lyketsos et al. 2002). The construct of "minor depression" (a mood disorder subsyndromal

for major depression) with comorbid dementia has been associated with significant psychological and functional impairment (Starkstein et al. 2005). Disinhibited social and sexual behavior, assaultiveness, and inappropriate laughter or tearfulness are common. Evening agitation ("sundowning") may be a notably disruptive symptom and has been linked to disturbed circadian rhythms and a phase delay of body temperature in DAT (Volicer et al. 2001). Other motor symptoms include motor slowing, extrapyramidal symptoms, gait disturbances, dysarthria, myoclonus, and seizures (Goldman et al. 1999; Rabins et al. 1997).

Psychosis is common in DAT; the early appearance of psychosis correlates with more rapid cognitive decline (Ropacki and Jeste 2005; Wilkosz et al. 2006). Visual hallucinations are the most common perceptual disturbance (Class et al. 1997). The prevalence of delusions in DAT is as high as 73%; delusions of persecution, theft, reference, and jealousy are common (Rao and Lyketsos 1998; Ropacki and Jeste 2005). The neuropathology of AD includes β-amyloid deposits, neuritic plaques, and neurofibrillary tangles (NFTs) (Felician and Sandson 1999; Jellinger 1996).

Diffuse plaques are β-amyloid depositions without surrounding neuronal degeneration (Felician and Sandson 1999). *Neuritic plaques* (a core of β-amyloid surrounded by dystrophic neurites) are surrounded by immune-activated microglia and reactive astrocytes (Felician and Sandson 1999; Smits et al. 2000). Neuritic plaque density is increased in several regions of the cortex, hippocampus, entorhinal cortex, amygdala, and cerebral vessels in AD and continues to increase with disease progression (Felician and Sandson 1999; Haroutunian et al. 1998).

NFTs—intraneuronal bundles of phosphorylated tau proteins—are an early pathological change in the hippocampus, amygdala, and entorhinal cortex (Felician and Sandson 1999). Dementia severity is proportional to the density of NFTs (Felician and Sandson 1999; Jellinger 1996). With accumulated neuron damage, presynaptic terminal density is decreased (Cummings et al. 1998).

The apolipoprotein E (APOE) ε4 allele on chromosome 19 affects the rate of β-amyloid production and the clinical manifestations of AD in a dose-dependent fashion; homozygotes have a higher risk, earlier onset, and faster rate of decline than do heterozygotes and noncarriers (Blennow et al. 2006; Caselli et al. 1999; Craft et al. 1998). Adults without dementia who carried the APOE ε4 allele were found to exhibit decreased verbal memory performance and minor hippocampal damage (Bottino and Almeida 1997; Small et al. 1999). The APOE ε2 allele may confer protection against AD, whereas the APOE ε3 allele appears to not change AD risk (Rebeck and Hyman 1999).

Frontotemporal dementia (FTD), including dementia due to Pick's disease, features an earlier age at onset than DAT, executive dysfunction, attentional deficits, loss of insight, aphasia, and personality changes (typically increased extraversion) with relatively spared memory and visuospatial functions (Boeve 2006; Kertesz and Munoz 2002; Mendez et al. 2006). Patients may exhibit "childlike" exuberance, "catastrophic" reactions to trivial events, decreased social awareness, disinhibition, distractibility, aphasia, perseveration, carbohydrate cravings, and frontal lobe release signs and may have a poorer response to cholinesterase inhibitors than do patients with AD (Duara et al. 1999; Kertesz and Munoz 2002). Consensus criteria for the diagnosis of FTD have been developed that include the following core diagnostic features: insidious onset and gradual progression, early decline in social interpersonal conduct, early impairment in regulation of personal conduct, early emotional blunting, and early loss of insight (Neary et al. 1998). Full neuropsychological assessment of FTD patients reveals deficits on tests of complex executive function, such as the Wisconsin Card Sorting Test and the Stroop Test (Kertesz and Munoz 2002). Neuropathological findings in FTD are restricted to the frontal and anterior temporal lobes and include characteristic Pick inclusion bodies, NFTs, and ballooned cells, all containing tau protein (Jellinger 1996; Kertesz and Munoz 2002).

Dementia due to Creutzfeldt-Jakob disease (CJD), also called "spongiform encephalopathy," is a prion-mediated infection. It manifests as a rapidly progressive cortical dementia accompanied by myoclonus and may first appear with psychosis (Dunn et al. 1999; Zerr et al. 2000). In patients with CJD, the EEG shows a characteristic pattern of repetitive sharp waves or slow spikes followed by synchronous triphasic sharp waves (Dunn et al. 1999; Zerr et al. 2000). In classic CJD, the cortex is diffusely affected, with a general loss of cortical substance and a spongy atrophic appearance (Dunn et al. 1999).

Dementia due to chronic subdural hematoma may present with focal neurological signs, personality changes, various cognitive impairments (including decreased memory, language disturbances, difficulty with abstraction, problems with calculation, and poor social judgment), lethargy, and/or agitation (G.W. Ross and Bowen 2002). The syndrome may have a relatively sudden onset and may show fluctuation in clinical status; a history of trauma may be absent in one-third of affected patients (G.W. Ross and Bowen 2002).

Subcortical Dementias

Dementia due to HIV initially manifests as decreases in psychomotor and information processing speed, verbal memory, learning efficiency, and fine motor function with later cortical symptoms of decreased executive function, aphasia, apraxia, and agnosia (J.L. Maldonado et al. 2000). In advanced stages, ataxia, spasticity, increased muscle tone, and incontinence may develop (J.L. Maldonado et al. 2000). Dementia has been reported in up to 30% of HIV-positive patients, may present early in the course of illness, increases suicide risk, and may compromise compliance with antiviral regimens (Cohen and Jacobson 2000; J.L. Maldonado et al. 2000). More recent estimates of the incidence of dementia due to HIV are somewhat lower, possibly due to the neuroprotective effects of early, aggressive antiviral treatment (d'Arminio Monforte et al. 2000; Goodkin et al. 2001). Dementia due to HIV results from neurotoxicity mediated by HIV-infected macrophages (which serve as the site for viral replication) (McDaniel et al. 2000; Smits et al. 2000).

Dementia due to Parkinson's disease (PD) is seen in as many as 60% of patients with PD and features bradyphrenia, apathy, poor retrieval memory, decreased verbal fluency, and attention deficits (Levy and Cummings 2000; Marsh 2000). Although dementia due to PD is classified as a primarily subcortical dementia, cortical symptoms of executive dysfunction, visuospatial impairment, agnosia, anomia, aphasia, and apraxia may be seen in patients with PD dementia who develop cortical Lewy bodies (Hurtig et al. 2000; Levy

and Cummings 2000). Increased age, greater severity of neurological symptoms, and the APOE ε2 allele have been associated with an increased risk of dementia in patients with PD (Harhangi et al. 2000; Hughes et al. 2000). Cognition may improve with treatment for the common comorbid mood disorders (Levy and Cummings 2000). Psychosis can be induced by antiparkinsonian treatment of the motor symptoms of PD. Dementia due to PD features deposition of α-synuclein or tau protein in the substantia nigra and commonly involves Lewy bodies in the substantia nigra, cortex, and subcortex, with resulting deficits in dopaminergic, noradrenergic, cholinergic, and serotonergic neurotransmission (Levy and Cummings 2000; Marsh 2000).

Dementia due to Huntington's disease features abulia and impairments in retrieval memory, cognitive speed, concentration, verbal learning, and cognitive flexibility (Boeve 2006; Ranen 2000). With progression, more global impairment in memory, visuospatial function, and executive function may follow (Ranen 2000). Comorbid mood disturbance, anxiety (including obsessive-compulsive symptoms), and psychotic symptoms are common (Boeve 2006; Tost et al. 2004). These patients have a high risk for personality change, irritability, aggressive behavior, and suicide (Ranen 2000; Rosenblatt and Leroi 2000). The dementia results from cell loss in primary sensory and association areas, entorhinal cortex, caudate nucleus, and putamen (Jellinger 1996; Ranen 2000).

Dementia due to multiple sclerosis is seen in as many as 65% of multiple sclerosis patients (Schwid et al. 2000). Clinical features include deficits in memory, attention, information processing speed, learning, and executive functions; language and verbal intelligence are relatively spared (Schwid et al. 2000). Cognitive impairment may present early in the course of multiple sclerosis, and progression is roughly proportional to the number of central nervous system (CNS) demyelinating lesions (Schwid et al. 2000).

Dementias With Cortical and Subcortical Features

Vascular dementia (VaD) broadly includes dementias resulting from vascular pathology that have as a final common pathway the loss of functional cortex. Because VaD exists on a continuum extending from the essentially subcortical pathology formerly described as multi-infarct dementia to the primarily cortical pathology in poststroke dementia (i.e., dementia following a single stroke), it is problematic to attempt to fit all VaDs (thus inclusively defined) into the "cortical versus subcortical" dichotomy.

Additionally, the boundary between AD and the broad category of VaD is itself quite permeable. The term *mixed dementia* is used to describe cases with coexisting DAT and VaD (Langa et al. 2004). It has been estimated that approximately 25% of DAT cases also feature concurrent vascular pathology and could be reasonably classified as mixed dementia (Langa et al. 2004). Cerebral infarcts in established AD are associated with greater overall severity of dementia and poorer neuropsychological testing performance (Heyman et al. 1999).

Multi-infarct VaD is characterized by abrupt onset, decreased executive functioning, gait disturbance, affective lability, and parkinsonian symptoms (Choi et al. 2000; Patterson et al. 1999). Risk factors include increased age, hypertension, diabetes mellitus, atherosclerotic heart disease, hypertriglyceridemia, and hyperlipidemia (Curb et al. 1999; G.W. Ross et al. 1999). Because the cognitive deficits follow a series of discrete lesions, progression is "stepwise," with relative stability of cognitive status between vascular insults as opposed to the gradual progression of deficits seen in AD. The progression of multi-infarct VaD may be affected by risk factor modification and antiplatelet therapy (Rabins et al. 1997). Lesions are generally located in the subcortical nuclei, frontal lobe white matter, thalamus, and internal capsule and are associated with a characteristic appearance on magnetic resonance imaging (MRI) of peri-ventricular hyperintensities on the T2 images (Choi et al. 2000). However, periventricular hyperintensities are also seen in normal aging and in other types of dementia and thus, in isolation, represent a nonspecific finding (Smith et al. 2000). Diffusion-weighted MRI has been shown to be a more sensitive method of evaluating small-vessel ischemic disease in VaD (Choi et al. 2000). The syndrome of cerebral autosomal dominant arteriopathy with subcortical infarcts and leukoencephalopathy is a syndrome of small-vessel vascular disease due to mutation in the *NOTCH3* gene and has been described as an archetype of pure subcortical VaD (Peters et al. 2005).

Poststroke VaD—dementia occurring as the acute or subacute consequence of a single stroke—may be difficult to clearly distinguish from multi-infarct VaD that follows a series of vascular events. Poststroke dementia is associated with apraxia, neglect, hemianopsia, facial paralysis, and extremity weakness (de Koning et al. 1998). Major dominant-hemisphere stroke, left-hemisphere location, internal carotid artery distribution, diabetes mellitus, prior cerebrovascular accident (CVA), older age, less education, and nonwhite race were found to be risk factors for poststroke dementia (Desmond et al. 2000). Major depression is common with poststroke dementia, with anterior left-hemisphere stroke posing the highest risk (Robinson 1998). The risk for poststroke dementia associated with major depression is highest in the first year (Robinson 1998). Deficits in orientation, language, visuoconstruction, and executive functions are common but may improve with treatment of the poststroke depression (Robinson 1998).

Lewy body variant (LBV) of AD and LBD have a significant degree of phenomenological overlap and may be difficult to differentiate clinically (Leverenz and McKeith 2002). The more general term *dementia with Lewy bodies* is often used to denote the continuum of LBV, LBD, and dementia due to PD (Boeve 2006; Gomez-Isla et al. 1999). A similar degree of overlap is seen in the neuropathology of LBV and LBD. Pathologically, LBV is characterized by the presence of Lewy bodies (intraneuronal eosinophilic inclusion bodies) in subcortical and cortical structures in addition to AD neuropathology (Gomez-Isla et al. 1999). LBV has a lower density of NFTs in the neocortex than does AD (Heyman et al. 1999). LBD also features subcortical and cortical Lewy bodies, with a relative absence of NFTs and other AD neuropathology (Litvan and McKee 1999).

Clinically, LBV and LBD share the common features of fluctuation of mental status, well-formed visual hallucinations, delusions, depression, apathy, anxiety, and extrapyramidal symptoms (Heyman et al. 1999; Lopez et al. 2000b). Visual hallucinations occur early in the course of illness, even with mild levels of cognitive impairment (Ballard et al. 2001; Leverenz and McKeith 2002). In comparison with AD, LBV exhibits greater deficits in attention, verbal fluency, and visuospatial functioning and increased parkinsonian symptoms (Lopez et al. 2000b; McKeith et al. 2000). LBV has also been associated with more rapid cognitive decline, earlier institutionalization, and shorter survival time (Lopez et al. 2000b; Serby et al. 2003). The clinical distinction between LBV and AD may be more apparent in the moderate/severe stages of dementia (Lopez et al. 2000a). LBD also features impaired executive functioning, disinhibited social behavior, syncope, and increased sensitivity to antipsychotic agents (manifested by drowsiness, further cognitive decline, and neuroleptic malignant syndrome) (Aarsland et al. 2005; McKeith et al. 2000). Progression is usually more rapid in LBD than in AD, although psychotic symptoms in LBV and LBD may be improved by treatment with cholinesterase inhibitors, whereas psychotic symptoms may paradoxically worsen with antipsychotic agents (Ballard et al. 2001; Leverenz and McKeith 2002; Levy and Cummings 2000). LBV and LBD are also associated with neuroleptic sensitivity, characterized by sedation, immobility, rigidity, postural instability, falls, and decreased cognitive status (Baskys 2004).

Dementia due to fragile X–associated tremor/ataxia syndrome (FXTAS) is a newly described syndrome that features frontal lobe and subcortical dementia symptoms in concert with motor anomalies in the grandfathers of children with the fragile X syndrome (Jacquemont et al. 2003). Patients experience amnesia, executive function deficits, and psychomotor slowing. Notable neurological symptoms include rigidity, tremor, and ataxia. Patients exhibit a progressive neurological and cognitive decline. Due to the prominent motor symptoms, this syndrome bears some resemblance to PD with dementia. Neuroimaging has revealed generalized cortical and cerebellar atrophy and increased signal intensity on the middle cerebellar peduncles (Brunberg et al. 2002). The laboratory test for FXTAS dementia is an alteration on the *FMR1* gene at Xq 27.3 on Southern blot and polymerase chain reaction.

Dementia due to normal pressure hydrocephalus is associated with amnesia, decreased psychomotor movement, gait apraxia (often described as a "magnetic" gait, where patients are unable to lift their feet to initiate walking), and incontinence (G.W. Ross and Bowen 2002). Neuroimaging reveals ventricular dilatation that is disproportionate to the sulcal widening. Cognitive and motor symptoms may improve following a tap of cerebrospinal fluid or shunting procedures.

Epidemiology

The risk of dementia increases exponentially with age, from 1% for those younger than 65 years to 25%–50% for those older than 85 years (Jorm and Jolley 1998). The annual risk of dementia is 0.5% between ages 60 and 69 years, 1% between 70 and 74 years, 2% between 75 and 79 years, 3% between 80 and 84 years, and 8% thereafter (Rabins et al. 1997). The prevalence of dementia was found to be 3.9% for patients older than 60 years in a general hospital population (Lyketsos et al. 2000a). The risk for patients between ages 60 and 64 years was 2.6%; this risk increased to

Table 3–8. Potentially reversible etiologies of dementia

Structural central nervous system factors
    Vascular dementia
    Head trauma
    Subdural hematoma
    Normal pressure hydrocephalus
    Multiple sclerosis

Psychiatric illnesses
    Major depression
    Substance dependence

Systemic/metabolic factors
    Hypothyroidism
    Hypercalcemia
    Hypoglycemia
    Thiamine, niacin, B_{12} deficiency
    Renal failure
    Hepatic failure
    Medications

Infectious diseases
    HIV
    Central nervous system infection

Table 3–9. Psychiatric differential diagnosis of dementia

Mild cognitive impairment

Delirium

Mood disorders

Amnestic disorders

Substance use disorders

Psychotic disorders

Mental retardation

8.9% for those older than 85 years. Reported estimates of the relative frequency of the different dementia types in study populations of dementia patients include 50%–90% DAT, 8%–20% VaD, and 7%–26% LBD, with other subtypes less common (Lyketsos et al. 2000b; Roman 2002). Poststroke VaD has been estimated in up to 41% of patients following stroke (Roman 2002). Reversible dementias are estimated to account for 1%–10% of dementias; examples of potentially reversible dementias are shown in Table 3–8 (Gliatto and Caroff 2001; Tager and Fallon 2001).

Comorbidity and Differential Diagnosis

The patient with cognitive impairment may have psychiatric illnesses other than or in addition to dementia. Clinical history and examination need to be focused to consider these other diagnostic possibilities. The psychiatric differential diagnosis of dementia is shown in Table 3–9.

Clinical Evaluation

History

A clinical history should first be obtained from the patient directly, initially without the presence of other family members. History taking should address recent cognitive function; examples include function at work, at home, while driving, and while performing other high-risk activities (Patterson et al. 1999). A complaint of memory loss may be predictive of a later diagnosis of DAT, even without demonstrable memory deficits on initial clinical examination (Geerlings et al. 1999). A personal and family history of psychiatric illness should be obtained, specifically to include dementia and neurological illness with high risk for dementia. Because the patient is most reliable in the early stages of illness, the physician should then separately interview family members and synthesize the separate histories obtained to derive the most balanced view of the patient's functioning.

The medical history should address all chronic systemic illnesses, with particular attention to conditions that increase risk for DAT, VaD, and other dementia types. Specific examples of such systemic illnesses include hypertension, diabetes mellitus, hyperlipidemia, PD, multiple sclerosis, and prior CVA (Geldmacher and Whitehouse 1997). Recent systemic illnesses that may put the patient at risk for delirium also need to be explored. The medication history should address both psychotropic and nonpsychotropic medications taken before the onset of the cognitive and behavioral symptoms (Doraiswamy et al. 1998). The use of nonprescription medications (especially antihistamines and sedatives) and herbal preparations also needs to be explored.

The social history should address the patient's living circumstances, presence of supportive family members and/or of other significant persons living nearby, financial and insurance resources, participation in social activities, and personal relationships. Collateral history obtained from family members should focus on concerns about the patient's cognitive function and overt behavior. Problematic symptoms such as paranoia, agitation, physical violence, and inattentive and reckless operation of dangerous machinery need to be addressed, as well as access to weapons and any threats made to self or others. Any complaint of neglect or abuse, or any physical examination findings suggestive of inappropriate care, should be reported promptly to the agency responsible for performing on-site evaluation of neglect or abuse of adults. Aggressive and/or delusional patients may be at greatest risk of such maltreatment (Cummings and Masterman 1998). Dementia patients are also at increased risk for syncope and loss of consciousness, which can result in head trauma, hip fracture, or other injuries. Any report of falls in dementia patients requires a full evaluation for injuries.

Mental Status Examination

Formal assessment of cognitive function must be added to routine evaluation of mood and affect, level of consciousness, psychomotor activity, speech production, thought content, and thought processes. It is recommended that the clinician use a cognitive assessment instrument such as the MMSE. A score of 24 or less on the MMSE, when correlated with clinical findings, is highly suggestive of dementia, but education and other patient-specific variables must be taken into close account (Patterson et al. 1999). A cutoff score of 22 is advised in the elderly nursing home

population; the MMSE may overestimate dementia in patients with less education, age older than 85, or a history of depression (Dufouil et al. 2000). Conversely, patients with high levels of education and other evidence of premorbid high intellectual function may score in the "unimpaired" range on the MMSE despite decreased functional status. Serial administrations of the MMSE can quantify the progress or stability of dementia; a typical decline in MMSE scores in DAT is 2–4 points per year in untreated patients (Folstein et al. 1975; Rabins et al. 1997). Adjunctive tests of cognitive function include clock drawing, category generation (e.g., having the patient name as many animals as possible in 1 minute; 16 is a cutoff score), and the "go, no-go" test (the patient is instructed to tap once if the examiner taps once, and to not tap if the examiner taps twice). The Neuropsychiatric Inventory is a 12-item behavioral rating scale to assess noncognitive symptoms of dementia (Aalten et al. 2003). A series of structured questions administered to the patient's caretaker are used to assess the following behavioral domains: delusions, hallucinations, agitation/aggression, dysphoria/depression, anxiety, apathy, irritability, euphoria, disinhibition, aberrant motor behavior, nighttime behavioral disturbance, and appetite/eating abnormalities (Aalten et al. 2003). For each item, severity is rated from 1 to 3 and frequency is rated from 1 to 4; these are summed for a total score. Depression rating scales (e.g., the Hamilton Rating Scale for Depression [Hamilton 1960], the Geriatric Depression Scale [Yesavage et al. 1983]) are recommended to assist in distinguishing dementia from depression and in monitoring response to antidepressants (Katz 1998).

Physical Examination

Assessment of vision and hearing should not be overlooked (Doraiswamy et al. 1998). Relative sensory deprivation due to uncorrected vision and/or hearing deficits can cause spuriously poor performance on formal cognitive testing. Loss of visual acuity and severe cognitive impairment in patients with DAT can increase visual hallucinations (Chapman et al. 1999). Neurological examination should include assessment of gait, frontal lobe release signs, movement disorders, sensory function, and focal neurological deficits (Doraiswamy et al. 1998). Physical examination should address blood pressure, orthostatic hypotension, cardiovascular disease, cerebrovascular disease, signs of metabolic illnesses, marginal hygiene, poor nutritional status, weight loss, and dehydration. Treatment of vascular risk factors has been shown to decrease the risk of dementia, including DAT and VaD (Alagiakrishnan et al. 2006; Peila et al. 2006).

Laboratory Tests

Laboratory tests may be modified on a case-by-case basis. Tests to consider are shown in Table 3–10 (Patterson et al. 1999; Rabins et al. 1997). Serum drug levels of medications associated with altered mental status (e.g., tricyclic antidepressants, anticonvulsants, digitalis, antiarrhythmics) should be obtained if clinically indicated. A 12-lead electrocardiogram should be considered, especially if there is a history of cardiac and/or vascular disease.

When CJD is suspected, cerebrospinal fluid samples should be obtained for testing for the neuronal proteins 14–3–3 and γ-enolase (Zerr et al. 2000). CJD is characterized by a classic electroencephalographic appearance of repetitive sharp waves or slow spikes followed by synchronous triphasic sharp waves, although the six different phenotypes of this illness may present with different combinations of EEG findings (Zerr et al. 2000). Lumbar puncture should also be considered if there is a clinical suspicion of normal pressure hydrocephalus, metastatic carcinoma, or unusually early onset and/or rapid progression of deficits (Small 1998). Other laboratory tests to consider in specific cases include serum ammonia, heavy metals, and cortisol; carotid Doppler studies; chest X ray; and mammography (Patterson et al. 1999; Rabins et al. 1997).

Table 3–10. Laboratory tests for dementia workup

Electrolytes, blood urea nitrogen, creatinine, calcium

Liver-associated enzymes

Glucose

Complete blood count

Thyroid profile with thyroid-stimulating hormone assay

Erythrocyte sedimentation rate, antinuclear antibody panel

Prothrombin time/partial thromboblastin time

B_{12} and folate

Syphilis serology

Urinalysis and urine toxicology

Pulse oximetry

Medication levels (e.g., tricyclic antidepressants, anticonvulsants, digitalis, antiarrhythmics)

HIV

Neuroimaging

Neuroimaging is increasingly routine in the evaluation of dementia. Computed tomography (CT) is generally more readily available and of lower cost than MRI, although MRI's superior resolution has led to its greater use in dementia evaluation (G. W. Ross and Bowen 2002). A diagnosis of VaD requires confirmatory neuroimaging (Roman 2002). In cases of suspected DAT, hippocampal atrophy may serve as a sensitive early marker for cognitive decline (Jack et al. 2000; Petersen et al. 2000). When more quantitative techniques for assessing hippocampal size and appearance become more widely available, they are likely to increase specificity.

Cortical atrophy and ventriculomegaly do not by themselves confirm dementia and, in isolation, are not specific findings (Doraiswamy et al. 1998; Small 1998a). Progressive cerebral atrophy and ventriculomegaly are more likely in DAT than in VaD and have been reported to correlate with declines in performance on the MMSE (Patterson et al. 1999). If initial neuroimaging reveals hippocampal and/or cortical atrophy that correlates with the clinical presentation and gradual course of DAT, then serial neuroimaging to follow progress is not routinely necessary. Periventricular hyperintensities on MRI may be seen in DAT as well as in VaD; their significance in DAT is unclear, because they may not correlate independently with cognitive changes (Doody et al. 1998; Smith et al. 2000). Decreased white matter volume has been associated with DAT (Smith et al. 2000). If initial imaging shows white matter lesions typical of VaD that correlate with clinical findings, a follow-up CT or MRI could be considered if the patient later presents with an abrupt decrease in mental status suggestive of delirium and/or a new CVA. Diffusion-weighted MRI, which has been shown to be more sensitive than CT in imaging the small-vessel ischemic disease in VaD, may be used to monitor progression of these patients (Choi et al. 2000). Functional neuroimaging (e.g., single photon emission computed tomography, positron emission tomography (PET) scanning, and in vivo proton MRS), although not currently widely available, holds promise in the evaluation of the cortical pathology of dementia, particularly when combined with genetic assessment of patients at risk for clinical dementia (Weiss et al. 2003). Functional neuroimaging techniques may reveal a specific pattern of parietal and temporal deficits in DAT that could lead the physician to consider earlier treatment with antidementia pharmacotherapy (Small and Leiter 1998).

Management

Clinical Management

Attention to comorbid systemic and neuropsychiatric illnesses is the first priority in clinical management of the dementia patient. Close collaboration with the patient's other physician(s) is essential for managing medical illnesses that increase the risk for cognitive deficits. Examples include the neurologist in the case of a patient with PD or multiple sclerosis and the internist in the case of a patient with VaD or HIV. Management of pain may decrease agitated behavior in patients with dementia. Psychopharmacological approaches to anxiety, psychotic, and mood disorders are discussed in detail later (see "Pharmacotherapy"). Substance abuse interventions consisting of medical detoxication, participation in Alcoholics Anonymous or other 12-Step recovery programs, judicious use of agonist therapies, and close attention to comorbid substance-induced mood and anxiety disorders are necessary in the dementia patient with comorbid substance abuse or dependence.

Early frank discussion of diagnosis, prognosis, and management, with clinical follow-ups scheduled at least every 3 months, are advised. Every visit should include an evaluation of whether the patient can still safely live at home. More frequent visits should be scheduled to monitor response and side effects when psychotropic medications are prescribed. Supportive psychotherapy may assist the patient in dealing with grief and loss. Admission to a psychiatry inpatient unit skilled in dealing with dementia patients may be needed for severely regressed, suicidal, violent, or psychotic patients, especially if complex psychopharmacological regimens and/or electroconvulsive therapy (ECT) is considered (Rabins et al. 1997).

Psychoeducation can be very valuable, especially for family caregivers (Grossberg and Lake 1998). *The 36-Hour Day: A Family Guide to Caring for Persons With Alzheimer's Disease, Related Dementing Illnesses, and Memory Loss in Later Life* (Mace and Rabins 1981) is often helpful to both patients and families. Support and advocacy groups are available through the Alzheimer's Association (1-800-621-0379; www.alz.org) (Rabins et al. 1997). The Alzheimer's Association can facilitate patient enrollment in the Safe Return program, a nationwide program that assists in the identification and return of dementia patients who wander. The patient should always carry and/or wear identification (e.g., a MedicAlert bracelet) and can be registered with the local police department. Physicians should inform caregivers of the increased risk of depression in primary caregivers of dementia patients and facilitate respite opportunities for caregivers (Grossberg and Lake 1998).

A major review of the psychological approaches to the neuropsychiatric disturbances in dementia demonstrated that behavior management strategies, caregiver and residential staff education, and (possibly) cognitive stimulation techniques had an adequate evidence base supporting their prolonged effectiveness (Livingston et al. 2005). Environmental and behavioral management may include provision of adequate lighting, music, access to pets, and appropriate levels of psychological stimulation. Because of the decreased psychological flexibility of the dementia patient, the home should be organized to allow for simplicity of routines, with prominent display of calendars, schedules, and the photographs and names of people close to the patient. Events that trigger problematic behaviors should be identified and minimized (Parnetti 2000). For safety, child-proofing devices may be considered. Vehicle keys, power tools, and sharp household objects should be secured. Weapons should be removed from the home or at least be secured in a locked cabinet.

Legal issues should be addressed early in the course of the illness, while the patient can still direct his or her wishes. These matters include the completion of medicolegal documents such as living wills, durable powers of attorney, and advance directives (Grossberg and Lake 1998). The physician may be asked to comment on the patient's capacity to make legally binding decisions. Neuropsychological testing may be of help. The capacity for medical decision making needs to be considered as well. The physician is advised to thoroughly evaluate the patient's clinical status at the time a medical decision is needed to ensure that the patient understands the implications of his or her medical choices. The capacity to vote is generally preserved in

mild DAT, whereas patients with moderate disease may require specific assessment of this capacity (Applebaum et al. 2005).

Driving or the operation of other dangerous machinery is often a point of great contention. Many patients will maintain the motor skills for driving despite showing substantial cognitive deficits on the clinical interview and on formal mental status testing (Rabins 1998). Even in mild dementia, the statistical risk of motor vehicle accidents is increased (Dubinsky et al. 2000). Physicians are advised to acquaint themselves with the disclosure laws regarding notification of dementia diagnoses to state motor vehicle departments. A road competency test may be advisable. A useful clinical guideline to consider is that driving is not advised whenever a dementia diagnosis leads the clinician to institute pharmacotherapy for dementia and/or when the MMSE score is less than 24. Other contraindications could be the presence of paranoia, agitation, or assaultive behavior.

Institutional placement is often a painful decision. To many patients, the loss of the home environment, even when clearly necessary to preserve safety, is a devastating experience that usually leads to further confusion, behavioral regression, and increased risk of depression. The lack of or loss of a primary caregiver may predict earlier institutionalization (Patterson et al. 1999). The physician should make every reasonable effort to maintain the patient in his or her home environment. An important intervention is respite care for caregivers. Various respite models to consider include in-home caregivers (e.g., the visiting nurse model) and adult day care centers/senior centers (in which the patient attends a supervised therapeutic environment for the business day and returns home at night).

Pharmacotherapy

Anticholinesterase agents act through inhibition of acetylcholinesterase, increasing the net amount of synaptic acetylcholine available for neurotransmission (Table 3–11). Anticholinesterase agents are advised early in the

Table 3–11. Dementia pharmacotherapy

Medication class	Target symptom(s)	Starting dosage	High dosage
Cholinesterase inhibitors	Decreased cognition, delusions, hallucinations		
Tacrine		10 mg qds	40 mg qds
Donepezil		5 mg/day	10 mg/day
Rivastigmine		1.5 mg bid	6 mg bid
Galantamine		4 mg bid	12 mg bid
NMDA antagonist	Decreased cognition		
Memantine		5 mg/day	10 mg bid
Antidepressants	Depression, irritability, anxiety		
Fluoxetine		10 mg/day	40 mg/day
Paroxetine		10 mg/day	40 mg/day
Sertraline		25 mg/day	200 mg/day
Citalopram		10 mg/day	40 mg/day
Escitalopram		5 mg/day	20 mg/day
Venlafaxine (extended release)		37.5 mg/day	350 mg/day
Mirtazapine		7.5 mg/day hs	45 mg/day hs
Duloxetine		20 mg bid	30 mg bid
Trazodone		25 mg/day hs	400 mg/day hs
Bupropion		37.5 mg bid	200 mg bid
Anxiolytic	Anxiety, irritability		
Buspirone		5 mg tid	20 mg tid
Anticonvulsants	Irritability, agitation		
Carbamazepine		100 mg/day	[a]
Valproate		125 mg/day	[b]
Oxcarbazepine		150 mg bid	600 mg bid
Antipsychotics	Delusions, hallucinations, disorganized thoughts, agitation		
Risperidone		0.25 mg/day hs	3 mg/day hs
Olanzapine		2.5 mg/day hs	10 mg/day hs
Quetiapine		25 mg/day hs	150 mg bid
Ziprasidone		20 mg/day hs	40 mg bid
Aripiprazole		5 mg/day	15 mg/day
Clozapine		25 mg bid	100 mg bid

Note. NMDA=*N*-methyl-D-aspartate.
[a]Upper limit of dosage to give serum drug level of 8–12 ng/mL.
[b]Upper limit of dosage to give serum drug level of 50–60 ng/mL.

course of DAT and may reduce the rate of cognitive decline (Blennow et al. 2006). Once initiated and well tolerated at the highest recommended dosages, anticholinesterase agents should be continued indefinitely, with regular monitoring of cognitive, emotional, and functional behavioral status. Although their effects may be relatively modest, more often involving a slowing of decline than a reversal of cognitive losses, they represent a major breakthrough in psychopharmacology (Bonner and Peskind 2002; Trinh et al. 2003). There is some early evidence that anticholinesterase agents may have a neuroprotective function on the hippocampus in DAT (Hashimoto et al. 2005; Krishnan et al. 2003).

Anticholinesterase agents should also be considered (along with antipsychotics) in managing dementia-related psychotic symptoms (Rao and Lyketsos 1998). These agents can also be safely combined with antidepressants, which may lead to greater symptomatic improvement, given that catecholamine abnormalities may be related to some of the symptoms of dementia (Tune and Sunderland 1998). Cholinergic side effects seen with anticholinesterase agents include nausea, abdominal discomfort, vomiting, loose stools, muscle cramps, muscle weakness, increased sweating, and bradycardia. Acetylcholinesterase inhibitors should be discontinued before surgery in which succinylcholine may be used because of the risk of prolonged paralysis.

Anticholinesterase agents may also be used for other dementing illnesses (e.g., dementia due to PD, LBV, LBD, and CJD; VaD; and mixed VaD and DAT); they may be particularly helpful with the psychotic symptoms of LBV and LBD (Roman et al. 2005; Simard and van Reekum 2004). Combination regimens consisting of an anticholinesterase agent and other agents more directly protective against neuronal degeneration (e.g., memantine, antioxidants, anti-inflammatory agents, hormones) with psychotropic medications (to address specific neuropsychiatric symptoms) are emerging as treatment for DAT. Tacrine, donepezil, rivastigmine, and galantamine are approved by the U.S. Food and Drug Administration (FDA) for DAT, although tacrine has been associated with hepatotoxicity and is now rarely used clinically.

Antidepressants should be used for comorbid depressive disorders, depressive and anxiety symptoms that do not qualify for a full depressive or anxiety disorder diagnosis, sleep disturbances, and agitation. Because of their generally benign side-effect profile and their effectiveness, selective serotonin reuptake inhibitors (SSRIs) are the preferred class of antidepressants in dementia patients and should be started at lower dosages than in healthy adults. Paroxetine has more clinically significant anticholinergic activity than the other SSRIs and should be used with caution. SSRIs may also have utility in managing sexual disinhibition in dementia (Stewart and Shin 1997).

Psychostimulants as adjunctive therapy with antidepressants may be considered for refractory mood symptoms and/or apathy; methylphenidate 2.5–5 mg/day is a recommended starting dosage (Rabins et al. 1997). An alternative agent is modafinil, with dosages starting at 100 mg to a maximum to 400 mg in the morning. ECT should be considered for cases of treatment-refractory depression; however, because of the risk for post-ECT delirium and amnesia, ECT treatments should be given no more frequently than twice per week, with unilateral electrode placement (Rabins et al. 1997).

Anxiolytics may be used for anxiety or agitation. Because of the high risk of further memory impairment, sedation, and falls, physicians should avoid the use of benzodiazepines in dementia patients (Rabins et al. 1997). Other agents to consider in managing agitated patients include carbamazepine, divalproex sodium, and β-blockers.

Antipsychotics are indicated for paranoid thinking, hallucinations, delirium, and agitation. Initial dosages in elderly patients with dementia should be less than those used in younger patients because of the risks of sedation and further cognitive decline. Although conventional antipsychotic agents are often used as first-line treatment for agitation, they are associated with frequent adverse side effects in patients with dementia (Alexopoulos et al. 1998; Daniel 2000).

The atypical antipsychotic agents risperidone, olanzapine, quetiapine, ziprasidone, and aripiprazole are recommended in dementia with agitation and psychosis because of their clinical efficacy and (when compared with conventional antipsychotics) greater tolerability and lower risk of extrapyramidal symptoms and neuroleptic malignant syndrome; clozapine is not generally recommended as a first-line antipsychotic in dementia due to the risk of agranulocytosis and its propensity to increase the risk of delirium and seizures (Carson et al. 2006; Mintzer et al. 2006; Sink et al. 2005). Reduced starting and maximum dosages (e.g., risperidone dosage range of 0.25–3 mg/day at bedtime) are recommended to minimize side effects (Daniel 2000). Nighttime dosing is preferred, because sleep is facilitated and the risk of daytime sedation is minimized.

Generally, olanzapine and quetiapine are more sedating than the other atypical antipsychotics. Olanzapine has been associated with gait disturbance in dementia patients (Lawlor 2004; Tariot et al. 2004). Quetiapine may minimize risk of motor side effects in psychosis with PD and LBD, as well as in other dementias, and be safer than clozapine (Baskys 2004; Keys and DeWald 2005b). Clozapine may be used in cases of PD and LBD (due to its relatively lower likelihood of exacerbating movement disorders) and in cases where psychosis is refractory to other agents (Keys and DeWald 2005b; Leverenz and McKeith 2002).

The atypical antipsychotics have been associated with weight gain, increased serum glucose, emergence of diabetes mellitus, and hyperlipidemia. This risk is particular high for olanzapine and clozapine (Keys and DeWald 2005b). Use of these medications of dementia should be accompanied by monitoring for these conditions (Keys and DeWald 2005a).

Recent concern has been raised over the increased risk of both CVA and death in de-

mentia patients who are treated with atypical antipsychotics; there does not seem to be a differential risk among the agents of this class (Schneider et al. 2005; Sink et al. 2005). This increased risk of adverse cerebrovascular events with atypical antipsychotics has not been seen in all studies (Herrmann et al. 2004; Liperoti et al. 2005). Risk for these complications may be greater in the immediate post-CVA period (Keys and DeWald 2005b). This concern has led to a 2005 Health Advisory Warning from the FDA (Sink et al. 2005). As a result, physicians should consider avoiding indefinite treatment with atypical antipsychotics for dementia-related psychosis and agitation and discontinue these medications promptly if clinical improvement is not seen (Sink et al. 2005).

Antiplatelet therapy and/or ergoloid mesylates (e.g., Hydergine 3 mg/day initially to a maximum of 9 mg/day) may be considered for cases of VaD and may stabilize or improve cognitive function (Meyer et al. 1995). Hydergine may be associated with nausea and other gastrointestinal symptoms; its use is contraindicated in patients with psychotic symptoms (Rabins et al. 1997). Other systemic interventions may be indicated in VaD, such as the statins, warfarin (in cases with atrial fibrillation), antihypertensives, calcium channel blockers, neuroprotective agents, and vascular surgery for hemodynamically significant carotid stenosis.

Highly active antiretroviral therapy for underlying HIV infection is an essential part of the management of HIV dementia and can reverse cognitive losses (Cohen and Jacobson 2000; McDaniel et al. 2000). The cognitive effects of this therapy may be further enhanced in combination with ibuprofen (Gendelman et al. 1998). Psychostimulants may be helpful in HIV-associated fatigue and decreased concentration and memory (J.L. Maldonado et al. 2000; McDaniel et al. 2000).

Dementia: Summary

The dementias are a heterogeneous group of clinical syndromes, unified by their common findings of deterioration in cognitive and executive functions. Physicians need to be alert to the need for a thorough history, targeted evaluation, and psychopharmacological and psychosocial management in patients with these clinical syndromes. Modern clinical interventions, including anticholinesterase agents in concert with other psychopharmacological agents, should be aggressively used early in the disease process to maintain the patient's cognitive functional status. Advances in basic science research point to possible new directions in the pathophysiology and psychopharmacological management of this major public health problem.

Amnestic and Other Cognitive Disorders
Amnestic Disorders

Amnestic disorders are characterized by a loss of memory due to the direct physiological effects of a general medical condition or due to the persisting effects of a substance. The amnestic disorders share a common symptom presentation of memory impairment but are differentiated by etiology. Amnestic disorders are secondary syndromes caused by systemic medical illness, primary cerebral disease or trauma, substance use disorders, or adverse medication effects. The impairment must be sufficient to compromise social and occupational functioning, and it should represent a significant decline from the previous level of functioning.

Epidemiology

Limited data are available on the prevalence and incidence of amnestic disorders (Harper et al. 1995). Memory impairment due to head trauma is probably the most common etiology, with more than 500,000 patients hospitalized annually in the United States for head injury. Alcohol abuse and associated thiamine deficiency are historically common etiologies, but some studies suggest that the incidence of alcohol-induced amnestic disor-

ders is decreasing, whereas that of amnestic disorders due to head trauma is increasing (Kopelman 1995).

Etiology

The DSM-IV-TR diagnostic classification for amnestic disorders is based on etiology. Amnestic disorders can be diagnosed as resulting from a general medical condition (Table 3–12), as due to the effects of a substance (Table 3–13), or as "not otherwise specified." The most common etiologies are listed in Table 3–14 and usually involve bilateral damage to areas of

---

Table 3–12.   DSM-IV-TR diagnostic criteria for amnestic disorder due to…[indicate the general medical condition]

A.   The development of memory impairment as manifested by impairment in the ability to learn new information or the inability to recall previously learned information.

B.   The memory disturbance causes significant impairment in social or occupational functioning and represents a significant decline from a previous level of functioning.

C.   The memory disturbance does not occur exclusively during the course of a delirium or a dementia.

D.   There is evidence from the history, physical examination, or laboratory findings that the disturbance is the direct physiological consequence of a general medical condition (including physical trauma).

Specify if:

Transient: if memory impairment lasts for 1 month or less

Chronic: if memory impairment lasts for more than 1 month

Coding note: Include the name of the general medical condition on Axis I, e.g., 294.0 amnestic disorder due to head trauma; also code the general medical condition on Axis III (see DSM-IV-TR Appendix G for codes).

Table 3–13. DSM-IV-TR diagnostic criteria for substance-induced persisting amnestic disorder

A. The development of memory impairment as manifested by impairment in the ability to learn new information or the inability to recall previously learned information.
B. The memory disturbance causes significant impairment in social or occupational functioning and represents a significant decline from a previous level of functioning.
C. The memory disturbance does not occur exclusively during the course of a delirium or a dementia and persists beyond the usual duration of substance intoxication or withdrawal.
D. There is evidence from the history, physical examination, or laboratory findings that the memory disturbance is etiologically related to the persisting effects of substance use (e.g., a drug of abuse, a medication).

Code [specific substance]–induced persisting amnestic disorder: (291.1 alcohol; 292.83 sedative, hypnotic, or anxiolytic; 292.83 other [or unknown] substance)

Table 3–14. Causes of amnestic disorders

Head trauma
Wernicke-Korsakoff syndrome
Alcohol-Induced blackouts
Benzodiazepines
Barbiturates
Intrathecal methotrexate
Methylenedioxymethamphetamine (MDMA; "Ecstasy")
Seizures
Herpes simplex encephalopathy
Klüver-Bucy syndrome
Electroconvulsive therapy
Carbon monoxide poisoning
Heavy metal poisoning
Hypoxia
Hypoglycemia
Cerebrovascular disorders
Cerebral neoplasms

the brain involved in memory. These areas include the dorsomedial and midline thalamic nuclei, the hippocampus, the amygdala, the fornix, and the mammillary bodies. Unilateral damage may sometimes be sufficient to produce memory impairment, particularly in the case of left-sided temporal lobe and thalamic structures (Benson 1978). Several iatrogenic causes, such as medication effects, ECT, and the ICU setting, lack clearly identified neuroanatomic damage (Jones et al. 2000).

Clinical Features

Patients with amnestic disorders either are impaired in their ability to learn and recall new information (anterograde amnesia) or are unable to recall previously learned material (retrograde amnesia). The deficits in short-term or recent memory seen in anterograde

amnesia can be assessed by asking the patient to recall three objects after a 5-minute distraction. Whereas anterograde amnesia is nearly always present, retrograde amnesia is more variable and depends on the location and severity of brain damage. Both immediate recall (as tested by digit span) and remote memory for distant past events are usually preserved. Memory for the physical traumatic event that caused the deficit is often lost. Orientation may be impaired, because it is dependent on the ability to store information regarding time, date, location, and circumstance. The patient may therefore present as confused and disoriented but without the fluctuation in level of consciousness associated with delirium. Orientation to self is nearly always preserved in amnestic disorders.

Most patients with amnestic disorders lack insight into their deficits and may vehemently deny the presence of memory impairment despite clear evidence to the contrary. This lack of insight may lead to anger, accusations, and occasionally agitation. More commonly, patients present with apathy, lack of initiative, and diminished affective expression suggestive of altered personality function.

Confabulation is often associated with amnestic disorders. Confabulation is characterized by responses to questions that not only are inaccurate but also are often so bizarre and unrealistic as to appear psychotic. Historically, confabulation was considered to represent an attempt by these patients to "cover up" their deficits in memory, but this explanation is probably overly simplistic. The presence and degree of confabulation are usually correlated not with the severity of memory deficits but rather with the loss of self-corrective and monitoring functions, as seen in bifrontal lobe disease (Mercer et al. 1977). Confabulation in amnestic disorders is usually seen during the early stages of the illness and tends to disappear over time.

The onset of amnesia may be sudden or gradual, depending on etiology. Head trauma, vascular events, and specific neurotoxic exposures such as carbon monoxide poisoning are associated with acute mental status changes. Prolonged substance use, sustained nutritional deficiency, and chronic neurotoxic exposures may produce a more gradual and sustained decline in memory function, eventually leading to a clinically diagnosable impairment.

Selected Amnestic Disorders

Head injury.   Severe neurological and psychiatric symptoms can result from head injury, even in the absence of radiological evidence of structural damage. Amnesia after head injury typically includes both anterograde (or ongoing) amnesia and retrograde amnesia for a period ranging from a few minutes to several years before the injury. As anterograde amnesia fades and the patient regains the ability to learn and recall new information, retrograde amnesia "shrinks," usually remaining only for the very short period (seconds to minutes) before the injury.

Wernicke-Korsakoff syndrome.   Wernicke-Korsakoff syndrome is an amnestic disorder caused by thiamine deficiency usually associated with excessive, prolonged ingestion of alcohol. It can occur in other malnourished conditions, such as marasmus, gastric carcinoma, and HIV (Kopelman 1995). The syndrome is associated with an acute phase of illness—known as Wernicke's encephalopathy—that presents with ophthalmoplegia, peripheral neuropathy, ataxia, nystagmus, and delirium. Although these acute neurological symptoms respond to aggressive thiamine repletion, a residual, persistent amnestic syndrome usually remains. The associated neuroanatomical abnormalities in Wernicke-Korsakoff syndrome include bilateral sclerosis of the mammillary bodies (Benson 1978) and punctate lesions of the gray nuclei in the periventricular regions of the third and fourth ventricles and the sylvian aqueduct (Victor et al. 1989).

Transient global amnesia.   Transient global amnesia (TGA) is a form of amnestic disorder characterized by an abrupt episode of profound anterograde amnesia and a variable inability to recall events that occur during the episode. These episodes typically last for only a few minutes or hours, ending with a rapid, spontaneous restoration of intact cognitive function. Mean duration of the amnestic period is 4.2 hours; periods greater than 12 hours are exceptional. The patient's level of consciousness and orientation to self are unaffected during the episode (Shuping et al. 1980). Patients are often bewildered and confused during the episodes and may ask repeated questions about their circumstances. The etiology is unclear, but most experts believe that it is associated with cerebrovascular disease and episodic vascular insufficiency of the mesial temporal lobe. Other etiologies of TGA, including brain tumors, cardiac arrhythmias, migraine, thyroid disorders, general anesthesia, sexual intercourse, polycythemia vera, epilepsy, and myxomatous mitral valvular disease, have also been reported (Hodges and Warlow 1990a; Pai and Yang 1999). TGA generally has a good prognosis, with only 8% of patients experiencing a second episode (Hodges and Warlow 1990b).

Benzodiazepine persisting amnestic disorder. Several medications have been associated with amnestic syndromes, with benzodiazepines receiving the most attention. Benzodiazepines can cause anterograde amnesia and may interfere with memory consolidation and retrieval. Risk factors include high dosage, intravenous administration, and use of high-potency, short-half-life agents such as triazolam (Scharf et al. 1987). These effects may be enhanced by the concurrent use of alcohol (Linnoila 1990). The resulting memory impairment is not associated with the degree of sedation or psychomotor impairment (Roache and Griffiths 1985). Amnestic sleep-related eating disorders can be seen, with transient amnesia for nocturnal eating (Morgenthaler and Silber 2002).

Differential Diagnosis

Memory deficits seen in amnestic syndromes are frequently a feature of delirium and dementia. In delirium, the memory disturbance is accompanied by a disturbed level of consciousness and usually fluctuates with time. More pervasive signs of cerebral dysfunction, such as difficulty focusing or sustaining attention, are present. In dementia, memory impairment is accompanied by additional cognitive impairments such as aphasia, apraxia, agnosia, and disturbances in executive functioning.

In dissociative or psychogenic forms of amnesia, the memory loss usually does not involve deficits in learning and recalling new information. Patients typically present with a circumscribed inability to recall previously learned and personal information, often regarding the patient's own identity or a traumatic or stressful event. These deficits persist even as the patient continues to function normally in the present. Patients with malingering or factitious disorders can present with amnestic symptoms that also fit the profile for dissociative amnesia. Systematic memory testing of these patients will often yield inconsistent results.

Treatment

As in delirium and dementia, the primary goal of treatment in amnestic disorders is to identify and treat the underlying cause or pathological process. There are no definitively effective treatments for amnestic disorder that are specifically aimed at reversing apparent memory deficits. Fortunately, these deficits are often temporary—as in transient amnestic syndromes—or are partially or completely reversible—as in head trauma, thiamine deficiency, or anoxia. Acute management should include continuous reorientation of the patient by means of verbal redirection, clocks, calendars, and familiar stimuli. Individual supportive psychotherapy for the patient, and family counseling to assist and educate caregivers, is also helpful. Chronic reversible amnestic syndromes may be managed with cognitive rehabilitation and therapeutic milieus intended to promote recovery from brain injury. More severe and permanent deficits may require supervised living environments to ensure appropriate care.

Mild Cognitive Impairment

Mild cognitive impairment (MCI) is a clinical syndrome defined as cognitive decline that is greater than expected for a patient's age and education level but that does not interfere with normal functioning. Prevalence in population-based epidemiological studies ranges from 3% to 19% in adults older than 65 years (Gauthier et al. 2006; G.W. Ross and Bowen 2002). Some patients with MCI remain stable or return to normal over time, but more than half progress to dementia within 5 years. The amnestic subtype in particular has a high probability of progressing to DAT (Ganguli et al. 2004) and could constitute a prodromal stage of this disorder, although the multiple-domain subtype has higher sensitivity for both DAT and VaD

(Rasquin et al. 2005). The rate of progression to DAT may be predicted by the severity of memory impairment at baseline, the severity of hippocampal atrophy, and the presence of an ε4 allele of the *APOE* gene (Geda et al. 2006). Comorbid depression with MCI more than doubles the risk of developing DAT, and patients with a poor response to antidepressants appear to be at an even greater risk (Modrego and Ferrandez 2004).

Postconcussion Syndrome

Postconcussion syndrome (PCS) is defined as a condition arising from traumatic brain injury that produces deficits in three areas of CNS function: somatic, psychological, and cognitive. The most common somatic symptom is headache, but fatigue, dizziness, blurred vision, and photophobia can also occur. Psychological symptoms include anxiety, depression, apathy, and emotional lability. Cognitive symptoms include decreased concentration, decreased verbal fluency, and impairments in working memory. The American Psychiatric Association's current criteria for postconcussional disorder (PCD), a similar diagnosis in Appendix B of DSM-IV-TR, require that there be an "acquired impairment in cognitive functioning, accompanied by specific neurobehavioral symptoms, that occurs as a consequence of closed head injury of sufficient severity to produce a significant cerebral concussion" (American Psychiatric Association 2000, p. 760). The most important differential diagnosis is usually malingering, and several psychiatric and neurological tests are available to assist the clinician. The Halstead-Reitan battery is reported to be 93.8% reliable in detecting patients who are intentionally trying to fake cognitive symptoms of head trauma (Mittenberg et al. 1996). Additional psychological testing that can be helpful includes the Minnesota Multiphasic Personality Inventory–2, the Dissimulation Scale, the Ego Strength Scale, and the Fake Bad Scale (Hall et al. 2005).

Neuropathological features of PCS probably relate to the primary pathological injury seen in brain trauma with axonal shearing and tensile strain damage to neurons due to rotational acceleration forces. Clinically significant concussions usually produce no detectable findings on neuroimaging because of the diffuse nature of the damage. Most symptoms of PCS resolve within 1 month, with only 7%–15% of patients having persistent symptoms after 1 year (McHugh et al. 2006). Risk factors for persistent PCS symptoms include female gender, age greater than 40 years, history of alcohol abuse, prior head injury, and significant comorbid medical or psychiatric illness (Ryan and Warden 2003). Treatment of PCS should be conservative, with education about PCS symptoms and positive prognoses associated with good outcomes (Corrigan et al. 2003).

Conclusion

The cognitive disorders represent a heterogeneous group of clinical syndromes that can generate incalculable agony from the threatened and often realized loss of a highly prized portion of our personhood: the capacity to think and remember. Psychiatrists need to be mindful of the broad differential diagnosis of patients presenting with cognitive impairment. It is advised that care of these patients be firmly grounded in the biopsychosocial-spiritual model; thorough history taking; directed mental status examinations; rational use of laboratory tests, electroencephalography, and neuroimaging; and comprehensive interventions. A commitment to remain current in the rapidly evolving knowledge base for the cognitive disorders is necessary to competently employ psychopharmacological and behavioral interventions. Tremendous and exciting research advances continue to build momentum and will yield improved options for the diagnosis, treatment, and prevention of cognitive impairment.

Key Points

Delirium

- Delirium is an acute brain disorder manifested by a syndromal array of neuropsychiatric symptoms.
- Delirium is epidemic among hospitalized patients, especially in the elderly.
- Numerous and widely varying precipitants can activate delirium in vulnerable patients.
- Delirium likely exerts an independent mortality risk for select populations and serves as a "medical alarm" for many others.
- Delirium can resolve completely, resolve gradually, or lead to a permanent cognitive disorder.
- The fundamental goal of treating delirium is to prevent and reverse delirium and thus mitigate associated morbidity and mortality risks.

Dementia

- Dementia is characterized by amnesia and one or more other impairment(s) in cognition.
- Cortical dementias feature notable aphasia, apraxia, agnosia, and visuospatial deficits plus amnesia that is not helped by cueing, whereas subcortical dementias feature apathy, affective lability, depressed mood, bradyphrenia, and decreased attention/concentration plus amnesia that is helped by cueing.
- Compared with dementia of the Alzheimer's type, frontotemporal dementia is characterized by executive dysfunction, disinhibition, attentional deficits, and personality changes with relatively preserved memory and visuospatial function.
- Lewy body dementia and Lewy body variant of Alzheimer's disease are characterized by fluctuations in mental status, well-formed visual hallucinations, delusions, depression, apathy, anxiety, extrapyramidal symptoms, and neuroleptic sensitivity.
- Neuroimaging is a routine expectation in the workup of dementia.

Amnestic and Other Cognitive Disorders

- Amnestic disorders are characterized by an inability to learn and recall new information (anterograde amnesia) or an inability to recall previously learned information (retrograde amnesia).
- Common causes of amnestic disorder include head injury, transient global amnesia, and benzodiazepines.
- Mild cognitive impairment (MCI) is defined as cognitive decline greater than expected for a patient's age and education level but without the deficits in normal functioning associated with dementia.
- MCI is a risk state for dementia, with more than half of patients with the amnestic subtype of MCI progressing to dementia within 5 years.
- Postconcussion syndrome is a constellation of somatic, psychological, and cognitive symptoms resulting from head trauma that usually resolve within 1 month, although persistent symptoms may continue for 1 year in 7%–15% of patients.

Suggested Readings

American Psychiatric Association: Practice guideline for the treatment of patients with Alzheimer's disease and other dementias of late life. Am J Psychiatry 154 (suppl): 1–39, 1997

American Psychiatric Association: Practice guideline for the treatment of patients with delirium. Am J Psychiatry 156 (suppl):1–20, 1999

Barber R, Ballard C, McKeith IG, et al: MRI volumetric study of dementia with Lewy bodies: a comparison with AD and vascular dementia. Neurology 54:1304–1309, 2000

Blesa R, Davidson M, Kurz A, et al: Galantamine provides sustained benefits in patients with "advanced moderate" Alzheimer's disease for at least 12 months. Dement Geriatr Cogn Disord 15:78–87, 2003

Bookheimer SY, Strojwas MH, Cohen MS, et al: Patterns of brain activation in people at risk for Alzheimer's disease. N Engl J Med 343:450–456, 2000

Brodaty H, Ames D, Snowdon J, et al: A randomized placebo-controlled trial of risperidone for the treatment of aggression, agitation, and psychosis of dementia. J Clin Psychiatry 64:134–143, 2003

Fontaine CS, Hynan LS, Koch K, et al: A double-blind comparison on olanzapine versus risperidone in the acute treatment of dementia-related behavioral disturbances in extended care facilities. J Clin Psychiatry 64:726–730, 2003

Fricchione G, Nejad S, Esses J, et al: Postoperative delirium. Am J Psychiatry 165:803–812, 2008

Grigoletto F, Zappala G, Anderson DW, et al: Norms for the Mini-Mental State Examination in a healthy population. Neurology 53:315–320, 1999

Folstein MF (ed): The Neurobiology of Primary Dementia. Washington, DC, American Psychiatric Publishing, 2005

ICU Delirium and Cognitive Impairment Study Group (http://www.icudelirium.org)

Kashima H, Kato M, Yoshimasu H, et al: Current trends in cognitive rehabilitation for memory disorders. Keio J Med 48:79–86, 1999

Levenson JL (ed): American Psychiatric Publishing Textbook of Psychosomatic Medicine. Washington, DC, American Psychiatric Publishing, 2005

Levy ML, Cummings JL, Fairbanks LA, et al: Longitudinal assessment of symptoms of depression, agitation, and psychosis in 181 patients with Alzheimer's disease. Am J Psychiatry 153:1438–1443, 1996

Nadler JD, Relkin NR, Cohen MS, et al: Mental status testing in the elderly nursing home population. J Geriatr Psychiatry Neurol 8:177–183, 1995

Olichney JM, Galasko D, Salmon DO, et al: Cognitive decline is faster in Lewy body variant than in Alzheimer's disease. Neurology 51:351–357, 1998

Paulsen JS, Salmon DP, Monsch AU, et al: Discrimination of cortical from subcortical dementias on the basis of memory and problem-solving tests. J Clin Psychol 51:48–58, 1995

Paulsen JS, Salmon DP, Thal LJ, et al: Incidence of and risk factors for hallucinations and delusions in patients with probable AD. Neurology 54:1965–1971, 2000

Perry RJ, Hodges JR: Differentiating frontal and temporal variant frontotemporal dementia from Alzheimer's disease. Neurology 54: 2277–2284, 2000

Pollock BG, Mulsant BH, Rosen J, et al: Comparison of citalopram, perphenazine, and placebo for the acute treatment of psychosis and behavioral disturbances in hospitalized, demented patients. Am J Psychiatry 159:460–465, 2002

Porter RJ, Lunn BS, Walker LLM, et al: Cognitive deficit induced by acute tryptophan depletion in patients with Alzheimer's disease. Am J Psychiatry 157:638–640, 2000

Rabinowitz J, Katz IR, De Deyn PP, et al: Behavioral and psychological symptoms in patients with dementia as a target for pharmacotherapy with risperidone. J Clin Psychiatry 65:1329–1334, 2004

Rainer MK, Masching AJ, Ertl MG, et al: Effect of risperidone on behavioral and psychological symptoms and cognitive function in dementia. J Clin Psychiatry 62:894–900, 2001

Starkstein SE, Petracca G, Chemerinski E, et al: Syndromic validity of apathy in Alzheimer's disease. Am J Psychiatry 158:872–877, 2001

Tariot PN, Erb R, Podgorski CA, et al: Efficacy and tolerability of carbamazepine for agitation and aggression in dementia. Am J Psychiatry 155:54–61, 1998

Tariot PN, Solomon PR, Morris JC, et al: A 5-month, randomized, placebo-controlled trial of galantamine in AD. Neurology 54:2269–2276, 2000

Terao T, Shimomura T, Izumi Y, et al: Two cases of quetiapine augmentation for donepezil-refractory visual hallucinations in dementia with Lewy bodies. J Clin Psychiatry 64:1520–1521, 2003

Terry RD, Katzman R, Bick KL, et al (eds): Alzheimer Disease, 2nd Edition. Philadelphia, PA, Lippincott Williams & Wilkins, 1999

Tschanz JT, Welsh-Bohmer KA, Skoog I, et al: Dementia diagnosis from clinical and neuropsychological data compared: the Cache County study. Neurology 54:1290–1296, 2000

Yudofsky SC, Hales RE (eds): American Psychiatric Publishing Textbook of Neuropsychiatry and Clinical Neurosciences, 4th Edition. Washington, DC, American Psychiatric Publishing, 2002

References

Aalten P, de Vugt ME, Lousberg R, et al: Behavioral problems in dementia: a factor analysis of the Neuropsychiatric Inventory. Dement Geriatr Cogn Disord 15:99–105, 2003

Aarsland D, Perry R, Larsen JP, et al: Neuroleptic sensitivity in Parkinson's disease and parkinsonian dementias. J Clin Psychiatry 66:633–637, 2005

Adamis D, Treloar A, Martin FC, et al: Recovery and outcome of delirium in elderly medical inpatients. Arch Gerontol Geriatr 43:289–298, 2006

Alagiakrishnan K, McCracken P, Feldman H: Treating vascular risk factors and maintaining vascular health: is this the way towards successful cognitive ageing and preventing cognitive decline? Postgrad Med J 82:101–105, 2006

Alexopoulos GS, Silver JM, Kahn DA, et al: Treatment of Agitation in Older Patients With Dementia: A Postgraduate Medicine Special Report. Minneapolis, MN, McGraw-Hill, 1998, pp 1–88

American Psychiatric Association: Practice guideline for the treatment of patients with delirium. Am J Psychiatry 156 (suppl):1–20, 1999

American Psychiatric Association: Diagnostic and Statistical Manual of Mental Disorders, 4th Edition, Text Revision. Washington, DC, American Psychiatric Association, 2000

Andrew MK, Freter SH, Rockwood K: Incomplete functional recovery after delirium in elderly people: a prospective cohort study. BMC Geriatr 5:1471–1423, 2005

Applebaum PS, Bonnie RJ, Karlawish JH: The capacity to vote of persons with Alzheimer's disease. Am J Psychiatry 162:2094–2100, 2005

Ballard CG, O'Brien JT, Swann AG, et al: The natural history of psychosis and depression in dementia with Lewy bodies and Alzheimer's disease: persistence and new cases over 1 year of follow-up. J Clin Psychiatry 62:46–49, 2001

Baskys A: Lewy body dementia: the litmus test for neuroleptic sensitivity and extrapyramidal symptoms. J Clin Psychiatry 65 (suppl):16–22, 2004

Bayindir O, Akpinar B, Can E, et al: The use of the 5-HT3-receptor antagonist ondansetron for the treatment of postcardiotomy delirium. J Cardiothorac Vasc Anesth 14:288–292, 2000

Bellelli G, Trabucchi M: Outcomes of older people admitted to postacute facilities with delirium. J Am Geriatr Soc 54:380–381, 2006

Benson DF: Amnesia. South Med J 71:1221–1227, 1231, 1978

Berger A-K, Fratiglioni L, Frosell Y, et al: The occurrence of depressive symptoms in the preclinical phase of AD: a population-based study. Neurology 53:1998–2002, 1999

Blennow K, de Leon MJ, Zetterberg H: Alzheimer's disease. Lancet 368:387–403, 2006

Boeve BF: A review of the non-Alzheimer dementias. J Clin Psychiatry 67:1983–2001, 2006

Bonner LT, Peskind ER: Pharmacological treatments of dementia. Med Clin North Am 86:657–674, 2002

Bottino CM, Almeida OP: Can neuroimaging techniques identify individuals at risk of developing Alzheimer's disease? Int Psychogeriatr 9:389–403, 1997

Bourdel-Marchasson I, Vincent S, Germain C, et al: Delirium symptoms and low dietary intake in older patients are independent predictors of institutionalization: a 1-year prospective population-based study. J Gerontol A Biol Sci Med Sci 59A:350–354, 2004

Bourgeois JA, Koike AK, Simmons JE, et al: Adjunctive valproic acid for delirium and/or agitation on a consultation-liaison service: a report of six cases. J Neuropsychiatry Clin Neurosci 17:232–238, 2005

Breitbart W, Marotta R, Platt MM, et al: A double-blind trial of haloperidol, chlorpromazine, and lorazepam in the treatment of delirium in hospitalized AIDS patients. Am J Psychiatry 153:231–237, 1996

Breitbart W, Rosenfeld B, Roth A, et al: The Memorial Delirium Assessment Scale. J Pain Symptom Manage 13:128–137, 1997

Breitbart W, Gibson C, Tremblay A: The delirium experience: delirium recall and delirium-related distress in hospitalized patients with cancer, their spouses/caregivers, and their nurses. Psychosomatics 43:183–194, 2002

Brown TM, Stoudemire A: Psychiatric Side Effects of Prescription and Over-the-Counter Medications. Washington, DC, American Psychiatric Press, 1998

Brunberg JA, Jacquemont S, Hagerman RJ, et al: Fragile X permutation carriers: characteristic MR imaging findings of adult male patients with progressive cerebellar and cognitive dysfunction. Am J Neuroradiol 23:1757–1766, 2002

Cameron DJ, Thomas RI, Mulvihill M, et al: Delirium: a test of the Diagnostic and Statistical Manual III criteria on medical inpatients. J Am Geriatr Soc 35:1007–1010, 1987

Carson S, McDonagh MS, Peterson K: A systematic review of the efficacy and safety of atypical antipsychotics in patients with psychological and behavioral symptoms of dementia. J Am Geriatr Soc 54:354–361, 2006

Caselli RJ, Graff-Radford NR, Reiman EM, et al: Preclinical memory decline in cognitively normal apolipoprotein E-epsilon4 homozygotes. Neurology 53:201–207, 1999

Cassem NH, Sos J: Intravenous use of haloperidol for acute delirium in intensive care settings. Paper presented at the 131st Annual Meeting of the American Psychiatric Association, Washington, DC, May 1978

Chapman FM, Dickinson J, McKeith I, et al: Association among visual hallucinations, visual acuity, and specific eye pathologies in Alzheimer's disease: treatment implications. Am J Psychiatry 156:1983–1985, 1999

Choi SH, Na DL, Chung CS, et al: Diffusion-weighted MRI in vascular dementia. Neurology 54:83–89, 2000

Class CA, Schneider L, Farlow MR: Optimal management of behavioural disorders associated with dementia. Drugs Aging 10:95–106, 1997

Cohen MAA, Jacobson JM: Maximizing life's potential in AIDS: a psychopharmacological update. Gen Hosp Psychiatry 22:375–388, 2000

Cole MG, Primeau FJ: Prognosis of delirium in elderly hospital patients. Can Med Assoc J 149:41–46, 1993

Corrigan JD, Wolfe M, Mysiw WF, et al: Early identification of mild traumatic brain injury in female victims of domestic violence. Am J Obstet Gynecol 188:71–76, 2003

Craft S, Teri L, Edland SD, et al: Accelerated decline in apolipoprotein E-epsilon 4 homozygotes with Alzheimer's disease. Neurology 51:149–153, 1998

Cummings JL, Masterman DL: Assessment of treatment-associated changes in behavior and cholinergic therapy of neuropsychiatric symptoms in Alzheimer's disease. J Clin Psychiatry 59 (suppl 13):23–30, 1998

Cummings JL, Vinters HV, Cole GM, et al: Alzheimer's disease: etiologies, pathophysiology, cognitive reserve, and treatment opportunities. Neurology 51 (1 suppl 1): S2–S17; discussion S65–S67, 1998

Curb JD, Rodriguez BL, Abbott RD, et al: Longitudinal association of vascular and Alzheimer's dementias, diabetes, and glucose tolerance. Neurology 52:971–975, 1999

Daniel DG: Antipsychotic treatment of psychosis and agitation in the elderly. J Clin Psychiatry 61 (suppl 14):49–52, 2000

d'Arminio Monforte A, Duca PG, Vago L, et al: Decreasing incidence of CNS AIDS-defining events associated with antiretroviral therapy. Neurology 54:1856–1859, 2000

de Koning I, van Kooten F, Dippel DW, et al: The CAMCOG: a useful screening instrument for dementia in stroke patients. Stroke 29:2080–2086, 1998

Desmond DW, Moroney JT, Paik MC, et al: Frequency and clinical determinants of dementia after ischemic stroke. Neurology 54:1124–1131, 2000

Doody RS, Massman PJ, Mawad M, et al: Cognitive consequences of subcortical magnetic resonance imaging changes in Alzheimer's disease: comparison to small-vessel ischemic vascular dementia. Neuropsychiatry Neuropsychol Behav Neurol 11:191–199, 1998

Doraiswamy PM, Steffens DC, Pitchumoni S, et al: Early recognition of Alzheimer's disease: What is consensual? What is controversial? What is practical? J Clin Psychiatry 59 (suppl):6–18, 1998

Duara R, Barker W, Luis CA: Frontotemporal dementia and Alzheimer's disease: differential diagnosis. Dement Geriatr Cogn Disord 10 (suppl):37–42, 1999

Dubinsky RM, Stein AC, Lyons K: Practice parameter: risk of driving and Alzheimer's disease (an evidence-based review). Neurology 54:2205–2211, 2000

Dufouil C, Clayton D, Brayne C, et al: Population norms for the MMSE in the very old: estimates based on longitudinal data. Mini-Mental State Examination. Neurology 55:1609–1613, 2000

Dunn NR, Alfonso CA, Young RA, et al: Creutzfeldt-Jakob disease appearing as paranoid psychosis. Am J Psychiatry 156:2016–2017, 1999

Dyer CB, Ashton CM, Teasdale TA: Postoperative delirium: a review of 80 primary data-collection studies. Arch Intern Med 155:461–465, 1995

Edelstein DM, Aharonoff GB, Karp A, et al: Effect of postoperative delirium on outcome after hip fracture. Clin Orthop Relat Res 1:195–200, 2004

Elie M, Cole MG, Primeau FJ, et al: Delirium risk factors in elderly hospitalized patients. J Gen Intern Med 13:204–212, 1998

Ely EW, Shintani A, Truman B, et al: Delirium as a predictor of mortality in mechanically ventilated patients in the intensive care unit. JAMA 291:1753–1762, 2004a

Ely EW, Stephens RK, Jackson JC, et al: Current opinions regarding the importance, diagnosis, and management of delirium in the intensive care unit: a survey of 912 healthcare professionals. Crit Care Med 32:106–112, 2004b

Engel GL, Romano J: Delirium: a syndrome of cerebral insufficiency. J Chronic Dis 9:260–277, 1959

Fayers PM, Hjermstad MJ, Ranhoff AH, et al: Which Mini-Mental State Exam items can be used to screen for delirium and cognitive impairment? J Pain Symptom Manage 30:41–50, 2005

Felician O, Sandson TA: The neurobiology and pharmacotherapy of Alzheimer's disease. J Neuropsychiatry Clin Neurosci 11:19–31, 1999

Fodale V, Santamaria LB: Drugs of anesthesia, central nicotinic receptors and postoperative cognitive dysfunction. Acta Anaesthesiol Scand 47:1180–1182, 2003

Folstein MF, Folstein SE, McHugh PR: "Mini-Mental State": a practical method for grading the cognitive state of patients for the clinician. J Psychiatr Res 12:189–198, 1975

Francis J, Kapoor WN: Prognosis after hospital discharge of older medical patients with delirium. J Am Geriatr Soc 40:601–606, 1992

Ganguli M, Dodge HH, Shen C, et al: Mild cognitive impairment, amnestic type: an epidemiologic study. Neurology 63:115–121, 2004

Gaudreau JD, Gagnon P: Psychogenic drugs and delirium pathogenesis: the central role of the thalamus. Med Hypotheses 64:471–475, 2005

Gaudreau JD, Gagnon P, Harel F, et al: Fast, systematic, and continuous delirium assessment in hospitalized patients: the nursing delirium screening scale. J Pain Symptom Manage 29:368–375, 2005

Gauthier S, Reisberg B, Zaudig M, et al: Mild cognitive impairment. Lancet 367:1262–1270, 2006

Geda YE, Knopman DS, Mrazek DA, et al: Depression, apolipoprotein E genotype, and the incidence of mild cognitive impairment: a prospective cohort study. Arch Neurol 63:435–440, 2006

Geerlings MI, Jonker C, Bouter LM, et al: Association between memory complaints and incident Alzheimer's disease in elderly people with normal baseline cognition. Am J Psychiatry 156:531–537, 1999

Geldmacher DS, Whitehouse PJ Jr: Differential diagnosis of Alzheimer's disease. Neurology 48 (5 suppl 6):S2–S9, 1997

Gendelman HE, Zheng J, Coulter CL, et al: Suppression of inflammatory neurotoxins by highly active antiretroviral therapy in human immunodeficiency virus–associated dementia. J Infect Dis 178:1000–1007, 1998

Gliatto MF, Caroff SN: Neurosyphilis: a history and clinical review. Psychiatr Ann 31:153–161, 2001

Goldman WP, Baty JD, Buckles VD, et al: Motor dysfunction in mildly demented AD individuals without extrapyramidal signs. Neurology 53:956–962, 1999

Gomez-Isla T, Growdon WB, McNamara M, et al: Clinicopathological correlates in temporal cortex in dementia with Lewy bodies. Neurology 53:2003–2009, 1999

Goodkin K, Baldewicz TT, Wilkie FL, et al: Cognitive-motor impairment and disorder in HIV-1 infection. Psychiatr Ann 31:37–44, 2001

Grossberg GT, Lake JT: The role of the psychiatrist in Alzheimer's disease. J Clin Psychiatry 59 (suppl 9):3–6, 1998

Gury C, Canceil O, Iaria P: Antipsychotic drugs and cardiovascular safety: current studies of prolonged QT interval and risk of ventricular arrhythmia (abstract). Encephale 26:62–72, 2000

Hall R, Hall R, Chapman M: Definition, diagnosis, and forensic implications of postconcussional syndrome. Psychosomatics 46:195–202, 2005

Hamilton M: A rating scale for depression. J Neurol Neurosurg Psychiatry 23:51–56, 1960

Han CS, Kim YK: A double-blind trial of risperidone and haloperidol for the treatment of delirium. Psychosomatics 45:297–301, 2004

Han L, McCusker J, Cole, M, et al: Use of medications with anticholinergic effect predicts clinical severity of delirium symptoms in older medical inpatients. Arch Intern Med 161:1099–1105, 2001

Harhangi BS, de Rijk MC, van Duijn CM, et al: APOE and the risk of PD with or without dementia in a population-based study. Neurology 54:1272–1276, 2000

Haroutunian V, Perl DP, Purohit DP, et al: Regional distribution of neuritic plaques in the nondemented elderly and subjects with very mild Alzheimer disease. Arch Neurol 55:1185–1191, 1998

Harper C, Fornes P, Duyckaerts C, et al: An international perspective on the prevalence of the Wernicke-Korsakoff syndrome. Metab Brain Dis 10:17–24, 1995

Hashimoto M, Kazui H, Matsumoto K, et al: Does donepezil treatment slow the progression of hippocampal atrophy in patients with Alzheimer's disease? Am J Psychiatry 162:676–682, 2005

Herrmann N, Mamdani M, Lanctot: Atypical antipsychotics and risk of cerebrovascular accidents. Am J Psychiatry 161:1113–1115, 2004

Heyman A, Fillenbaum GG, Gearing M, et al: Comparison of Lewy body variant of Alzheimer's disease with pure Alzheimer's disease. Neurology 52:1839–1844, 1999

Hodges JR, Warlow CP: Syndromes of transient global amnesia: towards a classification. A study of 153 cases. J Neurol Neurosurg Psychiatry 53:834–843, 1990a

Hodges JR, Warlow CP: The aetiology of transient global amnesia. A case-control study of 114 cases with prospective follow-up. Brain 113 (pt 3):639–657, 1990b

Hu H, Deng W, Yang H: A prospective random control study comparison of olanzapine and haloperidol in senile delirium. Journal of Chongqing Medical University 8:1234–1237, 2004

Hughes TA, Ross HF, Musa S, et al: A 10-year study of the incidence of and factors predicting dementia in Parkinson's disease. Neurology 54:1596–1602, 2000

Hurtig HI, Trojanowski JQ, Galvin J, et al: Alpha-synuclein cortical Lewy bodies correlate with dementia in Parkinson's disease. Neurology 54:1916–1921, 2000

Hy LX, Keller DM: Prevalence of AD among whites: a summary by levels of severity. Neurology 55:198–204, 2000

Ichikawa J, Dai J, O'Laughlin IA, et al: Atypical, but not typical, antipsychotic drugs increase cortical acetylcholine release without an effect in the nucleus accumbens or striatum. Neuropsychopharmacology 26:325–339, 2002

Ichikawa J, Chung YC, Dai J, et al: Valproic acid potentiates both typical and atypical antipsychotic-induced prefrontal cortical dopamine release. Brain Res 1052:56–62, 2005

Inouye SK: Current concepts: delirium in older persons. N Engl J Med 354:1157–1165, 2006

Inouye SK, Charpentier PA: Precipitating factors for delirium in hospitalized elderly persons: predictive model and interrelationship with baseline vulnerability. JAMA 275:852–857, 1996

Inouye SK, VanDyck CH, Alessi CA, et al: Clarifying confusion: the confusion assessment method: a new method for detection of delirium. Ann Intern Med 113:941–948, 1990

Inouye SK, Rushing JT, Foreman MD, et al: Does delirium contribute to poor hospital outcomes? A three-site epidemiologic study. J Gen Intern Med 13:234–242, 1998

Inouye SK, Bogardus ST, Charpentier PA, et al: A multicomponent intervention to prevent delirium in hospitalized older patients. N Engl J Med 340:669–676, 1999

Inouye SK, Foreman MD, Mikon LC, et al: Nurses' recognition of delirium and its symptoms: comparison of nurse and researcher ratings. Arch Intern Med 161:2467–2473, 2001

Jack CR, Petersen RC, Xu YC, et al: Prediction of AD with MRI-based hippocampal volume in mild cognitive impairment. Neurology 54:1397–1403, 2000

Jacquemont S, Hagerman RJ, Leehy, M, et al: Fragile X permutation tremor/ataxia syndrome: molecular, clinical, and neuroimaging correlates. Am J Hum Genet 72:869–878, 2003

Jellinger KA: Structural basis of dementia in neurodegenerative disorders. J Neural Transm 47 (suppl):1–29, 1996

Jones C, Griffiths R, Humphris G: Disturbed memory and amnesia related to intensive care. Memory 8:79–94, 2000

Jorm AF, Jolley D: The incidence of dementia: a meta-analysis. Neurology 51:728–733, 1998

Katz IR: Diagnosis and treatment of depression in patients with Alzheimer's disease and other dementias. J Clin Psychiatry 59 (suppl 9):38–44, 1998

Kelly KG, Zisselman M, Cutillo-Schmitter T, et al: Severity and course of delirium in medically hospitalized nursing facility residents. Am J Geriatr Psychiatry 9:72–77, 2001

Kennedy JS, Zager A, Bymaster F, et al: The central cholinergic system profile of olanzapine compared with placebo in Alzheimer's disease. Int J Geriatr Psychiatry 16:S24–S32, 2001

Kertesz A, Munoz DG: Frontotemporal dementia. Med Clin North Am 86:501–518, 2002

Keys MA, DeWald C: Clinical perspective on choice of atypical antipsychotics in elderly patients with dementia, part I. Annals of Long-Term Care: Clinical Care and Aging 13(2):26–32, 2005a

Keys MA, DeWald C: Clinical perspective on choice of atypical antipsychotics in elderly patients with dementia, part II. Annals of Long-Term Care: Clinical Care and Aging 13(3):30–38, 2005b

Kiely DK, Bergmann MA, Jones RN, et al: Characteristics associated with delirium persistence among newly admitted post-acute facility patients. J Gerontol A Biol Sci Med Sci 59A:344–349, 2004

Kopelman MD: The Korsakoff syndrome. Br J Psychiatry 166:154–173, 1995

Koponen H, Partanen J, Paakkonen A, et al: EEG spectral analysis in delirium. J Neurol Neurosurg Psychiatry 52:980–985, 1989a

Koponen H, Stenback U, Mattila E, et al: Delirium among elderly persons admitted to a psychiatric hospital: clinical course during the acute stage and one-year follow-up. Acta Psychiatr Scand 79:579–585, 1989b

Krishnan KRR, Charles HC, Doraiswamy PM, et al: Randomized, placebo-controlled trial of the effects of donepezil on neural markers and hippocampal volumes in Alzheimer's disease. Am J Psychiatry 160:2003–2011, 2003

Langa KM, Foster NL, Larson EB: Mixed dementia: emerging concepts and therapeutic implications. JAMA 292:2901–2908, 2004

Lawlor BA: Behavioral and psychological symptoms in dementia: the role of atypical antipsychotics. J Clin Psychiatry 65 (suppl): 5–10, 2004

Leslie DL, Zhang Y, Bogardus ST, et al: Consequences of preventing delirium in hospitalized older adults on nursing home costs. J Am Geriatr Soc 53:405–409, 2005

Leverenz JB, McKeith: Dementia with Lewy bodies. Med Clin North Am 86:519–535, 2002

Levy ML, Cummings JL: Parkinson's disease, in Psychiatric Management in Neurological Disease. Edited by Lauterbach EC. Washington, DC, American Psychiatric Press, 2000, pp 41–70

Linnoila MI: Benzodiazepines and alcohol. J Psychiatr Res 24 (suppl):121–127, 1990

Liperoti R, Gambassi G, Lapane KL, et al: Cerebrovascular events among elderly nursing home patients treated with conventional or atypical antipsychotics. J Clin Psychiatry 66:1090–1096, 2005

Lipowski ZJ: Transient cognitive disorders (delirium, acute confusional states) in the elderly. Am J Psychiatry 140:1426–1436, 1983

Lipowski ZJ: Delirium (acute confusional states). JAMA 258:1789–1792, 1987

Liptzin B, Levkoff SE: An empirical study of delirium subtypes. Br J Psychiatry 161:843–845, 1992

Litvan I, McKee A: Clinicopathological case report. Dementia with Lewy bodies (DLB). J Neuropsychiatry Clin Neurosci 11:107–112, 1999

Livingston G, Johnston K, Katona C, et al: Systemic review of psychological approaches to the management of neuropsychiatric symptoms of dementia. Am J Psychiatry 162:1996–2021, 2005

Lonergan E, Britton A, Luxenberg J, et al: Antipsychotics for delirium. Cochrane Database Syst Rev (2):CD005594, 2007

Lopez OL, Hamilton RL, Becker JT, et al: Severity of cognitive impairment and the clinical diagnosis of AD with Lewy bodies. Neurology 54:1780–1787, 2000a

Lopez OL, Wisniewski S, Hamilton RL, et al: Predictors of progression in patients with AD and Lewy bodies. Neurology 54:1774–1779, 2000b

Lyketsos CG, Sheppard JM, Rabins PV: Dementia in elderly persons in a general hospital. Am J Psychiatry 157:704–707, 2000a

Lyketsos CG, Steinberg M, Schantz JT, et al: Mental and behavioral disturbances in dementia: findings from the Cache County Study on Memory in Aging. Am J Psychiatry 157:708–714, 2000b

Lyketsos CG, Lopez O, Jones B, et al: Prevalence of neuropsychiatric symptoms in dementia and mild cognitive impairment: results from the Cardiovascular Health Study. JAMA 288:1475–1483, 2002

Mace NL, Rabins PV: The 36-Hour Day: A Family Guide to Caring for Persons With Alzheimer's Disease, Related Dementing Illnesses, and Memory Loss in Later Life. Baltimore, MD, Johns Hopkins University Press, 1981

Maldonado JL, Fernandez F, Levy JK: Acquired immunodeficiency syndrome, in Psychiatric Management in Neurological Disease. Edited by Lauterbach EC. Washington, DC, American Psychiatric Press, 2000, pp 271–295

Maldonado JR, VanDerStarre PJ, Wysong A: Postoperative sedation and the incidence of ICU delirium in cardiac surgery patients. ASA Annual Meeting Abstracts. Anesthesiology 99:A465, 2003

Marcantonio ER, Flacker JM, Michaels M, et al: Delirium is independently associated with poor functional recovery after hip fracture. J Am Geriatr Soc 48:618–624, 2000

Marcantonio ER, Kiely DK, Simon SE, et al: Outcomes of older people admitted to post-acute facilities with delirium. J Am Geriatr Soc 53:963–969, 2005

Marsh L: Neuropsychiatric aspects of Parkinson's disease. Psychosomatics 41:15–23, 2000

McCusker J, Cole M, Dendukuri N, et al: Delirium in older medical inpatients and subsequent cognitive and functional status: a prospective study. Can Med Assoc J 165:575–583, 2001

McDaniel JS, Chung JY, Brown L, et al: Practice guideline for the treatment of patients with

HIV/AIDS. Work Group on HIV/AIDS. American Psychiatric Association. Am J Psychiatry 157 (suppl):1–62, 2000

McHugh T, Laforce R, Gallagher P, et al: Natural history of the long-term cognitive, affective and physical sequelae of mild traumatic brain injury. Brain Cogn 60:209–211, 2006

McKeith IG, Ballard CG, Perry RH, et al: Prospective validation on consensus criteria for the diagnosis of dementia with Lewy bodies. Neurology 54:1050–1058, 2000

Meltzer HY: Mechanism of action of atypical antipsychotic drugs, in Neuropsychopharmacology: The Fifth Generation of Progress. Edited by Davis KL, Charney D, Coyle JT, et al. Philadelphia, PA, Lippincott Williams & Wilkins, 2002, pp 819–831

Mendez MF, Chen AK, Shapiro JS, et al: Acquired extroversion with bitemporal variant of frontotemporal dementia. J Neuropsychiatry Clin Neurosci 18:100–107, 2006

Mercer B, Wepner W, Gardner H, et al: A study of confabulation. Arch Neurol 34:429–433, 1977

Meyer JS, Muramatsu K, Mortel KF, et al: Prospective CT confirms differences between vascular and Alzheimer's dementia. Stroke 26:735–742, 1995

Milbrandt E, Deppen S, Harrison P, et al: Costs associated with delirium in mechanically ventilated patients. Crit Care Med 32:955–962, 2004

Mintzer J, Greenspan A, Caers I, et al: Risperidone in the treatment of Alzheimer disease: results from a prospective clinical trial. Am J Geriatr Psychiatry 14:280–291, 2006

Mirenda J, Broyles G: Propofol as used for sedation in the ICU. Chest 108:539–548, 1995

Mittenberg W, Rotholc A, Russell E, et al: Identification of malingered head injury on the Halstead-Reitan battery. Arch Clin Neuropsychol 11:271–281, 1996

Moceri VM, Kukull WA, Emanuel I, et al: Early life risk factors and the development of Alzheimer's disease. Neurology 54:415–420, 2000

Modrego PJ, Ferrandez J: Depression in patients with mild cognitive impairment increases the risk of developing dementia of Alzheimer type: a prospective cohort study. Arch Neurol 61:1290–1293, 2004

Monette J, Galbaud du Fort G, Fung SH, et al: Evaluation of the Confusion Assessment Method (CAM) as a screening tool for delirium in the emergency room. Gen Hosp Psychiatry 23:20–25, 2001

Morgenthaler TI, Silber MH: Amnestic sleep-related eating disorder associated with zolpidem. Sleep Med 3:323–327, 2002

Morita T, Hirai K, Sakaguchi Y, et al: Family perceived distress from delirium-related symptoms of terminally ill cancer patients. Psychosomatics 45:107–113, 2004

Morita T, Takigawa C, Onishi H, et al: Opioid rotation from morphine to fentanyl in delirious cancer patients: an open-label trial. J Pain Symptom Manage 30:96–103, 2005

Munford RS, Tracey KJ: Is severe sepsis a neuroendocrine disease? Mol Med 8:437–442, 2002

Neary D, Snowden JS, Gustafson L, et al: Frontotemporal lobar degeneration: a consensus on clinical diagnostic criteria. Neurology 51:1546–1554, 1998

Obrist WD: Electroencephalographic changes in normal aging and dementia, in Brain Function in Old Age. Edited by Hoffmeister F, Mhuller C. New York, Springer-Verlag, 1979, pp 102–111

O'Keeffe ST, Lavan J: The prognostic significance of delirium in older hospital patients. J Am Geriatr Soc 45:174–178, 1997

O'Keeffe ST, Mulkerrin EC, Nayeem K, et al: Use of serial Mini-Mental Status Examinations to diagnose and monitor delirium in elderly hospital patients. J Am Geriatr Soc 53:867–870, 2005

Pai M, Yang S: Transient global amnesia: a retrospective study of 25 patients. Chin Med J 62:140–144, 1999

Pandharipande P, Jackson J, Ely EW: Delirium: acute cognitive dysfunction in the critically ill. Curr Opin Crit Care 11:360–368, 2005

Pandharipande P, Shintani A, Peterson J, et al: Lorazepam is an independent risk factor for transitioning to delirium in intensive care unit patients. Anesthesiology 104:21–26, 2006

Parada MA, Hernandez L, Puig de Parada M, et al: Selective action of acute systemic clozapine on acetylcholine release in the rat prefrontal cortex by reference to the nucleus accumbens and striatum. J Pharmacol Exp Ther 281:582–588, 1997

Parnetti L: Therapeutic options in dementia. J Neurol 247:163–168, 2000

Patterson CJS, Gauthier S, Bergman H, et al: The recognition, assessment, and management of dementing disorders: conclusions from the Canadian Consensus Conference on Dementia. Can Med Assoc J 160 (suppl): S1–S14, 1999

Paulsen JS, Butters N, Sadek JR, et al: Distinct cognitive profiles of cortical and subcortical dementia in advanced illness. Neurology 45:951–956, 1995

Peila R, White LR, Masaki K, et al: Reducing the risk of dementia: efficacy of long-term treatment of hypertension. Stroke 37:1165–1170, 2006

Peters N, Opherk C, Danek A, et al: The pattern of cognitive performance in CADASIL: a monogenic condition leading to subcortical ischemic vascular dementia. Am J Psychiatry 162:2078–2085, 2005

Petersen RC, Jack CR, Xu Y-C, et al: Memory and MRI-based hippocampal volumes in aging and AD. Neurology 54:581–587, 2000

Peterson JF, Pun BT, Dittus RS, et al: Delirium and its motoric subtypes: a study of 624 critically ill patients. J Am Geriatr Soc 54:479–484, 2006

Pitkala KH, Laurila JV, Strandberg TE, et al: Prognostic significance of delirium in frail elderly people. Dement Geriatr Cogn Disord 19:158–163, 2005

Platt MM, Breitbart W, Smith M, et al: Efficacy of neuroleptics for hypoactive delirium. J Neuropsychiatry 6:66, 1994

Pratico C, Quattrone D, Lucanto T, et al: Drugs of anesthesia acting on central cholinergic system may cause postoperative cognitive dysfunction and delirium. Med Hypotheses 65:972–982, 2005

Rabins PV: Alzheimer's disease management. J Clin Psychiatry 59 (suppl 13):36–38, 1998

Rabins PV, Blacker D, Bland A, et al: Practice guideline for the treatment of patients with Alzheimer's disease and other dementias of late life. American Psychiatric Association. Am J Psychiatry 154 (suppl):1–39, 1997

Ranen NG: Huntington's disease, in Psychiatric Management in Neurological Disease. Edited by Lauterbach EC. Washington, DC, American Psychiatric Press, 2000, pp 71–92

Rao V, Lyketsos CG: Delusions in Alzheimer's disease: a review. J Neuropsychiatry Clin Neurosci 10:373–382, 1998

Rasquin SM, Lodder J, Visser PJ, et al: Predictive accuracy of MCI subtypes for Alzheimer's disease and vascular dementia in subjects with mild cognitive impairment: a 2-year follow-up study. Dement Geriatr Cogn Disord 19:113–119, 2005

Rebeck GW, Hyman BT: Apolipoprotein and Alzheimer's disease, in Alzheimer's Disease, 2nd Edition. Edited by Terry RD, Katzman R, Bick KL, et al. Philadelphia, PA, Lippincott Williams & Wilkins, 1999, pp 339–346

Riker RR, Fraser GL, Cox PM: Continuous infusion of haloperidol controls agitation in critically ill patients. Crit Care Med 22:433–440, 1994

Rizzo M, Anderson SW, Dawson J, et al: Visual attention impairments in Alzheimer's disease. Neurology 54:1954–1959, 2000

Roache JD, Griffiths RR: Comparison of triazolam and pentobarbital: performance impairment, subjective effects, and abuse liability. J Pharmacol Exp Ther 234:120–133, 1985

Robinson RG: The Clinical Neuropsychiatry of Stroke: Cognitive, Behavioral, and Emotional Disorders Following Vascular Brain Injury. New York, Cambridge University Press, 1998

Rockwood K, Cosway S, Carver, D, et al: The risk of dementia and death after delirium. Age Ageing 28:551–556, 1999

Roman GC: Vascular dementia revisited: diagnosis, pathogenesis, treatment, and prevention. Med Clin North Am 86:3477–3499, 2002

Roman GC, Wilkinson DG, Doody RS, et al: Donepezil in vascular dementia: combined analysis of two large-scale clinical trials. Dement Geriatr Cogn Disord 20:338–344, 2005

Romano J, Engel GL: Delirium, part 1: electroencephalographic data. Arch Neurol Psychiatry 51:356–377, 1944

Ropacki SA, Jeste DV: Epidemiology of and risk factors for psychosis of Alzheimer's disease:

a review of 55 studies published from 1990 to 2003. Am J Psychiatry 162:2022–2030, 2005

Rosenblatt A, Leroi I: Neuropsychiatry of Huntington's disease and other basal ganglia disorders. Psychosomatics 41:24–30, 2000

Ross CA, Peyser CE, Shapiro I, et al: Delirium: phenomenological and etiologic subtypes. Int Psychogeriatr 3:135–147, 1991

Ross GW, Bowen JD: The diagnosis and differential diagnosis of dementia. Med Clin North Am 86:455–476, 2002

Ross GW, Petrovitch H, White LR, et al: Characterization of risk factors for vascular dementia: the Honolulu–Asia Aging Study. Neurology 53:337–343, 1999

Royall DR, Cordes JA, Polk M: CLOX: an executive clock drawing task. J Neurol Neurosurg Psychiatry 64:588–594, 1998

Ryan LM, Warden DL: Post concussion syndrome. Int Rev Psychiatry 15:310–316, 2003

Scharf MB, Saskin P, Fletcher K: Benzodiazepine-induced amnesia: clinical laboratory findings. J Clin Psychiatry Monogr 5:14–17, 1987

Schneider LS, Dagerman KS, Insel P: Risk of death with atypical antipsychotic drug treatment for dementia: meta-analysis of randomized placebo-controlled trials. JAMA 294:1934–1943, 2005

Schwid SR, Weinstein A, Wishart HA, et al: Multiple sclerosis, in Psychiatric Management in Neurological Disease. Edited by Lauterbach EC. Washington, DC, American Psychiatric Press, 2000, pp 249–270

Seaman J: Seeing catatonia (letter). J Neuropsychiatry Clin Neurosci 17:558–559, 2005

Serby M, Brickman AM, Haroutunian V: Cognitive burden and excess Lewy-body pathology in the Lewy-body variant of Alzheimer's disease. Am J Geriatr Psychiatry 11:371–374, 2003

Serrano-Duenas M, Bleda MJ: Delirium in Parkinson's patients: a five year follow-up study. Parkinsonism Relat Disord 11:387–392, 2005

Sharma ND, Rosman HS, Padhi D, et al: Torsades de pointes associated with intravenous haloperidol in critically ill patients. Am J Cardiol 81:238–240, 1998

Shukry M, Clyde MC, Kalarickal PL, et al: Does dexmedetomidine prevent emergence delirium in children after sevoflurance-based general anesthesia? Pediatr Anesth 15:1098–1104, 2005

Shuping JR, Rollinson RD, Toole JF: Transient global amnesia. Ann Neurol 7:281–285, 1980

Siddiqi N, Stockdale R, Britton AM: Interventions for preventing delirium in hospitalized patients. Cochrane Database Syst Rev (2): CD005563, 2007

Simard M, van Reekum R: The acetylcholinesterase inhibitors for treatment of cognitive and behavioral symptoms in dementia with Lewy bodies. J Neuropsychiatry Clin Neurosci 16:409–425, 2004

Sink KM, Holden KF, Yaffe K: Pharmacological treatment of neuropsychiatric symptoms on dementia: a review of the evidence. JAMA 293:596–608, 2005

Small GW: Differential diagnosis and early detection of dementia. Am J Geriatr Psychiatry 6 (2 suppl 1):S26–S33, 1998

Small GW, Leiter F: Neuroimaging for diagnosis of dementia. J Clin Psychiatry 59 (suppl 11):4–7, 1998

Small GW, Chen ST, Komo S, et al: Memory self-appraisal in middle-aged and older adults with the apolipoprotein E-4 allele. Am J Psychiatry 156:1035–1038, 1999

Smith CD, Snowdon DA, Wang H, et al: White matter volumes and periventricular white matter hyperintensities in aging and dementia. Neurology 54:838–842, 2000

Smits HA, Boven LA, Pereira CF, et al: Role of macrophage activation in the pathogenesis of Alzheimer's disease and human immunodeficiency virus type 1-associated dementia. Eur J Clin Invest 30:526–535, 2000

Starkstein SE, Jorge R, Mizrahi R, et al: The construct of minor and major depression in Alzheimer's disease. Am J Psychiatry 162:2086–2093, 2005

Stewart JT, Shin KJ: Paroxetine treatment of sexual disinhibition in dementia. Am J Psychiatry 154:1474, 1997

Stumita PM, Baroletti SA, Anger KE, et al: Sedation and analgesia in the intensive care unit: evaluating the role of dexmedetomidine. Am J Health Syst Pharm 64:37–44, 2007

Tager FA, Fallon BA: Psychiatric and cognitive features of Lyme disease. Psychiatr Ann 31:173–181, 2001

Tariot PN, Profenno LA, Ismail MS: Efficacy of atypical antipsychotics in elderly patients with dementia. J Clin Psychiatry 65 (suppl): 11–15, 2004

Thomason JW, Shintani A, Peterson JF, et al: Intensive care unit delirium is an independent predictor of longer hospital stays: a prospective analysis of 261 nonventilated patients. Crit Care 9:R375–R381, 2005

Titier K, Canal M, Deridet E, et al: Determination of myocardium to plasma concentration ratios of five antipsychotic drugs: comparison with their ability to induce arrhythmia and sudden death in clinical practice. Toxicol Appl Pharmacol 199:52–60, 2004

Tost H, Wendt CS, Schmitt A, et al: Huntington's disease: phenomenological diversity of a neuropsychiatric condition that challenges traditional concepts in neurology and psychiatry. Am J Psychiatry 161:28–34, 2004

Trinh N-H, Hoblyn J, Mohanty S, et al: Efficacy of cholinesterase inhibitors in the treatment of neuropsychiatric symptoms and functional impairment in Alzheimer disease: a meta-analysis. JAMA 289:210–216, 2003

Trzepacz PT, Maue FR, Coffman G, et al: Neuropsychiatric assessment of liver transplantation candidates: delirium and other psychiatric disorders. Int J Psychiatry Med 7:101–111, 1986

Trzepacz PT, Baker RW, Greenhouse J: A symptom rating scale for delirium. Psychiatry Res 23:89–97, 1988a

Trzepacz PT, Brenner RP, Coffman G, et al: Delirium in liver transplantation candidates: discriminant analysis of multiple test variables. Biol Psychiatry 24:3–14, 1988b

Trzepacz PT, Leavitt M, Congioli K: An animal model for delirium. Psychosomatics 33:404–414, 1992

Trzepacz PT, Mulsant BH, Amanda Dew M, et al: Is delirium different when it occurs in dementia? A study using the delirium rating scale. J Neuropsychiatry Clin Neurosci 10:199–204, 1998

Trzepacz PT, Mittal D, Torres R, et al: Validation of the Delirium Rating Scale–Revised–98: comparison with the delirium rating scale and cognitive test for delirium. J Neuropsychiatry Clin Neurosci 13:229–242, 2001

Tune LE, Folstein MF: Postoperative delirium. Adv Psychosom Med 15:51–68, 1986

Tune LE, Sunderland T: New cholinergic therapies: treatment tools for the psychiatrist. J Clin Psychiatry 59 (suppl 13):31–35, 1998

Tune LE, Carr S, Hoag E, et al: Anticholinergic effects of drugs commonly prescribed for the elderly: potential means for assessing risk of delirium. Am J Psychiatry 149:1393–1394, 1992

Victor M, Adams RD, Collins GH: The Wernicke-Korsakoff Syndrome and Related Neurologic Disorders Due to Alcoholism and Malnutrition, 2nd Edition. Philadelphia, PA, FA Davis, 1989

Volicer L, Harper DG, Manning BC, et al: Sundowning and circadian rhythms in Alzheimer's disease. Am J Psychiatry 158:704–711, 2001

Voyer P, Cole MG, McCusker J, et al: Prevalence and symptoms of delirium superimposed on dementia. Clin Nurs Res 15:46–66, 2006

Weiss U, Bacher R, Vonbank H, et al: Cognitive impairment: assessment with brain magnetic resonance imaging and proton mass spectroscopy. J Clin Psychiatry 64:235–242, 2003

Wilkosz PA, Miyahara S, Lopez OL, et al: Prediction of psychosis onset in Alzheimer disease: the role of cognitive impairment, depressive symptoms, and further evidence of psychosis subtypes. Am J Geriatr Psychiatry 14:352–360, 2006

Yesavage JA, Brink TL, Rose TL, et al: Development and validation of a geriatric depression screening scale: a preliminary report. J Psychiatr Res 17:37–49, 1983

Zerr I, Schultz-Schaeffer WJ, Giese A, et al: Current clinical diagnosis in Creutzfeldt-Jakob disease: identification of uncommon variants. Ann Neurol 48:323–329, 2000

Zubenko GS, Zubenko WN, McPherson S: A collaborative study of the emergency and clinical features of the major depressive syndrome of Alzheimer's disease. Am J Psychiatry 160:857–866, 2003

4

SUBSTANCE-RELATED DISORDERS

Martin H. Leamon, M.D.
Tara M. Wright, M.D.
Hugh Myrick, M.D.

People have used psychoactive substances for millennia (Austin 1978). About half of the world population uses at least one psychoactive substance, and although most do so without difficulties, for others problems arise (United Nations Office on Drugs and Crime 2009). Nationally, 63% of American adults report that alcohol or drug addiction in themselves, family, or close friends has had an impact on their lives (Peter D. Hart Research Associates 2004).

Changes in the epidemiology of substance abuse are complex, and the interested reader is referred to the following U.S. annual surveys: Monitoring the Future (secondary school students; www.monitoringthefuture.org), National Survey on Drug Use and Health (adults; www.oas.samhsa.gov/nhsda.htm), and Treatment Episode Data Set (patients; www.drugabusestatistics.samhsa.gov/dasis.htm); and the following international survey: United Nations Office on Drugs and Crime *World Drug Report* (www.unodc.org/unodc/en/data-and-analysis/WDR.html). The National Epidemiologic Survey on Alcohol and Related Conditions (Grant and Dawson 2006) and the National Comorbidity Survey (adults; www.hcp.med.harvard.edu/ncs) may also be of interest.

Classification Systems

DSM-IV-TR (American Psychiatric Association 2000) describes substance-related disorders for 11 classes of substances and an additional class of other/unknown (for other medications or toxins). The specific sub-

Table 4–1. DSM-IV-TR classification of substance-related disorders

Substance use disorders
  Dependence
  Abuse

Substance-induced disorders
  Intoxication
  Withdrawal
  Others (see Table 4–6)

stance-related disorders are listed in Tables 4–1 through 4–6).

The World Health Organization's (2006) *International Statistical Classification of Diseases and Related Health Problems,* 10th Revision (ICD-10), is similar to DSM-IV-TR. Instead of the disorder of substance abuse, however, ICD-10 includes the disorder of harmful use (Table 4–7).

The National Institute on Alcohol Abuse and Alcoholism's (2005) classification system for alcohol defines high-risk and low-risk drinking (Table 4–8). This system focuses exclusively on volumetric and frequency criteria, based on the association of these parameters with risks of general medical sequelae to alcohol use (Rehm et al. 2003).

The words *dependence, abuse,* and *addiction* are often used with different meanings, potentially leading to confusion and misunderstanding (O'Brien et al. 2006). In this chapter, the uncapitalized terms *dependence* and *addiction* are used interchangeably, and the uncapitalized term *abuse* is used to refer to substance use that leads to problems at any level. In DSM-IV-TR, the diagnoses are capitalized, thus leading to the commonly encountered but somewhat paradoxical situation in which Substance Dependence and Substance Abuse are both forms of substance abuse. Finally, many clinicians and patients consider treatment for substance dependence to be a process that involves a reorientation of all areas of a patient's life—a process termed *recovery.* This chapter uses the terms *recovery* and *treatment* synonymously.

Table 4–2. DSM-IV-TR diagnostic criteria for substance intoxication

A. The development of a reversible substance-specific syndrome due to recent ingestion of (or exposure to) a substance.   **Note:** Different substances may produce similar or identical syndromes.

B. Clinically significant maladaptive behavioral or psychological changes that are due to the effect of the substance on the central nervous system (e.g., belligerence, mood lability, cognitive impairment, impaired judgment, impaired social or occupational functioning) and develop during or shortly after use of the substance.

C. The symptoms are not due to a general medical condition and are not better accounted for by another mental disorder.

Table 4–3. DSM-IV-TR diagnostic criteria for substance withdrawal

A. The development of a substance-specific syndrome due to the cessation of (or reduction in) substance use that has been heavy and prolonged.

B. The substance-specific syndrome causes clinically significant distress or impairment in social, occupational, or other important areas of functioning.

C. The symptoms are not due to a general medical condition and are not better accounted for by another mental disorder.

Neurobiology

Recent theories suggest that the process of becoming addicted to a substance includes a usurpation of the brain circuits involved in the pursuit and acquisition of normal "survival-relevant natural goals... [or] 'rewards,'" such as food or mating opportunities (Hyman

Table 4–4. DSM-IV-TR diagnostic criteria for substance abuse	Table 4–5. DSM-IV-TR diagnostic criteria for substance dependence
A. A maladaptive pattern of substance use leading to clinically significant impairment or distress, as manifested by one (or more) of the following, occurring within a 12-month period: (1) recurrent substance use resulting in a failure to fulfill major role obligations at work, school, or home (e.g., repeated absences or poor work performance related to substance use; substance-related absences, suspensions, or expulsions from school; neglect of children or household) (2) recurrent substance use in situations in which it is physically hazardous (e.g., driving an automobile or operating a machine when impaired by substance use) (3) recurrent substance-related legal problems (e.g., arrests for substance-related disorderly conduct) (4) continued substance use despite having persistent or recurrent social or interpersonal problems caused or exacerbated by the effects of the substance (e.g., arguments with spouse about consequences of intoxication, physical fights) B. The symptoms have never met the criteria for substance dependence for this class of substance.	A maladaptive pattern of substance use, leading to clinically significant impairment or distress, as manifested by three (or more) of the following, occurring at any time in the same 12-month period: (1) tolerance, as defined by either of the following: (a) a need for markedly increased amounts of the substance to achieve intoxication or desired effect (b) markedly diminished effect with continued use of the same amount of the substance (2) withdrawal, as manifested by either of the following: (a) the characteristic withdrawal syndrome for the substance (refer to criteria A and B of the criteria sets for withdrawal from the specific substances) (b) the same (or a closely related) substance is taken to relieve or avoid withdrawal symptoms (3) the substance is often taken in larger amounts or over a longer period than was intended (4) there is a persistent desire or unsuccessful efforts to cut down or control substance use (5) a great deal of time is spent in activities necessary to obtain the substance (e.g., visiting multiple doctors or driving long distances), use the substance (e.g., chain-smoking), or recover from its effects (6) important social, occupational, or recreational activities are given up or reduced because of substance use (7) the substance use is continued despite knowledge of having a persistent or recurrent physical or psychological problem that is likely to have been caused or exacerbated by the substance (e.g., current cocaine use despite recognition of cocaine-induced depression, or continued drinking despite recognition that an ulcer was made worse by alcohol consumption)

2005, p. 1414). These circuits, involving the neurotransmitters dopamine, glutamate, γ-aminobutyric acid (GABA), opioid neuropeptides, and perhaps others, have been well described by Kalivas and Volkow (2005).

The eventual circuitry changes resulting from the intracellular accumulation of gene transcription products and other neuronal modifications result in the substance use changing from intentional to compulsive and out of control (Nestler 2005). Interestingly, the circuitry involved with relapse (i.e., the reinstitution of substance use following a pe-

Table 4–6. DSM-IV-TR diagnoses associated with class of substances

	Dependence	Abuse	Intoxication	Withdrawal	Intoxication delirium	Withdrawal delirium	Dementia	Amnestic	Other disorders Psychotic	Mood	Anxiety	Sexual	Sleep
Alcohol	X	X	X	X	X	X	X	X	X	X	X	X	X
Amphetamines/ cocaine	X	X	X	X	X				X	X	X	X	X
Cannabis	X	X	X		X				X		X		
Hallucinogens	X	X	X		X				X*	X	X		
Inhalants	X	X	X		X		X		X	X	X		
Nicotine	X			X									
Opioids	X	X	X	X	X				X	X		X	X
Phencyclidine	X	X	X		X				X	X	X		
Sedative- hypnotics	X	X	X	X	X	X	X	X	X	X	X	X	X

Note. X indicates that the disorder is recognized in DSM-IV-TR.

*Includes hallucinogen persisting perception disorder (flashbacks).

Source. Adapted from American Psychiatric Association 2000, p. 193.

Table 4–7. ICD-10 classification of substance use disorders

Mental and behavioral disorders due to psychoactive substance use (F10–F19)

Acute intoxication

Harmful use
"A pattern of psychoactive substance use that is causing damage to health. The damage may be physical (e.g., hepatitis from self-administration of injected psychoactive substances) or mental (e.g., episodes of depressive disorder secondary to heavy consumption of alcohol)" (World Health Organization 2006).

Dependence syndrome

Withdrawal state

Others (e.g., withdrawal state with delirium, psychotic disorder, amnesic syndrome)

Table 4–8. Maximum alcohol consumption for low-risk drinking

For healthy men up to age 65 years
   No more than 4 drinks in a day *and*
   No more than 14 drinks in a week

For healthy women up to age 65 years
   No more than 3 drinks in a day *and*
   No more than 7 drinks in a week

For healthy adults older than 65 years
   No more than 1 drink in a day *and*
   No more than 7 drinks in a week

Recommend lower limits or abstinence as medically indicated

Source. Adapted from National Institute on Alcohol Abuse and Alcoholism 2005. Public domain.

riod of cessation of use in an addicted person) overlaps but is not identical to that involved in the initial addiction, and different pathways may be involved if the relapse is triggered by stress, exposure to substance-related cues, or direct substance use (Weiss 2005).

Susceptibility to addiction is influenced by multiple genes and is modulated by environmental influences (Kreek et al. 2005; Nader and Czoty 2005; Velleman et al. 2005). The questions of which genes are involved for which substances and what environmental factors increase or decrease susceptibility are matters of active research. One of the environmental factors may be the substance used. For example, calculations from the 2008 National Survey on Drug Use and Health revealed that the ratio of past-year dependent users to all past-year users was 3.6% for alcohol and 34.9% for heroin (Substance Abuse and Mental Health Services Administration 2009).

Approach to the Patient

A patient with a substance use disorder may present in a number of different ways, such as with complaints of mood problems, anxiety, sleep difficulties, or symptoms of another psychiatric disorder. For this reason, all patients should be routinely and consistently screened for substance use. Different instruments may be used depending on the specific clinical setting (Dyson et al. 1998; McPherson and Hersch 2000; Workgroup on Substance Use Disorders 2006). For example, with the CAGE-D (the CAGE questions adapted to include drugs), the patient's responses can lead to discussion of substance use (Brown and Rounds 1995). One should inquire about all classes of substances, including prescription medications, because a patient may not regard abuse of some substances to be as significant as that of others.

Because of stigma against people with substance use disorders, patients may be averse to acknowledging substance-related problems. Questions must be asked with nonjudgmental empathy and caring professional interest. Confrontational challenging may be countertherapeutic (Miller et al. 1993). Information from collateral sources (obtained with the patient's consent) and repeated assessments may be necessary to make accurate treatment recommendations. The basic areas of inquiry are listed in Table 4–9.

Assessment for intoxication and withdrawal varies according to substance, but a high degree of clinical vigilance should be maintained with inpatients. The first indication of a substance use disorder may occur several days into a hospital stay, with the emergence of agitation, confusion, or delirium due to an unanticipated withdrawal syndrome.

Treatment: General Principles

Substance-Induced Disorders: Intoxication and Withdrawal

Severe intoxications can be life threatening, requiring emergent general medical care. Treatment of nonemergent withdrawal is generally accomplished by one or a combination of two general methods (Center for Substance Abuse Treatment 2006). A cross-tolerant, less harmful, and longer-acting medication is substituted for the drug of abuse (e.g., methadone for heroin, nicotine for tobacco smoke, diazepam for alcohol). The dosage is adjusted until withdrawal symptoms are suppressed, and the medication is then gradually tapered. Alternatively, other medications may be used to reduce withdrawal-associated symptoms (e.g., clonidine for opioid withdrawal, bupropion for nicotine withdrawal). Because treatment focused on substance withdrawal alone does little to improve recovery outcomes, treatment of withdrawal should include initiation of treatment for the use disorder.

Substance Use Disorders: Dependence and Abuse

The Stages of Change model is useful for conceptualizing a patient's motivation to address substance use problems. The model di-

---

Table 4–9. Basic components of substance use disorder evaluation

1. Substance use history: onset, fluctuations over time, development of tolerance, episodes of withdrawal, periods of abstinence, resumption of use, most recent use

2. History of substance abuse treatment, including attendance at self-help meetings

3. Perceptions of substance-related difficulties, problems, or complications

4. Full psychiatric, general medical, and medication histories

5. Legal history, including substance-related legal problems

6. Family and social histories, including disorders in family members, diagnosed/treated or not

7. Screening for other psychiatric disorders and a mental status examination

8. General physical examination

9. Laboratory studies, as indicated by substances used

Source.   Adapted from Workgroup on Substance Use Disorders 2006. Used with permission.

---

vides the recovery process into sequential stages, with stage-specific goals to achieve before progression (Table 4–10) (Prochaska and DiClemente 1992).

At times, patients with substance-related criminal charges may be legally coerced into treatment. In most such situations, the treatment is to some extent voluntary or at least selected as an option by the entrant (Klag et al. 2005). Although the research base is diverse and incomplete, it does not appear that patients mandated into treatment by the legal system have particularly worse outcomes, and they may have better outcomes than similar groups of nonmandated patients (Kelly et al. 2005; Klag et al. 2005).

The intensity of treatment should match the severity of the problems. The Patient Placement Criteria algorithm developed by

Table 4–10. **Stages of change and stage-specific tasks**

Stage	Task
Precontemplation	Increase doubt and awareness of problem
Contemplation	Tip the decisional balance
Preparation	Determine best course of action
Action	Implement realistic plan
Maintenance	Develop new lifestyle Avoid relapse

Source. Adapted from Prochaska and DiClemente 1992.

the American Society of Addiction Medicine assigns patients to levels of care intensity based on ratings in six dimensions (Mee-Lee et al. 2001). Patients matched to treatment intensity have been shown to have better outcomes than mismatched patients, and the algorithm has been widely used (Magura et al. 2003). Unfortunately, treatment resources are often determined by financial constraints (Substance Abuse and Mental Health Services Administration 2009).

For some individuals, recovery occurs without formal treatment. Although the research base is developing, it is difficult to make conclusive generalizations about spontaneous or natural recovery at this time, other than to recognize that it happens (Dawson et al. 2007; Ellingstad et al. 2006; Moos and Moos 2006; Sobell et al. 2000).

Psychotherapies

Psychosocial, psychotherapeutic, or behavioral interventions are the mainstays for recovery from substance use disorders. Even opioid maintenance therapy for opioid dependence includes psychosocial intervention as an essential part of treatment (Workgroup on Substance Use Disorders 2006).

The most prevalent and widely used psychosocial interventions are the mutual self-help groups based on the 12 Steps of Alcoholics Anonymous (AA) (see resources listed in Table 4–11) (Peter D. Hart Research Associates 2001; Substance Abuse and Mental Health Services Administration 2009). More frequent AA attendance has been associated with better outcomes. For individuals who find the 12 Steps' emphasis on spirituality unacceptable, lay alternatives do exist, but there is much less evidence for their effectiveness.

A number of professional treatments have been shown to be effective in large studies in different clinical settings (Table 4–12). However, it is not yet clear exactly which type of psychotherapy is best for which individual patient.

Outcomes

Treatment outcomes in substance dependence are diverse, beyond the historical use of abstinence as the sole measure (McLellan et al. 2005). One optimal final goal for the in-

Table 4–11. **Examples of 12-Step group Web sites**

Alcoholics Anonymous	www.aa.org
Narcotics Anonymous	www.na.org
Dual Recovery Anonymous (co-occurring substance abuse and other psychiatric disorders)	www.draonline.org

Table 4–12. Empirically based psychosocial interventions

Type	Summary	Example
Motivational enhancement therapy	Directive client-centered approach focuses on uncovering and resolving ambivalence about changing substance use to increase motivation and commitment; avoids confrontation.	Miller WR, Zweben A, DiClemente CC, et al.: *Motivational Enhancement Therapy Manual.* Rockville, MD, U.S. Department of Health and Human Services, 1994
Cognitive-behavioral therapy	Focuses on relapse prevention and reversal of maladaptive thoughts and beliefs that support substance use.	Carroll KM: *A Cognitive-Behavioral Approach: Treating Cocaine Addiction.* Rockville, MD, U.S. Department of Health and Human Services, 1998
12-Step facilitation therapy	Reinforces the Alcoholics/Narcotics Anonymous approach to abstinence. Participation in 12-Step groups essential. May include couples sessions.	Nowinski J, Baker S, Carroll KM: *Twelve Step Facilitation Therapy Manual.* Rockville, MD, U.S. Department of Health and Human Services, 1995
Network therapy	Cognitive-behavioral approach combined with sessions with support network (family, friends, etc.). May be combined with disulfiram.	Galanter M: *Network Therapy for Alcohol and Drug Abuse.* New York, Guilford, 1999
Matrix model	A combination of cognitive-behavioral groups, family education groups, social support groups, individual counseling, regular drug testing, and optional 12-Step attendance.	Rawson RA, Marinelli-Casey P, Anglin MD, et al.: "A Multi-Site Comparison of Psychosocial Approaches for the Treatment of Methamphetamine Dependence." *Addiction* 99:708–717, 2004
Contingency management	Reinforces the achievement of interim goals (e.g., drug-free urine tests) with intermittent tangible rewards of increasing value.	Petry NM, Peirce JM, Stitzer ML, et al.: "Effect of Prize-Based Incentives on Outcomes in Stimulant Abusers in Outpatient Psychosocial Treatment Programs: A National Drug Abuse Treatment Clinical Trials Network Study." *Arch Gen Psychiatry* 62:1148–1156, 2005

Table 4–12. Empirically based psychosocial interventions *(continued)*

Type	Summary	Example
Brief advice or intervention	5- to 15-minute motivational/educational office-based intervention; may include one or more in-person or telephone follow-up contacts.	National Institute on Alcohol Abuse and Alcoholism: *Helping Patients Who Drink Too Much: A Clinician's Guide.* Rockville, MD, U.S. Department of Health and Human Services, 2007 (available at www.niaaa.nih.gov/guide) Fiore MC, Bailey WC, Cohen SJ, et al.: *Treating Tobacco Use and Dependence: Quick Reference Guide for Clinicians.* Rockville, MD, U.S. Department of Health and Human Services, 2000
Group and individual drug counseling	Strong emphasis on abstinence, preventing relapses, problem-solving, and involvement in 12-Step groups.	Boren JJ, Onken LS, Carroll KM (eds): *Approaches to Drug Abuse Counseling.* Rockville, MD, U.S. Department of Health and Human Services, 2000
Integrated treatment	Service delivery model for patients with chronic mental illness and substance abuse in which the same team delivers both mental health and substance abuse treatment.	Mueser KT, Noorsky DL, Drake RE, et al.: *Integrated Treatment for Dual Disorders: A Guide to Effective Practice.* New York, Guilford, 2003
Couples and family therapies	A number of different models.	Reviewed in Carroll KM, Onken LS: "Behavioral Therapies for Drug Abuse." *Am J Psychiatry* 162:1452–1460, 2005

Note. This listing is intended to be more representative than comprehensive. For general reviews, see Carroll and Onken 2005 or Woody 2003.

dividual patient should probably be abstinence from all non–medically supervised substance use. Treatment, however, may need to focus sequentially on more proximal objectives, such as decreased symptoms, decreased psychiatric hospitalizations, or more drug-free urine tests.

It is no longer debatable whether treatment is cost-effective. A large number of studies, using different methods and conducted at different times, have shown that $1 spent on treatment or intervention saves between $4 and $7 in direct, indirect, or combined costs. Clinical outcomes are nicely summarized by McLellan et al. (2000):

> Thus, 1-year postdischarge follow-up studies [of substance abuse treatment show that] 40% to 60% of discharged patients are continuously abstinent, although an additional 15% to 30% have not resumed dependent use during this period. Problems of low socioeconomic status, comorbid psychiatric conditions, and lack of family and social supports are among the most important predictors of poor adherence during addiction treatment and of relapse following treatment. (p. 1693)

Alcohol
Intoxication and Withdrawal

Impairment from alcohol intoxication is dependent on the individual's tolerance, the amount and type of alcoholic beverage ingested, and the amount absorbed. A rule of thumb is that the body metabolizes approximately one drink per hour, with a decrease in blood level of approximately 0.015 g/dL.

Alcohol withdrawal (Table 4–13) typically begins 6–8 hours after the last drink, peaks within 24–28 hours, and resolves within 7 days (Myrick and Anton 2004). Only about 5% of individuals with alcohol dependence will develop more than mild to moderate withdrawal symptoms.

Alcohol hallucinosis occurs in 3%–10% of patients with severe withdrawal. It presents as auditory, visual, or tactile hallucinations in the presence of a clear sensorium. Delirium tremens (DT), or alcohol withdrawal delirium, is characterized by agitation and tremulousness, autonomic instability, fevers, hallucinations, and disorientation. DT usually develops 2–4 days from the last drink, and lasts less than 1 week. DT occurs in about 5% of patients admitted for alcohol withdrawal (Mayo-Smith et al. 2004). It is an emergency; mortality can be as high as 20% without prompt treatment.

Alcohol withdrawal seizures, typically grand mal, occur in 5%–15% of patients. Usually occurring within 24 hours of the last drink, they can occur any time in the first 5 days. A past history of alcohol withdrawal seizures increases the risk for seizures in subsequent withdrawals.

Diagnosis

There are several questionnaires available for the detection of drinking-related problems, such as the CAGE and the Alcohol Use Disorders Identification Test (AUDIT; Babor et al. 2001).

Table 4–14 lists possible laboratory abnormalities in of alcohol abuse or dependence. The sensitivity of γ-glutamyltransferase (GGT) in detecting alcohol abuse is 40%–60%, with a specificity of about 80%. A newer test for heavy alcohol use is the relative percentage in serum of carbohydrate-deficient transferrin (%CDT). %CDT is a more sensitive and specific indicator of heavy drinking. The specificity of %CDT is significantly enhanced when used with a screening instrument (Kapoor et al. 2009).

Treatment

Acute Withdrawal

Detoxification includes treatment of comorbid medical problems, rehydration, electrolyte abnormalities (including hypomagnesemia, hypophosphatemia, and hypokalemia), and nutritional deficiencies. Oral multivitamins with folic acid are routinely administered. Thiamine replacement, particularly before

Table 4–13. DSM-IV-TR diagnostic criteria for alcohol withdrawal

A. Cessation of (or reduction in) alcohol use that has been heavy and prolonged.

B. Two (or more) of the following, developing within several hours to a few days after criterion A:

   (1) autonomic hyperactivity (e.g., sweating or pulse rate greater than 100)
   (2) increased hand tremor
   (3) insomnia
   (4) nausea or vomiting
   (5) transient visual, tactile, or auditory hallucinations or illusions
   (6) psychomotor agitation
   (7) anxiety
   (8) grand mal seizures

C. The symptoms in criterion B cause clinically significant distress or impairment in social, occupational, or other important areas of functioning.

D. The symptoms are not due to a general medical condition and are not better accounted for by another mental disorder.

Specify if: With perceptual disturbances

giving glucose, helps prevent Wernicke's encephalopathy.

Benzodiazepines—administered either on a fixed dosage and taper schedule or on an as-needed basis—are the gold standard for the treatment of alcohol withdrawal. The Clinical Institute Withdrawal Assessment Scale for Alcohol—Revised (Sullivan et al. 1989) is a 10-item assessment tool used to monitor and medicate patients going through withdrawal. Anticonvulsants such as valproate, carbamazepine, and perhaps gabapentin may also be used in alcohol detoxification.

Relapse Prevention

Maintaining recovery can be difficult—an estimated 50% of alcoholic individuals relapse within 3 months. Psychosocial support remains the cornerstone of treatment (see Table 4–12).

As of November 2009, four medications were approved by the U.S. Food and Drug Administration (FDA) for the maintenance treatment of alcohol dependence: disulfiram, two forms of naltrexone, and acamprosate (Table 4–15). These medications augment *but do not replace* concurrent psychosocial treat-

ment. Despite several large studies, the relative effectiveness of these medications, alone or in combination with behavioral interventions, is not fully elucidated, nor is it clear which patients are most likely to benefit from which treatments (e.g., Anton et al. 2006). Other medications, such as topiramate and baclofen, have been used but are not yet FDA approved (Garbutt 2009).

Table 4–14. Laboratory abnormalities associated with harmful levels of drinking

Blood alcohol level >0.3 mg/mL with minimal intoxication may indicate tolerance

Mean corpuscular volume >94 fL

Liver transaminases

γ-Glutamyltransferase >65 IU/L (more specific)

Aspartate aminotransferase >38 IU/L (less specific)

Alanine aminotransferase >45 IU/L (less specific)

Percentage carbohydrate-deficient transferrin >2.5%

Platelets <140 K/mm^3

Table 4–15. Comparison of U.S. Food and Drug Administration–approved medications for the treatment of alcohol dependence

	Disulfiram	Acamprosate	Naltrexone	Extended-release naltrexone injection
Mechanism of action	Alcohol deterrent Inhibits alcohol dehydrogenase, causing adverse reaction	Reduces craving Restores balance between excitatory glutamate and inhibitory γ-aminobutyric acid neurotransmitter systems	Opioid receptor antagonist; indirectly blocks alcohol-induced dopamine release Increases percentage of days abstinent, prolongs time to first heavy drinking, and reduces amount of alcohol consumed per drinking episode	
Interactions with alcohol	Reaction includes flushing, headache, nausea, and vomiting	None	None	None
Major advantages	Physical reaction is a disincentive to drinking	Generally well tolerated; few drug interactions; is not processed through liver	Generally well tolerated; recent large multisite study supports efficacy	Once-a-month injection can greatly enhance compliance
Major disadvantages	Cannot use in the setting of liver failure Patient must avoid *all* products containing alcohol	Dosing is two tablets three times daily	Cannot use in the setting of liver failure Cannot use concurrently with opioid analgesics	

Medical Complications

Heavy alcohol consumption can elevate blood pressure and increase the risk of myocardial infarction. There is an increased risk of cancer, particularly of the esophagus, head, neck, liver, stomach, colon, and lung. Chronic liver damage may lead to cirrhosis, requiring transplant for survival. Esophageal varices can rupture, leading to rapid, profuse, life-threatening bleeding.

Wernicke-Korsakoff syndrome is a result of chronic thiamine deficiency in alcoholism. Early symptoms include decreased concentration, apathy, mild agitation, and depressed mood. Confusion, amnesia, and confabulation are late signs of severe and prolonged thiamine deficit. The syndrome can be precipitated by the administration of glucose to asymptomatic individuals with thiamine deficiency. It is therefore of utmost importance to ensure that alcohol-dependent individuals receive supplemental thiamine *before* administration of glucose in an acute setting.

No amount of alcohol can be considered safe during pregnancy. Fetal alcohol syndrome is classically evident from congenital defects of wide-set eyes, short palpebral fissure, short and broad-bridged nose, hypoplastic philtrum, thinned upper lip, and flattened midface. Mental retardation is also common. Maternal alcohol use with breastfeeding has been shown to impair a child's motor, but not mental, development.

Cannabis

Intoxication and Withdrawal

Intoxication has been associated with increased risk of automobile accidents. Symptoms include relaxation, euphoria, altered time and sensory perception, and, at higher doses, hypervigilance or paranoia, anxiety, derealization, and hallucinations. Cannabis withdrawal is generally mild and begins 2–3 days after last use, but the duration has been variable in studies, from 1.5 to 7 weeks. Symptoms include craving, anxiety, irritability, insomnia, appetite changes, boredom, and memory improvement. Diaphoresis, tachycardia, gastrointestinal disturbances, and depression occur less frequently. No specific treatment is generally needed for either disorder.

Diagnosis and Treatment

Because patients often use cannabis in addition to other substances, careful history taking may be required to determine a diagnosis of a cannabis use disorder. Patients may believe that cannabis use is not "serious" and that abstinence is not worthwhile. Nevertheless, a relationship has consistently been shown between early, regular cannabis use and subsequent abuse of other drugs, although tobacco and alcohol use often precede cannabis use.

The modalities in Table 4-12 have been used for treatment, but there is little research (Budney et al. 2006). No medications have been shown to be consistently useful in treatment (Huestis et al. 2007).

Medical Complications

Chronic cannabis use has long been associated with increased risk of paranoia, but there is growing evidence (and debate) about associations between early onset of cannabis use and psychosis or schizophrenia (Moore et al. 2007). Additionally, as would be expected in a product that is burned and smoked, there is an increased risk of certain cancers and pulmonary complications.

Women who are pregnant or considering pregnancy should be strongly advised not to use cannabis. Fetal growth decreases, and subsequent cognitive and behavioral impairments and psychiatric symptoms in the child appear to be epidemiologically related to cannabis abuse during pregnancy (Workgroup on Substance Use Disorders 2006).

Stimulants
Intoxication and Withdrawal

Cocaine and amphetamine intoxication have similar symptoms, including physical effects such as tachycardia, bradycardia, arrhythmias, and elevated or lowered blood pressure in addition to the psychological symptoms. Chronic administration of either drug can induce a paranoid psychotic state that can be long-lasting and recurrent. Withdrawals are also similar, with dysphoric mood, fatigue, vivid dreams, changes in sleep, and psychomotor agitation or retardation. The differences in clinical presentation are due to the respective half-lives of the drugs—approximately 40–60 minutes for cocaine and 6–12 hours for methamphetamine. During the late withdrawal phase, a person may experience brief periods of intense, cue-induced drug craving and be at high risk for relapse.

Treatment

Psychosocial and behavioral approaches are the mainstays of treatment in stimulant-dependent individuals. There are currently no FDA-approved medications for the treatment of stimulant dependence, despite years of intensive research. A new approach currently in development is a vaccine for cocaine dependence (Martell et al. 2009).

Medical Complications

Cocaine-related myocardial ischemia and infarction are the most serious complications of cocaine abuse, and chest pain is the most common symptom in cocaine users presenting to the emergency department. Cardiac risks appear to be unrelated to the amount, route, or frequency of cocaine use.

Acute coronary syndrome and cardiac arrhythmias are common in individuals presenting to emergency departments after the use of methamphetamine, and intracerebral hemorrhage and stroke, even in younger people, have been associated with use (Turnipseed et al. 2003; Wadland and Ferenchick 2004).

Opioids
Intoxication

The characteristic symptoms of intoxication include euphoria, pupillary constriction, drowsiness, slurred speech, and impaired memory or attention. Nausea, vomiting, and severe itching can also occur. Onset and duration of symptoms depend on the opioid used and its dose and route of administration.

Opioid overdose is a life-threatening situation. Fatal respiratory depression can occur due to direct suppression of respiratory centers in the midbrain and medulla. It is crucial to obtain a blood/urine drug screen to identify not only the opioid but also the other unsuspected drugs. Benzodiazepines are frequently abused with opioids, and if indicated, the benzodiazepine component of the overdose can be reversed with flumazenil. Treatment of an opioid overdose includes general supportive management in addition to the use of naloxone, a pure opioid antagonist that can reverse the central nervous system effects of opioid intoxication and overdose.

Withdrawal

Table 4–16 outlines the most common signs and symptoms of opioid withdrawal. The timing of the withdrawal is dependent on the type of opioid used. With cessation of chronic heroin use, withdrawal symptoms begin about 8–12 hours after the last dose, peak between 36 and 72 hours, and subside over about 5 days. With methadone, which has a much longer half-life than heroin, the peak of the withdrawal syndrome is usually between days 4 and 6, with acute symptoms persisting for 14–21 days. With any opioid, after acute withdrawal symptoms have subsided, a protracted abstinence syndrome, including disturbances of mood and sleep, can persist for 6–8 months.

Treatment

Management of acute opioid withdrawal involves a combination of general supportive measures in conjunction with pharmacother-

Table 4–16. Signs and symptoms of opioid withdrawal

Early to moderate	Moderate to advanced
Anorexia	Abdominal cramps
Anxiety	Broken sleep
Craving	Hot or cold flashes
Dysphoria	Increased blood pressure
Fatigue	Increased pulse
Headache	Low-grade fever
Irritability	Muscle and bone pain
Lacrimation	Muscle spasm ("kicking the habit")
Mydriasis (mild)	Mydriasis (with fixed, dilated pupils at the peak)
Perspiration	Nausea and vomiting
Piloerection (gooseflesh; "cold turkey")	
Restlessness	
Rhinorrhea	
Yawning	

Source. Adapted from Collins and Kleber 2004.

apy (Table 4–17). In the outpatient setting, medication tapers usually have to be extended a good bit to decrease the likelihood of dropout and relapse.

Another option includes the use of a clonidine (an α_2-adrenergic agonist) taper for amelioration of tremor, diaphoresis, and agitation. Ultrarapid opioid detoxification under general anesthesia or conscious sedation is not recommended (Collins and Kleber 2004).

With all protocols, adjuvant medications may be used. Nonsteroidal anti-inflammatory drugs may be used for myalgias. Benzodiazepines or other hypnotics may be used for short-term management of insomnia. Cyclobenzaprine (a muscle relaxant) can be used to treat muscle cramps. Dicyclomine (an anticholinergic used to reduce the contraction of muscles in the intestine) is used to treat the gastrointestinal symptoms that occur in acute withdrawal.

Maintenance treatment with agonist therapy provides relief from opioid withdrawal symptoms and thereby allows psychosocial stabilization. Methadone has long been considered the gold standard treatment for maintenance treatment. In late 2002 the FDA also approved buprenorphine for both detoxification and maintenance treatment of opioid de-

pendence. Potential advantages of buprenorphine over methadone include a longer half-life, which decreases the frequency of clinic visits, and a high safety profile with less risk of respiratory depression in overdose. Training programs are available for physicians to become certified to prescribe buprenorphine in office-based settings, not just in the traditional methadone maintenance treatment program. Buprenorphine and methadone have both been shown to be effective maintenance treatments, although some patients report individual preferences for one or the other medication (Mattick et al. 2004).

Medical Complications

Opioid-induced respiratory depression can be fatal, especially when combined with benzodiazepine use. Infection with HIV and hepatitis B and C is a major concern. Opioid users also can experience decreased immune function, hyperalgesia, and bacterial infections, including abscesses and cellulitis of the skin. Mortality in heroin addicts can be 17 times higher than that in the general population (Hickman et al. 2003).

During pregnancy, opioid withdrawal, even when treated, can increase the risk of

---

Table 4–17. Opioid detoxification medication protocols

Methadone substitution and taper

- *Day 1:* Start with a dose of 10–20 mg. If withdrawal symptoms persist 1 hour after dosing, an additional 5–10 mg of methadone can be given. The initial dose should not exceed 30 mg, and the total 24-hour dose should not exceed 40 mg in the first few days unless there is clear documentation of the patient using opioids in excess of 40-mg methadone equivalents per day.
- *Days 2–4:* Maintain a stable dose for 2–3 days.
- *Days 5–Completion:* Slowly taper dose by 10%–15% per day.

Buprenorphine substitution and taper

- *Day 1:* Administer buprenorphine 4 mg sublingually after the emergence of mild to moderate withdrawal symptoms. If withdrawal symptoms persist after 1 hour, another 4-mg dose may be given.
- *Days 2–4:* On subsequent days, 8–12 mg may be sufficient to relieve withdrawal symptoms, although higher dosages may be required.
- *Days 5–Completion:* A slow taper has been shown be superior to rapid tapers in some studies, although the rate of taper is not clearly defined.

Clonidine taper

- *Day 1:* 0.1–0.2 mg orally every 4–6 hours up to 1 mg.
- *Days 2–4:* 0.2–0.4 mg orally every 4–6 hours up to 1.2 mg.
- *Days 5–Completion:* Reduce total daily dose by 0.2 mg daily, given in two to three divided doses (the nighttime dose should be reduced last).
- Adjunctive therapy, including nonsteroidal anti-inflammatory drugs for myalgias, benzodiazepines for insomnia, antiemetics, antimotility drugs for intestinal cramping, and muscle relaxants, may be necessary.

---

miscarriage and premature birth. In addition, there is a very high rate of relapse after detoxification, and risk of cycling between intoxication and withdrawal can be even more dangerous to the fetus. Methadone maintenance is the standard of care for a pregnant woman (Jarvis and Schnoll 1994). Buprenorphine maintenance is also increasingly being used. Coordinated care between the substance abuse treatment provider and the obstetrical team is of utmost importance.

Nicotine

Diagnosis

Although the diagnosis of nicotine dependence is made according to DSM-IV-TR criteria, other rating scales may be useful in treatment. The number of cigarettes smoked per day correlates negatively with ease in quitting. The Fagerstrom Test for Nicotine Dependence (Heatherton et al. 1991) similarly predicts difficulty in quitting.

Treatment

Treatment of nicotine dependence focuses on managing withdrawal and developing new behaviors that promote abstinence and prevent relapse. Withdrawal symptoms include dsyphoric or depressed mood, insomnia, difficulty concentrating, restlessness, decreased heart rate, and weight gain.

Although the long-term (e.g., 12-month) quit rates for a single attempt are less than 10%, the lifetime long-term quit rate is approximately 50%. Accordingly, one of the tasks for the treatment provider is to help the patient deal with relapse and maintain a sense of hope and self-efficacy.

Evidence-based clinical practice guidelines are readily available, as are self-help Web

---

Table 4–18. Smoking cessation information Web sites

- www.smokefree.gov (Tobacco Control Research Branch of the National Cancer Institute, National Institutes of Health)
- www.cancer.org/docroot/PED/content/PED_10_13X_Guide_for_Quitting_Smoking.asp (American Cancer Society Guide to Quitting Smoking)
- www.treatobacco.net (Society for Research on Nicotine and Tobacco)
- www.surgeongeneral.gov/tobacco (U.S. Office of the Surgeon General, Tobacco Cessation)

Note. Sites accessed November 13, 2009.

---

sites and helplines (Table 4–18). Treatment principles and pharmacotherapies are listed in Tables 4–19 and 4–20, respectively. The issue of concurrent versus sequential treatment of nicotine and other substance use disorders continues to be debated, with some groups recommending concurrent and others recommending sequential treatment (Kalman et al. 2005; Metz et al. 2005; Ziedonis et al. 2006).

Medical Complications

The nonnicotine components of tobacco smoke induce hepatic enzymes and drug metabolism. Nicotine-dependent patients hospitalized on nonsmoking units who are stabilized on medications such as valproate, clozapine, oxazepam, haloperidol, and others will have decreased blood levels of the medications if they resume smoking after discharge.

The cardiovascular, pulmonary, carcinogenic, and other medical complications of nicotine use are well described in the general medical literature and thus are not discussed here.

Sedative-Hypnotics

Intoxication

Signs and symptoms of intoxication are similar to those of alcohol intoxication. At more severe levels of intoxication, stupor and coma may develop. With barbiturates, tolerance may develop to the drug's therapeutic effects but not to its toxicity, and a barbiturate overdose can be fatal. An overdose on benzodiaz-

epines alone virtually never leads to death, but a polysubstance overdose can be fatal.

Withdrawal

Withdrawal symptoms are very similar to those of alcohol withdrawal (see Table 4–13) and can similarly be fatal. The time course and intensity depends on the particular drug. Withdrawal from short-acting drugs can begin 12–24 hours after the last dose and peak in 24–72 hours. With long-acting drugs, withdrawal symptoms may not peak until the fifth to eighth day.

For patients who were initially prescribed benzodiazepines for the treatment of psychiatric symptoms, those target symptoms may reemerge during withdrawal. Symptom reemergence is not uncommon, occurring in 60%–80% of benzodiazepine-dependent patients initially treated for anxiety and insomnia disorders. Symptom rebound is a brief, intensified return of the target symptoms and is the most common consequence of prolonged benzodiazepine use. Rebound symptoms usually resolve within a few weeks after discontinuation of the benzodiazepine. Protracted withdrawal can occur in a small proportion of patients, usually in the setting of long-term benzodiazepine use. Signs and symptoms of withdrawal can occur for weeks to months and consist of slowly abating symptoms of withdrawal.

Treatment

Management of severe benzodiazepine overdose includes careful monitoring of the patient's airway and ventilatory support when

---

Table 4–19. Principles of treatment for nicotine dependence

---

1. Every patient who uses tobacco should be offered treatment:
    - Patients *willing* to try to quit—evidence-based cessation treatment
    - Patients *unwilling* to try—brief intervention to increase motivation to quit
2. The intensity of counseling is directly related to its effectiveness.
    - Treatments involving person-to-person contact (e.g., individual, group, telephone) are consistently effective, with effectiveness increasing with treatment intensity (e.g., minutes of contact).
3. All patients attempting tobacco cessation should receive
    - Practical counseling (problem solving/skills training).
    - Social support as part of treatment (intratreatment social support).
    - Help in securing social support outside of treatment (extratreatment social support).
4. All patients attempting tobacco cessation should receive adjunctive pharmacotherapy unless contraindicated.
    - First-line pharmacotherapies include bupropion and nicotine gum, inhaler, nasal spray, and patch.
    - Second-line pharmacotherapies include clonidine and nortriptyline.
5. Tobacco dependence treatments are both clinically effective and cost-effective relative to other medical and disease prevention interventions.

Source.   Adapted from U.S. Department of Health and Human Services Public Health Service 2000. Public domain.

necessary. Flumazenil must be used carefully, because its abrupt induction of severe withdrawal can trigger seizures in benzodiazepine-dependent patients.

Several strategies can be used for sedative-hypnotic withdrawal. In the first-line protocol, a long-acting benzodiazepine or barbiturate (such as chlordiazepoxide or phenobarbital) is substituted for the abused drug and then gradually tapered (tables of cross-tolerant equivalents can be found in the Suggested Readings at the end of this chapter). In the second (and less-recommended) option, the dosage of the abused sedative-hypnotic is gradually tapered. A third (also less-established) option involves use of valproate or carbamazepine.

Hallucinogens

Intoxication

Lysergic acid diethylamide (LSD) interferes with serotonin neurotransporters. It typically induces euphoria in addition to delusions

and visual hallucinations; however, the psychological effects it induces can be unpredictable. The experience can be significantly influenced by the user's pre-intoxication mindset and also by the setting in which the drug is used. "Bad trips" can be marked by feelings of intense fear with avoidant responses. Physical effects include increased body temperature, heart rate, and blood pressure; sleeplessness; and loss of appetite.

Treatment

The treatment of acute intoxication with hallucinogens is largely supportive. Providing reassurance, support, and a calm, quiet environment are important. Benzodiazepines may be used for extreme feelings of panic or fear. Antipsychotics are rarely recommended. Mild withdrawal symptoms of fatigue, irritability, and anhedonia are reported by approximately 10% of users.

Medical Complications

A potential complication of hallucinogen use is hallucinogen persisting perception disor-

Table 4–20. First-line pharmacotherapies approved for use for smoking cessation by the U.S. Food and Drug Administration

Agent	Precautions/ contraindications	Side effects	Dosage	Duration	Availability
Bupropion sustained release	History of seizure History of eating disorders	Insomnia Dry mouth	150 mg every morning for 3 days, then 150 mg twice daily. (Begin treatment 1–2 weeks before quitting.)	7–12 weeks, maintenance up to 6 months	Prescription only
Nicotine gum		Mouth soreness Dyspepsia	1–24 cigarettes/day: 2-mg gum (up to 24 pieces/day) 25+ cigarettes/day: 4-mg gum (up to 24 pieces/day)	Up to 12 weeks	No prescription needed
Nicotine inhaler		Local irritation of mouth and throat	6–16 cartridges/day	Up to 6 months	Prescription only
Nicotine nasal spray		Nasal irritation	8–40 doses/day	3–6 months	Prescription only
Nicotine patch		Local skin reaction Insomnia	21 mg/24 hours 14 mg/24 hours 7 mg/24 hours 15 mg/16 hours	4 weeks 2 weeks 2 weeks 8 weeks	No prescription needed
Varenicline	May cause serious psychiatric symptoms	Nausea Sleep disturbance Constipation	Taper up to 1 mg twice a day by day 8. (Begin treatment 1 week before quitting.)	12–24 weeks	Prescription only

Note. The information contained within this table is not comprehensive. Please see package inserts for the individual medications for additional information.
Source. Adapted from Agency for Healthcare Research and Quality 2001.

der, or "flashbacks." The mechanism underlying flashbacks is not clearly understood, but they have reportedly been precipitated by selective serotonin reuptake inhibitors. Flashbacks are spontaneous experiences of the same effects that occurred while a person was intoxicated with a hallucinogen in the past. LSD users may manifest relatively long-lasting psychoses, although such severe reactions are not common.

Phencyclidine and Ketamine

Phencyclidine (PCP) selectively reduces the excitatory actions of glutamate on central nervous system neurons mediated by the *N*-methyl-D-aspartate (NMDA) receptor complex (Greydanus and Patel 2003).

Ketamine is a less-potent, shorter-acting derivative of PCP that is used as a dissociative anesthetic in humans and animals.

Intoxication and Withdrawal

Intoxication behaviors can include impulsiveness, unpredictability, psychomotor agitation, impaired judgment, and assaultiveness. Physical findings include hypertension, tachycardia, diminished pain sensation, ataxia, dysarthria, muscle rigidity, and seizures. PCP is the only drug that causes a vertical nystagmus, although it can also cause horizontal or rotatory nystagmus. Ketamine intoxication appears to be similar to that of PCP.

About 25% of heavy PCP users report withdrawal symptoms including depression, anxiety, irritability, hypersomnolence, diaphoresis, and tremor.

Treatment

The management of acute intoxication includes providing a calm environment with minimal stimuli. Objects that the patient could use to harm him- or herself should be removed. Diazepam or haloperidol may be useful for PCP-induced agitation. Use of

physical restraints may increase the risk of rhabdomyolysis, which may also occur spontaneously during intoxication.

Medical Complications

Death from severe hypertension or hypotension, hypothermia, seizures, or psychotic delirium can occur.

Club Drugs

"Club drugs," named after their popularization in dance clubs in the early 2000s, include methylenedioxymethamphetamine (MDMA), γ-hydroxybutyrate (GHB), and methamphetamine.

GHB, a Schedule I drug, is available as a Schedule III prescription medication, Xyrem, through a tightly controlled program solely for the treatment of narcoleptic cataplexy.

Intoxication

GHB is usually prepared in a liquid formulation that is colorless and odorless. It has a slightly bitter taste that is easy to disguise in drinks. Ingestion results in a "dreamy" stupor and amnesia. Because of these features, GHB has been used to incapacitate victims for sexual assault. Some users describe an alcohol-like buzz known as a "G-ber daze." Higher doses can result in unconsciousness, coma, and death.

MDMA is most commonly taken in tablet form, and its effects are similar to both an amphetamine and a hallucinogen. Users of MDMA report enhanced sensation, increased energy, and a strong sense of relatedness to others. Use also results in elevations of heart rate and blood pressure as well as dilated pupils. Symptoms that a patient reports after MDMA ingestion may also be due to other drugs, because street samples of MDMA have been found to contain caffeine, theophylline, methamphetamine, and other drugs in addition to or instead of actual MDMA.

Withdrawal

Individuals withdrawing from GHB report insomnia, anxiety, tremor, and intense craving. Acute symptoms usually resolve in 3–12 days. Withdrawal from MDMA can result in feelings of fatigue, dysphoria, and depression; loss of appetite; and trouble concentrating.

Treatment and Medical Complications

The management of acute intoxication with GHB is largely supportive, with close monitoring. There are numerous reports in the literature of overdose with GHB leading to coma, respiratory depression, and death. MDMA use has also resulted in death. Dysregulation of body temperature caused by MDMA ingestion, in addition to the high environmental temperatures at raves and increased muscular exertion from prolonged periods of dancing, has resulted in severe rhabdomyolysis. Dehydration is a very serious concern because the drug appears to depress the sense of thirst, and it is used in settings where one may be dancing for hours on end in a crowded, hot club. In addition, deaths involving MDMA use have also been related to cardiac arrhythmias, hypertensive crises, and acute renal failure. Treatment of acute intoxication involves rapid rehydration and core cooling. Lorazepam may be used for agitation, panic, and seizures. It is known that MDMA is a selective serotonergic neurotoxin. Long-term use of MDMA can result in problems with memory and mood.

Inhalants

Epidemiology

Inhalants are often among the first drugs that young children and adolescents experiment with. In 2005, 17.1% of eighth graders, 13.1% of tenth graders, and 11.4% of twelfth graders reported abusing inhalants at least once (National Institute on Drug Abuse 2005). Frequently termed "whippets," "poppers," or "snappers," inhalants are a diverse group of substances that can be easily purchased over the counter in most stores. Examples of use of common substances include sniffing glue, inhaling paints or sprays, and breathing contents of aerosol spray cans. The route of administration is often to soak a rag in the chemical and then either hold the rag near the face to inhale fumes or put it in a bag and inhale from the bag. Another common route of administration is to pour or spray the inhalant into a bag or balloon directly and then inhale the fumes.

Intoxication and Withdrawal

The National Institute on Drug Abuse (2009) has specified four categories of inhalants: volatile solvents, nitrites, gases, and aerosols. Most inhalants produce a rapid high that users report as similar to alcohol intoxication. There is no clearly documented withdrawal syndrome from inhalant use.

Treatment and Medical Complications

Consequences of inhalant use can include skin damage (burns and dermatitis). Cardiovascular complications can include arrhythmias, myocardial ischemia from hypoxia, myocardial fibrosis, and ventricular fibrillation. Pulmonary effects from inhalation range from coughing and wheezing to dyspnea, emphysema, and pneumonia. Long-term use of inhalants has also resulted in reports of liver toxicity, metabolic acidosis or alkalosis, acute renal failure, and bone marrow suppression leading to anemia and leukemia. Treatment is supportive and addresses the acute medical complications resulting from inhalant use. Death can result from anoxia, aspiration, asphyxia, cardiac arrhythmias, respiratory depression, and sudden trauma (Ridenour 2005). It has been noted that many AIDS patients with Kaposi's sarcoma had used volatile nitrites before the development of the sarcoma, but whether there is any causal relationship remains unclear. Neurotoxicity and neuropsychiatric complications are the most common reported consequences of inhalant use. Neurological damage can be manifested through ataxia, peripheral and sensorimotor neuropathy, speech problems, and tremor. Psychiatric symptoms resulting from inhalant use include apathy, delirium, dementia, depression, inattention, insomnia, memory loss, and psychosis (Anderson and Loomis 2003).

Polysubstance Use

Polysubstance use is common and can greatly complicate the treatment of intoxication and withdrawal. All substances must be addressed during treatment for abuse or dependence, and the patient may have different levels of motivation for recovery from different substances.

Co-Occurring Substance Use Disorders and Other Psychiatric Disorders

Substance use disorders and other psychiatric disorders commonly co-occur in children and adults, and the relationship is complex and bidirectional. The co-occurrence of psychiatric and substance use disorders is clinically important because comorbidity has a negative impact on the course, treatment outcome, and prognosis of both disorders. Screening patients presenting at either substance abuse or psychiatric treatment settings for both substance use disorders and other psychiatric disorders is essential.

Diagnostic Considerations

Accurate diagnosis and differentiation between substance-induced states, behaviors that are part of an addicted lifestyle, and symptoms attributable to other psychiatric disorders is one of the more difficult tasks in assessing patients with co-occurring psychiatric symptoms and substance use disorders.

Sustained psychiatric symptoms during lengthy periods of abstinence, a family history of the particular psychiatric disorder, and the onset of psychiatric symptoms before the onset of substance abuse and dependence all suggest a co-occurring psychiatric illness. There are minimal evidence-based guidelines on the requisite period of abstinence. Often, considerable patience, persistence, acceptance of ambiguity, and treatment experience with a patient are required to accurately diagnose and treat co-occurring disorders.

Treatment Considerations

Integrated psychiatric and substance abuse treatment results in better outcomes than parallel or sequential treatment (see Table 4–12).

Active substance abuse or relapse should not be considered an automatic contraindication for the continuance of medications for other psychiatric disorders. Similarly, medication may be indicated for the treatment of a substance-induced disorder with prolonged symptoms, such as alcohol-induced depressive disorder or methamphetamine-induced psychotic disorder.

Gender Considerations

One-third of the individuals with either alcohol abuse or dependence in the United States are women, as are more than one-third of the illicit drug users (Substance Abuse and Mental Health Services Administration 2002). Almost 5% of pregnant women are users of illicit drugs (Substance Abuse and Mental Health Services Administration 2005). Women may be more susceptible than men to interpersonal difficulties, trauma, and medical consequences stemming from substance abuse or dependence. Women are also more likely than men to be living with an addicted partner, with obvious treatment implications.

There are differences in the incidence, development, and consequences of alcohol dependence in women compared with men. Women have been shown to have higher blood alcohol levels than men when ingesting the same amount of alcohol. Lower levels of alcohol dehydrogenase in the gastric mucosa and liver of women compared with men may contribute to this, as may the lower adjusted total body water content and smaller volume of distribution. Women drink alone more often, binge less, have more regular drinking patterns, and drink smaller quantities compared with men. The faster onset of substance-related disorders and medical consequences from substance abuse in women compared with men has been termed the *telescoping effect* (Frezza et al. 1990): women move more quickly from drinking onset to dependence and progress more rapidly to liver disease and cirrhosis, with higher mortality.

Women with alcohol use disorders are more likely to present with problems other than substance use, such as marital or relationship difficulties, physical illness, or emotional problems, and are more likely to seek treatment in psychiatric or primary care settings. When identifying a woman with a substance use disorder and referring her for treatment, it is important to recognize gender-specific barriers to entry into and completion of treatment, such as lack of gender and cultural appropriateness in program content, fear of legal consequences (particularly loss of child custody), lack of child care and transportation, inadequate or no health insurance coverage, caretaker roles for dependent family members, and societal intolerance and stigmatization of substance-dependent women (Chasnoff 1991).

Considerations in Adolescents

Alcohol is the most common substance of abuse among adolescents, and marijuana is the most common illicit substance of abuse. Another key concern involves the rapidly growing high rates of nonmedical use of prescription opioids.

When evaluating an adolescent with possible substance use disorders, educational status, family functioning, peer relationships, legal status, and use of free time should be assessed, in addition to direct questions about the use of alcohol or drugs and possible psychiatric disorders. Patterns of use, negative consequences, and context and control of use may all be unique in adolescents in comparison with adults. The CRAFFT is a useful 6-item questionnaire to screen for substance disorders in adolescents (Knight et al. 2002).

Psychosocial treatments for substance use disorders in adolescents are similar to those used in adults, including 12-Step groups. If a family is available, their participation may be essential.

Considerations in Older Adults

Older adults (loosely defined as those 65 years or older) with substance abuse problems face particular challenges compared with younger adults (Oslin 2005). Changes in body composition and metabolism can lead to reversed tolerance, and social and occupational roles change with retirement. Treatment with age-appropriate components probably results in better outcomes (Blow 2003). Age-specific concerns to be addressed include the presence of multiple medical problems, resulting in multiple medications and multiple prescribing physicians; loss of independence, function, and social supports; and impaired mobility due to social isolation or general medical conditions, resulting in transportation difficulties.

Cultural/Ethnic Considerations

Culture is defined as "a set of meanings, norms, beliefs and values shared by a group of people" (Ton and Lim 2006, p. 6) and *ethnicity* as "an individual's sense of belonging to a group of people who have a common set of beliefs and customs (culture) and who share a common history and origin" (Ton and Lim 2006, p. 7). An individual's ethnic and cultural identification influences access to specific substances, socially acceptable patterns of substance use, and how someone who abuses substances is viewed in terms of deviancy, marginalization, or acceptance.

Diagnosing substance abuse or dependence requires the psychiatrist to be knowledgeable or acquire knowledge about a patient's culture, because culture may define the particulars of "major role obligations" and "social or interpersonal problems" (see Table 4–4) or of "important social, occupational, or recreational activities" (see Table 4–5) (American Psychiatric Association 2000).

Often addiction results in the abuser being marginalized or withdrawing from his or her original culture, and as part of treatment, the psychiatrist must know or gain knowledge of what mechanisms exist within the patient's culture that allow reintegration into endogenous support systems and roles. Additionally, a substance abuse treatment program must have ways of negotiating its institutionalized beliefs (e.g., about individuality, diagnoses and disorders, use of medications) with those of the patient to prevent the treatment from becoming more a debate about beliefs than a facilitated collaborative process of recovery (Edwards 1983).

Key Points

- Physicians should inquire about all classes of substances (e.g., alcohol, opioids, sedative-hypnotics, stimulants, cannabis, nicotine), including prescription medications, as well as legal and illegal substances, because a patient may not regard abuse of some substances to be as significant as that of others.

- Although psychosocial and behavioral approaches are the cornerstones of treatment for substance dependence, medications are increasingly used to augment the treatment of alcohol, opioid, and nicotine dependence. Developing medications for the treatment of stimulant dependence is a federal research priority.

- Although it may take several tries, the overall success rate in helping patients quit smoking is relatively good. The long-term (e.g., 12 months) quit rates for a single attempt are less than 10%, whereas the lifetime long-term quit rate is approximately 50%.

- If undetected, polysubstance abuse can complicate the treatment of substance intoxication, withdrawal, abuse, or dependence.

- Substance use disorders and other psychiatric disorders commonly co-occur, and the relationship is complex and bidirectional.

- The recent increase in the rates of nonmedical use of prescription pain killers (specifically opioids) in adolescents is notable and concerning.

Suggested Readings

Galanter M, Kleber HD (eds): The American Psychiatric Publishing Textbook of Substance Abuse Treatment, 4th Edition. Washington, DC, American Psychiatric Publishing, 2008

Kleber HD, Weiss RD, Anton RF Jr, et al: Practice Guidelines for the Treatment of Patients With Substance Use Disorders, 2nd Edition. Washington, DC, American Psychiatric Publishing, 2006

Ries RK, Miller SC, Fiellin DA, Saitz R (eds): Principles of Addiction Medicine, 4th Edition. Philadelphia, PA, Lippincott Williams & Wilkins, 2009

References

Agency for Healthcare Research and Quality: Suggestions for the Clinical Use of Pharmacotherapies for Smoking Cessation. Rockville, MD, U.S. Public Health Service, 2001. Available at: http://www.ahrq.gov/clinic/tobacco/clinicaluse.htm. Accessed July 7, 2006.

American Psychiatric Association: Diagnostic and Statistical Manual of Mental Disorders, 4th Edition, Text Revision. Washington, DC, American Psychiatric Association, 2000

Anderson CE, Loomis GA: Recognition and prevention of inhalant abuse. Am Fam Physician 68:869–874, 2003

Anton RF, O'Malley SS, Ciraulo DA, et al: Combined pharmacotherapies and behavioral interventions for alcohol dependence: the COMBINE study: a randomized controlled trial. JAMA 295:2003–2017, 2006

Austin G: Perspectives on the History of Psychoactive Substance Use (DHEW Publ No [ADM] 79-810). Bethesda, MD, National Institute on Drug Abuse, 1978

Babor TF, Higgins-Biddle JC, Saunders J, et al: AUDIT, the Alcohol Use Disorders Identification Test, 2nd Edition. Geneva, Switzerland, World Health Organization, 2001. Available at: http://whqlibdoc.who.int/hq/2001/WHO_MSD_MSB_01.6a.pdf. Accessed November 10, 2009.

Blow FC: Special issues in treatment: older adults, in Principles of Addiction Medicine,

3rd Edition. Edited by Graham AW, Schultz TK, Mayo-Smith MF, et al. Chevy Chase, MD, American Society of Addiction Medicine, 2003, pp 581–607

Brown RL, Rounds LA: Conjoint screening questionnaires for alcohol and drug abuse. Wis Med J 94:135–140, 1995

Budney AJ, Moore BA, Rocha HL, et al: Clinical trial of abstinence-based vouchers and cognitive-behavioral therapy for cannabis dependence. J Consult Clin Psychol 74:307–316, 2006

Carroll KM, Onken LS: Behavioral therapies for drug abuse. Am J Psychiatry 162:1452–1460, 2005

Center for Substance Abuse Treatment: Detoxification and Substance Abuse Treatment: Treatment Improvement Protocol (TIP) Series 45. DHHS Publ No (SMA) 06-4131. Rockville, MD, Substance Abuse and Mental Health Services Administration, 2006

Chasnoff IJ: Drugs, alcohol, pregnancy, and the neonate: pay now or pay later. JAMA 266:1567–1568, 1991

Collins ED, Kleber HD: Opioids: detoxification, in American Psychiatric Publishing Textbook of Substance Abuse Treatment, 3rd Edition. Edited by Galanter M, Kleber HD. Washington, DC, American Psychiatric Publishing, 2004, pp 265–289

Dawson DA, Goldstein RB, Grant BF: Rates and correlates of relapse among individuals in remission from DSM-IV alcohol dependence: a 3-year follow-up. Alcohol Clin Exp Res 31:2036–2045, 2007

Dyson V, Appleby L, Altman E, et al: Efficiency and validity of commonly used substance abuse screening instruments in public psychiatric patients. J Addict Dis 17:57–76, 1998

Edwards G: Countries differ in their treatment of drug problems, in Drug Use and Misuse: Cultural Perspectives. Edited by Edwards G, Arif A, Jaffe JH. New York, St. Martin's Press, 1983, pp 176–184

Ellingstad TP, Sobell LC, Sobell MB, et al: Self-change: a pathway to cannabis abuse resolution. Addict Behav 31:519–530, 2006

Frezza M, di Padova C, Pozzato G, et al: High blood alcohol levels in women: the role of decreased gastric alcohol dehydrogenase activity and first-pass metabolism. N Engl J Med 322:95–99, 1990

Garbutt JC: The state of pharmacotherapy for the treatment of alcohol dependence. J Subst Abuse Treat 36:S15–S23, 2009

Grant BF, Dawson DA: Introduction to the National Epidemiologic Survey on Alcohol and Related Conditions (NESARC). Alcohol Res Health 29:74–78, 2006

Greydanus DE, Patel DR: Substance abuse in adolescents: a complex conundrum for the clinician. Pediatr Clin North Am 50:1179–1223, 2003

Heatherton TF, Kozlowski LT, Frecker RC, et al: The Fagerström Test for Nicotine Dependence: a revision of the Fagerstrom Tolerance Questionnaire. Br J Addict 86:1119–1127, 1991

Hickman M, Carnwath Z, Madden P, et al: Drug-related mortality and fatal overdose risk: pilot cohort study of heroin users recruited from specialist drug treatment sites in London. J Urban Health 80:274–287, 2003

Huestis M, Boyd S, Heishman S, et al: Single and multiple doses of rimonabant antagonize acute effects of smoked cannabis in male cannabis users. Psychopharmacology, epub July 10, 2007. Available at: http://dx.doi.org/10.1007/s00213-007-0861-5. Accessed September 6, 2007.

Hyman SE: Addiction: a disease of learning and memory. Am J Psychiatry 162:1414–1422, 2005

Jarvis MA, Schnoll SH: Methadone treatment during pregnancy. J Psychoactive Drugs 26:155–61, 1994

Kalivas PW, Volkow ND: The neural basis of addiction: a pathology of motivation and choice. Am J Psychiatry 162:1403–1413, 2005

Kalman D, Morissette SB, George T: Comorbidity of smoking in patients with psychiatric and substance use disorders. Am J Addict 14:106, 2005

Kapoor A, Kraemer KL, Smith KJ, et al: Cost-effectiveness of screening for unhealthy alcohol use with % carbohydrate deficient transferrin: results from a literature-based decision analytic computer model. Alcohol Clin Exp Res 33:1440–1449, 2009

Kelly JF, Finney JW, Moos R: Substance use disorder patients who are mandated to treatment: characteristics, treatment process, and 1- and 5-year outcomes. J Subst Abuse Treat 28:213–223, 2005

Klag S, O'Callaghan F, Creed P: The use of legal coercion in the treatment of substance abusers: an overview and critical analysis of thirty years of research. Subst Use Misuse 40:1777–1795, 2005

Knight JR, Sherritt L, Shrier LA, et al: Validity of the CRAFFT substance abuse screening test among adolescent clinic patients. Arch Pediatr Adolesc Med 156:607–614, 2002

Kreek MJ, Nielsen DA, Butelman ER, et al: Genetic influences on impulsivity, risk taking, stress responsivity and vulnerability to drug abuse and addiction. Nat Neurosci 8:1450–1457, 2005

Magura S, Staines G, Kosanke N, et al: Predictive validity of the ASAM Patient Placement Criteria for naturalistically matched vs. mismatched alcoholism patients. Am J Addict 12:386–397, 2003

Martell BA, Orson FM, Poling J, et al: Cocaine vaccine for the treatment of cocaine dependence in methadone-maintained patients: a randomized, double-blind, placebo-controlled efficacy trial. Arch Gen Psychiatry 66:1116–1123, 2009

Mattick RP, Kimber J, Breen C, et al: Buprenorphine maintenance versus placebo or methadone maintenance for opioid dependence. Cochrane Database Syst Rev (3): CD002207, 2004

Mayo-Smith MF, Beecher LH, Fischer TL, et al: Management of alcohol withdrawal delirium: an evidence-based practice guideline. Arch Intern Med 164:1405–1412, 2004

McLellan AT, Lewis DC, O'Brien CP, et al: Drug dependence, a chronic medical illness: implications for treatment, insurance, and outcomes evaluation. JAMA 284:1689–1695, 2000

McLellan AT, McKay JR, Forman R, et al: Reconsidering the evaluation of addiction treatment: from retrospective follow-up to concurrent recovery monitoring. Addiction 100:447–458, 2005

McPherson TL, Hersch RK: Brief substance use screening instruments for primary care settings: a review. J Subst Abuse Treat 18:193–202, 2000

Mee-Lee D, Shulman G, Fishman M, et al (eds): ASAM Patient Placement Criteria for the Treatment of Substance-Related Disorders, 2nd Edition, Revised. Chevy Chase, MD, American Society of Addiction Medicine, 2001

Metz K, Kroger C, Buhringer G: Smoking cessation during treatment of alcohol dependence in drug and alcohol rehabilitation centers—a review [in German]. Deutsch Gesundheitsw 67:461–467, 2005

Miller WR, Benefield RG, Tonigan JS: Enhancing motivation for change in problem drinking: a controlled comparison of two therapist styles. J Consult Clin Psychol 61:455–461, 1993

Moore THM, Zammit S, Lingford-Hughes A, et al: Cannabis use and risk of psychotic or affective mental health outcomes: a systematic review. Lancet 370:319–328, 2007

Moos RH, Moos BS: Rates and predictors of relapse after natural and treated remission from alcohol use disorders. Addiction 101:212–222, 2006

Myrick H, Anton R: Recent advances in the pharmacotherapy of alcoholism. Curr Psychiatry Rep 6:332–338, 2004

Nader MA, Czoty PW: PET imaging of dopamine D2 receptors in monkey models of cocaine abuse: genetic predisposition versus environmental modulation. Am J Psychiatry 162:1473–1482, 2005

National Institute on Alcohol Abuse and Alcoholism: Helping Patients Who Drink Too Much: A Clinician's Guide. Rockville, MD, U.S. Department of Health and Human Services, 2005

National Institute on Drug Abuse: NIDA InfoFacts: High School and Youth Trends. Bethesda, MD, National Institute on Drug Abuse, 2005. Available at: http://www.drugabuse.gov/infofacts/HSYouthtrends.html. Accessed May 26, 2006.

National Institute on Drug Abuse: NIDA InfoFacts: Inhalants. Bethesda, MD, National Institute on Drug Abuse, June 2009. Available at: http://www.nida.nih.gov/Infofacts/Inhalants.html. Accessed March 5, 2010.

Nestler EJ: Is there a common molecular pathway for addiction? Nat Neurosci 8:1445–1449, 2005

O'Brien CP, Volkow N, Li TK: What's in a word? Addiction versus dependence in DSM-V. Am J Psychiatry 163:764–765, 2006

Oslin DW: Evidence-based treatment of geriatric substance abuse. Psychiatr Clin North Am 28:897–911, 2005

Peter D. Hart Research Associates: The Face of Recovery. Washington, DC, Peter D. Hart Research Associates, 2001. Available at: http://www.facesandvoicesofrecovery.org/pdf/hart_research.pdf. Accessed May 22, 2006.

Peter D. Hart Research Associates: Faces and Voices of Recovery Public Survey, Washington, DC, Peter D. Hart Research Associates, 2004. Available at: http://www.facesandvoicesofrecovery.org/pdf/2004_hart_survey_analysis.pdf. Accessed May 22, 2006.

Prochaska JO, DiClemente CC: Stages of change in the modification of problem behaviors. Prog Behav Modif 28:183–218, 1992

Rehm J, Room R, Graham K, et al: The relationship of average volume of alcohol consumption and patterns of drinking to burden of disease: an overview. Addiction 98:1209–1228, 2003

Ridenour TA: Inhalants: not to be taken lightly anymore. Curr Opin Psychiatry 18:243–247, 2005

Sobell LC, Ellingstad TP, Sobell MB: Natural recovery from alcohol and drug problems: methodological review of the research with suggestions for future directions. Addiction 95:749–764, 2000

Substance Abuse and Mental Health Services Administration: Results from the 2001 National Household Survey on Drug Abuse, Vol 1: Summary of National Findings. Rockville, MD, Office of Applied Studies, 2002

Substance Abuse and Mental Health Services Administration: Results from the 2008 National Survey on Drug Use and Health: National Findings (NSDUH Series H-36, HHS Publication No. SMA 09-4434). Rockville, MD, Office of Applied Studies, 2009. Available at: http://oas.samhsa.gov/nsduh/2k8nsduh/2k8Results.cfm#TOC. Accessed November 29, 2009.

Sullivan J, Sykora K, Schneiderman J, et al: Assessment of alcohol withdrawal: the Revised Clinical Institute Withdrawal Assessment for Alcohol scale (CIWA-Ar). Br J Addict 84:1353–1357, 1989

Ton H, Lim RF: The assessment of culturally diverse individuals, in Clinical Manual of Cultural Psychiatry. Edited by Lim RF. Washington, DC, American Psychiatric Publishing, 2006, pp 3–31

Turnipseed SD, Richards JR, Kirk JD, et al: Frequency of acute coronary syndrome in patients presenting to the emergency department with chest pain after methamphetamine use. J Emerg Med 24:369–373, 2003

United Nations Office on Drugs and Crime: World Drug Report 2009. Vienna, Austria, United Nations, 2009

U.S. Department of Health and Human Services Public Health Service: Agency for Health Care Policy and Research Supported Clinical Practice Guidelines: Treating Tobacco Use and Dependence (Revised 2000). Rockville, MD, U.S. Department of Health and Human Services, Public Health Service, 2000. Available at: http://www.ncbi.nlm.nih.gov/books/bv.fcgi?rid=hstat2.chapter.7644. Accessed July 1, 2006.

Velleman R, Templeton L, Copello A: The role of the family in preventing and intervening with substance use and misuse: a comprehensive review of family interventions, with a focus on young people. Drug Alcohol Rev 24:93, 2005

Wadland WC, Ferenchick GS: Medical comorbidity in addictive disorders. Psychiatr Clin North Am 27:675–687, 2004

Weiss F: Neurobiology of craving, conditioned reward and relapse. Curr Opin Pharmacol 5:9–19, 2005

Woody GE: Research findings on psychotherapy of addictive disorders. Am J Addict 12 (suppl):S19–S26, 2003

Workgroup on Substance Use Disorders: Practice Guideline for the Treatment of Patients With Substance Use Disorders, 2nd Edition. Washington, DC, American Psychiatric Publishing, 2006

World Health Organization: International Statistical Classification of Diseases and Related Health Problems, 10th Revision, Version for 2006. Geneva, Switzerland, World Health Organization, 2006. Available at: http://www.who.int/classifications/apps/icd/icd10online. Accessed May 18, 2006.

Ziedonis DM, Guydish J, Williams J, et al: Barriers and solutions to addressing tobacco dependence in addiction treatment programs. Alcohol Res Health 29:228–235, 2006

5

SCHIZOPHRENIA

Michael J. Minzenberg, M.D.
Jong H. Yoon, M.D.
Cameron S. Carter, M.D.

Schizophrenia is a serious and lifelong mental disorder that affects 1% of the population worldwide. It is characterized by symptoms of disruption in the experience of reality, such as hallucinations and delusions, which are grouped as positive symptoms. Signs of impoverishment in thinking, emotional experience, and social engagement are grouped as negative symptoms. Other signs and symptoms observed in this illness include disorganized thoughts and behaviors, negative mood states, and behavioral impulsivity.

Schizophrenia may be the most devastating mental illness that humans can experience (Mueser and McGurk 2004). Its onset is typically during adolescence or early adulthood, a period when individuals are just beginning to achieve a firm sense of self, to establish enduring relationships, and to make productive contributions to society. Schizophrenia has pervasive consequences for well-being, health (including physical health), and ability to function in society. Most patients with the illness are unable to maintain independent living or gainful employment for any significant period in their lives after the onset of the illness. Once a chronic course is established, patients generally have relapsing periods of overt psychotic symptoms, characterized by disruptions in the capacity to perceive the environment properly, maintain coherent thinking processes, or derive meaning in a manner that can properly guide thoughts, plans, and behaviors. During quiescent periods of the illness, patients continue to have cognitive and social disturbances that sharply limit their capacity for true recovery and reintegration into the community. Schizophrenia also has profound effects on the families who are forced to deal with the illness.

Overall, the public health effects of schizophrenia are staggering. Although the prevalence of the illness is approximately 1% in the United States (and consistent through out the world), patients with schizophrenia occupy 25% of all inpatient hospital beds (Terkelsen and Menikoff 1995) and represent 50% of all inpatient admissions (Geller 1992). The overall cost of schizophrenia in the U.S. in 2002 was estimated to be $62.7 billion (Wu et al. 2005). Schizophrenia is one of the top 10 causes of disability-adjusted life years (Murray and Lopez 1996), representing 2.3% of the total burden of disease in developed countries (the fourth leading cause among persons ages 15–44 years) and 0.8% in developing countries (U.S. Institute of Medicine 2001). In the United States (and probably to a lesser extent elsewhere in the world), patients with schizophrenia are also disproportionately found among the chronically homeless, those who undergo the "revolving door" of repeated brief hospitalizations with premature discharge and insufficient postdischarge care, and those languishing in jails and prisons, suggesting a pervasive failure in contemporary society to adequately meet the needs of these patients.

In recent years, many significant advances have been made in characterizing the disorder and its underpinnings in genetic, neurobiological, and environmental factors. This has led to incremental but steady progress in the development of treatment advances, as well as understanding the nature of factors that modify the course of this illness, all in an attempt to lessen the effect of the illness on both the afflicted and the larger society.

Historical Overview

John Haslam (1764–1844), and independently Philippe Pinel (1745–1826), both in early-nineteenth-century Europe, wrote the earliest descriptions of individuals afflicted with the illness that we now clearly recognize as schizophrenia according to the contemporary nosology.

Later in the eighteenth century, Bénédict Augustin Morel (1809–1873) first used the term *dementia praecox* to describe schizophrenia as a premature dementia, emphasizing the early onset and progressive clinical decline. This appears to be the first biological model of mental illness that explicitly considered hereditary factors (Palha and Esteves 1997). Wilhelm Griesinger (1817–1868) achieved an integration of psychiatric illness with other medical illness and explicitly proposed that these were disorders of the brain and suggested that diffuse cerebral pathology may form a unitary basis for a range of psychotic disorders. Karl Ludwig Kahlbaum (1828–1899), who is considered by some as the father of descriptive psychopathology, studied the course of illness in these patients, appropriating methods used to study medical illness.

Griesinger and Kahlbaum were followed in time by three individuals who have had an enduring influence on the description and understanding of schizophrenia throughout the modern era. Emil Kraepelin (1856–1926) has undoubtedly exerted the single greatest influence, evident in part by the "neo-Kraepelinian" orientation of the diagnostic criteria for schizophrenia found in recent editions of DSM (Compton and Guze 1995). He aimed to classify schizophrenia on the basis of a physical etiology and to establish the basis for mental illness in the natural sciences. Kraepelin's ultimate goal was to establish a nosology that would provide direction for prognosis, treatment, and prevention of mental illness. He initially appropriated the term *dementia praecox* from Morel's and Kahlbaum's descriptions of symptom complexes and catatonia. However, Kraepelin placed increasing emphasis on considerations of etiology, clinical course, and outcome. He noted that the age at onset, family history, premorbid personality, and a deteriorating clinical course were useful in the distinction of dementia praecox from manic-depressive illness. This was regarded at the time, and remains, one of the fundamental clinical distinctions in psychiatric nosology (Angst 2002). He emphasized hereditary factors, obstetrical complications, and physical abnormalities, which remain in consideration today as evidence for genetic and neurodevelopmental factors in the illness.

Among groups of symptoms, Kraepelin emphasized what are now considered negative symptoms as the fundamental disturbance in schizophrenia (Andreasen 1997), presaging the renewed attention to negative symptoms and cognitive dysfunction as the strongest determinants of functional impairment, treatment resistance, and prognosis.

Eugen Bleuler (1857–1939), a Swiss psychiatrist, introduced the term *schizophrenia.* He criticized the notion of dementia praecox, noting the late onset and stable course of illness seen in some patients. Nevertheless, he agreed with Kraepelin regarding the cerebral basis for the disease. Bleuler defined the primary features of schizophrenia as the "four *A*s": 1) looseness of associations, 2) affective flattening, 3) autism, and 4) ambivalence. This description is essentially an emphasis on cognition, apparent in the link between the term *schizophrenia* (or "split mind") and the formal thought disorder manifest in disturbed associations. Importantly, Bleuler also recognized disturbances in emotion and motivation that were largely neglected by earlier theorists. In contrast, he considered symptoms such as hallucinations, delusions, and catatonia to be "accessory" symptoms or psychological reactions to the existence of the primary symptoms.

Bleuler's dichotomy of symptoms parallels the distinction between positive and negative symptoms, which were later appropriated from John Hughlings Jackson's (1835–1911) approach to epilepsy and persisted until the recent addition of disorganized symptoms to the current empirically derived three-category scheme. Equally important, Bleuler's emphases on illness heterogeneity and the fundamental nature of cognitive dysfunction continue to exert wide influence on how schizophrenia is studied and understood. Bleuler's diagnostic scheme was broader than that of Kraepelin. This wider diagnostic net was endorsed in early editions

of DSM, but more recent editions have returned to the narrower Kraepelinian notion of schizophrenia as an illness with early onset and deteriorating course.

The other European figure whose work helped to shape modern notions of schizophrenia is Kurt Schneider (1887–1967), who outlined a set of "first-rank" symptoms that included many of the most extreme disruptions of reality, such as thought insertion and withdrawal, thought broadcasting, hallucinated voices in argument with each other, and other more severe delusional and passivity experiences reported by patients with schizophrenia. Schneider's scheme represented one of the first attempts at establishing a discrete criteria set for the diagnosis. This narrowed the diagnosis of schizophrenia because the first-rank symptoms were clearly pathological, in comparison to some of Bleuler's symptoms, which appeared to be more continuously distributed in the general population. Nevertheless, Schneider also was greatly interested in the subjective experience of the schizophrenic patient. The first-rank symptoms were of interest to Schneider because he thought that the loss of the boundaries of the self, and of psychological autonomy, was fundamental to the illness (Andreasen 1997). These symptoms were incorporated into a range of structured diagnostic interviews that were developed through DSM-III (American Psychiatric Association 1980).

Clinical Features

As is the case for other complex illnesses with an undefined pathophysiology, no single clinical feature is pathognomonic for schizophrenia, and there is no clear consensus regarding what constitutes the disorder's core symptoms. Schizophrenia's signs and symptoms cut across diverse domains of behavior and mental processes. The variability of clinical features over time for any particular patient with schizophrenia further adds

Table 5–1. Major symptoms in schizophrenia

Positive	Hallucinations	Perception of a real sensory experience in the absence of an external source
		Most often auditory but can occur in all sensory modalities
		Common attributes of auditory hallucinations:
		External source
		Commentary on patient's actions or thoughts
		Running dialogue between two or more voices
	Delusions	Fixed false beliefs
		Common types:
		Paranoid
		Grandiose
		Somatic
		Ideas of reference
Negative	Affect	Diminished expression of emotions (e.g., blunted affect)
		Apathy or amotivation
	Social	Withdrawal
		Lack of interest in social contacts
	Cognitive	Alogia/poverty of speech
Disorganized	Speech	Formal thought disorder (e.g., tangentiality)
	Behavior	Purposeless movements or sequence of actions

to this complexity. In this chapter, we mostly rely on a scheme that segregates clinical findings into positive, negative, and disorganized symptoms (Table 5–1). This system is simple and has received empirical validation in factor analytic studies (Bilder et al. 1985; Liddle 1987). The term *positive symptom* refers to the *presence* of abnormal mental processes, whereas *negative symptom* refers to the *absence* of normal mental function. The *disorganized* category refers to the linguistic and behavioral abnormalities.

Positive Symptoms

Three positive symptoms of schizophrenia are generally recognized: hallucinations, delusions, and disorganized speech or behavior.

Hallucinations

Hallucinations are defined as the perception of a real sensory process in the absence of an external source (e.g., hearing a voice when no one is talking). The perceptual qualities of hallucinations are variable. In some cases, hallucinations are perceived to be indistinguish-

able from real sensory experiences, whereas in other cases, they are described as only approximating real sensory experiences.

Hallucinations are most frequently reported in the auditory domain. Auditory hallucinations are manifest as voices or other common sounds in the environment such as dogs barking or objects clanging. Hallucinations can occur in all sensory modalities in schizophrenia, including visual, olfactory, gustatory, and tactile (Goodwin et al. 1971).

Delusions

The second core positive symptom is *delusions*, which are defined as fixed false beliefs. A belief is fixed when the individual cannot be dissuaded from believing in its veracity with contradictory evidence or arguments pointing out its implausibility. Another important feature of delusional thinking is the illogical manner in which a conviction is inferred. Delusions also may be vague or poorly formed, such as having a foreboding sense that others have ill intentions or plotting, or may be highly crystallized, such as the specific examples given later in this sub-section. The content of delusions also can be quite variable and may involve almost any subject. However, in general, delusions can be grouped into the following common types on the basis of their content: paranoid or per-secutory, grandiose, religious, and somatic.

Paranoid or persecutory delusions are perhaps the single most common variety. They involve the conviction that individuals, institutions, or forces are intending the pa-tient harm.

Grandiose delusions refer to self-aggran-dizing beliefs (e.g., that the patient has spe-cial powers or abilities), often but not neces-sarily of a bizarre or an unrealistic nature. Common examples of grandiose delusions include the belief that the patient holds a se-cret that is vital to national security and that the patient's special talents have led others to be jealous. Religious delusions involve reli-gious themes or concepts such as being the son of God.

Somatic delusions refer to false beliefs about the patient's own body parts or inter-nal organs. These delusions commonly in-volve the belief that a particular body part or organ is dysfunctional or causing the patient harm. Somatic delusions sometimes can tragically lead patients to commit grotesque self-injurious acts on the involved body part.

A special class of delusions, ideas of refer-ence, deserves special attention because of its high prevalence and historical importance. Patients with ideas of reference misperceive communications from other persons or enti-ties to be referring to them. Classic examples of this class of delusions include the belief that statements on television or passages in newspaper articles are actually coded mes-sages directed at the patient. Ideas of refer-ence are an important class of symptoms be-cause they were part of what Schneider referred to as "first-rank" symptoms. Other examples of first-rank symptoms include de-lusions of thought insertion, thought broad-casting, thought withdrawal, and external control of affect and motor acts.

The cultural context of these expressions is extremely important to the determination of whether they qualify as delusional. Even seemingly bizarre beliefs to an outsider should not be considered a delusion if that belief is commonly shared among the wider community.

Negative Symptoms

The negative symptoms of schizophrenia re-fer to clinical features putatively resulting from the absence of normal mental functions. These include deficits in affective, social, and cognitive realms. Once an acute psychotic state is stabilized with treatment, the nega-tive symptoms may be a stronger indicator of long-term disability.

Affective Deficits

One of the most apparent clinical manifesta-tions of negative symptoms in patients with schizophrenia is the disturbance of normal affective processes. *Blunting of affect* is a term describing the decrease in the amount and range of affective expressivity. Some research points to the possibility that patients with a predominance of paranoid delusions may have heightened sensitivity to negative or threatening situations.

Another common affective deficit is apa-thy, or apparent indifference of the patient to the consequences of his or her own or others' actions and decisions. This can manifest as lack of motivation to initiate or maintain ac-tivity. Patients with apathy spend an inordi-nate amount of time at home alone, unable to initiate and engage in a planned activity.

Social Deficits

Commonly, patients have little interest in participating in social events and interacting with people. Patients often describe not needing to spend much time with other peo-ple and preferring to be by themselves. They appear to have decreased social drive in that they do not derive pleasure from social inter-actions that most people experience.

Disorganization

The third symptom cluster is disorganization in language or other behavior. The phrase *formal thought disorder* has been defined in a variety of ways, but here we use a more restricted definition of this term, as in the disorganization of the form or flow of thoughts as evident in language output. Various terms can be used in the psychiatric mental status examination to describe formal thought disorder, including (in order of increasing severity) circumstantiality, derailment, tangentiality, and word salad. These terms attempt to capture the disruption of the normal processes governing the logical, syntactic, or semantic ordering or association of words and ideas. *Circumstantiality* refers to the preservation of a logical link between each consecutive sentence concomitant with a progressive drifting of ideas away from the original topic. *Derailment* describes a process in which a patient's response is initially topical and logical but then becomes not obviously related. *Tangentiality* refers to the immediate loss of connection between the patient's response and the initial question. Finally, *word salad* describes a complete absence of a logical link between adjacent words in an utterance.

Other common manifestations of formal thought disorder are distractibility (being easily distracted from a conversation by non-relevant sounds or events), echolalia (repeating verbatim words or statements directed at the patient), clang associations (stringing together words based on phonetic similarities; e.g., fair, share, tear, hair), perseverations (repeating words or phrases), blocking (unable to complete sentences because of apparent internal preoccupation, distraction, or inability to generate words), and neologisms (creation of new words).

Disorganization also can refer to non-linguistic behaviors such as disordered sequence of or bizarre actions lacking apparent purpose. For example, a patient may approach another person as if to engage in a conversation, but then, without apparent reason

or provocation, the patient pulls his sweater over his own head.

Cognitive Impairment

An important recent development has been the rediscovery of the importance of the cognitive deficits in schizophrenia, which earlier phenomenologists emphasized as a key clinical aspect of the illness.

As a group, patients with schizophrenia show a range of impaired higher cognitive functions, including problems with attention, long-term memory, working memory, abstraction and planning, and language comprehension and production. These cognitive deficits present significant barriers to maintaining occupational and everyday function. Research has shown that cognitive deficits may be the best predictor of functionality over other symptom clusters (M.F. Green 1996).

One of the most clinically apparent cognitive deficits is in attention. An individual with schizophrenia experiences difficulty maintaining focused attention on relevant tasks or events. Attentional problems also may manifest in patients as an inability to shift their focus of attention in an appropriate manner, expressed clinically as perseveration.

Working memory, the ability to store and manage information temporarily to rapidly guide thoughts and behavior, has been proposed as a fundamental cognitive deficit in schizophrenia. For example, thought disorder can be conceived as the inability to maintain a linguistic goal in mind. Problems with multitasking, distractibility, and planning also may involve working memory problems.

Long-term declarative memory deficits have been noted to be an important source of disability in schizophrenia. Common and clinically relevant manifestations of this impairment include forgotten appointments or medication directions, which may directly affect the treatment and stability of the patient.

Subtypes of Schizophrenia

Over the years, there has been increasing recognition that schizophrenia may constitute a heterogeneous collection of different conditions. Several schizophrenia subtype classification schemes have been proposed over the years. All of these are based on the assumptions that 1) clinically evident symptoms reflect underlying brain dysfunction and 2) grouping patients according to shared clinical characteristics will provide more homogeneous groups in terms of identifying underlying pathophysiology and predicting the course of treatment.

The DSM-IV-TR (American Psychiatric Association 2000) system is the most frequently used subtype classification system in clinical practice (Table 5–2). Empirical research has shown substantial instability over time in diagnostic subtypes, and significant overlap between subtype symptoms, indicating that the validity of this scheme remains to be determined. Nevertheless, it is still worthwhile to familiarize oneself with them, given the advantages of shared terminology conferred by the use of terms with near-universal recognition in psychiatry. DSM-IV-TR recognizes five subtypes of schizophrenia: paranoid, disorganized, catatonic, undifferentiated, and residual.

Paranoid Schizophrenia

The hallmark of paranoid schizophrenia is the relative prominence of paranoid delusions and auditory hallucinations compared with the other symptoms of schizophrenia. The presence of disorganized behavior or speech, catatonia, or flat or inappropriate affect precludes this diagnosis. These patients have better premorbid functioning, an older age at onset, higher social and occupational functioning after illness onset, and fewer cognitive and affective deficits.

Disorganized Schizophrenia

As the name implies, the disorganized subtype emphasizes the presence of clinical features related to disorganization. This subtype is thought to represent a more severe form of schizophrenia, with earlier onset, low levels of social and occupational functioning, and poor long-term prognosis. The presence of delusions or hallucinations does not exclude the diagnosis of this subtype, but these symptoms play a less prominent role in psychopathology. The older term *hebephrenic schizophrenia* is synonymous with the disorganized subtype.

Catatonic Schizophrenia

The term *catatonia* refers to extreme motor states of either stupor or overexcitement that can occur independently of schizophrenia. In catatonic stupor, the patient maintains one body position for a very long time without talking or reacting to others. In catatonic excitement, the patient engages in a series of apparently aimless and exaggerated rapid movements, which also may include acts of minimally directed violent behavior.

Undifferentiated Schizophrenia

Undifferentiated schizophrenia encompasses cases in which no one cluster of symptoms constituting the paranoid, disorganized, or catatonic subtypes predominates the clinical picture. Consequently, the diagnosis of undifferentiated schizophrenia is made when criterion A for schizophrenia (see Table 5–2) is met but the diagnostic criteria for the paranoid, disorganized, or catatonic subtypes are not met. This is the most frequently encountered subtype in clinical practice.

Residual Schizophrenia

The residual subtype is thought to represent a relatively attenuated state of schizophrenia in which the positive symptoms are relatively

Table 5–2. DSM-IV-TR diagnostic criteria for schizophrenia

A. *Characteristic symptoms:*   Two (or more) of the following, each present for a significant portion of time during a 1-month period (or less if successfully treated):
  (1) delusions
  (2) hallucinations
  (3) disorganized speech (e.g., frequent derailment or incoherence)
  (4) grossly disorganized or catatonic behavior
  (5) negative symptoms, i.e., affective flattening, alogia, or avolition
  Note: Only one criterion A symptom is required if delusions are bizarre or hallucinations consist of a voice keeping up a running commentary on the person's behavior or thoughts, or two or more voices conversing with each other.

B. *Social/occupational dysfunction:*   For a significant portion of the time since the onset of the disturbance, one or more major areas of functioning such as work, interpersonal relations, or self-care are markedly below the level achieved prior to the onset (or when the onset is in childhood or adolescence, failure to achieve expected level of interpersonal, academic, or occupational achievement).

C. *Duration:*   Continuous signs of the disturbance persist for at least 6 months. This 6-month period must include at least 1 month of symptoms (or less if successfully treated) that meet criterion A (i.e., active-phase symptoms) and may include periods of prodromal or residual symptoms. During these prodromal or residual periods, the signs of the disturbance may be manifested by only negative symptoms or two or more symptoms listed in criterion A present in an attenuated form (e.g., odd beliefs, unusual perceptual experiences).

D. *Schizoaffective and mood disorder exclusion:*   Schizoaffective disorder and mood disorder with psychotic features have been ruled out because either (1) no major depressive, manic, or mixed episodes have occurred concurrently with the active-phase symptoms; or (2) if mood episodes have occurred during active-phase symptoms, their total duration has been brief relative to the duration of the active and residual periods.

E. *Substance/general medical condition exclusion:*   The disturbance is not due to the direct physiological effects of a substance (e.g., a drug of abuse, a medication) or a general medical condition.

F. *Relationship to a pervasive developmental disorder:*   If there is a history of autistic disorder or another pervasive developmental disorder, the additional diagnosis of schizophrenia is made only if prominent delusions or hallucinations are also present for at least 1 month (or less if successfully treated).

Classification of longitudinal course (can be applied only after at least 1 year has elapsed since the initial onset of active-phase symptoms):
  Episodic with interepisode residual symptoms (episodes are defined by the reemergence of prominent psychotic symptoms); *also specify if:*   **With prominent negative symptoms**
  Episodic with no interepisode residual symptoms
  Continuous (prominent psychotic symptoms are present throughout the period of observation); *also specify if:*   **With prominent negative symptoms**
  Single episode in partial remission; *also specify if:*   **With prominent negative symptoms**
  Single episode in full remission
  Other or unspecified pattern

quiescent or less symptomatic. Like undifferentiated schizophrenia, this is a subtype diagnosis made by exclusion. The diagnosis is made when negative symptoms persist or two or more symptoms listed in DSM-IV-TR criterion A for schizophrenia (see Table 5–2) are present in an attenuated form, and prominent delusions, hallucinations, disorganized speech, and grossly disorganized or catatonic behavior are absent. Many patients achieve this relatively remitted clinical subtype after sustained effective treatment.

Diagnosis

The contemporary nosology of schizophrenia has been strongly influenced by Kraepelin but reflects emphases of Bleuler and Schneider as well. In DSM-IV-TR, the diagnostic manual currently in use in the United States, both cross-sectional and longitudinal criteria are emphasized, with a 6-month minimum duration (see Table 5–2). However, clinical courses that are episodic in manner, including single-episode cases that are followed by full remission, are now recognized. The positive symptom criteria reflect the influence of Schneider's first-rank symptoms as exemplars. The negative and disorganized symptom criteria reflect a renewed prominence given to features originally emphasized by Bleuler. The DSM-IV-TR criteria identify an individual as having schizophrenia if he or she experiences characteristic positive, negative, and/or disorganized symptoms for a significant portion of time during at least 1 month, unless the symptoms are successfully treated; these criterion A symptoms are referred to as *active-phase symptoms*. The patient must have impairment in psychosocial function (work, interpersonal relationships, or self-care). Continuous signs of disturbance must be evident for at least 6 months; this must include at least 1 month of active-phase symptoms but may include periods of prodromal or residual symptoms, which appear as attenuated criterion A symptoms. Major mood disorders (e.g., major depression, bipo-

lar disorder type I), schizoaffective disorder, and substance-related or medical etiologies of the symptoms are to be excluded, and if a pervasive developmental disorder (e.g., autism) is also found, the schizophrenia diagnosis is made only if prominent delusions or hallucinations are also present for at least 1 month. The longitudinal course is classified as episodic, continuous, or single episode, with remission, residual symptoms, and prominent negative symptoms further specified. In addition, subtypes are specified as outlined in the "Subtypes of Schizophrenia" section earlier in this chapter.

It is important to recognize that research into the illness has been furthered by the widespread use of a single straightforward and reasonably objective criteria set. However, these criteria sets were not intended to represent exhaustive sets of clinical features that fully described the illness or accounted for important individual variation that has consequences for treatment or prognosis. Clinicians therefore should not limit their knowledge of what constitutes the illness, much less how to understand the individual patient, to a brief set of diagnostic criteria (Andreasen 1997). In addition, recent diagnostic criteria sets (e.g., DSM-IV-TR) have not attained significant validity by identification of biological substrates of either individual criteria or the set as a whole. This suggests that although most clinicians are likely to agree on whether an individual patient is indeed experiencing a particular illness, advances in elucidating the etiology of the illness (and future treatment targets) must await more refined characterization of the expression of the illness in measures of clinical, behavioral, cognitive, or biological functions (Andreasen 2000). This forms the basis for the recent focus on endophenotypes.

Differential Diagnosis

The diagnosis of schizophrenia continues to rest solely on the history of illness and a thorough mental status examination (Table 5–3).

Table 5–3. Differential diagnosis of schizophrenia

Other disorders	Common clinical features	Distinctions from schizophrenia
Axis I diagnoses		
Schizoaffective disorder	Criterion A for schizophrenia, plus at least one lifetime major mood episode (unipolar and bipolar types)	On average, higher function but higher suicide risk; history of major mood episode not found in schizophrenia
Mood disorders with psychosis	Multiple symptoms of mood changes, vegetative symptoms, mood-congruent ideation, and other cognitive changes, with acute or subacute onset and often in response to psychosocial stressors	Mood symptoms are more enduring; more complete interepisodic recovery; psychosis only with severe mood episodes; fuller response to psychotherapy
Delusional disorder	Prominent delusions, with other cognitions and behavior organized around delusion but no other significant psychosis	Psychosis confined to one or more delusions, usually nonbizarre; function largely intact; minimal decline in function or change in symptoms over time; more refractory to treatment
Schizophreniform disorder	Duration of criterion A met for more than 1 month but less than 6 months	Shorter duration than schizophrenia; many ultimately receive schizophrenia diagnosis
Brief psychotic disorder	Psychosis with abrupt onset and duration less than 1 month; often in response to acute stressor	No prodrome; cognition generally intact; better prognosis
Drug-related psychosis	Significant history of drug use, with abuse and often dependence criteria met; associated cyclic impulsivity and interpersonal, occupational, and legal history	Psychosis typically during active periods of drug use, particularly psychostimulants; more complete recovery with sustained abstinence; characteristic medical comorbidity with chronic abuse
Axis II (personality) disorders		
Cluster A: schizotypal, paranoid, schizoid personality disorders	Subpsychotic (positive and/or negative) symptoms with mild to moderate cognitive and social impairment	Less functional decline than schizophrenia; cognition more intact, and rare impulsivity or need for hospitalization
Cluster B: borderline personality disorder	Instability in mood, impulse control, and interpersonal relationships	Less functional decline than schizophrenia; symptoms more sensitive to interpersonal factors; more unstable over time; psychosis only with significant stress

Table 5–3. Differential diagnosis of schizophrenia *(continued)*

Other disorders	Common clinical features	Distinctions from schizophrenia
Axis III (medical) disorders		
Dementias (cortical and subcortical)	Slow onset in middle to late adulthood, with progressive cognitive decline; some with prominent motor symptoms	Later onset; cognitive deficits more prominent compared with other symptoms; psychosis primarily in late stages
Acute confusional states (delirium; varied etiologies)	Abrupt onset with risk factors for neurological illness; clouded sensorium; transient psychosis can be in various sensory modes	Premorbid function intact; acute onset; psychotic symptoms less formed; full recovery possible with medical treatment
Iatrogenic psychosis (e.g., steroids, antibiotics, anticholinergics, antiparkinsonian medications)	Acute onset; transient psychosis can be in various sensory modes	Stable premorbid function; acute onset; psychotic symptoms less formed; associated somatic effects of medications; full recovery possible with medical treatment

No reliable laboratory tests have yet been established for this illness, but this remains an attainable goal in light of the consistent alterations shown by schizophrenic patients on biochemical, cognitive, and neuroanatomic measures. Along with the history taking and mental status examination, a full physical examination usually should be performed, particularly for new-onset cases, because medical causes of psychotic illness are varied. This list includes intracranial processes, metabolic disorders, and endocrine disorders. The dementias are often associated with psychotic features. Illicit substance use is also quite common in the community and can frequently lead to psychotic symptoms, not only with acute intoxication but also in an intermittent or even a persistent manner with chronic use, particularly with stimulant drugs. Many commonly prescribed medications can also cause psychosis, particularly those with direct effects on the brain, such as steroids, anticholinergics, and medications prescribed for Parkinson's disease. Those cases that present with atypical clinical features, such as late age at onset, clouding of the sensorium (i.e., confusional states), or findings on history or physical examination suggestive of concurrent medical problems should prompt the clinician to pursue alternative causes of illness. Routine laboratory tests that may aid the clinician in ruling out these etiologies include a complete blood count, renal and metabolic panels, liver enzymes, thyroid function, urinalysis, and serological tests for syphilis and HIV. Brain imaging such as magnetic resonance imaging (MRI) or computed tomography (CT) and electroencephalography may be indicated in atypical cases or when the history suggests the need to rule out intracranial pathology unrelated to psychiatric illness.

Although care should be taken to rule out medical causes of psychosis confidently, the major task in differential diagnosis will require distinction of schizophrenia from a range of other psychiatric disorders that also may involve psychotic symptoms. These include schizoaffective disorder; major mood disorders that can present with psychotic features, such as major depression and acute mania among bipolar affective disorder type I patients; delusional disorder; and personality disorders, particularly those in the A or B clusters. To rule out the major mood disorders or schizoaffective disorder, the active phase of psychosis should occur in the absence of an acute mood disorder episode, or alternatively, the mood episodes should be relatively brief in relation to the total duration of the psychotic episode. Most mood disorder patients also maintain or recover significant levels of psychosocial function in between episodes of illness because they do not experience continuous psychotic symptoms or persistently severe mood disturbance. Delusional disorder is distinguished by the lack of other psychotic symptoms, and the content of delusions tends not to be the bizarre thoughts or beliefs often observed in schizophrenia, such as beliefs that monitoring devices are implanted in the patient's body or that the patient is communicating with other species. Schizophreniform disorder and brief psychotic disorder are also characterized by overt psychotic symptoms. In some cases, a clinician may encounter the patient relatively early in the active psychotic phase of illness, and as a result, one of these diagnoses (both with a briefer duration criterion than that for schizophrenia) is most appropriate to assign initially. However, if psychotic symptoms persist beyond 6 months, then the diagnosis of schizophrenia is most appropriate.

Cluster A ("odd") personality disorders (schizoid, schizotypal, and paranoid) are often referred to as *schizophrenia spectrum disorders* and may be characterized by subthreshold or attenuated psychotic symptoms related to those of schizophrenia. Patients with these personality disorders may show symptoms of social withdrawal, anhedonia, and flat affect quite similar to, but more mild than, the negative symptoms of schizophrenia. However, overt psychotic symptoms are rare (and transient) in these individuals, and their level of function is typically higher, with gainful employment and independent living being the norm. Borderline personality disorder may present with acute, overt psychotic symptoms; however, in this personality disorder, in contrast to schizophrenia, interpersonal stressors are common precipitants of acute psychosis, emotional dysregulation (with lability, multiple negative mood states, and overt antagonism) is nearly ubiquitous, and behavioral impulsivity is present, often including dangerous or hazardous acts such as self injury and aggressive behavior. Other disorders such as depersonalization disorder, panic disorder, and obsessive-compulsive disorder may present with feelings of unreality or bizarre behavior; however, in each of these disorders, reality testing and social function are preserved, and overt delusions or hallucinations are rare. Finally, factitious disorder and malingering can be found in many clinical settings; the degree to which the clinical picture diverges from well-established profiles found in schizophrenia, along with the identification of secondary gains (e.g., material reward or avoidance of incarceration) attainable as a result of a psychiatric diagnosis or treatment, may call attention to the possibility of these last diagnoses.

Clinical Course
Premorbid Functioning

Any description of the clinical course of schizophrenia should address periods of development occurring well before the onset of overt psychotic symptoms. Good evidence indicates that in groups of individuals who will later develop schizophrenia, some signs are present long before onset of psychosis, as early as childhood. These signs tend to be subtle and do not warrant a diagnosis of any particular psychiatric disorder.

Nevertheless, children who later develop schizophrenia perform lower than their siblings and classmates who do not develop schizophrenia on tests of intelligence and achievement and have poorer grades in school (Jones et al. 1994). This deficit worsens in adolescence as test scores decline further between ages 13 and 16 years. In addition, children who go on to develop schizophrenia are less socially responsive, express less positively valenced emotion, and have poorer social adjustment than do children who maintain health into adulthood. Some of these deficits may be apparent as early as the first year of life. These children also have observable motor deficits, with an increased rate of delayed or abnormal motor development, which includes the attainment of walking. The motor dysfunction of childhood persists throughout the pre-illness period and into the clinical phase of overt illness. These children typically do not have a diagnosable mental disorder during childhood, even though childhood-onset schizophrenia does exist (Remschmidt 2002).

Prodrome to Schizophrenia

During adolescence, however, those who later develop schizophrenia often begin to undergo changes that are discernible to others, with the onset of significant overt psychiatric symptoms. These include symptoms of depression, social withdrawal, irritability, and antagonistic thoughts and behavior. In this period, these adolescents often come to the attention of school and community clinicians for conduct problems and academic decline. These symptoms are highly nonspecific because they are also characteristic of early symptoms of mood, anxiety, substance use, and personality disorders, all of which can have their onset during this same period. Nevertheless, these symptoms may be retrospectively identified as heralding the onset of the so-called prodrome of schizophrenia, a period of variable duration (usually lasting from several months to a few years) that precedes the onset of schizophrenia in most cases (Phillips et al. 2005). Several clinical signs that can be observed during this period have a high positive predictive value for the later onset of schizophrenia. These largely include subtle attenuated psychotic symptoms that differ from overt psychotic symptoms in frequency or severity. These symptoms may include suspiciousness or perceptual distortions that do not qualify as overtly psychotic. Reality testing is often intact at this stage because many individuals will doubt the veracity of these experiences.

Research into the phenomenology and course of individuals in the schizophrenia prodrome is an area of rapidly intensifying interest, given the importance of early and reliable identification of those who will develop schizophrenia. One issue in this work is how to make a positive identification of experiences as pathological within this range of experience, given the fact that it has been found that "psychotic-like" experiences can be commonly found in the general population at rates that are much higher than the rate of overt psychotic symptoms (Peters et al. 1999). This suggests that for some individuals, these symptoms must resolve without leading to overt psychotic symptoms. A second issue in this research is how to draw the boundary most appropriately between these symptoms and the symptoms of full-blown psychosis. Many experiences that patients endorse are on the cusp of psychosis, and it is often difficult to determine whether they should qualify as overtly psychotic. This distinction is important because antipsychotic medication has well-demonstrated efficacy against overt psychotic symptoms, and the use of these medications for psychotic symptoms is usually justified and advantageous. However, the use of these medications to treat symptoms that are below the threshold of psychosis has to date been poorly studied.

This issue takes on greater importance when one considers that early intervention may have potentially profound consequences for the course of illness in schizophrenia and even possibly for whether those individuals at risk for schizophrenia convert to the disorder.

Early Period of Psychotic Illness in Schizophrenia

The crossing of the boundary from the prodrome to schizophrenia proper is an event witnessed with great dismay by patients, families, and care providers alike. It remains an event with obscure causes for most patients, because the precipitants of overt psychosis have not been well established (Broome et al. 2005). In some cases, substance abuse may be a precipitant. Among persons at risk for schizophrenia, cannabis and amphetamines appear to be the most frequently abused substances around the time of onset of psychosis. However, in most cases, the cause of psychosis onset remains unknown. Both genetic and environmental origins have been considered (see section "Etiology and Pathophysiology" later in this chapter).

The onset of psychosis can be insidious or abrupt, and those who experience a rapid onset tend to have a more favorable prognosis. This active phase of initial psychotic symptoms is often referred to informally as the *first break*—that is, the break with reality that is a core feature of psychosis. Patients during this phase will experience florid symptoms of hallucinations, delusions, and occasionally disorganized thought and behavior and agitation. At this point, the distress experienced by the patient, family, or both often increases dramatically, prompting entry into treatment. Less often, the patient comes to the attention of the mental health system for involuntary evaluation, as the result of public disturbances or behaviors that are dangerous to the self or others. As treatment for first-episode psychosis proceeds, overt psychotic symptoms commonly abate in the days to few months thereafter. Ample evidence indicates that those patients who experience significant treatment delays have a worse prognosis even when illness severity at presentation is taken into account. This suggests that early intervention is an important treatment goal in schizophrenia.

Longitudinal studies of first-episode psychosis leading to a schizophrenia diagnosis find considerable heterogeneity at follow-up. For patients who do receive adequate treatment, a *residual phase* follows, during which the range and severity of symptoms can be quite similar to those seen in the prodrome. Over time, most patients will experience a series of acute exacerbations of symptoms occurring episodically as they go into and out of active-phase psychosis. These episodes are often precipitated by environmental stressors, substance abuse, or treatment discontinuation. The degree of remission between these episodes may vary, and there is a tendency in the early phase (the first 5–10 years after onset) of the overt illness for patients to progressively fail to attain the level of function observed prior to each episode (Lieberman et al. 2001). This describes the "clinical deterioration" associated with Kraepelin's construct of schizophrenia and particularly describes the course of patients identified in recent editions of DSM. Following this period, however, patients appear to attain a measure of stability in the severity of symptoms, rate of relapse, treatment responsivity, and general level of function.

In addition, a more severe early-onset form of schizophrenia (before age 12 years) has been described. It is quite rare and appears identical in both clinical and biological features to the more common adult-onset form (Nicolson and Rapoport 1999). In general, in comparison to the adult-onset form, childhood-onset schizophrenia has a worse prognosis. Nevertheless, those who experience a more acute onset, a rapid response to acute treatment, and relatively more positive than negative, cognitive, or depressive symptoms have a more favorable prognosis. In addition, a more benign course is observed among those childhood-onset patients who lack a family history of schizophrenia or who have greater family support (Remschmidt 2002).

Long-Term Outcome

Numerous studies have been conducted in an attempt to characterize the long-term outcome of patients with schizophrenia. Several studies have now been reported in which patients with schizophrenia were identified with contemporary diagnostic criteria and follow-up was obtained over at least 10 years (Jobe and Harrow 2005).

Only two long-term follow-up studies were fully prospective in design. The Chicago Follow-Up Study included 73 schizophrenic patients followed up to 20 years. This study found that schizophrenic patients generally fluctuated between moderate and severe disability, but more than 40% showed periods of recovery that often lasted for several years (Harrow and Jobe 2005). Some of these patients were able to function without the benefit of continuous antipsychotic treatment and had tended to have better premorbid function. In addition, a large percentage of the full sample of schizophrenic patients (65%) also had experienced at least one depressive syndrome at 20-year follow-up; the completed suicide rate was 10% at 10 years and higher than 12% at 20 years. The other long-term prospective study of schizophrenic patients, conducted by Carpenter and Strauss (1991), followed up 55 DSM-III-identified schizophrenic patients for 11 years and found no change in their relatively poorer outcome status at 5 and 10 years.

Several long-term follow-up studies have been conducted outside of North America. These studies have typically used International Classification of Diseases (ICD) criteria rather than DSM criteria to identify patients. Some of these studies have found women to have a relatively more benign course of illness compared with men (Angermeyer et al. 1989). One of these studies that is particularly important is the World Health Organization (WHO) study, referred to as the International Pilot Study of Schizophrenia. A total of 1,633 subjects from 14 incidence cohorts and 4 prevalence cohorts in 9 different nations were studied. The most dramatic finding was that outcome in schizophrenia was poorer in fully industrialized countries than in developing countries (Sartorius et al. 1977). Repeated psychotic episodes, for instance, were more common in the developed countries despite the greater availability of modern treatment. The range and severity of symptoms at initial enrollment were not significantly different between sites. This finding has been subject to a great deal of discussion. Some have suggested that a culture of tolerance and benevolence toward those with unusual thoughts and behaviors is more prevalent in developing countries, with a salutary effect of normalizing or "buffering" the patient's psychopathology and maintaining integration in the local community. However, this does not appear to account fully for the differences between these groups of nations (McGrath et al. 2004). Others have suggested that economies that are not fully market-oriented place fewer psychological and practical demands on schizophrenic patients, with less illness exacerbation and less downward social drift as a result. On the whole, in the WHO study, the strongest predictors of poor outcome were social isolation, duration of index episode, history of psychiatric treatment, unmarried status, and history of childhood behavior problems. These factors all may reflect a more severe form of illness at outset.

Etiology and Pathophysiology

The past five decades have borne witness to an impressive period of discovery in the neurobiological basis of schizophrenia. However, despite these advances, the full understanding of the causes and the biological pathways leading to schizophrenia remains one of the most enduring challenges facing modern medicine. This state of uncertainty is reflected by the presence of competing theories on the etiology of schizophrenia. The aim of this section is to review and synthesize these major theories and the evidence supporting them.

Two concepts describe the generally accepted framework reflecting the current understanding of the etiology and pathophysiology of schizophrenia. The first is the view that schizophrenia is a neurodevelopmental disorder—that disturbances in the normal growth and maturation of neurons and neural pathways give rise to schizophrenia. The other overarching framework is the diathesis stress model of schizophrenia. This model posits a dynamic interplay between heritable (diathesis) and environmental (stress) factors in determining whether any individual develops this illness. This model is consistent with available data showing that the risk of developing schizophrenia is strongly influenced by genetics, but the eventual development of this illness is also strongly modulated by environmental factors (D.A. Lewis and Levitt 2002; Lieberman et al. 2001).

Genetics

That schizophrenia has a strong genetic component is a readily accepted notion. The degree of risk is proportional to the degree of shared genes (Gottesman 1991). A review of twin studies showed concordance rates between 25% and 50% (Gottesman 1991). Adoption studies showed an elevated risk for schizophrenia among the offspring of mothers with schizophrenia (Kety et al. 1971).

The exact manner in which schizophrenia is heritable and the identity of the specific genes that may give rise to schizophrenia, however, remain topics of significant debate and uncertainty. Schizophrenia does not follow simple Mendelian principles of inheritance (McGue and Gottesman 1989). Complex diseases involve several genes, each with a modest effect on heritability, acting in concert, in either a linear or a synergistic manner, to confer an overall disease risk (Risch 1990). Additional complexity may arise from partial penetrance of these genes, interactions between genes, and epigenetic neurodevelopmental or environmental factors.

Twin adoption studies have been remarkably consistent in reporting approximately 50% concordance rate for monozygotic twins. This result accentuates the importance of both the genetic and the nongenetic factors in conferring disease risk. Consequently, nongenetic causes must account for this lack of full concordance. A 1994 study found that this elevated risk may be mediated in part by a stressful environment (Tienari et al. 1994). Similar models of gene–environment interaction leading to disease expression have received empirical validation in other psychiatric disorders (Moffitt et al. 2005).

The past 10 years have witnessed a tremendous proliferation in the number of putative schizophrenia risk genes, many of which are related to neurodevelopmental processes involved in the establishment of neural networks (e.g., neuronal migration and synapse formation or the regulation of synaptic transmission). One such gene that has received a great deal of attention is dysbindin (*DTNBP1*) (Straub et al. 2002). This gene product binds to components of the dystrophin complex, which are thought to be important in mediating neural synapse structure and function. Another putative schizophrenia gene is neuregulin (*NRG1*) (Stefansson et al. 2002). It is located on 8p21–22 and may have a diverse range of roles in neural transmission, axonal development, and synaptogenesis (Corfas et al. 2004). An important fact to keep in mind is that replications of findings from linkage studies have been relatively rare. However, this may be resolved by considering that several risk genes are involved, each with only modest effect. A meta-analysis of these linkage studies did show some support for the involvement of several regions (Badner and Gershon 2002; C.M. Lewis et al. 2003). Follow-up association studies in many of these regions have been promising, and they have identified several candidate schizophrenia risk genes (Owen et al. 2005).

Environmental Factors

In this section, we survey studies that have identified several environmental factors that may increase risk for schizophrenia.

A higher incidence of obstetric and perinatal complications was found in patients with schizophrenia in several studies. One meta-analytic review categorized these events as 1) complications of pregnancy, 2) abnormal fetal growth and development, and 3) complications of delivery (Cannon et al. 2002). The meta-analysis indicated that each of these categories was significantly associated with increased risk but that the effect sizes were generally modest. Another line of studies has found an association between maternal nutritional status and schizophrenia in the offspring. The Dutch famine study examined the prevalence of schizophrenia among a cohort of births that occurred during the winter of 1944–1945, a period of severe malnutrition for most citizens in a region of the Netherlands (Susser et al. 1996). The study showed a twofold increased risk for schizophrenia associated with extreme prenatal malnutrition.

Most epidemiological studies investigating environmental risk factors for schizophrenia are limited by the retrospective manner in which data are collected. The Prenatal Determinants of Schizophrenia Study addressed this limitation by relying on maternal serum obtained during prenatal visits and demographic information on the participants (Susser et al. 2000). From the cohort of approximately 12,000 pregnant women, potential cases of schizophrenia were identified. Of these potential cases, face-to-face diagnostic evaluations by research psychiatrists resulted in the identification of 71 subjects with schizophrenia. This study concluded that influenza infection in the first trimester is associated with a sevenfold increased risk for schizophrenia and related disorders (Brown et al. 2004). Other possible pathogens that were identified in the Prenatal Determinants of Schizophrenia Study include toxoplasmosis and lead.

Another line of research has pointed to the importance of the physical environment and fetal exposures during gestation. Seasonal variation in the prevalence of births leading to schizophrenia has been identified, with an excess of births in winter and spring months (G. Davies et al. 2003). Various theories attempting to account for this finding have been proposed—environmental factors that predisposed to schizophrenia development such as ambient temperature, exposure to infectious agents, and nutritional deficiencies; increased resistance to infections; and other insults conferred by schizophrenia, leading to increased survival in winter months.

Although the worldwide prevalence is thought to be equivalent across nations (Jablensky 2000; Sartorius et al. 1977), numerous findings and theories have suggested a direct relation between specific social and cultural factors and the development or severity of schizophrenia. Some of these factors include immigration status, urbanicity, and socioeconomic status.

Neurochemical Factors

The serendipitous discovery of the first neuroleptic ushered in the modern era of psychiatry. The finding that a pharmacological agent could ameliorate some of the symptoms of schizophrenia motivated researchers to identify the neurochemical pathways affected by these medications. Although most researchers now acknowledge that the etiology of schizophrenia cannot be understood solely in terms of neurotransmitter dysfunction, it is clear that dysregulation of neurotransmission is an important aspect in the expression of this disorder.

Dopamine

Chlorpromazine was originally synthesized in the 1950s as an antihistamine for use as a preanesthetic agent. After the French surgeon Henri Laborit noted a particularly calming effect on patients, he recommended chlorpromazine to his psychiatric colleagues for use with agitated patients. They quickly found it beneficial in patients with schizophrenia. They also noted parkinsonian side effects with higher doses. They coined the term *neuroleptic*, literally translated from the French as "seizing the neuron," to reflect their intuition that the mechanism of action somehow involved neural modulation.

The serendipitous discovery of the usefulness of chlorpromazine in schizophrenia led ultimately to the development of the dopamine hypothesis, one of the most influential theories on the etiology of schizophrenia. It posits that the symptoms of this illness are the by-products of dysfunction of dopamine neurotransmission. The main lines of evidence supporting this role for dopamine came from work in the 1960s and 1970s. Carlsson and Lindqvist (1963) determined that the administration of phenothiazines in animals blocks the behavioral effects of dopamine agonists (such as amphetamine) and results in increased turnover of dopamine. Conversely, the administration of amphetamine, which was known to increase synaptic levels of dopamine, resulted in behavioral abnormalities and symptoms reminiscent of schizophrenia. Later work further specified that the most important dopamine receptor may be the D_2 subtype in that clinical potency is best correlated with binding to this receptor subtype (Creese et al. 1976).

Neuroimaging has made significant contributions to our evolving understanding of the neurochemical basis for schizophrenia. Imaging modalities such as positron emission tomography (PET) and single photon emission computed tomography (SPECT) are allowing researchers to assess the functional status of neurotransmitter systems. PET studies have found that the dopaminergic tone associated with schizophrenia may be more complex than previously thought. This newer hypothesis proposes a hyperdopaminergic state in the striatal D_2 system (Abi-Dargham et al. 2000) that gives rise to positive symptoms and a hypodopaminergic state in the prefrontal D_1 system associated with higher-order cognitive deficits (Abi-Dargham et al. 2002).

The challenge to the dopamine hypothesis comes from primarily two lines of evidence. First, the dopamine hypothesis does not account for negative symptoms, which are now acknowledged to be essential components of this illness. Dopamine-blocking agents have not been shown to be effective in treating negative symptoms, nor have dopaminergic agents been shown to induce negative symptoms. The second challenge to the dopamine hypothesis comes from the efficacy of the so-called atypical antipsychotics, medications that are thought to act through multiple neurotransmitter systems in addition to dopamine.

Other Monoamines

It is hypothesized that other neurotransmitter systems may be involved in the pathophysiology of schizophrenia. One of the most important of these other neurotransmitters is serotonin. Serotonin has been implicated by the clinical efficacy of the many atypical agents with high affinity for its receptors. There are 14 known serotonin receptor subtypes, but some of the most important for schizophrenia include the 5-HT$_{2C}$, 5-HT$_{2A}$, and 5-HT$_{1A}$ subtypes.

The acetylcholine system was implicated in the pathophysiology of schizophrenia initially on the basis of the observation that patients with schizophrenia have high rates of use of tobacco products. This led to the hypothesis that the nicotine in tobacco provides some amelioration of symptoms through its action on the acetylcholine system. Nicotine has been found to normalize measures of deficient auditory gating in schizophrenia (L.E. Adler et al. 1992).

Glutamate and N-Methyl-D-Aspartate

Glutamate is the most prevalent excitatory neurotransmitter in the brain. Consequently, the function of glutamate is fundamentally different from that of dopamine and the other monoaminergic neurotransmitters, which are primarily modulators of excitatory or inhibitory neurotransmission. The involvement of the glutamate system in the pathophysiology of schizophrenia is inferred primarily from the observation that people intoxicated with agents acting on the glutamate receptor, such as phencyclidine (PCP) and ketamine, often exhibit a behavioral syndrome mimicking schizophrenia. Interestingly, this syndrome can include both positive and negative symptoms of schizophrenia (Javitt and Zukin 1991). PCP and ketamine bind to the N-methyl-D-aspartate (NMDA) class of glutamate receptors. The NMDA receptor regulation is highly complex with numerous sites of allosteric modulation. One of the most important in terms of psychopathology appears to be the glycine site. The results of clinical studies investigating the effects of glycine agonists have been mixed, with some studies showing benefit for both positive and negative symptoms.

Gamma-Aminobutyric Acid

The potential role for γ-aminobutyric acid (GABA) in the pathophysiology of schizophrenia follows two separate but related lines of research involving inhibitory interneurons. In the first line of research, the psychotomimetic effects of NMDA antagonists, such as PCP, are thought to be mediated through their action on GABA release. NMDA receptors are found on GABAergic inhibitory interneurons. Activation of these NMDA receptors results in increased GABA release, which then causes suppression of glutamate release from glutamatergic cells. The binding of an antagonist on the NMDA receptor on the inhibitory neurons ultimately results in a hyperglutamatergic state, which is presumed to cause symptoms of psychosis.

In the second line of research, alterations in the neural circuitry of the prefrontal cortex, involving GABA, are thought to give rise to the higher-order cognitive deficits in schizophrenia. Theories on GABA dysfunction in schizophrenia center on the parvalbumin-containing group of inhibitory interneurons. Studies showing a reduction in the number of parvalbumin cells and underexpression of glutamic acid decarboxylase, a key enzyme in GABA synthesis (Akbarian et al. 1995; Volk et al. 2000), point to a functional deficit in GABA in the prefrontal cortex. Taken together, the chandelier and wide arbor cells are thought to coordinate the fine control of the synchrony and spatial extent of pyramidal cell activity in the prefrontal cortex. The disruption of these functions in schizophrenia would be expected to lead to the loss of temporal and spatial organization in neuronal activity necessary for higher-order cognitive processes.

Anatomical and Histological Studies

The emergence of modern neuroimaging and molecular techniques has led to a renewed interest in the study of structural abnormalities in the brains of individuals with schizophrenia. Neuroimaging studies have shown consistent evidence of whole-brain volume deficits, and modern neuropathology studies have uncovered provocative clues pointing to alterations in the microscopic neuroanatomy in schizophrenia.

The advent of modern neuroimaging techniques has allowed detailed analysis of brain structures and has significantly shaped our understanding of the neural basis of schizophrenia. CT studies documenting significant enlargement of cerebral ventricles and decrease in overall brain volume in subjects with schizophrenia (relative to healthy control subjects) have provided the first compelling neuroimaging results indicating that schizophrenia is a brain-based disorder (Johnstone et al. 1976). More recent MRI volumetric studies have also identified several specific regions of decreased volume, including the prefrontal and medial temporal structures and lateral temporal cortex and thalamus (Harrison 1999). One meta-analysis of MRI studies involving first-episode subjects showed highly significant reductions in total brain volume and increased ventricular volume (Steen et al. 2006), suggesting that these findings are not just the result of disease chronicity or medication exposure.

Modern neuropathology studies have identified alterations not previously appreciated in the brains of individuals with schizophrenia. A review of the literature showed consistent findings, including reduction in cortical neuronal size, reduction in axonal and dendritic arborization, and reduction in the number of thalamic neurons. The latter finding involved loss of neurons in the mediodorsal nucleus of the thalamus, particularly in the subnucleus that projects to the dorsolateral prefrontal cortex (Popken et al. 2000).

The development of diffusion tensor imaging, a magnetic resonance–based technique, has allowed researchers to measure white fiber integrity in the brain, thereby testing the hypothesis that schizophrenia is a result of diminished connectivity between brain regions. A growing number of studies are finding loss of white fiber integrity in many areas, such as in tracts connecting the prefrontal and temporal cortices (for a review, see Kubicki et al. 2007).

Cognitive and Information Processing Deficits

Cognitive deficits have been recognized as an important feature of schizophrenia since the beginning of efforts to systematically study this condition. In the past 20 years, there has been renewed interest in studying cognitive dysfunction in schizophrenia as a way to understand its pathophysiology.

Evidence that cognition is a core feature of schizophrenia comes from many fronts. First, studies have documented a fairly strong correlation between cognitive deficits and functional status. This is in distinction to psychotic symptoms, which generally do not correlate well with functional status. Second, cognitive deficits are very common among individuals with schizophrenia. They predate the onset of psychotic symptoms, and they are present in unaffected first-degree relatives and identical twins.

Disturbances in cognitive control (the coordination of thought and actions), attention, language, and memory have been documented by several researchers who used diverse paradigms. Some investigators have attempted to develop comprehensive cognitive models of schizophrenia that could explain many of the behavioral deficits and symptoms of schizophrenia. Goldman-Rakic (1994) proposed that working memory, the maintenance of information "on-line" to guide behavior, is the fundamental disturbance in schizophrenia. She further proposed that the cognitive deficits and symptoms such as disorganization in speech and actions are manifestations of working memory deficits. Cohen et al. (1999) proposed the context-processing deficit model for schizophrenia. They defined *context* as the conjunction of items, rules, and goals required to guide behavior or decisions. According to the context-processing model, many of the diverse cognitive deficits seen in schizophrenia can be reduced to this inability to hold diverse representations in mind. Andreasen et al. (1998) proposed the cognitive dysmetria model of schizophrenia, in which the primary deficit is in the inability of patients to coordinate mental activity rapidly and efficiently in a task-appropriate manner.

Early Sensory-Processing Deficits

Dysfunction in higher-order cognitive processes has now been firmly established; however, another line of research is investigating the hypothesis that deficits in early sensory processing are a fundamental aspect of schizophrenia. Some have proposed that these early sensory deficits may contribute to higher-order cognitive deficits (Brenner et al. 2002; Javitt et al. 1997; Saccuzzo and Braff 1981). The visual and auditory systems have been the most well studied.

In the visual domain, studies examining the earliest processes in visual perception have detected deficits in schizophrenia.

In the auditory domain, early sensory deficits have been found with auditory evoked response potentials (ERPs). Patients have abnormalities in the so-called P50 suppression. This can be viewed as a type of habituation in which the repetition of a sensory event results in a dampening of the neural response. Patients do not show this P50 suppression with the second auditory stimulus.

This has been interpreted as the inability of patients to gate sensory information properly.

Affect Processing

Increasing attention is being paid to the study of affect and related processes in schizophrenia. These affect studies can be further categorized as those focusing on emotional expression, recognition of emotional signals, and the subjective experiencing of emotions.

Deficits in the emotional expressivity of patients (e.g., blunted or flat affect) are perhaps the single most visibly apparent symptom of schizophrenia. Other than the distressed expressions associated with psychosis, a marked decrease in the emotional expressivity and responsivity of the face occurs in schizophrenia (Berenbaum and Oltmanns 1992). Contrary to the belief that diminished expression of emotion reflects diminished experience of emotion, patients, in general, appear not to have a subjective experiential deficit (Berenbaum and Oltmanns 1992; Earnst and Kring 1999). This is true even in patients with the deficit syndrome or a predominance of blunted affect.

Social Cognition

As is the case with affect, the interest in examining deficits in social functioning in schizophrenia has greatly expanded. Abnormalities in social functions often occur during the prodromal phase (Davidson et al. 1999), at the time of initial diagnosis, and throughout the course of illness (Addington and Addington 2000). Studies on social cognition have identified two general areas of abnormality in schizophrenia: theory of mind and social perceptions (Pinkham et al. 2003). *Theory of mind* refers to the capacity to 1) understand that the mental state (beliefs, intentions, and perspectives) of others is separate and distinct from one's own and 2) make inferences about another's intentions. Studies have shown that patients with schizophrenia lack theory of mind skills (Corcoran et al. 1995; Frith and Corcoran 1996). *Social perception,* the ability to recognize information governing appropriate social behavior, also consistently has been shown to be abnormal in schizophrenia. The facial affect recognition deficits are an important example of a social perception dysfunction.

Functional Neuroimaging

Functional neuroimaging allows researchers to identify diseased brain regions and abnormal cognitive processes in schizophrenia by assessing the neural functional correlates of a given cognitive task. The identification of dysfunctional regions provides information that can inform and constrain hypotheses in studies that are using other research methods. For example, the discovery of abnormal engagement of the dorsolateral prefrontal cortex has been very important in guiding postmortem and genetic studies seeking the cellular and molecular basis of higher-order cognitive deficits in schizophrenia.

Functional Imaging Studies of Higher-Order Cognitive Deficits

Although modern functional neuroimaging studies are beginning to uncover the neural correlates of most clusters of clinical features of schizophrenia, including those associated with deficits in early sensory, affective, and social processes mentioned earlier, most functional neuroimaging studies have historically focused on higher-order cognitive deficits. These studies point to abnormalities in several multimodal associative brain regions. These include deficits in the anterior cingulate cortex, superior temporal gyrus, and medial temporal cortex. In the past 20 years, numerous neuroimaging studies have generally supported the notion of a dysfunctional dorsolateral prefrontal cortex in schizophrenia across different imaging modalities and cognitive paradigms (Callicott et al. 2000; Manoach et al. 2000; Perlstein et al. 2001).

Neural Basis of Symptoms

Functional neuroimaging has made significant contributions to our understanding of the neural basis of the clinical features of schizophrenia.

Broadly following the theories set forth by Goldman-Rakic and others, a series of functional imaging studies has determined that the degree of activation of the dorsolateral prefrontal cortex in schizophrenia is highly correlated with clinical measures of cognitive and behavioral disorganization (Perlstein et al. 2001).

Another series of studies is elucidating the neural basis of auditory hallucinations. Auditory hallucinations appear to be the result of abnormal activation of the neural system serving auditory sensory processing. In one study, the onset and offset of the hallucinations correlated with the engagement and disengagement of the primary auditory cortex (Dierks et al. 1999).

Functional neuroimaging studies have provided support for a novel treatment strategy targeting auditory hallucinations refractory to medications. Functional MRI (fMRI) studies have shown overactivation in the temporal-parietal cortex during auditory hallucinations. A large clinical study reported that repetitive transcranial magnetic stimulation (rTMS) of the left temporal-parietal region is a safe and effective method to reduce the severity of auditory hallucinations in medication-resistant subjects with schizophrenia (Hoffman et al. 2005).

Intervention and Management

Antipsychotic Medications

Mechanism of Action

To date, more than 30 medications from 11 different chemical classes have been introduced worldwide for the treatment of schizophrenia (Ban 2004). These are generally identified as first-generation antipsychotics or second-generation antipsychotics, also commonly known as "atypical" antipsychotics.

First-generation antipsychotics (typified by haloperidol) all have in common a high affinity for D_2 receptors, and the clinical efficacy of these medications is strongly related to binding affinity for these receptors (Seeman et al. 1976). Studies in which PET was used found that clinical antipsychotic effects occurred at doses at which striatal D_2 receptor occupancy was 65%–70%, whereas D_2 receptor occupancy greater than 80% was associated with a significantly increased incidence of extrapyramidal side effects (EPS) (Remington and Kapur 1999). These studies also have found that at therapeutic doses, first-generation antipsychotics block D_2-like receptors to an equal degree in limbic cortical areas and the striatum, which is also consistent with the relatively narrow range of antipsychotic efficacy in the absence of EPS (Xiberas et al. 2001). The precise cellular feature of altered dopaminergic activity that provides the basis for clinical efficacy remains an active area of investigation. A leading hypothesis suggests that acute administration of these medications is associated with antagonism of D_2 autoreceptors on dopaminergic nerve terminals, leading to a depolarization inactivation of ion channels at those terminals and a resulting incapacity of propagating action potentials to further depolarize the terminal, thus chronically blocking dopamine release into the synapse (Grace et al. 1997).

In contrast, the six second-generation antipsychotics that are currently available in the United States are more heterogeneous in their profile of dopamine receptor antagonism. Risperidone, for example, has D_2 antagonism that is within the range of that for first-generation antipsychotics and, consequently, at therapeutic doses is associated with rates of EPS intermediate between first-generation antipsychotics and other second-generation antipsychotics. Other second-generation antipsychotics, such as clozapine and quetiapine, show minimal D_2 receptor

binding at therapeutic doses (Miyamoto et al. 2005). These medications (including the other available second-generation antipsychotics olanzapine, ziprasidone, and aripiprazole) show very heterogeneous profiles of binding at other dopamine receptors.

A leading current hypothesis (the "fast-off" hypothesis) suggests that the relative lack of EPS stemming from the use of these medications may be a result of the relatively faster rate of dissociation of these agents from D_2 receptors. This faster dissociation rate would be expected to more optimally accommodate normal physiological dopamine transmission. In contrast, a competing hypothesis of what constitutes "atypicality" emphasizes the serotonergic receptor activity (5-HT_{2A} and 5-HT_{2C} antagonism and 5-HT_{1A} agonism) that is found among second-generation antipsychotics. These actions are associated with enhanced dopamine and glutamate in prefrontal relative to subcortical areas, and in particular, the ratio of 5-HT_{2A} to D_2 blockade may prevent EPS and remediate negative symptoms of schizophrenia in a manner superior to the first-generation antipsychotics (Meltzer et al. 2003). In addition, aripiprazole is unique as a D_2 partial agonist, which may stabilize elevated rates of dopamine transmission while avoiding a degree of dopamine blockade necessary for EPS.

It also should be emphasized here that all antipsychotics (first- and second-generation antipsychotics) have high-affinity binding at a range of other monoamine receptors in the brain, which may be partly responsible for their efficacy but is well established as the basis for many of their side effects. This includes antagonism at muscarinic, histaminergic, and α-adrenergic receptors, with predictable autonomic effects. In addition, the monoaminergic transporter–blocking effects and 5-HT_{1A} receptor partial agonism or antagonism shown by some second-generation antipsychotics suggest that these medications may exert antidepressant and anxiolytic effects as well.

Clinical Comparison of Second-Generation Antipsychotics With First-Generation Antipsychotics

Second-generation antipsychotics appear to have efficacy in treatment of positive symptoms that is comparable to that of first-generation antipsychotics (Miyamoto et al. 2005). However, they are consistently superior to first-generation antipsychotics (and placebo) in the treatment of negative symptoms, which, as indicated earlier, are important determinants of functional impairment among patients with schizophrenia. Some evidence indicates that second-generation antipsychotics (clozapine in particular) show greater efficacy in patients with treatment-refractory schizophrenia (McEvoy et al. 2006; Miyamoto et al. 2005). It remains unclear whether similar rates of response to first-generation antipsychotics would be seen after nonresponse to second-generation antipsychotics.

Second-generation antipsychotics also have been proposed to exert greater effects on the remediation of cognitive deficits in schizophrenia, and this constitutes a fundamental feature of atypicality. However, the empirical literature has been quite inconsistent on this question. The second-generation antipsychotics may have a lower liability for cognitive performance (compared with first-generation antipsychotics) rather than a greater efficacy. Furthermore, there has been a general lack of hypothesis development to lead investigators from the profile of neurochemical effects to the hypothesized cognitive efficacy of these medications. This is an important area of research because novel medications for schizophrenia are likely to be developed specifically to target cognitive dysfunction. Neurotransmitter systems under consideration as future therapeutic targets for both symptomatic and cognitive remediation currently include glutamate, GABA, acetylcholine, cannabinoid and peptide systems, and brain neurotrophic factors (Miyamoto et al. 2005).

In contrast, the differences between second- and first-generation antipsychotics in side-effect profiles have significant clinical implications. At present, the empirical literature strongly indicates that second-generation antipsychotics are superior to first-generation antipsychotics in the lower incidence of EPS resulting from their use. It appears likely that the incidence of tardive dyskinesia—a persistent, disfiguring, and treatment-refractory movement disturbance that emerges with chronic antipsychotic treatment and that represents an important cause of nonadherence—will be lower with second-generation antipsychotics. Other side effects of first-generation antipsychotic treatment that are lessened or nonexistent with second-generation antipsychotics include hyperprolactinemia and ocular effects in the lens and retina. In contrast, the second-generation antipsychotics as a group have been increasingly associated with significant weight gain, hyperlipidemia, insulin resistance and diabetes mellitus onset, prolonged QTc interval, and other cardiovascular complications (Newcomer 2004). These are important consequences of second-generation antipsychotic treatment and for some patients may lead to serious long-term health risks, as well as antipsychotic nonadherence and subsequent risk of relapse. Nevertheless, treatment with second-generation antipsychotics appears to be associated with a greater sense of well-being among patients, and this appears to be a major factor in the improved rates of compliance for these medications as a group, compared with first-generation antipsychotics (Naber et al. 2004). It remains to be adequately tested whether these two groups of medications have differential benefits for employment, productivity, or other measures of psychosocial function among patients with schizophrenia (Percudani et al. 2004).

In summary, several literature reviews have concluded that the overall clinical advantage of second-generation antipsychotics is either modest in magnitude or inadequately tested and that pharmaceutical industry influence on the study design, initiation, and reporting of clinical trials may have an inordinate effect on the state of the empirical literature (Miyamoto et al. 2005; Tandon and Fleischhacker 2005). This may be the case as well for determinations of comparative efficacy within the second-generation antipsychotic class (Heres et al. 2006). These investigators generally emphasize that both first- and second-generation antipsychotics are superior to placebo in the treatment of most features of schizophrenia, that the selection of medications for individual patients continues to be guided largely by side-effect profiles, and that the full antipsychotic pharmacopoeia should remain in consideration in the approach to an individual patient with schizophrenia.

Treatment of Acute Psychosis

The acute psychotic phase of schizophrenia is frequently accompanied by mood symptoms and behavioral activation such as agitation, which may appear as extreme states of anxiety, as well as hostility and aggressive and impulsive behavior. This phase of illness is encountered typically in the medical or psychiatric emergency department but is occasionally seen in outpatient clinic settings. The initial response should be a rapid and reliable determination of the acute risk that the patient poses to him- or herself or others, which may be influenced by virtually all of the presenting symptoms (as well as history, etiological factors, and so on). Immediate hospitalization may be indicated both to ensure physical safety and to facilitate the initiation of medications. In addition, the clinician should assess the possibility of other etiologies for psychosis, such as substance-induced and mood-related psychosis, because these disorders are common causes of acute psychosis, particularly when the diagnosis of schizophrenia has not been previously established.

Regardless of the etiology, pharmacological approaches to acute psychosis are well established in the rapid management of psychotic and behavioral symptoms. Repeated doses of antipsychotics are often necessary in the short term in inpatient settings; however, rapid loading or sustained high-dose antipsychotic treatment regimens do not confer added benefit and increase the risk of adverse side effects. Adjunctive medications such as benzodiazepines are frequently used both for their sedating effects and to permit the use of relatively lower doses of antipsychotics. Prophylaxis of EPS with the use of anticholinergic medications is also often indicated, particularly because EPS has a higher incidence in younger patients (i.e., those most likely to present with a first episode of acute psychosis) and is a common cause of early nonadherence to antipsychotics.

An increasingly used alternative to the first-generation antipsychotics in acute psychosis is the second-generation antipsychotics, particularly those for which therapeutic blood levels can be quickly attained (e.g., olanzapine, risperidone) or those for which parenteral formulations are available (olanzapine, ziprasidone). Current evidence indicates that these medications are probably as effective in acute psychosis as the first-generation antipsychotics and are much better tolerated.

Treatment of First-Episode Psychosis

An increasingly common approach in the outpatient setting is to initiate low to moderate doses of second-generation antipsychotics, primarily in light of the improved patient satisfaction and compliance that may be largely a function of reduced rates of EPS. It should be recalled that this approach largely trades the higher long-term risk of tardive dyskinesia for lower but significant metabolic and cardiovascular risks.

The clinical response rates to both first- and second-generation antipsychotics are high in a first psychotic episode, up to 75% in some well-designed studies (Robinson et al. 2005). To date, the few studies comparing second-generation antipsychotics with first-generation antipsychotics have not found differential response rates, and the comparative efficacy among individual second-generation antipsychotics for first-episode psychosis remains to be studied (Robinson et al. 2005). A large percentage of first-episode patients respond within the first week of treatment, with response rates reaching a plateau in the subsequent 3 months.

In general, the early diagnosis and intervention in schizophrenia have been increasingly advocated. Those who experience greater treatment delays tend to have a much worse long-term prognosis (Wyatt and Henter 1998). Others have suggested that individuals with a prolonged duration of untreated psychosis may be experiencing an inherently more severe form of psychopathology and that the treatment delay may reflect rather than cause the relatively worse prognosis (McGlashan 1999). The consensus is that the earliest possible intervention is most likely to lead to the most rapid and complete recovery.

Maintenance Treatment in Schizophrenia

With the resolution of an acute psychotic episode, patients with schizophrenia are transitioned to maintenance treatment to optimize prevention of relapse to acute psychosis and to improve psychosocial function and general recovery. Proper maintenance treatment also often requires considerable clinical attention to the numerous comorbid psychiatric and medical conditions that are prevalent in schizophrenia and an important cause of poor outcomes, including premature death (Escamilla 2001; A.I. Green et al. 2003). Continuous treatment with effective antipsychotic medications is a cornerstone of intervention in this phase, given the need to minimize relapse risk. With successive relapses following antipsychotic discontinuation, the time required to achieve remission on resumption of treatment lengthens, and ultimately a treatment-refractory state may supervene (Lieberman 1993).

Once the diagnosis of schizophrenia is certain, antipsychotic medication should be continued indefinitely, in a manner analogous to the lifelong pharmacological treatment indicated for disorders such as diabetes mellitus and hypertension. Sustained treatment with antipsychotics may modify the long-term course of this illness (Tandon 1998). Alternative strategies such as full antipsychotic withdrawal in schizophrenic patients are associated with significantly increased rates of relapse, as high as 98% at 2 years in one study (Gitlin et al. 2001). In another study, the rate of relapse among schizophrenic patients who self-discontinued their antipsychotic medications was increased fivefold over the rates in those who continued treatment (Robinson et al. 1999). In addition, intermittent dosing is probably less efficacious in preventing relapse in comparison with continuous dosing (Robinson et al. 2005). Baldessarini et al. (1988) found in a review of the older empirical literature that antipsychotic dosages between 50 and 150 mg of chlorpromazine equivalents per day are adequate for most outpatients with chronic schizophrenia.

Problems with treatment adherence are often a significant factor in this phase of treatment with schizophrenic patients. Often, many factors such as intolerable side effects to medication, cognitive dysfunction, social withdrawal, interpersonal conflict, comorbid substance abuse, financial hardship, and other barriers to treatment access sharply limit the capacity of some patients to continue adequate treatment (Fenton et al. 1997). Comprehensive psychosocial support may be necessary for those patients who experience great difficulty adhering to treatment regimens (Zygmunt et al. 2002). In addition, a pharmacological strategy that may be favorable for many of these patients is the transition to depot (long-acting injection) forms of antipsychotics. These forms offer comparable symptom relief (largely avoiding first-pass hepatic metabolism, for instance) while EPS, sedation, and other side effects are well controlled, possibly because of slower rates of absorption compared with oral forms of antipsychotics. Treatment adherence is improved as a result of both increased tolerability and less frequent dosing and may lead to lower relapse rates (Davis et al. 1993). At present, among first-generation antipsychotics, haloperidol and fluphenazine are available in decanoate forms for intramuscular administration (typically given at 4-week and 2-week intervals, respectively); among the second-generation agents, risperidone is available in depot form. Depot antipsychotics are widely and effectively used in Europe and elsewhere and are quite cost-effective; this strategy remains dramatically underused in the maintenance treatment of schizophrenia in the United States.

Treatment-Refractory Schizophrenia

A significant percentage of schizophrenic patients (up to 40%, depending on how they are identified) can be considered to be poorly responsive to standard antipsychotic medications (Kane et al. 1988). Treatment-refractory states emphasize poor response of positive symptoms to antipsychotic medications, which may increase over time in these patients. In contrast, refractory negative symptoms and cognitive impairment are usually present at the first episode (Meltzer and Pringuey 1998).

Evidence is still very minimal to indicate which clinical features should guide the choice of an individual antipsychotic agent. A typical approach to the patient with no antipsychotic treatment history is for the clinician to initiate one medication on the basis of an optimized side-effect profile, with an attempt to reach an adequate trial (typically defined in treatment guidelines as 4–6 weeks with adequate adherence to 400–600 mg of chlorpromazine equivalents per day) before switching, which may be done in favor of a second medication that is either within or across antipsychotic groups (first- or second-generation antipsychotic). After two such trials with an incomplete clinical response, the

rate of response to a standard third antipsychotic trial is quite low, and alternative strategies should be considered.

The available evidence favors clozapine as the most effective antipsychotic for treatment-refractory schizophrenia, although treatment-resistant schizophrenia may respond to other second-generation antipsychotics as well (possibly at lower response rates relative to clozapine) (Conley and Kelly 2001). Unfortunately, as many as 40%–70% of patients with treatment-refractory schizophrenia also experience an inadequate response to clozapine. The public health effect of managing these patients is enormous; one estimate suggests that as a group they may account for up to 97% of the cost of schizophrenia (L.M. Davies and Drummond 1994).

Patients with treatment-refractory schizophrenia have been found to have relatively greater cortical atrophy on MRI (Stern et al. 1993) and a higher likelihood of altered cortical cell migration (Kirkpatrick et al. 1999), compared with those with treatment-responsive schizophrenia.

Other Adjunctive Biological Treatments for Schizophrenia

A range of other medications are used together with antipsychotics in the various phases of treatment of schizophrenia. Anticholinergic medications are a mainstay of treatment, serving as effective prophylaxis for EPS found in response to not only first-generation antipsychotics but occasionally second-generation antipsychotics (especially risperidone). Some second-generation antipsychotics such as clozapine and olanzapine have significant intrinsic anticholinergic activity, which may be partly responsible for their lower rates of EPS and obviates the need for a second anticholinergic agent. Benzodiazepines are also well used in the treatment of acute psychosis and are effective in the treatment of akathisia associated with antipsychotics. They are often used in maintenance treatment of psychotic symptoms and in the treatment of anxiety and insomnia commonly found in these patients. It remains unclear if benzodiazepines allow for the effective use of relatively lower doses of antipsychotics generally across large samples of schizophrenic patients; however, this may be the case for individual patients (Wolkowitz and Pickar 1991). Other adjunctive treatments that target co-occurring symptoms in schizophrenic patients include anticonvulsants (Hosak and Libiger 2002), β-blockers, and lithium for aggressive and impulsive behaviors and antidepressants for both depressive and anxiety disorders that are commonly found in schizophrenia (Escamilla 2001). These important symptoms confer a significant portion of the morbidity and public health effect of schizophrenia, including significant rates of suicide, and adequate treatment of these symptoms is essential to achieve clinical stability and recovery in these patients. Clinicians should remain mindful that the rate of drug–drug interactions increases and adherence decreases with increasing complexity of medication regimens, as for the treatment of medical and psychiatric illness in general.

Electroconvulsive therapy (ECT) is another treatment modality that may continue to have a role in the rapid treatment of acute and subacute states that are refractory to pharmacological intervention, particularly catatonia (Tharyan and Adams 2005). ECT treatment has been refined considerably over the years and now is quite safely administered, with minimal short-term adverse events and no evidence for long-term morbidity associated with its use (Rasmussen et al. 2002). Nevertheless, access to ECT is limited in many treatment settings, and ECT has no apparent advantage over pharmacological treatment in the maintenance phase of schizophrenia. Another biologically based treatment modality currently being evaluated for patients with schizophrenia is rTMS, which has shown preliminary efficacy in reducing the severity of auditory hallucinations (Hoffman et al. 2000).

Psychosocial Treatments for Schizophrenia

Overview: The Importance of Integrated Treatment for Schizophrenia

Psychosocial treatment is an essential element of the treatment needs of all patients with schizophrenia. In general, all of the interventions described in this subsection are compatible not only with one another but also with pharmacological treatment (Lauriello et al. 2003). Because schizophrenia is a complex disorder that affects virtually every psychological and functional domain, a comprehensive treatment approach to schizophrenia must necessarily address a broad spectrum of problems. Lehman (1999) proposed a framework for evaluating outcomes in schizophrenia, which was based on the findings of a National Institute of Mental Health expert panel. Four domains were identified: clinical, rehabilitative, humanitarian, and public welfare. The clinical domain includes psychopathology and treatment issues. The rehabilitative domain includes social and vocational function. The humanitarian domain includes quality of life, subjective well-being, and other patient-centered measures, and the public welfare domain includes optimizing and resolving the rights of the patients with the welfare of the community at large. It is increasingly recognized that integration of care is associated with maximal benefit for patients with schizophrenia, particularly those who are the sickest and are the highest users of services (Lenroot et al. 2003). A cornerstone of this perspective is the establishment and maintenance of the alliance not only with the patient but also with families and other care and service providers. This is also of increasing importance given the progressive shifting of the locus of care for the most severely chronically disabled schizophrenic patients—from the large state hospitals of an earlier era to the community in the present.

Case Management and Assertive Community Treatment

Case management is fundamentally a method of coordinating services for the patient in the community. In this model, an individual case manager (typically, a licensed social worker) serves a role somewhat analogous to that of a primary care physician, assessing and prioritizing the needs of the patient, developing an integrated care plan, arranging for provision of this care, and serving as the patient's primary point of contact in the mental health system. Case managers interact with both social service agencies and clinicians to achieve and maintain access to entitlements, social services, and clinical care. Case management aims to maintain the patient in the system of care, to permit the most efficacious treatment in the least restrictive setting, and to optimize outcome, particularly quality of life and social function.

One particularly successful form of case management is referred to in the United States as Assertive Community Treatment (ACT). Candidates for this care are typically those with the highest service needs and are referred to a multidisciplinary team, often composed of the case manager (licensed social worker or psychologist), psychiatric nurse, psychiatrist, and other psychiatric support staff. ACT approaches have much the same goals as case management in general, with a more aggressive strategy targeted at a select population of the highest users of services. These approaches have been increasingly studied and in most studies appear to reduce the time spent in the hospital (Bustillo et al. 2001) and improve the stability of housing maintenance (Issakidis et al. 1999).

Cognitive-Behavioral Therapy

Some of the earliest documented experience with cognitive-behavioral therapy (CBT) addressed cases of schizophrenia. CBT remains more popular in the United Kingdom than in the United States for the treatment of schizophrenia (Turkington et al. 2006). Several features of CBT techniques are highly modified for use with schizophrenic patients. For instance, a relatively greater emphasis is placed on development of the therapeutic alliance as it arises from the patient's perspective. This may include a neutral stance with respect to the patient's delusional content to promote discovery and understanding. The clinician also works to identify and develop alternative explanations of symptoms that are acceptable to both patient and therapist. Another technique involves the use of "peripheral questioning," in which the therapist facilitates the patient to elaborate the belief system, and a related approach of "inference chaining," in which the personalized meaning and string of logic underlying a delusional structure are identified. These strategies are used together with a graded reality testing, with the goal of introducing doubt and possible alternative hypotheses. Cognitive-behavioral therapists attempt to normalize the patient's experience when it is appropriate and in general reduce the effect of positive symptoms. CBT is probably not advisable when the patient is too paranoid, withdrawn, or cognitively impaired to engage in treatment. However, CBT does not require that the patient accept the diagnosis of schizophrenia in order to be beneficial, because it is more focused on symptoms than on the diagnosis per se. It is also very compatible with biological approaches to the understanding and treatment of schizophrenia (Turkington et al. 2006).

CBT is generally very amenable to empirical research. Numerous randomized, controlled studies have shown that CBT is associated with greater improvement in symptom severity relative to both supportive therapy and treatment as usual (Dickerson and Lehman 2006; Turkington et al. 2006). In addition, patients with a first-episode psychosis do appear to benefit from CBT with reduced inpatient days, better treatment adherence, and reduced symptoms, relative to control treatments (Penn et al. 2005).

Cognitive Remediation and Rehabilitation

Cognitive remediation and rehabilitation emphasize the cognitive deficits that are readily evident in schizophrenia and are associated with functional impairment. Techniques include training exercises that have been successfully used in diverse clinical populations such as focal brain-injured and learning-disabled individuals. Computer-based or "pencil-and-paper" tasks guide patients through successive levels of skill in performing cognitive tasks of attention, memory, cognitive flexibility, problem solving, and other functions that are impaired in these patients. Treatment courses typically extend from 1 to 6 months with multiple sessions each week. The evidence to date suggests that certain cognitive functions (such as problem solving) may improve with this type of treatment, and modest effects on social function have been observed in some studies (Bellack et al. 1999).

Social Skills–Based Therapies

Social skills have been defined by Bellack and Mueser (1993) as "specific response capabilities necessary for effective social performance." Deficits in these functions are well established in schizophrenia. Social skills training aims to improve social function in patients by training the behavioral repertoire called on in social settings. One form of training, the basic model, decomposes complex social sequences into simpler components, with subsequent corrective training in which role-playing is used, and the settings should be as naturalistic as possible. In contrast, the social problem-solving model emphasizes improvements in cognitive functions that are thought to underlie social dysfunction. Deficits in receptive and expressive communicatory functions are addressed in the context of treatment adherence, basic social interactions, recreation, and general self-care. The social problem-solving model is associated with improvements in

measures of social adjustment that may last at least a few years (Liberman et al. 1998).

Vocational Rehabilitation

The rate of continuous employment in a competitive setting (outside of a rehabilitation or "sheltered" work setting) among patients with schizophrenia is probably much lower than 20% in most communities (Lehman 1995). This therefore represents an important goal for improved functional status in schizophrenia. Sheltered work settings provide an environment for patients in which the work and social demands are manageable and the interpersonal environment is accepting of limitations caused by the patient's illness. A contemporary example is the Compensated Work Therapy offered in Department of Veterans Affairs outpatient settings. Other vocational services include more formal job training programs. Individualized placement, with some accommodation of patient preferences; minimization of preemployment screening or pretraining; and sustained periods of support are important to the patient's success. Attainment of employment in competitive settings in the community does appear to be more frequent after these types of vocational rehabilitation compared with more traditional vocational rehabilitation (Bustillo et al. 2001).

Family Therapy

Interventions that involve working with the families of those with schizophrenia emphasize the importance of the family as the primary environment in which the disease is expressed and modified in a reciprocal manner and that the family is the first line of support for most patients. Intact, adequately functioning family environments offer an important buffer for the symptoms of schizophrenia and are associated with a relatively better prognosis for the patient. Reducing family distress and fostering a collaborative approach to treatment involving the patient, family, and treatment team are important goals for patients at all stages of illness. Approaches to these families often include psychoeducation and psychological support, which aid family members in anticipation of the patient's illness expression, and response strategies that help both patient and relatives optimally cope with the patient's illness.

The various forms of family therapy are probably equally efficacious (Penn and Mueser 1996) for all patients with schizophrenia and their families. An earlier review of 14 studies found that family therapy reduced relapse rates considerably (Carpenter 1996). Some of the benefit of family therapy may be derived from enhanced adherence to other concurrent treatments. This treatment approach appears cost-effective, may be useful in ethnic and cultural minority families, and in some cases has been structured in treatment manuals, suggesting a potential for wider application in the community (Bustillo et al. 2001).

Individual Psychotherapy

Following the landmark studies by May et al. (1981) and Gunderson et al. (1984), in which no benefit of individual psychoanalytically oriented psychotherapy was found for patients with schizophrenia, this treatment approach has been largely abandoned in the treatment of schizophrenia. At present, individual psychotherapy is generally considered to elevate the risk for psychotic decompensation, probably because of the unstructured and anxiety-provoking nature of this treatment. In contrast, supportive therapy approaches appear to be superior to treatment as usual in studies in which the primary focus is on the relative efficacy of CBT. Supportive therapy encompasses a diverse set of approaches to the patient, yet all have in common the goal of providing reassurance, guidance, and an interpersonal environment that is stable, predictable, and tolerant of the patient's expression, symptoms, and problems in living. It is generally less systematic and less symptom-focused than CBT. One particular approach has been termed *personal therapy*, which was developed by Hogarty et al.

(1995). It uses techniques that are individualized for the patient, with progressive focus on stress reduction first, followed by cognitive reframing, and later vocational rehabilitation, as the emphasis follows the patient's stage of recovery. Sessions are conducted weekly, with each session typically lasting 30–45 minutes. Empirical evaluation found personal therapy to exert relatively greater benefit for social adjustment compared with other forms of individual or family therapy (Hogarty et al. 1997).

Related Psychotic Disorders

Schizoaffective Disorder

The construct of schizoaffective disorder addresses individuals who have prominent features of both schizophrenia and major mood disorders.

The diagnosis of schizoaffective disorder has remained somewhat ambiguous, although it has nevertheless gained in recognition and is increasingly assigned to individuals in clinical settings. Several hypothetical ways to conceptualize these patients currently exist: 1) as having two coexisting disorders (schizophrenia and a mood disorder), 2) as having primarily schizophrenia with incidental mood symptoms, 3) as having primarily a mood disorder with some features of schizophrenia, or 4) as representing a distinct third group that has only phenomenological similarity to the two major diagnostic origins. Alternatively, patients with schizoaffective disorder may be a heterogeneous group in which some are more accurately deemed to have schizophrenia, whereas others have a mood disorder.

The epidemiological aspects of schizoaffective disorder largely remain to be determined. The base prevalence may be less than 1% in the community, although the disorder is found at much higher rates in clinical settings. The relatives of patients with schizoaffective disorder have an elevated risk for both schizophrenia and mood disorders.

Overall, the prognosis for schizoaffective patients is intermediate between that for patients with schizophrenia and that for patients with mood disorders. Predictors of poor prognosis in schizoaffective disorder include many of those also established for schizophrenia, including a family history of schizophrenia, poor premorbid function, insidious onset, early age at onset, lack of a clear precipitating factor, predominance of psychotic symptoms, and poor recovery between episodes. With regard to empirical studies of treatment, study samples composed solely of schizoaffective patients are rare; however, many studies of pharmacological treatment in schizophrenia include significant numbers of schizoaffective patients (C.M. Adler and Strakowski 2003). The treatment for schizoaffective disorder is largely consistent with that for schizophrenia and mood disorders—atypical antipsychotics, mood stabilizers, and antidepressants are used to target the same symptomatology when it is found in schizoaffective disorder (C.M. Adler and Strakowski 2003). Little evidence favors one combination regimen over another in this illness. Patients with treatment-refractory schizoaffective disorder should be approached in a manner similar to that for patients with treatment-refractory schizophrenia or mood disorders.

Delusional Disorder

Delusional disorder is characterized by the presence of one or more nonbizarre delusions in the relative absence of other symptoms of psychosis, and criterion A for schizophrenia has not been met. This is the central DSM-IV-TR diagnostic criterion and the only one that requires the presence of a particular symptom or sign. The delusions tend to be systematized, with associated affect that is consistent with the delusional belief. However, cognitive function and personality fea-

tures tend to remain intact (although the delusional belief itself may have circumscribed effects on interpersonal function). This diagnosis requires adequate exclusion of other more common psychotic disorders, such as schizophrenia, mood disorders, and dementia, and other medical etiologies.

Many patients will develop other psychotic symptoms leading to the diagnosis of schizophrenia. However, the pattern of clinical features and familial aggregation suggest that delusional disorder should not be classified as a subtype of schizophrenia or other psychotic disorders (Cardno and McGuffin 2006).

The pathophysiology of delusional disorder remains obscure. Most delusional disorder patients experience the delusional belief as "ego-syntonic," which means that the delusional thought is experienced as consistent with the patients' expectations, sense of self, and sense of reality in general. This sharply limits the capacity for insight into the nature of the belief, and as a result, patients generally do not have any incentive to enter mental health treatment because the subjective distress they feel is attributed to a rigid sense of the "state of affairs" in their environment rather than a psychological state in need of remediation. In addition, patients generally do not come to the attention of the mental health system because aggressive behavior or decline in self-care (which would prompt intervention from law enforcement, emergency medical, or social services) is not typical. However, a small percentage of these patients may be at significant risk for aggressive behavior, particularly those with persecutory delusions, which may prompt them to "defend" or retaliate against the perceived source of malevolence.

The empirical evidence for antipsychotic use in delusional disorder remains scant, and treatment of delusions in this disorder largely proceeds on the basis of established efficacy against delusions in schizophrenia (Smith and Buckley 2006).

Schizophreniform Disorder and Brief Psychotic Disorder

In DSM-IV-TR, the criteria for schizophreniform disorder are largely coincident with those for schizophrenia, except that the duration of symptoms in criterion A is shorter—in this case, longer than 1 month but less than 6 months. A large study of first-admission patients with a schizophreniform disorder diagnosis found that only 19% retained this diagnosis at 24-month follow-up, with 13% later receiving a mood disorder diagnosis. In contrast, 92% of the subsample who had initially received a schizophrenia diagnosis retained that diagnosis at follow-up (Naz et al. 2003). It appears likely that at the time of diagnosis with this disorder, patients in general are early in the course of overt illness, experiencing psychotic symptoms but without the duration criterion met for schizophrenia. The relatively better prognosis for these patients as a group, compared with patients identified as having schizophrenia at first encounter, may reflect the percentage who go on to identified mood disorders and also that, as a group, these patients have not endured repeated or sustained psychotic episodes and steady functional decline, as would a percentage of any group with a clearly established diagnosis of schizophrenia.

Brief psychotic disorder, on the other hand, is distinguished from schizophrenia as a DSM-IV-TR diagnostic category by the abrupt onset of overt psychotic symptoms (the same set of positive psychotic symptoms as in criterion A for schizophrenia), but the symptoms last for less than 1 month. Individuals whose symptoms meet the criteria for this disorder do not have a history of functional decline or signs that may be retrospectively attributed to a prodrome. In addition, the psychotic symptoms associated with the diagnosis tend to be precipitated more commonly by acute stressors, be associated with acute mood changes, and generally respond well to treatment. These patients as a group also have minimal negative symptoms and a

significantly better long-term prognosis than do patients with schizophrenia (on average). As with schizophreniform disorder, this diagnostic entity appears to be highly heterogeneous and reflects both the nonpathognomonic nature of psychotic symptoms and the fact that this diagnosis is established quite early in the course of illness, before certainty can be reached about a specific and enduring diagnosis with resulting implications for treatment and prognosis.

Conclusion

Our understanding of schizophrenia has evolved significantly in the era of modern medicine. This includes significant refinement in how it is identified and a deepened understanding of the natural course of illness, the relation of schizophrenia to boundary conditions, the disturbances in brain structure and function that underlie cognitive and functional deficits, and crucially the genetic and environmental factors that modify the appearance and clinical course of this illness. This progress has accelerated in recent years. The pathophysiology underlying this illness has yet to be definitively elucidated, but advances in neuroscience, genetics, and cognitive science are all being brought to bear on one of the most devastating illnesses to strike at human experience. The grail in this effort will be to attain a measure of effective primary or secondary prevention. For those who have the illness and those who care for them, advances in both psychopharmacological and psychological treatment approaches offer renewed hope that the effects of the illness can be mitigated and that patients may be increasingly able to retain a sense of well-being and a functional role in society. At the level of the individual, the family, and society, the effect of this illness remains enormous, and any breakthrough in prevention and treatment also stands to alleviate a global burden of one of humankind's most significant diseases.

Key Points

- Among medical illnesses, schizophrenia is one of the most serious for the afflicted individual, the family of the patient, and society at large.

- Schizophrenia, like psychiatric illness in general, occurs as a function of both a genetic predisposition and environmental factors.

- Schizophrenia is characterized by cognitive, perceptual, behavioral, and social disturbances and has profound consequences for the individual's capacity for autonomy and function in the community.

- Schizophrenia is currently conceived of as a neurodevelopmental disorder, with disturbances in development across a range of epochs, from early gestation through late adolescence.

- The pathophysiology of schizophrenia involves several anatomical regions and neurotransmitter and other functional systems in the brain.

- The various symptoms and problems in living that schizophrenic patients experience can be treated with the full range of treatment modalities currently available in psychiatry, including pharmacological and psychosocial approaches.

- Although many patients with schizophrenia endure relapsing and remitting periods of illness, with a significant decline in function over the early period of illness, many can retain a measure of well-being, symptom control, and autonomy in the community.

- Research into the causes, clinical course, and treatment of schizophrenia has shown considerable progress in recent times and shows promise for significant advances in the future treatment of this disorder.

Suggested Readings

Andreasen NC: Schizophrenia: the fundamental questions. Brain Res Brain Res Rev 31:106–112, 2000

Compton WM, Guze SB: The neo-Kraepelinian revolution in psychiatric diagnosis. Eur Arch Psychiatry Clin Neurosci 245:196–201, 1995

Lewis DA, Levitt P: Schizophrenia as a disorder of neurodevelopment. Annu Rev Neurosci 25:409–432, 2002

Miyamoto S, Duncan GE, Marx CE, et al: Treatments for schizophrenia: a critical review of pharmacology and mechanisms of action of antipsychotic drugs. Mol Psychiatry 10:79–104, 2005

Mueser KT, McGurk SR: Schizophrenia. Lancet 363:2063–2072, 2004

Online Resources

Schizophrenia.com: http://www.schizophrenia.com (general site, appropriate for families and lay public)

Schizophrenia Research Forum: http://www.schizophreniaforum.org (research-oriented site)

References

Abi-Dargham A, Rodenhiser J, Printz D, et al: Increased baseline occupancy of D2 receptors by dopamine in schizophrenia. Proc Natl Acad Sci U S A 97:8104–8109, 2000

Abi-Dargham A, Mawlawi O, Lombardo I, et al: Prefrontal dopamine D1 receptors and working memory in schizophrenia. J Neurosci 22:3708–3719, 2002

Addington J, Addington D: Neurocognitive and social functioning in schizophrenia: a 2.5 year follow-up study. Schizophr Res 44:47–56, 2000

Adler CM, Strakowski SM: Boundaries of schizophrenia. Psychiatr Clin North Am 26:1–23, 2003

Adler LE, Hoffer LJ, Griffith J, et al: Normalization by nicotine of deficient auditory sensory gating in the relatives of schizophrenics. Biol Psychiatry 32:607–616, 1992

Akbarian S, Kim JJ, Potkin SG, et al: Gene expression for glutamic acid decarboxylase is reduced without loss of neurons in prefrontal cortex of schizophrenics. Arch Gen Psychiatry 52:258–266, 1995

American Psychiatric Association: Diagnostic and Statistical Manual of Mental Disorders, 3rd Edition. Washington, DC, American Psychiatric Association, 1980

American Psychiatric Association: Diagnostic and Statistical Manual of Mental Disorders, 4th Edition, Text Revision. Washington, DC, American Psychiatric Association, 2000

Andreasen NC: The evolving concept of schizophrenia: from Kraepelin to the present and future. Schizophr Res 28:105–109, 1997

Andreasen NC: Schizophrenia: the fundamental questions. Brain Res Brain Res Rev 31:106–112, 2000

Andreasen NC, Paradiso S, O'Leary DS: "Cognitive dysmetria" as an integrative theory of schizophrenia: a dysfunction in cortical-subcortical-cerebellar circuitry? Schizophr Bull 24:203–218, 1998

Angermeyer MC, Goldstein JM, Kuehn L: Gender differences in schizophrenia: rehospitalization and community survival. Psychol Med 19:365–382, 1989

Angst J: Historical aspects of the dichotomy between manic-depressive disorders and schizophrenia. Schizophr Res 57:5–13, 2002

Badner JA, Gershon ES: Meta-analysis of whole-genome linkage scans of bipolar disorder and schizophrenia. Mol Psychiatry 7:405–411, 2002

Baldessarini RJ, Cohen BM, Teicher MH: Significance of neuroleptic dose and plasma level in the pharmacological treatment of psychoses. Arch Gen Psychiatry 45:79–91, 1988

Ban TA: Neuropsychopharmacology and the genetics of schizophrenia: a history of the diagnosis of schizophrenia. Prog Neuropsychopharmacol Biol Psychiatry 28:753–762, 2004

Bellack AS, Mueser KT: Psychosocial treatment for schizophrenia. Schizophr Bull 19:317–336, 1993

Bellack AS, Gold JM, Buchanan RW: Cognitive rehabilitation for schizophrenia: problems, prospects, and strategies. Schizophr Bull 25:257–274, 1999

Berenbaum H, Oltmanns TF: Emotional experience and expression in schizophrenia and depression. J Abnorm Psychol 101:37–44, 1992

Bilder RM, Mukherjee S, Rieder RO, et al: Symptomatic and neuropsychological components of defect states. Schizophr Bull 11:409–419, 1985

Brenner CA, Lysaker PH, Wilt MA, et al: Visual processing and neuropsychological function in schizophrenia and schizoaffective disorder. Psychiatry Res 111:125–136, 2002

Broome MR, Woolley JB, Tabraham P, et al: What causes the onset of psychosis? Schizophr Res 79:23–34, 2005

Brown AS, Begg MD, Gravenstein S, et al: Serologic evidence of prenatal influenza in the etiology of schizophrenia. Arch Gen Psychiatry 61:774–780, 2004

Bustillo J, Lauriello J, Horan W, et al: The psychosocial treatment of schizophrenia: an update. Am J Psychiatry 158:163–175, 2001

Callicott JH, Bertolino A, Mattay VS, et al: Physiological dysfunction of the dorsolateral prefrontal cortex in schizophrenia revisited. Cereb Cortex 10:1078–1092, 2000

Cannon M, Jones PB, Murray RM: Obstetric complications and schizophrenia: historical and meta-analytic review. Am J Psychiatry 159:1080–1092, 2002

Cardno AG, McGuffin P: Genetics and delusional disorder. Behav Sci Law 24:257–276, 2006

Carlsson A, Lindqvist M: Effect of chlorpromazine or haloperidol on formation of 3methoxytyramine and normetanephrine in mouse brain. Acta Pharmacol Toxicol (Copenh) 20:140–144, 1963

Carpenter WT Jr: Maintenance therapy of persons with schizophrenia. J Clin Psychiatry 57 (suppl 9):10–18, 1996

Carpenter WT Jr, Strauss JS: The prediction of outcome in schizophrenia, IV: eleven-year follow-up of the Washington IPSS cohort. J Nerv Ment Dis 179:517–525, 1991

Cohen JD, Barch DM, Carter C, et al: Context-processing deficits in schizophrenia: converging evidence from three theoretically motivated cognitive tasks. J Abnorm Psychol 108:120–133, 1999

Compton WM, Guze SB: The neo-Kraepelinian revolution in psychiatric diagnosis. Eur Arch Psychiatry Clin Neurosci 245:196–201, 1995

Conley RR, Kelly DL: Management of treatment resistance in schizophrenia. Biol Psychiatry 50:898–911, 2001

Corcoran R, Mercer G, Frith CD: Schizophrenia, symptomatology and social inference: investigating "theory of mind" in people with schizophrenia. Schizophr Res 17:5–13, 1995

Corfas G, Roy K, Buxbaum JD: Neuregulin 1-erbB signaling and the molecular/cellular basis of schizophrenia. Nat Neurosci 7:575–580, 2004

Creese I, Burt DR, Snyder SH: Dopamine receptor binding predicts clinical and pharmacological potencies of antischizophrenic drugs. Science 192:481–483, 1976

Davidson M, Reichenberg A, Rabinowitz J, et al: Behavioral and intellectual markers for schizophrenia in apparently healthy male adolescents. Am J Psychiatry 156:1328–1335, 1999

Davies G, Welham J, Chant D, et al: A systematic review and meta-analysis of Northern Hemisphere season of birth studies in schizophrenia. Schizophr Bull 29:587–593, 2003

Davies LM, Drummond MF: Economics and schizophrenia: the real cost. Br J Psychiatry Suppl (25):18–21, 1994

Davis JM, Kane JM, Marder SR, et al: Dose response of prophylactic antipsychotics. J Clin Psychiatry 54 (suppl): 24–30, 1993

Dickerson FB, Lehman AF: Evidence-based psychotherapy for schizophrenia. J Nerv Ment Dis 194:3–9, 2006

Dierks T, Linden DE, Jandl M, et al: Activation of Heschl's gyrus during auditory hallucinations. Neuron 22:615–621, 1999

Earnst KS, Kring AM: Emotional responding in deficit and non-deficit schizophrenia. Psychiatry Res 88:191–207, 1999

Escamilla MA: Diagnosis and treatment of mood disorders that co-occur with schizophrenia. Psychiatr Serv 52:911–919, 2001

Fenton WS, Blyler CR, Heinssen RK: Determinants of medication compliance in schizophrenia: empirical and clinical findings. Schizophr Bull 23:637–651, 1997

Frith CD, Corcoran R: Exploring "theory of mind" in people with schizophrenia. Psychol Med 26:521–530, 1996

Geller JL: A report on the "worst" state hospital recidivists in the US. Hosp Community Psychiatry 43:904–908, 1992

Gitlin M, Nuechterlein K, Subotnik KL, et al: Clinical outcome following neuroleptic discontinuation in patients with remitted recent-onset schizophrenia. Am J Psychiatry 158:1835–1842, 2001

Goldman-Rakic PS: Working memory dysfunction in schizophrenia. J Neuropsychiatry Clin Neurosci 6:348–357, 1994

Goodwin DW, Alderson P, Rosenthal R: Clinical significance of hallucinations in psychiatric disorders: a study of 116 hallucinatory patients. Arch Gen Psychiatry 24:76–80, 1971

Gottesman II: Schizophrenia Genesis: The Origins of Madness. New York, WH Freeman, 1991

Grace AA, Bunney BS, Moore H, et al: Dopamine-cell depolarization block as a model for the therapeutic actions of antipsychotic drugs. Trends Neurosci 20:31–37, 1997

Green AI, Canuso CM, Brenner MJ, et al: Detection and management of comorbidity in patients with schizophrenia. Psychiatr Clin North Am 26:115–139, 2003

Green MF: What are the functional consequences of neurocognitive deficits in schizophrenia? Am J Psychiatry 153:321–330, 1996

Gunderson JG, Frank AF, Katz HM, et al: Effects of psychotherapy in schizophrenia, II: comparative outcome of two forms of treatment. Schizophr Bull 10:564–598, 1984

Harrison PJ: The neuropathology of schizophrenia: a critical review of the data and their interpretation. Brain 122 (pt 4):593–624, 1999

Harrow M, Jobe TH: Longitudinal studies of outcome and recovery in schizophrenia and early intervention: can they make a difference? Can J Psychiatry 50:879–880, 2005

Heres S, Davis J, Maino K, et al: Why olanzapine beats risperidone, risperidone beats quetiapine, and quetiapine beats olanzapine: an exploratory analysis of head-to-head comparison studies of second-generation antipsychotics. Am J Psychiatry 163:185–194, 2006

Hoffman RE, Boutros NN, Hu S, et al: Transcranial magnetic stimulation and auditory hallucinations in schizophrenia. Lancet 355:1073–1075, 2000

Hoffman RE, Gueorguieva R, Hawkins KA, et al: Temporoparietal transcranial magnetic stimulation for auditory hallucinations: safety, efficacy and moderators in a fifty patient sample. Biol Psychiatry 58:97–104, 2005

Hogarty GE, Kornblith SJ, Greenwald D, et al: Personal therapy: a disorder-relevant psychotherapy for schizophrenia. Schizophr Bull 21:379–393, 1995

Hogarty GE, Greenwald D, Ulrich RF, et al: Three-year trials of personal therapy among schizophrenic patients living with or independent of family, II: effects on adjustment of patients. Am J Psychiatry 154:1514–1524, 1997

Hosak L, Libiger J: Antiepileptic drugs in schizophrenia: a review. Eur Psychiatry 17:371–378, 2002

Issakidis C, Sanderson K, Teesson M, et al: Intensive case management in Australia: a randomized controlled trial. Acta Psychiatr Scand 99:360–367, 1999

Jablensky A: Epidemiology of schizophrenia: the global burden of disease and disability. Eur Arch Psychiatry Clin Neurosci 250:274–285, 2000

Javitt DC, Zukin SR: Recent advances in the phencyclidine model of schizophrenia. Am J Psychiatry 148:1301–1308, 1991

Javitt DC, Strous RD, Grochowski S, et al: Impaired precision, but normal retention, of auditory sensory ("echoic") memory information in schizophrenia. J Abnorm Psychol 106:315–324, 1997

Jobe TH, Harrow M: Long-term outcome of patients with schizophrenia: a review. Can J Psychiatry 50:892–900, 2005

Johnstone EC, Crow TJ, Frith CD, et al: Cerebral ventricular size and cognitive impairment in chronic schizophrenia. Lancet 2:924–926, 1976

Jones P, Rodgers B, Murray R, et al: Child development risk factors for adult schizophrenia in the British 1946 birth cohort. Lancet 344:1398–1402, 1994

Kane JM, Honigfeld G, Singer J, et al: Clozapine in treatment-resistant schizophrenics. Psychopharmacol Bull 24:62–67, 1988

Kety SS, Rosenthal D, Wender PH, et al: Mental illness in the biological and adoptive families of adopted schizophrenics. Am J Psychiatry 128:302–306, 1971

Kirkpatrick B, Conley RC, Kakoyannis A, et al: Interstitial cells of the white matter in the inferior parietal cortex in schizophrenia: an unbiased cell-counting study. Synapse 34:95–102, 1999

Kubicki M, McCarley R, Westin CF, et al: A review of diffusion tensor imaging studies in schizophrenia. J Psychiatr Res 41(1–2):15–30, 2007

Lauriello J, Lenroot R, Bustillo JR: Maximizing the synergy between pharmacotherapy and psychosocial therapies for schizophrenia. Psychiatr Clin North Am 26:191–211, 2003

Lehman AF: Vocational rehabilitation in schizophrenia. Schizophr Bull 21:645–656, 1995

Lehman AF: Developing an outcomes-oriented approach for the treatment of schizophrenia. J Clin Psychiatry 60 (suppl 19):30–35; discussion 36–37, 1999

Lenroot R, Bustillo JR, Lauriello J, et al: Integrated treatment of schizophrenia. Psychiatr Serv 54:1499–1507, 2003

Lewis CM, Levinson DF, Wise LH, et al: Genome scan meta-analysis of schizophrenia and bipolar disorder, part II: schizophrenia. Am J Hum Genet 73:34–48, 2003

Lewis DA, Levitt P: Schizophrenia as a disorder of neurodevelopment. Annu Rev Neurosci 25:409–432, 2002

Liberman RP, Wallace CJ, Blackwell G, et al: Skills training versus psychosocial occupational therapy for persons with persistent schizophrenia. Am J Psychiatry 155:1087–1091, 1998

Liddle PF: The symptoms of chronic schizophrenia: a re-examination of the positive-negative dichotomy. Br J Psychiatry 151:145–151, 1987

Lieberman JA: Prediction of outcome in first-episode schizophrenia. J Clin Psychiatry 54 (suppl):13–17, 1993

Lieberman JA, Perkins D, Belger A, et al: The early stages of schizophrenia: speculations on pathogenesis, pathophysiology, and therapeutic approaches. Biol Psychiatry 50:884–897, 2001

Manoach DS, Gollub RL, Benson ES, et al: Schizophrenic subjects show aberrant fMRI activation of dorsolateral prefrontal cortex and basal ganglia during working memory performance. Biol Psychiatry 48:99–109, 2000

May PR, Tuma AH, Dixon WJ, et al: Schizophrenia: a follow-up study of the results of five forms of treatment. Arch Gen Psychiatry 38:776–784, 1981

McEvoy JP, Lieberman JA, Stroup TS, et al: Effectiveness of clozapine versus olanzapine, quetiapine, and risperidone in patients with chronic schizophrenia who did not respond to prior atypical antipsychotic treatment. Am J Psychiatry 163:600–610, 2006

McGlashan TH: Duration of untreated psychosis in first-episode schizophrenia: marker or determinant of course? Biol Psychiatry 46:899–907, 1999

McGrath J, Saha S, Welham J, et al: A systematic review of the incidence of schizophrenia: the distribution of rates and the influence of sex, urbanicity, migrant status and methodology. BMC Med 2:13, 2004

McGue M, Gottesman II: A single dominant gene still cannot account for the transmission of schizophrenia. Arch Gen Psychiatry 46:478–480, 1989

Meltzer HY, Pringuey D: Treatment-resistant schizophrenia: the importance of early detection and treatment. Introduction. J Clin Psychopharmacol 18 (2 suppl 1):1S, 1998

Meltzer HY, Li Z, Kaneda Y, et al: Serotonin receptors: their key role in drugs to treat schizophrenia. Prog Neuropsychopharmacol Biol Psychiatry 27:1159–1172, 2003

Miyamoto S, Duncan GE, Marx CE, et al: Treatments for schizophrenia: a critical review of pharmacology and mechanisms of action of antipsychotic drugs. Mol Psychiatry 10:79–104, 2005

Moffitt TE, Caspi A, Rutter M: Strategy for investigating interactions between measured genes and measured environments. Arch Gen Psychiatry 62:473–481, 2005

Mueser KT, McGurk SR: Schizophrenia. Lancet 363:2063–2072, 2004

Murray CJ, Lopez AD: Evidence-based health policy—lessons from the Global Burden of Disease Study. Science 274:740–743, 1996

Naber D, Lambert M, Karow A: Subjective well-being under antipsychotic treatment and its meaning for compliance and course of disease [in German]. Psychiatr Prax 31 (suppl 2): S230–232, 2004

Naz B, Bromet EJ, Mojtabai R: Distinguishing between first-admission schizophreniform disorder and schizophrenia. Schizophr Res 62:51–58, 2003

Newcomer JW: Metabolic risk during antipsychotic treatment. Clin Ther 26:1936–1946, 2004

Nicolson R, Rapoport JL: Childhood-onset schizophrenia: rare but worth studying. Biol Psychiatry 46:1418–1428, 1999

Owen MJ, Craddock N, O'Donovan MC: Schizophrenia: genes at last? Trends Genet 21:518–525, 2005

Palha AP, Esteves MF: The origin of dementia praecox. Schizophr Res 28:99–103, 1997

Penn DL, Mueser KT: Research update on the psychosocial treatment of schizophrenia. Am J Psychiatry 153:607–617, 1996

Penn DL, Waldheter EJ, Perkins DO, et al: Psychosocial treatment for first-episode psychosis: a research update. Am J Psychiatry 162:2220–2232, 2005

Percudani M, Barbui C, Tansella M: Effect of second-generation antipsychotics on employment and productivity in individuals with schizophrenia: an economic perspective. Pharmacoeconomics 22:701–718, 2004

Perlstein WM, Carter CS, Noll DC, et al: Relation of prefrontal cortex dysfunction to working memory and symptoms in schizophrenia. Am J Psychiatry 158:1105–1113, 2001

Peters E, Day S, McKenna J, et al: Delusional ideation in religious and psychotic populations. Br J Clin Psychol 38 (pt 1):83–96, 1999

Phillips LJ, McGorry PD, Yung AR, et al: Prepsychotic phase of schizophrenia and related disorders: recent progress and future opportunities. Br J Psychiatry Suppl 48:S33–44, 2005

Pinkham AE, Penn DL, Perkins DO, et al: Implications for the neural basis of social cognition for the study of schizophrenia. Am J Psychiatry 160:815–824, 2003

Popken GJ, Bunney WE Jr, Potkin SG, et al: Subnucleus-specific loss of neurons in medial thalamus of schizophrenics. Proc Natl Acad Sci U S A 97:9276–9280, 2000

Rasmussen KG, Sampson SM, Rummans TA: Electroconvulsive therapy and newer modalities for the treatment of medication-refractory mental illness. Mayo Clin Proc 77:552–556, 2002

Remington G, Kapur S: D2 and 5-HT2 receptor effects of antipsychotics: bridging basic and clinical findings using PET. J Clin Psychiatry 60 (suppl 10):15–19, 1999

Remschmidt H: Early onset schizophrenia as a progressive-deteriorating developmental disorder: evidence from child psychiatry. J Neural Transm 109:101–117, 2002

Risch N: Genetic linkage and complex diseases, with special reference to psychiatric disorders. Genet Epidemiol 7:3–16; discussion 17–45, 1990

Robinson D, Woerner MG, Alvir JM, et al: Predictors of relapse following response from a first episode of schizophrenia or schizoaffective disorder. Arch Gen Psychiatry 56:241–247, 1999

Robinson DG, Woerner MG, Delman HM, et al: Pharmacological treatments for first-episode schizophrenia. Schizophr Bull 31:705–722, 2005

Saccuzzo DP, Braff DL: Early information processing deficit in schizophrenia: new findings using schizophrenic subgroups and manic control subjects. Arch Gen Psychiatry 38:175–179, 1981

Sartorius N, Jablensky A, Shapiro R: Two-year follow-up of the patients included in the WHO International Pilot Study of Schizophrenia. Psychol Med 7:529–541, 1977

Seeman P, Lee T, Chau-Wong M, et al: Antipsychotic drug doses and neuroleptic/dopamine receptors. Nature 261:717–719, 1976

Smith DA, Buckley PF: Pharmacotherapy of delusional disorders in the context of offending and the potential for compulsory treatment. Behav Sci Law 24:351–367, 2006

Steen RG, Mull C, McClure R, et al: Brain volume in first-episode schizophrenia: systematic review and meta-analysis of magnetic resonance imaging studies. Br J Psychiatry 188:510–518, 2006

Stefansson H, Sigurdsson E, Steinthorsdottir V, et al: Neuregulin 1 and susceptibility to schizophrenia. Am J Hum Genet 71:877–892, 2002

Stern RG, Kahn RS, Davidson M: Predictors of response to neuroleptic treatment in schizophrenia. Psychiatr Clin North Am 16:313–338, 1993

Straub RE, Jiang Y, MacLean CJ, et al: Genetic variation in the 6p22.3 gene DTNBP1, the human ortholog of the mouse dysbindin gene, is associated with schizophrenia. Am J Hum Genet 71:337–348, 2002

Susser E, Neugebauer R, Hoek HW, et al: Schizophrenia after prenatal famine: further evidence. Arch Gen Psychiatry 53:25–31, 1996

Susser ES, Schaefer CA, Brown AS, et al: The design of the Prenatal Determinants of Schizophrenia Study. Schizophr Bull 26:257–273, 2000

Tandon R: In conclusion: does antipsychotic treatment modify the long-term course of schizophrenic illness? J Psychiatr Res 32:251–253, 1998

Tandon R, Fleischhacker WW: Comparative efficacy of antipsychotics in the treatment of schizophrenia: a critical assessment. Schizophr Res 79:145–155, 2005

Terkelsen KG, Menikoff A: Measuring the costs of schizophrenia: implications for the post-institutional era in the US. Pharmacoeconomics 8:199–222, 1995

Tharyan P, Adams CE: Electroconvulsive therapy for schizophrenia. Cochrane Database Syst Rev (2):CD000076, 2005

Tienari P, Wynne LC, Moring J, et al: The Finnish adoptive family study of schizophrenia: implications for family research. Br J Psychiatry Suppl (23):20–26, 1994

Turkington D, Kingdon D, Weiden PJ: Cognitive behavior therapy for schizophrenia. Am J Psychiatry 163:365–373, 2006

Volk DW, Austin MC, Pierri JN, et al: Decreased glutamic acid decarboxylase67 messenger RNA expression in a subset of prefrontal cortical gamma-aminobutyric acid neurons in subjects with schizophrenia. Arch Gen Psychiatry 57:237–245, 2000

U.S. Institute of Medicine: Neurological, Psychiatric, and Developmental Disorders: Meeting the Challenges in the Developing World. Washington, DC, National Academy of Sciences, 2001

Wolkowitz OM, Pickar D: Benzodiazepines in the treatment of schizophrenia: a review and reappraisal. Am J Psychiatry 148:714–726, 1991

Wu EQ, Birnbaum HG, Shi L, et al: The economic burden of schizophrenia in the United States in 2002. J Clin Psychiatry 66:1122–1129, 2005

Wyatt RJ, Henter ID: The effects of early and sustained intervention on the long-term morbidity of schizophrenia. J Psychiatr Res 32:169–177, 1998

Xiberas X, Martinot JL, Mallet L, et al: Extrastriatal and striatal D(2) dopamine receptor blockade with haloperidol or new antipsychotic drugs in patients with schizophrenia. Br J Psychiatry 179:503–508, 2001

Zygmunt A, Olfson M, Boyer CA, et al: Interventions to improve medication adherence in schizophrenia. Am J Psychiatry 159:1653–1664, 2002

6

MOOD DISORDERS

John A. Joska, M.D., M.Med.(Psych.), F.C.Psych.(S.A.)
Dan J. Stein, M.D., Ph.D.

Mood critically affects perception and appraisal of the self and the environment. Changes in mood occur as part of everyday experience, in response to multiple factors. In a proportion of people, mood states can become distressing, and psychopathology ensues. In this chapter, we describe the clinical features of mood disorders, summarize knowledge of their pathogenesis, and outline current approaches to management.

Phenomenology of Mood Disorders

Mood problems present in multiple ways, with variation across age, gender, culture, and medical setting. We summarize the current approaches to the phenomenology of mood disorders.

Classification of Mood Disorders

Both DSM-IV-TR (American Psychiatric Association 2000a) and ICD-10 (World Health Organization 1992) provide diagnostic criteria for mood disorders. These classifications reflect accumulated knowledge about distinctions between different mood disorders (e.g., unipolar vs. bipolar) and subtypes (e.g., typical vs. atypical).

Depression

Clinical Features of Depression

Mental state examination. Features of depression that may be present on the mental state examination include a downcast appearance, poor eye contact, and diminished or increased psychomotor activity. Speech may be slow and monotonous, with delays in the production of speech (so-called speech latency or speech pause time). The patient with depression may describe a low mood or may represent it by using particular cultural idioms. Affective expression in depression varies from bland and restricted to anxious, dysphoric, and agitated. Thought may range from slowed flow to poverty of ideation. In psychotic depression, the patient may have loosening of associations, delusions of nihilism ("I am worthless"; "I will be dying shortly"), perceptual disturbances (defamatory and command-type auditory hallucinations are commonest), and visual hallucinations. Cognitive impairment can occur, with disturbed memory, attention, and executive functions, especially in elderly individuals.

Depressed mood and anhedonia.   Together with low mood, a loss of pleasure—anhedonia—is the other essential feature of a DSM-IV-TR diagnosis of depression. In addition to the presence of depression, factors such as the duration, severity, and intensity of the depression must be considered. An inability to experience a lifting of mood in the presence of typically rewarding events is a key feature of melancholia (lack of "mood reactivity"). This subtype of depression includes the problems of early-morning awakening and diurnal variation in mood.

Cognitive, neurovegetative, and behavioral symptoms.   Cognitive impairment in depression includes the errors in information processing and distortions described by a cognitive-behavioral model. These include negative thoughts about the self, the world, and the future. Neuropsychological disturbances in depression include poor performance on tests of memory, concentration, and executive functions. Disturbances of sleep, appetite, and sexual behavior in depression are sometimes referred to as "neurovegetative." A small proportion of individuals sleep and eat excessively (hypersomnia and hyperphagia); these symptoms are part of the syndrome of atypical depression.

Duration, intensity, and episode specifiers.   The diagnosis of major depression requires depressive symptoms to be present for most days over a 2-week period. When symptoms have been present for a shorter period, a diagnosis of depressive disorder not otherwise specified or recurrent brief depression may be considered. When depression lasts 2 years or more, the diagnosis of dysthymic disorder is possible.

Although the characterization of an episode as mild, moderate, or severe may seem overly broad, it potentially helps inform management by suggesting which episode may require intensive, combined, or inpatient treatments. In addition, more severe depressive episodes have a tendency to recur more frequently and may require a longer duration of treatment (Kessler et al. 1994).

DSM-IV-TR includes several episode specifiers. Some, which have been mentioned earlier, include subtype specifiers, such as depression with melancholia, atypical features, or catatonic features. Other specifiers indicate when depression occurs: postpartum onset (occurring within 4 weeks of childbirth) or seasonal onset (occurring during a particular season, usually winter). The presence of psychotic symptoms should also be specified.

Major Depressive Disorder

Diagnostic criteria.   The DSM-IV-TR diagnostic criteria for major depressive episode are listed in Table 6–1.

Single-episode versus recurrent major depression.   Recurrence only follows a previously remitted episode and should not be diagnosed in the presence of residual symptoms of an inadequately treated episode. DSM-IV-TR allows for the addition of interepisode specifiers: with or without full interepisode recovery. This distinction usually depends on the degree of symptom remission assessed by the clinician. The use of rating scales such as the Hamilton Rating Scale for Depression may be useful (Hamilton 1960). Symptom scores of less than 75% of baseline, for example, are considered remitted.

Other Depressive Disorders

Dysthymic disorder.   Dysthymic disorder is a common depressive condition, with a

Table 6–1. DSM-IV-TR diagnostic criteria for major depressive episode

A. Five (or more) of the following symptoms have been present during the same 2-week period and represent a change from previous functioning; at least one of the symptoms is either (1) depressed mood or (2) loss of interest or pleasure.

Note: Do not include symptoms that are clearly due to a general medical condition, or mood-incongruent delusions or hallucinations.

  (1) depressed mood most of the day, nearly every day, as indicated by either subjective report (e.g., feels sad or empty) or observation made by others (e.g., appears tearful). **Note:** In children and adolescents, can be irritable mood.

  (2) markedly diminished interest or pleasure in all, or almost all, activities most of the day, nearly every day (as indicated by either subjective account or observation made by others)

  (3) significant weight loss when not dieting or weight gain (e.g., a change of more than 5% of body weight in a month), or decrease or increase in appetite nearly every day. **Note:** In children, consider failure to make expected weight gains.

  (4) insomnia or hypersomnia nearly every day

  (5) psychomotor agitation or retardation nearly every day (observable by others, not merely subjective feelings of restlessness or being slowed down)

  (6) fatigue or loss of energy nearly every day

  (7) feelings of worthlessness or excessive or inappropriate guilt (which may be delusional) nearly every day (not merely self-reproach or guilt about being sick)

  (8) diminished ability to think or concentrate, or indecisiveness, nearly every day (either by subjective account or as observed by others)

  (9) recurrent thoughts of death (not just fear of dying), recurrent suicidal ideation without a specific plan, or a suicide attempt or a specific plan for committing suicide

B. The symptoms do not meet criteria for a mixed episode.

C. The symptoms cause clinically significant distress or impairment in social, occupational, or other important areas of functioning.

D. The symptoms are not due to the direct physiological effects of a substance (e.g., a drug of abuse, a medication) or a general medical condition (e.g., hypothyroidism).

E. The symptoms are not better accounted for by bereavement; i.e., after the loss of a loved one, the symptoms persist for longer than 2 months or are characterized by marked functional impairment, morbid preoccupation with worthlessness, suicidal ideation, psychotic symptoms, or psychomotor retardation.

---

lifetime prevalence of up to 6% of the population (Moore and Bona 2001). It is characterized by milder depressive symptoms than in major depression that persist for at least 2 years (1 year in children and adolescents), with a symptom-free period of only 2 months in each year (Table 6–2). A major depressive episode may occur after onset of dysthymia ("double depression") (Moore and Bona 2001).

Psychotic depression. The presence of psychotic symptoms in depression is an indication of severity and a tendency to recurrence

(Coryell 1996). Inpatient treatment is usually required because of associated risk. Nihilistic or somatic delusions, together with auditory hallucinations, constitute the commonest psychotic symptoms in major depression. Significant impairment, distress, and sometimes suicide accompany this syndrome. The differential diagnosis includes schizophrenia and schizoaffective disorder.

Seasonal affective disorder. Seasonal affective disorder (SAD) is a relatively recent entry to the diagnostic system (Rosenthal et al. 1984). It is now classified as a mood disor-

---

Table 6–2. DSM-IV-TR diagnostic criteria for dysthymic disorder

---

A. Depressed mood for most of the day, for more days than not, as indicated by either subjective account or observation by others, for at least 2 years. **Note:** In children and adolescents, mood can be irritable and duration must be at least 1 year.

B. Presence, while depressed, of two (or more) of the following:
   (1) poor appetite or overeating
   (2) insomnia or hypersomnia
   (3) low energy or fatigue
   (4) low self-esteem
   (5) poor concentration or difficulty making decisions
   (6) feelings of hopelessness

C. During the 2-year period (1 year for children or adolescents) of the disturbance, the person has never been without the symptoms in criteria A and B for more than 2 months at a time.

D. No major depressive episode (see Table 6–1) has been present during the first 2 years of the disturbance (1 year for children and adolescents); i.e., the disturbance is not better accounted for by chronic major depressive disorder, or major depressive disorder, in partial remission. **Note:** There may have been a previous major depressive episode provided there was a full remission (no significant signs or symptoms for 2 months) before development of the dysthymic disorder. In addition, after the initial 2 years (1 year in children or adolescents) of dysthymic disorder, there may be superimposed episodes of major depressive disorder, in which case both diagnoses may be given when the criteria are met for a major depressive episode.

E. There has never been a manic episode (see Table 6–5), a mixed episode (see DSM-IV-TR p. 365), or a hypomanic episode (see DSM-IV-TR p. 368), and criteria have never been met for cyclothymic disorder.

F. The disturbance does not occur exclusively during the course of a chronic psychotic disorder, such as schizophrenia or delusional disorder.

G. The symptoms are not due to the direct physiological effects of a substance (e.g., a drug of abuse, a medication) or a general medical condition (e.g., hypothyroidism).

H. The symptoms cause clinically significant distress or impairment in social, occupational, or other important areas of functioning.

Specify if:
Early onset: if onset is before age 21 years
Late onset: if onset is age 21 years or older
Specify (for most recent 2 years of dysthymic disorder):
With atypical features (see DSM-IV-TR p. 420)

---

der specifier—with seasonal pattern. In major depressive disorder, a seasonal pattern may occur in up to one-third of cases. In addition to the usual treatments for depression, light therapy has been shown to be effective.

Recurrent brief depressive disorder and minor depressive disorder. Recurrent brief depressive disorder and minor depressive disorder are listed in the DSM-IV-TR research appendix. Individuals with recurrent brief depression have an increased risk for

suicide compared with the general population. This condition follows a different course from that of major depression (Pezawas et al. 2005). It may well represent a unique subtype of depression for this reason.

Premenstrual dysphoric disorder. Premenstrual mood symptoms are common, and about 3%–9% of women meet criteria for premenstrual dysphoric disorder (PMDD) (Halbreich et al. 2003). PMDD is characterized by the onset of severe symptoms, with at least one mood symptom, in the late luteal phase of the menstrual cycle, with remission during the early follicular phase. The association between depression and derangements of the hypothalamic-pituitary-gonadal (HPG) axis has been established, but the precise nature of the link is unclear. Treatment of PMDD with gonadal hormones has limited effectiveness, whereas intermittent treatment with selective serotonin reuptake inhibitors (SSRIs) is the current pharmacotherapy of choice (Dimmock et al. 2000).

Adjustment disorder and bereavement. The association between depression and loss is common. However, not all depressive episodes that follow a stressor develop into major depressive episodes. When a stressor has resulted in impaired function or distress, together with depressed mood, then the diagnosis of adjustment disorder with depressed mood is most appropriate.

Similarly, the normal human response to bereavement should not be diagnosed as depression. DSM-IV-TR allows for a 2-month bereavement period, but it does ask clinicians to exercise their judgment when assigning diagnoses. It is regarded as "normal" for bereaved individuals to experience the presence of their loved one in the time after bereavement. This may take the form of hallucinations or vivid dreams. Sleep disturbance, excessive crying, psychomotor changes, and thoughts of death also may occur. The clinician should be guided by the reactions of close family members, cultural norms, and the course of the bereavement. A clinically significant depression may follow in about 15% of people who are bereaved (Clayton 1990).

Differential Diagnosis of Depressive Disorders

Medical disorders. Many medical conditions may be associated with depression (Peveler et al. 2002). Some of these are listed in Table 6–3. The mechanism of association may be a result of the condition itself (such as hypothyroidism), a reaction to having a medi-

Table 6–3. Some medical conditions that may cause depression

Neurological disorders
    Epilepsies
    Parkinson's disease
    Multiple sclerosis
    Alzheimer's disease
    Cerebrovascular disease

Infectious disorders
    Neurosyphilis
    HIV/AIDS

Cardiac disorders
    Ischemic heart disease
    Cardiac failure
    Cardiomyopathies

Endocrine and metabolic disorders
    Hypothyroidism
    Diabetes mellitus
    Vitamin deficiencies
    Parathyroid disorders

Inflammatory disorders
    Collagen-vascular diseases
    Irritable bowel syndrome
    Chronic liver disorders

Neoplastic disorders
    Central nervous system tumors
    Paraneoplastic syndromes

cal condition, a result of the medical treatment of the condition, or a combination of these factors. In some instances, the medical disorder creates the appearance of depression with or without actually causing it. Examples include Parkinson's disease and cerebrovascular disease.

Depression secondary to substance use. The most widespread substance of abuse, alcohol, is a common and independent cause of depressive illness. Patients whose alcohol abuse leads to depression will commonly experience a remission of depressive symptoms after cessation of alcohol use without antidepressant treatment. Other causes of depression secondary to substance and medication use are listed in Table 6–4. The association between substance use and mood disorders has been established in several population surveys—in the Epidemiologic Catchment Area (ECA) study, the use of alcohol increased the likelihood of having major depression twofold and the likelihood of having bipolar disorder nearly fivefold (Regier et al. 1990).

In addition to the possibility that substance abuse leads to depression, depression may lead to substance use (i.e., "self-medication") (Khantzian 1985), or the two disorders may share a common diathesis (e.g., genetic loading). A careful clinical assessment must include a detailed substance use and mood disorder history, with a view to delineating whether mood symptoms occurred in the absence of a period of intoxication or withdrawal. The presence of severe or chronic symptoms, as well as comorbidity, also may help the clinician determine the primary disorder.

Depression and other psychiatric disorders. Other psychiatric disorders may be comorbid with depression or may need to be considered in the differential diagnosis. These include the prodrome of schizophrenia, schizoid personality disorder, pervasive developmental disorders, intellectual disability and dementia, and anxiety disorders.

Mania

Clinical Features of Mania

Mental state examination. The presentation of mania is varied. Central to mania, hypomania, or mixed episodes is the presence of elevated, irritable, or expansive mood. Mania may manifest in obvious ways (e.g., catatonic stupor; violent and aggressive behavior) or in more subtle ways (e.g., dressing in brighter clothing; agitated psychomotor function). Expansive mood may be elicited when the person describes his or her social interactions; a sense of being connected to the world is often expressed. Speech may be pressured. Affect is often euphoric but may be labile or hostile. Irritable or dysphoric mood may be difficult to

Table 6–4. Some substances and medications that may cause depression
Central nervous system depressants
Alcohol
Barbiturates
Benzodiazepines
Clonidine
Central nervous system medications
Amantadine
Bromocriptine
Levodopa
Phenothiazines
Phenytoin
Psychostimulants
Amphetamines
Systemic medications
Corticosteroids
Digoxin
Diltiazem
Enalapril
Ethionamide
Isotretinoin
Mefloquine
Methyldopa
Metoclopramide
Quinolones
Reserpine
Statins
Thiazides
Vincristine

distinguish from depression. *Dysphoria* describes a subjective sense of negative, labile, or irritable mood in the absence of persistently low mood and anhedonia. Problems with thought include excessive flow of ideas ("flight of ideas"); grandiose, religious, or persecutory delusions; and sometimes bizarre delusions. Perceptual disturbances range from auditory hallucinations (such as hearing the voice of God) to visions of religious and grandiose significance. These mood-congruent symptoms are most common, but incongruent psychosis has been described. Cognitive disturbances include distractibility, poor attention, and executive dysfunction (Table 6–5).

Cognitive, neurovegetative, and behavioral symptoms. Neurovegetative symptoms are usual in mania. Sleep disturbance is characterized by a decreased need for sleep. Libido and appetite are both often increased. Two types of behavior problems in mania may occur: increase in goal-directed behavior and behavior with potential for harm. In some cases, goal-directed behavior leads to increased productivity, increased self-esteem, and even an increase in earnings. This can hinder the patient's insight into the behavior as being abnormal. Harmful behaviors may include excessive spending, gambling, sexual promiscuity, traveling, drug use, or other risk-taking behavior.

Duration, intensity, and specifiers. Determining the duration of elevated mood episodes is key to establishing diagnosis. Short-lived episodes may reflect cyclothymic disturbance or rapid cycling, whereas longer episodes may result from treatment resistance or ongoing substance abuse. A life chart may be useful in depicting the nature and extent of mood episodes. Other specifiers include whether the episode was single or recurrent, whether it was postpartum in onset, and whether it was associated with psychosis.

Bipolar I Disorder

The diagnostic criteria for bipolar I disorder are listed in Table 6–6. The presence of any past or present manic episode is sufficient to meet criteria. The diagnosis of bipolar disorder should be considered in any patient who

---

Table 6–5. DSM-IV-TR diagnostic criteria for manic episode

A. A distinct period of abnormally and persistently elevated, expansive, or irritable mood, lasting at least 1 week (or any duration if hospitalization is necessary).

B. During the period of mood disturbance, three (or more) of the following symptoms have persisted (four if the mood is only irritable) and have been present to a significant degree:
   (1) inflated self-esteem or grandiosity
   (2) decreased need for sleep (e.g., feels rested after only 3 hours of sleep)
   (3) more talkative than usual or pressure to keep talking
   (4) flight of ideas or subjective experience that thoughts are racing
   (5) distractibility (i.e., attention too easily drawn to unimportant or irrelevant external stimuli)
   (6) increase in goal-directed activity (either socially, at work or school, or sexually) or psychomotor agitation
   (7) excessive involvement in pleasurable activities that have a high potential for painful consequences (e.g., engaging in unrestrained buying sprees, sexual indiscretions, or foolish business investments)

C. The symptoms do not meet criteria for a mixed episode (see DSM-IV-TR p. 365).

D. The mood disturbance is sufficiently severe to cause marked impairment in occupational functioning or in usual social activities or relationships with others, or to necessitate hospitalization to prevent harm to self or others, or there are psychotic features.

E. The symptoms are not due to the direct physiological effects of a substance (e.g., a drug of abuse, a medication, or other treatment) or a general medical condition (e.g., hyperthyroidism).

Note: Manic-like episodes that are clearly caused by somatic antidepressant treatment (e.g., medication, electroconvulsive therapy, light therapy) should not count toward a diagnosis of bipolar I disorder.

Table 6–6. DSM-IV-TR diagnostic criteria for bipolar I disorder, single manic episode

---

A. Presence of only one manic episode (see Table 6–5) and no past major depressive episodes.

   Note: Recurrence is defined as either a change in polarity from depression or an interval of at least 2 months without manic symptoms.

B. The manic episode is not better accounted for by schizoaffective disorder and is not superimposed on schizophrenia, schizophreniform disorder, delusional disorder, or psychotic disorder not otherwise specified.

Specify if:

Mixed: if symptoms meet criteria for a mixed episode (see DSM-IV-TR p. 365)

If the full criteria are currently met for a manic, mixed, or major depressive episode, *specify* its current clinical status and/or features:

Mild, moderate, severe without psychotic features/severe with psychotic features (see DSM-IV-TR p. 414)

With catatonic features (see DSM-IV-TR p. 417)

With postpartum onset (see DSM-IV-TR p. 422)

If the full criteria are not currently met for a manic, mixed, or major depressive episode, *specify* the current clinical status of the bipolar I disorder or features of the most recent episode:

In partial remission, in full remission (see DSM-IV-TR p. 414)

With catatonic features (see DSM-IV-TR p. 417)

With postpartum onset (see DSM-IV-TR p. 422)

---

presents with depressive symptoms. Certain features may suggest bipolarity: earlier age at onset of symptoms, family history of bipolarity, and presence of atypical depressive symptoms (Perlis et al. 2006).

The recurrence of mania requires a careful reevaluation of contributory factors, such as substance use, poor medication adherence, psychosocial stressors, and medical problems. In addition, a diagnosis of rapid-cycling bipolar disorder should be considered; this requires the presence of at least four discrete mood episodes in a 12-month period. Two additional subtypes of rapid cycling are included the nomenclature: ultra-rapid cycling (cycles lasting days to weeks) and ultradian cycling (abrupt mood changes over a 24-hour period) (Kramlinger and Post 1996).

Other Bipolar Disorders

Bipolar II disorder.   A diagnosis of bipolar II disorder requires the presence of hypomanic and major depressive episodes (Table 6–7). It is most usual for patients to present with severe depression. Bipolar II disorder should be considered in patients who have atypical features, who abuse substances as a form of self-medication, or who have chaotic relationships. A life chart may be helpful.

Cyclothymia.   Cyclothymia is characterized by a 2-year history of changing mood, with both depressive and hypomanic symptoms (Table 6–8). It occurs in about 0.5% of the general population (Weissman and Myers 1978). Some patients will later develop manic episodes (6%), and a quarter will go on to develop major depression (Akiskal et al. 1979). There may be a continuum between cyclothymia and intrinsic difficulties in affective regulation and borderline personality disorder, but patients with cyclothymia may respond particularly well to pharmacotherapy.

Bipolar spectrum disorders.   There is increasing recognition that many individuals with recurrent depressive episodes also may have subthreshold elevated mood states (Angst and Cassano 2005). The construct of

---

Table 6–7. DSM-IV-TR diagnostic criteria for bipolar II disorder

---

A. Presence (or history) of one or more major depressive episodes (see Table 6–1).

B. Presence (or history) of at least one hypomanic episode (see DSM-IV-TR p. 368).

C. There has never been a manic episode (see Table 6–5) or a mixed episode (see DSM-IV-TR p. 365).

D. The mood symptoms in criteria A and B are not better accounted for by schizoaffective disorder and are not superimposed on schizophrenia, schizophreniform disorder, delusional disorder, or psychotic disorder not otherwise specified.

E. The symptoms cause clinically significant distress or impairment in social, occupational, or other important areas of functioning.

Specify current or most recent episode:

Hypomanic: if currently (or most recently) in a hypomanic episode (see DSM-IV-TR p. 368)

Depressed: if currently (or most recently) in a major depressive episode (see Table 6–1)

If the full criteria are currently met for a major depressive episode, *specify* its current clinical status and/or features:

Mild, moderate, severe without psychotic features/severe with psychotic features (see DSM-IV-TR p. 412) **Note:** Fifth-digit codes specified on p. 413 cannot be used here because the code for bipolar II disorder already uses the fifth digit.

Chronic (see DSM-IV-TR p. 417)

With catatonic features (see DSM-IV-TR p. 417)

With melancholic features (see DSM-IV-TR p. 419)

With atypical features (see DSM-IV-TR p. 420)

With postpartum onset (see DSM-IV-TR p. 422)

If the full criteria are not currently met for a hypomanic or major depressive episode, *specify* the clinical status of the bipolar II disorder and/or features of the most recent major depressive episode (only if it is the most recent type of mood episode):

In partial remission, in full remission (see DSM-IV-TR p. 412) **Note:** Fifth-digit codes specified on p. 413 cannot be used here because the code for bipolar II disorder already uses the fifth digit.

Chronic (see DSM-IV-TR p. 417)

With catatonic features (see DSM-IV-TR p. 417)

With melancholic features (see DSM-IV-TR p. 419)

With atypical features (see DSM-IV-TR p. 420)

With postpartum onset (see DSM-IV-TR p. 422)

Specify:

Longitudinal course specifiers (with and without interepisode recovery) (see DSM-IV-TR p. 424)

With seasonal pattern (applies only to the pattern of major depressive episodes) (see DSM-IV-TR p. 425)

With rapid cycling (see DSM-IV-TR p. 427)

---

bipolar spectrum disorders emphasizes that symptoms of bipolar disorder occur in a diverse range of conditions more frequently than by chance—such as may occur in some personality disorders, eating disorders, or substance use disorders.

Differential Diagnosis of Bipolar Disorders

Both general medical disorders and other psychiatric disorders should be considered in the differential diagnosis of a manic episode.

Table 6–8. DSM-IV-TR diagnostic criteria for cyclothymic disorder

---

A. For at least 2 years, the presence of numerous periods with hypomanic symptoms (see DSM-IV-TR p. 368) and numerous periods with depressive symptoms that do not meet criteria for a major depressive episode.   **Note:** In children and adolescents, the duration must be at least 1 year.

B. During the above 2-year period (1 year in children and adolescents), the person has not been without the symptoms in criterion A for more than 2 months at a time.

C. No major depressive episode (see Table 6–1), manic episode (see Table 6–5), or mixed episode (see DSM-IV-TR p. 365) has been present during the first 2 years of the disturbance.
   Note: After the initial 2 years (1 year in children and adolescents) of cyclothymic disorder, there may be superimposed manic or mixed episodes (in which case both bipolar I disorder and cyclothymic disorder may be diagnosed) or major depressive episodes (in which case both bipolar II disorder and cyclothymic disorder may be diagnosed).

D. The symptoms in criterion A are not better accounted for by schizoaffective disorder and are not superimposed on schizophrenia, schizophreniform disorder, delusional disorder, or psychotic disorder not otherwise specified.

E. The symptoms are not due to the direct physiological effects of a substance (e.g., a drug of abuse, a medication) or a general medical condition (e.g., hyperthyroidism).

F. The symptoms cause clinically significant distress or impairment in social, occupational, or other important areas of functioning.

Medical disorders.   The emergence of mania or hypomania in the presence of a medical disorder may result from the disorder itself or the associated treatment (Table 6–9). The emergence of a manic episode in an individual older than 35 years should raise the level of suspicion for an underlying medical cause (Larson and Richelson 1988).

Mania secondary to substance use.   The use of substances early in the course of bipolar disorder is common (Table 6–10). Furthermore, the use of substances may predict an earlier onset of bipolar disorder and a worse course (Brady and Sonne 1995).

Mania and other psychiatric disorders. When dysphoria or hostility is prominent, diagnoses such as schizophrenia and other psychotic disorders, substance intoxication, antisocial or borderline personality disorder, impulse-control disorders, and intellectual disability should be considered in the differential diagnosis of manic episode. The nature of psychotic symptoms, if present, must be clarified, and a thorough substance misuse

---

Table 6–9. Some conditions that may cause mania

Neurological disorders
   Epilepsies
   Traumatic brain injury
   Multiple sclerosis
   Cerebrovascular disease

Infectious disorders
   Neurosyphilis
   HIV/AIDS

Neoplastic disorders
   Central nervous system tumors
   Paraneoplastic syndromes
   Traumatic brain injury

Endocrine disorders
   Hypo- and hyperthyroidism
   Diabetes mellitus
   Hypercortisolemia
   Vitamin deficiencies

Inflammatory disorders
   Collagen-vascular diseases

Table 6–10. **Some substances and medications that may cause mania**

Central nervous system depressants
  Alcohol

Psychostimulants
  Amphetamines
  Cocaine
  Methylphenidate
  Pseudoephedrine

Central nervous system medications
  Amantadine
  Antidepressants
  Baclofen
  Bromocriptine

Systemic medications
  Anabolic steroids
  Chloroquine
  Corticosteroids
  Dapsone
  Isoniazid
  Metoclopramide
  Theophylline

Comorbidity, Cultural Aspects, and Course of Mood Disorders

Comorbidity of Mood Disorders

The co-occurrence of mood disorders with anxiety is extremely common. For example, nearly 50% of individuals with depression will develop a lifetime anxiety disorder (de Graaf et al. 2003). Anxiety disorders usually precede depressive disorders in onset.

The coexistence of depression in persons with schizophrenia significantly increases the risk of suicide, with rates of up to 10%. The differential diagnosis should include mood disorder with psychotic features and schizoaffective disorder. Clinical symptoms that may assist in differentiating mood disorders with psychotic features from schizophrenia include bizarreness of delusions and severe thought disorder in schizophrenia

and mood congruency of delusions and hallucinations in mood disorders.

Personality disorders are commonly associated with mood disorders. Indeed, Cluster B personality disorders, particularly borderline personality disorder, may be characterized by a core disturbance in affect, with both decreased and elevated mood at times.

Mood Disorders Across the Life Span

Mood disorders in children and adolescents. Depression has a prevalence of up to 14% in adolescents (Birmaher et al. 1996). Depressed children may show irritability rather than depressed mood. Younger children may have more appetite changes and delusional thinking (Kovacs 1996). Associated features include low self-esteem, negative cognitions, and behavioral difficulties.

It is essential to screen for comorbid conditions, such as learning disability, attention-deficit/hyperactivity disorder (ADHD), disruptive behavior disorders, and anxiety disorders (Emslie et al. 1997). Children with chronic medical problems, including diabetes, asthma, and epilepsy, also have a high rate of depression (Grey et al. 2002).

The prevalence of bipolar disorder in children and adolescents is about 1% (Keller and Baker 1991). Although manic symptoms have been commonly reported in children, some maintain that bipolar disorder is difficult to diagnose in those younger than 10 years. Bipolar disorder in children is characterized by irritability, cyclical mood changes, and associated ADHD (Biederman et al. 2000). In addition, the clinical course may follow a more chronic, undulating pattern, with fewer discrete mood episodes. Adolescents are more likely to present with typical features of bipolar disorder (Carlson et al. 2003). Differential diagnosis includes ADHD—the presence of elevated mood, grandiosity, flight of ideas, and a decreased need for sleep are features unique to bipolar disorder.

Mood disorders in old age. The prevalence of depression rises with age. Rates approaching 25% in the elderly have been cited (Parmelee et al. 1989). First episodes also may occur in late life, as the result of life events, medical conditions, or treatment of these conditions or as a precursor to dementia. General medical conditions must be considered when a mood disorder first occurs in late life. Certain medical conditions, such as Parkinson's disease, other degenerative brain conditions, and endocrine problems, may present with features indistinguishable from depression. Antihypertensives, corticosteroids, and chemotherapies may lead to depression. Figures for completed suicide in elderly patients with depression approach 15%. Elderly patients who are unsupported, who are living with a terminal illness, or who live alone are especially at risk

Cultural Aspects of Depression

The core features of depression exist across cultures and ethnic groups, but the rates of reporting of these symptoms may differ (Kleinman and Good 1985). Idioms of distress may influence the expression of a variety of associated anxiety, psychosomatic, and dissociative symptoms.

Several well-conducted studies have found differing rates of depression across countries and cultures. The World Health Organization Cross-National Study of Mental Disorders in Primary Care found a point prevalence of depressive disorder of 29.5% in Santiago, Chile; 15.9% in Groningen, the Netherlands; and 4.0% in Shanghai, China (Sartorius et al. 1995). Weissman et al. (1996) found a lifetime prevalence of depression of 16.4% in Paris, France; 11.6% in Christchurch, New Zealand; and 4.3% in Puerto Rico. These figures may, however, reflect differences that are a consequence of the methodologies used. For example, rating scales used in these surveys may not have detected local idioms of distress.

The expression of distress across cultures and regions may reflect important differences in the way that the particular group views mental health, the concept of the body and the self, and the expression of emotion. Unique idioms of distress are recognized in

DSM-IV-TR and include feelings of loneliness and the sensation of a "hot or peppery feeling in the head."

Epidemiology of Mood Disorders

Mood disorders, and depression in particular, are among the most prevalent and disabling of all medical conditions. Although significant advances have been made in epidemiological studies, methodological issues affect our interpretation of the data. Diagnostic instruments differ a great deal in their reliability, validity, and comprehensiveness. Even when studies are carefully done, some data, such as lifetime prevalence, are affected by factors such as recall bias.

Current and lifetime prevalence rates. The 1-year prevalence rates of major depression in large published studies range from 2.7% in the ECA study (Regier et al. 1990) to 10.3% in the National Comorbidity Survey (NCS; Kessler et al. 2003). The lifetime prevalence rates for the same disorder range from 7.8% to 17.1%.

Fewer data are available for bipolar disorder. The ECA study found a prevalence of bipolar I disorder of 0.7%. Bijl et al. (1998) reported a 1-year prevalence of 1.1% and a lifetime prevalence of 1.8%. When validation studies used the Structured Clinical Interview for DSM-IV, adjusted rates of 0.9% were found (R. D. Goodwin et al. 2006). Higher rates may be seen depending on the diagnostic category used.

Sociodemographic correlates and risk factors. The mean age at onset of major depression has been found to be about 28 years (Regier et al 1990; de Graaf et al. 2003). In the replication of the National Comorbidity Survey (NCS-R), the median age at onset for mood disorders was 30 years (Kessler et al. 2003). People with bipolar disorder tend to develop symptoms in a bimodal distribution from ages 18 to 44 years (Kessler and Walters 1998).

Depression is twice as common in women (Kessler and Walters 1998), although this difference emerges only after adolescence. Reasons for this gender difference may include hormonal differences, social factors, or an unequal exposure to abuse and stressful life events (Klose and Jacobi 2004). In contrast, the rates of bipolar disorder among men and women appear to be similar (Kessler et al. 1994).

Depression is more common in unmarried compared with married persons (Kessler et al. (2003). This trend is similar for bipolar disorder. Higher rates of depression are reported in ethnic minorities (attributed to higher rates of poverty and lack of resources) and in people of low socioeconomic status (Kessler et al. 1994). Surveys of bipolar disorder in the general population have found a similar result. However, in clinical samples, bipolar disorder appears to be associated with a higher socioeconomic status.

Early childhood trauma and adverse life events (including loss of a parent) are associated with an increased risk for developing depression, particularly severe types. In adulthood, the presence of a negative life event has been shown consistently to be a risk factor for major depression.

The risk of developing major depression is significantly higher in relatives of patients with depression (see "Family, Twin, and Adoption Studies" below). Interactions between genes and the environment are becoming increasingly delineated. Variants in the gene coding for the serotonin transporter (5-HTT) and adverse life events, for example, appear to interact to predict higher rates of depression and anxiety disorders (Caspi et al. 2003). Similarly, the effect of personality on the development of depression has been examined in several studies, with high levels of neuroticism predicting a likelihood of developing depression (Kendler 1998). Data are too weak to categorically link stress as a direct risk factor for the development of bipolar disorder (R.D. Goodwin et al. 2006).

Course of Mood Disorders

Major depression tends to recur—figures range from 72.3% in the NCS (Kessler et al. 1994) to 40%–50% in the Netherlands Mental

Health Survey and Incidence Study (NEMESIS; Spijker et al. 2002). Factors that may affect the course of depression include family history, presence of comorbid anxiety, and the age at onset. Bipolar disorder also tends to be recurrent following the development of a first hypomanic or manic episode (Coryell and Winokur 1992).

Pathogenesis of Mood Disorders

Depression is likely to have multiple contributing factors.

Genetics and Inherited Factors

No single gene has been identified as a major cause of depression or bipolar disorder. Rather, genetic vulnerabilities may be the result of small, additive, and interactive effects of many genes.

Family, Twin, and Adoption Studies

Depression is two to four times more common in first-degree relatives of patients who have recurrent unipolar depression (Gershon et al. 1982; Sullivan and Kendler 2001). Factors that confer a greater degree of heritability include onset before 30 years, recurrence, presence of psychotic symptoms, and presence of certain comorbidities (such as panic disorder).

In families of bipolar patients, a spectrum of bipolar and unipolar disorders is found (Baron et al. 1983). These include bipolar I and II disorder, schizoaffective disorder, and recurrent major depression. There does not appear to be a risk of schizophrenia in relatives of bipolar probands. However, first degree relatives of schizophrenic patients are at increased risk for schizoaffective disorder and recurrent major depression (Gershon 1988).

Twin studies of recurrent major depression indicate that heritability is approximately 37%. The effect of the individual environment and the interaction between genes and the said environment probably account for a large portion of the remaining risk. In bipolar disorder, concordances range from 65.1% in monozygotic twins to 14.0% in dizygotic twins. Estimates of heritability of bipolar disorder in monozygotic twins are about 80% (McGuffin et al. 2003).

The risk of developing bipolar or unipolar disorder was found to be about 31% in adopted relatives of bipolar patients (Mendlewicz and Rainer 1977). This is similar to the risk of 26% seen in first-degree relatives of affected individuals who have not been adopted.

Neurochemistry

Early theories of mood disorders centered on the monoamine neurotransmitters serotonin (5-hydroxytryptamine [5-HT]); norepinephrine (NE; noradrenaline), and dopamine (DA). As the field has advanced, a range of other neurotransmitters and neurotrophic factors have been explored.

5-HT is synthesized from the essential amino acid tryptophan and metabolized by monoamine oxidase (MAO) to 5-hydroxyindoleacetic acid (5-HIAA). Synaptic serotonin is transported back into the neuron by a reuptake pump. Functions of the serotonin system in the brain include regulating neurovegetative functions, such as sleep, pain sensitivity, sexual function, and appetite (Maes and Meltzer 1995).

NE is synthesized from tyrosine via phenylalanine and DA in neuronal vesicles. Removal of released NE is by reuptake pumps for either NE or DA (into dopaminergic neurons) (Torres et al. 2003). The NE system is responsible for modulating behavior and attention, together with the prefrontal cortex. Firing of the locus coeruleus is stimulated by certain stressful situations. Together with the amygdala, NE neurons impart an emotional component to memory (Cahill et al. 2001). This may improve recall of emotionally charged material, but it also may provoke inappropriate memory cueing.

DA is synthesized in DA neurons from tyrosine. Synaptic DA is taken up by both NE and DA reuptake pumps (Torres et al. 2003). DA plays a role in reward processing and may be dysregulated in depression (Hasler et al. 2004) and mania. The role of DA in mania has been suggested by the manic illness following DA agonist use (e.g., amphetamine compounds). Similarly, DA releasers may be useful in depression, and DA antagonists are effective in treating mania.

Psychoneuroendocrinology

Hypothalamic-Pituitary-Adrenal Axis

Hypothalamic-pituitary-adrenal (HPA) axis stimulation modulates metabolism, reproduction, inflammation, immunity, and hippocampal neurogenesis (Plotsky et al. 1998). Patients with major depression have elevated plasma, cerebrospinal fluid, and urine cortisol levels, as well as elevated corticotropin-releasing hormone (CRH). In addition, the dexamethasone suppression test (DST) (failure to suppress cortisol release) is blunted in depression. The test is 90% sensitive to detecting depression but only 30%–50% specific (Copolov et al. 1989). In depression, CRH is hypersecreted, and early studies have suggested the efficacy of a CRH antagonist (Arborelius et al. 1999).

Thyroid Physiology in Depression

Hyperthyroid states are documented to produce emotional lability, irritability, insomnia, anxiety, weight loss, and agitation (Demet et al. 2002). Hypothyroidism typically induces fatigue, memory impairment, irritability, and loss of libido (Chueire et al. 2003), but not depression (Engum et al. 2002). In established depression, approximately one quarter of individuals have thyroid dysfunction—most commonly, an increase in free thyroxine (T_4) (Rubin 1989). Hypofunction of the hypothalamic-pituitary-thyroid (HPT) axis has been linked to poor antidepressant response and earlier recurrence (Joffe and

Marriott 2000). HPT axis abnormalities also have been reported in rapid-cycling bipolar disorder, although most first-line mood stabilizers decrease thyroid hormone levels (Baumgartner et al. 1995). The addition of thyroid hormone to tricyclic antidepressants (TCAs) may induce remission in some individuals with depression (Joffe 1997) and stabilize some patients with refractory bipolar disorder (Whybrow et al. 1992).

Cognitive Processing Models of Depression

Cognitive changes in depression include reduced speed of cognitive processing, impaired attention, and a bias toward negative stimuli (Williams 1997). Delayed recall is impaired more than recognition. Immediate recall seems to be relatively spared. Mood-congruent memory—the phenomenon whereby depressed individuals more readily recall memories when they are matched to negative emotional valence—is also affected. People with depression recall more negative memories (Matt et al. 1992).

Kindling and sensitization are important depressive phenomena. In kindling, people with prior depressive episodes are thought to be more likely to carry depressive thoughts and therefore activate subsequent episodes more readily (Post 1992). This theory is supported by evidence that people with recurrent depression develop subsequent episodes despite the absence of a stressor (Kendler et al. 2000).

Cognitive-behavioral studies of cognition in depression note the bias toward negative information, emotions, and memories. This selective attention may operate at schema level. In this way, negative thoughts and beliefs that prevail during depressive episodes are reinforced by underlying structures that have already been defined by previous negative experiences (Beck 1967).

Another aspect of cognition that needs to be addressed is the slow and effortful thought processing of the depressed individual (Hartlage et al. 1993). Homework tasks that involve mastering small problems and stepwise approaches may go some way to improve this deficit.

Management of Mood Disorders
Somatic Interventions for Mood Disorders
Antidepressants

Antidepressants are classified according to their activity at monoamine receptors (Table 6–11).

Tricyclics, tetracyclics, and monoamine oxidase inhibitors. The TCAs act by reuptake inhibition at both NE and 5-HT transporters. Activity at other receptors—such as adrenergic, histaminergic, muscarinic, and dopaminergic receptors—may produce many of the undesirable side effects. The anticholinergic side effects (dry mouth and constipation), together with hypotension, somnolence, and cardiac arrhythmias, make these less widely used. Other side effects include confusion, urinary retention, and blurred vision in the elderly; and increased appetite and weight gain.

TCAs may be more effective in major depression with melancholic features (Paykel 1972) than in depression with atypical features (Stewart et al. 2002). Care needs to be taken if TCAs are to be used in the elderly, and TCAs are generally not used in children and adolescents in view of lack of efficacy.

The TCAs generally should be administered in a slow, upward dosage titration. The measurement of plasma levels may be indicated in suspected overdose or poor adherence and to establish a minimum effective dose.

The monoamine oxidase inhibitors (MAOIs) increase the concentrations of monoamines through inhibition of the presynaptic enzyme MAO. The MAOIs are classified according to the degree of reversibility of binding to MAO and by their binding to

Table 6–11. Currently available antidepressants: activity, indications, adverse effects, and dosing

Antidepressant	Examples	Primary activity	Indications	Adverse effects	Dosing
Tricyclic antidepressants (TCAs)	Amitriptyline, desipramine, imipramine	SRI, NRI, ACh-M, Hist, α_1	Major depression, enuresis	Dry mouth, constipation, urinary retention, blurred vision, hypotension, cardiac toxicity, sedation	Commence at 25 mg, increase to 100–200 mg/day
Selective serotonin reuptake inhibitors (SSRIs)	Fluoxetine, paroxetine, sertraline	SRI	Major depression, anxiety disorders, impulse-control disorders, bulimia nervosa	Agitation, insomnia, headache, nausea and vomiting, sexual dysfunction, hyponatremia	Usually 20 mg/day (fluoxetine); may increase to 60 mg/day
Monoamine oxidase inhibitors (MAOIs)	Tranylcypromine, moclobemide	MAOI	Major depression, social phobia	Hypertensive crises for older agents, insomnia, nausea, agitation, confusion	Moclobemide: 150–600 mg twice daily after food
Serotonin–norepinephrine reuptake inhibitors (SNRIs)	Venlafaxine, duloxetine	NRI, SRI	Major depression, generalized anxiety disorder	Hypertension (venlafaxine), nausea, insomnia, dry mouth, sedation, sweating, agitation, headache, sexual dysfunction	Venlafaxine: commence at 75 mg/day; increase to 225 mg/day as needed
Norepinephrine and dopamine reuptake inhibitors (NDRIs)	Bupropion	NRI, DRI	Major depression, smoking cessation	Agitation, insomnia, headache, nausea and vomiting, seizures (0.4%)	150 mg twice daily
Serotonin antagonism and reuptake inhibitors (SARIs)	Nefazodone	SRI, 5-HT$_2$, α_1, NRI	Major depression	Sedation, hepatotoxicity, dizziness, hypotension, paresthesias; priapism (trazodone)	100–300 mg twice daily

Table 6–11. Currently available antidepressants: activity, indications, adverse effects, and dosing *(continued)*

Antidepressant	Examples	Primary activity	Indications	Adverse effects	Dosing
Norepinephrine and serotonin specific antidepressants (NASSAs)	Mirtazapine	α_2, 5-HT$_3$, 5-HT$_{2A}$, 5-HT$_{2C}$, Hist	Major depression	Weight gain, sedation, dizziness, headache; sexual dysfunction is rare	15–45 mg/day at night
Norepinephrine reuptake inhibitors (NRIs)	Reboxetine, atomoxetine	NRI	?Major depression, attention-deficit/hyperactivity disorder	Insomnia, sweating, dizziness, dry mouth, constipation, urinary hesitancy, tachycardia	Reboxetine: 4–6 mg twice daily

Note. SRI=serotonin reuptake inhibition; NRI=norepinephrine reuptake inhibition; MAOI=monoamine oxidase inhibition; DRI=dopamine reuptake inhibition; 5-HT$_2$=serotonin type 2 receptor antagonism; α_2=alpha-2 adrenergic blockade; 5-HT$_3$=serotonin type 3 receptor antagonism; 5-HT$_{2A}$=serotonin type 2A receptor antagonism; 5-HT$_{2C}$=serotonin type 2C receptor antagonism.

ACh-M=muscarinic anticholinergic; Hist=histamine blockade; α_1=alpha-1 adrenergic the respective isoforms—A or B. Tranyl-cypromine and phenelzine are irreversible inhibitors of both isoforms; selegiline is more selective for MAO-B; moclobemide is a reversible inhibitor of MAO-A (not available in the United States). The inhibition of MAO-A leads to an increase in NE, which may in turn precipitate a hypertensive crisis. For this reason, a diet free of the precursor tyramine is mandatory in patients taking these drugs. Transdermal selegiline may be better tolerated than older MAOIs in that it does not irreversibly inhibit gut or liver MAO-A, while binding to both forms of MAO in the brain (Thase 2006). Other adverse effects of the MAOIs include anticholinergic effects, dizziness, nausea, forgetfulness, and myoclonic jerks. Weight gain, muscle cramps, sexual dysfunction, and hypoglycemia are late effects. The MAOIs may interact with a range of medications, such as those that increase adrenergic tone or serotonin or dopamine concentrations. The MAOIs are useful in bipolar depression or atypical depression, but they are not commonly used in view of dietary restrictions and adverse events.

Selective serotonin reuptake inhibitors. The SSRIs are a group of drugs with similar but not identical effects. They are safer in overdose than are TCAs. Activities and dosing are shown in Table 6–12. In general, antidepressant response rates across studies vary from 60% to 75%, with no drug being more effective than another. Some studies have shown that SSRIs are less effective in melancholic depression (P.J. Perry 1996), whereas they are more effective in atypical depression.

Serotonin–norepinephrine reuptake inhibitors. Venlafaxine is an inhibitor of serotonin and NE transporters. It is prescribed in the dosage range of 75–225 mg/day. The extended-release preparation may be administered once daily (Gutierrez et al. 2003). Some elevation of blood pressure may be seen at higher doses, and this should be monitored in patients with a history of hypertension. Duloxetine is a more newly introduced sero-tonin–norepinephrine reuptake inhibitor, given in dosages ranging from 20 to 80 mg/day, that may be useful for individuals with comorbid pain or urinary incontinence.

Other antidepressants. Bupropion is an inhibitor of both NE and dopamine reuptake. It also may facilitate presynaptic release of these monoamines. It may spare depressed individuals from the sexual side effects commonly seen with serotonergic agents. It is regarded as having a lower tendency to induce rapid cycling or to induce mania compared with other antidepressants (Stoll et al. 1994). Bupropion is also approved for the treatment of smoking cessation. Adverse effects include anxiety, agitation, dizziness, and nausea. The risk of seizures may be significantly increased, and it should be used with caution in individuals with any predisposing factors for seizures. Dosages should not exceed 400 mg/day.

Mirtazapine is a novel tetracyclic that antagonizes the NE α_2 receptor, as well as the 5-HT_{2A} receptor (norepinephrine and serotonin specific antidepressant) (de Boer et al. 1996). In addition, it blocks 5-HT_2 and 5-HT_3 receptors, which contribute to anxiolysis. Antihistaminic effects include weight gain and sedation. Patients are given dosages between 15 and 45 mg/day.

Mood Stabilizers

In some ways, the term *mood stabilizer* is a misnomer because these drugs have wider uses than for mood disorders. Also, many other drugs (e.g., atypical antipsychotics) have mood-stabilizing properties.

Lithium. In acute mania, lithium remains effective across a range of domains of the illness (Hirschfeld et al. 2002). Treatment response usually can be seen within 5–14 days. Some evidence suggests that lithium is most effective when used in classic or euphoric mania or when the patient has had few lifetime episodes (Bowden 1995). In addition, efficacy appears to be accelerated when dose titration is rapid (Keck et al. 2001). Plasma monitoring is essential in lithium treatment.

Table 6–12. Selective serotonin reuptake inhibitors (SSRIs): activity, prescribing notes, and dosing

SSRI	Activity	Indications	Notes	Dosing
Fluoxetine	SRI, weak NRI and 5-HT$_{2C}$	Major depression, anxiety disorders, impulse-control disorders, bulimia nervosa	Long half-life (2 weeks), requires long washout before switching; highly protein bound	Usual dose 20 mg/day; increase gradually to 80 mg/day. Start 10 mg in young and old.
Paroxetine	SRI, weak ACh, Hist, and NRI	Major depression, panic disorder, generalized anxiety disorder, OCD	Produces sedation and anticholinergic effects; short half-life; discontinuation a problem	Start 20 mg/day; may increase to 60 mg/day
Sertraline	SRI, weak NRI and DRI	Major depression, PTSD		Start 50 mg/day; may increase to 200 mg/day
Fluvoxamine	NRI, SRI	OCD, depression		Start 50 mg/day; may increase to 200 mg/day
Citalopram	SRI, NRI (weak)	Major depression, panic disorder, and agoraphobia	Low inhibition of cytochrome P450 system; useful when drug interactions may be a problem	Start 20 mg/day; may increase to 60 mg/day
Escitalopram	SRI, NRI (weak)	Major depression, panic disorder, and agoraphobia	Low inhibition of cytochrome P450 system; useful when drug interactions may be a problem	Start 10 mg/day; may increase to 30 mg/day

Note. SRI=serotonin reuptake inhibition; NRI=norepinephrine reuptake inhibition; 5-HT$_2$=serotonin type 2 receptor antagonism; ACh= anticholinergic; Hist=histamine blockade; OCD=obsessive-compulsive disorder; DRI=dopamine reuptake inhibition; PTSD=posttraumatic stress disorder.

A range of 0.6–1.2 mEq/L is regarded as therapeutic. Higher levels may raise the risk of toxicity, with nausea, vomiting, confusion, myoclonus, seizures, hyperreflexia, and coma. Lower levels may increase the risk of relapse. Other adverse effects of lithium treatment include tremor, cognitive dulling, nausea, weight gain, and sedation.

In the maintenance phase of bipolar illness, lithium has been shown to reduce the risk of relapse (Burgess et al. 2001), although most patients require more than one drug to achieve stability (Grof 2003). In one study, the combination of lithium and valproate resulted in a significantly lower rate of relapse, compared with monotherapy (Solomon et al. 1997).

Lithium also has been shown to reduce the risk of suicide independently of its mood-stabilizing properties (Baldessarini et al. 2003). In acute bipolar depression, lithium is superior to placebo, although response is usually partial (Zornberg and Pope 1993). This finding often prompts the concomitant use of antidepressants. As in acute mania, plasma levels of lithium need to be greater than 0.8 mEq/L. In unipolar depression, lithium has proved useful in treatment-refractory cases. Rates of improvement of 56%–96% have been reported (M.P. Freeman et al. 2004).

Valproate and carbamazepine. The presence of depressive symptoms, impulsivity, hyperactivity, and multiple prior episodes may be associated with a better treatment response for valproate than for lithium (T.W. Freeman et al. 1992; Swann et al. 2002). The usual dose of valproate is 20 mg/kg but this can be increased to 30 mg/kg. Adverse effects include sedation, tremor, nausea and vomiting, hair loss, and weight gain. Rare problems include hepatotoxicity and pancreatitis.

Carbamazepine has been shown to be effective in acute mania (Weisler et al. 2004). Adverse effects of carbamazepine include diplopia, blurred vision, ataxia, sedation, and nausea. Rarer problems such as blood dyscrasias, hepatic failure, pancreatitis, and exfoliative dermatitis have been reported. Some data suggest that carbamazepine is effective in maintenance treatment (Dardennes et al. 1995). Small studies have shown some benefit for carbamazepine in acute bipolar and unipolar depression, but these were in treatment-refractory cases (Post et al. 1986). Oxcarbazepine is a similar agent with a lower incidence of side effects, but data on its efficacy are limited.

Other anticonvulsants. Several newer anticonvulsants have been studied in bipolar illness, including gabapentin, lamotrigine, and topiramate. To date, no trials have conclusively shown that any of these agents is effective in acute mania (Keck and McElroy 2006). In maintenance treatment, lamotrigine has been shown to reduce the incidence of depressive episodes but not manic ones (Bowden et al. 2003). Lamotrigine also has proved effective in acute bipolar depression (Calabrese et al. 1999). Adverse effects of lamotrigine include headache, nausea, and xerostomia. The risk of serious (but rare) rash is reduced with careful dose titration.

Antipsychotic Medications

The antipsychotics as a group have played a significant role in the treatment of mood disorders. They have been used both as adjunctive agents and (in the case of the second-generation antipsychotics) as primary agents.

In the United States, several antipsychotic agents are registered for use in acute mania as well as in maintenance treatment: olanzapine, risperidone, quetiapine, ziprasidone, aripiprazole, and chlorpromazine. In addition, olanzapine and aripiprazole are approved for maintenance treatment of bipolar disorder, and olanzapine is approved for acute bipolar depression. Although all first-generation agents are antimanic, chlorpromazine has been most studied in this respect (Keck et al. 1998). Likewise, the second-generation agents have been subjected to several controlled trials, and all were found to be effective in acute mania (Strakowski 2003), especially when added to a mood stabilizer.

Some second-generation antipsychotics are effective in acute bipolar depression; however, the first-generation agents are not useful in this regard, except when psychosis is present (Ahlfors et al. 1981; Keck et al. 2000). An emerging role for second-generation agents has also been found in treatment-resistant depression (Shelton et al. 2001). Risperidone is effective in combination with SSRIs in treatment-resistant unipolar depression. Olanzapine in combination with fluoxetine is safe and effective in patients with bipolar depression and those with fluoxetine-resistant depression. Ziprasidone and aripiprazole augmentation of SSRIs has been reported to be effective in treatment-resistant depression in open-label studies.

Electroconvulsive Therapy and Transcranial Magnetic Stimulation

Electroconvulsive therapy. Electroconvulsive therapy (ECT) remains an important part of treatment.

Mechanism of action. Possible mechanisms of ECT's action include downregulation of β-adrenergic receptors—a similar effect to antidepressant treatment (Kellar et al 1981); an increased density of 5-HT$_{2A}$ receptors (Kellar et al. 1981); and an increase in dopaminergic tone (Mann 1998). It has been suggested that ECT affects the HPA axis, particularly prolactin, with some authors stating that the magnitude of seizure is reflected in the postseizure prolactin level (Lisanby et al. 2000).

Indications. ECT should be considered if a rapid response is necessary, if medication has been ineffective, if psychotic features are present, or if the patient has had a history of good response to ECT (Nobler et al. 1997; Sackeim and Rush 1995). Other neurological indications for ECT include Parkinson's disease and intractable epilepsy.

The presence of intracranial pathology or any contraindication to anesthesia should prompt the clinician to seek alternative treatments. ECT is not contraindicated in elderly

persons and may be especially effective and safe in this population.

Adverse effects. Cognitive side effects after ECT are common, although most are transient. A brief period of postictal disorientation is usual. Anterograde amnesia usually resolves in 2–4 weeks (Sackeim 1994). Retrograde amnesia, however, may persist. It is temporally graded, being most dense for the time preceding the ECT. In rare cases, it may be more extensive and result in memory gaps dating back years (Squire and Slater 1983). The effect of amnesia may be reduced by right unilateral electrode placement, lower dose stimulation, and wider spacing of treatments.

Treatment considerations. The use of anticonvulsants and benzodiazepines during ECT may impede the treatment—these should be temporarily stopped or reduced. The use of lithium has been associated with prolonged delirium, and it also should be stopped or reduced before treatment. Most antidepressants, other than MAOIs, are safe during a course of ECT. ECT is usually given two to three times per week for between 6 and 12 treatments. Response is typically seen from the sixth treatment; an adequate trial requires at least 10 treatments.

Transcranial magnetic stimulation. Repetitive transcranial magnetic stimulation (rTMS) refers to the rapid pulse frequency application of a magnetic field to the head. This results in neuronal depolarization in a "subconvulsive" manner. Some stimulations can, however, produce seizures in vulnerable individuals (Pascual-Leone et al. 1993). The mechanisms of action are not well understood at present. rTMS appears to have antidepressant effects, although results have not always been consistent, and some uncertainties remain about optimal administration (Burt et al. 2002).

Novel and Other Somatic Treatments

Other novel treatment approaches to mood disorders include hormonal therapy, vagus nerve stimulation (VNS), and deep brain stimulation (DBS).

A range of antiglucocorticoids have been studied in depression, including ketoconazole, metyrapone, and mifepristone, with some evidence for their effects. Some studies have shown improvement in depressive symptoms in hypogonadal men treated with testosterone (Ehrenreich et al. 1999), but not all data are consistent. The effects on prostate enlargement must be considered. In women, estrogen is known to have mood-elevating properties, but this effect has not been shown in controlled studies in depression.

VNS involves stimulation of the vagus nerve in the neck. The vagus nerve carries both efferent and a large proportion of afferent fibers. The afferent portion is the target of VNS. In this technique, a generator is implanted into the left chest, and a lead is connected to the left cervical vagus nerve. Postulated mechanisms of action include changes in monoamine neurotransmitters, an antidepressant effect secondary to anticonvulsant effect, and longer-term changes in brain anatomy. VNS was initially used in epilepsy but was noted to have antidepressant effects in these patients (George et al. 2000). Although data on VNS are still at an early stage, VNS is now registered for use in the United States.

In DBS, an electrode is passed into brain tissue and connected to a generator in the chest. Like VNS, DBS was initially used in neurology settings, such as Parkinson's disease. In this patient population, mood changes were observed when brain stem structures were stimulated (Kumar et al. 1998).

Psychotherapy for Mood Disorders

Cognitive-Behavioral Therapy

The cognitive model.   Cognitive-behavioral aspects of depression were described earlier in this chapter (see section titled "Cognitive Processing Models of Depression"). The way in which negative automatic thoughts are structured can be defined in terms of differ-

ent types of cognitive distortion (Beck and Emery 1985). Examples include all-or-nothing thinking (e.g., "Either I am a success at this job or I am a total failure"); magnification (e.g., "This job is too big for me to do because I am incompetent); and jumping to conclusions (e.g., "If I cannot do this job, I will get fired"). Certain negative thoughts have an associated strong emotion, which amplifies the somatic and behavioral responses.

Cognitive-behavioral strategies and techniques.   Cognitive-behavioral therapy (CBT) is a brief, structured, and collaborative therapeutic intervention lasting from 12 to 20 sessions. Each session is structured to include a period of symptom review, intervention performance, and homework setting. Collaboration requires that the patient appreciate the need to give and receive feedback and that the patient–therapist team tackles assignments in a scientific and interactive manner. Psychoeducation is a crucial early component and usually makes use of a personally informed explanation of the condition and the therapy. Negative automatic thoughts are identified and then challenged in order to modify them. The Socratic technique offers an approach to challenge negative thoughts by means of reasoned inquiry (Beck et al. 1979).

As the therapy progresses, a pattern of thinking may emerge that reveals a series of underlying themes. These formative beliefs can be challenged. In some instances, they may be related to early experiences. The linking of a current belief system to a past experience may allow a patient to understand the source of negative feelings and thoughts. The introduction of behavioral techniques is particularly important when behavioral inactivation is present (Rehm 1977). Strategies aimed at improving a sense of competence through mastery by offering a series of graded exercises may be included. CBT usually does not require continuation, with relapse rates lower than 10% (Thase et al. 1992).

In a recent review of meta-analyses, CBT has been shown to produce consistently large effect sizes in the treatment of unipolar depression (Butler et al. 2006). In adults, this effect exceeds that of the antidepressants.

Cognitive-behavioral analysis. The cognitive-behavioral analysis system of psychotherapy was developed to treat chronic depression and dysthymia (McCullough 2000). In this therapy, the focus is on the patient's maladaptive style of social problem solving. By focusing on behaviors that produce positive outcomes, the therapist can reinforce more adaptive strategies. Four key strategies are used to achieve this goal: 1) situational analysis is used to identify the problematic behavior and then to modify it; 2) in a negative outcome situation, the patient may be offered options; 3) the positive thoughts and feelings that occur with a positive outcome are highlighted; and 4) the interpersonal discrimination exercise teaches the patient to examine expectations in relationships, including the therapeutic relationship, as a means to understand how negative feelings and attitudes may arise in relationships (McCullough 2000).

Interpersonal Psychotherapy

Interpersonal therapy (IPT) has its roots in the attachment theory of Bowlby (1969). Building on this approach, the interpersonal theorists noted that social events may be protective and also destructive, if negative in nature. Klerman et al. (1984) described interpersonal events in the social world as complicated bereavement, role disputes (relationship difficulties), role transitions (a loss of any kind), and interpersonal deficits (when social isolation is encountered). These events, when identified by the therapist, form the content of IPT. IPT differs from CBT in that it does not make use of homework assignments and differs from psychodynamic therapy in that the therapeutic relationship is not a focus of therapy. IPT has a wide range of indications within mood disorders, all of which have a strong evidence base. IPT has been shown to reduce depressive symptoms in

several different settings of major depression, including acute and recurrent major depression (Frank et al. 1990), depression in adolescents and elderly persons (Mufson et al. 1999), depression associated with HIV (Markowitz et al. 1998), depression in primary care (Schulberg et al. 1996), and dysthymia (Markowitz 2003).

IPT is a brief structured, collaborative therapy that usually lasts between 12 and 20 sessions. The early sessions are devoted to psychiatric assessment and formulation. A clear diagnosis is made, followed by feedback and psychoeducation. The analysis of the patient's interpersonal world is discussed, taking into account recent changes, patient expectations, and relationships that are proximal to the current depressive episode. In the middle phase, the therapist applies strategies (such as role-playing) to address the selected interpersonal focus area. During termination, the patient's competencies are reinforced, and an approach to identifying future depressive triggers is explored. IPT continues to be explored as an effective therapy for various psychiatric conditions.

Psychodynamic Psychotherapy

Psychodynamic therapy may be effective in mild depression and in depression in which personality factors are implicated (Gabbard 2000; Gallagher-Thompson and Steffen 1994). Patient factors predictive of success with psychodynamic therapy include motivation to understand, tolerance for frustration, significant suffering, and ability to hold a job. As with IPT, brief psychodynamic therapy seeks to define a focus for the therapy. This may involve a loss, a role confusion or change, or relationship stress. Longer-term psychodynamic therapy allows for the therapist to develop a psychodynamic formulation based on a detailed early and current account of events. Within the context of the therapeutic relationship, conflicts and anxieties (in the form of transference and resistance) emerge and offer the therapist an opportunity to analyze the issue. Much of the interaction must be carefully monitored by the therapist, so as to appreciate how he or she may be contributing to the dynamic relationship. Central to psychodynamic therapy is the therapeutic frame, which requires that the therapist retain relative anonymity, that sessions are set in time and place, and that extrasessional contact is dealt with in sessions.

In psychodynamic therapy for the treatment of depression, the therapist must listen carefully to experiences and themes that may have developed into depression. These may include ideas that the patient has internalized anger, has an overdeveloped superego or sense of responsibility, or feels helpless and dependent. Out of these thoughts and feelings, a range of defense mechanisms may have evolved, such as denial and projection. During the patient's account, patterns of relating may emerge. A core relationship theme may become prominent (Luborsky 1984). This conflict usually will repeat itself within the therapeutic relationship. This affords the therapist the opportunity to understand the patient's contribution to the conflict and a means by which to point out maladaptive defenses. The transference must be understood and brought into the therapy. The termination of psychodynamic therapy inevitably evokes earlier feelings of loss, and the therapist must deal with the unconscious sense of responsibility and anger.

Psychotherapy for Bipolar Disorder

Several therapeutic approaches may be of benefit to patients with bipolar disorder.

Psychoeducational therapy for bipolar disorder includes education about the illness and medication, training in recognition of the signs of early relapse, information about the value of seeking help, and promotion of regular sleep–wake cycles. A brief, focused psychoeducational therapy aimed at remitted patients with bipolar disorder was effective in reducing relapse rates (A. Perry et al. 1999).

CBT for bipolar disorder has made use of mood diaries, examination of negative thoughts about the illness, and addressing of

barriers to treatment adherence. When this type of CBT was added to routine care, the CBT group had fewer bipolar episodes, reduced episode duration, and reduced hospitalizations (Lam et al. 2003). CBT appears to have a greater advantage for depressive episodes than for manic episodes (Scott et al. 2001).

Family therapy for bipolar disorder makes use of psychoeducation, communication skills, and problem-solving skills (Miklowitz and Hooley 1998).

Integrative Management of Mood Disorders

An integrated approach to the treatment of mood disorders includes the use of medication, psychotherapies, and combined approaches.

Major Depressive Disorder

Treatment guidelines in major depression. Practice guidelines for the treatment of major depression include those published by the American Psychiatric Association (2000b), the Texas Medication Algorithm Project (Crismon et al. 1999), the Sequenced Treatment Alternatives to Relieve Depression (STAR*D) Study (Fava et al. 2003), and the National Institute for Health and Clinical Excellence (www.nice.org.uk).

Because no consistent evidence distinguishes between initial monotherapies at this time, a selection strategy might rather use other guides, such as a previously effective agent for that person or a first-degree relative or an agent with effectiveness for a comorbid condition. The goal of treatment is to achieve remission (absence of symptoms) rather than merely response (reduction of at least 50% of symptoms).

The duration of a first treatment trial is often debated. A response should be seen by 10 weeks. When response is partial, an augmentation or a combination strategy may be used. Fair evidence for lithium, thyroid hormone, and buspirone exists in this regard, and some of the atypical antipsychotics show promise as augmenting agents in major depression (Fava et al. 1994; Joffe and Singer 1990; Ostroff and Nelson 1999; Shelton et al. 2001; Smith 1998). Augmentation should result in response from 4 weeks. If response is adequate, then the strategy should be continued for 4–9 months.

Combined medication and psychotherapeutic approaches. The combination of medication and psychotherapy is indicated in chronic depressive conditions (Keller et al. 2000). Psychotherapy, particularly a cognitive-behavioral analysis system of psychotherapy, may be considered in early treatment if an individual with chronic depression presents for treatment (Schatzberg et al. 2005). Evidence indicates that individuals with chronic depression and a history of parental loss or abuse in childhood may respond well to psychotherapy (Nemeroff 2003).

Bipolar Disorder

It is useful to understand the management of bipolar disorder from acute-episode and maintenance-phase perspectives.

Treatment guidelines in bipolar disorder. Currently available guidelines include the practice guideline for the treatment of patients with bipolar disorder published by the American Psychiatric Association (2002), the guidelines published by the British Association for Psychopharmacology (G.M. Goodwin et al. 2003), and the Texas Medication Algorithm Project treatment algorithm for patients with bipolar disorder (Suppes et al. 2001). In addition, the prescriber must take into account whether the patient's symptoms have previously responded to an agent, whether rapid cycling is present (if so, use an anticonvulsant), and whether psychotic symptoms are present. The recommended duration of a trial of monotherapy is unclear. A response should be noted by 7–14 days, but remission may take considerably longer. Guidelines for the maintenance phase of the illness are less clear. Common practice and consensus suggest that most clinicians will

continue the mood stabilizer that the patient's symptoms responded to in the acute phase and will discontinue any antipsychotics that were used (Bowden et al. 2000).

In acute bipolar depression, the use of antidepressants alone generally should be avoided because of the risk of inducing rapid cycling. Fair evidence indicates that one of three treatment strategies—lithium, lamotrigine, or a fluoxetine–olanzapine combination—may be used. If the episode is severe, combinations of mood stabilizers, ECT, or an antidepressant–mood stabilizer combination could be considered. In all cases, thyroid abnormalities and comorbid substance abuse should be ruled out. In the maintenance phase of bipolar depression, there is good evidence for the effectiveness of lamotrigine when depressive episodes are recurrent (Bowden et al. 2003) and for lithium when both manic and depressive episodes recur (Prien et al. 1984). Long-term antidepressant use is associated with a higher risk of recurrence of mania.

Treatment of bipolar disorder in women of childbearing age. The clinician must pay special attention to a broad range of needs in women of childbearing age. It is best for women to plan pregnancies to allow for the possible withdrawal of mood stabilizers. In all instances, the clinician must make treatment decisions on the basis of benefits and risks to the fetus. All mood stabilizers are potentially teratogenic, and some may be harmful during lactation (American Psychiatric Association 2002). If drug therapy is considered essential, several strategies may be used to reduce risk to the fetus: using monotherapy at the lowest effective dose, using concomitant folate therapy, and avoiding medication during the first trimester of pregnancy (Iqbal et al. 2001).

Other Issues in Treatment of Mood Disorders

Treatment in children and adolescents. Much debate has surrounded the use of antidepressant medication in children and adolescents, with some negative trials of TCAs. To date, several trials have confirmed the effectiveness of SSRIs in childhood depression (Keller et al. 2001; Wagner et al. 2003). The first choice of monotherapy should be an SSRI. Controversy around the risk of suicide has emerged—the U.S. Food and Drug Administration found an increased risk of suicidality (defined as suicidal behavior or ideation) in children taking antidepressants compared with placebo, but no suicides were completed. Indeed, others have reported a decrease in the rates of suicide, possibly because of the increased use of antidepressants (Gould et al. 2003).

Treatment in the elderly.   In elderly patients with mood disorders, it is accepted practice to prescribe antidepressants initially at lower dosages and to titrate upward more slowly. Some investigators have argued that this strategy may not improve tolerability but rather may delay response (Roose et al. 1981). Treatment response is often slow, and a period of at least 2–3 months is necessary to ascertain whether treatment response has occurred (Young and Meyers 1992). Among the TCAs, some evidence suggests that nortriptyline may be better tolerated because it has less hypotensive effect (Roose et al. 1981). Some evidence (although limited) indicates that the SSRIs are effective in the elderly. The use of ECT also may need to be considered, and several studies have reported its effectiveness and safety.

Psychosocial treatment in the elderly is equally important. Clinicians may need to carefully consider hospital admission. The risk of displacing the individual may need to be weighed against the need for nursing care. Clearly targeted treatments such as music therapy, occupational therapy, and behavioral modification may need to be considered.

Conclusion

Mood disorders are among the most prevalent of all neuropsychiatric disorders, occurring in up to 20% of people in their lifetime. They are also among the most disabling of all medical conditions, and major depressive disorder in particular is predicted to become the second leading cause of medical disability by 2020. Understanding of the causes of depressive and bipolar disorders has grown, but remains elusive. At this stage, the contribution of several gene loci, together with the impact of life stress and the ensuing gene–environment interaction, could be seen to underpin most cases of depression. The differentiation of depressive syndromes is critical to understanding the course and clinical management of the condition: Individuals with a major depressive episode in the context of bipolar mood disorder will have a different course and treatment than those with a major depressive episode occurring in the course of unipolar depression. The integration of evidence-based psychotherapies into similarly proven somatic treatments may afford sufferers the best opportunity for recovery.

Key Points

- Depression is a symptom of a syndrome that may have many causes.

- Bipolar disorders can be difficult to diagnose because of the inability to detect past and future episodes.

- The clinical features of depression across cultures may vary, including expressions such as loneliness and somatic complaints.

- Major depression is common, with a lifetime prevalence of 7.8%–17.1%. It also causes about twice as much disability as any other medical condition.

- Major depression is a chronic and recurring illness, with relapses occurring in at least half of patients.

- The causes of depression are multifactorial and usually include genetic and environmental contributions.

- Treatment of major depression consists of selecting an appropriate antidepressant and giving consideration to an effective psychotherapy.

- Bipolar disorders should be treated with mood stabilizers first, with the addition of other agents if response is unsatisfactory.

References

Ahlfors UG, Baastrup PC, Dencker SJ: Flupenthixol decanoate in recurrent manic depressive illness. Acta Psychiatr Scand 64:226–237, 1981

Akiskal HS, Rosenthal RH, Rosenthal TL, et al: Differentiation of primary affective illness from situational, symptomatic, and secondary depressions. Arch Gen Psychiatry 36:635–643, 1979

American Psychiatric Association: Diagnostic and Statistical Manual of Mental Disorders, 4th Edition, Text Revision. Washington, DC, American Psychiatric Association, 2000a

American Psychiatric Association: Practice Guideline for the Treatment of Patients With Major Depressive Disorder, 2nd Edition. Washington, DC, American Psychiatric Association, 2000b

American Psychiatric Association: Practice guideline for the treatment of patients with bipolar disorder (revision). Am J Psychiatry 159 (4 suppl):1–50, 2002

Angst J, Cassano G: The mood spectrum: improving the diagnosis of bipolar disorder. Bipolar Disord 7 (suppl 4): 4–12, 2005

Arborelius L, Owens MJ, Plotsky PM, et al: The role of corticotropin-releasing factor in depression and anxiety disorders. J Endocrinol 160:1–12, 1999

Baldessarini RJ, Tondo L, Hennen J: Lithium treatment and suicide risk in major affective disorders: update and new findings. J Clin Psychiatry 64 (suppl 5):44–52, 2003

Baron M, Gruen R, Anis L, et al: Schizoaffective illness, schizophrenia and affective disorders: morbidity risk and genetic transmission. Acta Psychiatr Scand 65:253–262, 1983

Baumgartner A, von Stuckrad M, Muller-Oerlinghausen B, et al: The hypothalamic-pituitary-thyroid axis in patients maintained on lithium prophylaxis for years: high triiodothyronine serum concentrations are correlated to the prophylactic efficacy. J Affect Disord 34:211–218, 1995

Beck AT: Depression: Clinical, Experimental, and Theoretical Aspects. New York, Harper & Row, 1967

Beck AT, Emery G: Anxiety Disorders and Phobias: A Cognitive Perspective. New York, Basic Books, 1985

Beck AT, Rush AJ, Shaw BF, et al: Cognitive Therapy of Depression. New York, Guilford, 1979

Biederman J, Mick E, Faraone SV, et al: Pediatric mania: a developmental subtype of bipolar disorder? Biol Psychiatry 48:458–466, 2000

Bijl RV, Ravelli A, van Zessen G: Prevalence of psychiatric disorder in the general population: results of the Netherlands Mental Health Survey and Incidence Study (NEMESIS). Soc Psychiatry Psychiatr Epidemiol 33:587–595, 1998

Birmaher B, Ryan N, Williamson DE, et al: Childhood and adolescent depression: a review of the past 10 years, part I. J Am Acad Child Adolesc Psychiatry 35:1427–1439, 1996

Bowden CL: Predictors of response to divalproex and lithium. J Clin Psychiatry 56 (suppl 2):25–30, 1995

Bowden CL, Calabrese JR, McElroy SL, et al: Efficacy of divalproex versus lithium and placebo in maintenance treatment of bipolar disorder. Arch Gen Psychiatry 57:481–489, 2000

Bowden CL, Calabrese JR, Sachs GS, et al: A placebo-controlled 18-month trial of lamotrigine and lithium maintenance treatment in recently manic or hypomanic patients with bipolar I disorder. Arch Gen Psychiatry 60:392–400, 2003

Bowlby J: Attachment and Loss, Vol 1: Attachment. New York, Basic Books, 1969

Brady KT, Sonne SC: The relationship between substance abuse and bipolar disorder. J Clin Psychiatry 56 (suppl 3): 19–24, 1995

Burgess S, Geddes J, Hawton K, et al: Lithium for maintenance treatment of mood disorders. Cochrane Database Syst Rev (3):CD003013, 2001

Burt T, Lisanby SH, Sackeim HA: Neuropsychiatric applications of transcranial magnetic stimulation: a meta- analysis. Int J Neuropsychopharmacol 5:73–103, 2002

Butler AC, Chapman JE, Forman EM, et al: The empirical status of cognitive-behavioral therapy: a review of meta-analyses. Clin Psychol Rev 26:17–31, 2006

Cahill L, McGaugh JL, Weinberger NM: The neurobiology of learning and memory: some reminders to remember. Trends Neurosci 24:578–581, 2001

Calabrese JR, Bowden CL, Sachs GS, et al: A double-blind placebo-controlled study of lamotrigine monotherapy in outpatients with bipolar I depression. Lamictal 602 Study Group. J Clin Psychiatry 60:79–88, 1999

Carlson GA, Jensen PS, Findling RL, et al: Methodological issues and controversies in clinical trials with child and adolescent patients with bipolar disorder: report of a consensus conference. J Child Adolesc Psychopharmacol 13:13–27, 2003

Caspi A, Sugden K, Moffitt TE, et al: Influence of life stress on depression: moderation by a polymorphism in the 5-HTT gene. Science 301:386–389, 2003

Chueire VB, Silva ET, Perotta E, et al: High serum TSH levels are associated with depression in the elderly. Arch Gerontol Geriatr 36:281–288, 2003

Clayton PJ: Bereavement and depression. J Clin Psychiatry 51(suppl):34–38; discussion 39–40, 1990

Copolov DL, Rubin RT, Stuart GW, et al: Specificity of the salivary cortisol dexamethasone suppression test across psychiatric diagnoses. Biol Psychiatry 25:879–893, 1989

Coryell W: Psychotic depression. J Clin Psychiatry 57 (suppl 3): 27–31; discussion 49, 1996

Coryell W, Winokur G: Course and outcome, in Handbook of Affective Disorders, 2nd Edition. Edited by Paykel ES. New York, Guilford, 1992, pp 89–108

Crismon ML, Trivedi M, Pigott TA, et al: The Texas Medication Algorithm Project: report of the Texas Consensus Conference Panel on Medication Treatment of Major Depressive Disorder. J Clin Psychiatry 60:142–156, 1999

Dardennes R, Even C, Bange F: Comparison of carbamazepine and lithium in the prophylaxis of bipolar disorders: a meta-analysis. Br J Psychiatry 166:375–381, 1995

de Boer TH, Nefkens F, van Helvoirt A, et al: Differences in modulation of noradrenergic and serotonergic transmission by the alpha-2 adrenoceptor antagonists, mirtazapine, mianserin and idazoxan. J Pharmacol Exp Ther 277:852–860, 1996

de Graaf R, Bijl RV, Spijker J, et al: Temporal sequencing of lifetime mood disorders in relation to comorbid anxiety and substance use disorders—findings from the Netherlands Mental Health Survey and Incidence Study.

Soc Psychiatry Psychiatr Epidemiol 38:1–11, 2003

Demet MM, Ozmen B, Deveci A, et al: Depression and anxiety in hyperthyroidism. Arch Med Res 33:552–556, 2002

Dimmock PW, Wyatt KM, Jones PW, et al: Efficacy of selective serotonin reuptake inhibitors in premenstrual syndrome: a systematic review. Lancet 356:1131–1136, 2000

Ehrenreich H, Halaris A, Ruether E, et al: Psychoendocrine sequelae of chronic testosterone deficiency. J Psychiatr Res 33:379–387, 1999

Emslie GJ, Rush AJ, Weinberg WA, et al: Recurrence of major depressive disorder in hospitalized children and adolescents. J Am Acad Child Adolesc Psychiatry 36:785–792, 1997

Engum A, Bjoro T, Mykletun A, et al: An association between depression, anxiety and thyroid function—a clinical fact or an artefact? Acta Psychiatr Scand 106:27–34, 2002

Fava M, Rosenbaum JF, McGrath PJ, et al: Lithium and tricyclic augmentation of fluoxetine treatment for resistant major depression: a double-blind, controlled study. Am J Psychiatry 151:1372–1374, 1994

Fava M, Rush AJ, Trivedi MH, et al: Background and rationale for the Sequenced Treatment Alternatives to Relieve Depression (STAR*D) study. Psychiatr Clin North Am 26:457–494, 2003

Frank E, Kupfer DJ, Perel JM, et al: Three-year outcomes for maintenance therapies in recurrent depression. Arch Gen Psychiatry 47:1093–1099, 1990

Freeman MP, Wiegand C, Gelenberg AJ: Lithium, in The American Psychiatric Publishing Textbook of Psychopharmacology, 3rd Edition. Edited by Schatzberg AF, Nemeroff CB. Washington, DC, American Psychiatric Publishing, 2004, pp 547–565

Freeman TW, Clothier JL, Pazzaglia P, et al: A double-blind comparison of valproate and lithium in the treatment of acute mania. Am J Psychiatry 149:108–111, 1992

Gabbard GO: Psychodynamic Psychotherapy in Clinical Practice, 3rd Edition. Washington, DC, American Psychiatric Press, 2000

Gallagher-Thompson D, Steffen AM: Comparative effects of cognitive-behavioral and brief psychodynamic psychotherapies for depressed family caregivers. J Consult Clin Psychol 62:543–549, 1994

George MS, Sackeim HA, Marangell LB, et al: Vagus nerve stimulation: a potential therapy for resistant depression? Psychiatr Clin North Am 23:757–783, 2000

Gershon ES: Genetics, in Manic-Depressive Illness. Edited by Goodwin FK, Jamison KR. London, Oxford University Press, 1988, pp 373–401

Gershon ES, Hamovit J, Guroff JJ, et al: A family study of schizoaffective, bipolar I, bipolar II, unipolar, and normal control probands. Arch Gen Psychiatry 39:1157–1167, 1982

Goodwin GM, for the Consensus Group of the British Association for Psychopharmacology: Evidence-based guidelines for treating bipolar disorder: recommendations from the British Association for Psychopharmacology. J Psychopharmacol 17:149–173, 2003

Goodwin RD, Jacobi F, Bittner A, et al: Epidemiology of mood disorders, in The American Psychiatric Publishing Textbook of Mood Disorders. Edited by Stein DJ, Kupfer DJ, Schatzberg AF. Washington, DC, American Psychiatric Publishing, 2006, pp 33–54

Gould MS, Greenberg T, Velting DM, et al: Youth suicide risk and preventive interventions: a review of the past 10 years. J Am Acad Child Adolesc Psychiatry 42:386–405, 2003

Grey M, Whittemore R, Tamborlane W: Depression in type I diabetes in children: natural history and correlates. J Psychosom Res 53:907–911, 2002

Grof P: Selecting effective long-term treatment for bipolar patients: monotherapy and combinations. J Clin Psychiatry 64 (suppl 5):53–61, 2003

Gutierrez MA, Stimmel GL, Aiso JY: Venlafaxine: a 2003 update. Clin Ther 25:2138–2154, 2003

Halbreich U, Borenstein J, Pearlstein T, et al: The prevalence, impact, and burden of premenstrual dysphoric disorder. Psychoneuroendocrinology 28 (suppl 3):1–23, 2003

Hamilton M: A rating scale for depression. J Neurol Neurosurg Psychiatry 23:56–62, 1960

Hartlage S, Alloy LB, Vazquez C, et al: Automatic and effortful processing in depression. Psychol Bull 113:247–278, 1993

Hasler G, Drevets W, Manji H, et al: Discovering endophenotypes for major depression. Neuropsychopharmacology 29:1765–1781, 2004

Hirschfeld RM, Bowden CL, Gitlin MJ, et al: Practice guideline for the treatment of patients with bipolar disorder (revision). Am J Psychiatry 159:1–50, 2002

Iqbal MM, Gunlapalli SP, Ryan WG, et al: Effects of antimanic mood-stabilizing drugs on fetuses, neonates, and nursing infants. South Med J 94:304–322, 2001

Joffe RT: Refractory depression: treatment strategies, with particular reference to the thyroid axis. J Psychiatry Neurosci 22:327–331, 1997

Joffe RT, Marriott M: Thyroid hormone levels and recurrence of major depression. Am J Psychiatry 157:1689–1691, 2000

Joffe RT, Singer W: A comparison of triiodothyronine and thyroxine in the potentiation of tricyclic antidepressants. Psychiatry Res 32:241–251, 1990

Keck PE Jr, McElroy SL: Lithium and mood stabilizers, in The American Psychiatric Publishing Textbook of Mood Disorders. Edited by Stein DJ, Kupfer DJ, Schatzberg AF. Washington, DC, American Psychiatric Publishing, 2006, pp 281–290

Keck PE Jr, McElroy SL, Strakowski SM: Anticonvulsants and antipsychotics in the treatment of bipolar disorder. J Clin Psychiatry 59 (suppl 6):74–81; discussion 82, 1998

Keck PE Jr, Strakowski SM, McElroy SL: The efficacy of atypical antipsychotics in the treatment of depressive symptoms, hostility, and suicidality in patients with schizophrenia. J Clin Psychiatry 61 (suppl 3):4–9, 2000

Keck PE Jr, Strakowski SM, Hawkins JM, et al: Rapid lithium administration in the treatment of acute mania. Bipolar Disord 3:68–72, 2001

Kellar K, Cascio C, Bergstrom D, et al: Electroconvulsive shock and reserpine: effects on beta-adrenergic receptors in rat brain. J Neurochem 37:830–836, 1981

Keller MB, Baker L: Bipolar disorder: epidemiology, course, diagnosis, and treatment. Bull Menninger Clin 55:172–181, 1991

Keller MB, McCullough JP, Klein DN, et al: A comparison of nefazodone, the cognitive behavioral-analysis system of psychotherapy, and their combination for the treatment of chronic depression. N Engl J Med 342:1462–1470, 2000

Keller MB, Ryan N, Strober M, et al: Efficacy of paroxetine in the treatment of adolescent major depression: a randomized, controlled trial. J Am Acad Child Adolesc Psychiatry 40:762–772, 2001

Kendler KS: Major depression and the environment: a psychiatric genetic perspective. Pharmacopsychiatry 31:5–9, 1998

Kendler KS, Thornton LM, Gardner CO: Stressful life events and previous episodes in the etiology of major depression in women: an evaluation of the "kindling" hypothesis. Am J Psychiatry 157:1243–1251, 2000

Kessler RC, Walters EE: Epidemiology of DSM-III-R major depression and minor depression among adolescents and young adults in the National Comorbidity Survey. Depress Anxiety 7:3–14, 1998

Kessler RC, McGonagle KA, Zhao S, et al: Lifetime and 12-month prevalence of DSM-III-R psychiatric disorders in the United States. Results from the National Comorbidity Survey. Arch Gen Psychiatry 51:8–19, 1994

Kessler RC, Berglund P, Demler O, et al: The epidemiology of major depressive disorder results from the National Comorbidity Survey Replication (NCS-R). JAMA 289:3095–3105, 2003

Khantzian EJ: The self-medication hypothesis of addictive disorders: focus on heroin and cocaine dependence. Am J Psychiatry 142:1259–1264, 1985

Kleinman A, Good B: Culture and Depression: Studies in the Anthropology and Cross-Cultural Psychiatry of Affect and Disorder. Berkeley, University of California Press, 1985

Klerman GL, Weissman MM, Rounsaville BJ, et al: Interpersonal Psychotherapy of Depression. New York, Basic Books, 1984

Klose M, Jacobi F: Can gender differences in the prevalence of mental disorders be explained by sociodemographic factors? Arch Womens Ment Health 7:133–148, 2004

Kovacs M: Presentation and course of major depressive disorder during childhood and later years of the life span. J Am Acad Child Adolesc Psychiatry 35:705–715, 1996

Kramlinger KG, Post RM: Ultra-rapid and ultradian cycling in bipolar affective illness. Br J Psychiatry 168:314–323, 1996

Kumar A, Jin Z, Bilker W, et al: Late-onset minor and major depression: early evidence for common neuroanatomical substrates detected by using MRI. Proc Natl Acad Sci USA 95:7654–7658, 1998

Lam DH, Watkins ER, Hayward P, et al: A randomized controlled study of cognitive therapy for relapse prevention for bipolar affective disorder: outcome of the first year. Arch Gen Psychiatry 60:145–152, 2003

Larson EW, Richelson E: Organic causes of mania. Mayo Clin Proc 63:906–912, 1988

Lisanby SH, Maddox JH, Prudic J, et al: The effects of electroconvulsive therapy on memory of autobiographical and public events. Arch Gen Psychiatry 57:581–590, 2000

Luborsky L: Principles of Psychoanalytic Psychotherapy: A Manual for Supportive Expressive Treatment. New York, Basic Books, 1984

Maes M, Meltzer HY: The serotonin hypothesis of major depression, in Psychopharmacology: The Fourth Generation of Progress. Edited by Bloom FE, Kupfer DJ, Bunney BS, et al. New York, Raven, 1995, pp 933–944

Mann JJ: Neurobiological correlates of the antidepressant action of electroconvulsive therapy. J ECT 14:172–180, 1998

Markowitz JC: Interpersonal psychotherapy for chronic depression. J Clin Psychol 59:847–858, 2003

Markowitz JC, Kocsis JH, Fishman B, et al: Treatment of HIV-positive patients with depressive symptoms. Arch Gen Psychiatry 55:452–457, 1998

Matt GE, Vazquez C, Campbell WK: Mood-congruent recall of affectively toned stimuli: a meta-analytic review. Clin Psychol Rev 12:227–255, 1992

McCullough JP: Treatment for Chronic Depression: Cognitive Behavioral Analysis System of Psychotherapy. New York, Guilford, 2000

McGuffin P, Rijsdijk S, Andrew M, et al: The heritability of bipolar affective disorder and the genetic relationship to unipolar depression. Arch Gen Psychiatry 60:497–502, 2003

Mendlewicz J, Rainer JD: Adoption study supporting genetic transmission in manic-depressive illness. Nature 368:327–329, 1977

Miklowitz DJ, Hooley JM: Developing family psychoeducational treatments for patients with bipolar and other severe psychiatric disorders: a pathway from basic research to clinical trials. J Marital Fam Ther 24:419–435, 1998

Moore JD, Bona JR: Depression and dysthymia. Med Clin North Am 85:631–644, 2001

Mufson L, Weissman MM, Moreau D, et al: Efficacy of interpersonal psychotherapy for depressed adolescents. Arch Gen Psychiatry 56:573–579, 1999

Nemeroff C: The neurobiological consequences of child abuse. Paper presented at the 156th annual meeting of the American Psychiatric Association, San Francisco, CA, May 19, 2003

Nobler MS, Sackeim HA, Moeller JR, et al: Quantifying the speed of symptomatic improvement with electroconvulsive therapy: comparison of alternative statistical methods. Convuls Ther 13:208–221, 1997

Ostroff RB, Nelson JC: Risperidone augmentation of selective serotonin reuptake inhibitors in major depression. J Clin Psychiatry 60:256–259, 1999

Parmelee PA, Ketz IR, Lawton MP: Depression among institutionalized aged: assessment and prevalence estimation. J Gerontol 44: M22–M29, 1989

Pascual-Leone A, Houser CM, Reese K, et al: Safety of rapid-rate transcranial magnetic stimulation in normal volunteers. Electroencephalogr Clin Neurophysiol 89:120–130, 1993

Paykel ES: Correlates of a depressive typology. Arch Gen Psychiatry 27:203–210, 1972

Perlis RH, Brown E, Baker RW, et al: Clinical features of bipolar depression versus major depressive disorder in large multicenter trials. Am J Psychiatry 163:225–231, 2006

Perry A, Tarrier N, Morriss R, et al: Randomised controlled trial of efficacy of teaching patients with bipolar disorder to identify early symptoms of relapse and obtain treatment. BMJ 318:149–153, 1999

Perry PJ: Pharmacotherapy for major depression with melancholic features: relative efficacy of tricyclic versus selective serotonin reuptake inhibitor antidepressants. J Affect Disord 39:1–6, 1996

Peveler R, Carson A, Rodin G: Depression in medical patients. BMJ 325:149–152, 2002

Pezawas L, Angst J, Kasper S: Recurrent brief depression revisited. Int Rev Psychiatry 17:63–70, 2005

Plotsky PM, Owens MJ, Nemeroff CB: Psychoneuroendocrinology of depression: hypothalamic-pituitary-adrenal axis. Psychiatr Clin North Am 21:293–307, 1998

Post RM: Transduction of psychosocial stress into the neurobiology of recurrent affective disorder. Am J Psychiatry 149:999–1010, 1992

Post RM, Uhde TW, Roy-Byrne PP, et al: Antidepressant effects of carbamazepine. Am J Psychiatry 143:29–34, 1986

Prien RF, Kupfer DJ, Mansky PA, et al: Drug therapy in the prevention of recurrences in unipolar and bipolar affective disorders: report of the NIMH Collaborative Study Group comparing lithium carbonate, imipramine, and a lithium carbonate-imipramine combination. Arch Gen Psychiatry 41:1096–1104, 1984

Regier DA, Farmer ME, Rae DS, et al: Comorbidity of mental disorders with alcohol and other drug abuse: results from the Epidemiologic Catchment Area (ECA) Study. JAMA 264:2511–2518, 1990

Rehm LP: A self-control model of depression. Behav Ther 8:787–804, 1977

Roose SP, Glassman AH, Siris SG, et al: Comparison of imipramine and nortriptyline induced orthostatic hypotension: a meaningful difference. J Clin Psychopharmacol 1:316–319, 1981

Rosenthal NE, Sack DA, Gillin JC, et al: Seasonal affective disorder: a description of the syndrome and preliminary findings with light therapy. Arch Gen Psychiatry 41:72–80, 1984

Rubin RT: Pharmacoendocrinology of major depression. Eur Arch Psychiatry Neurol Sci 238:259–267, 1989

Sackeim HA: Magnetic stimulation therapy and ECT. Convuls Ther 10:255–258, 1994

Sackeim HA, Rush AJ: Melancholia and response to ECT (letter). Am J Psychiatry 152:1242–1243, 1995

Sartorius N, Ustun TB, Korten A, et al: Progress toward achieving a common language in psychiatry, II: results from the international field trials of the ICD-10 diagnostic criteria for research for mental and behavioral disorders. Am J Psychiatry 152:1427–1437, 1995

Schatzberg AF, Rush AJ, Arnow BA, et al: Chronic depression: medication (nefazodone) or psychotherapy (CBASP) is effective when the other is not. Arch Gen Psychiatry 62:513–520, 2005

Schulberg HC, Block MR, Madonia MJ, et al: Treating major depression in primary care practice: eight-month clinical outcomes. Arch Gen Psychiatry 53:913–919, 1996

Scott J, Garland A, Moorhead S: A pilot study of cognitive therapy in bipolar disorders. Psychol Med 31:459–467, 2001

Shelton RC, Tollefson GD, Tohen M, et al: A novel augmentation strategy for treating resistant major depression. Am J Psychiatry 158:131–134, 2001

Smith S: Tryptophan in the treatment of resistant depression: a review. Pharm J 261:819–821, 1998

Solomon DA, Ryan CE, Keitner GI: A pilot study of lithium carbonate plus divalproex sodium for the continuation and maintenance treatment of patients with bipolar I disorder. J Clin Psychiatry 58:95–99, 1997

Spijker J, de Graaf R, Bijl RV, et al: Duration of major depressive episodes in the general population: results from the Netherlands Mental Health Survey and Incidence Study. Br J Psychiatry 181:208–213, 2002

Squire LR, Slater PC: Electroconvulsive therapy and complaints of memory dysfunction: a prospective three-year follow-up study. Br J Psychiatry 142:1–8, 1983

Stewart JW, McGrath PJ, Quitkin FM: Do age of onset and course of illness predict different treatment outcome among DSM IV depressive disorders with atypical features? Neuropsychopharmacology 26:237–245, 2002

Stoll AL, Mayer PV, Kolbrener M, et al: Antidepressant-associated mania: a controlled comparison with spontaneous mania. Am J Psychiatry 151:1642–1645, 1994

Strakowski SM: Clinical update in bipolar disorders: second-generation antipsychotics in the maintenance therapy of bipolar disorder. Available at: http://www.medscape. com/viewprogram/2496. Release date June 26, 2003

Sullivan P, Kendler K: Genetic case-control studies in neuropsychiatry. Arch Gen Psychiatry 58:1015–1024, 2001

Suppes T, Swann AC, Dennehy EB, et al: Texas Medication Algorithm Project: development and feasibility testing of a treatment algorithm for patients with bipolar disorder. J Clin Psychiatry 62:439–447, 2001

Swann AC, Bowden CL, Calabrese JR, et al: Pattern of response to divalproex, lithium, or placebo in four naturalistic subtypes of mania. Neuropsychopharmacology 26:530–536, 2002

Thase ME: Novel transdermal delivery formulation of the monoamine oxidase inhibitor selegiline nearing release for treatment of depression. J Clin Psychiatry 67:671–672, 2006

Thase ME, Simons AD, McGeary J, et al: Relapse after cognitive-behavior therapy of depression: potential implications for longer courses of treatment? Am J Psychiatry 149:1046–1052, 1992

Torres GE, Gainetdinov RR, Caron MG: Plasma membrane monoamine transporters: structure, regulation and function. Nat Rev Neurosci 4:13–25, 2003

Wagner KD, Ambrosini PJ, Rynn M, et al: Efficacy of sertraline in the treatment of children and adolescents with major depressive disorder. JAMA 290:1033–1041, 2003

Weisler RH, Kalali AH, Ketter TA, the SPD417 Study Group: A multicenter, randomized, double-blind, placebo-controlled trial of beaded carbamazepine extended-release capsules (beaded-ERC-CBZ; SPD417) as monotherapy for bipolar patients with manic or mixed episodes. J Clin Psychiatry 65:478–484, 2004

Weissman MM, Myers J: Affective disorders in a U.S. urban community: the use of research diagnostic criteria in an epidemiological survey. Arch Gen Psychiatry 35:1304–1311, 1978

Weissman MM, Bland RC, Canino GJ, et al: Cross-national epidemiology of major depression and bipolar disorder. JAMA 276:293–299, 1996

Whybrow PC, Bauer MS, Gyulai L: Thyroid axis considerations in patients with rapid cycling affective disorder. Clin Neuropharmacol 15 (suppl 1, pt A):391A–392A, 1992

Williams JMG: Depression, in Science and Practice of Cognitive Behavior Therapy. Edited by Clark DM, Fairburn CG. Oxford, England, Oxford University Press, 1997, pp 259–283

World Health Organization: International Statistical Classification of Diseases and Related Health Problems, 10th Revision. Geneva, Switzerland, World Health Organization, 1992

Young RC, Meyers BS: Psychopharmacology, in Comprehensive Review of Geriatric Psychiatry. Edited by Sadavoy J, Lazarus LW, Jarvik LF. Washington, DC, American Psychiatric Press, 1992, pp 435–467

Zornberg GL, Pope HG Jr: Treatment of depression in bipolar disorder: new directions for research. J Clin Psychopharmacol 13:397–408, 1993

7

ANXIETY DISORDERS

Eric Hollander, M.D.

Daphne Simeon, M.D.

Anxiety disorders are the most common of all psychiatric illnesses and result in considerable functional impairment and distress. Recent research developments have had a broad impact on our understanding of the underlying mechanisms of illness and treatment response. Working with patients who have an anxiety disorder can be highly gratifying for the informed psychiatrist, because these patients, who are in considerable distress, often respond to proper treatment and return to a high level of functioning. The major anxiety disorders presented in this chapter are panic disorder, generalized anxiety disorder (GAD), social phobia (social anxiety disorder), specific phobias, obsessive-compulsive disorder (OCD), and posttraumatic stress disorder (PTSD). Table 7–1 presents a summary overview of the prevalence, gender ratio, and comorbidities of the major anxiety disorders.

Panic Disorder

Definition

The DSM-IV-TR (American Psychiatric Association 2000) definition of a *panic attack* is presented in Table 7–2. Panic disorder is subdivided into panic disorder with and without agoraphobia, depending on whether there is any secondary phobic avoidance (Table 7–3).

Clinical Description

Onset

In the typical onset of a case of panic disorder, individuals are engaged in some ordinary aspect of life when suddenly their heart begins to pound, and they cannot catch their breath. They feel dizzy, light-headed, and faint and are convinced they are about to die. Panic disorder patients are usually young adults,

Table 7–1. Approximate lifetime prevalence, gender ratio, and common comorbidities for the major anxiety disorders

Disorder	Prevalence	Females:Males	Comorbidity
Panic disorder	2%–4%	2+:1	Depression, other anxiety disorders
Generalized anxiety disorder	5%–7%	2:1	Overall, 90%; 50%–60%, major depression or another anxiety disorder
Social phobia	13%–16%	1+:1	Twofold risk of alcohol dependence, three- to sixfold risk of mood disorders
Specific phobias	10%	2:1	Depression and somatoform disorders
Agoraphobia	6%	2:1	
Obsessive-compulsive disorder	2%–3%	1:1	Anxiety, depression, tics, hypochondriasis, eating disorder, body dysmorphic disorder (childhood-onset more common in males)
Posttraumatic stress disorder	7%–9%	2:1	Depression, obsessive-compulsive disorder, panic, phobias

Table 7–2. DSM-IV-TR diagnostic criteria for panic attacks

Note: A panic attack is not a codable disorder. Code the specific diagnosis in which the panic attack occurs (e.g., 300.21 panic disorder with agoraphobia)

A discrete period of intense fear or discomfort, in which four (or more) of the following symptoms developed abruptly and reached a peak within 10 minutes:

(1) palpitations, pounding heart, or accelerated heart rate
(2) sweating
(3) trembling or shaking
(4) sensations of shortness of breath or smothering
(5) feeling of choking
(6) chest pain or discomfort
(7) nausea or abdominal distress
(8) feeling dizzy, unsteady, light-headed, or faint
(9) derealization (feelings of unreality) or depersonalization (being detached from oneself)
(10) fear of losing control or going crazy
(11) fear of dying
(12) paresthesias (numbness or tingling sensations)
(13) chills or hot flushes

most likely in the third decade, although onset may be as late as the sixth decade.

Although the first attack generally strikes during some routine activity, several events are often associated with the early presentation of panic disorder. Not uncommonly, the first panic attack occurs in the context of a life-threatening illness or accident, the loss of a close interpersonal relationship, or a separation from family (e.g., starting college or accepting a job out of town). Patients developing either hypo- or hyperthyroidism may

---

Table 7–3. DSM-IV-TR diagnostic criteria for panic disorder with or without agoraphobia

---

Diagnostic criteria for 300.01 panic disorder without agoraphobia

A. Both (1) and (2):
  (1) recurrent unexpected panic attacks
  (2) at least one of the attacks has been followed by 1 month (or more) of one (or more) of the following:
    (a) persistent concern about having additional attacks
    (b) worry about the implications of the attack or its consequences (e.g., losing control, having a heart attack, "going crazy")
    (c) a significant change in behavior related to the attacks

B. Absence of agoraphobia.

C. The panic attacks are not due to the direct physiological effects of a substance (e.g., a drug of abuse, a medication) or a general medical condition (e.g., hyperthyroidism).

D. The panic attacks are not better accounted for by another mental disorder, such as social phobia (e.g., occurring on exposure to feared social situations), specific phobia (e.g., on exposure to a specific phobic situation), obsessive-compulsive disorder (e.g., on exposure to dirt in someone with an obsession about contamination), posttraumatic stress disorder (e.g., in response to stimuli associated with a severe stressor), or separation anxiety disorder (e.g., in response to being away from home or close relatives).

Diagnostic criteria for 300.21 panic disorder with agoraphobia

A. Both (1) and (2):
  (1) recurrent unexpected panic attacks
  (2) at least one of the attacks has been followed by 1 month (or more) of one (or more) of the following:
    (a) persistent concern about having additional attacks
    (b) worry about the implications of the attack or its consequences (e.g., losing control, having a heart attack, "going crazy")
    (c) a significant change in behavior related to the attacks

B. The presence of agoraphobia.

C. The panic attacks are not due to the direct physiological effects of a substance (e.g., a drug of abuse, a medication) or a general medical condition (e.g., hyperthyroidism).

D. The panic attacks are not better accounted for by another mental disorder, such as social phobia (e.g., occurring on exposure to feared social situations), specific phobia (e.g., on exposure to a specific phobic situation), obsessive-compulsive disorder (e.g., on exposure to dirt in someone with an obsession about contamination), posttraumatic stress disorder (e.g., in response to stimuli associated with a severe stressor), or separation anxiety disorder (e.g., in response to being away from home or close relatives).

---

get the first flurry of attacks at this time. Attacks also begin in the immediate postpartum period. Finally, many patients have reported experiencing their first attacks while taking drugs of abuse, especially marijuana, lysergic acid diethylamide (LSD), sedatives, cocaine, and amphetamines. However, even when these concomitant conditions are resolved, the attacks often continue unabated. This situation gives the impression that some stressors may act as triggers to provoke the beginning of panic attacks in patients who are already predisposed.

Patients experiencing their first panic attack generally fear they are having a heart attack or losing their mind. Such patients often rush to the nearest emergency department, where routine laboratory tests, electrocardiography, and physical examination are performed. All that is found is an occasional case of sinus tachycardia, and the patients are reassured and sent home. These patients may indeed feel reassured, and at this point the diagnosis of panic disorder would be premature. However, perhaps a few days or even weeks later they will again have the sudden onset of severe anxiety with all of the associated physical symptoms. Again, they seek emergency medical treatment. At this point, they may be told the problem is psychological, be given a prescription for a benzodiazepine tranquilizer, or be referred for extensive medical workup.

Symptoms

Typically, during a panic attack, a patient will be engaged in a routine activity, perhaps reading a book, eating in a restaurant, driving a car, or attending a concert, when he or she will experience the sudden onset of overwhelming fear, terror, apprehension, and a sense of impending doom. Several of a group of associated symptoms, mostly physical, are also experienced: dyspnea, palpitations, chest pain or discomfort, choking or smothering sensations, dizziness or unsteady feelings, feelings of unreality (derealization and/or depersonalization), paresthesias, hot and cold flashes, sweating, faintness, trembling and shaking, and a fear of dying, going crazy, or losing control of oneself. It is clear that most of the physical sensations of a panic attack represent massive overstimulation of the autonomic nervous system.

Attacks usually last from 5 to 20 minutes and rarely as long as an hour. Patients who claim they have attacks that last a whole day may fall into one of four categories. Some patients continue to feel agitated and fatigued for several hours after the main portion of the attack has subsided. At times, attacks occur, subside, and occur again in a wave-like manner. Alternatively, the patient with so-called long panic attacks often has some other form of pathological anxiety, such as severe generalized anxiety, agitated depression, or obsessional tension states. Finally, in some cases, such severe anticipatory anxiety may develop with time in expectation of future panic attacks that the two may blend together in the patient's description and be difficult to distinguish.

Although many people experience an occasional unexpected attack of panic, the diagnosis of panic disorder is only made when the attacks occur with some regularity and frequency. However, patients with occasional unexpected panic attacks may be genetically similar to patients with panic disorder. A twin study found the best results for genetic linkage when patients with regular panic attacks were included together with patients who had only occasional attacks (Torgersen 1983).

Some patients do not progress in their illness beyond the point of continuing to have unexpected panic attacks. Most patients develop some degree of anticipatory anxiety consequent to the experience of repetitive panic attacks. The patient comes to dread experiencing an attack and starts worrying about doing so in the intervals between attacks. This can progress until the level of fearfulness and autonomic hyperactivity in the interval between panic attacks almost approximates the level during the actual attack itself. Such patients may be mistaken for GAD patients.

It is warranted to draw some further attention to what appears to be the cardinal symptom of panic. A number of lines of research evidence indicate that hyperventilation may be the central feature in the pathophysiology of panic attacks and panic disorder. Patients with panic disorder have been shown to be chronic hyperventilators who also acutely hyperventilate during spontaneous and induced panic. This hyperventilation then induces hypocapnia and alkalosis, leading to decreased cerebral blood flow and to the dizziness, confusion, and derealization characteristic of panic attacks. Indeed, signs and symptoms of hyperventilation seem to disappear once a patient with panic disorder has been successfully treated with antipanic medication. Also, behavioral breathing retraining treatments aimed at teaching the patient not to hyperventilate are successful in decreasing the frequency of panic attacks, presumably by dampening the ventilatory overreaction that may constitute the hallmark of panic.

Agoraphobia. Agoraphobia frequently develops in response to panic attacks, leading to the DSM-IV-TR diagnosis of panic disorder with agoraphobia. The clinical picture in agoraphobia consists of multiple and varied fears and avoidance behaviors that center around three main themes: 1) fear of leaving home, 2) fear of being alone, and 3) fear of being away from home in situations where one can feel trapped, embarrassed, or helpless. According to DSM-IV-TR, the fear is one of developing distressing symptoms in such situations where escape is difficult or help is unavailable. Typical agoraphobic fears are of using public transportation (e.g., buses, trains, subways, planes); being in crowds, theaters, elevators, restaurants, supermarkets, or department stores; waiting in line; or traveling a distance from home. In severe cases, patients may be completely housebound, fearful of leaving home without a companion or even of staying home alone.

Most cases of agoraphobia begin with a series of spontaneous panic attacks. If the attacks continue, the patient usually develops a constant anticipatory anxiety characterized by continued apprehension about the possible occasion and consequences of the next attack. Agoraphobic symptoms represent a tertiary phase in the illness. Many patients will causally relate their panic attacks to the particular situation in which the attacks have occurred. They then avoid these situations in an attempt to prevent further panic attacks.

Epidemiology

The National Institute of Mental Health Epidemiologic Catchment Area (ECA) study examined the population prevalence of DSM-III (American Psychiatric Association 1980)–

diagnosed panic disorder using the Diagnostic Interview Schedule (Regier et al. 1988). The 1-month, 6-month, and lifetime prevalence rates for panic disorder at all five study sites combined were 0.5%, 0.8%, and 1.6%, respectively. Women had a 1-month prevalence rate of 0.7%, which was significantly higher than the 0.3% rate found among men; women also tended to have a greater rise in panic disorder in the age range of 25 to 44 years, and their attacks tended to continue longer into older age (Regier et al. 1988).

More recently, the 2001–2002 National Epidemiologic Survey on Alcohol and Related Conditions (NESARC), which included about 43,000 participants, revealed a 1-year and lifetime prevalence of panic disorder of 2.1% and 5.1%, respectively (Grant et al. 2006); rates for panic disorder without agoraphobia were 1.6% and 4.0%, respectively, exceeding those of panic disorder with agoraphobia (0.6% and 1.1%, respectively). Being female, Native American, middle-aged, widowed/separated/divorced, and of low income increased risk for panic disorder, whereas being Asian, African American, or Hispanic decreased risk. Subjects with agoraphobia had an earlier age at onset, more severe symptoms, greater disability, and greater Axis I and II comorbidity compared with subjects without agoraphobia and were more likely to seek treatment early on. Thus, the overrepresentation of panic disorder with agoraphobia in treatment settings probably reflects greater treatment seeking and more severe disorder. On the other hand, agoraphobia without panic disorder was quite rare, with a 0.17% lifetime prevalence, raising questions about its standing as a distinct Axis I disorder. The National Comorbidity Survey Replication study reported highly similar findings, with a lifetime prevalence of 3.7% for panic disorder without agoraphobia and 1.1% with agoraphobia (Kessler et al. 2006), and again the presence of agoraphobia was associated with greater symptom severity, comorbidity, and impairment.

Table 7–4. Course and prognosis of panic disorder

Course
    Variable, typically with periods of
        exacerbations and remissions

Outcome
    About 33% recover, 50% have limited
        impairment, 20% or less have major
        impairment

Predictors of worse prognosis
    More severe initial panic attacks
    More severe initial agoraphobia
    Longer duration of illness
    Comorbid depression
    History of separation from parent (e.g.,
        death, divorce)
    High interpersonal sensitivity
    Single marital status

Course, Prognosis, Morbidity, and Mortality

The course of illness without treatment is highly variable and is summarized in Table 7–4.

Diagnosis

Physical Signs and Behavior

The diagnosis of panic disorder is made when a patient experiences recurrent panic attacks that are discrete and unexpected and followed by a month of persistent anticipatory anxiety or behavioral change. These panic attacks are characterized by a sudden crescendo of anxiety and fearfulness, in addition to the presence of at least four physical symptoms. Finally, these attacks are not secondary to a known organic factor or due to another mental disorder. However, these diagnoses are not always obvious, and a number of other psychiatric and medical disorders may mimic these conditions (Table 7–5).

Differential Diagnosis

Other psychiatric illnesses. Although the medical conditions that mimic anxiety disor-

Table 7–5. Differential diagnosis of panic disorder

Anxious depression
Somatization with panic-like physical
    complaints
Social phobia with socially cued panic
    attacks
Generalized anxiety with severe symptoms
    or during peak periods
Posttraumatic stress disorder with intense
    physiological response to reminders of the
    trauma
Agoraphobia secondary to conditions other
    than panic (depression, posttraumatic
    stress, paranoia, psychosis)
Obsessional anxiety of near-panic severity
Depersonalization disorder
Personality disorder with anxiety symptoms
Hyperthyroidism
Hypothyroidism
Mitral valve prolapse
Pheochromocytoma

der are usually easily ruled out, psychiatric conditions that involve pathological anxiety can make the differential diagnosis of panic disorder difficult. By far the most problematic is the differentiation of primary anxiety disorder from depression.

Patients with depression often manifest signs of anxiety and may even have frank panic attacks. On the other hand, patients with panic disorder, if untreated for significant amounts of time, routinely become demoralized as the impact of the illness progressively restricts their ability to enjoy a normal life. Further complicating the picture is the fact that some, but not all, studies have shown that patients with anxiety disorder have increased family history of affective disorder.

Although the differentiation of anxiety from depression can at times strain even the most experienced clinician, several points are helpful. Patients with panic disorder generally do not demonstrate the full range of vegetative symptoms seen in depression. Thus, anxious patients usually have trouble falling asleep—not early-morning awakening—and do not lose their appetite. Diurnal mood fluctuation is uncommon in anxiety disorder. Perhaps of greatest importance is the fact that most anxious patients do not lose the capacity to enjoy things or to be cheered up as endogenously depressed patients do.

The order of developing symptoms also differentiates depression from anxiety. In cases of panic disorder, anxiety symptoms usually precede any seriously altered mood. Patients can generally recall having anxiety attacks first, then becoming gradually more disgusted with life, and then feeling depressed. In depression, patients usually experience dysphoria first, with anxiety symptoms coming later. However, panic disorder can be complicated by secondary major depression and vice versa.

A few other psychiatric conditions often need to be differentiated from panic disorder. Patients with somatization disorder complain of a variety of physical ailments and discomforts, none of which are substantiated by physical or laboratory findings. Unlike panic disorder patients, somatizing patients present with physical problems that do not usually occur in episodic attacks but are virtually constant.

Patients with depersonalization disorder have episodes of derealization/depersonalization without the other symptoms of a panic attack. However, panic attacks not infrequently involve depersonalization and derealization as prominent symptoms.

Although patients with panic disorder often fear they will lose their minds or go crazy, psychotic illness is not an outcome of anxiety disorder. Reassuring the patient on this point is often the first step in a successful treatment.

Undoubtedly some patients with anxiety disorders abuse alcohol and drugs, such as sedatives, in attempts at self-medication. In one study, after successful detoxification a group of alcoholic patients with a prior history of panic disorder were treated with medication to block spontaneous panic attacks (Quitkin and Babkin 1982). These pa-

tients did not resume alcohol consumption once their panic attacks were eliminated.

With regard to the agoraphobic component of the disorder, widespread fears and avoidance of being alone or of leaving home can also be seen in paranoid and psychotic states, PTSD, and major depressive disorders. Psychotic states can be differentiated from agoraphobia by the presence of delusions, hallucinations, and thought process disorder. Although agoraphobic patients are frequently afraid that they are going crazy, they do not exhibit psychotic symptomatology. Patients with PTSD have a typical history of trauma, such as a fear of being or of traveling alone after an assault.

The distinction between depressive disorders and agoraphobia is more difficult. Both groups commonly experience spontaneous panic attacks. Patients with agoraphobia are frequently demoralized and will state that they feel depressed. Close questioning, however, usually does not reveal further vegetative symptoms or a loss of pleasure or interest in activities. Early-morning awakening and pervasive anhedonia, which are common symptoms in endogenous depression, are rare in agoraphobia. Agoraphobic individuals will usually say they would love to leave home and engage in a variety of activities, if only they could be sure of not panicking. In contrast, depressed individuals usually see no point in going out because nothing gives them any pleasure, and they believe that people will be better off without them.

Patients with atypical depression (i.e., depression characterized by hypersomnia, hyperphagia, extreme low energy, and depressed but reactive mood) frequently have panic attacks but rarely have agoraphobia as part of their life history or current symptomatology. Patients with atypical depression and a history of panic attacks may respond preferentially to monoamine oxidase inhibitors (MAOIs; Liebowitz et al. 1985).

Hyperthyroidism and hypothyroidism. Both hyper- and hypothyroidism can present with anxiety unaccompanied by other signs or symptoms. For this reason, it is imperative that all patients complaining of anxiety undergo routine thyroid function tests, including the evaluation of the level of thyroid-stimulating hormone. It should be remembered, however, that thyroid disease can act as one of the predisposing triggers to panic disorder, so that even when the apparently primary thyroid disease is corrected, panic attacks may continue until specifically treated.

Cardiac disease.   The relationship of mitral valve prolapse to panic disorder has attracted a great deal of attention over the years. This usually benign condition has been shown by a number of investigators to occur more frequently in patients with panic disorder than in normal subjects. However, screening of patients known to have mitral valve prolapse reveals no greater frequency of panic disorder than is found in the overall population.

Other medical illnesses.   Hyperparathyroidism occasionally presents as anxiety symptoms, warranting a serum calcium level before definitive diagnosis is made.

A variety of cardiac conditions can initially present as anxiety symptoms, although in most cases, the patient complains prominently of chest pain, skipped beats, or palpitations. Ischemic heart disease and arrhythmias, especially paroxysmal atrial tachycardia, should be ruled out by electrocardiography.

Pheochromocytoma is a rare, usually benign tumor of the adrenal medulla that secretes catecholamines in episodic bursts. During an active phase, the patient characteristically experiences flushing, tremulousness, and anxiety. Blood pressure is usually elevated during the active phase of catecholamine secretion but not at other times. Therefore, merely finding a normal blood pressure does not rule out a pheochromocytoma. If this condition is suspected, the diagnosis is made by collection of urine for 24 hours for determination of catecholamine metabolite concentration. In a study of patients with confirmed pheochromocytoma, about half met criteria for the physical symptoms of panic attacks, but none had panic disorder, because they did not experience terror during the attacks and did not develop anticipatory anxiety or agoraphobia (Starkman et al. 1990).

Disease of the vestibular nerve can cause episodic bouts of vertigo, light-headedness, nausea, and anxiety that mimic panic attacks. Rather than merely feeling dizzy, such patients often experience true vertigo in which the room seems to spin in one direction during each attack. Otolaryngology consultation is warranted when this condition is suspected. Some panic patients primarily complain of dizziness or unsteadiness. Whether they are a distinct subgroup with definite neurological abnormalities is currently under study.

Although many patients believe that their anxiety disorder is caused by reactive hypoglycemia, there is no scientific proof at present that this is ever a cause of any psychiatric disturbance. Glucose tolerance tests are not helpful in establishing hypoglycemia as the cause of anxiety, because up to 40% of the normal population has a random low blood-sugar level during a routine glucose tolerance test. The only convincing way to establish hypoglycemia as a cause of symptoms is to document a low blood-sugar level at the same time the patient is symptomatic. Studies with insulin tolerance tests in panic disorder have yielded negative results.

Treatment
Pharmacotherapy

Antidepressants.   When initiating a drug regimen for a patient with panic disorder, it is crucial for the patient to understand that the drug will block the panic attacks but may not necessarily decrease the amount of intervening anticipatory anxiety and avoidance, at least initially. For patients with severe anxiety, it can be helpful to initially prescribe a concomitant benzodiazepine that can be gradually tapered and discontinued after several weeks of antidepressant treatment. Also importantly, some patients with panic disorder display an initial hypersensitivity to antidepressants, whether tricyclic antidepressants (TCAs) or serotonin reuptake inhibitors, during which they complain of jitteriness, agitation, a speedy feeling, and insomnia. Although this is usually transient, it is one of the main reasons why patients unfortunately opt to discontinue medication early on. Therefore, it is strongly recommended that patients

with panic disorder be started on lower dosages of antidepressants than would be given to depressed patients. The central feature in the treatment of panic disorder is the pharmacological blockade of the spontaneous panic attacks. Several classes of medications have been shown to be effective in accomplishing this goal, and a summary of the pharmacological treatment of panic disorder is presented in Table 7–6.

Table 7–6. Pharmacological treatment of panic disorder

Selective serotonin reuptake inhibitors and serotonin–norepinephrine reuptake inhibitors

General indications: First-line, alone or in combination with benzodiazepines if needed. Also first choice with comorbid obsessive-compulsive disorder, generalized anxiety disorder, depression, and social phobia. Start with very low dosages and increase; response seen with low to moderate dosages.

Sertraline, paroxetine: FDA approved
Fluvoxamine, fluoxetine, citalopram, escitalopram: similarly efficacious
Venlafaxine extended-release: FDA approved

Tricyclic antidepressants

General indications: Established efficacy, second line if SSRIs fail or are not tolerated.

Imipramine: well studied
Clomipramine: high efficacy but not easily tolerated
Desipramine: if low tolerance of anticholinergic side effects
Nortriptyline: if prone to orthostatic hypotension, elderly

Monoamine oxidase inhibitors

General indications: Poor response to or tolerance of other antidepressants; comorbid atypical depression or social phobia.

Phenelzine: most studied
Tranylcypromine: less sedation

High-potency benzodiazepines

General indications: Poor response to or tolerance of antidepressants; prominent anticipatory anxiety or phobic avoidance; initial treatment phase until antidepressant begins to work.

Clonazepam: longer acting, less frequent dosing, less withdrawal, first choice
Alprazolam: well studied but short-acting
Alprazolam extended-release: once-daily dosing

Other medications

General indications: Particularly as augmentation in patients whose illness is refractory or who are intolerant of the above medications; not well tested to date.

Pindolol: effective augmentation in one controlled trial
Valproic acid: open trials only
Inositol: open trials only
Clonidine: initial response tends to fade in open trials
Atypical antipsychotics: open trials only

Note. FDA = U.S. Food and Drug Administration; SSRIs = selective serotonin reuptake inhibitors.

Benzodiazepines. Although clinicians prefer to use antidepressants for the first-line treatment of panic, high-potency benzodiazepines are also highly effective in treating the condition. These medications have fewer initial side effects than TCAs and serotonin reuptake inhibitors. However, the general treatment principle is that anxiolytics should be reserved until the different classes of antidepressants have failed, because they do pose some risk of tolerance, dependence, and withdrawal. For patients with severe acute distress and disability who may require immediate relief, it may be indicated to start with a benzodiazepine and then replace it with an antidepressant. There is evidence that benzodiazepines may be more effective, at least initially, in ameliorating the associated anticipatory anxiety and phobic avoidance, and this may be another indication for their initial use.

Clonazepam should generally be preferred as a first choice, because it is longer acting and thus has the advantage of less frequent twice-daily or even once-daily dosing and less risk of withdrawal symptoms than alprazolam. It should generally be started at 0.5 mg bid and increased only if needed, usually to a maximum dosage of 4 mg/day. Alprazolam is usually started at 0.5 mg qid and is gradually increased to an average dosage of 4 mg/day and a range of 2–10 mg/day according to the individual patient. Treatment of at least 6 months is recommended, as with the antidepressants. Patients' moods must be followed, because alprazolam may occasionally cause mania, and clonazepam may cause depression. Discontinuation must be gradual to prevent withdrawal: 15% of the total dosage weekly is generally a safe regimen, but an even slower rate may be required to prevent the recurrence of panic. In a controlled study, one-third of patients were unable to tolerate a 4-week taper off alprazolam after 8 months of maintenance treatment; the strongest predictor of taper failure was initial severity of panic attacks rather than alprazolam dosage (Rickels et al. 1993). The distinction between actual withdrawal and a simple recrudescence of the original anxiety symptom when the benzodiazepine is stopped remains controversial and can be difficult to make clinically. It has been convincingly shown that the introduction of cognitive-behavioral therapy (CBT) greatly increases the likelihood that panic patients will be able to successfully taper off benzodiazepines (Otto et al. 1993; Spiegel et al. 1994).

Although benzodiazepines are generally safe, with side effects limited mainly to sedation, there is a concern that some patients may become tolerant or even addicted to these medications. However, available data indicate that most patients are able to stop taking benzodiazepines without serious sequelae and that the problem of tolerance and dependence is overestimated and probably limited to an addiction-prone population or to patients with more refractory panic disorder who may escalate standard benzodiazepine usage in unsuccessful attempts at self-medication.

Psychotherapy

Psychodynamic psychotherapy. Even after medication has blocked the actual panic attacks, a subgroup of panic patients remain wary of independence and assertiveness. In addition to supportive and behavioral treatment, traditional psychodynamic psychotherapy might be helpful for some of these patients. Significant unconscious conflict over separations during childhood sometimes appears to operate in patients with panic disorder, leading to a reemergence of anxiety symptoms in adult life each time a new separation is imagined or threatened. Furthermore, it has been found that comorbid personality disorder is the major predictor of continued social maladjustment in patients otherwise treated for panic disorder (Noyes et al. 1990), suggesting that psychodynamic therapy may be an important additional treatment for at least some patients with panic.

Pharmacotherapy is in no way incompatible with behavioral or psychodynamic treatment for patients with panic disorder. The notion that reducing the symptoms of anxiety disorder with medication will disturb a successful psychotherapy has never been convincingly shown and is largely dogmatic. Indeed, successful psychotherapy often cannot take place until the more debilitating aspects of these syndromes have been eliminated pharmacologically.

Supportive psychotherapy. Despite adequate treatment of panic attacks with medication, phobic avoidance may remain. Supportive psychotherapy and education about the illness are necessary to urge the patient to confront the phobic situation. Patients who fail to respond may then need additional psychotherapy, either dynamic or behavioral. Encouragement from other patients with similar conditions is often quite helpful. Yet supportive psychotherapy alone is not an effective enough treatment for panic disorder.

Cognitive-behavioral therapy. CBTs have long focused on phobic avoidance, but more recently the techniques have been developed and shown to be effective for panic attacks. In recent years, interest in CBT for panic has surged, and it has become firmly established as a first-line treatment for this disorder and found to be comparable in effectiveness to first-line medication treatments (Table 7–7).

The major behavioral techniques for the treatment of panic attacks are breathing retraining, to control both acute and chronic hyperventilation; exposure to somatic cues, usually involving a hierarchy of exposure to feared sensations through imaginal and behavioral exercises; and relaxation training. Cognitive treatment of panic involves cogni-

tive restructuring, so as to give the uncomfortable affects and physical sensations associated with panic a more benign interpretation. These techniques can be administered in various combinations. The pure cognitive view is that panic attacks consist of normal physical sensations (e.g., palpitations, slight dizziness) to which panic disorder patients grossly overreact with catastrophic cognitions. A more middle-of-the-road view is that panic patients do have extreme physical sensations, such as bursts of tachycardia, but can still significantly help themselves by changing their interpretation of the event from "I am going to die of a heart attack" to "There go my heart symptoms again."

Several studies have shown that these various cognitive and behavioral techniques are successful in the treatment of panic disorder (Barlow et al. 1989; Beck et al. 1992; Michelson et al. 1990; Salkovskis et al. 1986). A study comparing CBT with in vivo exposure alone found similar efficacy for the two at the end of acute treatment and at 1-year follow-up (Ost et al. 2004).

Findings on long-term outcome of panic with CBT appear to be favorable, especially with combined cognitive restructuring and exposure. In addition, there is evidence that the introduction of CBT can reduce the risk of rebound panic in patients who are tapered off antipanic medications such as benzodiazepines or antidepressants (Schmidt et al. 2002). Conversely, there is evidence that in patients who do not benefit adequately from cognitive therapy alone, the addition of adjunctive selective serotonin reuptake inhibitor (SSRI) treatment can be beneficial (Kampman et al. 2002).

Table 7–7. Cognitive and behavioral approaches to treating panic disorder

Interoceptive exposure (to the somatic cues of panic attacks)
Situational exposure (to the settings that are phobically avoided)
Cognitive restructuring
Breathing retraining
Applied relaxation training

Generalized Anxiety Disorder

Definition and Clinical Description

DSM-IV-TR sharpened the distinction of GAD from "normal" anxiety by specifying that in GAD the worry must be clearly excessive, pervasive, difficult to control, and associated with marked distress or impairment. DSM-IV-TR also clarified that the diagnosis of GAD is excluded when occurring exclusively in relation to other major Axis I disorders, and the cumbersome somatic symptom list from the previous edition was simplified (Table 7–8).

GAD is the main diagnostic category for prominent and chronic anxiety in the absence of panic disorder. The essential feature of this syndrome, according to DSM-IV-TR, is persistent anxiety lasting at least 6 months. The symptoms of this type of anxiety fall within two broad categories: apprehensive expectation and worry, and physical symptoms. Patients with GAD are constantly worried over minor matters, fearful, and anticipating the worst. Muscle tension, restlessness, a "keyed up" feeling, difficulty concentrating, insomnia, irritability, and fatigue are typical signs of GAD and have become the symptom criteria for the disorder in DSM-IV-TR after a number of studies attempted to single out the physical symptoms that are the most distinctive and characteristic of GAD. Motor tension and hypervigilance better differentiate GAD from other anxiety states than autonomic hyperactivity. The diagnosis of GAD is made when a patient experiences at least 6 months of chronic anxiety and excessive worry. At least three of six physical symptoms must also be present. Finally, this chronic anxiety must not be secondary to another Axis I disorder or a specific organic factor.

The necessity of the "excessive worry" criterion in making the GAD diagnosis has been questioned and investigated in epidemiolog-ical samples, finding that the lifetime prevalence of GAD increases by about 40% when the excessiveness requirement is removed (Ruscio et al. 2005). Those who do have excessive worry have GAD onset earlier in life, a more chronic course, and greater symptom severity and comorbidity. However, even those without excessive worry manifest substantial persistence, impairment, comorbidity, and treatment seeking and share familial aggregation with those who do have excessive worry, bringing into question the validity of the excessiveness requirement and highlighting the need for more research (Ruscio et al. 2005).

Similarly, the 6-month duration criterion may be arbitrary and has come under scrutiny. The National Comorbidity Survey database has shown that a large number of people have a GAD-like syndrome of 1–5 months' duration, and they are similar to the DSM-IV-TR-defined group in onset, persistence, impairment, comorbidity, parental GAD, and sociodemographic correlates; thus the basis for excluding these individuals from the GAD diagnosis may need to be reexamined (Kessler et al. 2005). Finally, there are data that challenge the DSM-IV-TR hierarchy by which GAD cannot be diagnosed in the presence of concurrent major depression (Zimmerman and Chelminski 2003).

Epidemiology and Comorbidity

One epidemiological study using DSM-IV (American Psychiatric Association 1994) criteria found a 1.5% 1-year prevalence for threshold GAD and a 3.6% 1-year prevalence for subthreshold GAD (Carter et al. 2001). Higher rates of the disorder were found in women (2.7%) and the elderly (2.2%).

Despite its high comorbidity with substance use and other anxiety, mood, and personality disorders (Grant et al. 2005b), GAD stands on its own as a disorder with distinct onset, course, impairment, and prognosis. GAD and depression each show their own

Table 7–8. DSM-IV-TR diagnostic criteria for generalized anxiety disorder

A. Excessive anxiety and worry (apprehensive expectation), occurring more days than not for at least 6 months, about a number of events or activities (such as work or school performance).

B. The person finds it difficult to control the worry.

C. The anxiety and worry are associated with three (or more) of the following six symptoms (with at least some symptoms present for more days than not for the past 6 months).
   Note: Only one item is required in children.
   (1) restlessness or feeling keyed up or on edge
   (2) being easily fatigued
   (3) difficulty concentrating or mind going blank
   (4) irritability
   (5) muscle tension
   (6) sleep disturbance (difficulty falling or staying asleep, or restless unsatisfying sleep)

D. The focus of the anxiety and worry is not confined to features of an Axis I disorder, e.g., the anxiety or worry is not about having a panic attack (as in panic disorder), being embarrassed in public (as in social phobia), being contaminated (as in obsessive-compulsive disorder), being away from home or close relatives (as in separation anxiety disorder), gaining weight (as in anorexia nervosa), having multiple physical complaints (as in somatization disorder), or having a serious illness (as in hypochondriasis), and the anxiety and worry do not occur exclusively during posttraumatic stress disorder.

E. The anxiety, worry, or physical symptoms cause clinically significant distress or impairment in social, occupational, or other important areas of functioning.

F. The disturbance is not due to the direct physiological effects of a substance (e.g., a drug of abuse, a medication) or a general medical condition (e.g., hyperthyroidism) and does not occur exclusively during a mood disorder, a psychotic disorder, or a pervasive developmental disorder.

statistically significant and independent associations with impairment, of roughly equal magnitude, which cannot be accounted for by comorbidity or sociodemographic variables (Kessler et al. 1999a). Disability and impairment in pure GAD have been found to be equivalent to those of pure mood disorders and significantly greater than those of pure substance use and other anxiety and personality disorders (Grant et al. 2005b). On certain quality-of-life indexes, individuals with pure GAD actually fare worse than those with pure major depression (Wittchen et al. 2000).

Differential Diagnosis

The diagnosis of GAD is excluded when occurring exclusively in relation to other major Axis I disorders. We now know that clinicians must be cautious and conservative in applying this criterion, because as previously described, there are now compelling data demonstrating that even in the presence of high comorbidity of GAD with other anxiety and mood disorders, GAD is clearly a discrete disorder in terms of its onset, course, and associated impairment. Finally, the distinction between GAD and "normal" anxiety must be made; in GAD the worry must be clearly excessive, pervasive, difficult to control, and associated with marked distress or impairment. The differential diagnosis of GAD is summarized in Table 7–9.

Treatment

Pharmacotherapy

The pharmacological treatment of GAD is summarized in Table 7–10. Although the major changes in diagnostic criteria in consecu-

Table 7–9.   Differential diagnosis of generalized anxiety disorder

Anxious depression
Panic attacks or anticipatory anxiety
Social anxiety
Posttraumatic stress disorder–related
  hyperarousal symptoms
Obsessional fearfulness
Hypochondriasis
Paranoid anxiety associated with psychosis
  or personality disorder

tive editions of DSM, the presence of frequent comorbidity, and a tendency to view GAD as a secondary or minor condition hampered past treatment research, pharmacotherapy options have blossomed in recent years.

Benzodiazepines.   In past years, benzodiazepines were the first-line treatment of GAD. Currently, however, newer medication choices such as buspirone, SSRIs, and serotonin–norepinephrine reuptake inhibitors (SNRIs) have replaced the benzodiazepines as first-line treatments. A number of controlled studies clearly show that chronically anxious patients respond well to benzodiazepines, and all benzodiazepines are probably similarly efficacious in treating GAD. There is some evidence that benzodiazepines may be more effective in treating the physical symptoms of anxiety, whereas antidepressants, whether TCAs or SSRIs, may be more effective in treating the psychic symptoms (Rocca et al. 1998). Although benzodiazepines are generally safe, with side effects limited mainly to sedation and slowed mentation, there is a concern that some patients may become tolerant or even addicted to these medications. However, available data indicate that the concern over benzodiazepine abuse in chronically anxious populations is overestimated, and in reality most patients continue to derive clinical benefits without developing abuse or dependence (Romach et al. 1995). Concerns over addiction are probably justified, for the most part, in individuals with histories of addiction proneness.

Buspirone.   Buspirone is a 5-hydroxytryptamine (serotonin) type 1A (5-HT$_{1A}$) agonist, nonbenzodiazepine antianxiety agent. Treatment with buspirone is usually started at 5 mg tid, and the dosage can be increased until a maximum dosage of 60 mg/day is reached. A twice-daily regimen is probably as efficacious as a thrice-daily regimen and easier to comply with. There has existed a suggestion in the literature that patients previously treated with benzodiazepines may not respond successfully to buspirone. However, a controlled treatment study has refuted this, finding that patients who gradually discontinued lorazepam and were then treated with buspirone in a double-blind fashion did not exhibit benzodiazepine withdrawal or rebound anxiety and did as well with buspirone as they had done with lorazepam (Delle Chiaie et al. 1995). There is some evidence, via a controlled trial (Rickels et al. 2000), that in long-term benzodiazepine users, a successful strategy may be to start buspirone or an antidepressant for 1 month prior to undertaking a gradual 4- to 6-week taper of the benzodiazepine. Other independent predictors of successful benzodiazepine taper were lower initial dosages and less severe and chronic anxiety symptoms.

Antidepressants.   Over the past few years, newer antidepressants have become established as first-line treatments for GAD, because controlled trials have documented their efficacy and because they tend to be well tolerated, require only once-daily dosing, and do not risk abuse and dependence. Several large controlled trials to date have established the efficacy of extended-release venlafaxine, an SNRI, in treating GAD (Rickels et al. 2000). Venlafaxine has been found effective in dosages ranging from 75 to 225 mg/day. Response rate is approximately 70%, with benefits appearing as early as the first 2 weeks of treatment. Venlafaxine is generally well tolerated, with nausea, somno-

---

Table 7–10. Pharmacological treatment of generalized anxiety disorder

---

Venlafaxine extended-release
General indications: First-line treatment; approved by FDA, with proven efficacy in large controlled trials; generally well tolerated; once-daily dosing; recommended starting dosage is 75 mg/day, which may be adequate for a number of patients.

Selective serotonin reuptake inhibitors (SSRIs)
General indications: First-line treatment; paroxetine is FDA approved; generally well tolerated; once-daily dosing; recommended starting dosage is 20 mg/day, which may be adequate for many patients; other SSRIs also efficacious.

Benzodiazepines
General indications: Well-known efficacy and widely used; all appear similarly efficacious; issues with dependence and withdrawal in certain patients; may be more effective for the physical rather than cognitive symptoms of generalized anxiety disorder.

Buspirone
General indications: Proven efficacy; well tolerated; a trial is generally indicated in all patients; compared with benzodiazepines, takes longer to take action and is not associated with a "high"; may have less efficacy and compliance with very recent benzodiazepine use.

Tricyclic antidepressants (TCAs)
General indications: Demonstrated efficacy in few trials; more side effects than benzodiazepines, buspirone, and newer antidepressants; delayed action compared with benzodiazepines; may be more effective for cognitive rather than physical symptoms of anxiety.
   Imipramine: demonstrated efficacy
   Trazodone: demonstrated efficacy

Other medications
Clonidine: tends to lose initial response
Propranolol: may be useful adjuvant in patients with pronounced palpitations and tremor
Atypical antipsychotics
Riluzole: open trials
Tiagabine: randomized controlled trial; mixed results
Pregabalin: not marketed in United States

Note. FDA=U.S. Food and Drug Administration.

---

lence, and dry mouth being the most common side effects.

SSRIs are also efficacious in treating GAD. The SSRI paroxetine has been studied in several controlled trials. One trial showed paroxetine at fixed dosages of both 20 mg and 40 mg daily to be superior to placebo over an 8-week treatment period, with approximately two-thirds of patients considered responders (Bellew et al. 2000). Sertraline has also been found to be superior to placebo in decreasing both the psychic and somatic symptoms of GAD during a 12-week treatment (Dahl et al.

2005) at flexible dosages of 50–150 mg/day (Allgulander et al. 2004), and one study showed comparable efficacy and tolerability for paroxetine and sertraline (Ball et al. 2005). Three pooled similar placebo-controlled trials of the SSRI escitalopram, administered for 8 weeks at a dosage of 10–20 mg/day, reported significant improvement in GAD with good tolerability in more than 800 patients (Goodman et al. 2005).

Several older studies have shown TCAs to be effective in treating chronically anxious patients independent of the presence of depressive symptoms, although TCA use has largely fallen out of favor in favor of the newer antidepressants. A recent open trial reported that mirtazapine, at a daily dosage of 30 mg for 12 weeks, resulted in at least 50% improvement in 80% of 44 patients (Gambi et al. 2005).

Other medications. β-Adrenergic–blocking drugs such as propranolol may only be rarely indicated as an adjuvant in patients who experience significant palpitations or tremor. Clonidine, which inhibits locus coeruleus discharge, would seem for theoretical reasons to be a good antianxiety drug. A tendency to lose clinical response, plus a number of bothersome side effects, makes clonidine a poor initial choice for treatment.

Psychotherapy

Research into the psychotherapy of GAD has not been as extensive as for other anxiety disorders. Still, a number of studies exist that clearly show that a variety of psychotherapies are helpful in treating GAD (Table 7–11).

Given the previously described cognitive profile of GAD, several aspects of the disorder can serve as the foci of psychotherapeutic interventions. These include the heightened tendency to perceive threat; the expectation of low-likelihood catastrophic outcomes; poor problem solving, especially in the face of ambivalence or ambiguity; the central feature of worry; and the physical symptoms of anxiety. A variety of treatments have been developed for GAD, including cognitive restructuring; behavioral anxiety management, such as relaxation and rebreathing techniques; exposure therapy with or without a cognitive component; and psychodynamic treatment.

Combined Pharmacotherapy and Psychotherapy

In a meta-analysis of 65 CBT and pharmacological treatment studies of GAD, overall similar efficacy was reported for the two treatment approaches, with lower attrition rates for psychotherapy (Mitte 2005). There are minimal data on the use of combined

Table 7–11. Cognitive and behavioral approaches to treating generalized anxiety disorder

Exposure
Cognitive restructuring
Breathing retraining
Applied relaxation training

psychotherapy and medication in the treatment of GAD.

Social Phobia (Social Anxiety Disorder)

Definition and Clinical Description

The central feature of social phobia is a marked, persistent fear of social situations in which public humiliation or embarrassment is possible. DSM-IV-TR criteria for social phobia are presented in Table 7–12.

Socially phobic individuals fear and/or avoid a variety of situations in which they would be required to interact with others or to perform a task in front of other people. Typical social phobias are of speaking, eating, or writing in public; using public lavatories; and attending parties or interviews. In addition, a common fear of socially phobic individuals is that other people will detect and ridicule their anxiety in social situations. An individual may have one, limited, or numerous social fears. Social phobia is described as generalized if the social fear encompasses most social situations as opposed to being present in circumscribed ones. Generalized social phobia is overall a more serious and impairing condition. Generalized social phobia can be reliably diagnosed as a subtype; it has an earlier onset, and affected individuals are more often single and have more interactional fears and greater comorbidity with atypical depression and alcoholism (Mannuzza et al. 1995).

Table 7–12. DSM-IV-TR diagnostic criteria for social phobia

A. A marked and persistent fear of one or more social or performance situations in which the person is exposed to unfamiliar people or to possible scrutiny by others. The individual fears that he or she will act in a way (or show anxiety symptoms) that will be humiliating or embarrassing. **Note:** In children, there must be evidence of the capacity for age-appropriate social relationships with familiar people and the anxiety must occur in peer settings, not just in interactions with adults.

B. Exposure to the feared social situation almost invariably provokes anxiety, which may take the form of a situationally bound or situationally predisposed panic attack. **Note:** In children, the anxiety may be expressed by crying, tantrums, freezing, or shrinking from social situations with unfamiliar people.

C. The person recognizes that the fear is excessive or unreasonable. **Note:** In children, this feature may be absent.

D. The feared social or performance situations are avoided or else are endured with intense anxiety or distress.

E. The avoidance, anxious anticipation, or distress in the feared social or performance situation(s) interferes significantly with the person's normal routine, occupational (academic) functioning, or social activities or relationships, or there is marked distress about having the phobia.

F. In individuals under age 18 years, the duration is at least 6 months.

G. The fear or avoidance is not due to the direct physiological effects of a substance (e.g., a drug of abuse, a medication) or a general medical condition and is not better accounted for by another mental disorder (e.g., panic disorder with or without agoraphobia, separation anxiety disorder, body dysmorphic disorder, a pervasive developmental disorder, or schizoid personality disorder).

H. If a general medical condition or another mental disorder is present, the fear in criterion A is unrelated to it, e.g., the fear is not of stuttering, trembling in Parkinson's disease, or exhibiting abnormal eating behavior in anorexia nervosa or bulimia nervosa.

Specify if:

Generalized: if the fears include most social situations (also consider the additional diagnosis of avoidant personality disorder)

As in specific phobias, the anxiety in social phobia is stimulus bound. When forced or surprised into the phobic situation, the individual experiences profound anxiety accompanied by a variety of somatic symptoms. Interestingly, different anxiety disorders tend to be characterized by their own constellation of most prominent somatic symptoms. For example, palpitations and chest pain or pressure are more common in panic attacks, whereas sweating, blushing, and dry mouth are more common in social anxiety. Actual panic attacks may also occur in individuals with social phobia in response to feared social situations. Blushing is the cardinal physical symptom characteristic of social phobia, whereas commonly encountered cognitive constellations include tendencies for self-focused attention, negative self-evaluation regarding social performance, difficulty gauging nonverbal aspects of one's behavior, discounting of social competence in positive interactions, and a positive bias toward appraising others' social performance (Alden and Wallace 1995).

Individuals who have only limited social fears may be functioning well overall and be relatively asymptomatic unless confronted with the necessity of entering their phobic situation. When faced with this necessity, they are often subject to intense anticipatory anxiety. Multiple social fears, on the other hand, can lead to chronic demoralization, social isolation, and disabling vocational and interpersonal impairment. Alcohol and sedative drugs are often utilized to alleviate at least the anticipatory component of this anxiety disorder, possibly leading to abuse. In a study that systematically compared individuals with a public speaking phobia with those with generalized social phobia, the latter were found to be younger, less educated, and have greater anxiety, depression, fears of negative social evaluation, and unemployment (Heimberg et al. 1990).

Epidemiology and Comorbidity

In the National Comorbidity Survey (Kessler et al. 1994; Magee et al. 1996), which employed DSM-III-R (American Psychiatric Association 1987) criteria, social phobia had a lifetime occurrence of 13.3%, 1-year incidence of 7.9%, and 1-month incidence of 4.5% and was somewhat more common in women than in men (lifetime, 15.5% vs. 11.1%). Of those affected, about one-third reported exclusively public speaking fears, whereas the rest were characterized by at least one other social fear. About one-third had multiple fears qualifying for the generalized type of social phobia, which was found to be more persistent, impairing, and comorbid than the specific public speaking type.

The NESARC found a 1-year and lifetime prevalence of DSM-IV social anxiety disorder of 2.8% and 5.0%, respectively (Grant et al. 2005a). Being Native American, being young in age, or having low income increased risk, whereas being male; being Asian, Hispanic, or African American; or living in urban settings reduced risk. Mean age at onset was 15 years. The disorder was chronic; mean age at first treatment was about 12 years later, and 80% had never received treatment. There was significant comorbidity with other psychiatric disorders, especially GAD, bipolar I, and avoidant and dependent personality disorders.

Epidemiological studies have consistently found significant comorbidity between lifetime social phobia and various mood disorders, with an approximately three- to sixfold higher risk for dysthymia, depression, and bipolar disorder (Kessler et al. 1999b). Social phobia almost always predated the mood disorder and was a predictor not only of a higher likelihood of future mood disorder but also of more severity and chronicity.

Social phobia can be associated with a variety of personality disorders, particularly avoidant personality disorder. In epidemiologically identified probands with social phobia alone, avoidant personality disorder alone, or both, a similarly elevated familial risk of social phobia has been found, suggesting that the Axis I and II disorders may represent dimensions of social anxiety rather than discrete conditions (Tillfors et al. 2001). Indeed, a review of the literature comparing generalized social phobia, avoidant personality disorder, and shyness concluded that all three may exist on a continuum (Rettew 2000) or may even be alternative conceptualizations of the same underlying condition (Ralevski et al. 2005).

Social phobia is a highly disabling disorder whose impact on functioning and quality of life has probably been greatly underestimated and hidden in past years. Socially phobic persons are impaired on a broad spectrum of measures, ranging from dropping out of school to experiencing significant disability in whatever their main activities are. They describe dissatisfaction with many aspects of life, and the quality of their life is rated as quite low. Importantly, comorbid depression seems to contribute only modestly to these outcomes. Even in preadolescent children, pervasive and serious functional impairment can already be found.

Course and Prognosis

Social phobia is clearly a chronic and potentially highly impairing condition; course and prognosis are summarized in Table 7–13.

Table 7–13. Course and prognosis of social phobia

Course

Typically early onset at or before adolescence and very chronic course

Outcome

About one-half found to be recovered after 25 years of illness

Predictors of poorer prognosis

Onset before age 8–11 years
Psychiatric comorbidity
Lower educational status
More symptoms at baseline
Comorbid health problems

Differential Diagnosis

Differential diagnosis of social phobia is summarized in Table 7–14. Before the diagnosis of social phobia can be made, the presence of other disorders that may cause irrational fear of people and avoidance behaviors must be ruled out. Avoidance of social situations is seen as part of avoidant, schizoid, and paranoid personality disorders; agoraphobia; OCD; depressive disorders; schizophrenia; and paranoid disorders.

Table 7–14. Differential diagnosis of social phobia

Personality disorder, such as avoidant, schizoid, paranoid

Axis I paranoid disorder such as paranoid schizophrenia or paranoid delusional disorder

Depression-related social withdrawal secondary to anhedonia or feelings of defectiveness

Obsessive-compulsive disorder–related fears exacerbated in social settings (e.g., contamination)

Panic disorder with phobic avoidance not limited to social situations

Deficits/impaired social skills associated with schizophrenia and related disorders

---

Persons with paranoid disorders fear that something unpleasant will be done to them by others. In contrast, those with social phobia fear that they themselves will act inappropriately and cause their own embarrassment or humiliation.

In avoidant personality disorder the central fear is also rejection, ridicule, or humiliation by others. The distinction between this entity and generalized social phobia may be conceptual and semantic, and its validity is a subject of dispute. Automatically labeling such patients as having avoidant personalities may lead practitioners away from potentially useful pharmacotherapy and behavioral treatment efforts.

Some agoraphobic patients say that they are afraid they will embarrass themselves by losing control if they panic while in a social situation. These patients are distinguished from patients with social phobia by the presence of panic attacks that also occur in situations not involving scrutiny or evaluation by others.

Interpersonal anxiety or fears of humiliation leading to social avoidance are not diagnosed as social phobia when occurring in the context of schizophrenia, schizophreniform or brief reactive psychoses, and major depressive disorder. Patients with psychotic vulnerabilities and massive social isolation or poor interpersonal skills may occasionally be mistaken as having social phobia if seen when they are in nonpsychotic or prepsychotic phases of illness.

Social withdrawal seen in depressive disorders is usually associated with a lack of interest or pleasure in the company of others rather than a fear of scrutiny. In contrast, individuals with social phobia generally express the wish to be able to interact appropriately with others and anticipate pleasure in this eventuality.

Treatment

Pharmacotherapy

The pharmacological treatment of social phobia is summarized in Table 7–15. There

---

Table 7–15. Pharmacological treatment of social phobia

Selective serotonin reuptake inhibitors (SSRIs) and other newer antidepressants

General indications: First-line treatment; shown efficacy; well tolerated; once-daily dosing; effective for comorbid depression, panic, generalized anxiety disorder, or obsessive-compulsive disorder.

    Paroxetine: best studied in large controlled trials; FDA approved; average dosage 40 mg/day
    Other SSRIs: also efficacious
    Venlafaxine: also efficacious
    Mirtazapine: also efficacious, fewer data

Benzodiazepines

General indications: Clinically widely used and reportedly efficacious in open trials; generally well tolerated; concerns about dependence and withdrawal in certain patients.

    Clonazepam: long-acting; efficacy demonstrated in controlled trial

Beta-blockers

General indications: Highly effective for performance anxiety, taken on an as-needed basis about 1 hour before event. For the most part not helpful in patients with generalized social phobia.

    Propranolol, atenolol

Monoamine oxidase inhibitors (MAOIs)

General indications: Demonstrated high effectiveness; may be difficult to tolerate and require dietary restrictions; effective for several comorbid conditions including atypical depression, social phobia, and panic; well worth trying in patients with otherwise refractory illness.

    Phenelzine: most studied
    Tranylcypromine: also effective

Other medications

Gabapentin: effective in one controlled trial
Buspirone: well tolerated; effective in open trial but not in controlled trial
Bupropion: effective in open trial
Topiramate: open trial
Pregabalin: controlled trial
Atypical neuroleptics: open trials
D-*cycloserine:* used in conjunction with exposure therapy

Note. FDA=U.S. Food and Drug Administration.

are a number of medication options that are clearly helpful.

Beta-blockers. In performance-type social phobia, several analogue (i.e., nonclinical samples with performance or social anxiety) studies have shown β-blocker efficacy, particularly when these agents are used acutely prior to a performance. Many performing artists or public speakers find that β-blockers, taken orally a few hours before stage time, reduce palpitations, tremor, and the "butterflies feeling." Although a variety of β-blockers have been used in studies and are probably efficacious for performance anxiety, the most common ones used are propranolol, 20 mg, or atenolol, 50 mg, taken about 45 minutes before a performance. It also seems that they are more effective in controlling stage fright, with minimal or no side effects, than are benzodiazepines, which may decrease subjective anxiety but not optimize performance and may have an adverse effect on "sharpness."

Newer antidepressants. In the past few decades, SSRIs have been tested and have shown efficacy in treating social phobia; as a result, SSRIs have become the first-line treatment for the disorder. They are generally well tolerated, easy to dispense and monitor, and used in standard dosages comparable with those used in depression.

Newer antidepressants other than SSRIs are also efficacious in treating social phobia. A 12-week extended-release venlafaxine study, using dosages of 75–225 mg/day, demonstrated significant benefit over placebo in social anxiety symptoms and social impairment, with good tolerability (Rickels et al. 2004). A placebo-controlled trial of mirtazapine in 66 women with social phobia also reported efficacy (Muehlbacher et al. 2005). Bupropion is the least studied antidepressant to date, but it may have some efficacy in social phobia (Emmanuel et al. 1991).

Benzodiazepines. Benzodiazepines can also be helpful in treating generalized social phobia, despite the usual concerns about their chronic use. Several open trials have reported positive results, and in one controlled study clonazepam at dosages of 0.5–3.0 mg/day (mean dosage, 2.4 mg/day) was found to be superior to placebo, with a response rate of 78% and improvement in social anxiety, avoidance, performance, and negative self-evaluation (Davidson et al. 1993). Alprazolam has also been found to be superior to placebo, with results comparable with those for phenelzine and CBT. However, the alprazolam group had the highest relapse rate 2 months after treatment discontinuation (Gelernter et al. 1991). Given its longer half-life, clonazepam is a better choice than alprazolam. Both have advantages, such as relatively rapid onset of action and good tolerability. Disadvantages are the potential for abuse, withdrawal, relapse, and lack of efficacy for comorbid depression. The benzodiazepines would not be considered a first-line treatment for social phobia.

Monoamine oxidase inhibitors. MAOIs were the medications proven most effective in treating generalized social phobia until recently. Liebowitz et al. (1992) conducted a controlled study comparing phenelzine, atenolol, and placebo in the treatment of patients with DSM-III social phobia. About two-thirds of patients had a marked response to phenelzine, at dosages of 45–90 mg/day, whereas atenolol was not superior to placebo. Tranylcypromine in dosages of 40–60 mg/day was also associated with significant improvement in about 80% of patients with DSM-III social phobia treated openly for 1 year (Versiani et al. 1988).

Cognitive and Behavioral Therapies

Three major cognitive-behavioral techniques are used in the treatment of social phobia: exposure, cognitive restructuring, and social skills training (Table 7–16).

Exposure treatment involves imaginal or in vivo exposure to specific feared performance and social situations. Although patients with very high levels of social anxiety may need to start out with imaginal exposure until a certain degree of habituation is attained, therapeutic results are not gained until in vivo exposure to the real-life feared situations is done. Cognitive restructuring focuses on poor self-concepts, the fear of negative evaluation by others, and the attribution of positive outcomes to chance or circumstance

---

Table 7–16. Cognitive and behavioral approaches to treating social phobia

---

Exposure (imaginal and/or in vivo)

Cognitive restructuring

Social skills training (modeling, rehearsal, role-playing, practice)

Virtual reality exposure

Exposure preceded by D-cycloserine administration

---

and negative outcomes to one's own short-comings. It consists of a variety of homework identifying negative thoughts, evaluating their accuracy, and reframing them in a more realistic way. Social skills training employs modeling, rehearsal, role-playing, and assigned practice to help individuals learn appropriate behaviors and decrease anxiety in social situations, with an expectation that this will lead to more positive responses from others. This type of training is not necessary for all individuals with social phobia and is more applicable to those who have actual deficits in social interacting above and beyond their anxiety or avoidance of social situations.

Exposure, cognitive restructuring, and social skills training may all be of significant benefit to patients with social phobia. In addition, these techniques appear superior to non-specific supportive therapy, as shown in a randomized, controlled study comparing supportive therapy with initial individual cognitive therapy followed by group social skills training (Cottraux et al. 2000). The success of CBTs appears to be mediated, at least in part, by a decrease in self-focused attention (Woody et al. 1997). Decreases in negative self-focused thoughts and social anxiety symptoms were significantly intercorrelated in patients treated with CBT but not with exposure, despite the comparable improvement of the two groups (Hofmann et al. 2004).

It has been suggested that cognitive aspects may be of greater importance in social phobia than in other anxiety or phobic conditions, and therefore cognitive restructuring may be a necessary component to maximize treatment gains. Although long-term outcome is more difficult to assess, studies suggest that CBT leads to long-lasting gains (Turner et al. 1995) and therefore may be of particular significance in social phobia, which tends to have a chronic, often lifetime, course.

Very recently, virtual reality therapy techniques have surfaced as an interesting and potentially powerful alternative to standard exposure therapies in treating phobias, including social phobia.

Other Types of Psychotherapy

The successful use of medication and/or behavioral treatments has resulted in psychodynamic therapy for phobias falling out of favor (Gabbard 1990).

Combination Treatment

Combination treatment with CBT and medication has also received some attention. It appears that medication alone compared with CBT alone has comparable results in the acute treatment of social phobia (Heimberg et al. 1998; Otto et al. 2000).

Specific Phobias
Definition and Clinical Description

Specific phobias are circumscribed fears of specific objects, situations, or activities. The syndrome has three components: an anticipatory anxiety that is brought on by the possibility of confrontation with the phobic stimulus, the central fear itself, and the avoidance behavior by which the individual minimizes anxiety. In specific phobia, the fear is usually not of the object itself but of some dire outcome that the individual believes may result from contact with that object. For example, persons with driving phobia are afraid of accidents; those with snake phobia, that they will be bitten; and those who are claustrophobic, that they will suffocate or be trapped in an enclosed space. These fears are excessive, unreasonable, and enduring; although most individuals with specific phobias will readily acknowledge that they know there is really nothing to be afraid of, reassuring them of this does not diminish their fear.

In DSM-IV, for the first time, types of specific phobias were adopted: natural environment (e.g., storms); animal (e.g., insects); blood-injury-injection; situational (e.g., cars, elevators, bridges); and other (e.g., choking, vomiting). The validity of such distinctions is supported by data showing that these types

---

Table 7–17. DSM-IV-TR diagnostic criteria for specific phobia

A. Marked and persistent fear that is excessive or unreasonable, cued by the presence or anticipation of a specific object or situation (e.g., flying, heights, animals, receiving an injection, seeing blood).

B. Exposure to the phobic stimulus almost invariably provokes an immediate anxiety response, which may take the form of a situationally bound or situationally predisposed panic attack.   **Note:** In children, the anxiety may be expressed by crying, tantrums, freezing, or clinging.

C. The person recognizes that the fear is excessive or unreasonable.   **Note:** In children, this feature may be absent.

D. The phobic situation(s) is avoided or else is endured with intense anxiety or distress.

E. The avoidance, anxious anticipation, or distress in the feared situation(s) interferes significantly with the person's normal routine, occupational (or academic) functioning, or social activities or relationships, or there is marked distress about having the phobia.

F. In individuals under age 18 years, the duration is at least 6 months.

G. The anxiety, panic attacks, or phobic avoidance associated with the specific object or situation are not better accounted for by another mental disorder, such as obsessive-compulsive disorder (e.g., fear of dirt in someone with an obsession about contamination), posttraumatic stress disorder (e.g., avoidance of stimuli associated with a severe stressor), separation anxiety disorder (e.g., avoidance of school), social phobia (e.g., avoidance of social situations because of fear of embarrassment), panic disorder with agoraphobia, or agoraphobia without history of panic disorder.

Specify type:

Animal type
Natural environment type (e.g., heights, storms, water)
Blood-injection-injury type
Situational type (e.g., airplanes, elevators, enclosed places)
Other type (e.g., fear of choking, vomiting, or contracting an illness; in children, fear of loud sounds or costumed characters)

---

tend to differ with respect to age at onset, mode of onset, familial aggregation, and physiological responses to the phobic stimulus (Fyer et al. 1990). A comparable structure has been found in child and adolescent specific phobia, clustering into three subtypes (Muris et al. 1999). DSM-IV and DSM-IV-TR make the diagnosis of phobic disorder only when single or multiple phobias are the predominant aspect of the clinical picture, a source of significant distress to the individual, and not the result of another mental disorder. The diagnostic criteria for specific phobia are presented in Table 7–17.

Epidemiology

In the National Comorbidity Survey (Magee et al. 1996), which employed DSM-III-R crite-

ria, specific phobias had the same lifetime prevalence of 11.3%, with a median age of illness onset of 15, and women were affected more than twice as often as men. In a community study of adolescents, the prevalence of specific phobias was found to be 3.5%, higher in girls than boys, and to have significant comorbidity with depressive and somatoform disorders in about one-third of the sample (Essau et al. 2000). It is rare for individuals to seek treatment for this disorder.

Treatment

The treatment of choice for specific phobias is exposure, aimed at fear extinction. The problem lies in persuading the patient that exposure is worth trying and will be beneficial. Exposure treatments may be divided into two groups depending on whether exposure to the phobic object is "in vivo" or "imaginal." In vivo exposure involves the patient in real-life contact with the phobic stimulus. Imaginal techniques confront the phobic stimulus through the therapist's descriptions and the patient's imagination.

The method of exposure in both the in vivo and imaginal techniques can be graded or ungraded. Graded exposure uses a hierarchy of anxiety-provoking events varying from least to most stressful. The patient begins at the least stressful level and gradually progresses up the hierarchy. Ungraded exposure begins with the patients confronting the most stressful items in the hierarchy. Exposure can be accompanied by varying degrees and types of cognitive interventions that decatastrophize the phobic stimulus and encourage risk taking.

Most exposure techniques have been used in both individual and group settings. In a group setting, both the example and the encouragement of other members are often particularly helpful in persuading the patient to reenter the phobic situation. Techniques may include systematic desensitization, imaginal flooding, prolonged in vivo exposure, and participant modeling and reinforced practice.

In recent years, promising computer-aided self-help exposure programs via the Internet, with brief telephone support from a therapist, have been developed for those who are unable to travel due to their phobias (Kenwright and Marks 2004). Another new and exciting development in the treatment of all phobias, including specific phobias, is the development of virtual reality exposure techniques, which permit "virtual exposure" in a clinical setting, greatly facilitating the ease of administration of many in vivo–type exposures. One virtual reality study of driving phobia reported positive results (Wald and Taylor 2003). Similarly promising results were reported in a virtual reality treatment study of spider phobia (Garcia-Palacios et al. 2002) and one of flying phobia (Banos et al. 2002).

Medications have not generally been shown to be effective in treating specific phobias. TCAs, benzodiazepines, and β-blockers generally do not appear useful for specific phobias based on the limited number of studies available to date.

There has been a recent surge in interest in the combination of medication and exposure therapy (traditional or virtual reality) in treating anxiety and fear, including specific phobias.

Obsessive-Compulsive Disorder

Definition

The essential features of OCD are obsessions or compulsions. DSM-IV-TR criteria for OCD are presented in Table 7–18.

The terminology of "obsessions" or "compulsions" is sometimes used more broadly to characterize conditions that are not true OCD. Although some activities, such as eating, sexual behavior, gambling, or drinking, when engaged in excessively may be referred to as "compulsive," these activities are distinguished from true compulsions in that they are experienced as pleasurable and ego-syntonic, although their consequences may become increasingly unpleasant and ego-dystonic over time. Obsessive brooding, ruminations, or preoccupations, typically characteristic of depression, may be unpleasant but are distinguished from true obsessions because they are not as senseless or intrusive and the individual regards them as meaningful, although possibly excessive and painful.

There are several presentations of OCD based on symptom clusters. One group includes patients with obsessions about dirt and contamination, whose rituals center around compulsive washing and avoidance of contaminated objects. A second group includes patients with pathological counting and compulsive checking. A third group includes purely obsessional patients with no compulsions. Primary obsessional slowness

---

Table 7–18. DSM-IV-TR diagnostic criteria for obsessive-compulsive disorder

A. Either obsessions or compulsions:

Obsessions as defined by (1), (2), (3), and (4):

(1) recurrent and persistent thoughts, impulses, or images that are experienced, at some time during the disturbance, as intrusive and inappropriate and that cause marked anxiety or distress

(2) the thoughts, impulses, or images are not simply excessive worries about real-life problems

(3) the person attempts to ignore or suppress such thoughts, impulses, or images, or to neutralize them with some other thought or action

(4) the person recognizes that the obsessional thoughts, impulses, or images are a product of his or her own mind (not imposed from without as in thought insertion)

Compulsions as defined by (1) and (2):

(1) repetitive behaviors (e.g., hand washing, ordering, checking) or mental acts (e.g., praying, counting, repeating words silently) that the person feels driven to perform in response to an obsession, or according to rules that must be applied rigidly

(2) the behaviors or mental acts are aimed at preventing or reducing distress or preventing some dreaded event or situation; however, these behaviors or mental acts either are not connected in a realistic way with what they are designed to neutralize or prevent or are clearly excessive

B. At some point during the course of the disorder, the person has recognized that the obsessions or compulsions are excessive or unreasonable. **Note:** This does not apply to children.

C. The obsessions or compulsions cause marked distress, are time consuming (take more than 1 hour a day), or significantly interfere with the person's normal routine, occupational (or academic) functioning, or usual social activities or relationships.

D. If another Axis I disorder is present, the content of the obsessions or compulsions is not restricted to it (e.g., preoccupation with food in the presence of an eating disorder; hair pulling in the presence of trichotillomania; concern with appearance in the presence of body dysmorphic disorder; preoccupation with drugs in the presence of a substance use disorder; preoccupation with having a serious illness in the presence of hypochondriasis; preoccupation with sexual urges or fantasies in the presence of a paraphilia; or guilty ruminations in the presence of major depressive disorder).

E. The disturbance is not due to the direct physiological effects of a substance (e.g., a drug of abuse, a medication) or a general medical condition.

Specify if:

With poor insight: if, for most of the time during the current episode, the person does not recognize that the obsessions and compulsions are excessive or unreasonable

---

is evident in another group, in whom slowness is the predominant symptom. Patients may spend many hours every day washing, getting dressed, and eating breakfast, and life goes on at an extremely slow speed. Some OCD patients, called "hoarders," are unable to throw anything out for fear they might someday need something they discarded.

In DSM-IV-TR, OCD is classified among the anxiety disorders because 1) anxiety is often associated with obsessions and resistance to compulsions, 2) anxiety or tension is often immediately relieved by yielding to compulsions, and 3) OCD often occurs in association with other anxiety disorders. However, compulsions decrease anxiety only transiently, and the nature of the fears in OCD is distinct from those of other anxiety disorders.

Clinical Description

Onset

OCD usually begins in adolescence or early adulthood but can begin prior to that time; 31% of first episodes occur between ages 10 and 15 years, with 75% developing OCD by age 30. In most cases, no particular stress or event precipitates the onset of OCD symptoms, and after an insidious onset there is a chronic and often progressive course. However, some patients describe a sudden onset of symptoms. This is particularly true of patients with a neurological basis for their illness. There is evidence of OCD associated with the 1920s encephalitis epidemic, abnormal birth events, and onset following head injury or seizures. Of interest are reports of new onset of OCD during pregnancy (Neziroglu et al. 1992).

Symptoms

Obsessions. Obsessive and compulsive symptoms have been recognized for centuries and were first described in the psychiatric literature by Esquirol in 1838 (Rachman and Hodgson 1980). *Obsessional thoughts* were defined by Karl Westphal in 1878 as ideas that in an otherwise intact intelligence, without being caused by an emotional or affect-like state, and against the will of the person come into the foreground of the consciousness (Westphal 1878).

An *obsession* is an intrusive, unwanted mental event usually evoking anxiety or discomfort. Obsessions may be thoughts, ideas, images, ruminations, convictions, fears, or impulses and are often of an aggressive, sexual, religious, disgusting, or nonsensical content. Obsessional ideas are repetitive thoughts that interrupt the normal train of thinking, whereas obsessional images are often vivid visual experiences. Much obsessive thinking involves horrific ideas. The person may think of doing the worst possible thing (e.g., blasphemy, rape, murder, child molestation). Ob-

sessional convictions are often characterized by an element of magical thinking, such as "step on a crack, break your mother's back." Obsessional ruminations may involve prolonged, excessive, and inconclusive thinking about metaphysical questions. Obsessional fears often involve dirt or contamination and differ from phobias because they are present in the absence of the phobic stimulus. Other common obsessional fears involve harm coming to oneself or to others as a consequence of the patient's misdoings, such as one's home catching on fire because the stove was not checked or running over a pedestrian because of careless driving. Obsessional impulses may be aggressive or sexual, such as intrusive impulses of stabbing one's spouse or raping one's child.

Attributing these obsessions to an internal source, the patient resists or controls them to a variable degree, and significant impairment in functioning can result. *Resistance* is the struggle against an impulse or intrusive thought, and *control* is the patient's actual success in diverting his or her thinking. Obsessions are usually accompanied by compulsions but may also occur as the main or only symptom. Approximately 10%–25% of OCD patients are purely obsessional or predominantly experience obsessions (Akhtar et al. 1975; Rachman and Hodgson 1980).

Another hallmark of obsessive thinking involves lack of certainty or persistent doubting. In contrast to manic or psychotic patients, who manifest premature certainty, OCD patients are unable to achieve a sense of certainty between incoming sensory information and internal beliefs. Are my hands clean? Is the door locked? Is the fertilizer poisoning the water supply? Compulsive rituals such as excessive washing or checking appear to arise from this lack of certainty and consist of a misguided attempt to increase certainty.

Compulsions. A *compulsive ritual* is a behavior that usually reduces discomfort but is carried out in a pressured or rigid fashion. Such behavior may include rituals involving washing, checking, repeating, avoiding, striving for completeness, and being meticulous. "Washers" represent about 25%–50% of most OCD samples (Akhtar et al. 1975; Rachman and Hodgson 1980). These individuals are concerned with dirt, contaminants, or germs and may spend many hours a day washing their hands or showering. They may also attempt to avoid contaminating themselves with feces, urine, or vaginal secretions.

"Checkers" have pathological doubt and thus compulsively check to see if they have, for example, run over someone with their car or left the door unlocked. Checking often fails to resolve the doubt and, in some cases, may actually exacerbate it. In the DSM-IV field trial, washing and checking were the two most common groups of compulsions.

Although slowness results from most rituals, it is the major feature of the rare and disabling syndrome of primary obsessional slowness. It may take several hours for the obsessionally slow individual to get dressed or get out of the house. This slowness may be a response to a lack of certainty as well. These patients may have little anxiety despite their obsessions and rituals.

Mental compulsions are also quite common and should be inquired about directly, because they could go undetected if the clinician only asks about behavioral rituals. Such patients, for example, may replay over and over in their minds past conversations with others to make sure they did not somehow incriminate themselves. In the DSM-IV OCD field trials, 80% of patients had both behavioral and mental compulsions, and mental compulsions were the third most common type after checking and washing.

Although distinct symptom clusters exist (washers, checkers, those who are purely obsessional, hoarders, and those with primary slowness), these symptoms may overlap or develop sequentially.

Epidemiology

The ECA study (described earlier in this chapter) suggested that OCD is quite com-

mon, with a 1-month prevalence of 1.3%, a 6-month prevalence of 1.5%, and a lifetime rate of 2.5% (Regier et al. 1988). In clinical samples of adult OCD, there is a roughly equal ratio of men to women (Black 1974). However, in childhood-onset OCD, about 70% of patients are male (Swedo et al. 1989). This difference seems to be accounted for by the earlier age at onset in males, and it may suggest partly differing etiologies or vulnerabilities in the two sexes.

There are reports demonstrating comorbidity of OCD with schizophrenia, depression, other anxiety disorders such as panic disorder and simple and social phobia, eating disorders, autism, and Tourette's syndrome. Epidemiologically, the OCD comorbidity risk for other major psychiatric disorders was found to be fairly high but nondistinctive (Karno et al. 1988).

Course and Prognosis

The course and prognosis of OCD is summarized in Table 7–19.

Table 7–19. Course and prognosis of obsessive-compulsive disorder

Course
  Less than 15% phasic with periods of complete remission
  One-fourth to one-third have fluctuating course
  Half (50%) have constant or progressive illness

Outcome
  80% improve over 40 years

Predictors of worse prognosis
  Early age at onset
  Longer duration of illness
  Presence of both obsessions and compulsions
  Poorer baseline social functioning
  Magical thinking

Differential Diagnosis

Although a variety of biological and neuro-psychiatric markers have been associated with OCD, the diagnosis rests purely on the psychiatric examination and history. DSM-IV-TR defines OCD as the presence of either obsessions or compulsions that cause marked distress, are time-consuming, or interfere with social or occupational functioning. Although all other Axis I disorders are allowed to be comorbidly present, the OCD symptoms must not be just secondary to another disorder (e.g., thoughts about food in the presence of an eating disorder or guilty thoughts in the presence of major depression). The diagnosis is usually clear-cut, but occasionally it can be more difficult to distinguish OCD from depression, psychosis, phobias, or severe obsessive-compulsive personality disorder.

The differential diagnosis of OCD is summarized in Table 7–20.

Treatment

Pharmacotherapy

Advances in recent decades in the pharmacotherapy of OCD have been quite dramatic and have generated a great deal of excitement for successful treatment of this disorder. What was previously thought to be a rare, psychodynamically laden, and difficult-to-treat illness now appears to have a strong biological component and to respond well to potent serotonin reuptake blockers. The pharmacological approach to treatment of OCD is summarized in Table 7–21.

Serotonin reuptake inhibitors.   The most extensively studied medication for the treatment of OCD is clomipramine, a potent serotonin reuptake inhibitor with weak norepinephrine reuptake blockade. In a multicenter trial comparing clomipramine (average dosage: 200–250 mg/day) with placebo in more than 500 patients with OCD, the average reduction in OCD symptoms was about 40%, and about 60% of patients were clinically much or very much improved (Clomipra-

Table 7–20. Differential diagnosis of obsessive-compulsive disorder

Eating disorder with obsessions surrounding food and weight

Body dysmorphic disorder with obsessions about body appearance other than weight

Hypochondriasis with obsessions related to feared illnesses

Panic disorder or generalized anxiety (if obsessional anxiety is severe)

Obsessive ruminations of depression (typically mood congruent)

Severe obsessive-compulsive personality disorder

Paranoid psychosis (e.g., delusions of poisoning rather than contamination fears)

Social phobia (if avoiding social situations because they exacerbate illness)

mine Collaborative Study Group 1991). Patients should typically be started on 25 mg of clomipramine at nighttime, and the dosage then should be gradually increased by 25 mg every 4 days or 50 mg every week until a maximum dosage of 250 mg is reached. Some patients are unable to tolerate the highest dosage and may be stabilized at 150 mg or 200 mg. Improvement with clomipramine is relatively slow, with maximal response occurring after 5–12 weeks of treatment. Some of the more common side effects reported by patients are dry mouth, tremor, sedation, nausea, and ejaculatory failure in men. The seizure risk is comparable with that of TCAs and is acceptable for dosages up to 250 mg/day in the absence of prior neurological history. Clomipramine is equally effective for OCD patients with pure obsessions and those with rituals, in contrast to behavioral treatments, which are less useful for patients who predominantly experience obsessions. Controlled studies have also demonstrated that clomipramine is effective in treating OCD when other antidepressants, such as amitriptyline, nortriptyline, desipramine, and the MAOI clorgiline, have no therapeutic effect.

Table 7–21. Pharmacological treatment of obsessive-compulsive disorder

---

Serotonin reuptake inhibitors

General indications: First-line treatments; moderate to high dosages.

Fluoxetine, fluvoxamine, sertraline: efficacy shown in large controlled trials

Paroxetine, citalopram: less studied, similar efficacy

Clomipramine: efficacy shown in multiple controlled trials; may have small superiority over SSRIs, however, typically not used until at least two SSRIs have failed secondary to side-effect profile; can be used in low dosages in combination with SSRIs in patients with more refractory illness; clomipramine plus desmethylclomipramine levels must be closely followed for toxicity

Venlafaxine, mirtazapine: less studied

Augmentation strategies

General indications: Partial response to serotonin reuptake inhibitors; presence of other target symptoms.

Atypical antipsychotics: several studies show additional benefit

Pindolol: effective in controlled trial

Clonazepam: effective in controlled trial; comorbid very high anxiety

Buspirone: one positive trial, three negative

Lithium: ineffective in controlled trial

Trazodone: ineffective in controlled trial

Monoamine oxidase inhibitors: hardly any evidence; possibly phenelzine in symmetry obsessions

Topiramate

Riluzole

Other medications

Intravenous clomipramine: efficacy in controlled trial of oral clomipramine–refractory patients

Plasma exchange and intravenous immunoglobulin: effective in children with streptococcus-related obsessive-compulsive disorder

---

Note. SSRIs = selective serotonin reuptake inhibitors.

This finding strongly suggests that improvement in OCD symptoms is mediated through the blockade of serotonin reuptake.

Numerous controlled trials since the early 1990s have documented the efficacy of all SSRIs for OCD. Fluvoxamine has been found to have a significant antiobsessional effect in several controlled studies (Hollander et al. 2003; Jenike et al. 1990). Sertraline's efficacy in OCD has been established at daily dosages ranging from 50 to 200 mg (Greist et al. 1995; Kronig et al. 1999). Paroxetine and citalopram are also efficacious in treating OCD, generally at dosages of 20–60 mg/day.

One issue with SSRI treatment is how high to push the dosage, beyond the standard recommended OCD treatment dosage, in an attempt to get a response. One study examined this question in subjects who did not respond to 16 weeks of treatment with sertraline 200 mg/day and found that increasing to a mean dosage of 350 mg/day did result in some symptom improvement but no change in responder status (Ninan et al. 2006).

The SNRI venlafaxine also appears effective in treating OCD. Although clomipramine appears to have an edge over SSRIs in treating OCD, satisfactory systematic comparisons of the various serotonin reuptake blockers, balancing benefits and side effects, have not been conducted.

Medication combination and augmentation. It is important to keep in mind that the medication response in OCD is not as dramatic as in, for example, major depression: a considerable number of patients show a negligible or partial response to the first-line medications. As a helpful rule of thumb, it is useful to remember that approximately 40%–60% of OCD patients improve by about 30%–60% with a first-line drug. Thus, various combination and augmentation strategies are often needed to attain a satisfactory response. The most commonly used augmenting agents in OCD are buspirone, clonazepam, atypical antipsychotics, inositol, and glutamatergic agents. As these augmentation strategies are more rigorously tested, they often do not look as promising as was initially thought. Still, given the relatively limited treatment options, these strategies are worth undertaking sequentially, beginning with the most compelling ones.

Antipsychotics are the main medication class used to augment partial response to serotonin reuptake blockers in OCD. The combination of clomipramine with an SSRI is also a commonly used strategy for treating refractory patients and is generally well tolerated, although lower dosages of clomipramine should be used with monitoring of blood levels to avoid toxicity because clomipramine levels can become markedly elevated. In one small randomized trial in patients with refractory OCD, citalopram combined with clomipramine led to significantly greater improvement than citalopram alone (Pallanti et al. 1999).

Maintenance treatment. OCD tends to be a chronic illness, and many patients may require indefinite drug treatment to stay well. Long-term continuation of medication treatment generally maintains a good treatment response.

Cognitive-Behavioral Therapy

Behavioral treatments of OCD (Table 7–22) can be highly effective and involve two main components: 1) exposure procedures that aim to decrease the anxiety associated with obsessions and 2) response prevention techniques that aim to decrease the frequency of rituals or obsessive thoughts. Exposure techniques

Table 7–22. Cognitive and behavioral approaches to treating obsessive-compulsive disorder

Graded exposure (imaginal and/or in vivo)
Flooding
Response prevention
Cognitive restructuring

range from systematic desensitization with brief imaginal exposure to flooding, in which prolonged exposure to the real-life ritual-evoking stimuli causes profound discomfort. Exposure techniques aim to ultimately decrease the discomfort associated with the eliciting stimuli through habituation. In exposure therapy, the patient is assigned homework exercises that must be adhered to, and he or she may require assistance from the therapist (in a home visit) or from family members to achieve exposure at home. Response prevention involves having patients face feared stimuli (e.g., dirt, chemicals) without excessive hand washing or tolerate doubt (e.g., "Is the door really locked?") without excessive checking. Initial work may involve delaying performance of the ritual, but ultimately the patient works to fully resist the compulsions. The psychoeducation and support of family members can be pivotal to the success of the behavioral therapy, because family dysfunction is very prevalent and the majority of parents or spouses accommodate to or are involved in the patients' rituals, possibly as a way to reduce the anxiety or anger that patients may direct at their family members.

It is generally agreed upon that combined behavioral techniques—that is, exposure and response prevention (ERP)—yield the greatest improvement. It is also generally reported that patients who primarily experience obsessions and have few rituals are the least responsive to behavioral treatment, although new behavioral techniques for obsessions may also be promising. Cognitive therapy has also been more recently advocated and is efficacious in the treatment of OCD, centering on cognitive reformulation of themes related to the perception of danger, estimation of catastrophe, expectations about anxiety and its consequences, excessive responsibility, thought–action fusion, and illogical inferences.

Several studies have directly compared cognitive versus behavioral therapy for OCD in randomized trials and have reported similar efficacy (Cottraux et al. 2001; van Oppen et al. 1995; Whittal et al. 2005). A meta-analysis of cognitive versus behavioral treatment trials for OCD reported that behavioral treatment was somewhat more effective in clinically significant improvement (about 50%–60% of participants), whereas for full remission the two approaches had a similar effectiveness of about 25% (Fisher and Wells 2005).

Combination Pharmacotherapy and Psychotherapy

The relative efficacy of pharmacotherapy versus psychotherapy for OCD is an important question in deciding what first-line treatment to undertake. A meta-analytic comparison study of OCD treatments, after controlling for a number of confounding variables, found that clomipramine, SSRIs, and ERP all had comparable results (Kobak et al. 1998). Similarly in children, a study comparing behavioral treatment versus clomipramine found that both were similarly helpful, suggesting that nonpharmacological options are a reasonable first-line option in the younger population in an initial attempt to avoid medication (de Haan et al. 1998). A more recent 12-week multicenter study suggested that behavior therapy may have an edge over medication therapy (Foa et al. 2005; Simpson et al. 2005). The study compared ERP alone, clomipramine alone, their combination, and a placebo pill in 122 adults with OCD and found that both ERP and combination treatment were superior to medication alone (response rates for all groups were 62%, 42%, 70%, and 8%, respectively). ERP and combination treatment had a greater edge over clomipramine alone for remission

compared with response; a sizable number of patients did not achieve remission by the end of treatment regardless of the type of treatment. Similarly, a large pediatric trial found that combination treatment was superior both to CBT and to sertraline alone and therefore recommended that this age group start treatment with CBT or combined treatment (Pediatric OCD Treatment Study Team 2004). There is also evidence that in the short term (12 weeks) after treatment discontinuation, patients who were treated with ERP relapsed significantly less than those treated with medication alone (Simpson et al. 2004). However a longer-term (5-year) follow-up study has reported that long-term outcome did not differ among patients initially treated with cognitive therapy alone, ERP alone, or psychotherapy combined with medication, with an overall remission rate of about 50%; patients initially treated with medication were more likely to be taking medication at follow-up (van Oppen et al. 2005). So, in sum, medication and CBT are approximately equal first-line treatment choices.

Despite the similar efficacy of pharmacotherapy and CBT for OCD, given the common failure of either treatment to achieve a strong enough response or remission, combination therapy, either concurrent or sequential, is commonly used and recommended in the treatment of OCD. A common approach used in clinical practice, especially by psychiatrists, is to start out with medication, attain a degree of clinical improvement that will allow better utilization of CBT, and then possibly attempt some degree of medication taper once CBT has been mastered and effective.

Posttraumatic Stress Disorder

Definition

PTSD was first introduced in DSM-III, spurred in part by the increasing recognition of posttraumatic conditions in veterans of the

Vietnam War. The current DSM-IV-TR diagnostic criteria for PTSD are presented in Table 7–23.

In acknowledgment of the spectrum of disorders stemming from severe stress, DSM-IV added acute stress disorder to the anxiety disorders. Acute stress disorder is similar to PTSD in the precipitating traumatic event and in symptomatology, but it is time limited, up to 1 month after the event. In addition, dissociative symptoms figure prominently in the definition of acute stress disorder, whereas they are not addressed in the PTSD description. It has now been well established by a number of studies, including prospective ones, that acute stress disorder is a highly reliable predictor of developing PTSD down the road; it may well be that the two should not be defined as discrete disorders.

Clinical Description

A soldier participates in the torture and murder of civilians. A passenger is the sole survivor of the crash of a commercial airliner. A woman is raped and severely beaten by an unknown assailant. The characteristic features that may develop after traumatic events such as these include psychic numbing, reexperiencing of the trauma, and increased autonomic arousal. The trauma is reexperienced in recurrent painful and intrusive recollections, daydreams, or nightmares. Dissociative states may occur, lasting from minutes to days, in which there is a dreamlike, unreal state with hazy memory and a distorted sense of time. Psychic numbing or emotional anesthesia is manifest by diminished responsiveness to the external world, with feelings of being detached from other people, loss of interest in usual activities, and inability to feel emotions such as intimacy, tenderness, or sexual interest. Symptoms of excessive autonomic arousal may include hyperactivity and irritability, an exaggerated startle response, difficulty concentrating, and sleep abnormalities. Rape or mugging victims sometimes become afraid to venture forth alone for variable periods of time. Situations reminiscent of the original trauma may be systematically avoided.

Other symptoms may include guilt about having survived, guilt about not having prevented the traumatic experience, depression, anxiety, panic attacks, shame, and rage. There may be prolonged episodes of intense affect; increased irritability; explosive, hostile behavior; and impulsive behavior. Other accompanying or complicating symptoms associated with PTSD may include substance abuse, self-injurious behavior and suicide attempts, occupational impairment, and interference with interpersonal relationships.

Epidemiology

Although there are marked individual differences in how people react to stress, when stressors become extreme, such as in concentration camp situations or in extended combat, the rate of morbidity rapidly increases. In a large randomized community survey of young adults, the lifetime prevalence of PTSD was found to be 9.2% (Breslau et al. 1991). The prevalence was higher in women (11.3%) than in men (6%). In the National Comorbidity Survey, the lifetime prevalence of PTSD was similarly found to be 7.8% and was again more common in women. The most common stressors were combat exposure in men and sexual assault in women (Kessler et al. 1995).

Symptoms of PTSD, too few in number to meet the full diagnostic criteria, are quite common in the general population. In a Canadian community survey, full PTSD was found in 2.7% of women and 1.2% of men, whereas partial PTSD was found in an additional 3.4% of women and 0.3% of men. Such individuals, seemingly women in particular, may be important to identify because they experience clinically meaningful distress and functional impairment (M. B. Stein et al. 1997).

A high rate of comorbid disorders is found in PTSD. In the Breslau et al. (1991) survey, a high comorbidity risk was found for OCD, agoraphobia, panic, and depression, whereas the association with drug or alcohol abuse was weaker. The comorbidity of PTSD

Table 7–23. DSM-IV-TR diagnostic criteria for posttraumatic stress disorder

A. The person has been exposed to a traumatic event in which both of the following were present:
   (1) the person experienced, witnessed, or was confronted with an event or events that involved actual or threatened death or serious injury, or a threat to the physical integrity of self or others
   (2) the person's response involved intense fear, helplessness, or horror.   **Note:** In children, this may be expressed instead by disorganized or agitated behavior.

B. The traumatic event is persistently reexperienced in one (or more) of the following ways:
   (1) recurrent and intrusive distressing recollections of the event, including images, thoughts, or perceptions.   **Note:** In young children, repetitive play may occur in which themes or aspects of the trauma are expressed.
   (2) recurrent distressing dreams of the event. **Note:** In children, there may be frightening dreams without recognizable content.
   (3) acting or feeling as if the traumatic event were recurring (includes a sense of reliving the experience, illusions, hallucinations, and dissociative flashback episodes, including those that occur on awakening or when intoxicated).   **Note:** In young children, trauma-specific reenactment may occur.
   (4) intense psychological distress at exposure to internal or external cues that symbolize or resemble an aspect of the traumatic event
   (5) physiological reactivity on exposure to internal or external cues that symbolize or resemble an aspect of the traumatic event

C. Persistent avoidance of stimuli associated with the trauma and numbing of general responsiveness (not present before the trauma), as indicated by three (or more) of the following:
   (1) efforts to avoid thoughts, feelings, or conversations associated with the trauma
   (2) efforts to avoid activities, places, or people that arouse recollections of the trauma
   (3) inability to recall an important aspect of the trauma
   (4) markedly diminished interest or participation in significant activities
   (5) feeling of detachment or estrangement from others
   (6) restricted range of affect (e.g., unable to have loving feelings)
   (7) sense of a foreshortened future (e.g., does not expect to have a career, marriage, children, or a normal life span)

D. Persistent symptoms of increased arousal (not present before the trauma), as indicated by two (or more) of the following:
   (1) difficulty falling or staying asleep
   (2) irritability or outbursts of anger
   (3) difficulty concentrating
   (4) hypervigilance
   (5) exaggerated startle response

E. Duration of the disturbance (symptoms in criteria B, C, and D) is more than 1 month.

F. The disturbance causes clinically significant distress or impairment in social, occupational, or other important areas of functioning.

Specify if:
Acute: if duration of symptoms is less than 3 months
Chronic: if duration of symptoms is 3 months or more
Specify if:
With delayed onset: if onset of symptoms is at least 6 months after the stressor

with depression is a very consistent one, and the nature of the relationship between the two conditions is controversial. Epidemiological analyses suggest that in trauma victims the vulnerabilities for PTSD and depression are not separate, but rather the risk for depression is highly elevated in just those trauma victims who manifest PTSD (Breslau et al. 2000).

Risk Factors and Predictors

There is agreement that a variety of premorbid risk factors predispose to the development of PTSD (Table 7–24). Although the disorder can certainly develop in people without significant preexisting psychopathology, a number of biological and psychological variables have been identified that render individuals more vulnerable to the development of PTSD.

Course and Prognosis

The course and prognosis of PTSD are summarized in Table 7–25.

Differential Diagnosis

The diagnosis of PTSD is usually not difficult if there is a clear history of exposure to a traumatic event, followed by symptoms of intense anxiety lasting at least 1 month, with arousal and stimulation of the autonomic nervous system, numbing of responsiveness, and avoidance or reexperiencing of the traumatic event. However, a wide variety of anxiety, depressive, somatic, and behavioral symptoms for which the relationship between their onset and the traumatic event is less clear-cut may easily lead to misdiagnosis.

The differential diagnosis of PTSD is described in Table 7–26.

Major Depression

There is much overlap between PTSD and major mood disorders. Symptoms such as psychic numbing, irritability, sleep disturbance, fatigue, anhedonia, impairments in family and social relationships, anger, concern with physical health, and pessimistic outlook

Table 7–24. Risk factors for posttraumatic stress disorder (PTSD)

Past history of trauma prior to the index trauma

Past history of PTSD

Past history of depression

Past history of anxiety disorders

Comorbid Axis II disorders (predictive of greater chronicity)

Family history of anxiety (including parental PTSD)

Disrupted parental attachments

Severity of exposure to trauma (more predictive of acute symptoms)

High premorbid intelligence may be protective

may occur in both disorders. In some veteran outreach populations, 70%–80% of patients meet diagnostic criteria for both disorders. Major depression is a frequent complication of PTSD; when it occurs, it must be treated aggressively, because comorbidity carries an increased risk of suicide. If major depression

Table 7–25. Course and prognosis of posttraumatic stress disorder (PTSD)

Course
  80% longer than 3 months
  75% longer than 6 months
  50% 2 years' duration

Outcome
  Minority can remain symptomatic for years or decades

Predictors of worse outcome
  Greater number of PTSD symptoms
  Psychiatric history of other anxiety and mood disorders
  Higher numbing or hyperarousal to stressors
  Comorbid medical illnesses
  Female sex
  Childhood trauma
  Alcohol abuse

Table 7–26. Differential diagnosis of posttraumatic stress disorder (PTSD)

Depression after trauma (numbing and avoidance may be present, but not hyperarousal and intrusive symptoms)

Panic disorder if the panic attacks are not limited to reminders/triggers of the trauma

Generalized anxiety disorder (may have similar symptoms to PTSD hyperarousal)

Agoraphobia (if avoidance not directly trauma related)

Specific phobia (if avoidance not directly trauma related)

Adjustment disorder (usually less severe stressor and different symptoms)

Acute stress disorder (if less than 1 month has elapsed since trauma)

Dissociative disorders (if prominent dissociative symptoms)

Factitious disorders or malingering (especially if there could be apparent secondary gain)

---

develops secondary to PTSD, both disorders should be diagnosed. Dysthymic symptoms are frequently secondary to PTSD, but if of sufficient severity, the additional diagnosis of dysthymic disorder should be made.

Phobic Disorders

Following a traumatic event, patients may be aversively conditioned to the surroundings of the trauma and develop a phobia of objects, surroundings, or situations that remind them of the trauma itself. Phobic patients experience anxiety in the feared situation, whereas avoidance is accompanied by anxiety reduction that reinforces the avoidant behavior. In PTSD, the phobia may be symptomatically similar to specific phobia, but the nature of the precipitant and the symptom cluster of PTSD distinguish this condition from simple phobia.

Generalized Anxiety Disorder

The symptoms of GAD, such as motor tension, autonomic hyperactivity, apprehensive expectation, and vigilance and scanning, are also present in PTSD. However, the onset and course of the illness differ: GAD has an insidious or gradual onset and a course that fluctuates with environmental stressors, whereas PTSD has an acute onset often followed by a chronic course. Phobic symptoms, which are absent in GAD, are often present in PTSD. DSM-IV-TR does not allow for the diagnosis of GAD if PTSD is present.

Panic Disorder

Patients with PTSD may also experience panic attacks. In some patients, panic attacks predate the PTSD or do not occur exclusively in the context of stimuli reminiscent of the traumatic event. In some patients, however, panic attacks develop after the PTSD and are cued solely by traumatic stimuli.

Adjustment Disorder

Adjustment disorders are maladaptive reactions to identifiable psychosocial pressures. Signs and symptoms may include a wide variety of disturbances and emerge within 3 months of the stressful event. If symptoms are of sufficient severity to meet other Axis I criteria, then the diagnosis of adjustment disorder is not made. Adjustment disorder differs from PTSD in that the stressor is usually less severe and within the range of common experience, and the characteristic symptoms of PTSD, such as reexperiencing the trauma, are absent. The prognosis of full recovery in adjustment disorder is usually excellent.

Compensation Neurosis (Factitious Disorder and Malingering)

Both factitious disorder and malingering involve conscious deception and feigning of illness, although the motivation for each condition differs. Factitious disorder may present with physical or psychological symptoms; the feigning of symptoms is under voluntary control, and the motivation is to assume the "patient" role. Chronic factitious disorder with physical symptoms (i.e., Munchausen's syndrome) involves frequent doctor visits and surgical interventions. PTSD differs from this by its absence of fabricated symptoms, acute onset after a trauma, and absence of a bizarre pretraumatic medical history.

Malingering involves the conscious fabrication of an illness for the purpose of achieving a definite goal such as money, compensation, and so forth. Malingerers often reveal an inconsistent history, unexpected symptom clusters, a history of antisocial behavior and substance abuse, and chaotic lifestyle, and there is often a discrepancy between history, claimed distress, and objective data.

Postconcussion Syndrome

Mental disorders secondary to head injury are influenced by physiological, psychological, and environmental factors. Psychological symptoms are extremely common after mild closed head injuries, even without loss of consciousness. The so-called postconcussion syndrome comprises the symptoms of headache, dizziness, irritability, and emotional la-

bility after a head injury with concussion. Depression and lethargy are the affective symptoms that occur most commonly. These symptoms bear no relation to the degree of physical injury.

Treatment

Pharmacotherapy

A variety of different psychopharmacological agents have been used in the treatment of PTSD by clinicians and reported in the literature as case reports, open clinic trials, and controlled studies. These are summarized in the following sections; in recent years, SSRIs and other serotonergic agents have emerged as the first-line pharmacological treatment of PTSD (Table 7–27).

Serotonin reuptake inhibitors. SSRIs have become established as first-line medications for PTSD treatment (D.J. Stein et al. 2006).

Table 7–27.   Pharmacotherapy of posttraumatic stress disorder (PTSD)

Selective serotonin reuptake inhibitors (SSRIs) and newer antidepressants
General indications: First-line treatment; well-tolerated; once/day dosing; documented efficacy.
   Sertraline: FDA approved, large controlled trials
   Other SSRIs: similar efficacy
   Venlafaxine, mirtazapine

Other antidepressants
Tricyclic antidepressants: overall modest results when tested in double-blind fashion
Monoamine oxidase inhibitors: may be superior to tricyclics, especially for intrusive symptoms

Other medications
General indications: When response to first-line options not adequate; additional treatment of specific PTSD symptoms or comorbid disorders.
   Prazosin: nightmares and daytime intrusions
   Atypical antipsychotics: several studies documenting some benefit
   Clonidine: some efficacy in open treatment
   Lithium: improvement in intrusive symptoms and irritability in open trial
   Anticonvulsants (carbamazepine, valproate, lamotrigine, tiagabine, topiramate, levetiracetam, phenytoin): mostly open trials showing some efficacy
   Buspirone: efficacy in an open trial
   Triiodothyronine: improvement in small open trial, possibly antidepressant response
   Trazodone, benzodiazepines, diphenhydramine: sleep disturbance

---

Note.   FDA = U.S. Food and Drug Administration.

Newer serotonergic antidepressants other than SSRIs may also be beneficial. There may also be benefit to continuing SSRI treatment beyond the initial 6-month period.

Adrenergic blockers.   Kolb et al. (1984) treated 12 Vietnam veterans with PTSD in an open trial of the β-blocker propranolol over a 6-month period. Dosage ranged from 120 to 160 mg daily. Eleven patients reported a positive change in self-assessment at the end of the 6-month period, with less explosiveness, fewer nightmares, improved sleep, and a decrease in intrusive thoughts, hyperalertness, and startle.

Recently, the α_1-adrenergic antagonist prazosin has emerged as a very promising agent in the treatment of PTSD. Evidence supporting its use is mostly available for bedtime administration, but benefits can also occur for daytime symptoms. There is also recent interest in using β-blockers in the acute aftermath of a trauma in order to diminish the consolidation of traumatic memories and attenuate the course of posttraumatic symptoms and evolving PTSD.

Psychotherapy

It is generally agreed that some form of psychotherapy is necessary in the treatment of posttraumatic pathology. Crisis intervention shortly after the traumatic event is effective in reducing immediate distress and possibly preventing chronic or delayed responses, and if the pathological response is still tentative, it may allow for briefer intervention.

Brief dynamic psychotherapy has been advocated both as an immediate treatment procedure and as a way of preventing chronic disorder. The therapist must establish a working alliance that allows the patient to work through his or her reactions.

Group psychotherapy can also serve as an important adjunctive treatment, or as the central treatment mode, in traumatized patients (van der Kolk 1987). Because of past experiences, such patients are often mistrustful and reluctant to depend on authority figures, whereas the identification, support, and

hopefulness of peer settings can facilitate therapeutic change.

Drug treatment has been impressionistically reported to have a positive impact on psychotherapy in 70% of cases, with improvements in symptom severity leading to a more positive and motivated approach to psychotherapy and an enhancement of accessibility to uncovering and working through (Bleich et al. 1986).

Cognitive and Behavioral Therapies

A variety of cognitive and behavioral techniques have gained increasing popularity and validation in the treatment of PTSD (Table 7–28).

People involved in traumatic events such as accidents frequently develop phobias or phobic anxiety related to or associated with these situations. When a phobia or phobic anxiety is associated with PTSD, systematic desensitization or graded exposure has been found to be effective. This is based on the principle that when patients are gradually exposed to a phobic or anxiety-provoking stimulus, they will become habituated or deconditioned to the stimulus. Variations of this treatment include using imaginal techniques (i.e., imaginal desensitization) and exposure to real-life situations (i.e., in vivo desensitization). Prolonged exposure, a form of extended repeat exposure to the same trau-

---

Table 7–28.   Cognitive and behavioral approaches to treating posttraumatic stress disorder

Graded exposure (imaginal and/or in vivo)

Prolonged exposure

Virtual reality exposure

Cognitive reprocessing

Stress inoculation training

Hypnosis

Affect management

Eye movement desensitization and reprocessing

---

matic memory over a series of sessions, if tolerated, is an effective technique first reported to be successful in the treatment of Vietnam veterans (Fairbank and Keane 1982) and has become established as a first-line treatment of PTSD (Foa et al. 2000). Virtual reality exposure is another computer-based exposure technique that has been piloted in Vietnam veterans and appears promising (Rothbaum et al. 2001).

Relaxation techniques produce the beneficial physiological result of reducing motor tension and lowering the activity of the autonomic nervous system, effects that may be particularly efficacious in PTSD. Progressive muscle relaxation involves contracting and relaxing various muscle groups to induce the relaxation response. This is useful for symptoms of autonomic arousal such as somatic symptoms, anxiety, and insomnia. Hypnosis has also been used to induce the relaxation response with success in PTSD. Relaxation, combined with elements of distraction, thought-stopping, and self-guided dialogue, is a technique known as stress inoculation training.

Cognitive therapy, also referred to as cognitive reprocessing or restructuring, involves various cognitive formulations and corrections of patients' traumatic recollections—that is, identifying distorted and maladaptive cognitions and replacing them with more realistic ones (Resick et al. 2002). Cognitive processing therapy was shown to be more efficacious than wait-list control in a study of women with childhood sexual abuse (Chard 2005). CBT appears to also be highly beneficial for children and adolescents.

Eye movement desensitization and reprocessing (EMDR) is a technique that has been extensively applied to the treatment of trauma-related pathology. There continues to be some controversy in the literature regarding the efficacy of EMDR as well as its underlying mechanisms of action.

Conclusion

The anxiety disorders are a diverse collection of psychiatric conditions that have high rates of comorbidity with each other and with depression, somatoform disorders, and alcohol abuse. The anxiety disorders are the psychiatric illnesses most frequently encountered in primary care settings, with prevalence rates ranging from 2% to 16%. Because anxiety disorders present so commonly and with other disorders, clinicians need to be familiar with their diverse presentations and the range of effective pharmacological and psychosocial therapies available to treat them.

Key Points

- Anxiety disorders are prevalent in the general population, with lifetime prevalence ranging from about 2%–3% for panic disorder and obsessive-compulsive disorder to 15% for social phobia (social anxiety disorder).

- Anxiety disorders are highly treatable: medication and/or cognitive-behavioral therapy constitute first-line treatments for all these disorders.

- Serotonin reuptake inhibitors are the first-line treatment for all anxiety disorders.

- Exposure, relaxation, and cognitive restructuring are the main types of psychotherapies helpful in treating the anxiety disorders.

Suggested Readings

Barlow DH: Clinical Handbook of Psychological Disorders: A Step-by-Step Treatment Manual, 3rd Edition. New York, Guilford, 2001

Hollander E, Bakalar N: Coping With Social Anxiety: The Definitive Guide to Effective Treatment Options. New York, Henry Holt and Company, 2005

Hollander E, Simeon D: Concise Guide to the Anxiety Disorders. Washington, DC, American Psychiatric Publishing, 2003

Hollander E, Stein DJ (eds): Obsessive Compulsive Disorders. New York, Marcel Dekker, 1997

Horowitz MJ: Treatment of Stress Response Syndromes. Washington, DC, American Psychiatric Publishing, 2003

Stein DJ, Hollander E: The American Psychiatric Publishing Textbook of Anxiety Disorders. Washington, DC, American Psychiatric Publishing, 2002

Yehuda R: Treating Trauma Survivors With PTSD. Washington, DC, American Psychiatric Publishing, 2002

References

Akhtar S, Wig NN, Varma VK, et al: A phenomenological analysis of symptoms in obsessive-compulsive neurosis. Br J Psychiatry 127:342–348, 1975

Alden LE, Wallace ST: Social phobia and social appraisal in successful and unsuccessful social interactions. Behav Res Ther 33:497–505, 1995

Allgulander C, Dahl AA, Austin C, et al: Efficacy of sertraline in a 12-week trial for generalized anxiety disorder. Am J Psychiatry 161:1642–1649, 2004

American Psychiatric Association: Diagnostic and Statistical Manual of Mental Disorders, 3rd Edition. Washington, DC, American Psychiatric Association, 1980

American Psychiatric Association: Diagnostic and Statistical Manual of Mental Disorders, 3rd Edition, Revised. Washington, DC, American Psychiatric Association, 1987

American Psychiatric Association: Diagnostic and Statistical Manual of Mental Disorders, 4rd Edition. Washington, DC, American Psychiatric Association, 1994

American Psychiatric Association: Diagnostic and Statistical Manual of Mental Disorders, 4rd Edition, Text Revision. Washington, DC, American Psychiatric Association, 2000

Ball SG, Kuhn A, Wall D, et al: Selective serotonin reuptake inhibitor treatment for generalized anxiety disorder: a double-blind, prospective comparison between paroxetine and sertraline. J Clin Psychiatry 66:94–99, 2005

Banos RM, Botella C, Perpina C, et al: Virtual reality in treatment of flying phobia. IEEE Trans Inf Technol Biomed 6:206–212, 2002

Barlow DH, Craske MG, Cerny JA, et al: Behavioral treatment of panic disorder. Behav Ther 20:261–282, 1989

Beck AT, Sokol L, Clark DA, et al: A crossover study of focused cognitive therapy for panic disorder. Am J Psychiatry 149:778–783, 1992

Bellew KM, McCafferty JP, Iyengar M, et al: Paroxetine treatment of GAD: a double-blind, placebo-controlled trial. Presented at the 153rd annual meeting of the American Psychiatric Association, Chicago, IL, 2000

Black A: The natural history of obsessional neurosis, in Obsessional States. Edited by Beech HK. London, England, Methuen, 1974, pp 19–54

Bleich A, Siegel B, Garb R, et al: Post-traumatic stress disorder following combat exposure: clinical features and psychopharmacological treatment. Br J Psychiatry 149:365–369, 1986

Breslau N, Davis GC, Andreski P, et al: Traumatic events and posttraumatic stress disorder in an urban population of young adults. Arch Gen Psychiatry 48:216–222, 1991

Breslau N, Davis GC, Peterson EL, et al: A second look at comorbidity in victims of trauma: the posttraumatic stress disorder–major depression connection. Biol Psychiatry 48:902–909, 2000

Carter RM, Wittchen HU, Pfister H, et al: One-year prevalence of subthreshold and threshold DSM-IV generalized anxiety disorder in a nationally representative sample. Depress Anxiety 13:78–88, 2001

Chard KM: An evaluation of cognitive processing therapy for the treatment of posttraumatic stress disorder related to childhood sexual abuse. J Consult Clin Psychol 73:965–971, 2005

Clomipramine Collaborative Study Group: Clomipramine in the treatment of patients with obsessive-compulsive disorder. Arch Gen Psychiatry 48:730–738, 1991

Cottraux J, Note I, Albuisson E, et al: Cognitive behavior therapy versus supportive therapy in social phobia: a randomized controlled trial. Psychother Psychosom 69:137–146, 2000

Cottraux J, Note I, Yao SN, et al: A randomized controlled trial of cognitive therapy versus intensive behavior therapy in obsessive compulsive disorder. Psychother Psychosom 70:288–297, 2001

Dahl AA, Ravindran A, Allgulander C, et al: Sertraline in generalized anxiety disorder: efficacy in treating the psychic and somatic anxiety factors. Acta Psychiatr Scand 111:429–435, 2005

Davidson J, Potts N, Richichi E, et al: Treatment of social phobia with clonazepam and placebo. J Clin Psychopharmacol 13:423–428, 1993

de Haan E, Hoogduin KA, Buitelaar JK, et al: Behavior therapy versus clomipramine for the treatment of obsessive-compulsive disorder in children and adolescents. J Am Acad Child Adolesc Psychiatry 37:1022–1029, 1998

Delle Chiaie R, Pancheri P, Casacchia M, et al: Assessment of the efficacy of buspirone in patients affected by generalized anxiety disorder, shifting to buspirone from prior treatment with lorazepam: a placebo-controlled, double-blind study. J Clin Psychopharmacol 15:12–19, 1995

Emmanuel NP, Lydiard BR, Ballenger JC: Treatment of social phobia with bupropion. J Clin Psychopharmacol 1:276–277, 1991

Essau CA, Conradt J, Petermann F: Frequency, comorbidity, and psychosocial impairment of specific phobia in adolescents. J Clin Child Psychol 29:221–231, 2000

Fairbank TA, Keane TM: Flooding for combat-related stress disorders: assessment of anxiety reduction across traumatic memories. Behav Ther 13:499–510, 1982

Fisher PL, Wells A: How effective are cognitive and behavioral treatments for obsessive compulsive disorder? A clinical significance analysis. Behav Res Ther 43:1543–1558, 2005

Foa EB, Keane TM, Friedman MJ: Effective Treatments for PTSD: Practice Guidelines From the International Society for Traumatic Stress Studies. New York, Guilford, 2000

Foa EB, Liebowitz MR, Kozak MJ, et al: Randomized, placebo controlled trial of exposure and ritual prevention, clomipramine, and their combination in the treatment of obsessive compulsive disorder. Am J Psychiatry 162:151–161, 2005

Fyer AJ, Mannuzza S, Gallops MS, et al: Familial transmission of simple phobias and fears: a preliminary report. Arch Gen Psychiatry 47:252–256, 1990

Gabbard GO: Psychodynamic Psychiatry in Clinical Practice. Washington, DC, American Psychiatric Press, 1990

Gambi F, De-Berardis D, Campanella D, et al: Mirtazapine treatment of generalized anxiety disorder: a fixed dose, open label study. J Psychopharmacol 19:483–487, 2005

Garcia-Palacios A, Hoffman H, Carlin A, et al: Virtual reality in the treatment of spider phobia: a controlled study. Behav Res Ther 40:983–993, 2002

Gelernter CS, Uhde TW, Cimbolic P, et al: Cognitive-behavioral and pharmacological treatments of social phobia: a controlled study. Arch Gen Psychiatry 48:938–945, 1991

Goodman WK, Bose A, Wang Q: Treatment of generalized anxiety disorder with escitalopram: pooled results from double-blind, placebo-controlled trials. J Affect Discord 87:161–167, 2005

Grant BF, Hasin DS, Blanco C, et al: The epidemiology of social anxiety disorder in the United States: results from the National Epidemiologic Survey on Alcohol and Related Conditions. J Clin Psychiatry 66:1351–1361, 2005a

Grant BF, Hasin DS, Stinson FS, et al: Prevalence, correlates, comorbidity, and comparative disability of DSM-IV generalized anxiety disorder in the USA: results from the

National Epidemiologic Survey on Alcohol and Related Conditions. Psychol Med 35:1747–1759, 2005b

Grant BF, Hasin DS, Stinson FS, et al: The epidemiology of DSM-IV panic disorder and agoraphobia in the United States: results from the National Epidemiologic Survey on Alcohol and Related Conditions. J Clin Psychiatry 67:363–374, 2006

Greist JH, Chouinard G, DuBoff E, et al: Double-blind parallel comparison of three dosages of sertraline and placebo in outpatients with obsessive-compulsive disorder. Arch Gen Psychiatry 52:289–295, 1995

Heimberg RG, Hope DA, Dodge CS, et al: DSM-III-R subtypes of social phobia: comparison of generalized social phobics and public speaking phobics. J Nerv Ment Dis 178:172–179, 1990

Heimberg RG, Liebowitz MR, Hope DA, et al: Cognitive behavioral group therapy vs phenelzine therapy for social phobia: a 12-week outcome. Arch Gen Psychiatry 55:1133–1141, 1998

Hofmann SG, Moscovitch DA, Kim HJ, et al: Changes in self perception during treatment of social phobia. J Consult Clin Psychol 72:588–596, 2004

Hollander E, Koran LM, Goodman WK, et al: A double blind, placebo controlled study of the efficacy and safety of controlled release fluvoxamine in patients with obsessive compulsive disorder. J Clin Psychiatry 64:640–647, 2003

Jenike MA, Hyman S, Baer L, et al: A controlled trial of fluvoxamine in obsessive-compulsive disorder: implications for a serotonergic theory. Am J Psychiatry 147:1209–1215, 1990

Kampman M, Keijers GP, Hoogduin CA, et al: A randomized, double-blind, placebo-controlled study of the effects of adjunctive paroxetine in panic disorder patients unsuccessfully treated with cognitive-behavioral therapy alone. J Clin Psychiatry 63:772–777, 2002

Karno M, Golding JM, Sorenson SB, et al: The epidemiology of obsessive-compulsive disorder in five US communities. Arch Gen Psychiatry 45:1094–1099, 1988

Kenwright M, Marks IM: Computer aided self help for phobia/panic via Internet at home: a pilot study. Br J Psychiatry 184:448–449, 2004

Kessler RC, McGonagle KA, Zhao S, et al: Lifetime and 12-month prevalence of DSM-III-R psychiatric disorders in the United States: results from the National Comorbidity Survey. Arch Gen Psychiatry 51:8–19, 1994

Kessler RC, Sonnega A, Bromet E, et al: Posttraumatic stress disorder in the National Comorbidity Survey. Arch Gen Psychiatry 52:1048–1060, 1995

Kessler RC, DuPont RL, Berglund P, et al: Impairment in pure and comorbid generalized anxiety disorder and major depression at 12 months in two national surveys. Am J Psychiatry 156:1915–1923, 1999a

Kessler RC, Stang P, Wittchen HU, et al: Lifetime comorbidities between social phobia and mood disorders in the US National Comorbidity Survey. Psychol Med 29:555–567, 1999b

Kessler RC, Brandenburg N, Lane M, et al: Rethinking the duration requirement for generalized anxiety disorder: evidence from the National Comorbidity Survey Replication. Psychol Med 35:1073–1082, 2005

Kessler RC, Chiu WT, Jin R, et al: The epidemiology of panic attacks, panic disorder, and agoraphobia in the National Comorbidity Survey Replication. Arch Gen Psychiatry 63:415–424, 2006

Kobak KA, Greist JH, Jefferson JW, et al: Behavioral versus pharmacological treatments of obsessive compulsive disorder: a meta-analysis. Psychopharmacology (Berl) 136:205–216, 1998

Kolb LC, Burris BC, Griffiths S: Propranolol and clonidine in treatment of the chronic posttraumatic stress disorders of war, in Post-Traumatic Stress Disorder: Psychological and Biological Sequelae. Edited by van der Kolk BA. Washington, DC, American Psychiatric Press, 1984, pp 97–105

Kronig MH, Apter J, Asnis G, et al: Placebo-controlled, multicenter study of sertraline treatment for obsessive-compulsive disorder. J Clin Psychopharmacol 19:172–176, 1999

Liebowitz MR, Gorman JM, Fyer AJ, et al: Social phobia: review of a neglected anxiety disorder. Arch Gen Psychiatry 42:729–736, 1985

Liebowitz MR, Schneier F, Campeas R, et al: Phenelzine vs atenolol in social phobia: a placebo-controlled comparison. Arch Gen Psychiatry 49:290–300, 1992

Magee WJ, Eaton WW, Wittchen HU, et al: Agoraphobia, simple phobia, and social phobia in the National Comorbidity Survey. Arch Gen Psychiatry 53:159–168, 1996

Mannuzza S, Schneier FR, Chapman TF, et al: Generalized social phobia: reliability and validity. Arch Gen Psychiatry 52:230–237, 1995

Michelson L, Marchione K, Greenwald M, et al: Panic disorder: cognitive-behavioral treatment. Behav Res Ther 28:141–151, 1990

Mitte K: Meta-analysis of cognitive-behavioral treatments for generalized anxiety disorder: a comparison with pharmacotherapy. Psychol Bull 131:785–795, 2005

Muehlbacher M, Nickel MK, Nickel C, et al: Mirtazapine treatment of social phobia in women: a randomized, double-blind, placebo-controlled study. J Clin Psychopharmacol 25:580–583, 2005

Muris P, Schmidt H, Meckelbach H: The structure of specific phobia symptoms among children and adolescents. Behav Res Ther 37:863–868, 1999

Neziroglu F, Anemone R, Yaryura-Tobias JA: Onset of obsessive-compulsive disorder in pregnancy. Am J Psychiatry 149:947–950, 1992

Ninan PT, Koran LM, Kiev A, et al: High-dose sertraline strategy for nonresponders to acute treatment for obsessive-compulsive disorder: a multicenter double-blind trial. J Clin Psychiatry 67:15–22, 2006

Noyes R Jr, Reich JH, Christiansen J, et al: Outcome of panic disorder: relationship to diagnostic subtypes and comorbidity. Arch Gen Psychiatry 47:809–818, 1990

Ost LG, Thulin U, Ramnero J: Cognitive behavior therapy vs. exposure in vivo in the treatment of panic disorder with agoraphobia. Behav Res Ther 42:1105–1127, 2004

Otto MW, Pollack MH, Sachs GS, et al: Discontinuation of benzodiazepine treatment: efficacy of cognitive-behavioral therapy for patients with panic disorder. Am J Psychiatry 150:1485–1490, 1993

Otto MW, Pollack MH, Gould RA, et al: A comparison of the efficacy of clonazepam and cognitive-behavioral group therapy for the treatment of social phobia. J Anxiety Disord 14:345–358, 2000

Pallanti S, Quercioli L, Paiva RS, et al: Citalopram for treatment-resistant obsessive-compulsive disorder. Eur Psychiatry 14:101–106, 1999

Pediatric OCD Treatment Study Team: Cognitive behavior therapy, sertraline, and their combination for children and adolescents with obsessive compulsive disorder: the Pediatric OCD Treatment Study (POTS) randomized controlled trial. JAMA 292:1969–1976, 2004

Quitkin F, Babkin J: Hidden psychiatric diagnosis in the alcoholic, in Alcoholism and Clinical Psychiatry. Edited by Soloman J. New York, Plenum, 1982, pp 129–140

Rachman SJ, Hodgson RJ: Obsessions and Compulsions. Englewood Cliffs, NJ, Prentice-Hall, 1980

Ralevski E, Sanislow CA, Grilo CM, et al: Avoidant personality disorder and social phobia: distinct enough to be separate disorders? Acta Psychiatr Scand 112:208–214, 2005

Regier DA, Boyd JH, Burke JD Jr, et al: One-month prevalence of mental disorders in the United States, based on five Epidemiologic Catchment Area sites. Arch Gen Psychiatry 45:977–986, 1988

Resick PA, Nishith P, Weaver TL, et al: A comparison of cognitive processing therapy with prolonged exposure and a waiting condition for the treatment of chronic posttraumatic stress disorder in female rape victims. J Consult Clin Psychol 70:867–879, 2002

Rettew DC: Avoidant personality disorder, generalized social phobia, and shyness: putting the personality back into personality disorders. Harv Rev Psychiatry 8:283–297, 2000

Rickels K, Downing R, Schweizer E, et al: Antidepressants for the treatment of generalized anxiety disorder: a placebo-controlled comparison of imipramine, trazodone, and diazepam. Arch Gen Psychiatry 50:884–895, 1993

Rickels K, DeMartinis N, Garcia-Espana F, et al: Imipramine and buspirone in treatment of patients with generalized anxiety disorder who are discontinuing long-term benzodiazepine therapy. Am J Psychiatry 157:1973–1979, 2000

Rickels K, Mangano R, Khan A: A double blind placebo controlled study of a flexible dose of venlafaxine ER in adult outpatients with generalized social anxiety disorder. J Clin Psychopharmacol 24:488–496, 2004

Rocca P, Beoni AM, Eva C, et al: Peripheral benzodiazepine receptor messenger RNA is decreased in lymphocytes of generalized anxiety disorder patients. Biol Psychiatry 43:767–773, 1998

Romach M, Busto U, Somer G, et al: Clinical aspects of chronic use of alprazolam and lorazepam. Am J Psychiatry 152:1161–1167, 1995

Rothbaum BO, Hodges LF, Ready D, et al: Virtual reality exposure therapy for Vietnam veterans with posttraumatic stress disorder. J Clin Psychiatry 62:617–622, 2001

Ruscio AM, Lane M, Roy-Byrne P, et al: Should excessive worry be required for a diagnosis of generalized anxiety disorder? Results from the U.S. National Comorbidity Survey Replication. Psychol Med 35:1761–1772, 2005

Salkovskis PM, Jones DRO, Clark DM: Respiratory control in the treatment of panic attacks: replication and extension with concurrent measurement of behaviour and pCO2. Br J Psychiatry 148:526–532, 1986

Schmidt NB, Wollaway-Bickel K, Trakowski JH, et al: Antidepressant discontinuation in the context of cognitive behavioral treatment for panic disorder. Behav Res Ther 40:67–73, 2002

Simpson HB, Liebowitz MR, Foa EB, et al: Post treatment effects of exposure therapy and clomipramine in obsessive compulsive disorder. Depress Anxiety 19:225–233, 2004

Simpson HB, Huppert JD, Petkova E, et al: Response versus remission in obsessive compulsive disorder. J Clin Psychiatry 67:269–276, 2005

Spiegel DA, Bruce TJ, Gregg SF, et al: Does cognitive behavior therapy assist slow-taper alprazolam discontinuation in panic disorder? Am J Psychiatry 151:876–881, 1994

Starkman MN, Cameron OG, Nesse RM, et al: Peripheral catecholamine levels and the symptoms of anxiety: studies in patients with and without pheochromocytoma. Psychosom Med 52:129–142, 1990

Stein DJ, Ipser JC, Seedat S: Pharmacotherapy for post traumatic stress disorder. Cochrane Database Syst Rev (1):CD002795, 2006

Stein MB, Walker JR, Hazen AL, et al: Full and partial posttraumatic stress disorder: findings from a community survey. Am J Psychiatry 154:1114–1119, 1997

Swedo SE, Rapoport JL, Leonard H, et al: Obsessive-compulsive disorder in children and adolescents: clinical phenomenology of 70 consecutive cases. Arch Gen Psychiatry 46:335–341, 1989

Tillfors M, Furmark T, Ekselius L, et al: Social phobia and avoidant personality disorder as related to parental history of social anxiety: a general population study. Behav Res Ther 39:289–298, 2001

Torgersen S: Genetic factors in anxiety disorders. Arch Gen Psychiatry 40:1085–1089, 1983

Turner SM, Beidel DC, Cooley-Quille MR: Two-year follow-up of social phobias treated with social effectiveness therapy. Behav Res Ther 33:553–555, 1995

van der Kolk BA: The role of the group in the origin and resolution of the trauma response, in Psychological Trauma. Edited by van der Kolk BA. Washington, DC, American Psychiatric Press, 1987, pp 153–171

van Oppen P, de Haan E, van Balkom AJ, et al: Cognitive therapy and exposure in vivo in the treatment of obsessive compulsive disorder. Behav Res Ther 33:379–390, 1995

van Oppen P, van Balkom AJ, de Haan E, et al: Cognitive therapy and exposure in vivo alone and in combination with fluvoxamine in obsessive compulsive disorder: a 5 year follow up. J Clin Psychiatry 66:1415–1422, 2005

Versiani M, Mundim FD, Nardi AE, et al: Tranylcypromine in social phobia. J Clin Psychopharmacol 8:279–283, 1988

Wald J, Taylor S: Preliminary research on the efficacy of virtual reality exposure therapy to treat driving phobia. Cyberpsychol Behav 6:459–465, 2003

Westphal K: Ueber Zwangsverstellungen [obsessional thoughts]. Arch Psychiatr Neurol 8:734–750, 1878

Whittal ML, Thordarson DS, McLean PD, et al: Treatment of obsessive compulsive disorder: cognitive behavior therapy vs. exposure and response prevention. Behav Res Ther 43:1559–1576, 2005

Wittchen HU, Carter RM, Pfister H, et al: Disabilities and quality of life in pure and comorbid generalized anxiety disorder and major depression in a national survey. Int Clin Psychopharmacol 15:319–328, 2000

Woody SR, Chambless DL, Glass CR: Self-focused attention in the treatment of social phobia. Behav Res Ther 35:117–129, 1997

Zimmerman M, Chelminski I: Generalized anxiety disorder in patients with major depression: is DSM-IV's hierarchy correct? Am J Psychiatry 160:504–512, 2003

8

SOMATOFORM DISORDERS

Sean H. Yutzy, M.D.
Brooke S. Parish, M.D.

The somatoform disorders were first delineated as a class of psychiatric disorders in DSM-III (American Psychiatric Association 1980). The class was created to facilitate the differential diagnosis of disorders characterized primarily by "physical symptoms suggesting physical disorder (hence somatoform) for which there are no demonstrable organic findings or known physiological mechanisms and for which there is positive evidence, or a strong presumption, that the symptoms are linked to psychological factors or conflicts" (American Psychiatric Association 1980, p. 241). With minor modifications, this grouping and its underlying concept were retained in DSM-III-R (American Psychiatric Association 1987) and, after some debate (Martin 1995), in DSM-IV (American Psychiatric Association 1994) as well as DSM-IV-TR (American Psychiatric Association 2000). (Noteworthy here was that the explicit diagnostic criteria from DSM-IV remained the same in DSM-IV-TR.) In contrast to factitious disorders and malingering, somatoform disorder symptoms are not under voluntary control. The stipulation in DSM-IV-TR that symptoms are not fully accounted for by known physiological mechanisms distinguishes somatoform disorders from disorders formerly designated as psychophysiological disorders, some of which are included in DSM-IV-TR under "Psychological Factors Affecting Medical Condition." Beliefs involving preoccupations with symptoms are not of delusional intensity, except possibly for body dysmorphic disorder. Symptoms are not better accounted for by other mental disorders.

In DSM-IV-TR, the disorders included under the somatoform rubric are somatization disorder, undifferentiated somatoform disorder, conversion disorder, pain disorder, hypochondriasis, body dysmorphic disorder, and the residual category somatoform disorder not otherwise specified (NOS). The grouping is based on the clinical utility of a shared diagnostic concern rather than assumptions regarding shared etiology or mechanism—that is, occult "physical" or "organic" pathology underlying the symptoms is excluded. In DSM-IV-TR terminology, such etiologies are referred to as "general medical conditions" or the "direct effects of a substance." General medical conditions include all conditions not included in the mental disorders section of ICD-10 (World Health Organization 1992). As examples, all infectious and parasitic, endocrine, nutritional, metabolic, immunological, and congenital disorders affecting virtually any organ system (including the nervous system) are considered general medical conditions. This terminology was adopted to avoid the implication that mental (i.e., psychiatric) conditions do not have organic causes and to underscore the view that psychiatric disorders are also medical conditions.

The utility of grouping disorders on the basis of a shared clinical concern was endorsed by the symptom-driven *Diagnostic and Statistical Manual of Mental Disorders, 4th Edition, Primary Care Version* (American Psychiatric Association 1995), which included "unexplained physical symptoms" as the basis of 1 of its 10 algorithms. Likewise, the *Diagnostic and Management Guidelines for Mental Disorders in Primary Care: ICD-10 Chapter V Primary Care Version* (World Health Organization 1996) was organized with a diagnostic category for "unexplained somatic complaint."

Historically, many overlapping, conflicting, and even contradictory diagnostic conventions have been used to identify and distinguish somatoform disorders. For the sake of consistency, this chapter uses DSM-IV-TR criteria and terminology, with other systems reviewed and contrasted when appropriate.

Given the heterogeneity of the somatoform disorder class, extensive discussion of the class in general is not particularly useful. The specific somatoform disorders are best discussed individually. Thus, we review the somatoform disorders included in DSM-IV-TR. For convenience, the disorders are discussed in the order in which they appear in DSM-IV-TR.

Somatization Disorder
Definition and Clinical Description

The core features of somatization disorder are recurrent multiple physical complaints that are not fully explained by physical factors and that result in medical attention or significant impairment.

A patient with somatization disorder is typified by the following example:

> An internist referred a married, 35-year-old woman to a psychiatrist because of the physician's inability to establish a clear longitudinal history and medical explanation for her numerous physical complaints. Physical examination and laboratory testing had been completely unrevealing. The physician had treated her for anxiety and depressive complaints; however, the pharmacotherapy, which was initially apparently effective, subsequently failed.
>
> On presentation to the psychiatrist, the patient offered a laundry list of physical complaints in a dramatic yet vague manner. The patient often went into elaborate and flamboyant discussions of her marital, social, and occupational problems. Careful review of the presentation identified a long history of chronic physical complaints without medical explanation. Furthermore, the physical problems appeared to be temporally associated with multiple psychosocial stressors.

Somatization disorder is the most pervasive somatoform disorder. By definition, somatization disorder is a polysymptomatic disorder affecting multiple body systems. Symptoms of other specific somatoform disorders (e.g., conversion disorder and pain disorder) are included in the diagnostic criteria for somatization disorder. Undifferentiated somatoform disorder, in essence, represents a syndrome similar to somatization disorder but with a less extensive symptomatology. From a hierarchical perspective, none of these disorders is diagnosed if symptoms occur exclusively during the course of somatization disorder.

Somatization disorder has been the most rigorously studied somatoform disorder and is the best validated in terms of diagnostic reliability, stability over time, prediction of medical utilization, and even heritability. Yet its validity as a discrete syndrome has been challenged (Bass and Murphy 1990). Vaillant (1984), noting that most of the research on this disorder has emanated from four academic centers in the midwestern United States, went so far as to state that the diagnosis "lies in the eyes of the beholder."

Diagnosis

DSM-IV-TR Criteria

In an attempt to address these issues for DSM-IV, a comprehensive reassessment of the extant literature and preexisting data sets was coordinated by the American Psychiatric Association. On the basis of this review, Cloninger and Yutzy (1993) suggested a diagnostic strategy that simplified the criteria for somatization disorder and appeared useful in routine practice. Data from a sample of 500 psychiatric outpatients were reanalyzed, leading to the development of an empirically derived algorithm to diagnose somatization disorder. This algorithm required four pain symptoms, two nonpain gastrointestinal symptoms, one nonpain sexual or reproductive symptom, and one pseudoneurological (conversion or dissociative) symptom. This approach was adopted for DSM-IV (Table 8–1). The data reanalysis criteria identified nearly the same patients as did both the original Feighner criteria (Feighner et al. 1972) for hysteria and the DSM-III-R criteria for somatization disorder ($\kappa=0.79$; sensitivity = 81%, specificity = 96%) (Yutzy et al. 1992).

The new criteria were tested in a multicenter field trial designed to examine their concordance with previous diagnostic criteria. The findings supported the DSM-IV diagnostic strategy for somatization disorder.

Differential Diagnosis

The symptom picture encountered in somatization disorder is frequently nonspecific and can overlap with a multitude of medical disorders. According to Cloninger (1994), three features are useful in discriminating between somatization disorder and physical illness: 1) involvement of multiple organ systems, 2) early onset and chronic course without development of physical signs of structural abnormalities, and 3) absence of characteristic laboratory abnormalities of the suggested physical disorder. These features should be considered in cases for which careful analysis leaves the etiology unclear. The clinician also should be aware that several medical disorders may be confused with somatization disorder (Table 8–2). Patients with multiple sclerosis or systemic lupus erythematosus (SLE) may have vague functional and sensory disturbances with unclear physical signs. Patients with acute intermittent porphyria may have a history of episodic pain and various neurological disturbances, and patients with hemochromatosis often have vague and diffuse pains that may be confused with those described by patients who have somatization disorder.

According to Cloninger (1994), three psychiatric disorders must be carefully considered in the differential diagnosis of somatization disorder: anxiety disorders (in particular, panic disorder), mood disorders, and schizophrenia.

Individuals with antisocial, borderline, and/or histrionic personality disorder may have an associated somatization disorder (Cloninger et al. 1997; Hudziak et al. 1996; Stern et al. 1993). Antisocial personality disorder has been shown to cluster both within individuals and within families (Cloninger and Guze 1970; Cloninger et al. 1975) and may have a common etiology in many cases.

Patients with somatization disorder often complain of psychological or interpersonal

---

Table 8–1. DSM-IV-TR diagnostic criteria for somatization disorder

---

A. A history of many physical complaints beginning before age 30 years that occur over a period of several years and result in treatment being sought or significant impairment in social, occupational, or other important areas of functioning.

B. Each of the following criteria must have been met, with individual symptoms occurring at any time during the course of the disturbance:

   (1) *four pain symptoms:* a history of pain related to at least four different sites or functions (e.g., head, abdomen, back, joints, extremities, chest, rectum, during menstruation, during sexual intercourse, or during urination)

   (2) *two gastrointestinal symptoms:* a history of at least two gastrointestinal symptoms other than pain (e.g., nausea, bloating, vomiting other than during pregnancy, diarrhea, or intolerance of several different foods)

   (3) *one sexual symptom:* a history of at least one sexual or reproductive symptom other than pain (e.g., sexual indifference, erectile or ejaculatory dysfunction, irregular menses, excessive menstrual bleeding, vomiting throughout pregnancy)

   (4) *one pseudoneurological symptom:* a history of at least one symptom or deficit suggesting a neurological condition not limited to pain (conversion symptoms such as impaired coordination or balance, paralysis or localized weakness, difficulty swallowing or lump in throat, aphonia, urinary retention, hallucinations, loss of touch or pain sensation, double vision, blindness, deafness, seizures; dissociative symptoms such as amnesia; or loss of consciousness other than fainting)

C. Either (1) or (2):

   (1) after appropriate investigation, each of the symptoms in criterion B cannot be fully explained by a known general medical condition or the direct effects of a substance (e.g., a drug of abuse, a medication)

   (2) when there is a related general medical condition, the physical complaints or resulting social or occupational impairment are in excess of what would be expected from the history, physical examination, or laboratory findings

D. The symptoms are not intentionally produced or feigned (as in factitious disorder or malingering).

Table 8–2. General medical conditions that may be confused with somatization disorder

---

Multiple sclerosis
Systemic lupus erythematosus
Acute intermittent porphyria
Hemochromatosis

---

problems in addition to somatic symptoms. Wetzel et al. (1994) summarized these as "psychoform symptoms." In this study, Minnesota Multiphasic Personality Inventory (Hathaway and McKinley 1943) profiles of somatization disorder patients mimicked multiple psychiatric disorders (Wetzel et al. 1994).

Commonly, individuals with somatization disorder are inconsistent historians, and obtaining the medical records often will be necessary to definitively establish the diagnosis.

Natural History

E. Robins and O'Neal (1953) found somatization disorder to be unusual in children younger than 9 years. In most cases, characteristic symptoms begin during adolescence, and the criteria are satisfied by the mid-20s (Guze and Perley 1963; Purtell et al. 1951).

Somatization disorder is a chronic illness with fluctuations in the frequency and diversity of symptoms, but it rarely, if ever, totally remits (Guze and Perley 1963; Guze et al. 1986). The most active symptomatic phase is usually early adulthood, but aging does not lead to total remission (Goodwin and Guze 1996). Pribor et al. (1994) found that patients with somatization disorder age 55 years and older did not differ from younger patients in terms of the number of somatization symptoms or the use of health care services. Longitudinal prospective studies have confirmed that 80%–90% of the patients diagnosed with somatization disorder maintain a consistent clinical syndrome and retain the same diagnosis over many years (Cloninger et al. 1986; Guze et al. 1986; Perley and Guze 1962).

According to Goodwin and Guze (1996), the most frequent and important complications of somatization disorder are repeated surgical operations, drug dependence, suicide attempts, and marital separation or divorce. These authors suggested that the first two complications are preventable if the disorder is recognized and the patient's symptoms are managed appropriately. Generally, because of awareness that somatization disorder is an alternative explanation for various pains and other symptoms, invasive techniques can be withheld or postponed when objective indications are absent or equivocal. There is no evidence of excess mortality in patients with somatization disorder.

Avoiding the prescribing of habit-forming or addictive substances for persistent or recurrent complaints of pain should be paramount in the mind of the treating physician. Suicide attempts are common, but completed suicide is not (Martin et al. 1985; Murphy and Wetzel 1982). It is unclear whether marital or occupational dysfunction can be minimized through psychotherapy.

Epidemiology

The lifetime risk, prevalence, and incidence of somatization disorder are unclear. The lifetime risk for somatization disorder was estimated at about 2% in women when age at onset and method of assessment were taken into account (Cloninger et al. 1975). This risk is similar to the previously noted 2% prevalence rate identified by Woodruff et al. (1971). Cloninger et al. (1984), using complete lifetime medical records, found a 3% frequency of somatization disorder in 859 Swedish women in the general population.

Somatization disorder is diagnosed predominantly in women and rarely in men. Some have suggested that this sex difference may be artifactual, because somatization disorder criteria are biased against making the diagnosis in men because of the inapplicability of pregnancy and menstrual complaints. Also, men tend to report fewer symptoms than do women. Some investigators have suggested an adjustment for this discrepancy (Temoshok and Attkisson 1977). DSM-III reduced the number of symptoms required to diagnose somatization disorder from 14 (in women) to 12 in men, compensating for the inapplicable gynecological symptoms but not for the response bias in the number of somatic complaints. Diagnosis of somatization disorder remains much less frequent in men than in women unless the number of somatic complaints required for diagnosis in men is reduced to half (i.e., 7) of the 14 required in women (Cloninger 1994).

Etiology

The etiology of somatization disorder is unknown, but it is clearly a familial disorder. In several studies, approximately 20% of the female first-degree relatives of patients with somatization disorder also met criteria for the disorder (Cloninger and Guze 1970; Guze et al. 1986; Woerner and Guze 1968). Guze et al. (1986) demonstrated the familial nature of somatization disorder in a "blind" family study and documented an association between somatization disorder and antisocial personality disorder in male and female relatives. In addition, several studies have suggested that male relatives of female patients with somatization disorder have an increased risk of antisocial personality disorder and alcoholism (Cloninger et al. 1975; Woerner and Guze 1968). Cloninger et al. (1986) found that men with multiple somatic complaints were clinically heterogeneous and did not aggregate in families with either male or female somatizing subjects. Overall, these findings suggest that somatization disorder in women shares a common etiology with antisocial personality disorder, whereas somatization disorder in men may be related more to anxiety disorders (Cloninger et al. 1984, 1986).

A relation between somatization disorder and certain personality disorders has been posited. Hudziak et al. (1996) and Cloninger et al. (1997) identified similarities and even overlap between somatization disorder and borderline personality disorder, as did Stern et al. (1993) with personality disorders broadly. These studies support interpretations that somatization disorder is more of a personality (Axis II) disorder than an Axis I disorder, considering its early onset, nonremitting nature, and pervasiveness, which in some cases results in chronic dysfunctional states.

Experimental neuropsychological testing has indicated that individuals with somatization disorder have difficulty with information processing related to problems with attention and memory (Almgren et al. 1978; Bendefeldt et al. 1976; Ludwig 1972).

Other theories attempt to explain the characteristics of patients with somatization disorder. In particular, Shapiro (1965) and Horowitz (1977) suggested that "hysterical" information processing may be responsible for many of the clinical features. The information-processing deficit may be the basis for the somatic complaints, mental status findings of vagueness and circumstantiality, and many social, interpersonal, and occupational problems prominent in these patients and their biological relatives (Cloninger 1978; Flor-Henry et al. 1981; Horowitz 1977). Ford (1983) and Quill (1985) postulated a social communication model based on the theory that individuals with somatization disorder learn to somatize as a means of expressing emotion (i.e., distress) in their family constellation, evoking support and care from significant individuals. Further work needs to be done to evaluate these theories.

Treatment

Somatization disorder is difficult to treat, and there appears to be no single superior treatment approach (Murphy 1982). Primary care physicians generally can manage patients with somatization disorder adequately, but the expertise of at least a consulting psychiatrist has been shown to be useful. In a prospective, randomized, controlled study, Smith et al. (1986) found a reduction in health care costs for patients with somatization disorder who received a psychiatric consultation as opposed to those who did not receive a consultation. Reduced expenditures were largely the result of decreased rates of hospitalization. These gains were accomplished with no decrement in medical status or in patient satisfaction, suggesting that many of the evaluations and treatments otherwise provided to patients with somatization disorder are unnecessary. Smith et al. (1986) suggested that treatment include regularly scheduled visits with an appropriate physician. The frequency of visits should be determined on the basis of support for the patient, not in response to the frequency or severity of complaints.

Scallet et al. (1976) reviewed the earlier psychiatric literature on treatment of hysteria and reported the success rates of various approaches. Although most of the studies were uncontrolled and otherwise methodologically flawed, one study by Luff and Garrod (1935) noted a 51% improvement rate at 3-year follow-up in patients treated with an "eclectic approach." As summarized by Scallet et al. (1976), this treatment involved "reeducation, reassurance and suggestion." These techniques were also described by Carter (1949) as being effective in the treatment of acute conversion.

An eclectic approach accords well with the general principles of treatment recommended by Quill (1985), Cloninger (1994), and Smith et al. (1986). Three important suggestions emerge from review of these reports: 1) establish a firm therapeutic alliance with the patient, 2) educate the patient about the manifestations of somatization disorder, and 3) provide consistent reassurance. Implementation of these principles may greatly facilitate clinical management of somatization disorder and prevent potentially serious complications, including the effects of unnecessary diagnostic and therapeutic procedures. The superiority of more specific treatment approaches has not yet been documented in controlled trials (Kellner 1989).

During the late 1990s and early 2000s, cognitive-behavioral approaches embodying some of the principles just described were applied to "somatization" patients and yielded tentatively positive results in small studies (Kroenke and Swindle 2000; Lidbeck 1997). In 2001 the National Institute of Mental Health funded a single-blind, active-control, parallel-assignment interventional study of cognitive-behavioral therapy (CBT) for somatization disorder in the primary care setting. In this study, Allen et al. (2006) found that CBT with psychiatric consultation was more effective in producing symptom improvement and functioning than psychiatric consultation alone.

The clinician should develop a relationship with the patient's family. This facilitates attaining a better appreciation of the patient's social structure, which may be crucial to understanding and managing the patient's often chaotic personal lifestyle. When appropriate, the clinician must place firm limits on excessive demands, manipulations, and attention seeking (Murphy 1982; Murphy and Guze 1960).

Undifferentiated Somatoform Disorder

Definition and Clinical Description

The essential aspect of undifferentiated somatoform disorder is the presence of one or more clinically significant, medically unexplained somatic symptoms with a duration of 6 months or more that are not better accounted for by another mental disorder (Table 8–3). In effect, this category serves to capture syndromes that resemble somatization disorder but do not meet the full criteria. Symptoms that may be seen include those also considered for somatization disorder.

Diagnosis

DSM-IV-TR Criteria

After some debate, minor changes in the category *undifferentiated somatoform disorder* were made in DSM-IV. Because of perceived low use of the undifferentiated somatoform disorder diagnosis by clinicians, which was attributed to ambiguity of the term *undifferentiated disorder*, the term *multisomatoform disorder* was suggested. However, because the scarce empirical data available seemed to indicate a variable course, with unclear boundaries with normality and other mental disorders (especially anxiety and depressive disorders), this term was not adopted. As a result, the only changes involved substituting the standard "general medical condition" for DSM-III-R's "organic pathology." A threshold for diagnosis also was added, requiring clinically significant distress or impairment. Instead of excluding the diagnosis on the basis of "occurrence exclusively during the course of another mental disorder," exclusion in DSM-IV was on the basis of "not better accounted for by another mental disorder."

Kroenke et al. (1997) used improved diagnostic criteria with inclusion and exclusion criteria and found that the proposed multisomatoform disorder had a large and independent effect on impairment in a study of 1,000 patients from four primary care sites. In terms of validity of the proposed disorder, evidence of temporal stability is still lacking.

Differential Diagnosis

Principal considerations in the differential diagnosis include the question of whether, with follow-up, criteria for somatization disorder will be met. Patients with somatization disor-

---

Table 8–3. DSM-IV-TR diagnostic criteria for undifferentiated somatoform disorder

---

A. One or more physical complaints (e.g., fatigue, loss of appetite, gastrointestinal or urinary complaints).

B. Either (1) or (2):

    (1) after appropriate investigation, the symptoms cannot be fully explained by a known general medical condition or the direct effects of a substance (e.g., a drug of abuse, a medication)

    (2) when there is a related general medical condition, the physical complaints or resulting social or occupational impairment is in excess of what would be expected from the history, physical examination, or laboratory findings

C. The symptoms cause clinically significant distress or impairment in social, occupational, or other important areas of functioning.

D. The duration of the disturbance is at least 6 months.

E. The disturbance is not better accounted for by another mental disorder (e.g., another somatoform disorder, sexual dysfunction, mood disorder, anxiety disorder, sleep disorder, or psychotic disorder).

F. The symptom is not intentionally produced or feigned (as in factitious disorder or malingering).

---

der are typically inconsistent historians. During one evaluation, they may report many symptoms and fulfill criteria for the full syndrome, whereas during another, they may report fewer symptoms, perhaps only fulfilling criteria for an abridged syndrome (Martin et al. 1979). Another consideration is whether the somatic symptoms qualifying a patient for the diagnosis of undifferentiated somatoform disorder are the manifestation of a depressive or an anxiety disorder. Indeed, high rates of major depression and anxiety disorders have been found in somatizing patients attending family medicine clinics (Kirmayer et al. 1993).

Epidemiology

Some investigators have argued that undifferentiated somatoform disorder is the most common somatoform disorder. Escobar et al. (1991) used a construct requiring six somatic symptoms for women and four for men and reported that in the United States 11% of non-Hispanic whites and Hispanics, as well as 15% of blacks, fulfilled the criteria. In Puerto Rico, 20% met the criteria. A preponderance of women was evident in all groups except the Puerto Rican sample.

Etiology

If undifferentiated somatoform disorder is simply an abridged form of somatization disorder, etiological theories reviewed under that diagnosis should also apply to undifferentiated somatoform disorder. Of theoretical interest would be the question of why the syndrome is fully expressed in some and only partially in others. Some investigators postulate theories of etiology involving primarily the concept of somatization, for which there are numerous explanations. As reviewed by Kirmayer and Robbins (1991), somatization can be viewed as a pattern of illness behavior by which bodily idioms of distress may serve as symbolic means of social regulation as well as protest or contestation. As yet, there is little, if any, empirical evidence for such theories.

Treatment

Existing data have been derived from studies fraught with methodological problems, including the use of diverse groups with only a certain number of chronic somatic complaints in common. Several studies suggested that improvement is accelerated with psychotherapy of a supportive, rather than a nondirective, type. However, a substantial proportion of patients improve or recover with no formal psychotherapy. Judicious use of pharmacotherapy appears to be beneficial, with trials of antidepressant medications indicated for patients with depressive symptoms and trials of buspirone, benzodiazepines, and propranolol for patients with anxiety symptoms. Again, definitive recommendations await a more extensive empirical database.

Conversion Disorder
Definition and Clinical Description

The essential features of conversion disorder are the nonintentionally produced symptoms or deficits affecting voluntary motor or sensory function that suggest but are not fully explained by a neurological or general medical condition, by the direct effects of a substance, or by a culturally sanctioned behavior or experience. Specific symptoms mentioned as examples in DSM-IV-TR include motor symptoms such as impaired coordination or balance, paralysis or localized weakness, difficulty swallowing or lump in throat (e.g., "globus hystericus"), aphonia, and urinary retention; sensory symptoms, including hallucinations, loss of touch or pain sensation, double vision, blindness, and deafness; and seizures or convulsions with voluntary motor or sensory components. Single episodes usually involve one symptom, but longitudinally, other conversion symptoms will be evident as well. Psychological factors generally appear to be involved, because symptoms often occur in the context of a conflictual situation that may in some way be resolved with the development of the symptom.

Diagnosis
DSM-IV-TR Criteria

As defined in DSM-IV-TR, nonintentional "symptoms or deficits affecting voluntary motor or sensory function" (American Psychiat-

ric Association 2000, p. 498) are central to conversion disorder (Table 8–4). The majority of such symptoms will suggest a neurological condition (i.e., are pseudoneurological), but other general medical conditions may be suggested as well. Pseudoneurological symptoms remain the classic symptomatology. By definition, symptoms limited to pain or disturbance in sexual functioning are not included.

In conversion disorder, as in the other somatoform disorders, the symptom cannot be fully explained by a known physical disorder. This criterion is perhaps the most imperative diagnostic consideration. In addition, the symptom is defined as not fully explained by a culturally sanctioned behavior or experience. Symptoms such as seizurelike episodes occurring in conjunction with certain religious ceremonies and culturally expected responses, such as women swooning in response to excitement, would qualify as examples.

DSM-IV-TR specifies that the symptoms in conversion disorder are not intentionally produced, thus distinguishing conversion symptoms from those of a factitious disorder or malingering. Although this judgment is difficult to make, it is an important one because the recommended management and expected outcome of factitious disorder and malingering are markedly different.

Clinical judgment also is required in determining whether psychological factors are etiologically related to the symptom. Inclusion of this criterion is perhaps a holdover from the initial conceptualization of conversion symptoms as representing the conversion of unconscious psychic conflict into a physical symptom. As reviewed by Cloninger (1987), such determination is virtually impossible except in cases in which there is a temporal relationship between a psychosocial stressor and the symptom or in cases in which similar situations led to conversion symptoms in the past.

Differential Diagnosis

Conversion symptoms suggest physical illness, and nonpsychiatrists are generally seen

---

Table 8–4. DSM-IV-TR diagnostic criteria for conversion disorder

---

A. One or more symptoms or deficits affecting voluntary motor or sensory function that suggest a neurological or other general medical condition.

B. Psychological factors are judged to be associated with the symptom or deficit because the initiation or exacerbation of the symptom or deficit is preceded by conflicts or other stressors.

C. The symptom or deficit is not intentionally produced or feigned (as in factitious disorder or malingering).

D. The symptom or deficit cannot, after appropriate investigation, be fully explained by a general medical condition, or by the direct effects of a substance, or as a culturally sanctioned behavior or experience.

E. The symptom or deficit causes clinically significant distress or impairment in social, occupational, or other important areas of functioning or warrants medical evaluation.

F. The symptom or deficit is not limited to pain or sexual dysfunction, does not occur exclusively during the course of somatization disorder, and is not better accounted for by another mental disorder.

Specify type of symptom or deficit:

With motor symptom or deficit
With sensory symptom or deficit
With seizures or convulsions
With mixed presentation

---

initially. Neurologists are frequently consulted by primary care physicians for such symptoms because most suggest neurological disease. It has been estimated that 1% of the patients admitted to the hospital for neurological problems have conversion symptoms (Marsden 1986), and up to one-third of new neurology clinic patients have medically unexplained symptoms (Carson et al. 2003; Stone et al. 2003). One major problem with conversion symptoms is that they suggest neurological or general medical conditions, and a conversion (mis-) diagnosis may be applied when a true illness is present. Some older studies found that significant proportions of patients initially diagnosed with conversion symptoms had neurological illnesses on follow-up. Slater and Glithero (1965) found a misdiagnosis rate of 50% during a 7- to 11-year follow-up; Gatfield and Guze (1962) reported a rate of 21%. In 1996 Mace and Trimble observed a rate of 15%. However, other recent studies have suggested a misdiagnosis rate of around 4%, which has been stable since 1970 (Stone et al. 2005). Also

noteworthy is the fact that misdiagnosis may happen in reverse, with patients with multiple sclerosis ultimately being diagnosed with conversion disorder (Hankey and Stewart-Wynne 1987). The trend toward less misdiagnosis may reflect increasing sophistication in neurological diagnosis. Nevertheless, one needs to be tentative in making a diagnosis of conversion disorder.

Symptoms of various neurological illnesses may seem to be inconsistent with known neurophysiology or neuropathology and may suggest conversion. Diseases to be considered include multiple sclerosis (consider blindness secondary to optic neuritis with initially normal fundi), myasthenia gravis, periodic paralysis, myoglobinuric myopathy, polymyositis, other acquired myopathies (all of which may include marked weakness in the presence of normal deep tendon reflexes), and Guillain-Barré syndrome, in which early weakness of the arms and legs may be inconsistent (Cloninger 1994). As reviewed by Ford and Folks (1985), more than 13% of actual neurological cases are diagnosed as "functional" before the elucidation of a neurological illness. Initial evidence of some neurological disease is predictive of a subsequent neurological explanation (Mace and Trimble 1996).

Complicating diagnosis is the fact that physical illness and conversion (or other apparent psychiatric overlay) are not mutually exclusive. Patients with incapacitating and frightening physical illnesses may appear to exaggerate their symptoms. Patients with actual neurological illness also may have "pseudosymptoms." For example, patients with actual seizures often have pseudoseizures (Desai et al. 1982).

Longitudinal studies indicate the most reliable predictor that a patient with apparent conversion symptoms will not later be shown to have a physical disorder is a history of conversion or other unexplained symptoms (Cloninger 1994). Conversion symptoms first occurring in middle age or later should increase suspicion of an occult physical illness.

Natural History

Onset of conversion disorder is generally from late childhood to early adulthood. Conversion disorder is rare before age 10 years (Maloney 1980) and seldom first presents after age 35 years, but it has been reported to begin as late as the ninth decade (Weddington 1979). When onset is in middle or late age, the possibility of a neurological or other medical condition is increased.

Onset of conversion disorder is generally acute, but it may be characterized by gradually increasing symptomatology. The typical course of individual conversion symptoms is generally short; half (Folks et al. 1984) to nearly all (Carter 1949) patients show a disappearance of symptoms by the time of hospital discharge. However, 20%–25% will relapse within 1 year. Factors traditionally associated with good prognosis include acute onset, presence of clearly identifiable stress at the time of onset, short interval between onset and institution of treatment, and good intelligence (Toone 1990). One study noted a better

outcome for patients with affective illnesses and a poor prognosis for those with personality disorders (Mace and Trimble 1996). The study also reported that a diagnosis of somatization disorder at follow-up was especially associated with chronicity. Symptoms of blindness, aphonia, and paralysis have been noted to have a relatively good prognosis, whereas seizures and tremor were identified to be more persistent (Toone 1990). However, these findings were not supported in the Mace and Trimble (1996) study. When followed up longitudinally, some patients initially diagnosed only with conversion disorder will subsequently meet the criteria for somatization disorder (Kent et al. 1995; Mace and Trimble 1996).

Generally, individual conversion symptoms are self-limited and do not lead to physical changes or disabilities. Occasionally, physical sequelae such as atrophy may occur, but this is rare. Morbidity in terms of marital and occupational impairment appears to be less than that in somatization disorder (Kent et al. 1995; Tomasson et al. 1991). In a long-term follow-up study (up to 44 years) of a small number ($N=28$) of individuals with conversion disorder, excess mortality by unnatural causes was observed (Coryell and House 1984). None of the deaths in this study was by suicide.

Epidemiology

Conclusions regarding the epidemiology of conversion disorder are compromised by methodological differences in diagnostic boundaries as well as by ascertainment procedures from study to study. Vastly different estimates have been reported. Lifetime prevalence rates of treated conversion symptoms in general populations have ranged from 11 in 100,000 to 500 in 100,000 (Ford and Folks 1985; Toone 1990). A marked excess of women compared with men develop conversion symptoms. More than 25% of healthy postpartum and medically ill women report having had conversion symptoms sometime during their lives (Cloninger 1994).

Approximately 5%–24% of psychiatric outpatients, 5%–14% of general hospital patients, and 1%–3% of outpatient psychiatric referrals have a history of conversion symptoms (Cloninger 1994; Ford 1983; Toone 1990). Conversion is associated with lower socioeconomic status, lower education, lack of psychological sophistication, and rural setting (Folks et al. 1984; Guze and Perley 1963; Lazare 1981; Stefansson et al. 1976; Weinstein et al. 1969). Consistent with this finding, much higher rates (nearly 10%) of outpatient psychiatric referrals in developing countries are for conversion symptoms. As countries develop, there may be a declining incidence over time, which may relate to increasing levels of education and sophistication (Stefanis et al. 1976).

Conversion disorder appears to be diagnosed more often in women than in men, with ratios varying from 2:1 (Ljundberg 1957; Stefansson et al. 1976) to 10:1 (Raskin et al. 1966). In part, this variance may relate to referral patterns, but it also appears that indeed a predominance of women compared with men develop conversion symptoms.

Etiology

An etiological hypothesis is implicit in the term *conversion*. The term, in fact, is derived from the hypothesized conversion of psychological conflict into a somatic symptom. Several psychological factors have been implicated in the pathogenesis, or at least pathophysiology, of conversion disorder. However, as the following discussion will show, such etiological relationships are difficult to establish. (Refer to Table 8–5 for definitions.)

In primary gain, anxiety is theoretically reduced by keeping an internal conflict or need out of awareness by symbolic expression of an unconscious wish as a conversion symptom. However, individuals with active conversion symptoms often continue to show marked anxiety, especially on psychological tests (Lader and Sartorius 1968; Meares and Horvath 1972). Symbolism is infrequently evident, and its evaluation in-

Table 8–5. Key terms related to conversion disorder

Conversion: Hypothesized conversion of a psychological conflict into a somatic complaint.

Primary gain: Anxiety is theoretically reduced by keeping an internal conflict or need out of conscious awareness through production of a symptom; the symptom is involuntarily produced and not under conscious control.

Secondary gain: The symptom is voluntarily produced and under conscious control; production is for the purpose of a goal, such as avoiding work, obtaining money (i.e., malingering).

La belle indifférence: The individual seems indifferent or disinterested in personal medical issues that should concern anyone.

volves highly inferential and unreliable judgments (Raskin et al. 1966). Interpretation of symbolism in persons with occult medical disorder has been noted to contribute to misdiagnosis. Secondary gain, whereby conversion symptoms allow avoidance of noxious activities or the obtaining of otherwise unavailable support, also may occur in persons who have medical conditions, who often take advantage of such benefits (Raskin et al. 1966; Watson and Buranen 1979).

Individuals with conversion disorder may show a lack of concern, in keeping with the nature or implications of the symptom (the so-called *la belle indifférence*). However, such indifference to symptoms is not invariably present in conversion disorder (Lewis and Berman 1965; Sharma and Chaturvedi 1995), and it also can be seen in individuals with general medical conditions (Raskin et al. 1966), sometimes as denial or stoicism (Pincus 1982). Conversion symptoms may be revealed in a dramatic or histrionic fashion. A minority of individuals with conversion disorder fulfill criteria for histrionic personality disorder.

Limited data suggest that conversion symptoms are more frequent in relatives of individuals with conversion disorder (Toone 1990). Rates that were 10 times greater than similarly derived general population estimates in female relatives and approximately 5 times the corresponding rate in male relatives were reported in a nonblind study (Ljundberg 1957).

If not directly etiological, many factors have been suggested as predisposing individuals to conversion disorder. In many instances, preexisting personality disorders are diagnosable and may predispose some individuals to conversion disorder. Several psychosocial factors in addition to a history of abuse may be involved. Preliminary functional imaging studies postulate an association among conversion disorder, depression, and posttraumatic stress disorder (Ballmaier and Schmidt 2005). Individuals from rural backgrounds and those who are psychologically and medically unsophisticated appear to be predisposed to conversion disorder, as are those with existing neurological disorders. In the last case, a tendency to conversion symptoms has been attributed to "modeling"—that is, patients with neurological disorders are likely to observe in others, as well as in themselves, various neurological symptoms that they at other times simulate as conversion symptoms.

Treatment

Generally, the initial aim in treating conversion disorder is the removal of the symptom. The pressure behind accomplishing this goal depends on the distress and disability associated with the symptom (Merskey 1989). If the patient is not in particular discomfort and the need to regain function is not great, direct attention may not be necessary. In any situation, direct confrontation is not recommended. Such a communication may cause a patient to feel even more isolated. A conservative approach of reassurance and relaxation is effective. Reassurance need not come from a psychiatrist but can be performed effectively by the primary physician. After physical illness is excluded, prognosis for

conversion symptoms is good. Folks et al. (1984), for example, found that half of 50 general hospital patients with conversion symptoms showed complete remission by the time of discharge.

If symptoms do not resolve with a conservative approach and there is an immediate need for symptom resolution, several techniques, including narcoanalysis (e.g., amobarbital interview), hypnosis, and behavior therapy, may be tried (Merskey 1989). It does appear that prompt resolution of conversion symptoms is important in that the duration of conversion symptoms is associated with greater risk of recurrence and chronic disability (Cloninger 1994).

Anecdotal reports exist of positive response to somatic treatments such as phenothiazines, lithium, and even electroconvulsive therapy (ECT). Of course, in some cases, such a response again may be attributable to suggestion. In others, it may be that symptom removal occurred because of resolution of another psychiatric disorder, especially a mood disorder. Interestingly, even without a diagnosable mood disorder, antidepressants may be helpful (Bourgeois et al. 2002; Hurwitz 2004).

Thus far, the discussion on treatment of conversion disorder has centered on acute treatment primarily for symptom removal. Longer-term approaches would include strategies that were previously discussed for somatization disorder. These involve a pragmatic, conservative approach that entails support for and exploration of various areas of conflict, particularly interpersonal relationships. Ford (1995) suggested a treatment strategy based on "three Ps," whereby predisposing factors, precipitating stressors, and perpetuating factors are identified and addressed. A certain degree of insight may be attained, at least in terms of appreciating relationships between various conflicts and stressors and the development of symptoms. More ambitious goals have been adopted by some in terms of long-term, intensive, insight-oriented psychotherapy, especially of a psychodynamic nature. Reports of such approaches date from Freud's work with Anna O. Three studies involving a series of patients treated with psychoanalytic psychotherapy have reported success (Merskey 1989).

Hypochondriasis

Definition and Clinical Description

The essential feature in hypochondriasis is preoccupation not with symptoms themselves but rather with the fear or idea of having a serious disease, based on the misinterpretation of bodily signs and sensations. The preoccupation persists despite evidence to the contrary and reassurance from physicians. Some degree of preoccupation with disease is apparently quite common. As reviewed by Kellner (1987), 10%–20% of "normal" and 45% of "neurotic" persons have intermittent, unfounded worries about illness, with 9% of patients doubting reassurances given by physicians. In another review, Kellner (1985) estimated that 50% of all patients attending physicians' offices "suffer either from primary hypochondriacal syndromes or have 'minor somatic disorders with hypochondriacal overlay'" (p. 822). How these estimates relate to hypochondriasis as a disorder is difficult to assess because they do not appear to distinguish between preoccupation with symptoms (as is present in somatization disorder) and preoccupation with the implications of the symptoms (as is the case in hypochondriasis).

Diagnosis

DSM-IV-TR Criteria

Specific criteria for the diagnosis of hypochondriasis are presented in Table 8–6.

Hypochondriasis is not diagnosed if symptoms occur exclusively during the course of generalized anxiety disorder, obsessive-compulsive disorder (OCD), panic disorder, a major depressive episode, separation anxiety, or another somatoform disorder.

Table 8–6. DSM-IV-TR diagnostic criteria for hypochondriasis

A. Preoccupation with fears of having, or the idea that one has, a serious disease based on the person's misinterpretation of bodily symptoms.

B. The preoccupation persists despite appropriate medical evaluation and reassurance.

C. The belief in criterion A is not of delusional intensity (as in delusional disorder, somatic type) and is not restricted to a circumscribed concern about appearance (as in body dysmorphic disorder).

D. The preoccupation causes clinically significant distress or impairment in social, occupational, or other important areas of functioning.

E. The duration of the disturbance is at least 6 months.

F. The preoccupation is not better accounted for by generalized anxiety disorder, obsessive-compulsive disorder, panic disorder, a major depressive episode, separation anxiety, or another somatoform disorder.

Specify if:

With poor insight: if, for most of the time during the current episode, the person does not recognize that the concern about having a serious illness is excessive or unreasonable

---

Differential Diagnosis

The first step in evaluating patients with hypochondriasis is to assess the possibility of physical disease. The list of serious diseases associated with the type of complaints seen in hypochondriacal patients is extensive, yet certain general categories emerge (Kellner 1985, 1987). These include neurological diseases, such as myasthenia gravis and multiple sclerosis; endocrine diseases; systemic diseases, such as SLE, that affect several organ systems; and occult malignancies.

If, after appropriate assessment, the probability of physical illness appears low, the condition should be considered relative to other psychiatric disorders (i.e., whether the hypochondriacal symptoms represent a primary disorder or are secondary to another psychiatric illness). One useful criterion is whether the belief is of delusional proportions. Patients with hypochondriasis as a primary disorder, although extremely preoccupied, are generally able to acknowledge the possibility that their concerns are unfounded. Delusional patients, on the other hand, are not. Hypochondriasis with poor insight would lie somewhere in between, with the patient not recognizing that the concern is unwarranted for most of the episode. Somatic delusions of serious illness are seen in some cases of major depressive disorder and in schizophrenia. A useful discriminator is the presence of other psychiatric symptoms. A patient with hypochondriacal concerns secondary to depression should show other symptoms of depression such as sleep and appetite disturbance, feelings of worthlessness, and self-reproach, although elderly patients particularly may deny sadness or other expressions of depressed mood. Generally, schizophrenic patients will have bizarre delusions of illness (e.g., "I have congenital Hodgkin's caused by a snail hormone imbalance") and will show other signs of schizophrenia such as looseness of associations, peculiarities of thought and behavior, hallucinations, and other delusions. A confounding feature is the fact that hypochondriacal patients often will develop anxiety or depression in association with their hypochondriacal concerns. In general, characterizing the chronology of the episode will separate such patients from those with hypochondriasis.

Treatment trials also may have diagnostic significance. Depressed patients who are hypochondriacal may respond to antidepressant medication or ECT (often necessary in reversing a depressive state of sufficient severity to lead to such profound symptoms), with resolution of the hypochondriacal as well as the depressive symptoms. In schizophrenic patients, a disease-related delusion may show improvement with neuroleptic treatment. Although if questioned carefully the patient still may report a somatic delusion, preoccupation with the delusion will have diminished.

Natural History

Traditionally, limited data suggested that approximately one-fourth of the patients with a diagnosis of hypochondriasis do poorly, two-thirds show a chronic but fluctuating course, and one-tenth recover. However, such predictions may not reflect advances in psychopharmacology. It also must be remembered that such findings pertain to the full syndrome. A much more variable course is seen in patients with some hypochondriacal concerns.

Epidemiology

Estimates of the frequency of hypochondriacal symptoms warranting a diagnosis are somewhat compromised because DSM-III-R did not provide threshold criteria, other than requiring a duration of more than 6 months. The ECA study (L. N. Robins et al. 1984) did not assess for hypochondriasis. One study reported prevalences ranging from 3% to 13% in different cultures (Kenyon 1965), but it is not clear whether this range represented the full syndrome or just hypochondriacal symptoms. More recent studies suggest a prevalence in general medical practice of 3%–9% (Barsky et al. 1990; Escobar et al. 1998; Kellner et al. 1983/1984). As previously mentioned, many patients have such symptoms as part of other psychiatric disorders, particularly depressive and anxiety disorders, whereas others develop transient hypochondriacal symptoms in response to stress, particularly serious physical illness.

Etiology

In considering hypochondriasis as an aspect of depression or anxiety disorders, it has been posited that these conditions create a state of hypervigilance to insult, including overperception of physical problems (Barsky and Klerman 1983). Hypochondriasis has been discussed extensively in the psychoanalytic literature.

More recently, hypochondriasis has been classified by some within the posited obsessive-compulsive spectrum disorders, which include, in addition to OCD, body dysmorphic disorder, anorexia nervosa, Tourette's disorder, and certain impulsive disorders (e.g., trichotillomania and pathological gambling; Hollander 1993). This clustering is based, in part, on the phenomenological similarity of repetitive thoughts and behaviors that are difficult or impossible to delay or inhibit (Martin and Yutzy 1997).

Treatment

Patients referred early for psychiatric evaluation and treatment of hypochondriasis appear to have a better prognosis than those continuing with only medical evaluations and treatments (Kellner 1983). Psychiatric referral should be performed with sensitivity. Perhaps the best guideline to follow is for the referring physician to stress that the patient's distress is serious and that psychiatric evaluation will be a supplement to, not a replacement for, continued medical care.

Hypochondriacal symptoms secondary to depressive and anxiety disorders may improve with successful treatment of the primary disorder. However, until recently, hypochondriasis as a primary condition was not considered to be responsive to known psychopharmacological medications. Early results of placebo-controlled, double-blind studies are pending, but anecdotal case reports, open-label trials, and review of preliminary data show some promise for the selective serotonin reuptake inhibitors (SSRIs; Fallon et al. 1996). Interestingly, these medications have been shown to be effective in OCD, and preliminary data are promising for their use in other obsessive-compulsive spectrum disorders, including body dysmorphic disorder and anorexia nervosa.

Investigators have tried many psychotherapeutic approaches in treating hypo-

chondriasis. These may be summarized as supportive, rational, ventilative, and educative (Kellner 1987).

Stoudemire (1988) suggested an approach that includes consistent treatment, generally by the same primary physician, with supportive, regularly scheduled office visits not based on the evaluation of symptoms. Hospitalization, medical tests, and medications with addictive potential are to be avoided if possible. Focus during the office visits gradually should be shifted from symptoms to social or interpersonal problems. Psychotherapeutic approaches may be enhanced greatly by the promising potential of effective pharmacotherapy. Of note, CBT has recently been found to be effective in one study in which 57% of CBT-treated patients at 12-month follow-up had a lessening of hypochondriacal beliefs (Barsky and Ahern 2004). There is increasing hope for attaining the overriding goal in treating hypochondriacal patients: preventing adoption of the sick role and chronic invalidism (Kellner 1987).

Body Dysmorphic Disorder
Definition and Clinical Description

The essential feature of body dysmorphic disorder is a preoccupation with some imagined defect in appearance or markedly excessive concern with a minor physical anomaly (Table 8–7). Such preoccupation persists even after reassurance. Common complaints include a diversity of imagined flaws of the face or head, such as various defects in the hair (too much or too little), skin, shape of the face, or facial features. However, any body part may be the focus, including genitals, breasts, buttocks, extremities, shoulders, and even overall body size. De Leon et al. (1989) stated that the nose, ears, face, and sexual organs are most often involved. It is not surprising, then, that patients with body dys-

---

Table 8–7. DSM-IV-TR diagnostic criteria for body dysmorphic disorder

A. Preoccupation with an imagined defect in appearance. If a slight physical anomaly is present, the person's concern is markedly excessive.

B. The preoccupation causes clinically significant distress or impairment in social, occupational, or other important areas of functioning.

C. The preoccupation is not better accounted for by another mental disorder (e.g., dissatisfaction with body shape and size in anorexia nervosa).

---

morphic disorder are found most commonly among persons seeking cosmetic surgery.

Diagnosis

DSM-IV-TR Criteria

In DSM-IV-TR, the essential feature of body dysmorphic disorder is preoccupation with an imagined defect in appearance or markedly excessive concern for a slight anomaly (see Table 8–7). This criterion represents a slight change from that in DSM-III-R, in which the phrase "in a normal-appearing person" was included. Because a person with some defect may have a preoccupation with a different imagined or exaggerated defect, this phrase was dropped.

As in other somatoform disorders, diagnosis requires that the preoccupation causes clinically significant distress or impairment, thus excluding those individuals with trivial symptoms. As is explained in the following discussion, body dysmorphic disorder is not diagnosed if the preoccupation is better accounted for by another mental disorder. On the other hand, DSM-IV dropped the exclusion on the basis of the preoccupation being delusional.

Differential Diagnosis

By definition, body dysmorphic disorder is not diagnosed when the body preoccupation is better accounted for by another mental disorder. Anorexia nervosa, in which there is dissatisfaction with body shape and size, is specifically mentioned in the criteria as an example of such an exclusion. In DSM-III-R, transsexualism (gender identity disorder in DSM-IV-TR) also was mentioned as such a disorder. Although not specifically mentioned in DSM-IV and DSM-IV-TR, if a preoccupation is limited to discomfort or a sense of inappropriateness of one's primary and secondary sex characteristics, coupled with a strong and persistent cross-gender identification, body dysmorphic disorder would not be diagnosed. Diagnostic problems may develop when a patient has the mood-congruent ruminations of major depression (e.g., preoccupation with a perceived unattractive appearance in association with poor self-esteem). However, such concerns generally lack the focus on a particular body part that is seen in body dysmorphic disorder. Somatic obsessions and even grooming or cleaning rituals in OCD may suggest body dysmorphic disorder; however, in such cases, other obsessions and compulsions are seen as well. In body dysmorphic disorder, the preoccupations are limited to concerns with appearance. Preoccupations in body dysmorphic disorder may reach delusional proportions, and patients with this disorder may show ideas of reference regarding defects in their appearance, which may lead to consideration of the diagnosis of schizophrenia. However, bizarre delusions and hallucinations are not seen in patients with body dysmorphic disorder. From the other perspective, schizophrenic patients with somatic delusions generally do not focus on a specific defect in appearance.

Unlike the diagnostic guideline for hypochondriasis, if the preoccupation is of psychotic proportions, a diagnosis of body dysmorphic disorder still can be made. De Leon et al. (1989) pointed out the difficulties in determining whether a dysmorphophobic concern is delusional. They suggest that cases be classified as "primary dysmorphophobia" without attempting to distinguish between delusional and nondelusional concerns, as long as schizophrenia, major depression, and organic mental disorders are excluded. This point of view was adopted in DSM-IV (Phillips and Hollander 1996). In body dysmorphic disorder, it appears that a continuum exists between preoccupations and delusions, and thus it is difficult, if not impossible, to draw a discrete boundary between body dysmorphic disorder and delusional disorder, somatic type. Furthermore, individual patients seem to move along this continuum. Thus, it was decided to allow both diagnoses if a dysmorphic preoccupation was delusional. This decision was controversial, and the debate continues.

Natural History

Onset of body dysmorphic disorder usually begins in adolescence or early adulthood (Phillips 1991). The disorder is generally a chronic condition, with a waxing and waning of intensity but rarely full remission (Phillips et al. 1993). Over a lifetime, multiple preoccupations are typical. (In their study, Phillips et al. [1993] found an average of four preoccupations.) In some people, the preoccupation remains unchanged; in others, preoccupations with newly perceived defects are added to the original ones. In some individuals, symptoms remit only to be replaced by others.

Recent studies of special populations have revealed varying findings regarding outcomes, with one study finding that at 4-year follow-up, 58% of patients were in full remission and 84% were in partial remission (Phillips et al. 2005). A second study found that only 9% experienced full remission, with 21% experiencing partial remission (Phillips et al. 2006). Body dysmorphic disorder is highly incapacitating. Almost all persons with this disorder show marked impairment in social and occupational activities. About 75% will never marry, and among those who do, most will divorce (Phillips 1995). Perhaps a third become housebound. Most attribute their limitations to embarrassment concern-

ing their "defect." The precise extent to which patients with body dysmorphic disorder receive surgery or medical treatments is unknown. Of interest, Phillips (2001) found that nearly one-half of adolescents studied had received medical or surgical treatment that was usually ineffective in relieving the symptoms of body dysmorphic disorder. Superimposed depressive episodes are common, as are suicidal ideation and suicide attempts. The estimated lifetime risk of depression is 76% (Gunstad and Phillips 2003). The lifetime suicide attempt rate has been estimated at 22%–24% (Phillips and Diaz 1997; Veale et al. 1996). The completed suicide rate is unknown.

Epidemiology

The lifetime risk of body dysmorphic disorder in the general population is unknown, but it is thought to be underdiagnosed even when patients are in psychiatric care. Often patients will not mention their concerns unless directly asked. Studies have reported prevalences varying from 0.7% to 5% in special populations (Bohne et al. 2002; Otto et al. 2001; Rief et al. 2006). Grant et al. (2001) found a prevalence rate of 13% in psychiatric inpatients. Although body dysmorphic disorder is seldom reported in psychiatric settings, Andreasen and Bardach (1977) estimated that 2% of the patients seeking corrective cosmetic surgery have this disorder. Generally, patients with body dysmorphic disorder are seen psychiatrically only after referral from plastic surgery, dermatology, and otorhinolaryngology clinics (De Leon et al. 1989). The male-to-female ratio is about 1:1 (Phillips 1995).

Etiology

Although the etiology of body dysmorphic disorder remains elusive, there has been significant nosological debate recently in several areas. First, the possibility that the label represents a spectrum of disorders as opposed to simply psychotic versus nonpsychotic variants has been raised. Although not a settled issue, the general consensus appears to support this position (Castle and Rossel 2006). The second issue is whether body dysmorphic disorder should be classified as an anxiety disorder, particularly a variant of OCD. This is problematic because patients with body dysmorphic disorder tend to be younger, more socially dysfunctional, and nonresponsive to antipsychotics.

Treatment

Simply recognizing that a complaint derives from body dysmorphic disorder may have therapeutic benefit by interrupting an unending procession of repeated evaluations by physicians and eliminating the possibility of needless surgery. Surgery actually has been recommended as a treatment for this disorder, but there is no clear evidence that it is helpful. There is a long history of anecdotal reports suggesting the value of diverse treatments, including behavior therapy, dynamic psychotherapy, and pharmacotherapy. Recommended medications include neuroleptics and antidepressants (De Leon et al. 1989). Response to neuroleptic treatment has been suggested as a diagnostic test to distinguish body dysmorphic disorder from delusional disorder, somatic type (Riding and Munro 1975). Delusional syndromes, in general, may respond to neuroleptics, whereas in body dysmorphic disorder, even when the bodily preoccupations are psychotic, there is less likelihood of success. Pimozide has been singled out as a neuroleptic having specific effectiveness for somatic delusions, but this drug does not appear to be any more effective than other neuroleptics in treating body dysmorphic disorder.

In earlier reports, it was not clear if reported response to antidepressant drugs or ECT was due to amelioration of dysmorphic symptoms per se or to improvement in depressive symptoms. Several studies have suggested that SSRIs, including fluoxetine, fluvoxamine, and clomipramine, have been effective in treating the disorder (Hollander et al. 1993; Phillips et al. 1993). Patients showing

a partial response to the SSRI may benefit further from augmentation with buspirone. Improvement with SSRIs seems to be a primary effect in that response was not predicted on the basis of coexisting major depression or OCD. Also of note are observations that patients with somatic delusions may respond to SSRIs.

Somatoform Disorder Not Otherwise Specified

Definition and Clinical Description

Somatoform disorder NOS is the true residual category for the somatoform disorders. By definition, conditions included under this category are characterized by somatoform symptoms that do not meet the criteria for any of the specified somatoform disorders. DSM-IV-TR gives several examples, but syndromes potentially included under this category are not limited to those examples. Unlike undifferentiated somatoform disorder, no minimum duration is required. In fact, some disorders may be relegated to the NOS category because they do not meet the time requirements for a specified somatoform disorder.

Diagnosis

DSM-IV-TR Criteria

The basic DSM-IV-TR requirement for a diagnosis of somatoform disorder NOS is that a disorder with somatoform symptoms does not meet criteria for a specified somatoform disorder (Table 8–8). The first example of such a disorder listed in DSM-IV-TR is pseudocyesis.

Differential Diagnosis

As mentioned in the preceding discussion, DSM-IV-TR lists several syndromes that, if not for their short duration, would qualify for a diagnosis as the specified somatoform disorder that they resemble.

Table 8–8.   DSM-IV-TR diagnostic criteria for somatoform disorder not otherwise specified

---

This category includes disorders with somatoform symptoms that do not meet the criteria for any specific somatoform disorder. Examples include

1. Pseudocyesis: a false belief of being pregnant that is associated with objective signs of pregnancy, which may include abdominal enlargement (although the umbilicus does not become everted), reduced menstrual flow, amenorrhea, subjective sensation of fetal movement, nausea, breast engorgement and secretions, and labor pains at the expected date of delivery. Endocrine changes may be present, but the syndrome cannot be explained by a general medical condition that causes endocrine changes (e.g., a hormone-secreting tumor).
2. A disorder involving nonpsychotic hypochondriacal symptoms of less than 6 months' duration.
3. A disorder involving unexplained physical complaints (e.g., fatigue or body weakness) of less than 6 months' duration that are not due to another mental disorder.

Epidemiology, Etiology, and Treatment

Discussion of epidemiology, etiology, and treatment for a residual category such as somatoform disorder NOS would not be meaningful, given that the category represents a grouping of diverse disorders. Conditions that would warrant diagnosis of a specified somatoform disorder except for their insufficient duration (less than 6 months) are probably best considered to be in the spectrum of the resembled disorder. Thus, the epidemiological, etiological, and treatment considerations pertaining to the specified disorder should be reviewed because these may apply, at least in part, to the shorter-duration syndromes.

Conclusion

Syndromes now subsumed under the rubric "somatoform disorders" have had a tortuous course in the evolution of psychiatric nosology and therapy. Yet they are extremely important because they are disorders that must be differentiated from conditions with identifiable, and often treatable, physical bases.

Ultimately it may prove possible to obtain a better understanding of the somatoform disorders, a group of complex, incapacitating disorders. Better understanding should facilitate more effective treatments. Already there has been some preliminary discussion regarding the development of practice guidelines for somatoform disorders. Consideration of guidelines would have been highly unlikely even a few years ago.

Key Points

- The somatoform disorders are grouped because they suggest a physical disorder for which there are no organic findings or known physiological mechanism or there is a strong presumption that the symptoms are linked to psychological issues.

- Somatization disorder is uncommon, but it is considered one of very few valid and reliable mental illnesses.

- Conversion disorder is a diagnosis that should be applied only after significant effort has been expended to eliminate any possible treatable organic disorder.

- Hypochondriasis is a rather uncommon disorder that usually follows a fluctuating course.

- Body dysmorphic disorder is a diagnosis in evolution, with conflicting data regarding amenability to treatment.

Suggested Readings

Castle DJ, Phillips KA: Obsessive-compulsive spectrum disorders: a defensible construct. Aust N Z J Psychiatry 40:114–120, 2006

Castle DJ, Rossell SL: An update on body dysmorphic disorder. Curr Opin Psychiatry 19:74–78, 2006

Hurwitz TA: Somatization and conversion disorder. Can J Psychiatry 49:172–178, 2004

Lamberg L: New mind/body tactics target medically unexplained physical symptoms and fears. JAMA 294:2152–2154, 2005

Phillips KA: Body dysmorphic disorder: recognizing and treating imagined ugliness. World Psychiatry 3:12–17, 2004

References

Allen L, Woolfolk R, Escobar J, et al: Cognitive-behavioral therapy for somatization disorder. Arch Intern Med 166:1512–1518, 2006

Almgren P-E, Nordgren L, Skantze H: A retrospective study of operationally defined hysterics. Br J Psychiatry 132:67–73, 1978

American Psychiatric Association: Diagnostic and Statistical Manual of Mental Disorders, 3rd Edition. Washington, DC, American Psychiatric Association, 1980

American Psychiatric Association: Diagnostic and Statistical Manual of Mental Disorders, 3rd Edition, Revised. Washington, DC, American Psychiatric Association, 1987

American Psychiatric Association: Diagnostic and Statistical Manual of Mental Disorders, 4th Edition. Washington, DC, American Psychiatric Association, 1994

American Psychiatric Association: Diagnostic and Statistical Manual of Mental Disorders, 4th Edition, Primary Care Version. Washington, DC, American Psychiatric Association, 1995

American Psychiatric Association: Diagnostic and Statistical Manual of Mental Disorders, 4th Edition, Text Revision. Washington, DC, American Psychiatric Association, 2000

Andreasen NC, Bardach J: Dysmorphophobia: symptom or disease? Am J Psychiatry 134:673–676, 1977

Ballmaier M, Schmidt R: Conversion disorder revisited. Funct Neurol 20:105–113, 2005

Barsky AJ, Ahern DK: Cognitive behavior therapy for hypochondriasis. JAMA 291:1464–1470, 2004

Barsky AJ, Klerman GL: Overview: hypochondriasis, bodily complaints, and somatic styles. Am J Psychiatry 140:273–283, 1983

Barsky AJ, Wyshak G, Klerman GL, et al: The prevalence of hypochondriasis in medical outpatients. Soc Psychiatry Psychiatr Epidemiol 25:89–94, 1990

Bass CM, Murphy MR: Somatization disorder: critique of the concept and suggestions for future research, in Somatization: Physical

Symptoms and Psychological Illness. Edited by Bass C. Oxford, England, Blackwell Scientific, 1990, pp 301–332

Bendefeldt F, Miller LL, Ludwig AM: Cognitive performance in conversion hysteria. Arch Gen Psychiatry 33:1250–1254, 1976

Bohne A, Wilhelm S, Keuthen N, et al: Prevalence of body dysmorphic disorder in a German college student sample. Psychiatry Res 109:101–104, 2002

Bourgeois JA, Chang CH, Hilty DM, et al: Clinical manifestations and management of conversion disorders. Curr Treat Options Neurol 4:487–497, 2002

Carson A, Best S, Postma K, et al: The outcome of neurology patients with medically unexplained symptoms: a prospective study. J Neurol Neurosurg Psychiatry 74:897–900, 2003

Carter AB: The prognosis of certain hysterical symptoms. BMJ 1:1076–1079, 1949

Castle DJ, Rossell SL: An update on body dysmorphic disorder. Curr Opin Psychiatry 19:74–78, 2006

Cloninger CR: The link between hysteria and sociopathy: an integrative model based on clinical, genetic, and neurophysiological observations, in Psychiatric Diagnosis: Explorations of Biological Predictors. Edited by Akiskal HS, Webb WL. New York, Spectrum, 1978, pp 189–218

Cloninger CR: Diagnosis of somatoform disorders: a critique of DSM-III, in Diagnosis and Classification in Psychiatry: A Critical Appraisal of DSM-III. Edited by Tischler GL. New York, Cambridge University Press, 1987, pp 243–259

Cloninger CR: Somatoform and dissociative disorders, in The Medical Basis of Psychiatry, 2nd Edition. Edited by Winokur G, Clayton P. Philadelphia, PA, WB Saunders, 1994, pp 169–192

Cloninger CR, Guze SB: Psychiatric illness and female criminality: the role of sociopathy and hysteria in the antisocial woman. Am J Psychiatry 127:303–311, 1970

Cloninger CR, Yutzy S: Somatoform and dissociative disorders: a summary of changes for DSM-IV, in Current Psychiatric Therapy. Edited by Dunner DL. Philadelphia, PA, WB Saunders, 1993, pp 310–313

Cloninger CR, Reich T, Guze SB: The multifactorial model of disease transmission, III: familial relationship between sociopathy and hysteria (Briquet's syndrome). Br J Psychiatry 127:23–32, 1975

Cloninger CR, Sigvardsson S, von Knorring A-L, et al: An adoption study of somatoform disorders, II: identification of two discrete somatoform disorders. Arch Gen Psychiatry 41:863–871, 1984

Cloninger CR, Martin RL, Guze SB, et al: A prospective follow-up and family study of somatization in men and women. Am J Psychiatry 143:873–878, 1986

Cloninger CR, Bayon C, Przybeck TR: Epidemiology and Axis I comorbidity of antisocial personality, in Handbook of Antisocial Behavior. Edited by Stoff DM, Breiling J, Maser JD. New York, Wiley, 1997, pp 12–21

Coryell W, House D: The validity of broadly defined hysteria and DSM-III conversion disorder: outcome, family history, and mortality. J Clin Psychiatry 45:252–256, 1984

De Leon J, Bott A, Simpson GM: Dysmorphophobia: body dysmorphic disorder or delusional disorder, somatic subtype? Compr Psychiatry 30:457–472, 1989

Desai BT, Porter RJ, Penry K: Psychogenic seizures: a study of 42 attacks in six patients, with intensive monitoring. Arch Neurol 39:202–209, 1982

Escobar JI, Swartz M, Rubio-Stipec M, et al: Medically unexplained symptoms: distribution, risk factors, and comorbidity, in Current Concepts of Somatization: Research and Clinical Perspectives. Edited by Kirmayer LJ, Robbins JM. Washington, DC, American Psychiatric Press, 1991, pp 63–78

Escobar JL, Gara MA, Waitzkins H, et al: DSM-IV Hypochondriasis in primary care. Gen Hosp Psychiatry 20:155–159, 1998

Fallon BA, Schneir FR, Narshall R, et al: The pharmacotherapy of hypochondriasis. Psychopharmacol Bull 32:607–611, 1996

Feighner JP, Robins E, Guze SB, et al: Diagnostic criteria for use in psychiatric research. Arch Gen Psychiatry 26:57–63, 1972

Flor-Henry P, Fromm-Auch D, Tapper M, et al: A neuropsychological study of the stable syndrome of hysteria. Biol Psychiatry 16:601–626, 1981

Folks DG, Ford CV, Regan WM: Conversion symptoms in a general hospital. Psychosomatics 25:285–295, 1984

Ford CV: The Somatizing Disorders: Illness as a Way of Life. New York, Elsevier, 1983

Ford CV: Conversion disorder and somatoform disorder not otherwise specified, in Treatment of Psychiatric Disorders, 2nd Edition. Edited by Gabbard GO. Washington, DC, American Psychiatric Press, 1995, pp 1737–1753

Ford CV, Folks DG: Conversion disorders: an overview. Psychosomatics 26:371–383, 1985

Gatfield PD, Guze SB: Prognosis and differential diagnosis of conversion reactions (a follow-up study). Dis Nerv Syst 23:623–631, 1962

Goodwin DW, Guze SB: Psychiatric Diagnosis, 5th Edition. New York, Oxford University Press, 1996

Grant JE, Kim SU, Crow SJ: Prevalence and clinical features of body dysmorphic disorder in adolescents and adult psychiatric inpatients. J Clin Psychiatry 62:517–522, 2001

Gunstad J, Phillips KA: Axis I comorbidity in body dysmorphic disorder. Compr Psychiatry 44:270–276, 2003

Guze SB, Perley MJ: Observations on the natural history of hysteria. Am J Psychiatry 119:960–965, 1963

Guze SB, Cloninger CR, Martin RL, et al: A follow-up and family study of Briquet's syndrome. Br J Psychiatry 149:17–23, 1986

Hankey GJ, Stewart-Wynne EG: Pseudo-multiple sclerosis: a clinico-epidemiological study. Clin Exp Neurol 24:11–19, 1987

Hathaway SR, McKinley JC: Minnesota Multiphasic Personality Schedule. Minneapolis, MN, University of Minnesota Press, 1943

Hollander E: Obsessive-compulsive spectrum disorders: an overview. Psychiatr Ann 23:355–358, 1993

Hollander E, Cohen LJ, Simeon D: Body dysmorphic disorder. Psychiatr Ann 23:359–364, 1993

Horowitz MJ: Hysterical Personality. New York, Jason Aronson, 1977

Hudziak JJ, Boffeli TJ, Kreisman JJ, et al: Clinical study of the relation of borderline personality disorder to Briquet's syndrome (hysteria), somatization disorder, antisocial personality disorder, and substance abuse disorders. Am J Psychiatry 153:1598–1606, 1996

Hurwitz TA: Somatization and conversion disorder. Can J Psychiatry 49:172–178, 2004

Kellner R: The prognosis of treated hypochondriasis: a clinical study. Acta Psychiatr Scand 67:69–79, 1983

Kellner R: Functional somatic symptoms and hypochondriasis: a survey of empirical studies. Arch Gen Psychiatry 42:821–833, 1985

Kellner R: Hypochondriasis and somatization. JAMA 258:2718–2722, 1987

Kellner R: Somatization disorder, in Treatments of Psychiatric Disorders: A Task Force Report of the American Psychiatric Association, Vol 3. Washington, DC, American Psychiatric Association, 1989, pp 2166–2171

Kellner R, Abbott P, Pathak D, et al: Hypochondriacal beliefs and attitudes in family practice and psychiatric patients. Int J Psychiatry Med 13:127–139, 1983/1984

Kent D, Tomasson K, Coryell W: Course and outcome of conversion and somatization disorders: a four-year follow-up. Psychosomatics 36:138–144, 1995

Kenyon FE: Hypochondriasis: a survey of some historical, clinical, and social aspects. Br J Psychiatry 138:117–133, 1965

Kirmayer LJ, Robbins JM: Introduction: concepts of somatization, in Current Concepts of Somatization: Research and Clinical Perspectives. Edited by Kirmayer LJ, Robbins JM. Washington, DC, American Psychiatric Press, 1991, pp 1–19

Kirmayer LJ, Robbins JM, Dworkind M, et al: Somatization and the recognition of depression and anxiety in primary care. Am J Psychiatry 150:734–741, 1993

Kroenke K, Swindle R: Cognitive-behavioral therapy for somatization and symptom syndromes: a critical review of controlled clinical trials. Psychother Psychosom 9:205–215, 2000

Kroenke K, Spitzer RL, de Gruy FV, et al: Multisomatoform disorder: an alternative to undifferentiated somatoform disorder for the somatizing patient in primary care. Arch Gen Psychiatry 54:352–358, 1997

Lader M, Sartorius N: Anxiety in patients with hysterical conversion symptoms. J Neurol Neurosurg Psychiatry 31:490–495, 1968

Lazare A: Conversion symptoms. N Engl J Med 305:745–748, 1981

Lewis WC, Berman M: Studies of conversion hysteria, I: operational study of diagnosis. Arch Gen Psychiatry 13:275–282, 1965

Lidbeck J: Group therapy for somatization disorders in general practice: effectiveness of a short cognitive-behavioral treatment model. Acta Psychiatr Scand 196:14–24, 1997

Ljundberg L: Hysteria: clinical, prognostic and genetic study. Acta Psychiatr Scand Suppl 32:1–162, 1957

Ludwig AM: Hysteria: a neurobiological theory. Arch Gen Psychiatry 27:771–777, 1972

Luff MC, Garrod M: The after-results of psychotherapy in 500 adult cases. BMJ 2:54–59, 1935

Mace CJ, Trimble MR: Ten-year prognosis of conversion disorder. Br J Psychiatry 169:282–288, 1996

Maloney MJ: Diagnosing hysterical conversion disorders in children. J Pediatr 97:1016–1020, 1980

Marsden CD: Hysteria: a neurologist's view. Psychol Med 16:277–288, 1986

Martin RL: DSM-IV changes in the somatoform disorders. Psychiatr Ann 25:29–39, 1995

Martin RL, Yutzy SH: Somatoform disorders, in Psychiatry. Edited by Tasman A, Kay J, Lieberman JA. Philadelphia, PA, WB Saunders, 1997, pp 1119–1155

Martin RL, Cloninger CR, Guze SB: The evaluation of diagnostic concordance in follow-up studies, II: a blind prospective follow-up of female criminals. J Psychiatr Res 15:107–125, 1979

Martin RL, Cloninger CR, Guze SB, et al: Mortality in a follow-up of 500 psychiatric outpatients, II: cause-specific mortality. Arch Gen Psychiatry 42:58–66, 1985

Meares R, Horvath TB: "Acute" and "chronic" hysteria. Br J Psychiatry 121:653–657, 1972

Merskey H: Conversion disorder, in Treatments of Psychiatric Disorders: A Task Force Report of the American Psychiatric Association, Vol 3. Washington, DC, American Psychiatric Association, 1989, pp 2152–2159

Murphy GE: The clinical management of hysteria. JAMA 247:2559–2564, 1982

Murphy GE, Guze SB: Setting limits. Am J Psychother 14:30–47, 1960

Murphy GE, Wetzel RD: Family history of suicidal behavior among suicide attempters. J Nerv Ment Dis 170:86–90, 1982

Otto M, Wilhelm S, Cohen L, et al: Prevalence of body dysmorphic disorder in a community sample of women. Am J Psychiatry 158:2061–2063, 2001

Perley M, Guze SB: Hysteria: the stability and usefulness of clinical criteria: a quantitative study based upon a 6- to 8-year follow-up of 39 patients. N Engl J Med 266:421–426, 1962

Phillips KA: Body dysmorphic disorder: the distress of imagined ugliness. Am J Psychiatry 148:1138–1149, 1991

Phillips KA: Body dysmorphic disorder: clinical features and drug treatment. CNS Drugs 3:30–40, 1995

Phillips KA: Body dysmorphic disorder, in Somatoform and Factitious Disorders (Review of Psychiatry Series, Vol 20, No 3; Oldham JM, Riba MB, series eds). Edited by Phillips KA. Washington, DC, American Psychiatric Publishing, DC, 2001, pp 67–94

Phillips KA, Diaz SF: Gender differences in body dysmorphic disorder. J Nerv Ment Dis 185:570–577, 1997

Phillips KA, Hollander E: Body dysmorphic disorder, in DSM-IV Sourcebook, Vol 2. Edited by Widiger TA, Frances AJ, Pincus HA, et al. Washington, DC, American Psychiatric Press, 1996, pp 949–960

Phillips KA, McElroy SL, Keck PE Jr, et al: Body dysmorphic disorder: 30 cases of imagined ugliness. Am J Psychiatry 150:302–308, 1993

Phillips KA, Grant JE, Siniscalchi JM, et al: A retrospective follow-up study of body dysmorphic disorder. Compr Psychiatry 46:315–321, 2005

Phillips KA, Pagano ME, Menard W, et al: A 12-month follow-up study of the course of body dysmorphic disorder. Am J Psychiatry 163:907–912, 2006

Pincus J: Hysteria presenting to a neurologist, in Hysteria. Edited by Roy A. London, England, Wiley, 1982, pp 131–144

Pribor EF, Smith DS, Yutzy SH: Somatization disorder in the elderly. Am J Geriatr Psychiatry 2:109–117, 1994

Purtell J, Robins E, Cohen M: Observations on clinical aspects of hysteria: a quantitative study of 50 hysteria patients and 156 control subjects. JAMA 146:902–909, 1951

Quill TE: Somatization disorder: one of medicine's blind spots. JAMA 254:3075–3079, 1985

Raskin M, Talbott JA, Meyerson AT: Diagnosis of conversion reactions: predictive value of psychiatric criteria. JAMA 197:530–534, 1966

Riding J, Munro A: Pimozide in the treatment of monosymptomatic hypochondriacal psychosis. Acta Psychiatr Scand 52:23–30, 1975

Rief W, Buhlmann U, Wilhelm A, et al: The prevalence of body dysmorphic disorder in a population based survey. Psychol Med 36:877–885, 2006

Robins E, O'Neal P: Clinical features of hysteria in children. The Nervous Child 10:246–271, 1953

Robins LN, Helzer JE, Weissman MM, et al: Lifetime prevalence of specific psychiatric disorders in three sites. Arch Gen Psychiatry 41:949–958, 1984

Scallet A, Cloninger CR, Othmer E: The management of chronic hysteria: a review and double-blind trial of electrosleep and other relaxation methods. Dis Nerv Syst 37:347–353, 1976

Shapiro D: Neurotic Styles. New York, Basic Books, 1965

Sharma P, Chaturvedi SK: Conversion disorder revisited. Acta Psychiatr Scand 92:301–304, 1995

Slater ETO, Glithero C: A follow-up of patients diagnosed as suffering from "hysteria." J Psychosom Res 9:9–13, 1965

Smith GR Jr, Monson RA, Ray DC: Psychiatric consultation in somatization disorder: a randomized controlled study. N Engl J Med 314:1407–1413, 1986

Stefanis C, Markidis M, Christodoulou G: Observations on the evolution of the hysterical symptomatology. Br J Psychiatry 128:269–275, 1976

Stefansson JH, Messina JA, Meyerowitz S: Hysterical neurosis, conversion type: clinical and epidemiological considerations. Acta Psychiatr Scand 59:119–138, 1976

Stern J, Murphy M, Bass C: Personality disorders in patients with somatization disorder: a controlled study. Br J Psychiatry 163:785–789, 1993

Stone J, Sharpe M, Rothwell PM, et al: The 12 year prognosis of unilateral functional weakness and sensory disturbance. J Neurol Neurosurg Psychiatry 74:591–596, 2003

Stone J, Smyth R, Carson A, et al: Systematic review of misdiagnosis of conversion symptoms and "hysteria." BMJ 331:989, 2005

Stoudemire GA: Somatoform disorders, factitious disorders, and malingering, in American Psychiatric Press Textbook of Psychiatry. Edited by Talbott JA, Hales RE, Yudofsky SC. Washington, DC, American Psychiatric Press, 1988, pp 533–556

Temoshok L, Attkisson CC: Epidemiology of hysterical phenomena: evidence for a psychosocial theory, in Hysterical Personality. Edited by Horowitz MJ. New York, Jason Aronson, 1977, pp 143–222

Tomasson K, Kent D, Coryell W: Somatization and conversion disorders: comorbidity and demographics at presentation. Acta Psychiatr Scand 84:288–293, 1991

Toone BK: Disorders of hysterical conversion, in Physical Symptoms and Psychological Illness. Edited by Bass C. London, England, Blackwell Scientific, 1990, pp 207–234

Vaillant GE: The disadvantages of DSM-III outweigh its advantages. Am J Psychiatry 141:542–545, 1984

Veale D, Boocock A, Gournay K, et al: Body dysmorphic disorder: a survey of fifty cases. Br J Psychiatry 169:196–201, 1996

Watson CG, Buranen C: The frequency and identification of false positive conversion reactions. J Nerv Ment Dis 167:243–247, 1979

Weddington WW: Conversion reaction in an 82-year-old man. J Nerv Ment Dis 167:368–369, 1979

Weinstein EA, Eck RA, Lyerly OG: Conversion hysteria in Appalachia. Psychiatry 32:334–341, 1969

Wetzel RD, Guze SB, Cloninger CR, et al: Briquet's syndrome (hysteria) is both a somatoform and a "psychoform" illness: an MMPI study. Psychosom Med 56:564–569, 1994

Woerner PI, Guze SB: A family and marital study of hysteria. Br J Psychiatry 114:161–168, 1968

Woodruff RA, Clayton PJ, Guze SB: Hysteria: studies of diagnosis, outcome, and prevalence. JAMA 215:425–428, 1971

World Health Organization: International Statistical Classification of Diseases and Related Health Problems, 10th Revision. Geneva, Switzerland, World Health Organization, 1992

World Health Organization: Diagnostic and Management Guidelines for Mental Disorders in Primary Care: ICD-10 Chapter V Primary Care Version. Gottingen, Germany, Hogrefe & Huber, 1996

Yutzy SH, Pribor EF, Cloninger CR, et al: Reconsidering the criteria for somatization disorder. Hosp Community Psychiatry 43:1075–1076, 1149, 1992

9

ADJUSTMENT DISORDERS

James J. Strain, M.D.
Kimberly G. Klipstein, M.D.
Jeffrey H. Newcorn, M.D.

The issue of defining boundaries is especially problematic in subthreshold diagnoses such as the adjustment disorders, for which there are no symptom checklists, algorithms, or guidelines for the "quantification of attributes." According to DSM-IV (American Psychiatric Association 1994), "[t]he essential feature of an adjustment disorder is the development of clinically significant emotional or behavioral symptoms in response to an identifiable psychosocial stressor or stressors" (p. 623). Less phenomenological and more etiological in nature, this definition differs from most Axis I disorders in DSM-IV in that it was to remain atheoretical. In DSM-IV-TR (American Psychiatric Association 2000; Table 9–1), the term *psychosocial stressor* was changed to the broader concept of stres-

sor. Emotional reactions to physical stress, such as the Chernobyl reactor incident (Havenaar et al. 1996) or cardiac surgery (Oxman et al. 1994), are well documented in the literature and suggest that a psychosocial stressor as a criterion is too restrictive.

Critics of the adjustment disorder diagnosis present a threefold argument. They state that the symptom complex is too subjective or "depends structurally on clinical judgment" as opposed to sound, operational criteria (Casey et al. 2001). Second, the idea of a "clinically significant" emotional reaction to a particular stressor is also fraught with subjectivity. Powell and McCone (2004) made this point in their case report of the treatment of a patient with adjustment disorder secondary to the September 11th terrorist

This work was funded by The Malcolm Gibbs Foundation, Inc., New York, New York.

Table 9–1. DSM-IV-TR diagnostic criteria for adjustment disorders

A. The development of emotional or behavioral symptoms in response to an identifiable stressor(s) occurring within 3 months of the onset of the stressor(s).

B. These symptoms or behaviors are clinically significant as evidenced by either of the following:

   (1) marked distress that is in excess of what would be expected from exposure to the stressor

   (2) significant impairment in social or occupational (academic) functioning

C. The stress-related disturbance does not meet the criteria for another specific Axis I disorder and is not merely an exacerbation of a preexisting Axis I or Axis II disorder.

D. The symptoms do not represent bereavement.

E. Once the stressor (or its consequences) has terminated, the symptoms do not persist for more than an additional 6 months.

   Specify if:

   Acute: if the disturbance lasts less than 6 months

   Chronic: if the disturbance lasts for 6 months or longer

Adjustment disorders are coded based on the subtype, which is selected according to the predominant symptoms. The specific stressor(s) can be specified on Axis IV.

   309.0 **With depressed mood**

   309.24 **With anxiety**

   309.28 **With mixed anxiety and depressed mood**

   309.3 **With disturbance of conduct**

   309.4 **With mixed disturbance of emotions and conduct**

   309.9 **Unspecified**

attacks. Because there has never before been a large-scale terrorist attack in America, how are clinicians to know what a "normal" response to such an event would be? Finally, the concept of the "stressor" lacks quantifiable and qualifiable guidelines, thus contributing to the vague and nonspecific nature of the adjustment disorder diagnosis.

The lack of specificity in the diagnosis of adjustment disorders may alternatively be considered an advantage. It allows clinicians to "tag" early or temporary mental states when the clinical picture is vague and indistinct but the morbidity is more than expected in a normal reaction. This clinical picture may be the earliest sign of an evolving major mental disorder. Therefore, the adjustment disorders occupy an essential place in the psychiatric taxonomic spectrum (Strain et al. 1998a).

The updated "Associated Features and Disorders" section in DSM-IV-TR served to clarify comorbidity with other disorders.

Adjustment disorders are associated with suicide attempts, suicide, excessive substance use, and somatic complaints. Adjustment disorder has been reported in individuals with preexisting mental disorders in selected samples, such as children and adolescents and in general medical and surgical patients. The presence of an adjustment disorder may complicate the course of illness in individuals who have a general medical condition (e.g., decreased compliance with the recommended medical regimen or increased length of hospital stay).

With regard to specific culture, age, and gender issues, it is necessary to take these attributes into account when making the clinical judgment of whether the individual's response to the stressor is maladaptive or in excess of that which normally would be expected. Women are given the diagnosis of adjustment disorder twice as often as men. In children and adolescents, however, the gender assignment of adjustment disorder is equivalent.

The DSM-IV-TR "Prevalence" section includes rates in children, adolescents, and the elderly (2%–8% in community samples). Adjustment disorder "has been diagnosed in up to 12% of general hospital inpatients who are referred for a mental health consultation, in 10%–30% of those in mental health outpatient settings, and in as many as 50% in special populations that have experienced a specific stressor (e.g., following cardiac surgery)" (American Psychiatric Association 2000, p. 681). Those populations with increased stressors (e.g., indigent patients, medically ill patients) are at higher risk for adjustment disorder.

As indicated in the "Course" section in DSM-IV-TR, adjustment disorder may progress to more severe mental disorders in children and adolescents more frequently than in adults (Andreasen and Hoenk 1982). However, this increased risk may be secondary to the co-occurrence of other mental disorders or the fact that the subthreshold presentation was an early phase of a more pernicious illness.

The adjustment disorder diagnosis can be used with another Axis I diagnosis if the symptoms of that diagnosis meet criteria for a major diagnosis (e.g., major depressive disorder), even if a stressor had precipitated that major depressive disorder. If the symptoms extant are secondary to the direct physiological effects of a general medical condition and/or its treatment, adjustment disorder should not be diagnosed. Additionally, demoralization has been suggested as another V-code category and should be distinguished from adjustment disorder and other pathological conditions (Slavney 1999).

Definition and History

The literature review and the Western Psychiatric Institute and Clinic data reanalysis supported by a MacArthur grant prompted the American Psychiatric Association Task Force on Psychological System Interface Disorders to recommend that specific changes to the adjustment disorders be included in DSM-IV and DSM-IV-TR:

1. Enhance the clarity of the language.
2. Describe the time of the reaction to reflect duration: acute (less than 6 months) or chronic (6 months or longer).
3. Allow for the continuation of the stressor for an indefinite period.
4. Eliminate the subtypes of mixed emotional features, work (or academic) inhibition, withdrawal, and physical complaints. (These subtypes were rarely being employed.)

The lack of specificity that characterizes the adjustment disorder diagnoses makes it often difficult to distinguish them from other psychiatric syndromes. Spalletta et al. (1996) observed that assessment of suicidal behavior is an important tool in differentiating major depression, dysthymia, and adjustment disorder. Patients with adjustment disorder were among the most common recipients of a deliberate self-harm diagnosis, with the majority involving self-poisoning (Vlachos et al. 1994). Deliberate self-harm is more common in these patients (Vlachos et al. 1994), whereas the percentage of suicidal behavior was higher in depressed patients (Spalletta et al. 1996). Casey et al. (2006) examined variables that might distinguish adjustment disorder from other depressive episodes. Patients were screened for depression severity with the Beck Depression Inventory (BDI) and then interviewed with Schedules for Clinical Assessment in Neuropsychiatry, which includes questions assessing the presence of adjustment disorder. The authors were unable to find any independent variables that distinguished adjustment disorder from other depressive episodes, including the severity of the BDI score at the outset.

Epidemiology

Andreasen and Wasek (1980) reported that 5% of an inpatient and outpatient sample were labeled as having adjustment disorder. Fabrega et al. (1987) observed that 2.3% of a sample of patients at a walk-in clinic (diagnostic and evaluation center) met criteria for adjustment disorder, with no other diagnoses on Axis I or Axis II; 20% had the diagnosis of adjustment disorder when patients with other Axis I diagnoses (i.e., Axis I comorbidities) also were included. In general hospital psychiatric consultation populations, adjustment disorder was diagnosed in 21.5% (Popkin et al. 1990), 18.5% (Foster and Oxman 1994), and 11.5% (Snyder and Strain 1989).

Strain et al. (1998b) examined the consultation-liaison data from seven university teaching hospitals in the United States, Canada, and Australia. The sites had all used a common computerized clinical database to examine 1,039 consecutive referrals—the MICRO-CARES software system (Strain et al. 1998b). Adjustment disorder was diagnosed in 125 patients (12.0%); it was the sole diagnosis in 81 (7.8%) and comorbid with other Axis I and II diagnoses in 44 (4.2%). It had been considered as a "rule-out" diagnosis in an additional 110 (10.6%). Adjustment disorder with depressed mood, anxious mood, or mixed emotions were the most common subcategories used. Adjustment disorder was diagnosed comorbidly most frequently with personality disorder and organic mental disorder. Sixty-seven subjects (6.4%) were assigned a V-code diagnosis only. Patients with adjustment disorder were referred significantly more often for problems of anxiety, coping, and depression; had less past psychiatric illness; and were rated as functioning better than those patients with major mental disorders—all consistent with the construct of adjustment disorder as a maladaptation to a psychosocial stressor. Interventions prescribed for this general hospital inpatient cohort were similar to those for other Axis I and II diagnoses, in particular, the prescription of antidepressant medications. Patients with adjustment disorder required a similar amount of clinical time and resident supervision when compared with patients with other Axis I and II disorders.

Oxman et al. (1994) observed that 50.7% of elderly patients (age 55 years or older) receiving elective surgery for coronary artery disease developed adjustment disorder related to the stress of surgery. Thirty percent had symptomatic and functional impairment 6 months after surgery. Kellermann et al. (1999) reported that 27% of elderly patients examined 5–9 days after a cerebrovascular accident fulfilled the criteria for adjustment disorder. Research indicates that half of all cancer patients have a psychiatric disorder, usually an adjustment disorder with depression (Spiegel 1996). Adjustment disorder is frequently diagnosed in patients undergoing head and neck surgery (16.8%; Kugaya et al. 2000), patients with HIV (73% with psychological morbidity, most commonly dementia or adjustment disorder; Pozzi et al. 1999), patients with cancer (27% in a multicenter survey of consultation-liaison psychiatry in oncology; Grassi et al. 2000), dermatology patients (29% of the 9% who had a psychiatric diagnosis; Pulimood et al. 1996), and suicide attempters examined in emergency departments (22%; Schnyder and Valach 1997). In other studies, a diagnosis of adjustment disorder was found in more than 60% of burn inpatients (Perez-Jimenez et al. 1994), in 20% of patients in early stages of multiple sclerosis (Sullivan et al. 1995), and in 40% of poststroke patients (Shima et al. 1994).

D. Schafer (personal communication, April 1990) noted that up to 70% of children in the psychiatric setting may be given the diagnosis of adjustment disorder in a variety of mental health care settings. Faulstich et al. (1986) reported a 12.5% prevalence of DSM-III (American Psychiatric Association 1980) adjustment disorder and conduct issues in adolescent psychiatric inpatients.

Etiology

Stress has been described as the etiological agent for adjustment disorders. However, diverse variables and modifiers are involved regarding who will experience an adjustment disorder following stress. Cohen (1981) argued that 1) acute stresses are different from chronic ones in both psychological and physiological terms, 2) the meaning of the stress is affected by "modifiers" (e.g., ego strengths, support systems, prior mastery), and 3) the manifest and latent meanings of the stressor(s) must be differentiated (e.g., loss of job may be a relief or a catastrophe). Adjustment disorder with maladaptive denial of pregnancy, for example, can be a consequence of a stressor such as separation from a partner (Brezinka et al. 1994). An objectively overwhelming stress may have little effect on one individual, whereas a minor one could be regarded as cataclysmic by another. A recent minor stress superimposed on a previous underlying (major) stress that has no observable effect on its own may have a significant additive effect (i.e., concatenation of events; B. Hamburg, personal communication, April 1990).

Andreasen and Wasek (1980) described the differences between the types of stressors found in adolescents and those found in adults: 59% and 35%, respectively, of the precipitants had been present for 1 year or more and 9% and 39% for 3 months or less. Fabrega et al. (1987) reported that their adjustment disorder group had greater registration of stressors compared with the specific-diagnosis and the no-illness cohorts. There was a significant difference in the amount of stressors reported relevant to the clinical request for evaluation: the group with adjustment disorder, compared with the specific-diagnosis and the no-illness patients, was overrepresented in the "higher stress category." Popkin et al. (1990) reported that in 68.6% of the cases in their consultation cohort, the medical illness itself was judged to be the primary psychosocial stressor. Snyder and Strain (1989)

observed that stressors as assessed on Axis IV were significantly higher ($P=0.0001$) for consultation patients with adjustment disorder than for patients with other diagnostic disorders.

Recent research highlights the role of childhood experiences in the later development of adjustment disorders. Studies of young male soldiers with adjustment disorder secondary to conscription revealed that stress at a young age, such as abusive and overprotective parenting or adverse early family events, is a risk factor for the later development of adjustment disorder (For-Wey et al. 2002; Hansen-Schwartz et al. 2005). In a similar cohort, a history of childhood separation anxiety was found to be correlated with the later development of adjustment disorder (Giotakos and Konstantakopoulos 2002).

Clinical Features

DSM-IV-TR recognizes six subtypes of adjustment disorder, classified according to their clinical features: with depressed mood, with anxiety, with mixed anxiety and depressed mood, with disturbance of conduct, with mixed disturbance of emotions and conduct, and unspecified (Table 9–2).

Treatment

Psychotherapy

Treatment of adjustment disorder rests primarily on psychotherapeutic measures that enable reduction of the stressor, enhanced coping with the stressor that cannot be reduced or removed, and establishment of a support system to maximize adaptation. The first goal is to note significant dysfunction secondary to a stressor and to help the patient moderate this imbalance. Many stressors may be avoided or minimized (e.g., taking on more responsibility than can be managed by the individual or putting oneself at risk by having unprotected sex with an unknown partner). Other stressors may elicit an

Table 9–2. Types of DSM-IV-TR adjustment disorder

With depressed mood	The predominant symptoms are those of a minor depression. For example, the symptoms might be depressed mood, tearfulness, and hopelessness.
With anxiety	This type of adjustment disorder is diagnosed when anxiety symptoms are predominant, such as nervousness, worry, and jitteriness. The differential diagnosis would include anxiety disorders.
With mixed anxiety and depressed mood	This category should be used when the predominant symptoms are a combination of depression and anxiety or other emotions. An example would be an adolescent who, after moving away from home and parental supervision, reacts with ambivalence, depression, anger, and signs of increased dependence.
With disturbance of conduct	The symptomatic manifestations are those of behavioral misconduct that violate societal norms or the rights of others. Examples are fighting, truancy, vandalism, and reckless driving.
With mixed disturbance of emotions and conduct	This diagnosis is made when the disturbance combines affective and behavioral features of adjustment disorder with mixed emotional features and adjustment disorder with disturbance of conduct.
Unspecified	This is a residual diagnosis within the diagnostic category. This diagnosis can be used when a maladaptive reaction that is not classified under other adjustment disorders occurs in response to stress. An example would be a patient who, when given a diagnosis of cancer, denies the diagnosis of malignancy and is noncompliant with treatment recommendations.

overreaction on the part of the patient (e.g., abandonment by a lover). The patient may attempt suicide or become reclusive, damaging his or her source of income. In this situation, the therapist would attempt to help the patient put his or her rage and other feelings into words rather than into destructive actions and assist more optimal adaptation and mastery of the trauma–stressor. The role of verbalization cannot be overestimated in an attempt to reduce the pressure of the stressor and enhance coping. The therapist also needs to clarify and interpret the meaning of the stressor for the patient. For example, a mastectomy may have devastated a patient's feelings about her body and herself. It is necessary to clarify that the patient is still a woman, capable of having a fulfilling relationship, including a sexual one, and that the patient can have the cancer removed or treated and not have a recurrence. Otherwise, the patient's pernicious fantasies—"all is lost"—may take over in response to the stressor (i.e., the mastectomy) and make her dysfunctional in work and/or sex and precipitate a painful disturbance of mood that is incapacitating.

Counseling, psychotherapy, medical crisis counseling, crisis intervention, family therapy, and group treatment may be used to encourage the verbalization of fears, anxiety, rage, helplessness, and hopelessness related to the stressors imposed on a patient. The goals of treatment in each case are to expose the concerns and conflicts that the patient is experiencing, identify means to reduce the stressors, enhance the patient's coping skills, and help the patient gain perspective on the adversity and establish relationships (i.e., a support network) to assist in the management of the stressors and the self. Cognitive-behavioral therapy, for example, was successfully used in young military recruits (Nardi et al. 1994).

Interpersonal psychotherapy was applied to depressed HIV-positive outpatients and found to be useful (Markowitz et al. 1992). Markowitz et al.'s (1992) description of the mechanisms of interpersonal psychotherapy is important in understanding psychotherapeutic approaches to the adjustment disorders. These mechanisms include psychoeducation about the sick role, a here-and-now framework, formulation of the problems from an interpersonal perspective, exploration of options for changing dysfunctional behavior patterns, identification of focused interpersonal problem areas, and the confidence that therapists gain from a systematic approach to problem formulation and treatment.

Elderly patients are particularly vulnerable to the development of adjustment disorders as the stress of medical illness abounds. Additionally, life transitions such as relocating to a nursing home or losing one's driving privileges are commonly experienced as stressors in the elderly. Frankel (2001) has described a type of psychotherapy called "ego-enhancing therapy" for the treatment of adjustment disorders in late life.

Support groups have also been employed in patients with adjustment disorders (Fawzy et al. 2003; Spiegel et al. 1989). Although studies looking at the survival benefits of psychosocial group interventions have been mixed and show (at most) questionable benefits, improvements in mood, distress level, and overall quality of life in cancer patients who attend support groups are very well documented (Goodwin et al. 2001; Newell et al. 2002).

Another therapeutic modality, eye movement desensitization and reprocessing, has been studied in patients with adjustment disorder. Results showed significant improvement in patients with anxious or mixed features but not in those with depressed mood. Additionally, those with ongoing stressors did not show improvement (Mihelich 2000).

A search of the Cochrane database revealed only two randomized, controlled trials of specific psychotherapeutic treatment of adjustment disorders. Gonzalez-Jaimes and Turnbull-Plaza (2003) showed that "mirror psychotherapy" for patients with adjustment disorder with depressed mood secondary to a myocardial infarction was both an efficient and effective treatment compared with two other treatments, Gestalt psychotherapy or medical conversation.

In another randomized, controlled trial, an "activating intervention" was carried out for the treatment of adjustment disorders resulting in occupational dysfunction. Employees ($N = 192$) were randomly assigned to receive either the intervention or care as usual (van der Klink and van Dijk 2003). The intervention consisted of an individual cognitive-behavioral approach to a graded activity, similar to stress inoculation training. Goals of treatment emphasized the acquisition of coping skills and the regaining of control. The treatment proved to be effective in decreasing sick leave duration and shortening long-term absenteeism when compared with the control group. This study formed the basis for the "Dutch Practice Guidelines for the Treatment of Adjustment Disorders in Primary and Occupational Health Care" (van der Klink et al. 2003).

Pharmacotherapy

Although psychotherapy has historically been the mainstay of treatment for the adjustment disorders, Stewart et al. (1992) emphasized the importance of including psychopharmacological interventions in the treatment of minor depression. These authors argued that pharmacotherapy is generally recommended, but data do not support this contention. Despite the lack of rigorous scientific evidence, Stewart and colleagues advocated successive trials with antidepressants in any depressed patient (major or minor disorders), particularly if he or she has not benefited from psychotherapy or other supportive measures for 3 months. In a randomized, controlled trial in the treatment of minor depressive disorder, fluoxetine proved superior to placebo in reducing depressive symptoms, improving overall psychosocial functioning, and alleviating suffering (Judd 2000). The question remains, does this also apply to adjustment disorders with depressed mood?

Randomized, controlled pharmacological trials of the use of pharmacotherapy in patients with adjustment disorder are rare. Tricyclic antidepressants or buspirone was recommended in place of benzodiazepines for patients with current or past heavy alcohol use because of the greater risk of dependence in these patients (Uhlenhuth et al. 1995). In a 25-week multicenter randomized, placebo-controlled, double-blind trial, WS 1490 (a special extract from kava kava) was reported to be effective in adjustment disorder with anxiety and did not have the tolerance issues associated with tricyclics and benzodiazepines (Volz and Kieser 1997). In a similar randomized, controlled trial, Bourin et al. (1997) randomly assigned patients to receive either Euphytose—a preparation containing a combination of plant extracts (*Crataegus*, *Ballota*, *Passiflora*, and *Valeriana*, which have mild sedative effects, and *Cola* and *Paullinia*, which mainly act as mild stimulants)—or placebo. Patients taking the experimental drugs improved significantly more than those taking placebo. In another study, tianeptine, alprazolam, and mianserin were found to be equally effective in symptom improvement in patients with adjustment disorder with anxiety (Ansseau et al. 1996). In a randomized, double-blind study, trazodone was more effective than clorazepate in cancer patients for the relief of anxious and depressed symptoms (Razavi et al. 1999). Similar findings were observed in HIV-positive patients with adjustment disorder (DeWit et al. 1999).

It is important to note that there are no randomized, controlled trials employing selective serotonin reuptake inhibitors (SSRIs), mixed SSRI atypicals (nefazodone and venlafaxine), buspirone, or mirtazapine. In a study of medically ill patients with depressive disorders (unspecified), Rosenberg et al. (1991) reported that 16 of 29 patients (55%) improved within 2 days of treatment with the maximal dosage of amphetamine derivatives. The presence of delirium was associated with a decreased response. Whether methylphenidate would be useful in adjustment disorders with depressed mood remains to be investigated.

Schatzberg (1990) recommended that therapists consider both psychotherapy and pharmacotherapy in adjustment disorders with anxious mood and that anxiolytics should be part of psychiatrists' armamentarium. Nguyen et al. (2006), using a double-blind randomized, controlled trial, compared the efficacies of etifoxine, a nonbenzodiazepine anxiolytic drug, and lorazepam, a benzodiazepine, in the treatment of adjustment disorder with anxiety in a primary care setting. Efficacy was evaluated on days 7 and 28 using the Hamilton Rating Scale for Anxiety. The two drugs were found to be equivalent in anxiolytic efficacy on day 28. However, overall more etifoxine recipients responded to the treatment. Moreover, 1 week after stopping treatment, fewer patients taking etifoxine experienced rebound anxiety compared with lorazepam patients.

Treatment of Adjustment Disorders in Primary Care

The Agency for Health Care Policy and Research (1993) developed guidelines for the treatment of depression in primary care. It would seem that if any depressive disorders could be treated in primary care, the adjustment disorders—subthreshold—would be the most likely candidates. A randomized, controlled trial was conducted at the University of Washington, Seattle, to determine the specificity and intensity of mental health training programs that are necessary to ensure the sufficient transfer of knowledge from psychiatrists to primary care physicians (Katon and Gonzales 1994). This trial included providing education to the patient and the physician as well as changing the structure of medical care delivery to enhance the primary care physician's capacity to adequately treat depressive disorders.

Optimal therapeutic outcome in the primary care setting depends on three actions: 1) sufficient patient education, 2) conjoint sessions with the psychiatrist and the primary care physician, and 3) sufficient follow-up by the psychiatrist during the course of treatment (Katon and Gonzales 1994).

Strain et al. (1998b) observed in multiple settings that adjustment disorder patients seen in psychiatric consultation in the general hospital setting required just as much of the psychiatric consultant's time and were just as likely to receive medication as were patients with major psychiatric disorders. The adjustment disorders are currently thought to require talking treatment (psychotherapy and/or counseling), which takes time and is poorly reimbursed for primary care physicians. Because talking effectively may require more skill than prescribing drugs, treatment of adjustment disorders in the primary care setting remains problematic.

Hameed et al. (2005) in a retrospective chart review sought to determine if there was a difference in antidepressant efficacy in the treatment of major depressive disorder versus adjustment disorder in a primary care setting. Patients were prescribed mostly SSRIs. DSM-IV-TR symptoms, Patient Health Questionnaire–9 depression rating scale scores, and functional disability reports were systematically used to assess patients' response. Results showed that neither depressed nor adjustment disorder patients demonstrated a difference in clinical response to any particular antidepressant. Patients with a diagnosis of adjustment disorder, however, were twice as likely to respond to standard antidepressant treatment as depressed patients. This study suggests that antidepressants are very effective in treating depression in the primary care setting and may be even more effective in the treatment of adjustment disorder with depressed mood.

Course and Prognosis

Andreasen and Hoenk's (1982) landmark study demonstrated that the prognosis was favorable for adjustment disorder in adults but that in adolescents, many major psychiatric illnesses eventually occur. At 5-year follow-up, 71% of the adults were completely well, 8% had an intervening problem, and 21% had developed a major depressive disorder or alcoholism. In adolescents at 5-year follow-up, only 44% were without a psychiatric diagnosis, 13% had an intervening psychiatric illness, and 43% had gone on to develop major psychiatric morbidity (e.g., schizophrenia, schizoaffective disorder, major depression, bipolar disorder, substance abuse, personality disorders). The presence of behavioral symptoms in the adolescents were the strongest predictors for major pathology at the 5-year follow-up. The number and type of symptoms were less useful than the length of treatment and chronicity of symptoms as predictors of future outcome.

Mezzich et al. (1981) and Strain et al. (1998a) observed that many of the subtypes of adjustment disorder were infrequently used (e.g., "with mixed emotional features"), whereas "with physical complaints," a DSM-III-R (American Psychiatric Association 1987) category, had insufficient time to be observed. Both subtypes were deleted in DSM-IV-TR.

As Chess and Thomas (1984) reported, it is important to note that adjustment disorder with disturbance of conduct, regardless of age, has a more guarded outcome. Just as Andreasen and Wasek (1980) observed, Chess and Thomas (1984) underscored that a significant number of adjustment disorder patients either do not improve or grow worse in adolescence and early adult life.

Despland et al. (1997) observed 52 patients with adjustment disorder at the end of treatment or after 3 years of treatment. Results showed the occurrence of psychiatric comorbidity (31%), suicide attempts (14%), development of a more serious psychiatric disorder (29%), and an unfavorable clinical state (23%). Adjustment disorder is an important disorder requiring follow-up and observation. Spalletta et al. (1996) stated that suicidal behavior and deliberate self-harm are important predictors in diagnosis of adjustment disorder. These symptoms can lead to the most distressing consequence—death.

Kovacs et al. (1994) also examined children and youth (ages 8–13 years) for up to 8 years and found that, controlling for the effects of comorbidity, adjustment disorder does not predict later dysfunction. A more recent report by Jones et al. (2002) examined 10 years of readmission data for various psychiatric diagnoses, including the adjustment disorders. They found that admission diagnosis was a significant predictor of readmission and that adjustment disorders had the lowest readmission rates. Furthermore, initial psychological recovery from an adjustment disorder may in large part be attributable to removal of the stressor. This was found to be the case in prisoners who developed adjustment disorders after being placed in solitary confinement and whose symptoms resolved shortly after their release (Andersen et al. 2000).

Many studies investigating the association between suicide and adjustment disorder underscore the importance of monitoring patients closely for suicidality. Runeson et al. (1996) observed from psychological autopsy methods that the median interval between first suicidal communication and suicide was very short in the patients with adjustment disorder (<1 month) compared with patients who have major depression (3 months), borderline personality disorder (30 months), or schizophrenia (47 months).

Conclusion

The issues of diagnostic rigor and clinical utility seem at odds for the adjustment disorders. Clinicians need a "wild card" (Robert Spitzer, personal communication, 1954), and field studies need to use reliable and valid instruments (e.g., depression or anxiety rating scales, stress assessments, length of disability, treatment outcome, family patterns) to determine more exact specification of the parameters of the diagnosis. Identification of the time course, remission or evolution to another diagnosis, and evaluation of stressors (characteristics, duration, and nature of adaptation to stress) would enhance the understanding of the concept of a stress-response illness.

Studies with adequate symptom checklists rated independently from the establishment of the diagnosis would help clarify the threshold between major and minor depression and anxiety, as well as help guide an entry cutoff point for adjustment disorder. Although the upper threshold is established by the criteria for the major syndromes, the lower threshold between an adjustment disorder and problems of living/normality is bereft of operational criteria that would define an entry "boundary." The careful examination of associated demographic and treatment outcome variables also would enable clinicians to describe more specifically the boundaries between diagnoses. Associated features such as family history, biological correlates, treatment response, and long-term course are all critical to establishing the authenticity of a diagnosis—that is, construct and criterion validity. The theory and practice of medicine have documented the need for a comprehensive multidimensional formulation of multiple physiological and functional variables and mechanisms to describe an illness.

Because of the subjective nature of the adjustment disorder diagnosis, diagnostic tools to aid clinicians in identifying this condition are significantly lacking. Maercker et al. (2006) identified three central processes/symptoms characteristic of patients with adjustment disorder in a medical setting: recurrent intrusions of upsetting images, avoidance of reminders, and failure to adapt. Many widely used screening instruments (e.g., Clinical Interview Schedule—Revised, Composite International Diagnostic Interview) utilized in psychiatric research today fail to incorporate the diagnosis (Casey 2001; Casey et al. 2001). Although the Hospital Anxiety and Depression Scale, a commonly used self-report screen for psychological distress in hospitalized patients, does not screen for adjustment disorders specifically, a study of terminally ill cancer patients found it to be a useful predictor of adjustment disorders and major depression in

patients who did not show clinical evidence of psychological distress at baseline (Akechi et al. 2004). Brief screening instruments have also recently been developed to help in the detection of adjustment disorders in cancer patients. The one-question interview and the impact thermometer are two such instruments that appear efficacious in identifying patients (Akizuki et al. 2003, 2005). Although they have shown to be valid tools, they lack the ability to distinguish between adjustment disorder and other depressive disorders, thus limiting their usefulness in promoting the concept of adjustment disorder as a separate and meaningful diagnostic entity.

Key Points

- Adjustment disorders are of two forms: acute (less than 6 months) and chronic (6 months or longer).

- In children, adjustment disorders are predictive of more serious mental illnesses for late adolescence and adulthood.

- An adjustment disorder diagnosis can be used concurrently with another Axis I diagnosis.

- The adjustment disorders have a clear threshold for when they are supplanted by another Axis I diagnosis, because the other diagnoses have established thresholds and symptom guidelines. The point at which the patient crosses the threshold between normal behavior and an adjustment disorder is less clear, however, because the symptom guidelines for entry are less specific.

- It has been suggested that adjustment disorders could be placed with other diagnoses identified by the mood and behavior; for example, adjustment disorder with depressed mood could be positioned as an affective disorder.

Suggested Readings

Newcorn JH, Strain J: Adjustment disorder in children and adolescents, in DSM-IV Source Book, Vol 3. Washington, DC, American Psychiatric Association, 1997, pp 291–301

Sadock BJ, Sadock VA: Kaplan and Sadock's Pocket Handbook of Clinical Psychiatry, 4th Edition. Philadelphia, PA, Lippincott Williams & Wilkins, 2005, pp 2055–2062

Strain JJ, Klipstein K: Adjustment disorder, in Treatments of Psychiatric Disorders, 4th Edition (TPD-IV). Edited by Gabbard GO. Washington, DC, American Psychiatric Publishing, 2006, pp 419–426

Strain JJ, Wolf D, Newcorn J, et al: Adjustment disorder, in DSM-IV Source Book, Vol 2. Washington, DC, American Psychiatric Association, 1996, pp 1033–1049

Strain JJ, Newcorn J, Mezzich J, et al: Adjustment disorder: the MacArthur reanalysis, in DSM-IV Source Book, Vol 4. Washington, DC, American Psychiatric Association, 1998, pp 403–424

References

Agency for Health Care Policy and Research: Depression Guideline Panel: Depression in Primary Care, Vol 1: Diagnosis and Detection; Vol 2: Treatment of Major Depression. Clinical Practice Guideline No. 5 (AHCPR publications 93-0550, 93-0551). Rockville, MD, U.S. Department of Health and Human Services, Public Health Service, Agency for Health Care Policy and Research, 1993

Akechi T, Okuyama T, Sugawara Y, et al: Major depression, adjustment disorders, and posttraumatic stress disorder in terminally ill cancer patients: associated and predictive factors. J Clin Oncol 22:1957–1965, 2004

Akizuki N, Akechi T, Nakanishi T, et al: Development of a brief screening interview for adjustment disorders and major depression in patients with cancer. Cancer 97:2605–2613, 2003

Akizuki N, Yamawaki S, Akechi T, et al: Development of an impact thermometer for use in combination with the distress thermometer as a brief screening tool for adjustment disorders and/or major depression in cancer patients. J Pain Symptom Manage 29:91–99, 2005

American Psychiatric Association: Diagnostic and Statistical Manual of Mental Disorders, 3rd Edition. Washington, DC, American Psychiatric Association, 1980

American Psychiatric Association: Diagnostic and Statistical Manual of Mental Disorders, 3rd Edition, Revised. Washington, DC, American Psychiatric Association, 1987

American Psychiatric Association: Diagnostic and Statistical Manual of Mental Disorders, 4th Edition. Washington, DC, American Psychiatric Association, 1994

American Psychiatric Association: Diagnostic and Statistical Manual of Mental Disorders, 4th Edition, Text Revision. Washington, DC, American Psychiatric Association, 2000

Andersen HS, Sestoft D, Lillebaek T, et al: A longitudinal study of prisoners on remand: psychiatric prevalence, incidence and psychopathology in solitary vs. non-solitary confinement. Acta Psychiatr Scand 102:19–25, 2000

Andreasen NC, Hoenk PR: The predictive value of adjustment disorders: a follow-up study. Am J Psychiatry 139:584–590, 1982

Andreasen NC, Wasek P: Adjustment disorders in adolescents and adults. Arch Gen Psychiatry 37:1166–1170, 1980

Ansseau M, Bataille M, Briole G, et al: Controlled comparison of tianeptine, alprazolam and mianserin in the treatment of adjustment disorders with anxiety and depression. Hum Psychopharmacol 11:293–298, 1996

Bourin M, Bougerol T, Guitton B, et al: A combination of plant extracts in the treatment of outpatients with adjustment disorder with anxious mood: controlled study versus placebo. Fundam Clin Pharmacol 11:127–132, 1997

Brezinka C, Huter O, Biebl W, et al: Denial of pregnancy: obstetrical aspects. J Psychosom Obstet Gynaecol 15:1–8, 1994

Casey P: Adult adjustment disorder: a review of its current diagnostic status. J Psychiatr Pract 7:32–40, 2001

Casey P, Dowrick C, Wilkinson G: Adjustment disorders fault line in the psychiatric glossary. Br J Psychiatry 179:479–481, 2001

Casey P, Maracy M, Kelly BD, et al: Can adjustment disorder and depressive episode be distinguished? J Affect Disord 92:291–297, 2006

Chess S, Thomas A: Origins and Evolution of Behavior Disorders: From Infancy to Early Adult Life. New York, Brunner/Mazel, 1984

Cohen F: Stress and bodily illness. Psychiatr Clin North Am 4:269–286, 1981

Despland JN, Monod L, Ferrero F: Etude clinique du trouble de l'adaptation selon le DSM-III-R [in French]. Schweiz Arch Neurol Neurochir Psychiatr 148:19–24, 1997

DeWit S, Cremers L, Hirsch D, et al: Efficacy and safety of trazodone versus clorazepate in the treatment of HIV-positive subjects with adjustment disorders: a pilot study. J Int Med Res 27:223–232, 1999

Fabrega H Jr, Mezzich JE, Mezzich AC: Adjustment disorder as a marginal or transitional illness category in DSM-III. Arch Gen Psychiatry 44:567–572, 1987

Faulstich ME, Moore JR, Carey MP, et al: Prevalence of DSM-III conduct and adjustment disorders for adolescent psychiatric inpatients. Adolescence 21:333–337, 1986

Fawzy FI, Canada AL, Fawzy NW: Malignant melanoma: effects of a brief, structured psychiatric intervention on survival and recurrence at 10-year follow-up. Arch Gen Psychiatry 60:100–103, 2003

For-Wey L, Fei-Yin L, Bih-Ching S: The relationship between life adjustment and parental bonding in military personnel with adjustment disorder in Taiwan. Mil Med 167:678–682, 2002

Foster P, Oxman T: A descriptive study of adjustment disorder diagnoses in general hospital patients. Ir J Psychol Med 11:153–157, 1994

Frankel M: Ego enhancing treatment of adjustment disorders of later life. J Geriatr Psychiatry 34:221–223, 2001

Giotakos O, Konstantakopoulos G: Parenting received in childhood and early separation anxiety in male conscripts with adjustment disorder. Mil Med 167:28–33, 2002

Gonzalez-Jaimes EI, Turnbull-Plaza B: Selection of psychotherapeutic treatment for adjustment disorder with depressive mood due to acute myocardial infarction. Arch Med Res 34:298–304, 2003

Goodwin PJ, Leszcz M, Ennis M, et al: The effects of group psychosocial support on survival in metastatic breast cancer. N Engl J Med 345:1719–1726, 2001

Grassi L, Gritti P, Rigatelli M, et al: Psychosocial problems secondary to cancer: an Italian multicenter survey of consultation-liaison psychiatry in oncology. Italian Consultation-Liaison Group. Eur J Cancer 36:579–585, 2000

Hameed U, Schwartz TL, Malhotra K, et al: Antidepressant treatment in the primary care office: outcomes for adjustment disorder versus major depression. Ann Clin Psychiatry 17:77–81, 2005

Hansen-Schwartz J, Kijne B, Johnsen A, et al: The course of adjustment disorder in Danish male conscripts. Nord J Psychiatry 59:193–196, 2005

Havenaar JM, Van den Brink W, Van den Bout J, et al: Mental health problems in the Gomel region (Belarus): an analysis of risk factors in an area affected by the Chernobyl disaster. Psychol Med 26:845–855, 1996

Jones R, Yates WR, Zhou MD: Readmission rates for adjustment disorders: comparison with other mood disorders. J Affect Disord 71:199–203, 2002

Judd LL: Diagnosis and treatment of minor depressive disorders. Int J Neuropsychopharmacol 3 (suppl):S66, 2000

Katon W, Gonzales J: A review of randomized trials of psychiatric consultation-liaison studies in primary care. Psychosomatics 35:268–278, 1994

Kellermann M, Fekete I, Gesztelyi R, et al: Screening for depressive symptoms in the acute phase of stroke. Gen Hosp Psychiatry 21:116–121, 1999

Kovacs M, Gatsonis C, Pollock M, et al: A controlled prospective study of DSM-III adjustment disorder in childhood: short-term prognosis and long-term predictive validity. Arch Gen Psychiatry 51:535–541, 1994

Kugaya A, Akechi T, Okuyama T, et al: Prevalence, predictive factors, and screening for psychological distress in patients with newly diagnosed head and neck cancers. Cancer 88:2817–2823, 2000

Maercker A, Einsle F, Kollner V: Adjustment disorders as a stress response syndromes: a new diagnostic concept and its exploration in a medical sample. Psychopathology 627:135–146, 2006

Markowitz JC, Klerman GL, Perry SW: Interpersonal psychotherapy of depressed HIV-positive outpatients. Hosp Community Psychiatry 43:885–890,1992

Mezzich JE, Dow JT, Rich CL, et al: Developing an efficient clinical information system for a comprehensive psychiatric institute, II: initial evaluation form. Behavioral Research Methods and Instrumentation 13:464–478, 1981

Mihelich ML: Eye movement desensitization and reprocessing treatment of adjustment disorder. Dissertation Abstracts International 61:1091, 2000

Nardi C, Lichtenberg P, Kaplan Z: Adjustment disorder of conscripts as a military phobia. Mil Med 159:612–616, 1994

Newell SA, Sanson-Fisher RW, Savolainen NJ: Systematic review of psychological therapies for cancer patients: overview and recommendations for future research. J Natl Cancer Inst 94:558–584, 2002

Nguyen N, Fakra E, Pradel V, et al: Efficacy of etifoxine compared to lorazepam monotherapy in the treatment of patients with adjustment disorders with anxiety: a double-blind controlled study in general practice. Hum Psychopharmacol 21:139–149, 2006

Oxman TE, Barrett JE, Freeman DH, et al: Frequency and correlates of adjustment disorder relates to cardiac surgery in older patients. Psychosomatics 35:557–568, 1994

Perez-Jimenez JP, Gomez-Bajo GJ, Lopez-Catillo JJ, et al: Psychiatric consultation and post-traumatic stress disorder in burned patients. Burns 20:532–536, 1994

Popkin MK, Callies AL, Colon EA, et al: Adjustment disorders in medically ill patients referred for consultation in a university hospital. Psychosomatics 31:410–414, 1990

Powell S, McCone D: Treatment of adjustment disorder with anxiety: a September 11, 2001, case study with a 1-year follow-up. Cogn Behav Pract 11:331–336, 2004

Pozzi G, Del Borgo C, Del Forna A, et al: Psychological discomfort and mental illness in patients with AIDS: implications for home care. AIDS Patient Care STDS 13:555–564, 1999

Pulimood S, Rajagopalan B, Rajagopalan M, et al: Psychiatric morbidity among dermatology inpatients. Natl Med J India 9:208–210, 1996

Razavi D, Kormoss N, Collard A, et al: Comparative study of the efficacy and safety of trazodone versus clorazepate in the treatment of adjustment disorders in cancer patients: a pilot study. J Int Med Res 27:264–272, 1999

Rosenberg PB, Ahmed I, Hurwitz S: Methylphenidate in depressed medically ill patients. J Clin Psychiatry 52:263-267, 1991

Runeson BS, Beskow J, Waern M: The suicidal process in suicides among young people. Acta Psychiatr Scand 93:35–42, 1996

Schatzberg AF: Anxiety and adjustment disorder: a treatment approach. J Clin Psychiatry 51 (suppl):20–24, 1990

Schnyder U, Valach L: Suicide attempters in a psychiatric emergency room population. Gen Hosp Psychiatry 19:119–129, 1997

Shima S, Kitagawa Y, Kitamura T, et al: Post-stroke depression. Gen Hosp Psychiatry 16:286–289, 1994

Slavney PR: Diagnosing demoralization in consultation psychiatry. Psychosomatics 40:325–329, 1999

Snyder S, Strain JJ: Differentiation of major depression and adjustment disorder with depressed mood in the medical setting. Gen Hosp Psychiatry 12:159–165, 1989

Spalletta G, Troisi A, Saracco M, et al: Symptom profile: Axis II comorbidity and suicidal behaviour in young males with DSM-III-R depressive illnesses. J Affect Disord 39:141–148, 1996

Spiegel D: Cancer and depression. Br J Psychiatry 168 (suppl):109–116, 1996

Spiegel, D, Bloom JR, Kramer HJC, et al: Effect of psychosocial treatment on survival of patients with metastatic breast cancer. Lancet 14:88–89, 1989

Stewart JW, Quitkin FM, Klein DF: The pharmacotherapy of minor depression. Am J Psychother 46:23–36, 1992

Strain JJ, Newcorn JH, Mezzich JE, et al: Adjustment disorder: the MacArthur reanalysis, in DSM-IV Sourcebook, Vol 4. Washington, DC, American Psychiatric Association, 1998a, pp 403–424

Strain JJ, Smith GC, Hammer JS, et al: Adjustment disorder: a multisite study of its utilization and interventions in the consultation-liaison psychiatry setting. Gen Hosp Psychiatry 20:139–149, 1998b

Sullivan MJ, Winshenker B, Mikail S: Screening for major depression in the early stages of multiple sclerosis. Can J Neurol Sci 22:228–231, 1995

Uhlenhuth EH, Balter MB, Ban TA, et al: International study of expert judgment on therapeutic use of benzodiazepines and other psychotherapeutic medications, III: clinical features affecting experts' therapeutic recommendations in anxiety disorders. Psychopharmacol Bull 31:289–296, 1995

van der Klink JJL, van Dijk FJH: Dutch practice guidelines for managing adjustment disorders in occupational and primary health care. Scand J Work Environ Health 29:478–487, 2003

van der Klink JJL, Blonk RWB, Schene AH, et al: Reducing long term sickness absence by an activating intervention in adjustment disorders: a cluster randomized controlled design. Occup Environ Med 60:429–437, 2003

Vlachos IO, Bouras N, Watson JP, et al: Deliberate self-harm referrals. Eur Psychiatry 8:25–28, 1994

Volz HP, Kieser M: Kava-kava extract WS 1490 versus placebo in anxiety disorders: a randomized placebo-controlled 25-week outpatient trial. Pharmacopsychiatry 30:1–5, 1997

10

IMPULSE-CONTROL DISORDERS NOT ELSEWHERE CLASSIFIED

Eric Hollander, M.D.

Heather A. Berlin, Ph.D., M.P.H.

Dan J. Stein, M.D., Ph.D.

Whereas impulse-control disorders (ICDs) were once conceptualized as either addictive or compulsive behaviors, they are now classified within the DSM-IV-TR (American Psychiatric Association 2000) ICD category. These include intermittent explosive disorder (IED; failure to resist aggressive impulses), kleptomania (failure to resist urges to steal items), pyromania (failure to resist urges to set fires), pathological gambling (failure to resist urges to gamble), and trichotillomania (failure to resist urges to pull one's hair) (Table 10–1). However, behaviors characteristic of these disorders may be notable in individuals as symptoms of another mental disorder. If the symptoms progress to such a point that they occur in distinct, fre-

quent episodes and begin to interfere with the person's normal functioning, they may then be classified as a distinct ICD.

There are also a number of other disorders that are not included as a distinct category but are categorized as ICDs not otherwise specified in DSM-IV-TR. These include sexual compulsions (impulsive-compulsive sexual disorder), compulsive shopping (impulsive-compulsive buying disorder), skin picking (impulsive-compulsive self-injurious disorder), and Internet addiction (impulsive-compulsive Internet usage disorder). One proposal for the research agenda leading up to DSM-V is to include these emerging disorders as new and unique ICDs rather than lumping them together as ICDs not oth-

Table 10–1. DSM-IV-TR impulse-control disorders

Impulse-control disorders not elsewhere classified
Intermittent explosive disorder
Kleptomania
Pyromania
Pathological gambling
Trichotillomania

Impulse-control disorders not otherwise specified
Impulsive-compulsive sexual disorder
Impulsive-compulsive self-injurious
   disorder
Impulsive-compulsive Internet usage
   disorder
Impulsive-compulsive buying disorder

Source. American Psychiatric Association 2000.

erwise specified. These disorders are unique in that they share features of both impulsivity and compulsivity and might be labeled as ICDs. Patients afflicted with these disorders engage in the behavior to increase arousal. However, there is a compulsive component in which the patient continues to engage in the behavior to decrease dysphoria. An area of discussion for DSM-V may include whether these disorders should be recognized as distinct ICDs.

In DSM-IV-TR, ICDs are characterized by five stages of symptomatic behavior (Table 10–2). First is the increased sense of tension or arousal, followed by the failure to resist the urge to act. During the act, the person may feel pleasure, gratification, or relief. Once the act has been completed, there is a sense of release from the urge. Finally, the patient experiences guilt and remorse at having committed the act.

Impulsivity—the failure to resist an impulse, drive, or temptation that is potentially harmful to oneself or others—is both a common clinical problem and a core feature of human behavior. An impulse is rash and lacks deliberation. It may be sudden and ephemeral, or a steady rise in tension may reach a climax in an explosive expression of the impulse, which may result in careless actions without regard for self or others. Impulsivity is evidenced behaviorally as carelessness; an underestimated sense of harm; extraversion; impatience, including the inability to delay gratification; and a tendency toward risk taking, pleasure, and sensation seeking (Hollander 2002). What makes an impulse pathological is an inability to resist it and its expression. The nature of impulsivity as a core symptom domain within the ICDs allows it to be distinguished as either a symptom or a distinct disorder, much in the same way as anxiety or depression.

Impulsivity research has been conducted both in disorders characterized by impulsivity (e.g., borderline personality disorder, antisocial personality disorder, conduct disorder) and in traditional ICDs (e.g., IED). For this reason, the basic tenets of impulsivity can be applied both to the ICDs and to other related psychiatric conditions.

Table 10–2. Core features of impulse-control disorders

Essential feature	Failure to resist an impulse, drive, or temptation to perform an act that is harmful to the person or to others
Before the act	The individual feels an increasing sense of tension or arousal. The individual is unable to resist the urge to act.
At the time of committing the act	The individual experiences pleasure, gratification, or relief.
After the act	The individual experiences a sense of release from the urge. The individual may or may not feel regret, self-reproach, or guilt.

Source. American Psychiatric Association 2000.

Intermittent Explosive Disorder

Definition and Diagnostic Criteria

IED is a DSM diagnosis used to describe people with pathological impulsive aggression (Table 10–3). Many clinicians and researchers rarely consider this diagnosis, although impulsive aggressive behavior is relatively common. In community surveys, 12%–25% of men and women in the United States reported engaging in physical fights as adults, a frequent manifestation of impulsive aggression (Robins and Regier 1991). Impulsive aggressive behavior usually is pathological and causes substantial psychosocial distress or dysfunction (McElroy et al. 1998). Being on the receiving end of impulsive aggressive behavior can lead to similar behavior in a child who grows up in this environment (Huesmann et al. 1984).

Table 10–3. DSM-IV-TR diagnostic criteria for intermittent explosive disorder

A. Several discrete episodes of failure to resist aggressive impulses that result in serious assaultive acts or destruction of property.

B. The degree of aggressiveness expressed during the episodes is grossly out of proportion to any precipitating psychosocial stressors.

C. The aggressive episodes are not better accounted for by another mental disorder (e.g., antisocial personality disorder, borderline personality disorder, a psychotic disorder, a manic episode, conduct disorder, or attention-deficit/hyperactivity disorder) and are not due to the direct physiological effects of a substance (e.g., a drug of abuse, a medication) or a general medical condition (e.g., head trauma, Alzheimer's disease).

IED-R and DSM-IV Criteria: Defining Integrated Research Criteria for Intermittent Explosive Disorder

Due to difficulties with the DSM criteria, until recently little research was done using categorical expressions of impulsive aggression. To use an IED diagnosis in research studies, research criteria were created. The research criteria for IED—Revised (IED-R) contain five criteria for IED, emphasizing the severity, impulsive nature, frequency, and pathology of the impulsive aggressive behavior.

Although DSM-IV (American Psychiatric Association 1994) made some changes to the IED criteria, it still did not provide criteria useful for research. The "aggressive impulses" of criterion A are not specific in terms of the type or number of acts or the time frame during which the acts must occur. Apparently, no official guidelines for these items had been determined or considered by the DSM-IV subcommittee.

When the subjects from the original IED-R series were reassessed with research criteria for IED-R and DSM-IV IED criteria, 69% met both IED-R and DSM-IV IED diagnoses, 20% met criteria for only DSM-IV IED, and 11% met criteria for only IED-R (Coccaro 2003). Because the two criteria sets did not differentiate groups with different aggression and impulsivity levels, and each alone left a number of subjects undiagnosed, integrated research criteria for IED (IED-IR) were created to allow subjects from any or both of these groups to be identified.

Epidemiology

DSM-IV-TR describes IED as "apparently rare." However, clinical interview or survey data give a different picture. A number of studies have looked at clinical populations, and one community survey has been done to determine the prevalence of IED. Numbers range between 1.1% and 6.3%. The evaluation of studies is complicated by the variety of defining criteria used, from DSM-III (American Psychiatric Association 1980) to current research criteria and IED-IR. More recently, Zimmerman et al. (1998) used the Structured Clinical Interview for DSM-IV to study current or lifetime IED in 411 outpatient psychiatric subjects. They reported a rate of 3.8% for current IED and 6.2% for lifetime IED using DSM-IV criteria. A recent reanalysis of a much larger sample from the same population revealed similar rates of IED (Coccaro et al. 2005). Further, data from a pilot community sample study revealed a community rate of lifetime IED by DSM-IV-TR criteria at 4% and by IED-IR criteria at 5.1% (Coccaro et al. 2004). Considering the rates found in these more recent studies, IED could be as common as other major psychiatric disorders such as schizophrenia or bipolar illness. Most of the limited published data on gender differences suggest that males outnumber females with IED. However, more recent data suggest that the male-to-female ratio is approximately 1:1 (Coccaro et al. 2005).

Comorbidity

Subjects with IED most frequently have other Axis I and II disorders. The Axis I diagnoses most commonly comorbid with IED include mood, anxiety, substance, eating, and other impulse-control disorders, ranging in frequency from 7% to 89% (Coccaro et al. 1998; McElroy et al. 1998). Such Axis I comorbidity rates raise the question of whether IED constitutes a separate disorder. However, recent data indicating earlier onset of IED compared with all disorders except for phobic-type anxiety disorders suggest that IED is not secondary to these other disorders (Coccaro et al. 2005).

Bipolar Disorder

McElroy et al. (1998) reported that the aggressive episodes observed in their subjects resembled "microdysphoric" manic episodes. Symptoms in common with both manic and IED episodes included irritability (79%–92%), increased energy (83%–96%), racing thoughts (62%–67%), anxiety (21%–42%), and depressed (dysphoric) mood (17%–33%). However, this finding may not be surprising, because 56% of the subjects in question had a comorbid bipolar diagnosis of some type (bipolar I, 33%; bipolar II, 11%; bipolar not otherwise specified or cyclothymia, 11%). The Rhode Island Hospital Study (Coccaro et al. 2005) suggests a much lower rate of comorbid bipolar illness, with a rate of 11% (bipolar I, 5%; bipolar II, 5%; bipolar not otherwise specified, 1%). Regardless, clinicians should fully evaluate for bipolar disorder prior to determining treatment for IED because mood stabilizers, rather than selective serotonin reuptake inhibitors (SSRIs), would be the first-line treatment for IED comorbid with bipolar disorder.

Other Impulse-Control Disorders

McElroy et al. (1998) reported that up to 44% of their IED subjects had another ICD, such as compulsive buying (37%) or kleptomania (19%). However, in the Coccaro et al. (1998) study, few IED subjects had a comorbid ICD, and in the Rhode Island Hospital Study, only 5% of IED subjects had another ICD (Coccaro et al. 2005).

Borderline and Antisocial Personality Disorders

Coccaro et al. (1998) reported the rate of BPD and/or antisocial personality disorder in IED subjects to be 38%. However, rates of IED in subjects with BPD have been noted at 78% and in subjects with antisocial personality disorder at 58% (Coccaro et al. 1998). A review of unpublished data (E. Hollander, 2005) from the first author's research program suggests that these rates are lower among subjects not seeking treatment and are lowest in the community (23% for BPD and/or antisocial personality disorder; see also Coccaro et al. 2004). Regardless, BPD and antisocial personality disorder subjects with a comorbid diagnosis of IED do appear to have higher scores for aggression and lower scores for general psychosocial function than do BPD/antisocial personality disorder subjects without IED (Coccaro et al. 2005).

Pathogenesis

Our understanding of the pathogenesis of IED has been informed by various approaches, including family and twin studies, molecular genetic studies, biological correlates of serotonin and other neurotransmitters, and imaging and brain localization studies.

Course

Limited research is available concerning the age at onset and natural course of IED. However, according to DSM-IV-TR, the onset appears to be from childhood to the early 20s. The age at onset and course of IED distinguish it as separate from its comorbid diagnoses. The course of IED is variable, with an episodic course in some and a more chronic course in others. A mean age at onset of 16 years and an average duration of about 20 years have been described (McElroy et al. 1998). Preliminary data (Coccaro et al. 2005) confirm these findings and indicate that onset of DSM-IV-TR IED occurs by the end of the first decade in 31%, by the end of the second decade in 44%, by the end of the third decade in 19%, and by the end of the fourth decade in only 6%.

The mode of onset of IED is abrupt and without a prodromal period. Episodes typically last less than 30 minutes and involve physical assault, verbal assault, and/or destruction of property. If provocation is involved, it is usually from a known person and is seemingly minor in nature (McElroy et al. 1998). Many individuals frequently have minor aggressive episodes in the interim between severely aggressive/destructive episodes. Considerable distress and social, financial, occupational, or legal consequences typically result from these episodes.

Treatment

There are few studies in which subjects with IED have been the focus of treatment. There are, however, a number of studies concerning the treatment of impulsive aggression in related subjects.

Pharmacotherapy

A number of medications have been used to treat impulsive aggression, such as tricyclic antidepressants, benzodiazepines, mood stabilizers, and neuroleptics. Recently, pharmacotherapy studies of aggression have turned to SSRIs and mood stabilizers as first-line treatments. Fluoxetine and other SSRIs have been studied in impulsive aggressive subjects and IED patients. In a treatment trial of subjects meeting IED-IR criteria, impulsive aggressive behavior did respond to fluoxetine (Coccaro and Kavoussi 1997), but nonserotonin-specific antidepressants had little benefit for impulsive aggression and many side effects in treatment studies. Soloff et al. (1986) found that affective symptoms improved with amitriptyline in some BPD and schizotypal personality disorder inpatients, but impulsivity and aggression worsened in a set of patients, perhaps due to the noradrenergic effects of tricyclic antidepressants (Links et al. 1990). Thus, clinicians should be cautious when using the new dual-action antidepressants in these patients.

Psychotherapy

Anger treatment studies focus on treatment of anger as a component of other psychiatric illnesses such as substance abuse, posttraumatic stress disorder, depression, and domestic violence and in forensic and mentally impaired populations. Therapy for anger and aggression focuses on cognitive-behavioral group therapy. In a few rare cases, anger is addressed as the primary or only problem, and a limited number of treatments have been described. Imaginal exposure therapy, used frequently in anxiety disorders, was studied in a noncontrolled pilot study of anger treatment (Grodnitzky and Tafrate 2000). Subjects habituated to anger-provoking scenarios, and the treatment was felt to be useful.

Kleptomania

Definition and Diagnostic Criteria

Kleptomania was officially designated a psychiatric disorder in 1980 in DSM-III, and in DSM-III-R (American Psychiatric Association 1987) it was grouped under the category "disorders of impulse control not elsewhere classified." Kleptomania is currently classified in DSM-IV-TR as an ICD, but it is still poorly understood and has received very little empirical study. The DSM-IV-TR criteria for kleptomania are listed in Table 10–4.

Epidemiology

Although preliminary evidence suggests that the lifetime prevalence of kleptomania may be approximately 0.6% (Goldman 1991), this figure may be an underestimate. The shame and embarrassment associated with stealing prevent most people from voluntarily reporting kleptomania symptoms (Grant and Kim 2002b). No national epidemiological studies of kleptomania have been performed, but studies of kleptomania in various clinical samples suggest a higher prevalence. A recent study in the United States of 204 adult psychiatric inpatients with multiple disorders revealed that kleptomania may in fact be fairly common. The study found that 7.8% ($n=16$) endorsed current symptoms consistent with a diagnosis of kleptomania and 9.3% ($n=19$) had a lifetime diagnosis of kleptomania (Grant et al. 2005). Kleptomania appeared equally common in patients with mood, anxiety, substance use, or psychotic disorders.

The literature clearly suggests that the majority of patients with kleptomania are women (e.g., Grant and Kim 2002a; McElroy et al. 1991b; Presta et al. 2002). One explanation for this is that kleptomania occurs more frequently in women, but another reason may be that women are more likely to present for psychiatric evaluation. The courts may send male shoplifters to prison while sending female shoplifters for psychiatric evaluation (Goldman 1991). The severity of kleptomania symptoms and the clinical presentation of symptoms do not appear to differ based on gender (Grant and Kim 2002a).

Comorbidity

High rates of other psychiatric disorders have been found in patients with kleptomania and have sparked debate over the proper characterization of this disorder. Rates of lifetime comorbid affective disorders range from 59% (Grant and Kim 2002a) to 100% (McElroy et al. 1991b). The rate of lifetime comorbid bipolar disorder has been reported as ranging from 9% (Grant and Kim 2002a) to 27% (Bayle et al. 2003) to 60% (McElroy et al. 1991b). Studies have also found high lifetime rates of comorbid anxiety disorders (60%–80%; McElroy et al. 1991b, 1992), ICDs (20%–46%; Grant and Kim 2003), substance use disorders (23%–50%; Grant and Kim 2002a; McElroy et al. 1991b), and eating disorders (60%; McElroy et al. 1991b). Personality disorders have been found in 43%–55% of patients with kleptomania, the most common being paranoid personality disorder and histrionic personality disorder (Bayle et al. 2003; Grant 2004).

Table 10–4. DSM-IV-TR diagnostic criteria for kleptomania

A. Recurrent failure to resist impulses to steal objects that are not needed for personal use or for their monetary value.

B. Increasing sense of tension immediately before committing the theft.

C. Pleasure, gratification, or relief at the time of committing the theft.

D. The stealing is not committed to express anger or vengeance and is not in response to a delusion or a hallucination.

E. The stealing is not better accounted for by conduct disorder, a manic episode, or antisocial personality disorder.

Pathogenesis

Biological theories of kleptomania have focused on serotonin and inhibition, dopamine and reward deficiency, and the opioid system and craving and pleasure, in addition to other psychological theories of kleptomania.

Course

Kleptomania may begin in childhood, adolescence, or adulthood and sometimes in late adulthood. However, most patients have an onset of symptoms before age 21 years (i.e., by late adolescence; Goldman 1991; Grant and Kim 2002a; McElroy et al. 1991a, 1991b; Presta et al. 2002). Onset beyond 50 years of age is unusual, and in some of these cases, remote histories of past kleptomania can be elicited (Goldman 1991). Most clinical samples of kleptomania patients report shoplifting for more than 10 years prior to entering treatment (Goldman 1991; Grant and Kim 2002b; McElroy et al. 1991b).

Due to the sparse data on the course of kleptomania and the unavailability of longitudinal studies, the prognosis is not clearly known. However, without treatment the behavior may persist for decades, despite multiple convictions for shoplifting (arrest or imprisonment), with transient periods of remission. Three typical courses have been described: sporadic with brief episodes and long periods of remission; episodic with protracted periods of stealing and periods of remission; and chronic with varying intensity (American Psychiatric Association 2000). Fifteen or 16 years may pass before an individual seeks treatment (Goldman 1991; McElroy et al. 1991a). At peak frequency, McElroy et al. (1991a) found a mean of 27 episodes of theft per month, with one patient reporting as many as 4 thefts per day.

Treatment

Studies of treatment approaches for kleptomania are quite limited and principally involve SSRIs.

Pharmacotherapy

No medication is currently approved by the U.S. Food and Drug Administration for treating kleptomania, so it is important to inform patients of "off-label" uses of medications for this disorder and the empirical basis for considering medication treatment.

Psychotherapy

Many different kinds of psychotherapy have been tried in the treatment of kleptomania. The success of these therapies exists only in case reports, with no published controlled trials of therapy.

Because few empirical studies are available, research is needed to guide the selection of which psychotherapy to utilize and to investigate the combination of medication and psychotherapy in treating patients with kleptomania.

Pyromania
Definition and Diagnostic Criteria

The essential feature of pyromania is multiple deliberate and purposeful (rather than accidental) fire setting (Table 10–5). The firesetting behavior is primary, unrelated to another psychiatric state or to ideology, vengeance, or criminality, and does not result from impaired judgment (e.g., in dementia or mental retardation). DSM-IV-TR also excludes "communicative arson," by which some individuals with mental disorders or personality disorders use fire to communicate a desire or need.

Another important clinical feature of pyromania is the fascination of subjects with fire. People with pyromania like watching fire. They are often recognized as regular "watchers" at fires in their neighborhoods. They may like setting off false fire alarms. Their fascination with fire leads some to seek employment or to volunteer as a firefighter. Patients may be indifferent to the conse-

Table 10–5. DSM-IV-TR diagnostic criteria for pyromania

A. Deliberate and purposeful fire setting on more than one occasion.

B. Tension or affective arousal before the act.

C. Fascination with, interest in, curiosity about, or attraction to fire and its situational contexts (e.g., paraphernalia, uses, consequences).

D. Pleasure, gratification, or relief when setting fires, or when witnessing or participating in their aftermath.

E. The fire setting is not done for monetary gain, as an expression of sociopolitical ideology, to conceal criminal activity, to express anger or vengeance, to improve one's living circumstances, in response to a delusion or hallucination, or as a result of impaired judgment (e.g., in dementia, mental retardation, substance intoxication).

F. The fire setting is not better accounted for by conduct disorder, a manic episode, or antisocial personality disorder.

quences of the fire for life or property or may get satisfaction from the resulting destruction. Their behaviors may lead to property damage, legal consequences, or injury or loss of life to themselves or others.

Recent diagnostic classifications include pyromania among the ICDs. Although the fire setting results from a failure to resist an impulse, significant preparation of the fire may take place (Wise and Tierney 1999). The person may leave obvious clues of his or her fire preparation. Pyromania, however, is considered an uncontrolled and most often impulsive behavior.

Epidemiology

Most epidemiological studies have not directly focused on pyromania. These studies include various populations of arsonists or fire setters. Most reveal a preponderance of males with a history of fire fascination (Barker 1994). They also suggest that true pyromania is rare. Fire setting for profit or revenge or secondary to delusions or hallucinations is more frequent than "authentic" ICD. Fire setting is frequent in children and in adolescents. "True" pyromania in childhood rarely appears. Juvenile fire setting is most often associated with conduct disorder, attention-deficit/hyperactivity disorder (ADHD), or adjustment disorder.

The classic study *Pathological Fire-Setting (Pyromania)* by Lewis and Yarnell (1951) is one of the largest epidemiological studies of this topic and includes approximately 2,000 records from the National Board of Fire Underwriters and cases provided through fire departments, psychiatric clinics and institutions, and police departments near New York City. Thirty-nine percent of the fire setters from the study received the diagnosis of pyromania. Twenty-two percent had borderline to dull normal intelligence, and 13% had between dull and low average intelligence. The authors also described the fire setter as a "pale and yellow, insignificant creature" driven by an irresistible impulse to set fires. The peak incidence of fire setting was between the ages of 16 and 18 years, but this observation has not been confirmed by more recent studies. Pyromania is found in adolescents and is also present at any age. Among females, the diversity of ages is particularly apparent (Barker 1994).

The high prevalence rates of pyromania have not been confirmed by more recent studies. Koson and Dvoskin (1982) found no cases of pyromania in a population of 26 arsonists. Ritchie and Huff (1999) identified only 3 cases of pyromania in 283 cases of arson. According to DSM-IV-TR, pyromania occurs more often in males, especially those with poorer social skills and learning difficulties. This notation confirms the Lewis and Yarnell (1951) data that only 14.8% of those with pyromania are female.

Comorbidity

Pyromania and Depression

Lejoyeux et al. (2002) assessed ICDs, using the Minnesota Impulsive Disorders Interview, in 107 depressed inpatients who met DSM-IV-TR criteria for major depressive episodes. Thirty-one depressed patients met criteria for ICDs: 18 had IED, 3 had pathological gambling, 4 had kleptomania, 3 had pyromania, and 3 had trichotillomania. Patients with comorbid ICDs were significantly younger (mean age, 37.7 vs. 42.8 years). Patients with pyromania had a higher number of previous depressions (3.3 vs. 1.3, $P=0.01$). Bipolar disorders were more frequent in the ICD group than in the group without ICDs (19% vs. 1.3%, $P=0.002$). The findings of this study may suggest higher prevalence rates of ICDs than are found in a less severely ill population. There were no significant gender differences among patients presenting with ICDs, and in all cases the ICD appeared when patients no longer had mania or hypomania.

Pyromania and Alcohol Dependence

Laubichler et al. (1996) compared the files ($n=103$) of criminal fire setters and subjects with pyromania. Subjects with pyromania were younger (average age, 20 years) than criminal fire setters (average age, 30 years). Seventy of the 103 subjects had consumed alcohol before setting a fire. Fifty-four presented with alcohol dependence. The authors suggested a correlation between the amount of alcohol consumed and the frequency of fire setting. Rasanen et al. (1995) found that young arsonists have frequent alcohol problems: 82% had alcoholism and 82% were intoxicated at the time of committing the crime. The excessive consumption of alcohol had a close connection with the arson committed.

Lejoyeux et al. (1999) searched for ICDs among consecutive admissions for detoxification of alcohol-dependent patients in a French department of psychiatry. They found 30 alcohol-dependent persons presenting with at least one ICD (19 with IED, 7 with pathological gambling, 3 with kleptomania, and 1 case of trichotillomania), but none of the patients presented with two or more ICDs, and no patient presented with pyromania. However, it cannot be concluded from such a limited population that pyromania is not associated with alcohol dependence. Further studies are clearly needed to corroborate or refute this preliminary result.

Fire Setting and Psychiatric Disorders

In most cases, fire-setting behavior is not directly related to pyromania. On the other hand, fire setting in subjects who do not have pyromania appears frequent and often underrecognized. Among psychiatric patients, some research found that 26% of the subjects had a history of fire-setting behavior. Sixteen percent of these patients had actually set fires (Geller and Bertsch 1985). Ritchie and Huff (1999) reviewed mental health records and prison files from 283 arsonists, 90% of whom had a recorded history of mental health problems. Thirty-six percent had schizophrenia or bipolar disorder, and 64% were misusing alcohol or drugs at the time of their fire setting.

Pathogenesis

In addition to a number of psychodynamic models, pyromania has been suggested to be associated with reactive hypoglycemia, low concentrations of 3-methoxy-4-hydroxyphenylglycol (MHPG) and cerebrospinal fluid 5-hydroxyindoleacetic acid (5-HIAA), alcoholism, and a family history of alcoholism and violence.

Course

According to DSM-IV-TR, there are insufficient data to establish a typical age at onset of pyromania and to predict the longitudinal course. In individuals with pyromania, fire-setting incidents are episodic and may wax and wane in frequency. Studies indicate that the recidivism rate for fire setters ranges from

4.5% (Mavromatis and Lion 1977) to 28% (Lewis and Yarnell 1951). Barnett et al. (1997, 1999) compared mentally ill and mentally "healthy" fire setters from trial records in Germany in a cross-sectional and 10-year follow-up study. Mentally disordered arsonists were more likely than those with no disorder to have a history of arson before their trial. They also were more often convicted of arson again (11% relapse compared with 4%), had fewer registrations of common offenses such as theft as well as traffic violations and alcohol-related offenses, had a higher rate of recurrence, and committed fewer common offenses other than fire setting. Among all arsonists who committed crimes other than arson, those who were found to be partly responsible for their arson committed the highest number of offenses, followed by those who were deemed not responsible for their actions and those who were fully responsible.

Treatment

Treatment for fire setters is problematic because they frequently refuse to take responsibility for their acts, are in denial, have alcoholism, and lack insight (Mavromatis and Lion 1977). Behavioral treatments such as aversive therapy have helped fire setters (Koles and Jenson 1985; McGrath and Marshall 1979). Other methods of treatment rely on positive reinforcement with threats of punishment, stimulus satiation, and operant structured fantasies (Bumpass et al. 1983). Bumpass et al. (1983) treated 29 child fire setters and used a graphing technique that sequentially correlated external stress, behavior, and feelings on graph paper. After treatment (average follow-up, 2.5 years), only 2 of the 29 children continued to set fires.

Franklin et al. (2002) confirmed the positive effect of a prevention program for pyromania. In 1999, they developed the Trauma Burn Outreach Prevention Program. All subjects arrested and convicted after setting a fire received 1 day of information. The program's interactive content focused on the medical, financial, legal, and societal impacts of fire-setting behavior. The rate of recidivism was less than 1% in the group who attended the program compared with 36% in the control group.

Pathological Gambling

Definition and Diagnostic Criteria

Pathological gambling has been considered a distinct diagnostic entity since 1980, when it was first included in DSM-III and similarly in ICD-9-CM (World Health Organization 1978). DSM-IV-TR currently classifies pathological gambling as an ICD not elsewhere classified. The essential feature of pathological gambling is recurrent gambling behavior that is maladaptive (e.g., loss of judgment, excessive gambling) and in which personal, family, or vocational endeavors are disrupted (Table 10–6).

Epidemiology

Prevalence estimates for pathological gambling range from 1% to 3% of the U.S. population (American Psychiatric Association 1994). A U.S. national survey suggested that 68% of the general population participated in some form of gambling and that 0.77% of American adults are considered probable pathological gamblers (Commission on the Review of the National Policy Toward Gambling 1976). Prevalence estimates of probable pathological gambling from state surveys range from 1.2% to 3.4%, with increased rates in states that provide greater opportunity for legal gambling (Commission on the Review of the National Policy Toward Gambling 1976; Volberg 1990; Volberg and Steadman 1988, 1989).

A meta-analysis of 120 published studies indicated that the lifetime prevalence of serious gambling (meeting DSM criteria for pathological gambling) among adults is 1.6% (Shaffer et al. 1999). Among those younger than 18 years, the prevalence is 3.9%, with

---

Table 10–6. DSM-IV-TR diagnostic criteria for pathological gambling

---

A. Persistent and recurrent maladaptive gambling behavior as indicated by five (or more) of the following:

   (1) is preoccupied with gambling (e.g., preoccupied with reliving past gambling experiences, handicapping or planning the next venture, or thinking of ways to get money with which to gamble)

   (2) needs to gamble with increasing amounts of money in order to achieve the desired excitement

   (3) has repeated unsuccessful efforts to control, cut back, or stop gambling

   (4) is restless or irritable when attempting to cut down or stop gambling

   (5) gambles as a way of escaping from problems or of relieving a dysphoric mood (e.g., feelings of helplessness, guilt, anxiety, depression)

   (6) after losing money gambling, often returns another day to get even ("chasing" one's losses)

   (7) lies to family members, therapist, or others to conceal the extent of involvement with gambling

   (8) has committed illegal acts such as forgery, fraud, theft, or embezzlement to finance gambling

   (9) has jeopardized or lost a significant relationship, job, or educational or career opportunity because of gambling

   (10) relies on others to provide money to relieve a desperate financial situation caused by gambling

B. The gambling behavior is not better accounted for by a manic episode.

---

past-year rates for adults and adolescents being 1.1% and 5.8%, respectively (Shaffer and Hall 1996).

Prevalence estimates of pathological gambling in the general population differ from estimates in a treatment-seeking population. In a New York State epidemiological survey, relative to gamblers identified in treatment programs, there were higher rates of pathological or probable pathological gamblers who were female (36% vs. 7%, respectively), younger (<30 years; 38% vs. 18%, respectively), and nonwhite (43% vs. 9%, respectively) (Volberg and Steadman 1988). Female pathological gamblers clearly represent an understudied and underserved group, because they account for approximately one-third of pathological gamblers (Lesieur 1988). Prevalence estimates of pathological gambling among high school students range from 1.7%–3.6% (Ladouceur and Mireault 1988) to as high as 5.7% (Lesieur and Klein 1987).

Comorbidity

The literature to date strongly suggests that three Axis I disorders frequently co-occur with pathological gambling: substance abuse or dependence, affective disorders (i.e., bipolar spectrum disorders), and ADHD (Figure 10–1).

There appears to be a strong relationship between pathological gambling and substance abuse, as evidenced by the high rates of comorbid substance abuse and dependence with pathological gambling (Lesieur 1988; Lesieur et al. 1986; Linden et al. 1986; McCormick et al. 1984). Failure to treat comorbid substance use disorders in gamblers may lead to higher relapse rates (Maccallum and Blaszczynski 2002). Pathological gambling is also highly comorbid with affective disorders among inpatient (McCormick et al. 1984) and outpatient (Linden et al. 1986) samples.

Pathological gambling has been associated with ADHD (Carlton and Goldstein

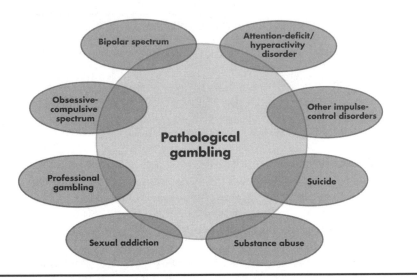

Figure 10–1. Pathological gambling: comorbidity and issues in classification.

Source. Reprinted from Pallanti S, Baldini Rossi N, Hollander E: "Pathological Gambling," in *Clinical Manual of Impulse-Control Disorders.* Edited by Hollander E, Stein DJ. Washington, DC, American Psychiatric Publishing, 2006, pp. 251–289. Copyright 2006, American Psychiatric Publishing. Used with permission.

1987) and has been described as being part of the obsessive-compulsive spectrum and sharing features with both obsessive-compulsive disorder (OCD) and the impulsive cluster of obsessive-compulsive spectrum disorders (Bienvenu et al. 2000; Dell'Osso et al. 2005). Compulsive sexual behavior, compulsive buying disorder, and IED are relatively frequent, as are personality disorders (Taber et al. 1987).

Pathogenesis

There is evidence of serotonergic, noradrenergic, and dopaminergic dysfunction in pathological gambling. Molecular genetic studies in pathological gamblers have also reported findings consistent with the involvement of these neurotransmitter systems, which may play a unique role in the mechanisms that underlie the arousal, behavioral initiation, behavioral disinhibition, and reward or reinforcement evident in pathological gambling, in line with neuropsychological studies showing executive function deficits in pathological gamblers.

Course

The course of pathological gambling tends to be chronic, but the pattern of gambling may be regular or episodic. Chronicity is usually associated with increases in the frequency of gambling and the amount gambled. Gambling may increase during periods of increased stress. Gambling behavior frequently leads to severe personal, familial, financial, social, and occupational impairment.

Psychiatric disorders such as major depression and alcohol or substance abuse and dependence may develop from or be exacerbated by pathological gambling. There is also a mortality risk associated with pathological gambling. Estimates of suicide attempts in pathological gamblers range from 17% to 24% (Ciarrochi and Richardson 1989; Hollander et al. 2000a). One study found that the suicide rate in cities where gambling has been legalized is four times higher than the rate in cities without legal gambling (Phillips et al. 1997). Younger patients are more likely to have suicidal tendencies and major depressive disorders (McCormick et al. 1984).

Because most pathological gamblers begin gambling during adolescence (Hollander et al. 2000a), early identification and intervention are critical.

Gender differences have been described in the course of pathological gambling. In males, the disorder usually begins in adolescence (Hollander et al. 2000a) and may remain undiagnosed for years; male pathological gamblers often present with a 20- to 30-year gambling history, with gradual development of dependence. In contrast, onset of pathological gambling in females is more likely to occur later in life. Prior to their seeking treatment, the duration of pathological gambling in women is approximately 3 years. Thus, as a result of the differences in onset and duration, female pathological gamblers generally have a better prognosis than male pathological gamblers (Rosenthal 1992). Female pathological gamblers also tend to be depressed and may use gambling as an anesthetic, accompanied by excitement, to escape from life's problems (i.e., as in a dissociative state [Jacobs 1988]).

Treatment

There is a relative lack of effective treatments for pathological gambling reported in the literature. The uncontrolled and few controlled treatment studies in the literature, although helpful in providing preliminary direction, are frequently methodologically flawed.

Pharmacotherapy

Currently there are only a few controlled pharmacological treatment studies of pathological gambling, although this is a recently developing area of research. Pharmacological treatment studies of pathological gambling have demonstrated some promising results with the use of serotonin reuptake inhibitors (de la Gandara 1999; Hollander et al. 1992, 1998, 2000b; Kim et al. 2002; Zimmerman et al. 2002), serotonin antagonists (Pallanti et al. 2002a), mood stabilizers (Haller and Hinterhuber 1994; Hollander et al. 2002; Pallanti et al. 2002b), opiate antagonists (Kim et al.

2001), and atypical antipsychotics (Potenza and Chambers 2001). However, some studies have not reported significant findings, primarily due to small samples, high placebo response rates, or high rates of discontinuation (Blanco et al. 2002; Grant et al. 2003).

These data suggest the need for conducting well-designed controlled clinical trials of various pharmacological agents in the treatment of pathological gambling, according to different clinical presentations and comorbidities. Treatment should ultimately target all symptom domains within the individual patient that contribute to compulsive gambling, including common comorbid conditions such as bipolar spectrum disorder, ADHD, and substance abuse/dependence disorders.

Psychotherapy

Treatment modalities for pathological gambling are similar to those of other substance abuse disorders and were created based on the addiction model, such as self-help groups, inpatient treatment programs, and rehabilitation programs. Essential features of any therapeutic intervention for pathological gambling include the need to establish both a therapeutic alliance and network, address the underlying pathology, interrupt the behavior and maintain abstinence, problem-solve, and improve quality of life.

The most popular intervention for problem gambling is Gamblers Anonymous (GA), which is similar to Alcoholics Anonymous and Narcotics Anonymous. However, evidence suggests that GA may not be very effective when used without other treatment modalities (Petry and Armentano 1999). Retrospective studies show a dropout rate of up to 70% within the first year (Stewart and Brown 1988), and overall dropout rates range from 75% to 90% (Moody 1990). Only 8% of GA members report total abstinence at 1-year follow-up and 7% at 2-year follow-up (Brown 1985). Although participation in GA's spousal component, Gam-Anon, may be helpful for some family members, little evidence suggests that it reduces disordered gambling (Petry and Armentano 1999).

Behavioral, cognitive, and combined cognitive-behavioral methods have been used in treating pathological gambling. Aversive therapy has been employed to reach the goal of total abstinence of gambling, as have behavior monitoring, contingency management, contingency contracting, covert sensitization, systematic desensitization, imaginal desensitization, in vivo exposure, imaginal relaxation, psychoeducation, cognitive restructuring, problem-solving skills training, social skills training, and relapse prevention. Use of cognitive restructuring facilitates a decrease in the frequency of gambling and irrational verbalizations associated with gambling (Ladouceur 1990).

Trichotillomania

Definition and Diagnostic Criteria

Trichotillomania is a chronic ICD characterized by repetitive pulling out of one's own hair, resulting in noticeable hair loss. The DSM-IV-TR criteria for trichotillomania are listed in Table 10–7.

Approximately 75% of adult trichotillomania patients report that most of their hair-pulling behavior takes place "automatically" or outside of awareness, whereas the remaining 25% describe themselves as primarily focused on hair pulling when they pull (Christenson and Mackenzie 1994). However, some patients engage in both types of hair pulling. Compared with unfocused hair pullers, the subset who primarily engage in focused hair pulling are more likely to pull hair from the pubic area and to report shame as a result of their hair pulling (du Toit et al. 2001). Some suggest that trichotillomania patients who engage primarily in focused hair pulling are more similar to patients with OCD and may be more responsive to pharmacological interventions found effective for OCD (Christenson and O'Sullivan 1996; du Toit et al.

Table 10–7. DSM-IV-TR diagnostic criteria for trichotillomania

A. Recurrent pulling out of one's hair resulting in noticeable hair loss.

B. An increasing sense of tension immediately before pulling out the hair or when attempting to resist the behavior.

C. Pleasure, gratification, or relief when pulling out the hair.

D. The disturbance is not better accounted for by another mental disorder and is not due to a general medical condition (e.g., a dermatological condition).

E. The disturbance causes clinically significant distress or impairment in social, occupational, or other important areas of functioning.

2001). The issue of trichotillomania subtyping is one of both considerable importance and ongoing debate, and no formal subtyping system incorporating affective correlates of pulling has been advanced.

The few published data on how trichotillomania presents in children and adolescents suggest similarities to adult hair pulling. As with adults, the scalp is the most common pulling site in children and adolescents, followed by eyelashes and eyebrows (Hanna 1997; Reeve 1999).

Epidemiology

Early clinical studies suggested that trichotillomania was extremely rare; however, survey research with nonclinical samples has indicated that hair pulling is more common than originally suggested. In studies involving college samples, 10%–13% of students reported hair pulling, with the prevalence of clinically significant pulling ranging between 1% and 3.5% (Christenson et al. 1991b; Rothbaum et al. 1993). A large epidemiological study of trichotillomania and skin picking using self-report instruments is under way in a large sample of college freshmen (Hajcak et al. 2006). Epidemiological research on trichotillomania is extremely limited both in terms of the number of studies and methodology. One epidemiological survey of 17-year-old adolescents in Israel suggests a prevalence rate of 1% for current or past hair pulling, with fewer reporting noticeable hair loss or distress from these symptoms (King et al. 1995). There is a need for more epidemiological research on trichotillomania.

Comorbidity

Psychiatric comorbidity is quite common among adults with trichotillomania. Christenson et al. (1991a) found that approximately 82% of an adult sample with trichotillomania met criteria for a past or current comorbid Axis I disorder, the most common being affective, anxiety, and addictive disorders. Of the patients with comorbid disorders, there was a lifetime prevalence rate of 65% for mood disorders, 57% for anxiety disorders, 22% for substance abuse disorders, 20% for eating disorders, and 42% for personality disorders. The most frequently cited comorbid personality disorders are histrionic, borderline, and obsessive-compulsive (Christenson et al. 1992; Schlosser et al. 1994; Swedo and Leonard 1992). In a larger sample of adults seeking treatment for trichotillomania, Christenson (1995) found comorbidity rates of 57% for major depression, 27% for generalized anxiety disorder, 20% for eating disorders, 19% for alcohol abuse, and 16% for other substance abuse. In a mixed sample of children, adolescents, and adults with trichotillomania, Swedo and Leonard (1992) found comorbidity rates of 39% for unipolar depression, 32% for generalized anxiety disorder, 16% for OCD, and 15% for substance abuse.

A key debate in the field is whether trichotillomania should be conceptualized as an ICD or a variant of OCD. In support of the classification as an obsessive-compulsive spectrum disorder is the apparent similarity between compulsions and the repetitive and perceived uncontrollable nature of hair pulling and accompanying anxiety relief (Swedo 1993; Swedo and Leonard 1992), the possible selective responsiveness of trichotillomania to serotonin reuptake inhibitors, and the elevated rates of OCD in patients with trichotillomania (Christenson et al. 1991a). Others argue that trichotillomania and OCD are separate diagnoses because trichotillomania is not characterized by persistent intrusive thoughts regarding hair pulling, hair pulling often occurs outside awareness, and the repetitive behavior in trichotillomania is generally limited to hair pulling whereas compulsions in OCD often consist of a variety of anxiety-relieving behaviors. Those with OCD also describe their compulsions as unpleasant but necessary to reduce negative affect (i.e., maintained by negative reinforcement), whereas most subjects with trichotillomania describe hair pulling as pleasurable or satisfying (i.e., maintained by positive reinforcement). Furthermore, OCD patients' age at onset is generally later (Himle et al. 1995; Swedo 1993; Tukel et al. 2001), they report higher levels of overall anxiety (Himle et al. 1995; Tukel et al. 2001), and they have a more restricted range of affective states than trichotillomania patients (Stanley and Cohen 1999). The proposed difference between OCD and trichotillomania has led to the use of disparate cognitive-behavioral strategies for each.

Many authors (e.g., Christenson and Mansueto 1999) have noted similarities among skin picking and severe nail biting as well as common co-occurrence. If the skin picking and nail biting appear to be largely negatively reinforcing—reducing anxiety associated with specific obsessional thoughts and/or reducing the likelihood of feared outcomes—they may be better conceptualized as OCD behaviors. Clinical experience suggests these conditions are much more likely to formally resemble trichotillomania. More research is needed to determine whether they are all one entity or distinct conditions.

Pathogenesis

While experimental and descriptive psychopathology research in trichotillomania is sparse, preliminary data are converging on a tentative biopsychosocial model in which biologically vulnerable individuals become trapped in cycles of hair pulling that are triggered by internal and contextual discriminative cues and subsequently reinforced because the behavior reduces a variety of negative internal stimuli or elicits positive sensations. This cycle persists despite clear negative social and emotional consequences because such consequences are delayed and thus are outweighed by more immediate and salient reinforcers.

Course

Age at onset usually ranges from early childhood to young adulthood. Initial onset after young adulthood is uncommon, but there have been reports of onset as early as 14 months and as late as 61 years. Peak age at onset in children is about age 5–8 years, whereas for patients who present to clinicians in adulthood, the mean age at onset is about 13 years (Rothbaum et al. 1993; Swedo et al. 1989).

Transient periods of hair pulling in early childhood may be considered benign and usually have a self-limited course, with most cases remitting spontaneously by the teenage years. Circumscribed periods of hair pulling (weeks to months) followed by complete remission are common among children. This may be because it usually represents a "habit" without the presence of an obvious precipitant or a transient behavior in response to a psychosocial stressor.

Trichotillomania in adolescents and adults typically follows a chronic course, involves multiple hair sites, and is associated with high rates of psychiatric comorbidity (Christenson et al. 1991a). The chronic course may take one of two patterns: in one, the frequency and severity of hair pulling wax and wane over months, without any true remissions; in the other, episodes are characterized by frequent hair pulling separated by long periods of remission (Moore and Jefferson 2004). Some have continuous symptoms for decades. For others, the disorder may come and go for weeks, months, or years. Sites of hair pulling may vary over time. Progression of the condition seems to be unpredictable.

Treatment

The treatment literature for trichotillomania is generally made up of case studies, with progressively more controlled investigation in recent years. In general, knowledge about trichotillomania treatments is limited by small sample sizes, lack of specificity regarding sample characteristics, nonrandom assignment to treatment, dearth of long-term follow-up data, exclusive reliance on patient self-report measures, and lack of information regarding rates of treatment refusal and dropout. Treatment approaches to trichotillomania have included SSRIs, naltrexone, cognitive-behavioral therapy (CBT), and behavior therapy.

Pharmacotherapy

Of the six randomized, controlled trials evaluating the efficacy of pharmacotherapy conducted to date, five involved serotonin reuptake inhibitors. This may reflect the previously prevailing view that trichotillomania is a variant of OCD and thus ought to be responsive to the same pharmacological agents proven successful in OCD. Interestingly, naltrexone, an opioid antagonist thought to decrease positive reinforcement, has also been found superior to placebo in reducing trichotillomania symptoms (Christenson et al. 1994).

Although no double-blind discontinuation studies have been conducted in trichotillomania, evidence from open studies suggests that treatment response gained from pharmacotherapy may not be maintained in the long run (Iancu et al. 1996; Pollard et al. 1991). The absence of a single randomized, controlled trial in pediatric trichotillomania limits treatment recommendations for this population.

Psychotherapy

With respect to behavioral approaches and CBT, a variety of specific techniques have been applied, including awareness training, self-monitoring, aversion, covert sensitization, negative practice, relaxation training, habit reversal, competing response training, stimulus control, and overcorrection. Although the state of the CBT literature justifies only cautious recommendations, habit reversal, awareness training, and stimulus control are generally purported as the core efficacious interventions for trichotillomania.

Successful outcome has been reported with several of the aforementioned interventions. However, because the vast majority of the literature consists of uncontrolled case reports or small case series, confident conclusions cannot be drawn about the specificity of the observed reductions. The limited and equivocal treatment literature suggests that there is neither a universal nor a complete response to any treatment for trichotillomania. Controlled studies examining the efficacy of CBT treatments involving habit reversal, pharmacotherapy, and their combination are needed.

Conclusion

This chapter has focused on disorders found in the DSM-IV-TR section on ICDs not otherwise classified: IED, kleptomania, pyromania, pathological gambling, and trichotillomania. Nevertheless, pathological impulsivity may be a crucial construct in understanding a broad range of psychiatric disorders, ranging from common psychotic disorders (e.g., bipolar disorder) to a range of conditions that have emerged together with new lifestyles and technologies (e.g., compulsive shopping, Internet addiction). The development of reliable diagnostic criteria for ICDs has been extremely useful in promoting research on these disorders and has provided a basis for epidemiological work demonstrating the prevalence of these disorders, their high comorbidity and morbidity, and their significant social costs. At the same time, advances in basic research on impulsivity and addiction, together with new methods in clinical research, have led to increased understanding of the overlapping neurocircuitry and neurochemistry that may be involved in a range of these conditions, and this in turn may ultimately lead to a revised nosology of these conditions. Developments in psychometrics and psychobiology have in turn encouraged researchers to conduct rigorous randomized clinical trials of a range of medications and psychotherapies in the ICDs, and a number of effective strategies are now available. Nevertheless, the range of clinical trials in this area remains comparatively limited, and for now clinicians are required to adopt a flexible approach that includes multiple modalities of intervention in the management of the ICDs. Although many patients can be helped by such an approach, much further work is needed to delineate fully the psychobiology of these disorders and to develop effective treatments. There is also a need to develop coordinated approaches to the prevention of disorders, such as pathological gambling, which are influenced greatly by the availability of particular facilities or technologies.

Key Points

- Pathological impulsivity is a useful construct in understanding a broad range of psychiatric symptoms and disorders, including the impulse-control disorders (ICDs) not otherwise specified (NOS).

- ICDs are highly prevalent and associated with significant disability and costs but receive disproportionately little attention from clinicians and researchers.

- Ultimately, a better understanding of the psychobiological underpinnings of impulsivity, behavior addiction, and other related constructs may lead to changes in our classification of these disorders.

- Although no medication is registered for the treatment of ICDs, a number of randomized, controlled trials have demonstrated the potential value of pharmacotherapy.

- Current clinical practice also emphasizes the need for a comprehensive approach to management that includes psychotherapy and family intervention. Additional work is needed to improve efficacy.

Suggested Readings

Coccaro E (ed): Aggression: Psychiatric Assessment and Treatment. New York, Informa Healthcare, 2003

Coccaro E: Intermittent explosive disorder. Curr Psychiatry Rep 2:67–71, 2005

Dell'Osso B, Altamura AC, Allen A, et al: Epidemiologic and clinical updates on impulse control disorders: a critical review. Eur Arch Psychiatry Clin Neurosci 256:464–475, 2006

Grant JE, Potenza MN (eds): Pathological Gambling: A Clinical Guide to Treatment. Washington, DC, American Psychiatric Publishing, 2004

Grant JE, Potenza MN: Impulse-control disorders: clinical characteristics and pharmacological management. Ann Clin Psychiatry 16:27–34, 2004

Hollander E, Evers M: New developments in impulsivity. Lancet 358:949–950, 2001

Hollander E, Stein DJ (eds): Impulsivity and Aggression. Sussex, England, Wiley, 1995

Hollander E, Stein DJ (eds): Clinical Manual of Impulse-Control Disorders. Washington, DC, American Psychiatric Publishing, 2006

Stein DJ, Christenson G, Hollander E: Trichotillomania. Washington, DC, American Psychiatric Press, 1999

References

American Psychiatric Association: Diagnostic and Statistical Manual of Mental Disorders, 3rd Edition. Washington, DC, American Psychiatric Association, 1980

American Psychiatric Association: Diagnostic and Statistical Manual of Mental Disorders, 3rd Edition, Revised. Washington, DC, American Psychiatric Association, 1987

American Psychiatric Association: Diagnostic and Statistical Manual of Mental Disorders, 4th Edition. Washington, DC, American Psychiatric Association, 1994

American Psychiatric Association: Diagnostic and Statistical Manual of Mental Disorders, 4th Edition, Text Revision. Washington, DC, American Psychiatric Association, 2000

Barker AF: Arson: A Review of the Psychiatric Literature (Institute of Psychiatry, Maudsley Monographs No 35). Oxford, England, Oxford University Press, 1994

Barnett W, Richter P, Sigmund D, et al: Recidivism and concomitant criminality in pathological firesetters. J Forensic Sci 42:879–883, 1997

Barnett W, Richter P, Renneberg B: Repeated arson: data from criminal records. Forensic Sci Int 101:49–54, 1999

Bayle FJ, Caci H, Millet B, et al: Psychopathology and comorbidity of psychiatric disorders in patients with kleptomania. Am J Psychiatry 160:1509–1513, 2003

Bienvenu OJ, Samuels JF, Riddle MA, et al: The relationship of obsessive-compulsive disorder to possible spectrum disorders: results from a family study. Biol Psychiatry 48:287–293, 2000

Blanco C, Petkova E, Ibanez A, et al: A pilot placebo-controlled study of fluvoxamine for pathological gambling. Ann Clin Psychiatry 14:9–15, 2002

Brown RI: The effectiveness of Gamblers Anonymous, in The Gambling Studies: Proceedings of the 6th National Conference on Gambling and Risk-Taking. Edited by Eadington WR. Reno, University of Nevada, 1985

Bumpass ER, Fagelman FD, Brix RJ: Intervention with children who set fires. Am J Psychother 37:328–345, 1983

Carlton PL, Goldstein L: Physiological determinants of pathological gambling, in A Handbook of Pathological Gambling. Edited by Glaski T. Springfield, IL, Charles C Thomas, 1987, pp 657–663

Christenson GA: Trichotillomania: from prevalence to comorbidity. Psychiatr Times 12:44–48, 1995

Christenson GA, Mackenzie TB: Trichotillomania, in Handbook of Prescriptive Treatments for Adults. Edited by Hersen M, Ammerman RT. New York, Plenum, 1994, pp 217–235

Christenson GA, Mansueto CS: Trichotillomania: descriptive characteristics and phenomenology, in Trichotillomania. Edited by Stein DJ, Christenson GA, Hollander E. Washington, DC, American Psychiatric Press, 1999, pp 1–41

Christenson GA, O'Sullivan RL: Trichotillomania: rational treatment options. CNS Drugs 6:23 34, 1996

Christenson GA, Mackenzie TB, Mitchell JE: Characteristics of 60 adult chronic hair pullers. Am J Psychiatry 148:365–370, 1991a

Christenson GA, Pyle RL, Mitchell JE: Estimated lifetime prevalence of trichotillomania in college students. J Clin Psychol 52:415–417, 1991b

Christenson GA, Chernoff-Clementz E, Clementz BA: Personality and clinical characteristics in patients with trichotillomania. J Clin Psychiatry 53:407–413, 1992

Christenson GA, Crow SJ, Mackenzie TB: A placebo controlled double blind study of naltrexone for trichotillomania. Paper presented at the 147th annual meeting of the American Psychiatric Association, Philadelphia, PA, May 1994

Ciarrochi J, Richardson R: Profile of compulsive gamblers in treatment: update and comparisons. Journal of Gambling Behavior 5:53–65, 1989

Coccaro EF: Intermittent explosive disorder, in Aggression: Psychiatric Assessment and Treatment. Edited by Coccaro EF. New York, Marcel Dekker, 2003, pp 149–166

Coccaro EF, Kavoussi RJ: Fluoxetine and impulsive aggressive behavior in personality disordered subjects. Arch Gen Psychiatry 54:1081–1088, 1997

Coccaro EF, Kavoussi RJ, Berman ME, et al: Intermittent explosive disorder-revised: devel

opment, reliability and validity of research criteria. Compr Psychiatry 39:368–376, 1998

Coccaro EF, Schmidt CA, Samuels JF, et al: Lifetime and 1-month prevalence rates of intermittent explosive disorder in a community sample. J Clin Psychiatry 65:820–824, 2004

Coccaro EF, Posternak MA, Zimmerman M: Prevalence and features of intermittent explosive disorder in a clinical setting. J Clin Psychiatry 66:1221–1227, 2005

Commission on the Review of the National Policy Toward Gambling: Gambling in America. Washington, DC, U.S. Government Printing Office, 1976

de la Gandara JJ: Fluoxetine: open-trial in pathological gambling. Paper presented at the 152nd annual meeting of the American Psychiatric Association, Washington, DC, May 1999

Dell'Osso B, Allen A, Hollander E. Comorbidity issues in the pharmacological treatment of pathological gambling: a critical review. Clin Pract Epidemiol Ment Health 10:1–21, 2005

du Toit PL, van Kradenburg J, Niehaus DHJ, et al: Characteristics and phenomenology of hair-pulling: an exploration of subtypes. Compr Psychiatry 42:247–256, 2001

Franklin GA, Pucci PS, Arbabi S, et al: Decreased juvenile arson and firesetting recidivism after implementation of a multidisciplinary prevention program. J Trauma 53:260–266, 2002

Geller J, Bertsch G: Fire-setting behavior in the histories of a state hospital population. Am J Psychiatry 142:464–468, 1985

Goldman MJ: Kleptomania: making sense of the nonsensical. Am J Psychiatry 148:986–996, 1991

Grant JE: Co-occurrence of personality disorders in persons with kleptomania: a preliminary investigation. J Am Acad Law Psychiatry 34:395–398, 2004

Grant JE, Kim SW: Clinical characteristics and associated psychopathology of 22 patients with kleptomania. Compr Psychiatry 43:378–384, 2002a

Grant JE, Kim SW: An open label study of naltrexone in the treatment of kleptomania. J Clin Psychiatry 63:349–356, 2002b

Grant JE, Kim SW: Comorbidity of impulse-control disorders among pathological gamblers. Acta Psychiatr Scand 108:207–213, 2003

Grant JE, Kim SW, Potenza MN, et al: Paroxetine treatment of pathological gambling: a multi-centre randomized controlled trial. Int Clin Psychopharmacol 18:243–249, 2003

Grant JE, Levine L, Kim D, et al: Impulse-control disorders in adult psychiatric inpatients. Am J Psychiatry 162:2184–2188, 2005

Grodnitzky GR, Tafrate RC: Imaginal exposure for anger reduction in adult outpatients: a pilot study. J Behav Ther Exp Psychiatry 31:259–279, 2000

Hajcak G, Franklin ME, Simons RF, et al: Hair-pulling and skin picking in relation to affective distress and obsessive-compulsive symptoms. J Psychopathol Behav Assess 28:177–185, 2006

Haller R, Hinterhuber H: Treatment of pathological gambling with carbamazepine. Pharmacopsychiatry 27:129, 1994

Hanna GL: Trichotillomania and related disorders in children and adolescents. Child Psychiatry Hum Dev 27:255–268, 1997

Himle JA, Bordnick PS, Thyer BA: A comparison of trichotillomania and obsessive-compulsive disorder. J Psychopathol Behav Assess 17:251–260, 1995

Hollander E: Impulsive and compulsive disorders, in Neuropsychopharmacology: The Fifth Generation of Progress. Edited by Davis K, Charney D, Coyle J, et al. New York, American College of Neuropsychopharmacology, 2002, pp 1591–1757

Hollander E, Frenkel M, DeCaria C, et al: Treatment of pathological gambling with clomipramine (letter). Am J Psychiatry 149:710–711, 1992

Hollander E, DeCaria CM, Mari E, et al: Short-term single-blind fluvoxamine treatment of pathological gambling. Am J Psychiatry 155:1781–1783, 1998

Hollander E, Buchalter AJ, DeCaria CM: Pathological gambling. Psychiatr Clin North Am 23:629–642, 2000a

Hollander E, DeCaria CM, Finkell JN, et al: A randomized double-blind fluvoxamine/placebo crossover trial in pathological gambling. Biol Psychiatry 47:813–817, 2000b

Hollander E, Pallanti S, Baldini Rossi N, et al: Sustained release lithium/placebo treatment response in bipolar spectrum pathological gamblers. Paper presented at the New Clinical Drug Evaluation (NCDEU) Annual Meeting, Boca Raton, FL, June 2002

Huesmann LR, Leonard E, Lefkowitz M, et al: Stability of aggression over time and generations. Dev Psychopathol 20:1120–1134, 1984

Iancu I, Weizman A, Kindler S, et al: Serotonergic drugs in trichotillomania: treatment results in 12 patients. J Nerv Ment Dis 184:641–644, 1996

Jacobs DF: Evidence for a common dissociative-like reaction among addicts. Journal of Gambling Behavior 4:27–37, 1988

Kim SW, Grant JE, Adson DE, et al: Double-blind naltrexone and placebo comparison study in the treatment of pathological gambling. Biol Psychiatry 49:914–921, 2001

Kim SW, Grant JE, Adson DE, et al: A double-blind placebo-controlled study of the efficacy and safety of paroxetine in the treatment of pathological gambling. J Clin Psychiatry 63:501–507, 2002

King RA, Scahill L, Vitulano LA, et al: Childhood trichotillomania: clinical phenomenology, comorbidity, and family genetics. J Am Acad Child Adolesc Psychiatry 34:1451–1459, 1995

Koles MR, Jenson WR: Comprehensive treatment of chronic fire setting in a severely disordered boy. J Behav Ther Exp Psychiatry 16:81–85, 1985

Koson DF, Dvoskin J: Arson: a diagnostic study. Bull Am Acad Psychiatry Law 10:39–49, 1982

Ladouceur R: Cognitive activities among gamblers. Paper presented at the Association for Advancement of Behavior Therapy (AABT) Convention, San Francisco, CA, November 1990

Ladouceur R, Mireault C: Gambling behavior among high school students in the Quebec area. Journal of Gambling Behavior 4:3–12, 1988

Laubichler W, Kuhberger A, Sedlmeier P: "Pyromania" and arson: a psychiatric and criminological data analysis [in German]. Nervenarzt 67:774–780, 1996

Lejoyeux M, Feuché N, Loi S, et al: Study of impulse-control disorders among alcohol-dependent patients. J Clin Psychiatry 40:302–305, 1999

Lejoyeux M, Arbaretaz M, McLoughlin M, et al: Impulse-control disorders and depression. J Nerv Ment Dis 190:310–314, 2002

Lesieur HR: The female pathological gambler, in Gambling Studies: Proceedings of the 7th International Conference on Gambling and Risk-Taking. Edited by Eadington WR. Reno, University of Nevada, 1988, pp 230–258

Lesieur HR, Klein R: Pathological gambling among high school students. Addict Behav 12:129–135, 1987

Lesieur H, Blume S, Zoppa R: Alcoholism, drug abuse, and gambling. Alcohol Clin Exp Res 10:33–38, 1986

Lewis NDC, Yarnell H: Pathological Firesetting (Pyromania) (Nervous and Mental Disease Monograph, No 82). New York, Coolidge Foundation, 1951

Linden RD, Pope HG, Jonas JM: Pathological gambling and major affective disorders: preliminary findings. J Clin Psychiatry 47:201–203, 1986

Links PS, Steiner M, Boiago I, et al: Lithium therapy for borderline patients: preliminary findings. J Personal Disord 4:173–181, 1990

Maccallum F, Blaszczynski A: Pathological gambling and comorbid substance use. Aust N Z J Psychiatry 36:411–415, 2002

Mavromatis M, Lion JR: A primer on pyromania. Dis Nerv Syst 38:954–955, 1977

McCormick RA, Russo AM, Ramirez LF, et al: Affective disorders among pathological gamblers seeking treatment. Am J Psychiatry 141:215–218, 1984

McElroy SL, Hudson JI, Pope HG, et al: Kleptomania: clinical characteristics and associated psychopathology. Psychol Med 21:93–108, 1991a

McElroy SL, Pope HG, Hudson JI, et al: Kleptomania: a report of 20 cases. Am J Psychiatry 148:652–657, 1991b

McElroy SL, Hudson JI, Pope HG, et al: The DSM-III-R impulse-control disorders not elsewhere classified: clinical characteristics and relationship to other psychiatric disorders. Am J Psychiatry 149:318–327, 1992

McElroy SL, Soutullo CA, Beckman DA, et al: DSM-IV intermittent explosive disorder: a report of 27 cases. J Clin Psychiatry 59:203–210, 1998

McGrath P, Marshall PG: A comprehensive treatment program for a fire-setting child. J Behav Ther Exp Psychiatry 10:69–72, 1979

Moody G: Quit Compulsive Gambling. London, Thorsons, 1990

Moore DP, Jefferson JW: Handbook of Medical Psychiatry, 2nd Edition. St. Louis, MO, Mosby, 2004

Pallanti S, Baldini Rossi N, Sood E, et al: Nefazodone treatment of pathological gambling: a prospective open-label controlled trial. J Clin Psychiatry 63:1034–1039, 2002a

Pallanti S, Quercioli L, Sood E, et al: Lithium and valproate treatment of pathological gambling: a randomized single-blind study. J Clin Psychiatry 63:559–564, 2002b

Petry NM, Armentano C: Prevalence, assessment, and treatment of pathological gambling: a review. Psychiatr Serv 50:1021–1027, 1999

Phillips DP, Welty WR, Smith MM: Elevated suicide levels associated with legalized gambling. Suicide Life Threat Behav 27:373–378, 1997

Pollard CA, Ibe IO, Krojanker DN, et al: Clomipramine treatment of trichotillomania: a follow-up report on four cases. J Clin Psychiatry 52:128–130, 1991

Potenza MN, Chambers RA: Schizophrenia and pathological gambling. Am J Psychiatry 158:497–498, 2001

Presta S, Marazziti D, Dell'Osso L, et al: Kleptomania: clinical features and comorbidity in an Italian sample. Compr Psychiatry 43:7–12, 2002

Rasanen P, Hirvenoja R, Hakko H, et al: A portrait of a juvenile arsonist. Forensic Sci Int 73:41–47, 1995

Reeve E: Hair pulling in children and adolescents, in Trichotillomania. Edited by Stein DJ, Christenson GA, Hollander E. Washington, DC, American Psychiatric Press, 1999, pp 201–224

Ritchie EC, Huff TG: Psychiatric aspects of arsonists. J Forensic Sci 44:733–740, 1999

Robins LN, Regier DA: Psychiatric Disorders in America. New York, Free Press, 1991

Rosenthal RJ: Pathological gambling. Psychiatr Ann 22:72–78, 1992

Rothbaum BO, Shaw L, Morris R, et al: Prevalence of trichotillomania in a college freshman population (letter to the editor). J Clin Psychiatry 54:72, 1993

Schlosser S, Black DW, Blum N, et al: The demography, phenomenology, and family history of 22 persons with compulsive hair pulling. Ann Clin Psychiatry 6:147–152, 1994

Shaffer HJ, Hall MN: Estimating the prevalence of adolescent gambling disorders: a quantitative synthesis and guide toward standard gambling nomenclature. J Gambl Stud 12:193–214, 1996

Shaffer HJ, Hall MN, Vanderbilt J: Estimating the prevalence of disordered gambling behavior in the United States and Canada: a research synthesis. Am J Public Health 89:1369–1376, 1999

Soloff PH, George A, Nathan RS, et al: Paradoxical effects of amitriptyline in borderline patients. Am J Psychiatry 143:1603–1605, 1986

Stanley MA, Cohen LJ: Trichotillomania and obsessive-compulsive disorder, in Trichotillomania. Edited by Stein DJ, Christenson GA, Hollander E. Washington, DC, American Psychiatric Press, 1999, pp 225–261

Stewart R, Brown RIF: An outcome study of Gamblers Anonymous. Br J Psychiatry 152:284–288, 1988

Swedo SE: Trichotillomania. Psychiatr Ann 23:402–407, 1993

Swedo SE, Leonard HL: Trichotillomania: an obsessive compulsive spectrum disorder? Psychiatr Clin North Am 15:777–790, 1992

Swedo SE, Leonard HL, Rapoport JL, et al: A double-blind comparison of clomipramine and desipramine in the treatment of trichotillomania hair pulling. N Engl J Med 321:497–501, 1989

Taber JI, McCormick RA, Russo AM, et al: Follow-up of pathological gamblers after treatment. Am J Psychiatry 144:757–761, 1987

Tukel R, Keser V, Karali NT, et al: Comparison of clinical characteristics in trichotillomania and obsessive-compulsive disorder. J Anxiety Disord 15:433–441, 2001

Volberg RA: Estimating the prevalence of pathological gambling in the United States. Paper presented at the 8th International Conference on Risk and Gambling, London, England, August 1990

Volberg RA, Steadman HJ: Refining prevalence estimates of pathological gambling. Am J Psychiatry 145:502–505, 1988

Volberg RA, Steadman HJ: Prevalence estimates of pathological gambling in New Jersey and Maryland. Am J Psychiatry 146:1618–1619, 1989

Wise MG, Tierney JG: Impulse-control disorders not elsewhere classified, in The American Psychiatric Press Textbook of Psychiatry, 3rd Edition. Edited by Hales RE, Yudofsky SC, Talbott JA. Washington, DC, American Psychiatric Press, 1999, pp 773–794

World Health Organization: International Classification of Diseases, 9th Revision, Clinical Modification. Ann Arbor, MI, Commission on Professional and Hospital Activities, 1978

Zimmerman M, Mattia J, Younken S, et al: The prevalence of DSM-IV impulse-control disorders in psychiatric outpatients (NR265), in 1998 New Research Program and Abstracts, American Psychiatric Association 151st Annual Meeting, Toronto, Ontario, Canada, May 30–June 4, 1998

Zimmerman M, Breen RB, Posternak MA: An open-label study of citalopram in the treatment of pathological gambling. J Clin Psychiatry 63:44–48, 2002

11

PERSONALITY DISORDERS

Andrew E. Skodol, M.D.
John G. Gunderson, M.D.

Clinicians frequently encounter patients with personality disorders in both outpatient and inpatient settings. Studies indicate that at least 50% of patients evaluated in clinical settings have a personality disorder (Zimmerman et al. 2005), often comorbid with an Axis I disorder, making personality disorders among the most frequently seen by mental health professionals. Personality disorders are also common in the general population, with an estimated prevalence of about 10% (Torgersen 2009).

Patients with personality disorders are among the most complex and clinically challenging. Some patients intensely desire relationships with others but fearfully avoid them because they anticipate rejection. Others endlessly seek admiration and are engrossed with grandiose fantasies of limitless power, brilliance, or ideal love. Still others have self-concepts so disturbed that they feel they embody evil or do not exist and, consequently, engage in self-mutilation or attempt suicide.

General Considerations

What Is a Personality Disorder?

According to DSM-IV-TR (American Psychiatric Association 2000), personality disorders are patterns of inflexible and maladaptive personality traits and behaviors that cause subjective distress, significant impairment in social or occupational functioning, or both. These patterns deviate markedly from the culturally expected and accepted range and are manifest in two or more of the following areas: cognition, affectivity, control over impulses and need gratification, and ways of relating to others. The maladaptive traits and behaviors are pervasive—that is, they are exhibited across a broad range of contexts and situations rather than in only one specific triggering situation or in response to a particular stimulus or person. Finally, the patterns must have been stably present and enduring since adolescence or early adulthood.

Classification Issues

Since DSM-III (American Psychiatric Association 1980), the personality disorders have been grouped into three clusters: the *odd or eccentric Cluster A* (paranoid, schizoid, and schizotypal); the *dramatic, emotional, or erratic Cluster B* (antisocial, borderline, histrionic, and narcissistic); and the *anxious or fearful Cluster C* (avoidant, dependent, and obsessive-compulsive) (Table 11–1). Although these clusters were originally based on face validity alone, they have since received some empirical support (Sanislow et al. 2002). Nonetheless, these clusters are limited because they are based on descriptive similarities rather than on similarities in etiology or external validators such as familial aggregation or treatment response. Recently, interest in personality disorders in Cluster A has increased because neurobiological abnormalities found in patients with schizotypal personality disorder and in patients with chronic schizophrenia suggest common vulnerabilities as well as factors that protect vulnerable patients from developing frank psychosis (Siever and Davis 2004).

A pressing issue is whether the personality disorders are best classified as dimensions or categories (Widiger and Samuel 2005). Do personality disorders exist along dimensions that reflect extreme variants of general personality functioning, or are they distinct categories that are qualitatively different, and clearly demarcated, from normal personality traits and one another? Categorical diagnoses of personality disorders have been increasingly criticized for a number of reasons. First, excessive diagnostic co-occurrence between personality disorders has been observed in many studies: most patients with personality disorders meet criteria for more than one disorder. Second, there is considerable heterogeneity of features among patients receiving the same diagnosis. Finally, despite the fact that 10 specific personality disorder types are listed in DSM-IV-TR, the residual category of *personality disorder not otherwise specified* may be the most commonly applied in clinical practice (Ver-

heul and Widiger 2004), which suggests inadequate coverage of personality psychopathology by the DSM classification—or else reflects the secondary importance assigned to personality disorders and the inadequate time allotted to accurately diagnose them.

Many different dimensional approaches to personality disorder assessment have been proposed as alternatives to DSM-IV-TR categories (Widiger and Simonsen 2005). The simplest has been to simply transform the categories into dimensions by counting criteria or rating the degree to which patients meet criteria on a continuous scale (Oldham and Skodol 2000). This approach has been shown to increase the strength of the relationship of personality disorder representations with external validators such as functional impairment (Skodol et al. 2005a). Another "person-centered" dimensional approach is the prototype-matching approach proposed by Westen et al. (2006). Using this approach, clinicians rate the degree to which patients meet written descriptions of a prototypical patient with each personality disorder on continuous scales. This approach has also been shown to have clinical utility and is very "clinician friendly." Other dimensional approaches rate pathological personality traits on scales of severity (Livesley and Jackson 2000), whereas still other "spectrum" models attempt to bring together Axis I and Axis II disorders that seem to share fundamental underlying dimensions of psychopathology, such as internalization versus externalization (Krueger et al. 2005) or cognitive/perceptual versus affective disturbances (Siever and Davis 1991).

The most widely used dimensional approaches describe personality according to a number of broad factors and more narrow trait dimensions and assess the degree to which traits are present for a given patient. These may more comprehensively cover both normal and pathological personality traits. Indeed, one of the recent large-scale efforts in personality research has been to describe DSM personality disorder types in terms of dimensions of general personality function-

Table 11–1. DSM-IV-TR personality clusters, specific types, anc their defining clinical features

Cluster	Type	Characteristic features
A (odd or eccentric)		
	Paranoid	Pervasive distrust and suspiciousness of others such that their motives are interpreted as malevolent
	Schizoid	Pervasive pattern of detachment from social relationships and restricted range of expression of emotions in interpersonal settings
	Schizotypal	Pervasive pattern of social and interpersonal deficits marked by acute discomfort wi:h, and reduced capacity for, close relationships as well as by cognitive or perceptual distortions and eccentricities of behavior
B (dramatic, emotional, or erratic)		
	Antisocial	History of conduct disorder before age 15 years; pervasive pattern of disregard for anc violation of the rights of ot:ers; current age at least 18 years
	Borderline	Pervasive pattern of instability of interpersonal relationships, self-image, and affects and marked impulsivity
	Histrionic	Pervasive pattern of excessive emotionality and attention seeking
	Narcissistic	Pervasive pattern of grandiosity (in fantasy or behavior), need for admiration, and lac< of empathy
C (anxious or fearful)		
	Avoidant	Pervasive pattern of social inhibition, feelings of inadequacy, and hypersensitivity to negative evaluation
	Dependent	Pervasive and excessive need to be taken care of that leads to submissive and clinging behavior and fears of separation
	Obsessive-compulsive	Pervasive pattern of preoccupation with orderliness, perfectionism, and mental and interpersonal control at the expense of flexibility, openness, and efficiency

Source. Adapted from American Psychiatric Association 2000.

ing (Widiger 2000). Of special significance are the widely heralded "Big Five" dimensions of the Five-Factor Model of Personality: neuroticism, extraversion, openness, agreeableness, and conscientiousness. Cloninger's seven-dimension psychobiological model of temperament and character (Cloninger et al. 1993), which was theoretically linked to abnormalities in specific neurotransmitter systems, has generated a large body of research, but the data have generally not supported these neurobiological hypotheses (Paris 2005).

Dimensional models vary in the empirical support each has received. The broad domains of most trait-based models can be integrated, however, into a common structure consisting of four basic personality dimensions: 1) extraversion versus introversion, 2) antagonism versus compliance, 3) constraint versus impulsivity, and 4) emotional dysregulation versus emotional stability (Markon et al. 2005; Widiger and Mullins-Sweatt 2005). Furthermore, the genetic and phenotypic structure of the basic traits delineating personality disorders has been shown to be consistent (Livesley et al. 1998). Dimensional approaches are, nonetheless, unfamiliar to those trained in a medical model of diagnosis; are complex to use (up to 30 dimensions to describe personality by the facets of the Five-Factor Model); and have limited empirical data to support their utility for clinical decision making (First et al. 2004; Verheul 2005). Given that clinicians already overlook personality disorders in their diagnostic assessments (Zimmerman and Mattia 1999), it seems unlikely that they would embrace a more demanding assessment model.

The categorical model, in contrast, better reflects how clinicians think—that is, in terms of pathological syndromes that a person either has or does not have. The use of categories also makes it possible for clinicians to summarize patients' difficulties succinctly and facilitates communication about them. Although DSM-IV-TR is based primarily on the categorical model, it also incorporates a dimensional approach to a limited extent in that it encourages clinicians to identify problematic personality traits that are subthreshold for any particular diagnosis.

In 2007, a Personality and Personality Disorders Work Group was appointed to consider the future of personality disorder assessment and classification in DSM-V. Key questions were articulated to inform potential revisions: what is the core definition of a personality disorder that distinguishes it from other types of psychopathology; is personality psychopathology better described by dimensional representations of diagnostic categories or by extremes on dimensions of general personality functioning than by the categories themselves; is a separate Axis II for personality assessment valuable; and what is the clinical importance (for risk, treatment, or prognosis) of assessing personality or personality disorders in other diagnostic domains, such as mood, anxiety, substance use, or eating disorders?

The current proposal under consideration for the DSM-V assessment of personality and personality disorders consists of five parts: 1) an overall rating of personality (self and interpersonal) functioning ranging from normal to severely impaired; 2) prototype descriptions of major personality (disorder) types; 3) personality trait assessment, on which the prototypes are based, but which can also be used to describe major personality characteristics of patients who either do not have a personality disorder or have a personality disorder that does not conform to one of the prototypes; 4) generic criteria for personality disorder consisting of severe deficits in self differentiation and integration and in the capacity for interpersonal relatedness; and 5) measures of adaptive functioning (Skodol and Bender 2009).

Assessment Issues and Methods

The assessment of Axis II disorders is in some ways more complex than that of Axis I disorders. It can be difficult to assess multiple domains of experience and behavior (i.e., cognition, affect, impulse control, and interpersonal interactions) and to determine that traits are distressing or impairing, of early onset, pervasive, and sufficiently enduring (Skodol 2005). Nonetheless, a personality disorder assessment is essential to the comprehensive evaluation and adequate treatment of all patients.

Comprehensiveness of Evaluation

A skilled clinical interview is the mainstay of personality disorder diagnosis and requires the clinician to be familiar with DSM criteria, take a longitudinal view, and use multiple sources of information. However, because an open-ended approach may provide insufficient information to assess all Axis II disorders, the addition of a self-report or semistructured (i.e., interviewer-administered) personality disorder assessment instrument may be used to augment a clinical interview (Kaye and Shea 2000; McDermut and Zimmerman 2005). Such instruments systematically assess each personality disorder criterion with standard questions or probes. Although self-report instruments have the advantage of saving interviewer time and being free of interviewer bias, they often yield false-positive diagnoses and allow contamination of Axis II traits by Axis I states. Semistructured interviews—which require the interviewer to use certain questions, but allow further probing—facilitate accurate diagnosis in several ways: they ensure coverage of relevant domains of personality psychopathology, allow the interviewer to attempt to differentiate Axis II traits from Axis I states, encourage clarification of contradictions or ambiguities in the patient's response, and provide the opportunity to determine that traits are pervasive (i.e., by eliciting multiple examples of trait expression) rather than limited to a specific situation.

Nonetheless, even with the use of a semistructured interview, the interviewer must use his or her judgment. For example, is a given

trait present in enough situations to be considered pervasive? How extreme/severe must the trait be, and how much distress or impairment is necessary to consider the criterion present? Is a given characteristic a personality trait or a symptom of an Axis I disorder (i.e., a mental state secondary to depression or substance abuse, for example)?

Ego-Syntonic Traits

Some patients are unaware of the traits that reflect their disorder or may not perceive them as problematic. This limited self-awareness can interfere with personality disorder assessment, especially if the questions asked have negative or unflattering implications. This problem can be reduced by the use of multiple sources of information (e.g., medical records and informants who know the patient well). Still, because studies have shown low concordance rates between patient-based and informant-based interviews (Klonsky et al. 2002), interviewers will also need to rely on their personal experience with the patient to reach a conclusion (Westen 1997). Which source of information—the patient, the informant, or the interviewer's firsthand experience with the patient—is most useful for a specific clinical purpose, such as choosing a treatment or predicting outcome, has yet to be definitively determined.

State Versus Trait

The presence of an Axis I disorder can complicate the assessment of Axis II traits. For example, a person with social withdrawal, low self-esteem, and lack of motivation or energy due to major depression might appear to have avoidant or dependent personality disorder, when in fact these features reflect the Axis I condition. A hypomanic person with symptoms of grandiosity or hypersexuality might appear narcissistic or histrionic. In some cases, assessment of Axis II disorders may need to wait until the Axis I condition, such as severe depression or a manic episode, has subsided. However, the clinician can often differentiate personality traits from

Axis I states during an Axis I episode by asking the patient to describe his or her usual personality at times not in an Axis I episode; the use of informants who have observed the patient over time with and without an Axis I disorder can also be helpful. Systematic assessment of Axis I conditions before turning attention to Axis II is invaluable in alerting the clinician to which Axis II traits will need particularly careful assessment.

Medical Illness Versus Trait

Similarly, the interviewer must ascertain that apparent personality traits are not symptoms of a medical illness. For example, aggressive outbursts caused by a seizure disorder should not be attributed to borderline or antisocial personality disorder, nor should the unusual perceptual experiences that can accompany temporal lobe epilepsy be attributed to schizotypal personality disorder. A medical evaluation should be included if a medical causation is suspected.

Situation Versus Trait

The interviewer should also determine that personality disorder features are pervasive—that is, not limited to only one situation or occurring in response to only one specific trigger or person. Similarly, personality traits should be relatively enduring rather than transient. Asking the patient for behavioral examples of the expression of traits can help determine that the trait is indeed present in a wide variety of situations and is expressed in many relationships. Specific behaviors, such as suicidal or other self-destructive behaviors, may only be evident at specific times or in specific situations, but the trait of impulsivity should be more persistent.

Sex and Cultural Bias

Although most research suggests that existing personality disorder criteria are relatively free of sex bias (Morey et al. 2005), interviewers can unknowingly allow such bias to affect their assessments. It is important, for example, that histrionic, borderline, and dependent personality disorders be assessed as carefully in men as in women and that obsessive-compulsive, antisocial, and narcissistic personality disorders be assessed as carefully in women as in men. Interviewers should also be careful to avoid cultural bias when diagnosing personality disorders, especially when evaluating such traits as diffidence, passivity, emotionality, suspiciousness, or recklessness; emphasis on work and productivity; or unusual beliefs and rituals that may reflect different norms in different cultures (Alarcon 2005).

Diagnosis of Personality Disorders in Children and Adolescents

Because the personalities of children and adolescents are still developing, personality disorders should be diagnosed with care in this age group. Although children and early adolescents frequently manifest significant personality disorder characteristics (Johnson et al. 2000), it is often preferable to defer diagnoses until early adulthood, at which time a personality disorder diagnosis may be appropriate if the features appear to be pervasive, stable, and likely to be enduring. Early diagnosis may prove to be wrong as stage-specific difficulties of adolescence resolve and as the person matures (Cohen and Crawford 2005). A meta-analysis of 152 longitudinal studies of personality traits showed that change was the rule up until about the age of 22 (Roberts and DelVecchio 2000). Nonetheless, adolescents with high levels of personality psychopathology are at greater risk for developing personality disorders in early adulthood (Kasen et al. 1999).

Clinical Significance of Personality Disorders

By definition, personality disorders cause significant problems for those who have them. Persons with these disorders often suffer, and their relationships with others are typically problematic. They have difficulty responding flexibly and adaptively to the environment and to the changes and demands of life, and they lack resilience when under stress. Instead, their usual ways of responding tend to perpetuate and intensify their difficulties. However, these individuals may blame others for their difficulties or even deny that they have any problems at all.

A number of studies have compared patients with personality disorders with patients with no personality disorder or with Axis I disorders and have found that patients with personality disorders were more likely to be separated, divorced, or never married and to have had more unemployment, frequent job changes, or periods of disability. Studies that have examined quality of functioning found poorer social functioning or interpersonal relationships and poorer work functioning or occupational achievement and satisfaction. Among the different personality disorders, those with severe types, such as schizotypal and borderline, have been found to have significantly more impairment at work, in social relationships, and at leisure than patients with less severe types, such as obsessive-compulsive, or with an impairing Axis I disorder, such as major depressive disorder in the absence of personality disorder. Even the less impaired patients with personality disorders (e.g., obsessive-compulsive), however, have moderate to severe impairment in at least one area of functioning (or a Global Assessment of Functioning rating of 60 or less) (Skodol et al. 2002). Thus, patients with specific personality disorders differ from each other not only in the degree of associated functional impairment but also in the breadth of impairment across functional domains.

Impairment in functioning in patients with personality disorders tends to be persistent even beyond apparent improvement in personality disorder psychopathology itself (Seivewright et al. 2004; Skodol et al. 2005b). The persistence of impairment is understandable because personality disorder psychopathology has usually been relatively long-standing and therefore has disrupted a person's work and social development over a period of time (Roberts et al. 2003).

Personality disorders also often cause problems for others and are costly to society. They are associated with elevated rates of separation, divorce, conflict with family members and romantic partners, child custody proceedings, homelessness, high-risk sexual behavior, and perpetration of child abuse. Those with personality disorders also have increased rates of accidents; police contacts; emergency department visits; medical hospitalization and treatment utilization; violence and criminal behavior, including homicide; self-injurious behavior; attempted suicide; and completed suicide. A high percentage of individuals with criminal convictions, alcoholism, and drug abuse have a personality disorder.

Finally, personality disorders should be identified because of their treatment implications. Personality disorders often need to be a focus of treatment or, at the very least, need to be taken into account when comorbid Axis I disorders are treated, because their presence often affects an Axis I disorder's prognosis and treatment response. For example, patients with depressive disorders, bipolar disorder, panic disorder, obsessive-compulsive disorder, and substance abuse often respond less well to pharmacotherapy when they have a comorbid personality disorder. The presence of a comorbid personality disorder is also associated with poor compliance with pharmacotherapy. Furthermore, personality disorders have been shown to predict the development and relapse of major depression (Johnson et al. 2005b), and individuals with a personality disorder are less likely to remit from major depression (Grilo et al. 2005), bipolar disorder (Dunayevich et al. 2000), and generalized anxiety disorder (Yonkers et al. 2000). As most clinicians are well aware, the characteristics of patients with personality disorders are likely to be manifested in the treatment relationship regardless of whether the personality disorder is the focus of treatment. For example, some patients may be overly dependent on the clinician, others may not follow treatment recommendations, and still others may experience significant conflict about getting well. Although individuals with personality disorders tend to use psychiatric services extensively (Bender et al. 2001), they are more likely to be dissatisfied with the treatment they receive (Kent et al. 1995).

Etiology and Pathogenesis

What causes personality disorders remains the central and most challenging question relevant to this group of complex disorders. As is the case with other psychiatric disorders, the answer is not likely to be simple. All available data suggest that personality disorders (as well as normal personality traits) result from a complex combination of, and interactions between, temperament (genetic and other biological contributions) and psychological (developmental or environmental) factors. Although the degree to which genetic and environmental factors contribute to etiology may vary for different personality disorders, twin studies show that both factors are important in all of these disorders (Kendler et al. 2008; Reichborn-Kjennerud et al. 2006; Torgersen et al. 2000). Of relevance, too, are studies showing that approximately half of the observed variance in personality traits such as neuroticism, introversion, callousness, and even identity problems can be traced to genetic variation (Carey and DiLalla 1994; Jang et al. 1996).

Investigation of the underlying neurobiology of personality disorders is rapidly increasing. A growing body of evidence supports the importance of various neurobiological abnormalities in persons with personality disorders.

Increasing numbers of studies of environmental antecedents of personality disorders, such as family environment and sexual and/or physical abuse, are substantiating a likely role for such factors in the development of certain disorders, particularly borderline personality disorder (Zanarini 1997). Of note has been the growing literature on the relationship of disturbed early attach-

ment to later development of personality disorders (Fonagy et al. 2007; Schore 2002). Research in these areas is expected to continue to increase rapidly. In addition to providing information about the origins of the personality disorders, such investigations are expected to open new avenues for treating these often difficult-to-treat patients.

Treatment

Personality disorders have been thought to consist of deeply ingrained attitudes and behavior patterns that consolidate during development, have endured since early adulthood, and are very resistant to change. Moreover, as noted previously, treatment efforts are further confounded by the degree to which patients with personality disorders do not recognize their maladaptive personality traits as undesirable or in need of change. Despite this general wariness about the treatability of patients with personality disorders, increasing evidence has accumulated from longitudinal studies that personality disorders are quite variable in their course (Grilo and McGlashan 2005) and much more malleable and treatable than had been thought (Leichsenring and Leibing 2003).

Psychoanalysts pioneered the notion that persons with personality disorders could respond to treatment. Seminal contributions from Wilhem Reich (1949) and Maxwell Jones (1953) illustrated that patients with personality disorders needed to first learn to identify how their ego-syntonic traits were maladaptive—that is, how those traits contributed to creating the problems that patients perceived as originating from outside of themselves—and that in order for patients to do this, therapists or group therapy participants needed to challenge or confront patients, often repeatedly. This general principle was subsequently adopted by other forms of sociotherapy, notably those within hospital milieus and in family therapies.

Families or couples may present complications because the designated patient's disordered interpersonal and behavioral patterns may serve functions for, or be complementary to, the disordered patterns of persons with whom the patient is closely associated. For example, a dependent person is apt to bond with an overly authoritarian partner, or an emotionally constricted and obsessional person may find an emotionally expressive, hysterical person particularly attractive. Under these circumstances, treatment is primarily directed not at confronting the maladaptive aspects of one person's character traits but rather at identifying the ways in which these aspects may be welcomed and reinforced in one relationship but maladaptive and impairing in others (Sholevar 2005).

Significant developments in the treatment of personality disorders include the use of multiple modalities, the growth of an empirical base of the results of treatment studies, and greater optimism about treatment effectiveness. Reviews of psychotherapy outcome studies, including psychodynamic/interpersonal, cognitive-behavioral, mixed, and supportive therapies, have found that psychotherapy was associated with a significantly faster rate of recovery compared with the natural course of personality disorders (Leichsenring and Leibing 2003; Perry et al. 1999). Therapeutic nihilism has yielded to widespread but very inconsistent use of the spectrum of potentially valuable treatment modalities.

A significant development has been the emergence of cognitive-behavioral strategies, which are generally more focused and structured than those used in psychodynamic therapies. Cognitive strategies involve identifying specific internal mental schemes by which patients typically misunderstand certain situations or misrepresent themselves and then learning how to modify those internal schemes (Beck et al. 2004; Young et al. 2003). Cognitive therapy for personality disorders is more complicated than that for most Axis I disorders because of the unique challenges (e.g., cognitive and affective avoidance, lack of psychological flexibility, pervasiveness of problems, and ambivalence about

having problems and getting treatment for them) that character pathology presents. Behavioral strategies involve efforts to diminish traits such as impulsivity or to increase assertiveness by using relaxation techniques, role-playing exercises, and other behavioral techniques.

Although psychotherapy remains the mainstay of personality disorder treatment, the utility of pharmacotherapy has begun to be explored as biological dimensions of personality psychopathology are identified. For example, research has increasingly suggested that impulsivity and aggression may respond to serotonergic medications; mood instability and lability may respond to serotonergic or dopaminergic medications; and psychotic-like experiences may respond to antipsychotics (Soloff 2005).

A clinically oriented overview of each DSM-IV-TR personality disorder follows. These descriptions, based on clinical tradition, have also been informed by the growing body of empirically based knowledge. This research has focused on many different aspects of personality disorders, such as their descriptive features, family history, course, treatment response, and etiology.

Specific Personality Disorders

Paranoid Personality Disorder

Epidemiology

The median prevalence of paranoid personality disorder in 12 general population studies was 1.7% (Torgersen 2009). Whether it is more common among men than among women is uncertain (Grant et al. 2004; Zimmerman and Coryell 1990).

Clinical Features

Persons with paranoid personality disorder have a pervasive, persistent, and inappropriate mistrust of others. They are suspicious of others' motives and assume that others intend to exploit, harm, or deceive them. Thus, they may question, without justification, the loyalty or trustworthiness of friends or romantic partners, and they are reluctant to confide in others for fear the information will be used against them. Persons with paranoid personality disorder appear guarded, tense, and hypervigilant, and they frequently scan their environments for clues of possible attack, deception, or betrayal. They often find "evidence" of such malevolence by misinterpreting benign events (such as a glance in their direction) as demeaning or threatening. In response to perceived or actual insults or betrayals, these individuals overreact quickly, becoming excessively angry and responding with counterattacking behavior. They are unable to forgive or forget such incidents and instead bear long-term grudges against their supposed betrayers; some persons with paranoid personality disorder are extremely litigious. Whereas individuals with this disorder can appear quietly and tensely aloof and hostile, others are overtly angry and combative. Persons with this disorder are usually socially isolated and, because of their paranoia, often have difficulties with bosses and co-workers.

Differential Diagnosis

Unlike paranoid personality disorder, the Axis I disorders *paranoid schizophrenia* and *delusional disorder, persecutory type*, are both characterized by prominent and persistent paranoid delusions of psychotic proportions; paranoid schizophrenia is also accompanied by hallucinations and other core symptoms of schizophrenia. The hypervigilance and feelings of threat or danger seen in posttraumatic stress disorder (PTSD) and the fearfulness and social avoidance of social phobia may resemble symptoms of paranoid personality disorder. In PTSD, the symptoms are in reaction to a severely stressful event. In social phobia, the fear is of humiliation or embarrassment rather than of exploitation, harm, or deceit. Although paranoid and schizotypal personality disorders both involve suspiciousness, paranoid personality

disorder does not include magical thinking, perceptual distortions, or odd thinking or speech. Borderline personality disorder may include transient, stress-related paranoid ideation, but not the pervasive and persistent distrust or suspiciousness of paranoid personality disorder. The jealousy and envy of narcissistic personality disorder may be confused or overlap with the pathology of paranoid personality disorder.

Etiology

Paranoid personality disorder is among the least studied personality disorders. Negative childhood experiences, including physical, sexual, and emotional abuse, have been strongly associated with paranoid personality disorder (Bierer et al. 2003).

Family history studies have found a greater morbid risk of paranoid personality disorder in the first-degree relatives of delusional disorder probands than in relatives of probands with schizophrenia or medical illness (Kendler and Gruenberg 1982). Several studies have found paranoid personality disorder in the relatives of probands with schizophrenia (Kendler et al. 1993, 1995), but others have not (Webb and Levinson 1993). The estimated heritability of paranoid personality disorder was 0.28 in a twin study using a clinical sample (Torgersen et al. 2000) and 0.21–0.66 in a twin study using a population-based sample (Kendler et al. 2006). Heritability estimates were higher when self-report rather than interviewer assessments were made (Kendler et al. 2006).

Treatment

Because they mistrust others, persons with paranoid personality disorder usually avoid psychiatric treatment. If they do seek treatment, the therapist immediately encounters the challenge of engaging them and keeping them in treatment. This can best be accomplished by maintaining an unusually respectful, straightforward, and unintrusive style aimed at building trust. If a rupture develops in the treatment relationship—for example, the patient accuses the therapist of some fault—it is best simply to offer a straightforward apology, if warranted, rather than to respond evasively or defensively. It is also best to avoid an overly warm style, because excessive warmth and expression of interest can intensify the patient's thoughts about the therapist's motives (Appelbaum 2005). A supportive individual psychotherapy that incorporates such approaches may be the best treatment for these patients (Gabbard 2000).

Although group treatment or cognitive-behavioral treatment aimed at anxiety management and the development of social skills can occasionally be of benefit, these patients tend to resist such approaches because of their suspiciousness, hypersensitivity to criticism, and misinterpretation of others' comments (Piper and Ogrodniczuk 2005).

Although seldom studied, antipsychotic medications may be sometimes useful in the treatment of paranoid personality disorder. Patients may view such treatment with mistrust; however, these medications are more clearly indicated in the treatment of the overtly psychotic decompensations that these patients sometimes experience.

Schizoid Personality Disorder

Epidemiology

Schizoid personality disorder is one of the rarest personality disorders, occurring in less than 1% of the general population (Torgersen 2009). Schizoid personality disorder is more common among men than women (Torgersen et al. 2001; Zimmerman and Coryell 1990).

Clinical Features

Schizoid personality disorder is characterized by a profound defect in the ability to relate to others in a meaningful way. Persons with this disorder have little or no desire for relationships with others and, as a result, are extremely socially isolated. They prefer to engage in solitary, often intellectual, activities, such as computer games or puzzles, and they often create an elaborate fantasy world that they retreat into and that substitutes for relationships with real people. As a result of their lack of interest in relationships, they have few or no close friends or confidants. They date infrequently, seldom marry, and have little interest in sex, and they often work at jobs requiring little interpersonal interaction (e.g., as a night watchman). These individuals are also notable for their lack of emotional expression or affect. They usually appear cold, detached, aloof, and constricted, and they have particular discomfort with warm feelings. Few, if any, activities or experiences give them pleasure, resulting in chronic anhedonia.

Differential Diagnosis

Schizoid personality disorder shares the features of social isolation and restricted emotional expression with schizotypal personality disorder, but it lacks the latter disorder's characteristic cognitive and perceptual distortions. Unlike individuals with avoidant personality disorder, who intensely desire relationships but avoid them because of exaggerated fears of rejection, persons with schizoid personality disorder have little or no apparent interest in developing relationships with others. Schizoid individuals can be distinguished from those with paranoid personality disorder by the lack of suspiciousness and mistrust. They can be differentiated from milder forms of autistic disorder or Asperger's disorder by the more severely impaired social interactions and stereotyped behavior and interests seen in the latter.

Etiology

Schizoid personality disorder has rarely been studied. There is reason to believe that constitutional factors contribute to the childhood pattern of shyness that often precedes the disorder. Introversion (intimacy problems, inhibition), which characterizes schizoid (as well as avoidant and schizotypal) personality disorder, appears to be substantially heritable (DiLalla et al. 1996). Prenatal exposure to famine has also been shown to increase the risk for schizoid personality disorder, suggesting a role for environmental factors very early in development (Hoek et al. 1996). The heritability of schizoid personality disorder has been estimated as 0.28 (Torgersen et al. 2000) and 0.29 (Kendler et al. 2006) in two Norwegian twin studies.

Treatment

Persons with schizoid personality disorder, like those with paranoid personality disorder, rarely seek treatment. They do not perceive the formation of any relationship—including a therapeutic relationship—as potentially valuable or beneficial. They may, however, occasionally seek treatment for an associated problem, such as depression, or they may be brought for treatment by others. Whereas some patients can tolerate only a supportive therapy or treatment aimed at the resolution of a crisis or associated Axis I disorder, others may actually do well with insight-oriented psychotherapy aimed at bringing about a basic shift in their comfort with intimacy and affects.

Development of a therapeutic alliance may be difficult and can be facilitated by an interested and caring attitude to address the possibility of underlying neediness (Bender 2005) and by avoidance of early interpretation or confrontation. Some authors have suggested the use of so-called inanimate bridges, such as writing and artistic productions, to ease the patient into a therapy relationship. Incorporation of cognitive-behavioral approaches that encourage gradually increasing social involvement may be of value (Beck et al. 2004). Although many patients may be unwilling to participate in a group, group therapy may also facilitate the development of social skills and relationships (Piper and Ogrodniczuk 2005).

Schizotypal Personality Disorder

Epidemiology

Schizotypal personality disorder occurs in less than 1% of the general population (Torg-ersen 2009). Unlike the other two Cluster A personality disorders, no gender difference in prevalence has been found for this disorder (Torgersen et al. 2001; Zimmerman and Coryell 1990).

Clinical Features

Schizotypal personality disorder, like schizophrenia, is characterized by positive, psychotic-like symptoms and negative, deficit-like symptoms. Persons with schizotypal personality disorder experience cognitive or perceptual distortions (positive), behave in an eccentric manner, and are socially withdrawn and anxious (negative). Common cognitive and perceptual distortions include ideas of reference, bodily illusions, and unusual telepathic and clairvoyant experiences. These distortions, which are inconsistent with subcultural norms, occur frequently and are an important and pervasive component of the person's experience. They help explain the odd and eccentric behavior characteristic of this disorder. Individuals with schizotypal personality disorder may, for example, talk to themselves in public, gesture for no apparent reason, or dress in a peculiar or unkempt fashion. Their speech is often odd and idiosyncratic—for example, unusually circumstantial, metaphorical, or vague—and their affect is constricted or inappropriate. Such a person may, for example, laugh inappropriately when discussing his or her problems.

Persons with schizotypal personality disorder are socially uncomfortable and isolated, with few friends. This isolation is often due to their eccentric cognitions and behavior, as well as their lack of desire for relationships, which stems in part from their suspiciousness of others. If they develop relationships, they tend to remain distant or may end them because of their persistent social anxiety and paranoia.

Differential Diagnosis

Schizotypal personality disorder shares the feature of suspiciousness with paranoid personality disorder and that of social isolation with schizoid personality disorder, but the latter two disorders lack the markedly peculiar behavior and significant cognitive and perceptual distortions typical of schizotypal personality disorder. The symptoms of schizotypal personality disorder appear to be attenuated versions of the symptoms of schizophrenia, but enduring periods of overt psychosis and social deterioration over time are not characteristic.

Etiology

Schizotypal personality disorder is considered a schizophrenia spectrum disorder—that is, related to Axis I schizophrenia (Siever and Davis 2004). Phenomenological as well as genetic, biological, treatment, and outcome data support this link. For example, family history studies show an increased risk for schizophrenia-related disorders in relatives of schizotypal probands and, conversely, an increased risk for schizotypal personality disorder in relatives of probands with schizophrenia (Kendler et al. 1993; Torgersen et al. 1993). Both the positive and the negative components of schizotypal personality are moderately heritable (Linney et al. 2003), although only the deficit symptoms may be genetically related to schizophrenia (Fanous et al. 2001; Torgersen et al. 2002). In addition, at least some forms of schizotypal personality disorder involve abnormalities of brain structure, physiology, chemistry, and functioning characteristic of schizophrenia. Because of this evidence, the *International Statistical Classification of Diseases and Related Health Problems*, 10th Revision (ICD-10; World Health Organization 2006) classifies schizotypal personality disorder with schizophrenia rather than with the personality disorders. Differences between the disorders also exist, however, particularly with respect to frontal lobe structure and functioning, which may account for the absence of overt psychosis in schizotypal patients (Suzuki et al. 2005). Genetic or environ-mental factors that promote greater frontal lobe capacity and reduced striatal dopaminergic reactivity might protect persons with schizotypal personality disorder from developing psychosis and the severe social and cognitive deterioration of chronic schizophrenia (Siever and Davis 2004).

Treatment

Because they are socially anxious and somewhat paranoid, persons with schizotypal personality disorder usually avoid psychiatric treatment. They may, however, seek such treatment—or be brought for treatment by concerned family members—when they become depressed or overtly psychotic. As with patients with paranoid personality disorder, it is difficult to establish an alliance with schizotypal patients, and they are unlikely to tolerate exploratory techniques that emphasize interpretation or confrontation. A supportive relationship that counters cognitive distortions and ego-boundary problems may be useful (Stone 1985). This may involve an educational approach that fosters the development of social skills or encourages risk-taking behavior in social situations or, if these efforts fail, encourages the development of activities with less social involvement. If the patient is willing to participate, cognitive-behavioral therapy and highly structured educational groups with a social skills focus may also be helpful.

Several studies support the usefulness of low-dosage antipsychotic medications in the treatment of schizotypal personality disorder, including atypical antipsychotics such as risperidone (double-blind, placebo-controlled study; Koenigsberg et al. 2003) and olanzapine (Keshavan et al. 2004). These medications may ameliorate the anxiety and psychotic-like features associated with this disorder, and they are particularly indicated in the treatment of the more overt psychotic decompensations that these patients can experience.

Antisocial Personality Disorder

Epidemiology

Antisocial personality disorder occurs in about 1.1% of the general population (Torgersen 2009). It is much more common among men than women (Torgersen et al. 2001; Zimmerman and Coryell 1989).

Clinical Features

The central feature of antisocial personality disorder is a long-standing pattern of socially irresponsible behaviors that reflects a disregard for the rights of others. Many persons with this disorder engage in repeated unlawful acts. The more prevailing personality characteristics include a lack of interest in or concern for the feelings of others, deceitfulness, and, most notably, a lack of remorse for the harm they may cause others. These characteristics generally make antisocial individuals fail in roles requiring fidelity (e.g., as a spouse), honesty (e.g., as an employee), or reliability (e.g., as a parent). Some antisocial persons possess a glibness and charm that can be used to seduce, outwit, and exploit others. Although most antisocial persons are indifferent to their effects on others, a notable subgroup takes sadistic pleasure in doing harm (Stone 2005). Recent research has demonstrated that psychopathy is multidimensional and that each dimension may have distinct developmental trajectories (Edens et al. 2006) and may be variants of normal personality traits and behaviors (Hare and Neumann 2005). Antisocial personality syndromes are associated with high rates of substance abuse (Compton et al. 2005), which may contribute to the persistence of antisocial behavior over time (Malone et al. 2004).

Differential Diagnosis

The primary differential diagnostic issue involves narcissistic personality disorder. Indeed, these two disorders may be variants of the same basic type of psychopathology (Hare et al. 1991). However, the antisocial person, unlike the narcissistic person, is likely to be reckless and impulsive. In addition, narcissistic individuals' exploitiveness and disregard for others are attributable to their sense of uniqueness and superiority rather than to a desire for materialistic gains.

Etiology

Twin and adoption studies indicate that genetic factors predispose to the development of antisocial personality disorder (Grove et al. 1990; Lyons et al. 1995). Nonetheless, it is unclear how much variance is accounted for by genetic factors and whether the nature of the predisposition is relatively specific or is best conceptualized in terms of relatively nonspecific traits such as impulsivity, excitability, or hostility. Conduct problems (56%), stimulus seeking (40%), and callousness (56%) are antisocial traits that have substantial heritability (Jang et al. 1996). Psychopathic traits of fearless dominance and impulsive antisociality also show significant genetic influences (Blonigen et al. 2005). Growing evidence indicates that the impulsive and aggressive behaviors may be mediated by abnormal serotonin transporter functioning in the brain (Coccaro et al. 1996).

In addition to biological factors, it is also clear that the early family lives of these persons often pose severe environmental handicaps in the form of absent, inconsistent, or abusive parenting. Indeed, many family members also have significant action-oriented psychopathology, such as substance abuse or antisocial personality disorder itself. Modern behavioral genetic research is focusing on interactions between genes and the environment to explain the genesis of antisocial behavior (Moffitt 2005; Reiss et al. 1995).

Treatment

It is clinically important to recognize antisocial personality disorder, because an uncritical acceptance of these individuals' glib or shallow statements of good intentions and collaboration can permit them to have disruptive influences on treatment teams and other patients. However, there is little evidence to suggest that this disorder can be successfully treated by usual psychiatric interventions. Of interest, nonetheless, are reports suggesting that in confined settings, such as the military or prisons, depressive and introspective concerns may surface. Under these circumstances, confrontation by peers may bring about changes in the antisocial person's social behaviors. It is also notable that some antisocial patients demonstrate an ability to form a therapeutic alliance with psychotherapists, which augurs well for these patients' future course (Woody et al. 1985). These findings contrast with the clinical tradition that emphasizes such persons' inability to learn from harmful consequences. Yet longitudinal follow-up studies have shown that the prevalence of this disorder diminishes with age as these individuals become more aware of the social and interpersonal maladaptiveness of their most harmful social behaviors.

Borderline Personality Disorder

Epidemiology

Borderline personality disorder (BPD) is present in 1%–1.6% of the general population (Torgersen 2009) and in about 20% of hospital and clinical admissions (Gunderson and Links 2007). Although BPD is more common among women than men in clinical settings, this difference is not found in community-based studies (Grant et al. 2008; Lenzenweger et al. 2007; Torgersen et al. 2001; Zimmerman and Coryell 1990).

Clinical Features

BPD is characterized by instability and dysfunction in affective, behavioral, and interpersonal domains. Central to the psychopathology of this disorder are a severely impaired capacity for attachment (Levy et al. 2005) and predictably maladaptive behavior patterns related to separation (Gunderson 1996). When borderline patients feel cared for, held on to, and supported, depressive

features (notably loneliness and emptiness) are most evident. When the threat of losing such a sustaining relationship arises, the idealized image of a beneficent caregiver is replaced by a devalued image of a cruel persecutor. This shift between idealization and devaluation is called *splitting*. An impending separation also evokes intense abandonment fears. To minimize these fears and to prevent the separation, rageful accusations of mistreatment and cruelty and angry self-destructive behaviors may occur. These behaviors often elicit a guilty or fearful protective response from others.

Another central feature of this disorder is extreme affective instability that often leads to impulsive and self-destructive behaviors. These episodes are usually brief and reactive and involve extreme alternations between angry and depressed states. The experience and expression of anger can be particularly difficult for the borderline patient. During periods of unusual stress, dissociative experiences, ideas of reference, or desperate impulsive acts (including substance abuse and promiscuity) commonly occur.

Roughly half of borderline patients have significant remissions of their overt psychopathology within 2 years. Levels of social dysfunction, severity of childhood trauma, and persistence of substance abuse are predictive of a worse prognosis (Gunderson et al. 2006). Overall, the longer-term course of BPD may be more benign than previously thought and may be predicted from historical, clinical, functional, and personality features (Zanarini et al. 2006). About 10% of patients with the disorder commit suicide, however (Oldham 2006).

Differential Diagnosis

The most common differential diagnosis involves the interface of BPD with bipolar disorder—particularly bipolar II. The major distinctions are that bipolar patients have periods of elation and borderline patients have abandonment fears and repeated episodes of self-harm when alone. This diagnostic issue has been magnified by the widespread overutilization of bipolar diagnoses for anyone with affective instability (Goldberg et al. 2008) and by the equally misleading reluctance of clinicians to assign patients the BPD diagnosis (Zimmerman and Mattia 1999).

Borderline patients' intense feelings of being bad or evil are distinctly different from the idealized self-image of narcissistic persons. Patients with BPD differ from those with antisocial personality disorder in that the impulsive behaviors of borderline patients are primarily interpersonally oriented and aimed toward obtaining support rather than materialistic gains. Paranoid ideas may also occur in patients with schizotypal or paranoid personality disorders, but these symptoms are more transient, interpersonally reactive, and responsive to external structuring in borderline patients. Patients with dependent personality disorder are characterized by fear of abandonment, but they react to such threats by efforts at appeasement and submissiveness rather than with feelings of emptiness and rage.

Etiology

Psychoanalytic theories have emphasized the importance of early parent–child relationships in the etiology of BPD. These theories are gradually being explored and modified by direct observation of early dyads with long-term follow-up. This research has generally confirmed that inconsistent or absent feedback from caretakers predicts insecure attachment and also that infants themselves have traits that significantly shape their caretakers' responses (Gunderson and Lyons-Ruth 2008). A considerable body of empirical research has also documented a high frequency of traumatic early abandonment, physical abuse, and sexual abuse (Johnson et al. 2005a). These experiences have enduring traumatic effects when they occur in particularly sensitive children or in children who do not have opportunities to process the events (Paris 1998). The lack of reliably involved attachment to caretakers during development is a source of borderline patients' inability to maintain stable senses of themselves or of others without ongoing contact (Bender and Skodol 2007).

Twin study evidence of 69% overall heritability for BPD (Torgersen et al. 2000) has mobilized efforts to identify genetic contributions to the etiology of specific borderline traits. Siever and Davis (1991) posited fundamental dimensions of affective instability and impulsive aggression underlying BPD. Livesley et al. (1993) found heritability of about 50% for borderline traits such as affective lability and insecure attachment and later for the broader domains of emotional dysregulation and dissocial behavior (Livesley et al. 1998). There is evidence of serotonergic dysfunction in the borderline trait of impulsivity.

All modern theories about the etiology of BPD posit a genetic vulnerability underlying poor emotional, behavioral, and interpersonal controls, with recognition that whether these vulnerabilities are expressed—whether children with these vulnerabilities develop BPD—depends on adverse childhood environments and on triggering stressors. Thus, although the specific factors in the etiology of BPD are yet to be determined, the pathways to this illness are complex and multifactorial (Gunderson 2009).

Treatment

Borderline patients are high utilizers of psychiatric outpatient, inpatient, partial hospital, and psychopharmacological treatment. Almost all modalities can be helpful. The extensive literature on the treatment of BPD universally notes the extreme difficulties that clinicians encounter with these patients. These problems derive from the patients' appeals to their treaters' wishes to rescue and from their angry accusations when they perceive their treaters to have failed them. Many clinicians do not like working with these patients despite their generally good prognosis. Often therapists develop intense countertransference reactions that lead them to attempt to re-parent or, conversely, to reject borderline patients. Many borderline patients can get better—even much better—without long-term therapy. Regardless of the treatment approach used, personal maturity and considerable clinical experience are important assets.

Treatment of borderline patients typically requires good case management (American Psychiatric Association 2001). Essential aspects include skills in managing suicidal or self-destructive threats and behaviors alongside calm and knowledgeable psychoeducational discussion of the diagnosis and its treatment. Such interventions frame realistic goals and a good alliance. Case management is usually accompanied by psychotherapeutic and pharmacological interventions.

Much of the early treatment literature focused on the value of intensive exploratory psychotherapies directed at modifying borderline patients' basic character structure. However, this literature has increasingly suggested that improvement may be related not to the acquisition of insight but to the corrective experience of developing a stable, trusting relationship with a therapist who fails to retaliate in response to these patients' angry and disruptive behaviors. Paralleling this development has been the suggestion that supportive psychotherapies or group therapies may bring about similar changes (Appelbaum 2005; Piper and Ogrodniczuk 2005). Evidence has provided support for the effectiveness of two forms of psychoanalytic treatment. The first, called "mentalization-based treatment" (MBT), involves a nondirective discussion of the interactions between the patient and therapist (Bateman and Fonagy 1999). The second, called "transference-focused psychotherapy" (TFP), involves more traditional interventions (Clarkin et al. 1999). Both attribute change to improved abilities to mentalize.

Linehan et al. (2006) have shown that behavioral treatment consisting of a once-weekly individual and twice-weekly group regimen can effectively diminish the self-destructive behaviors and hospitalizations of borderline patients. The success and cost benefits of this treatment, called *dialectical behavior therapy*, have led to its widespread adoption and to modifications that can be used in a variety of settings. *Schema-focused therapy* is a newer cognitive therapy that has also been shown to be efficacious (Giesen-Bloo et al. 2006).

Although no one medication has been found to have dramatic or predictable effects, studies indicate that many medications may diminish specific problems such as impulsivity, affective lability, or intermittent cognitive and perceptual disturbances, as well as irritability and aggressive behavior (Hollander et al. 2005; Soloff 2005). In general, the profusion of options and the often unclear benefits have encouraged polypharmacy, with sometimes unfortunate side effects (Zanarini et al. 2004).

Histrionic Personality Disorder

Epidemiology

Histrionic personality disorder occurs in about 1.5% of the general population (Torgersen 2009). Those with histrionic personality disorder are more often women (Torgersen et al. 2001; Zimmerman and Coryell 1990).

Clinical Features

Central to histrionic personality disorder is an overconcern with attention and appearance. Persons with this disorder spend an excessive amount of time seeking attention and making themselves attractive. The desire to be found attractive may lead to inappropriately seductive or provocative dress and flirtatious behavior, and the desire for attention may lead to other flamboyant acts or self-dramatizing behavior. Persons with histrionic personality disorder also display an effusive, but labile and shallow, range of feelings. They are often overly impressionistic and given to hyperbolic descriptions of others. More generally, these persons do not attend to detail or facts, and they are reluctant or unable to make reasoned critical analyses of problems or situations. Persons with this disorder often present with complaints of depression, somatic problems of unclear origin, and a history of disappointing romantic relationships.

Differential Diagnosis

Histrionic personality disorder can be confused with dependent, borderline, and narcissistic personality disorders. Histrionic individuals are often willing, even eager, to have others make decisions and organize their activities for them. However, unlike persons with dependent personality disorder, histrionic persons are uninhibited and lively companions who willfully forgo appearing autonomous because they believe that this attracts others. Unlike persons with BPD, those with histrionic personality do not perceive themselves as bad, and they lack ongoing problems with rage or willful self-destructiveness. Persons with narcissistic personality disorder also seek attention to sustain their self-esteem but differ in that their self-esteem is characterized by grandiosity, and the attention they crave must be admiring.

Etiology

Research suggests that qualities such as emotional expressiveness (Jang et al. 1996) and egocentricity (Torgersen et al. 1993) are heritable temperaments. From this perspective, histrionic personality disorder would consist of extreme variants of temperamental dispositions, the environmental contributions of which remain to be determined.

Treatment

Individual psychodynamic psychotherapy, including psychoanalysis, remains the cornerstone of most treatment for persons with histrionic personality disorder (Gabbard 2005). This treatment is directed at increasing patients' awareness of 1) how their self-esteem is maladaptively tied to their ability to attract attention at the expense of developing other skills, and 2) how their shallow relationships and emotional experience reflect unconscious fears of real commitments. Much of this increase in awareness occurs through analysis of the here-and-now doctor–patient relationship rather than through the reconstruction of childhood experiences. Therapists should be aware that the typical idealization and eroticization that such patients bring into treatment are the material for exploration, and thus therapists should be aware of countertransferential gratification.

Narcissistic Personality Disorder

Epidemiology

Narcissistic personality disorder had a median prevalence of 0.5% in 12 community studies (Torgersen 2009). The disorder appears to be more common among men (Stinson et al. 2008; Torgersen et al. 2001; Zimmerman and Coryell 1990).

Clinical Features

Persons with narcissistic personality disorder lack empathy for others. In relationships, narcissistic persons are often quite distant and try to sustain "an illusion of self-sufficiency" (Modell 1975). This allows them to unknowingly treat others insensitively while pursuing their self-serving goals. The DSM-IV-TR definition emphasizes these individuals' grandiose self-esteem, fantasies of unlimited potential, a sense of entitlement, and extreme needs for admiration. Persons with narcissistic personality disorder are vulnerable to intense reactions when their self-image is damaged. They respond with strong feelings of hurt or anger to even small slights, rejections, defeats, or criticisms. Serious depression can ensue, which is the usual precipitant for their seeking clinical help. There are other less arrogant, socially conspicuous forms of narcissistic personality disorder, however, in which a conviction of personal superiority is hidden behind social withdrawal and a fa-cade of self-sacrifice and even humility.

Differential Diagnosis

Narcissistic personality disorder can be most readily confused with antisocial and histri-onic personality disorders. Like persons with antisocial personality disorder, those with narcissistic personality disorder are capable of exploiting others, but narcissistic persons usually rationalize their behavior on the basis of the specialness of their goals or their per-sonal virtue. In contrast, antisocial persons' goals are materialistic, and their rationaliza-tions, if offered, are based on a view that oth-ers would do the same to them. The narcissis-tic person's excessive pride in achievements, relative constraint in expression of feelings, and disregard for other people's rights and sensitivities help distinguish him or her from persons with histrionic personality disorder. Perhaps the most difficult differential diag-nostic problem is whether a person who meets criteria for narcissistic personality dis-order has a stable personality disorder or is in an episode of an Axis I disorder, such as an adjustment reaction. If the emergence of nar-cissistic traits has been defensively triggered by experiences of failure or rejection, these traits may diminish radically and self-esteem may be restored when new relationships or successes occur. When manic, patients with bipolar disorder can appear quite similar to those with narcissistic personality disorder.

Etiology

Little scientific evidence is available about the pathogenesis of narcissistic personality disor-der. Reconstructions based on developmental history and observations in psychotherapeutic treatment indicate that this disorder develops in persons who have had their fears, failures, or dependency responded to with criticism, disdain, or neglect during their childhood years. Such experiences leave them contemp-tuous of such reactions in themselves and oth-ers and inexperienced in viewing others as sources of comfort and support. They develop a veneer of invulnerability and self-sufficiency that masks their underlying emptiness and constricts their capacity to feel deeply.

Treatment

Individual psychodynamic psychotherapy, including psychoanalysis, is the cornerstone of treatment for persons with narcissistic per-sonality disorder (Gabbard 2005). Following Kohut's (1971) lead, some therapists believe that the vulnerability to narcissistic injury in-dicates that intervention should be directed at conveying empathy for the patient's sensi-tivities and disappointments. This approach, in theory, allows a positive idealized transfer-ence to develop that will then be gradually disillusioned by the inevitable frustrations encountered in therapy—disillusionment that will clarify the excessive nature of the patient's reactions to frustrations and disap-pointments. An alternative view, explicated by Kernberg (1975), is that the vulnerability should be addressed earlier and more di-rectly by interpretations and confrontations through which these persons will come to recognize their grandiosity and its maladap-tive consequences. With either approach, the psychotherapeutic process usually requires a relatively intensive schedule over a period of years in which the narcissistic patient's hy-persensitivity to slights and tendency to mea-sure others' worth by whether they gratify his or her needs must be foremost in the ther-apist's mind and interventions.

Avoidant Personality Disorder

Epidemiology

The prevalence of avoidant personality disor-der based on epidemiological studies is about 1.7% (Torgersen 2009). This is in part due to the frequency with which it was found in a Scandinavian study (Torgersen et al. 2001), which illustrates how culture may contribute to the form a personality disorder may take. Avoidant personality disorder may be more common among women (Grant et al. 2004; Zimmerman and Coryell 1989, 1990).

Clinical Features

Persons with avoidant personality disorder experience excessive and pervasive anxiety and discomfort in social situations and in intimate relationships. Although strongly desiring relationships, they avoid them because they fear being ridiculed, criticized, rejected, or humiliated. These fears reflect their low self-esteem and hypersensitivity to negative evaluation by others. When they do enter into social situations or relationships, they feel inept and are self-conscious, shy, awkward, and preoccupied with being criticized or rejected. Their lives are constricted in that they tend to avoid not only relationships but also any new activities because they fear that they will embarrass or humiliate themselves. Patients with avoidant personality disorder may engage in deliberate self-harm (Klonsky et al. 2003) and experience disability in social, educational, and physical realms (Kessler 2003).

Differential Diagnosis

Schizoid personality disorder also involves social isolation, but the schizoid person does not desire relationships, whereas the avoidant person desires them but avoids them because of anxiety and fears of humiliation and rejection. Whereas avoidant personality disorder is characterized by avoidance of situations and relationships involving possible rejection, disappointment, ridicule, or shame, Axis I social phobia usually consists of specific fears related to social performance (e.g., a fear of saying something inappropriate or of being unable to answer questions in front of other people). Furthermore, patterns of avoidance in persons with avoidant personality disorder often extend beyond social situations to include emotional and novelty avoidance (Taylor et al. 2004). Some avoidant persons are actually vulnerable subtypes of narcissistic character styles (Dickinson and Pincus 2003).

Etiology

Research on childhood experiences of avoidant persons reveals negative childhood memories (e.g., of isolation, rejection) (Meyer and Carver 2000); poorer athletic performance, less involvement in hobbies, and less popularity (Rettew et al. 2003); and parental neglect (Joyce et al. 2003). Research in the biological sphere has implicated the importance of inborn temperament in the development of avoidant behavior. Kagan (1989) found that some children as young as 21 months manifest increased physiological arousal and avoidant traits in social situations (e.g., retreat from the unfamiliar and avoidance of interaction with strangers) and that this social inhibition tends to persist for many years. Family studies have demonstrated elevated rates of trait and social anxiety, as well as personality traits such as harm avoidance, in the first-degree relatives of individuals with generalized social phobia, suggesting that social anxiety lies on a continuum that may be influenced by familial factors (Stein et al. 2001).

Treatment

Because of their excessive fear of rejection and criticism and their reluctance to form relationships, individuals with avoidant personality disorder may be difficult to engage in treatment. Engagement in psychotherapy may be facilitated by the therapist's use of supportive techniques, sensitivity to the patient's hypersensitivity, and gentle interpretation of the defensive use of avoidance. Although early in treatment these patients may tolerate only supportive techniques, they may eventually respond well to all kinds of psychotherapy (Gabbard 2005). Clinicians should be aware of the potential for countertransference reactions such as overprotectiveness, hesitancy to adequately challenge the patient, or excessive expectations for change.

Although few data exist, it seems likely that assertiveness and social skills training may increase patients' confidence and willingness to take risks in social situations. Cognitive techniques that gently challenge patients' pathological assumptions about their sense of ineptness may also be useful (Beck et al. 2004). Group experiences—perhaps, in particular, homogeneous supportive groups that emphasize the development of social skills—may prove useful for avoidant patients (Piper and Ogrodniczuk 2005).

Promising preliminary data suggest that avoidant personality disorder may improve with treatment with monoamine oxidase inhibitors or serotonin reuptake inhibitors. Anxiolytics sometimes help patients better manage anxiety (especially severe anxiety) caused by facing previously avoided situations or trying new behaviors.

Dependent Personality Disorder

Epidemiology

Dependent personality disorder occurs in about 0.7% of the general population (Torgersen 2009) and is much more common among women (Grant et al. 2004; Torgersen et al. 2001; Zimmerman and Coryell 1989, 1990).

Clinical Features

Dependent personality disorder is characterized by an excessive need to be cared for by others, which leads to submissive and clinging behavior and excessive fears of separation. Although these individuals are able to care for themselves, they doubt their abilities and judgment, and they view others as much stronger and more capable than they are. These persons excessively rely on "powerful" others to initiate and do things for them, make their decisions, assume responsibility for their actions, and guide them through life. Low self-esteem and doubts about their effectiveness lead them to avoid positions of responsibility. Because they feel unable to function without excessive guidance, they go to great lengths to maintain dependent relationships. They may, for example, always agree with those on whom they depend, and they tend to be excessively passive and self-sacrificing. Because they feel incapable of caring for themselves when relationships end, these individuals feel helpless and fearful. They may indiscriminately begin another relationship so that they can be provided with direction and nurturance—an unfulfilling or even abusive relationship may seem better than being on their own.

Differential Diagnosis

Although persons with BPD also dread being alone and need ongoing support, dependent persons want others to assume a controlling function that would frighten the borderline patient. Moreover, persons with dependent personality disorder become appeasing rather than rageful or self-destructive when threatened with separation. Although both avoidant and dependent personality disorders are characterized by low self-esteem, rejection sensitivity, and an excessive need for reassurance, persons with dependent personality disorder seek out rather than avoid relationships, and they quickly and indiscriminately replace ended relationships instead of further withdrawing from others.

Etiology

Genetic or constitutional factors, such as innate submissiveness, may contribute to this disorder's etiology; a twin study found heritability of 45% on a scale measuring submissiveness (Jang et al. 1996). Another twin study found no heritability for submissiveness, based on DSM-III-R (American Psychiatric Association 1987) criteria, 4% for insecurity, and 63% for self-effacing behavior (Torgersen et al. 1993).

Cultural and social factors may also play a role in the development of dependent personality disorder. Dependency is considered not only normative but desirable in certain cultures, including our own. Thus, dependent personality disorder may represent an exaggerated and maladaptive variant of normal dependency; that is, it may—along with histrionic, obsessive-compulsive, and avoidant personality disorders—best be conceptualized as a "trait" disorder (i.e., occurring on a continuum with normal personality traits). It is important to recognize that to qualify for a diagnosis of dependent personality disorder, dependent traits should be so extreme that they cause significant distress or impairment in functioning.

Treatment

Patients with dependent personality disorder often enter therapy with complaints of depression or anxiety that may be precipitated by the threatened or actual loss of a dependent relationship. They often respond well to various types of individual psychotherapy. Treatment may be particularly helpful if it explores the patients' fears of independence; uses the transference to explore their dependency; and is directed toward increasing patients' self-esteem, sense of effectiveness, assertiveness, and independent functioning. These patients often seek an excessively dependent relationship with the therapist, which can lead to countertransference problems that may actually reinforce their dependence. The therapist may, for example, overprotect or be overly directive with the patient, give inappropriate reassurance and support, or prolong the treatment unnecessarily. He or she may also have excessive expectations for change or withdraw from a patient who is perceived as too needy.

Group therapy (Piper and Ogrodniczuk 2005) and cognitive-behavioral therapy (Beck et al. 2004) aimed at increasing independent functioning, including assertiveness and social skills training, may be useful for some patients. If the patient is in a relationship that is maintaining and reinforcing his or her excessive dependence, couples or family therapy may be helpful.

Obsessive-Compulsive Personality Disorder

Epidemiology

Obsessive-compulsive personality disorder (OCPD) is one of the most common in the general population, with a prevalence of about 2.1% (Torgersen 2009). OCPD is more common in men than in women (Torgersen et al. 2001; Zimmerman and Coryell 1989, 1990).

Clinical Features

Persons with OCPD are excessively orderly. They are neat, punctual, overly organized, and overly conscientious. Although these traits might be considered virtues, to qualify as OCPD the traits must be so extreme that they cause significant distress or impairment in functioning. For example, attention to detail is so excessive or time-consuming that the point of the activity is lost, conscientiousness is so extreme that it causes rigidity and inflexibility, and perfectionism interferes with task completion. Although these individuals tend to work extremely hard, they do so at the expense of leisure activities and relationships. The most characteristic thought of persons with OCPD is "I should"—a phrase that aptly captures their overly high standards, drivenness, conscientiousness, perfectionism, rigidity, and devotion to work and duties.

These individuals also tend to be overly concerned with control—not only over the details of their own lives but also over their emotions and other people. They have difficulty expressing warm and tender feelings, often using stilted, distant phrasing that reveals little of their inner experience. They may be obstinate and reluctant to delegate tasks or to work with others unless others submit exactly to their ways of doing things, which reflects their needs for interpersonal control as well as their fears of making mistakes. Their tendency to doubt and worry also manifests itself in their inability to discard worn-out or worthless objects that might be needed in the future.

Differential Diagnosis

OCPD differs from Axis I obsessive-compulsive disorder in that the latter disorder is characterized by specific repetitive thoughts and ritualistic behaviors rather than the personality traits of orderliness, perfectionism, and control.

Etiology

Constitutional factors may play a role in the formation of OCPD. Compulsivity (37%), oppositionality (46%), restricted expression of emotion (50%, Jang et al. 1996), and perfectionism (30%; Torgersen et al. 1993) have all been shown to be moderately heritable. An increase in serotonin activity has been associated with perfectionism and compulsivity. As is the case with other personality disorders, more empirical studies are needed to clarify this disorder's sources.

Treatment

Persons with OCPD may seem difficult to treat because of their excessive intellectualization and difficulty expressing emotion. However, these patients often respond well to psychoanalytic psychotherapy or psychoanalysis (Gabbard 2005). Therapists usually need to be relatively active in treatment. They should also avoid being drawn into interesting but affectless discussions that are unlikely to have therapeutic benefit. In other words, rather than intellectualizing with patients, therapists should focus on the feelings these patients usually avoid. Power struggles that may occur in treatment offer opportunities to address the patient's excessive need for control.

Cognitive techniques may also be used to diminish the patient's excessive need for control and perfection (Beck et al. 2004). Although patients may resist group treatment because of their need for control, dynamically oriented groups that focus on feelings may provide insight and increase patients' comfort with exploring and expressing new affects.

Other Personality Disorders

The following three personality disorders were considered for inclusion on DSM-IV (American Psychiatric Association 1994) Axis II on the basis of their historical tradition, clinical utility, and/or empirical support. However, they were thought to require further study.

Depressive Personality Disorder

Persons with depressive personality disorder are persistently gloomy, burdened, worried, serious, pessimistic, and incapable of enjoyment or relaxation. They also tend to be guilty, moralistic, self-denying, passive, unassertive, and introverted. They have low self-esteem and are excessively sensitive to criticism and rejection. Although they may be critical of others, they have difficulty directing criticism or any form of aggression toward others and find it easier to criticize themselves. They are also overly dependent on the love and acceptance of others, but they inhibit the expression of this dependency and may instead appear counterdependent.

Although concern has been expressed that this personality disorder may overlap excessively with Axis I depressive disorders—in particular, dysthymia—available data suggest that its overlap with dysthymia, major depression, and other personality disorders is far from complete and that depressive personality disorder appears to be a separate construct (Klein and Shih 1998). This disorder should not be diagnosed, however, if it occurs only during major depressive episodes. Although depressive personality disorder appears distinct from Axis I depressive disorders, family history and other data suggest that it may be related to these disorders.

Depressive personality disorder is thought to respond well to psychoanalytic psychotherapy and psychoanalysis.

Negativistic Personality Disorder

Negativistic personality disorder describes a pervasive pattern of passive resistance to demands for social and occupational performance, encompassing a wide range of negativistic attitudes and behaviors, such as anger, pessimism, and cynicism; sullenness and argumentativeness; criticism of others; and envy of those who are perceived as more fortunate. In addition, these individuals tend to alternate between hostile self-assertion and contrite submission. A factor-analytic study found that negativistic personality disorder is a unidimensional construct that is associated with narcissistic personality disorder (Fossati et al. 2000). The clinical features of this disorder and its distinctiveness from other personality disorders remain to be empirically confirmed.

Self-Defeating Personality Disorder

Self-defeating personality disorder applies to persons who exhibit a pervasive pattern of self-defeating behavior that does not occur only in response to, or in anticipation of, physical, sexual, or psychological abuse. Persons with this disorder feel unworthy of being treated well and, as a result, treat themselves poorly and unwittingly encourage others to make them suffer. They may, for example, reject opportunities for pleasure, choose people or situations that lead to mistreatment or failure, and incite others to become angry with them or reject them. If things do go well for them, they attempt to undermine themselves by, for example, becoming depressed or causing themselves pain.

The treatment of the disorder is complicated by the patient's self-defeating tendencies; patients may unknowingly sabotage the treatment and their progress because they feel undeserving of improvement or happiness. Exploring the patient's need to be victimized and making his or her investment in

suffering ego-dystonic may allow a successful outcome with insight-oriented psychotherapy or psychoanalysis (Gabbard 2005).

Conclusion

Clinical interest and research in the personality disorders have grown enormously since 1980, when these disorders were put on a separate axis in DSM-III. The ensuing period has brought to light more specific and effective treatment strategies and a better understanding of these disorders' prognosis and etiology. Even more dramatic than the knowledge gained is the heightened awareness of the clinical impact and potential research significance of personality disorders and the new and more informed questions that this awareness has generated. Remaining challenges include a resolution of the boundaries between personality disorders and both normal personality and Axis I conditions, the discovery of biogenetic bases for personality traits underlying disorders, and the development of even more effective treatments. There is good reason to believe that with continued inquiry by clinical and basic-science investigators, the classification of personality disorders will continue to change so that it becomes even more tightly linked to etiology, treatment, and outcome.

Key Points

- Personality disorders are common in clinical settings and in the community.

- Personality disorders can be challenging to diagnose.

- Personality disorders cause significant problems for those who have them and for others and are costly to society.

- Personality disorders often complicate the treatment of other mental disorders.

- Personality disorders result from an interaction between temperamental (genetic/biological) and psychological (developmental/environmental) factors.

Suggested Readings

Beck AT, Freeman A, Davis DD, et al: Cognitive Therapy of Personality Disorders, 2nd Edition. New York, Guilford, 2004

Cloninger CR (ed): Personality and Psychopathology. Washington, DC, American Psychiatric Press, 1999

Costa PT, Widiger TA (eds): Personality Disorders and the Five-Factor Model of Personality, 2nd Edition. Washington, DC, American Psychological Association, 2001

Gunderson JG: Borderline Personality Disorder: A Clinical Guide. Washington, DC, American Psychiatric Press, 2001

Livesley WJ (ed): Handbook of Personality Disorders: Theory, Research, and Treatment. New York, Guilford, 2001

Oldham JM, Skodol AE, Bender DS (eds): Essentials of Personality Disorders. Washington, DC, American Psychiatric Publishing, 2009

Paris J: Personality Disorders Over Time: Precursors, Course, and Outcome. Washington, DC, American Psychiatric Publishing, 2003

Pervin L, John O (eds): Handbook of Personality: Theory and Research, 2nd Edition. New York, Guilford, 1999

Plomin R, Caspi A: Behavioral Genetics and Personality. New York, Guilford, 1999

Stone MH: Personality-Disordered Patients: Treatable and Untreatable. Washington, DC, American Psychiatric Publishing, 2006

References

Alarcon RD: Cross-cultural issues, in The American Psychiatric Publishing Textbook of Personality Disorders. Edited by Oldham JM, Skodol AE, Bender DS. Washington, DC, American Psychiatric Publishing, 2005, pp 561–578

American Psychiatric Association: Diagnostic and Statistical Manual of Mental Disorders, 3rd Edition. Washington, DC, American Psychiatric Association, 1980

American Psychiatric Association: Diagnostic and Statistical Manual of Mental Disorders, 3rd Edition, Revised. Washington, DC, American Psychiatric Association, 1987

American Psychiatric Association: Diagnostic and Statistical Manual of Mental Disorders, 4th Edition. Washington, DC, American Psychiatric Association, 1994

American Psychiatric Association: Diagnostic and Statistical Manual of Mental Disorders, 4th Edition, Text Revision. Washington, DC, American Psychiatric Association, 2000

American Psychiatric Association: Practice guideline for the treatment of patients with borderline personality disorder. Am J Psychiatry 158 (suppl):1–52, 2001

Appelbaum AH: Supportive therapy, in The American Psychiatric Publishing Textbook of Personality Disorders. Edited by Oldham JM, Skodol AE, Bender DS. Washington, DC, American Psychiatric Publishing, 2005, pp 335–346

Bateman A, Fonagy P: Effectiveness of partial hospitalization in the treatment of borderline personality disorder: a randomized controlled trial. Am J Psychiatry 156:1563–1569, 1999

Beck AT, Freeman A, Davis DD, et al: Cognitive Therapy of Personality Disorders, 2nd Edition. New York, Guilford, 2004

Bender DS: Therapeutic alliance, in The American Psychiatric Publishing Textbook of Personality Disorders. Edited by Oldham JM, Skodol AE, Bender DS. Washington, DC, American Psychiatric Publishing, 2005, pp 405–420

Bender DS, Skodol AE: Borderline personality as a self-other representational disturbance. J Personal Disord 21:500–517, 2007

Bender DS, Dolan RT, Skodol AE, et al: Treatment utilization by patients with personality disorders. Am J Psychiatry 158:295–302, 2001

Bierer LM, Yehuda R, Schmeidler J, et al: Abuse and neglect in childhood: relationship to personality disorder diagnoses. CNS Spectr 8:737–754, 2003

Blonigen DM, Hicks BM, Krueger RF, et al: Psychopathic personality traits: heritability and genetic overlap with internalizing and externalizing psychopathology. Psychol Med 35:637–648, 2005

Carey G, DiLalla DL: Personality and psychopathology: genetic perspectives. J Abnorm Psychol 103:32–43, 1994

Clarkin JF, Yeomans FE, Kernberg OF: Psychotherapy for Borderline Personality. New York, John Wiley & Sons, 1999

Cloninger CR, Svrakic DM, Przybeck TR: A psychobiological model of temperament and character. Arch Gen Psychiatry 50:975–990, 1993

Coccaro EF, Kavoussi RJ, Sheline YI, et al: Impulsive aggression in personality disorder: correlates with tritiated paroxetine binding in the platelet. Arch Gen Psychiatry 53:531–536, 1996

Cohen P, Crawford T: Developmental issues, in The American Psychiatric Publishing Textbook of Personality Disorders. Edited by Oldham JM, Skodol AE, Bender DS. Washington, DC, American Psychiatric Publishing, 2005, pp 171–185

Compton WM, Conway KP, Stinson FS, et al: Prevalence, correlates, and comorbidity of DSM-IV antisocial personality syndromes and alcohol and specific drug use disorders in the United States: results from the national epidemiologic study on alcohol and related conditions. J Clin Psychiatry 66:677–685, 2005

Dickinson KA, Pincus AL: Interpersonal analysis of grandiose and vulnerable narcissism. J Personal Disord 17:188–207, 2003

DiLalla DL, Carey G, Gottesman II, et al: Heritability of MMPI personality indicators of psychopathology in twins reared apart. J Abnorm Psychol 105:491–499, 1996

Dunayevich E, Sax KW, Keck PE Jr, et al: Twelve-month outcome in bipolar patients with and without personality disorders. J Clin Psychiatry 61:134–139, 2000

Edens JF, Marcus DK, Lillienfeld SO, et al: Psychopathic, not psychopath: taxometric evidence for the dimensional structure of psychopathy. J Abnorm Psychol 115:131–144, 2006

Fanous A, Gardner C, Walsh D, et al: Relationship between positive and negative symptoms of schizophrenia and schizotypal symptoms in nonpsychotic relatives. Arch Gen Psychiatry 58:669–673, 2001

First M, Pincus H, Levine J, et al: Clinical utility as a criterion for revising psychiatric diagnoses. Am J Psychiatry 161:949–954, 2004

Fonagy P, Gergely G, Target M: The parent-infant dyad and the construction of the subjective self. J Child Psychol Psychiatry 48:288–328, 2007

Fossati A, Maffei C, Bagnato M, et al: A psychometric study of DSM-IV passive-aggressive (negativistic) personality disorder criteria. J Personal Disord 14:72–83, 2000

Gabbard GO: Psychodynamic Psychiatry in Clinical Practice, 3rd Edition. Washington, DC, American Psychiatric Publishing, 2000

Gabbard GO: Psychoanalysis, in The American Psychiatric Publishing Textbook of Personality Disorders. Edited by Oldham JM, Skodol AE, Bender DS. Washington, DC, American Psychiatric Publishing, 2005, pp 257–273

Giesen-Bloo J, van Dyck R, Spinhoven P, et al: Outpatient psychotherapy for borderline personality disorder: randomized trial of schema-focused therapy vs. transference-focused psychotherapy. Arch Gen Psychiatry 63:649–658, 2006

Goldberg JF, Garno JL, Callahan AM, et al: Overdiagnosis of bipolar disorder among substance use disorder patients with mood instability. J Clin Psychiatry 8:e1–e7, 2008

Grant BF, Hasin DS, Stinson FR, et al: Prevalences, correlates, and disability of personality disorders in the United States: results from the National Epidemiologic Survey on Alcohol and Related Conditions. J Clin Psychiatry 65:948–958, 2004

Grant BF, Chon P, Goldstein RB, et al: Prevalence, correlates, disability, and comorbidity of DSM-IV borderline personality disorder: results from the Wave 2 National Epidemiologic Survey on Alcohol and Related Conditions. J Clin Psychiatry 69:533–537, 2008

Grilo CM, McGlashan TH: Course and outcome of personality disorders, in The American Psychiatric Publishing Textbook of Personality Disorders. Edited by Oldham JM, Skodol AE, Bender DS. Washington, DC, American Psychiatric Publishing, 2005, pp 103–115

Grilo CM, Sanislow CA, Shea MT, et al: Two-year prospective naturalistic study of remission from major depressive disorder as a function of personality disorder co-morbidity. J Consult Clin Psychol 73:78–85, 2005

Grove WM, Eckert ED, Heston L, et al: Heritability of substance abuse and antisocial behavior: a study of monozygotic twins reared apart. Biol Psychiatry 27:1293–1304, 1990

Gunderson JG: The borderline patient's intolerance of aloneness: insecure attachment and therapist availability. Am J Psychiatry 153:752–758, 1996

Gunderson JG: Borderline personality disorder: ontogeny of a diagnosis. Am J Psychiatry 166:530–539, 2009

Gunderson JG, Links P: Borderline personality disorder, in Treatment of Psychiatric Disorders, 4th Edition. Edited by Gabbard GO. Washington, DC, American Psychiatric Publishing, 2007, pp 795–821

Gunderson JG, Lyons-Ruth K: BPD's interpersonal hypersensitivity phenotype: a gene-environment-developmental model. J Personal Disord 22:22–41, 2008

Gunderson JG, Daversa MT, Grilo CM, et al: Predictors of 2-year outcome for patients with borderline personality disorder. Am J Psychiatry 163:822–826, 2006

Hare RD, Neumann CS: Structural models of psychopathy. Curr Psychiatry Rep 7:57–64, 2005

Hare RD, Hart SD, Harpur TJ: Psychopathy and the DSM-IV criteria for antisocial personality disorder. J Abnorm Psychol 100:391–398, 1991

Hoek HW, Susser E, Buck KA, et al: Schizoid personality disorder after prenatal exposure to famine. Am J Psychiatry 153:1637–1639, 1996

Hollander E, Swann AC, Coccaro EF, et al: Impact of trait impulsivity and state aggression on divalproex versus placebo response in borderline personality disorder. Am J Psychiatry 162:621–624, 2005

Jang KL, Livesley WJ, Vernon PA, et al: Heritability of personality disorder traits: a twin study. Acta Psychiatr Scand 94:438–444, 1996

Johnson JG, Cohen P, Kasen S, et al: Age-related change in personality disorder trait levels between early adolescence and adulthood: a community-based longitudinal investigation. Acta Psychiatr Scand 102:265–275, 2000

Johnson JG, Bromley E, McGeoch PG: Role of childhood experiences in the development of maladaptive and adaptive personality traits, in The American Psychiatric Publishing Textbook of Personality Disorders. Edited by Oldham JM, Skodol AE, Bender DS. Washington, DC, American Psychiatric Publishing, 2005a, pp 209–221

Johnson JG, First MB, Cohen P, et al: Adverse outcomes associated with personality disorder not otherwise specified in a community sample. Am J Psychiatry 162:1926–1932, 2005b

Jones M: The Therapeutic Community: A New Treatment in Psychiatry. New York, Basic Books, 1953

Joyce PR, McKenzie JM, Luty SE, et al: Temperament, childhood environment and psychopathology as risk factors for avoidant and borderline personality disorders. Aust N Z J Psychiatry 37:756–764, 2003

Kagan J: Temperamental influences on the preservation of styles of social behavior. McLean Hospital Journal 14:23–34, 1989

Kasen S, Cohen P, Skodol AE, et al: The influence of child and adolescent psychiatric disorders on young adult personality disorder. Am J Psychiatry 156:1529–1535, 1999

Kaye AL, Shea MT: Personality disorders, personality traits, and defense mechanisms measures, in Handbook of Psychiatric Measures. Edited by Task Force for the Handbook of Psychiatric Measures. Washington, DC, American Psychiatric Association, 2000, pp 713–749

Kendler KS, Gruenberg AM: Genetic relationship between paranoid personality disorder and the "schizophrenic spectrum" disorders. Am J Psychiatry 139:1185–1186, 1982

Kendler KS, McGuire M, Gruenberg AM, et al: The Roscommon Family Study, III: schizophrenia-related personality disorders in relatives. Arch Gen Psychiatry 50:781–788, 1993

Kendler KS, Neale MC, Walsh D: Evaluating the spectrum concept of schizophrenia in the Roscommon Family Study. Am J Psychiatry 152:749–754, 1995

Kendler KS, Czajkowski N, Tambs K, et al: Dimensional representations of DSM-IV cluster A personality disorders in a population-based sample of Norwegian twins: a multivariate study. Psychol Med 36:1583–1591, 2006

Kendler KS, Myers J, Torgersen S, et al: The heritability of cluster A personality disorders assessed by both personal interview and questionnaire. Psychol Med 37:655–665, 2008

Kent S, Fogarty M, Yellowlees P: A review of studies of heavy users of psychiatric services. Psychiatr Serv 46:1247–1253, 1995

Kernberg OF: Borderline Conditions and Pathological Narcissism. New York, Jason Aronson, 1975

Keshavan M, Shad M, Soloff P, et al: Efficacy and tolerability of olanzapine in the treatment of schizotypal personality disorder. Schizophr Res 71:97–101, 2004

Kessler RC: The impairments caused by social phobia in the general population: implications for intervention. Acta Psychiatr Scand Suppl (417):19–27, 2003

Klein DN, Shih JH: Depressive personality: associations with DSM-III-R mood and personality disorders and negative and positive affectivity, 30-month stability, and prediction of course of Axis I depressive disorders. J Abnorm Psychol 107:319–327, 1998

Klonsky ED, Oltmanns TF, Turkheimer E: Informant-reports of personality disorder: relation to self-reports and future directions. Clin Psychol Sci Pract 9:300–311, 2002

Klonsky ED, Oltmanns TF, Turkheimer E: Deliberate self-harm in a nonclinical population: prevalence and psychological correlates. Am J Psychiatry 160:1501–1508, 2003

Koenigsberg HW, Reynolds D, Goodman M, et al: Risperidone in the treatment of schizotypal personality disorder. J Clin Psychiatry 64:628–634, 2003

Kohut H: The Analysis of the Self: A Systematic Approach to the Psychoanalytic Treatment of Narcissistic Personality Disorders. New York, International Universities Press, 1971

Krueger RF, Markon KE, Patrick CJ, et al: Externalizing psychopathology in adulthood: a dimensional-spectrum conceptualization and its implications for DSM-V. J Abnorm Psychol 114:537–550, 2005

Leichsenring F, Leibing E: The effectiveness of psychodynamic therapy and cognitive behavior therapy in the treatment of personality disorders: a meta-analysis. Am J Psychiatry 160:1223–1232, 2003

Lenzenweger MF, Lane MC, Loranger AW, et al: DSM-IV personality disorders in the national comorbidity survey replication. Biol Psychiatry 62:553–564, 2007

Levy KN, Meehan KB, Weber M, et al: Attachment and borderline personality disorder: implications for psychotherapy. Psychopathology 38:64–74, 2005

Linehan MM, Comtois KA, Murray AM, et al: Two-year randomized controlled trial and follow-up of dialectical behavior therapy vs. therapy by experts for suicidal behaviors and borderline personality disorder. Arch Gen Psychiatry 63:757–766, 2006

Linney YM, Murray RM, Peters ER, et al: A quantitative genetic analysis of schizotypal personality traits. Psychol Med 33:803–816, 2003

Livesley J, Jackson D: Dimensional Assessment of Personality Pathology. Port Huron, MI, Sigma, 2000

Livesley WJ, Jang KL, Jackson DN, et al: Genetic and environmental contributions to dimensions of personality disorder. Am J Psychiatry 150:1826–1831, 1993

Livesley WJ, Jang KL, Vernon PA: Phenotypic and genetic structure of traits delineating personality disorder. Arch Gen Psychiatry 55:941–948, 1998

Lyons MJ, True WR, Eisen SA, et al: Differential heritability of adult and juvenile antisocial traits. Arch Gen Psychiatry 52:906–915, 1995

Malone SM, Taylor J, Marmorstein NR, et al: Genetic and environmental influences on antisocial behavior and alcohol dependence from adolescence to early adulthood. Dev Psychopathol 16:943–966, 2004

Markon KE, Krueger RF, Watson D: Delineating the structure of normal and abnormal personality: an integrative hierarchical approach. J Personal Soc Psychol 88:139–157, 2005

McDermut W, Zimmerman M: Assessment instruments and standardized evaluation, in The American Psychiatric Publishing Textbook of Personality Disorders. Edited by Oldham JM, Skodol AE, Bender DS. Washington, DC, American Psychiatric Publishing, 2005, pp 89–101

Meyer B, Carver CS: Negative childhood accounts, sensitivity, and pessimism: a study of avoidant personality disorder features in college students. J Personal Disord 14:233–248, 2000

Modell AH: A narcissistic defense against affects and the illusion of self-sufficiency. Int J Psychoanal 56:275–282, 1975

Moffitt TE: The new look of behavioral genetics in developmental psychopathology: gene-environment interplay in antisocial behaviors. Psychol Bull 131:533–554, 2005

Morey LC, Alexander GM, Boggs C: Gender, in The American Psychiatric Publishing Textbook of Personality Disorders. Edited by Oldham JM, Skodol AE, Bender DS. Washington, DC, American Psychiatric Publishing, 2005, pp 541–559

Oldham J: Borderline personality disorder and suicidality. Am J Psychiatry 163:20–26, 2006

Oldham JM, Skodol AE: Charting the future of Axis II. J Personal Disord 14:17–29, 2000

Paris J: Working with Traits: Psychotherapy of Personality Disorders. Northvale, NJ, Jason Aronson, 1998

Paris J: Neurobiological dimensional models of personality: a review of the models of Cloninger, Depue, and Siever. J Personal Disord 19:156–170, 2005

Perry JC, Banon E, Ianni F: Effectiveness of psychotherapy for personality disorders. Am J Psychiatry 156:1312–1321, 1999

Piper WE, Ogrodniczuk JS: Group treatment, in The American Psychiatric Publishing Textbook of Personality Disorders. Edited by Oldham JM, Skodol AE, Bender DS. Washington, DC, American Psychiatric Publishing, 2005, pp 347–357

Reich W: On the technique of character analysis, in Character Analysis, 3rd Edition. New York, Simon & Schuster, 1949, pp 39–113

Reichborn-Kjennerud T, Czajkowski N, Neal MC, et al: Genetic and environmental influences on dimensional representations of DSM-IV cluster C personality disorders: a population-based multivariate twin study. Psychol Med 37:645–653, 2006

Reiss D, Hetherington EM, Plomin R, et al: Genetic questions for environmental studies: differential parenting and psychopathology in adolescence. Arch Gen Psychiatry 52:925–936, 1995

Rettew DC, Zanarini MC, Yen S, et al: Childhood antecedents of avoidant personality disorder: a retrospective study. J Am Acad Child Adolesc Psychiatry 42:1122–1130, 2003

Roberts BW, DelVecchio WF: The rank-order consistency of personality traits from childhood to old age: a quantitative review of longitudinal studies. Psychol Bull 126:3–25, 2000

Roberts BW, Caspi A, Moffitt TE: Work experiences and personality development in young adulthood. J Personal Soc Psychol 84:582–593, 2003

Sanislow CA, Morey LC, Grilo CM, et al: Confirmatory factor analysis of DSM-IV borderline, schizotypal, avoidant, and obsessive-compulsive personality disorders: findings from the Collaborative Longitudinal Personality Study. Acta Psychiatr Scand 105:28–36, 2002

Schore AN: Dysregulation of the right brain: a fundamental mechanism of traumatic attachment and the psychopathogenesis of posttraumatic stress disorder. Aust N Z J Psychiatry 36:9–30, 2002

Seivewright H, Tyrer P, Johnson T: Persistent social dysfunction in anxious and depressed patients with personality disorder. Acta Psychiatr Scand 109:104–109, 2004

Sholevar GP: Family therapy, in The American Psychiatric Publishing Textbook of Personality Disorders. Edited by Oldham JM, Skodol AE, Bender DS. Washington, DC, American Psychiatric Publishing, 2005, pp 359–373

Siever LJ, Davis KL: A psychobiological perspective on the personality disorders. Am J Psychiatry 148:1647–1658, 1991

Siever LJ, Davis KL: The pathophysiology of schizophrenia disorders: perspectives from the spectrum. Am J Psychiatry 161:398–413, 2004

Skodol AE: Manifestations, clinical diagnosis, and comorbidity, in The American Psychiatric Publishing Textbook of Personality Disorders. Edited by Oldham JM, Skodol AE, Bender DS. Washington, DC, American Psychiatric Publishing, 2005, pp 57–87

Skodol AE, Bender DS: The future of personality disorders in DSM-V? Am J Psychiatry 166:388–391, 2009

Skodol AE, Gunderson JG, McGlashan TH, et al: Functional impairment in patients with schizotypal, borderline, avoidant, or obsessive-compulsive personality disorder. Am J Psychiatry 159:276–283, 2002

Skodol AE, Oldham JM, Bender DS, et al: Dimensional representations of DSM-IV personality disorders: relationships to functional impairment. Am J Psychiatry 162:1919–1925, 2005a

Skodol AE, Pagano MP, Bender DS, et al: Stability of functional impairment in patients with schizotypal, borderline, avoidant, or obsessive-compulsive personality disorder over two years. Psychol Med 35:443–451, 2005b

Soloff PH: Somatic treatments, in The American Psychiatric Publishing Textbook of Personality Disorders. Edited by Oldham JM, Skodol AE, Bender DS. Washington, DC, American Psychiatric Publishing, 2005, pp 387–403

Stein MB, Chartier MJ, Lizak MV, et al: Familial aggregation of anxiety-related quantitative traits in generalized social phobia: clues to understanding "disorder" heritability? Am J Med Genet 105:79–83, 2001

Stinson FS, Dawson DA, Goldstein RB, et al: Prevalence, correlates, disability, and comorbidity of DSM-IV narcissistic personality disorder. Results from the Wave 2 National Epidemiologic Survey of Alcohol and Related Conditions. J Clin Psychiatry 69:1033–1045, 2008

Stone M: Schizotypal personality: psychotherapeutic aspects. Schizophr Bull 11:576–589, 1985

Stone M: Violence, in The American Psychiatric Publishing Textbook of Personality Disorders. Edited by Oldham JM, Skodol AE, Bender DS. Washington, DC, American Psychiatric Publishing, 2005, pp 477–491

Suzuki M, Zhou S-Y, Takahashi T, et al: Differential contributions of prefrontal and temporolimbic pathology to mechanisms of psychosis. Brain 128:2109–2122, 2005

Taylor CT, Laposa JM, Alden LE: Is avoidant personality disorder more than just social avoidance? J Personal Disord 18:571–594, 2004

Torgersen S: Prevalence, sociodemographics, and functional impairment, in Essentials of Personality Disorders. Edited by Oldham JM, Skodol AE, Bender DS. Washington, DC, American Psychiatric Publishing, 2009, pp 83–102

Torgersen S, Onstad S, Skre I, et al: "True" schizotypal personality disorder: a study of co-twins and relatives of schizophrenic probands. Am J Psychiatry 150:1661–1667, 1993

Torgersen S, Lygren S, Øien PA, et al: A twin study of personality disorders. Compr Psychiatry 41:416–425, 2000

Torgersen S, Kringlen E, Cramer V: The prevalence of personality disorders in a community sample. Arch Gen Psychiatry 58:590–596, 2001

Torgersen S, Edvardsen J, Øien PA, et al: Schizotypal personality disorder inside and outside the schizophrenia spectrum. Schizophr Res 54:33–38, 2002

Verheul R: Clinical utility of dimensional models for personality pathology. J Personal Disord 19:283–302, 2005

Verheul R, Widiger TA: A meta-analysis of the prevalence and usage of the personality disorder not otherwise specified (PDNOS) diagnosis. J Personal Disord 18:309–319, 2004

Webb CT, Levinson DF: Schizotypal and paranoid personality disorder in the relatives of patients with schizophrenia and affective disorders: a review. Schizophr Res 11:81–92, 1993

Westen D: Divergences between clinical and research methods for assessing personality disorders: implications for research and the evolution of Axis II. Am J Psychiatry 154:895–903, 1997

Westen D, Shedler J, Bradley R: A prototype approach to personality disorder diagnosis. Am J Psychiatry 163:846–856, 2006

Widiger TA: Personality disorders in the 21st century. J Personal Disord 14:3–16, 2000

Widiger TA, Mullins-Sweatt SN: Categorical and dimensional models of personality disorders, in The American Psychiatric Publishing Textbook of Personality Disorders. Edited by Oldham JM, Skodol AE, Bender DS. Washington, DC, American Psychiatric Publishing, 2005, pp 35–53

Widiger TA, Samuel DB: Diagnostic categories or dimensions? A question for the Diagnostic and Statistical Manual of Mental Disorders—Fifth Edition. J Abnorm Psychol 114:494–504, 2005

Widiger TA Simonsen E: Alternative dimensional models of personality disorder: finding a common ground. J Personal Disord 19:110–130, 2005

Woody GE, McLellan AT, Luborsky L, et al: Sociopathy and psychotherapy outcome. Arch Gen Psychiatry 42:1081–1086, 1985

World Health Organization: International Statistical Classification of Diseases and Related Health Problems, 10th Revision, Version for 2006. Geneva, Switzerland, World Health Organization, 2006. Available at: http://www.who.int/classifications/apps/icd/icd10online. Accessed May 18, 2006.

Yonkers KA, Dyck IR, Warshaw M, et al: Factors predicting the clinical course of generalised anxiety disorder. Br J Psychiatry 176:544–549, 2000

Young JE, Klosko J, Weishaar ME: Schema Therapy: A Practitioner's Guide. New York, Guilford, 2003

Zanarini M: Role of Sexual Abuse in the Etiology of Borderline Personality Disorder. Washington, DC, American Psychiatric Press, 1997

Zanarini MC, Frankenburg FR, Yong L, et al: Borderline psychopathology in the first-degree relatives of borderline and Axis II comparison probands. J Personal Disord 18:439–447, 2004

Zanarini MC, Frankenberg FR, Hennen J, et al: Prediction of the 10-year course of borderline personality disorder. Am J Psychiatry 163:827–832, 2006

Zimmerman M, Coryell W: DSM-III personality disorder diagnoses in a nonpatient sample: demographic correlates and comorbidity. Arch Gen Psychiatry 46:682–689, 1989

Zimmerman M, Coryell W: Diagnosing personality disorders in the community: a comparison of self-report and interview measures. Arch Gen Psychiatry 47:527–531, 1990

Zimmerman M, Mattia JI: Differences between clinical and research practices in diagnosing borderline personality disorder. Am J Psychiatry 156:1570–1574, 1999

Zimmerman M, Rothchild L, Chelminski I: The prevalence of DSM-IV personality disorders in psychiatric outpatients. Am J Psychiatry 162:1911–1918, 2005

DISORDERS USUALLY FIRST DIAGNOSED IN INFANCY, CHILDHOOD, OR ADOLESCENCE

Amy M. Ursano, M.D.

Paul H. Kartheiser, M.D.

L. Jarrett Barnhill, M.D.

In recent years, it has become increasingly recognized that many psychiatric disorders have their onset in youth. Like many experiences of childhood, these disorders can have enduring effects, and they may affect an individual's sense of satisfaction with relationships, occupation, or self and ultimately play a significant role in the development of adult psychopathology. Variations in the presentation of psychiatric diagnoses can often be attributed to an individual's developmental stage. In fact, disorders such as separation anxiety or elimination disorder represent normal behavior at an early age, although contin-

ued symptoms inappropriate to a patient's developmental level become diagnosable and thereby a focus of treatment. Despite limited research, we have effective treatments for many childhood psychiatric illnesses.

This chapter focuses on the DSM-IV-TR (American Psychiatric Association 2000) category "Disorders Usually First Diagnosed in Infancy, Childhood, or Adolescence," which includes conditions that not only begin in childhood but also are typically diagnosed during childhood (Table 12–1). Other disorders may also have an onset of symptoms during childhood.

Table 12–1. **DSM-IV-TR disorders usually first diagnosed in infancy, childhood, or adolescence**

Mental retardation
Mild mental retardation
Moderate mental retardation
Severe mental retardation
Profound mental retardation
Mental retardation, severity unspecified

Learning disorders
Reading disorder
Mathematics disorder
Disorder of written expression
Learning disorder not otherwise specified

Motor skills disorder
  Developmental coordination disorder

Communication disorders
  Expressive language disorder
  Mixed receptive–expressive language
    disorder
  Phonological disorder
  Stuttering
  Communication disorder not otherwise
    specified

Pervasive developmental disorders
Autistic disorder
Rett's disorder
Childhood disintegrative disorder
Asperger's disorder
Pervasive developmental disorder not
  otherwise specified

Attention-deficit and disruptive behavior disorders
  Attention-deficit/hyperactivity disorder
    Predominantly inattentive type
    Predominantly hyperactive–impulsive
      type
    Combined type
    Not otherwise specified
  Conduct disorder
  Oppositional defiant disorder
  Disruptive behavior disorder not otherwise
    specified

Table 12–1. **DSM-IV-TR disorders usually first diagnosed in infancy, childhood, or adolescence** *(continued)*

Feeding and eating disorders of infancy or early childhood
Pica
Rumination disorder
Feeding disorder of infancy or early childhood

Tic disorders
Tourette's disorder
Chronic motor or vocal tic disorder
Transient tic disorder
Tic disorder not otherwise specified

Elimination disorders
Encopresis
Enuresis

Other disorders of infancy, childhood, or adolescence
Separation anxiety disorder
Selective mutism
Reactive attachment disorder of infancy or
  early childhood
Stereotypic movement disorder
Disorder of infancy, childhood, or
  adolescence not otherwise specified

Source. American Psychiatric Association 2000.

Mental Retardation
Clinical Description

Intellectual disability (previously called *mental retardation*) is a developmental disorder with onset prior to age 18 years characterized by impairments in measured intellectual performance and adaptive skills across multiple domains (Table 12–2). DSM-IV-TR classifies mental retardation as an Axis II disorder and reminds clinicians that intellectual disability is not synonymous with psychiatric illness (Harris 2006).

Table 12–2. DSM-IV-TR diagnostic criteria for mental retardation

---

A. Significantly subaverage intellectual functioning: an IQ of approximately 70 or below on an individually administered IQ test (for infants, a clinical judgment of significantly subaverage intellectual functioning).

B. Concurrent deficits or impairments in present adaptive functioning (i.e., the person's effectiveness in meeting the standards expected for his or her age by his or her cultural group) in at least two of the following areas: communication, self-care, home living, social/interpersonal skills, use of community resources, self-direction, functional academic skills, work, leisure, health, and safety.

C. The onset is before age 18 years.

Code based on degree of severity reflecting level of intellectual impairment:

317 **Mild mental retardation:** IQ level 50–55 to approximately 70

318.0 **Moderate mental retardation:** IQ level 35–40 to 50–55

318.1 **Severe mental retardation:** IQ level 20–25 to 35–40

318.2 **Profound mental retardation:** IQ level below 20 or 25

319 **Mental retardation, severity unspecified:** when there is strong presumption of mental retardation but the person's intelligence is untestable by standard tests

---

Epidemiology

Intellectual disability is operationally defined by scores on tests of measured intelligence that are 2 standard deviations below the mean (with the mean equal to 100 IQ points and each standard deviation equal to 15 points). According to a symmetrical bell-shape curve, 3% of the population should be intellectually disabled. Yet prevalence studies from community samples consistently report rates of 1.5%. This discrepancy may be due to age and socioeconomic status of the population surveyed; early loss of infants with severe illness; unexplained death in individuals with epilepsy, congenital abnormalities, or associated diseases; and "disappearance" of individuals with mild disability and good adaptive skills once their school careers are over (Aman et al. 2003).

Across the spectrum of intellectual disability, there is a 1.4:1.0 male-to-female ratio. The preponderance of males is also observed in many developmental disorders. Sources of this gender bias include vulnerability to chromosomal and genetic aberrances (X-linked disorders) and increased susceptibility to prenatal and perinatal insults among males. For some genetic disorders and autism, affected females may have more severe

subtypes of the disorder (Guthrie et al. 1999; Joy et al. 2003).

Individuals classified as having mild intellectual disability comprise nearly 89%, those with moderate disability comprise 7%, and those with severe to profound disability approximately 3%–4% of those identified (Table 12–3).

Etiology

The more common biological causes of intellectual disability include prenatal exposure to toxins or infectious agents, genetic and chromosomal abnormalities, disturbances in normal brain development, nutritional factors, and early postnatal insults. The most common sources of prenatal neurotoxicity are alcohol and other substances of abuse. A similar pattern of risk factors exists for most infectious disease: type of infection, inherent neurotropism of the virus or bacteria, timing of exposure (e.g., first trimester in rubella), and time of recognition and treatment. Postnatal exposures tend to be most devastating to infants and very young children (Joy et al. 2003). In the developing world, exposure to pre- and postnatal infectious diseases and environmental neurotoxins (e.g., HIV and waterborne pollutants) remains a major etiol-

Table 12–3.　Clinical features of mental retardation

	Mild	Moderate	Severe	Profound
IQ	50–55 to approximately 70	35–40 to 50–55	20–25 to 35–40	<20 or 25
Age at death (years)	50s	50s	40s	About 20
Percentage of mentally retarded population	89	7	3	1
Socioeconomic class	Low	Less low	No skew	No skew
Academic level achieved by adulthood	Sixth grade	Second grade	Below first-grade level in general	Below first-grade level in general
Education	Educable	Trainable (self-care)	Untrainable	Untrainable
Residence	Community	Sheltered	Mostly living in highly structured and closely supervised settings	Mostly living in highly structured and closely supervised settings
Economic	Makes change; manages a job; budgets money with effort or assistance	Makes small change; is usually able to manage change well	Can use coin machines; can take notes to shop owner	Is dependent on others for money management

Source.　Reprinted from American Psychiatric Association: *Diagnostic and Statistical Manual of Mental Disorders*, 4th Edition, Text Revision. Washington, DC, American Psychiatric Association, 2000. Used with permission.

ogy of developmental disabilities in children (Harris 2006). Starvation and malnutrition have a profound impact on brain development. Postnatal injuries can have catastrophic consequences. As with toxic exposure, the timing of the insults is crucial to the impact and prognosis. Severe brain trauma during infancy can produce severe intellectual disability due to adverse effects on basic skill acquisition. Children from chaotic and understimulating environments are at greater risk for cognitive and educational deficits. Academic performance is also adversely affected by poverty, parental attitudes, substance abuse, psychopathology, and neglect or abuse (Harris 2006).

Individuals with severe intellectual disability have greater prevalence rates for genetic disorders, severe prenatal insults, complicated and medically refractory forms of symptomatic epilepsies, and serious developmental brain anomalies. The confluence of both genetic and developmental anomalies, motor disorders, sensory impairments, and language communication deficits further limits adaptive skills in this population (Joy et al. 2003).

Diagnostic Evaluation

The diagnosis of intellectual disability often begins with parent or teacher concerns. Formal diagnosis requires a multidisciplinary process that incorporates familial, genetic, developmental, and educational history within a thorough medical neurological examination. To accurately assess adaptive skills, it is essential to collect data from multiple sources. Medical and neurological evaluations should be comprehensive and look specifically for treatable conditions. Detailed neuroimaging and neurophysiological, genetic, and metabolic studies are needed if there is a high index of suspicion for structural anomalies, seizures, or genetic-metabolic disorders (Joy et al. 2003).

Children with mild disability may not be diagnosed until they have poor academic performance. Early recognition can also be delayed by sociocultural factors such as disruptive behaviors, diminished suspicion among teachers, and relatively high levels of social and adaptive skills. Workup includes an assessment of psychosocial factors and adaptive skills, measures of intellectual abilities, and psychoeducational testing. If questions arise, referrals should be made for more extensive medical and neurological evaluations (Harris 2006).

Detailed genetic testing is often not practical, but children from families with histories of developmental disorders, mental retardation, or specific syndromes such as fragile X syndrome warrant a more extensive workup (Harris 2002). Specifically, such a workup should be pursued in the presence of significant dysmorphology, multiorgan or multisystem involvement, and other comorbid medical or neurological conditions, including poorly controlled mixtures of complex and simple partial or myoclonic seizures (Guthrie et al. 1999).

Due to significant delays in sensorimotor and language development, children with severe to profound intellectual disability are often recognized at a younger age. They are more likely to have prenatal developmental motor disorders, perinatal trauma, congenital infections, and genetic or chromosomal disorders. Syndromal diagnoses can help define treatment approaches and alert clinicians to the presence of associated behavioral and cognitive phenotypes (Moldavsky et al. 2001).

Behavioral Phenotypes

In recent years, there has been growing interest in the behavioral phenotypes associated with specific genetic syndromes. Behavioral phenotypes are patterns of cognition and behavior that have a greater probability of expression within a specific disorder (Harris 2002). The likelihood of specific emotional responses and behaviors occurring in these syndromes is greater than in the general population of individuals with intellectual disability. Although patients with specific behavioral phenotypes do not meet the criteria for major psychiatric disorders, and the boundary between known behavioral phenotypes and psychiatric disorders is still unsettled, behavioral phenotypes do provide clues about the complex nature of gene–behavior interactions. For example, nearly one-third of children with velocardiofacial syndrome (22q deletions) develop symptoms consistent with adolescent-onset bipolar disorder and psychosis (Goldstein and Reynolds 1999; Harris 2002).

Comorbid Psychiatric Disorders

All psychiatric diagnoses may co-occur with intellectual disability. Comorbid diagnoses include depression, bipolar and anxiety disorders, autistic spectrum disorders, learning disorders (LDs), and psychotic disorders. These individuals may have disruptive behavior disorders, and up to 50% may have attention-deficit/hyperactivity disorder (ADHD).

The accurate diagnosis of primary psychiatric disorders in individuals with intellectual disability requires an understanding of the degree of their intellectual disability and of their verbal and communicative abilities, as well as a knowledge of comorbid medical or neurological conditions. The clinician must also appreciate that severe behavioral disorganization may be a response to environmental challenges. It is difficult for many clinicians to reliably diagnose comorbid disorders because psychiatrists generally depend on an individual's self-report of mental or emotional states. Nonverbal patients require additional tools, including instruments standardized for patients with intellectual disability. It is important for the clinician to directly examine or observe the individual and to review reports from multiple sources familiar with the person as well as objective behavioral data (Aman et al. 2003; Einfield and Aman 1995).

Once adequate information is obtained, it may still be difficult to distinguish symptoms related to intellectual disability (e.g., baseline aggression) from those secondary to a psychiatric disorder (e.g., increase in base-line aggression in an individual with comorbid bipolar disorder). Diagnosis is further complicated in patients with moderate to severe intellectual disability because they may present with atypical or subsyndromal symptoms of mood or anxiety disorders, phobias, or even prodromal schizophrenia. These complexities partly explain the reason so many patients with intellectual disability are classified with "not otherwise specified" diagnoses (Barnhill 2003; Harris 2006).

Treatment

There is no cure for intellectual disability. Prevention and early intervention remain the most effective treatments. This includes bypassing of enzymatic defects in metabolic disorders, better prenatal care, treatments for infectious diseases, and early recognition and treatment of seizure disorders (Aman et al. 2003). The most effective early intervention strategies employ child-specific ecological modifications (e.g., environmental enrichment) and developmentally focused education and behavioral interventions. In addition, focused efforts directed at temperamental vulnerabilities or behavioral phenotypes may impact the emergence of challenging behaviors. These intervention strategies allow for accommodation and skill training that are specific to the individual neurobiological, cognitive, or emotional needs and vulnerabilities of the child (Harris 2006).

Setting

Most treatment plans involve some form of habilitation that enhances adaptive or social skills or provides training for specific vocational or educational niches. These programs usually include school-based training, assisted employment, communication enhancement, and daily living skill training. Other community-based programs focus on enhancing family supports, respite services, and developmental centers (Griffiths et al. 1998).

Many individuals with intellectual disability do well in either family or community settings as opposed to institutional placement. These individuals tend to have few problematic behaviors and minimal neurological or psychiatric symptoms. Those with mild intellectual disabilities and no significant behavioral or psychiatric disorders may rarely come to attention once their school careers end. These individuals may use clinical services when crises emerge, but rates of challenging behaviors and psychiatric disorders are at most moderately elevated. Those with histories of abuse, childhood behavioral or emotional problems, and family histories of addiction or major psychiatric disorders may require higher levels of care (Griffiths et al. 1998; Harris 2006).

Psychotherapy

Psychotherapy can be an important part of the treatment plan. For individuals with mild intellectual disability, verbal and cognitive skills may be adequate for modified forms of several psychotherapies. There is growing evidence that modified forms of traditional supportive, dynamic, cognitive, and dialectical behavior therapy can be extremely effective. The availability of qualified or skilled therapists is frequently the limiting factor to their use (Harris 2006). In individuals with severe intellectual disability, impaired or absent language and communication skills and severe cognitive deficits prevent the use of many forms of psychotherapy. Behavioral interventions remain the most common form of therapy. The goal of behavioral therapy is to reduce unwanted behaviors by modifying environmental or antecedent factors or by changing the contingencies of maladaptive behaviors. Successful strategies can range from extinction procedures, differential reinforcement of alternative or incompatible behaviors, or skill building through shaping techniques. (See Chapter 18, "Cognitive Therapy," for further discussion of behavioral therapy.)

Pharmacotherapy

Pharmacotherapy has a complicated history in the management of individuals with intel-

lectual disability. In the past, medications were used to effect behavioral control or to compensate for overcrowding and lack of programming in custodial institutions. Unfortunately, even today, psychotropics are often used in lieu of effective behavioral programs, and polypharmacy has become the new form of maintaining community-based "behavioral management" (Harris 2006).

Even with effective behavioral programming, many individuals with intellectual disability continue to show challenging behaviors. In order to maintain a least restrictive placement, there is a frequent need for well-monitored pharmacotherapy. The decision to proceed with medication management is the result of a careful review of the neurobiology and etiology of intellectual disability, the presence of a specific behavioral phenotype, the history of past treatment, and a medical-neurological workup. The clinician needs to integrate available behavioral data and consult with all members of the treatment team about special environmental or interpersonal factors (Aman et al. 2003).

It is not uncommon to see individuals with severe intellectual disability taking extremely high dosages of multiple medications. There seems to be a growing trend toward polypharmacy based on treatment models extrapolated from basic research or inaccurately diagnosed psychiatric disorders. At the root of this trend is a preference for selecting pharmacological agents based on a single symptom (e.g., a patient who is crying or appears sad must be depressed) or hypothetical neurotransmitter abnormality (e.g., all aggression is related to reductions in serotonin activity). The basic problem with this approach is the failure to recognize the heterogeneity of challenging behaviors (Barnhill 2003).

Even the treatment of clearly defined psychiatric disorders is confounded by comorbidities in individuals as well as possible drug-related or iatrogenic symptoms in patients who may be prescribed medications by several physicians. Much of our limited evidence base for the use of pharmacological agents does not account for these comorbid conditions. A full understanding of a patient's presentation comes from integrating this information with knowledge of the patient's developmental, neurological, and medical history (Aman et al. 2003; Harris 2006).

There has been an explosion in the use of second- and third-generation antipsychotic drugs, antidepressant or antianxiety drugs (e.g., selective serotonin reuptake inhibitors [SSRIs], serotonin–norepinephrine reuptake inhibitors (SNRIs), atypical antidepressants), and antiepileptic mood stabilizers. These medications are used to treat primary psychiatric disorders as well as challenging behaviors. When compared with previous approaches, these newer agents appear to reduce some of the intolerable side effects of older agents (e.g., extrapyramidal symptoms, risk of tardive dyskinesia, sedation, and anticholinergic side effects). However, the new treatments are not without side effects. Dermatological, hematological, endocrinological, and cardiac side effects are still problematic. In every situation, the clinician must use a limited evidence base to make risk–benefit judgments. Unfortunately many treatment approaches are "off-label" or extrapolated from data in typical children or adults (Aman et al. 2003; Joy et al. 2003; see Chapter 19, "Treatment of Children and Adolescents").

Clinicians face three basic issues when considering pharmacotherapy in individuals with intellectual disability. The first involves the focus of treatment. Typically, symptoms (as opposed to syndromes or disorders) are the target of medication interventions. The goal is to establish accurate psychiatric diagnoses and direct treatment at the problematic symptoms. Response can be monitored through available assessment and treatment instruments. Those designed for or adapted to people with intellectual disability are preferred. If there is no diagnosable disorder but challenging behaviors remain resistant to behavioral interventions, then pharmacother-

apy should proceed based on the best available evidence-based data. If such evidence is lacking, the best practices or expert consensus data can help with clinical decision making.

The second issue relates to the difficulty in making reliable psychiatric diagnoses in patients with intellectual disability. These disorders may affect the clinical course, prognosis, and treatment of the presenting syndrome. There is also the degree of heterogeneity within diagnostic categories, such as differences in sleep disturbance within mood disorders. This heterogeneity is compounded among patients with severe intellectual disability, who often have additional neurological, developmental, metabolic, and neurophysiological disorders (Barnhill 2003).

The third issue involves the heterogeneity of intellectual disability itself. There are many subgroups of intellectual disability based on severity, comorbid neurological disorders, genetic etiology, and underlying developmental brain abnormalities. For example, individual patients with fragile X syndrome vary from the lengths of CGG repeats and degree of DNA methylation to such epigenetic phenomena as intellectual ability and presence and severity of stereotypies or self-injury. Individuals with trisomy 21 and mood disorders need to be evaluated for thyroid dysfunction, basal ganglia abnormalities, or the emergence of apathy and seizures in conjunction with the cognitive decline of evolving dementia. The clinician must account for these variables in order to match treatment to psychiatric diagnosis and to determine and monitor the pre-illness baseline (and assess recovery or remission) as well as anticipate potential adverse drug effects (Joy et al. 2003).

Intellectual Disability Summary

Intellectual disability is a complex, heterogeneous collection of disorders characterized by deficits in measured intelligence and adaptive abilities and onset during the developmental period. Depending on the severity of the intellectual disability, there is a considerable range of comorbid neurological, metabolic, and genetic disorders that can confound psychiatric care. Challenging behaviors emerge in the context of medical, neurological, and ecological variables that are manifestations of a mismatch between the individual's needs and abilities and his or her living environment. These individuals challenge our understanding of the relationships between brain development and behavior. In essence, the understanding of intellectual disability requires a thorough working knowledge of developmental neuropsychiatry and an appreciation of the multiple factors that influence human behavior.

The treatment of challenging behaviors and neuropsychiatric disorders requires a team. There is probably no single treatment modality that fits each individual. Combined treatments often are needed. The ultimate goal of treatment is to maximize the quality of life for individuals with intellectual disability. Many individuals with intellectual disability are subject to daily stressors that seriously tax their capacity to adapt. In order to be helpful, clinicians need to approach each individual from a biopsychosocial frame of reference.

Learning Disorders and Motor Skills Disorder

Clinical Description

Learning disorders involve deficits in acquiring and performing basic academic skills. Currently, LDs are categorized into disorders of reading, mathematics, and written expression (Tables 12–4, 12–5, and 12–6). Developmental coordination disorder (DCD), the only motor skills disorder in DSM, is defined in DSM-IV-TR by significant impairment in gross or fine motor coordination, including delays in motor milestones or difficulty with other expected motor tasks during development (Table 12–7).

Table 12–4. DSM-IV-TR diagnostic criteria for reading disorder

A. Reading achievement, as measured by individually administered standardized tests of reading accuracy or comprehension, is substantially below that expected given the person's chronological age, measured intelligence, and age-appropriate education.

B. The disturbance in criterion A significantly interferes with academic achievement or activities of daily living that require reading skills.

C. If a sensory deficit is present, the reading difficulties are in excess of those usually associated with it.

Coding note: If a general medical (e.g., neurological) condition or sensory deficit is present, code the condition on Axis III.

Table 12–5. DSM-IV-TR diagnostic criteria for mathematics disorder

A. Mathematical ability, as measured by individually administered standardized tests, is substantially below that expected given the person's chronological age, measured intelligence, and age-appropriate education.

B. The disturbance in criterion A significantly interferes with academic achievement or activities of daily living that require mathematical ability.

C. If a sensory deficit is present, the difficulties in mathematical ability are in excess of those usually associated with it.

Coding note: If a general medical (e.g., neurological) condition or sensory deficit is present, code the condition on Axis III.

Reading Disorder

Reading is crucial to academic performance and functioning in societies with significant education-based social stratification. Historically, reading disorders were considered

Table 12–6. DSM-IV-TR diagnostic criteria for disorder of written expression

A. Writing skills, as measured by individually administered standardized tests (or functional assessments of writing skills), are substantially below those expected given the person's chronological age, measured intelligence, and age-appropriate education.

B. The disturbance in criterion A significantly interferes with academic achievement or activities of daily living that require the composition of written texts (e.g., writing grammatically correct sentences and organized paragraphs).

C. If a sensory deficit is present, the difficulties in writing skills are in excess of those usually associated with it.

Coding note: If a general medical (e.g., neurological) condition or sensory deficit is present, code the condition on Axis III.

Table 12–7. DSM-IV-TR diagnostic criteria for developmental coordination disorder

A. Performance in daily activities that require motor coordination is substantially below that expected given the person's chronological age and measured intelligence. This may be manifested by marked delays in achieving motor milestones (e.g., walking, crawling, sitting), dropping things, "clumsiness," poor performance in sports, or poor handwriting.

B. The disturbance in criterion A significantly interferes with academic achievement or activities of daily living.

C. The disturbance is not due to a general medical condition (e.g., cerebral palsy, hemiplegia, or muscular dystrophy) and does not meet criteria for a pervasive developmental disorder.

D. If mental retardation is present, the motor difficulties are in excess of those usually associated with it.

Coding note: If a general medical (e.g., neurological) condition or sensory deficit is present, code the condition on Axis III.

perceptual disorders. In recent years the focus has shifted to the relationship between reading speed and accuracy and morpheme–phoneme and visual grapheme processing speed and factors related to reading comprehension. Currently the literature supports the idea that reading is hierarchically organized and requires the functional integrity of multiple interconnected brain circuits (Ramus et al. 2003).

Developmentally, reading progresses from sight recognition of words and the use of contextual cues (e.g., pictures) to increased use of rapid phonetic analysis and syntactical cues. Clinically, reading correlates with the speed and efficiency of processing and responding to phonemes (i.e., speed and accuracy of processing).

Mathematics Disorder

Mathematics disorder represents a derailment of the progression of skills, a failure to move from counting to basic math operations (arithmetic) and then on to advanced mathematics that require sequential reasoning, significant verbal skills, and abstract reasoning (Fletcher 2005). Mathematical reasoning may be deficient. An interesting deficit involves poor estimating ability or a difficulty recognizing math errors or the validity of answers. Even more intriguing are math savants. Those with autism can sometimes perform unbelievable arithmetic computations but are unable to use these skills in making change or to enhance occupational functioning (Lachiewicz et al. 2006).

Written Expression and Motor Skills Disorders

Although distinct disorders, disorder of written expression and DCD are interrelated. Writing is a motor skill, and some problems described in disorders of written language are shared with other motor dyspraxias. Writing, however, involves combining these motor skills with reading language. Handwriting and motor dyscoordination are commonly problematic in nonverbal LDs, tic disorders, and other developmental disorders. Delays in written language may co-occur with other motor skill disorders but are often recognized later, when demands for written expression increase (Peters et al. 2001).

In some respects, written language is a subset of motor skill disorders, which are disorders of planning, organization, and implementation of motor programs. They differ from paralysis or paresis based on the level of motor impairment. Clumsiness is one example of DCD.

Epidemiology

Learning disorders are the most prevalent developmental disorders of childhood. Although standardized definitions exist, the prevalence rates vary. The inconsistency among reported prevalence rates may be due to the clinical heterogeneity and the evolving nature of these diagnoses.

The most common LD, reading disorder, is thought to occur in 2%–10% of all children. It accounts for up to 80% of children diagnosed with an LD (Shaywitz et al. 2000). Reading disorders tend to have the greatest impact on education levels and occupational achievement, but many children learn to compensate to some degree. Mathematics disorders are thought to occur in 1%–6%, and disorders of written expression have a prevalence of 2%–8% (American Academy of Child and Adolescent Psychiatry 1998). DCD is estimated to occur in up to 6% of children 5–11 years old (American Psychiatric Association 2000). Perhaps the most devastating LD involves a combination of academic skill deficits. The global disabilities overlap and are frequently confused with intellectual disability or pervasive developmental disorder (PDD) (Lachiewicz et al. 2006; Rourke et al. 2003).

There are gender differences in the prevalence rates for LDs and DCD. As is the case for many developmental disorders, males are most often affected by DCD and LDs, except for mathematics disorder, which affects more girls than boys. There are also gender differences in the types of comorbid psychiatric disorders that may affect LDs. Males more frequently present with disruptive behaviors such as ADHD, oppositional defiant disorder (ODD), and conduct disorder (CD; Connors and Schulte 2002). Females with LDs more typically demonstrate internalizing disorders. Additionally, those with LDs are at increased risk for substance use disorders (Klein and Mannuzza 2000).

Etiology

Although most LDs are either language or nonverbally based, the differences in functional neuroimaging studies make clear that no single area represents the reading or mathematics "center." Instead, a network that integrates both hemispheres and multiple regions and subcortical circuitries develops. This degree of coherence and integration follows a developmental trajectory that changes with neuronal maturation, myelinization of key interconnecting pathways, and prefrontal/executive supervision (Litt et al. 2005; Rourke et al. 2003). These processes appear to be disrupted in children with LD.

Course and Prognosis

There is considerable variability in the developmental course of LDs and DCD. A subset of children presents with delays in skill acquisition that suggest an aberrant trajectory for brain maturation that improves with maturity. Others appear to have a developmental deficit or functional "lesion" that requires more extensive remedial training or habilitation. Many of these children may have lifelong problems or display only partial compensation (Litt et al. 2005).

Diagnostic Evaluation

Determining a child's intellectual capacity is essential to evaluation of an LD. The assessment instruments for LDs are developmental tests designed and standardized based on a child's age and intelligence level. There are general tests of academic skills (e.g., Wide Range Achievement Test, Woodcock-Johnson tests) that provide an overview of major areas of academic performance. More specialized instruments focus on specific domains such as written expression, mathematical abilities, or subtypes of reading disorders. Neuropsychological assessments help define functional domains that underlie learning and can be quite helpful in planning cognitive remediation (Connors and Schulte 2002; Rourke et al. 2003; Weinberg and McLean 1986). Each subtest provides a piece of the puzzle but may not entirely explain an individual's struggles in school. It is important to listen to the life story of each child because determination, motivation, talents, and passions all affect learning (Rourke et al. 2003).

In the evaluation of DCD, one must obtain a careful history, including prenatal and perinatal history, as well as a review of developmental milestones and specific behaviors such as grasping, drawing, and dressing (Denckla and Roeltgen 1992). DCD requires a medical evaluation to rule out neurological conditions or PDDs. If mental retardation is present, the motor difficulties must be greater than those usually associated with the level of retardation. Consultation with an occupational therapist may be appropriate.

Treatment

Like other chronic illnesses in children, LDs are probably not curable. Treatment consists primarily of compensatory techniques or technologies to minimize the impact of these disorders on educational and social function. The importance of an individualized education plan with tailored treatment by communicative providers supported by involved, interested parents cannot be overstressed. Behavioral techniques attempt to develop effective strategies to assist learning and ultimately promote self-esteem. Even with compensatory techniques and functional improvement, the underlying neurocognitive substrates may

continue to influence brain development and increase the risk for comorbid behavioral and psychiatric disorders (Fletcher 2005; Litt et al. 2005).

There are no pharmacological cures for LD. At best, medications may help reduce the impact of co-occurring disorders, such as ADHD or mood disorders, that can have profound effects on symptom manifestation. Medications, notably anticonvulsant drugs, may impede learning in complex ways.

The most significant intervention for a child with DCD who meets criteria for special education in the public school is the implementation of an individualized education plan with annual goals for improvement. The primary treatment for DCD is occupational therapy either individually or with a group.

Communication Disorders

Communication disorders, as defined in DSM-IV-TR, are characterized by delays in expressive or receptive language in excess of the difficulties expected given an individual's intelligence and that result in significant scholastic, work, or social interference. These disorders have an enormous impact on concurrent and subsequent development, social functioning, and psychiatric outcomes.

Expressive Language Disorder and Mixed Receptive–Expressive Language Disorder

Clinical Description

In expressive language disorder, language understanding is intact, but the individual cannot express him- or herself adequately. This impairment often results in brief verbal responses and incorrect sentences and use of words. Seemingly regressive or immature speech is common and is consistent with the slow acquisition of skills (Table 12–8). In

Table 12–8. DSM-IV-TR diagnostic criteria for expressive language disorder

A. The scores obtained from standardized individually administered measures of expressive language development are substantially below those obtained from standardized measures of both nonverbal intellectual capacity and receptive language development. The disturbance may be manifest clinically by symptoms that include having a markedly limited vocabulary, making errors in tense, or having difficulty recalling words or producing sentences with developmentally appropriate length or complexity.

B. The difficulties with expressive language interfere with academic or occupational achievement or with social communication.

C. Criteria are not met for mixed receptive–expressive language disorder or a pervasive developmental disorder.

D. If mental retardation, a speech–motor or sensory deficit, or environmental deprivation is present, the language difficulties are in excess of those usually associated with these problems.

Coding note: If a speech–motor or sensory deficit or a neurological condition is present, code the condition on Axis III.

Table 12–9. DSM-IV-TR diagnostic criteria for mixed receptive–expressive language disorder

A. The scores obtained from a battery of standardized individually administered measures of both receptive and expressive language development are substantially below those obtained from standardized measures of nonverbal intellectual capacity. Symptoms include those for expressive language disorder as well as difficulty understanding words, sentences, or specific types of words, such as spatial terms.

B. The difficulties with receptive and expressive language significantly interfere with academic or occupational achievement or with social communication.

C. Criteria are not met for a pervasive developmental disorder.

D. If mental retardation, a speech–motor or sensory deficit, or environmental deprivation is present, the language difficulties are in excess of those usually associated with these problems.

Coding note: If a speech–motor or sensory deficit or a neurological condition is present, code the condition on Axis III.

mixed receptive–expressive language disorder, the impaired expressive communication is compounded by deficits in comprehension of aspects of language (Table 12–9). Given the disparate abilities between intellect and expressive skills, significant frustration is common and can be conceptualized as an etiology for the social difficulties and dysphoria individuals with these disorders often experience.

Epidemiology

Prevalences for the communication disorders are difficult to determine given the variable definitions that have been, and continue to be, used. The U.S. Department of Educa-

tion reported in 2002 that 18.9% of the nearly 5.8 million children in the public schools receiving special education are treated for "speech and language impairments," although this number may be limited by the availability of services. Male predominance of 3–4:1 is evident.

Etiology

Etiologies for communication disorders are often found in combination and appear to be cumulative. Biological factors such as prenatal exposures, perinatal adversity, early childhood illness (e.g., otitis media), and known genetic or metabolic disorders have been shown to be important. Environmental risk factors such as abuse, neglect, and poverty have also been implicated.

Psychiatric comorbidity is common. The possibility of a common etiology between the language disorders and ADHD has been proposed. Disruptive behavior disorders, anxiety disorders, and substance use disorders are frequently comorbid in these individuals.

Course and Prognosis

Approximately one-half of young children with expressive and mixed receptive–expressive language disorders develop normal language abilities by adolescence. Those with persistent disorders typically demonstrate greater severity of symptoms at the time of initial presentation. A diagnosis of mixed receptive–expressive language disorder may have a poorer prognosis than that of expressive language disorder.

Diagnostic Evaluation

In addition to documenting the developmental history, careful assessment of language can occur in the context of a clinical examination. Rutter (1987) proposed special attention to inner language (the use of symbolization), language production, phonation, and pragmatic communication. Should concerns arise, a referral for further assessment involving cognitive and language testing should be made.

Treatment

Specialized treatment for children identified as having a communication disorder is available through special education services in the public school system. The interventions available vary from system to system but should follow from an individualized assessment and plan. Specific approaches are roughly categorized as behavioral, child-centered, or a combination of these approaches (Paul 2001).

Phonological Disorder

Clinical Description and Symptoms

Very common in pediatric populations, phonological disorder is characterized by im-

Table 12–10. DSM-IV-TR diagnostic criteria for phonological disorder

A. Failure to use developmentally expected speech sounds that are appropriate for age and dialect (e.g., errors in sound production, use, representation, or organization such as, but not limited to, substitutions of one sound for another [use of /t/ for target /k/ sound] or omissions of sounds such as final consonants).

B. The difficulties in speech sound production interfere with academic or occupational achievement or with social communication.

C. If mental retardation, a speech–motor or sensory deficit, or environmental deprivation is present, the speech difficulties are in excess of those usually associated with these problems.

Coding note: If a speech–motor or sensory deficit or a neurological condition is present, code the condition on Axis III.

pairment in the ability to produce and use developmentally appropriate speech sounds. Typically, this results in poor intelligibility or gives the appearance of persistent "baby talk" (Table 12–10). Most children do grow out of their symptoms; however, in moderate to severe cases, difficulties may persist.

Epidemiology

Occurring in nearly 20% of preschool and approximately 6% of school-age children, phonological disorder's prevalence decreases with advancing age. Milder forms are more common than moderate and severe cases. Phonological disorder affects males more frequently than females and is associated with LDs, enuresis, neurological soft signs, DCD, and scholastic difficulty (American Psychiatric Association 2000).

Etiology

Speech production impairments due solely to intellectual disability, hearing impairment, or problems with the speech mechanism are excluded from the diagnosis. As in the other communication disorders, biological and environmental factors are likely.

Diagnostic Evaluation

Again, as in the other communication disorders, screening can occur during initial interviews, paying special attention to developmental history and school difficulties. Given the high rates of comorbidity with additional communication disorders and LDs, assessments of intelligence and hearing and a full speech/language assessment are often warranted.

Treatment

Amelioration of symptoms can be gained through the use of speech therapy. Appropriate treatment of associated difficulties is important.

Stuttering

Clinical Description

Stuttering is the interruption of normal flow of speech. It is characterized by frequent repetitions or prolongations of sounds or syllables, involuntary and irregular hesitation, broken words, and silent or audible blocking (Table 12–11). Stuttering typically begins between 2 and 7 years of age, with a peak onset at age 5 years. Stuttering must be distinguished from normal dysfluencies that occur frequently in young children but generally last less than 6 months. The onset is typically insidious, and the child is usually unaware. Anxiety commonly aggravates the disturbance. About two-thirds of individuals who stutter ultimately are able to make effective use of treatment techniques and overcome the difficulty. Some individuals recover spontaneously, typically before the age of 16 years.

Epidemiology

Approximately 1% of young children stutter, and increased rates of comorbid communication disorders such as phonological disorder are often found. The male-to-female ratio is approximately 3:1 (American Psychiatric Association 2000). This may be secondary to the fact that females demonstrate higher rates of recovery compared with males. The effect of stuttering on self-esteem may be linked with increased impairments in social functioning as well as academic and occupational difficulties.

Table 12–11. DSM-IV-TR diagnostic criteria for stuttering

A. Disturbance in the normal fluency and time patterning of speech (inappropriate for the individual's age), characterized by frequent occurrences of one or more of the following:
   (1) sound and syllable repetitions
   (2) sound prolongations
   (3) interjections
   (4) broken words (e.g., pauses within a word)
   (5) audible or silent blocking (filled or unfilled pauses in speech)
   (6) circumlocutions (word substitutions to avoid problematic words)
   (7) words produced with an excess of physical tension
   (8) monosyllabic whole-word repetitions (e.g., "I-I-I-I see him")
B. The disturbance in fluency interferes with academic or occupational achievement or with social communication.
C. If a speech–motor or sensory deficit is present, the speech difficulties are in excess of those usually associated with these problems.
Coding note: If a speech–motor or sensory deficit or a neurological condition is present, code the condition on Axis III.

Etiology

Genetic mechanisms for stuttering are strongly implicated given the strong familial association and high rates of affected first-degree relatives. Stuttering may also be acquired by stroke or degenerative disorder located in the cerebellum, basal ganglia, or cortex.

Diagnostic Evaluation

In addition to the comprehensive interview that is appropriate when concern for a communication disorder is raised, potential organic (i.e., brain-based) causes of stuttering need to be considered and ruled out. Assessments of speech, language, and hearing are needed, and referral to a speech/language specialist is typically made.

Treatment

Behavioral interventions are the cornerstone of treatment for stuttering. These include specific speech therapy as well as elements of relaxation, rhythm control, feedback, modification of environmental triggers, role-playing, and assertiveness training. Pharmacotherapy and psychotherapy can be considered for associated amenable symptoms (e.g., performance anxiety, self-esteem).

Pervasive Developmental Disorders

The PDDs are a heterogeneous group of neuropsychiatric disorders characterized by recognizable patterns of deviation in typical development during the first years of life. These deviations typically arise in the areas of 1) social understanding and interest, 2) communication, and 3) cognitive abilities; however, additional domains of development are frequently involved. Assessment of the affected individual is often complicated by the nonuniform degree of disruption within specific areas of development, and highly individualized profiles of abilities, interests, and difficulties are typical.

Autistic Disorder

Clinical Description

First formally described by Kanner (1943), "early infantile autism" was characterized by autistic disinterest in the social environment and obsessive insistence on sameness. Additional features included speech delay, echolalia and pronoun reversal, and unusual repetitive motor behaviors (or stereotypies). In 1968, Rutter proposed four essential characteristics that emanated from the existing evidence and were present in nearly all children with autism: 1) lack of social interest and responsiveness, 2) impaired language, 3) bizarre motor behavior, and 4) onset prior to the age of 30 months. In 1980, with the development of DSM-III (American Psychiatric Association 1980), the diagnosis of infantile autism was included with the new class of "pervasive developmental disorders." In DSM-IV (American Psychiatric Association 1994), the diagnosis of autistic disorder was established via a large multisite study (Volkmar et al. 1994), and emphasis was placed on developmental aspects of the disorder. Minor adjustments to the diagnostic criteria were made in DSM-IV-TR in an attempt to facilitate clinical use (Table 12–12).

Individuals with autistic disorder may present at any age although most often in the first few years of life. Widely varying levels of relative strengths and weaknesses in specific areas of functioning are typical, and when the diagnosis co-occurs with intellectual disability (mental retardation), this intellectual profile can help to distinguish the diagnosis from the often uniform pattern of difficulties seen in intellectual disability alone.

Approximately two-thirds to three-fourths of individuals with autism also have intellectual disability. Clinicians should be aware that individuals with autism seem to be especially disadvantaged when it comes to performance on standardized assessments of cognitive ability due to the condition's inherent difficulties in verbal and reading comprehension, sequencing, feature extraction, and

---

Table 12–12. DSM-IV-TR diagnostic criteria for autistic disorder

---

A. A total of six (or more) items from (1), (2), and (3), with at least two from (1), and one each from (2) and (3):
   (1) qualitative impairment in social interaction, as manifested by at least two of the following:
      (a) marked impairment in the use of multiple nonverbal behaviors such as eye-to-eye gaze, facial expression, body postures, and gestures to regulate social interaction
      (b) failure to develop peer relationships appropriate to developmental level
      (c) a lack of spontaneous seeking to share enjoyment, interests, or achievements with other people (e.g., by a lack of showing, bringing, or pointing out objects of interest)
      (d) lack of social or emotional reciprocity
   (2) qualitative impairments in communication as manifested by at least one of the following:
      (a) delay in, or total lack of, the development of spoken language (not accompanied by an attempt to compensate through alternative modes of communication such as gesture or mime)
      (b) in individuals with adequate speech, marked impairment in the ability to initiate or sustain a conversation with others
      (c) stereotyped and repetitive use of language or idiosyncratic language
      (d) lack of varied, spontaneous make-believe play or social imitative play appropriate to developmental level
   (3) restricted repetitive and stereotyped patterns of behavior, interests, and activities, as manifested by at least one of the following:
      (a) encompassing preoccupation with one or more stereotyped and restricted patterns of interest that is abnormal either in intensity or focus
      (b) apparently inflexible adherence to specific, nonfunctional routines or rituals
      (c) stereotyped and repetitive motor mannerisms (e.g., hand or finger flapping or twisting, or complex whole-body movements)
      (d) persistent preoccupation with parts of objects
B. Delays or abnormal functioning in at least one of the following areas, with onset prior to age 3 years: (1) social interaction, (2) language as used in social communication, or (3) symbolic or imaginative play.
C. The disturbance is not better accounted for by Rett's disorder or childhood disintegrative disorder.

---

executive function. The presence of extraordinary abilities or savant skills is rare.

Social Interaction

Individuals with autistic disorder demonstrate wide ranges of interest and ability in social interaction. Kanner's (1943) original description of infantile autism, which described an aloof disinterest in others and avoidance of eye contact, represents only a portion of the autistic population. Many accurately diagnosed individuals with autistic disorder demonstrate social interest but lack the understanding necessary for typical reciprocal interaction. Early on there is often a lack of social referencing, and others exist solely as objects. Attachment to unusual things may be evident, whereas attachment to and affection for others typically demonstrate significant delay. Social interest may grow with time; however, a lack of reciprocity and an inability to appreciate others' perceptions may cause increasing problems with maturing peers, and frustration over friendships is common.

Communication Impairment

Individuals with autism typically demonstrate impaired verbal comprehension, delayed and unusual speech, and limited nonverbal communication. Mutism is very common among people with autism, and even in bright individuals, speech can be slow to develop (or appear to explode fully developed after an initial period of delay). Gestures are infrequently used. Echolalia, pronoun reversals, and abnormal or absent intonation can make the speech of individuals with autism difficult to understand. The subtleties of humor and imaginative or abstract thought typically remain elusive. Topics of discussion tend to be limited to the autistic person's areas of special interest. Often, high-functioning people with autism develop and rely on scripted bits of dialogue, which can prove surprisingly effective during superficial or initial social interactions.

Patterns of Behavior

Individuals with autism are uncommonly resistant to change, and seemingly minor alterations to an expected pattern can provoke significant distress and anxiety. This often results in the routinization of activities. Ritualized compulsive thoughts and behavior are commonplace and may be manifest in preoccupations, repetitive questioning, and physical mannerisms (e.g., hand flapping, spinning). Unusual responses to sensory stimuli are commonplace, with many people with autism becoming "overwhelmed" by sounds, smells, or levels of light that are tolerable for others or in turn tolerating (even enjoying) stimuli that nonautistic individuals find noxious. Associated physical observations often include poor motor imitation, gait and tone abnormalities, and neurological soft signs and may include hyperactivity and self-injurious behavior (SIB). "Impulsivity," upon careful assessment, frequently becomes explicable in light of an understanding of the individual's special interests or anxieties.

Epidemiology

Autism appears to occur in approximately 10–20 per 10,000 births (Fombonne et al. 2006; Gillberg and Wing 1999), although widely varying prevalences have been reported (0.15–34.00 per 10,000; see Tsai 2004). Prevalences have consistently increased since the mid-1990s, and this has raised public concern. It is difficult to ascertain whether a true increase in incidence exists or whether it is a reflection of expanding awareness and ascertainment. A male predominance of approximately 4:1 exists, although females tend to be more severely affected and may have greater cognitive impairment. Approximately 70% have intellectual disability, although this percentage has declined in recent years, likely due to increased popular awareness of autism as well as the widening acceptance of the concept of a spectrum of dysfunction in the disorder. Early suggestions that autism is associated with higher socioeconomic class were the result of ascertainment bias.

Psychiatric comorbidities have been difficult to quantify given the significant symptom overlap between autism, mental retardation, and other psychiatric disorders. Careful consideration and, ideally, comparison with a large population of individuals with autism are necessary to distinguish, for example, the anxiety, obsessive and compulsive behaviors, or impulsivity common in autism from anxiety disorders, obsessive-compulsive disorder (OCD), and impulse-control disorders, respectively.

Seizure disorder is more common in individuals with autism and demonstrates an apparent bimodal distribution of onset, with new seizures appearing more frequently in the first year of life and again during adolescence.

Severe environmental deprivation can result in a presentation that demonstrates many features consistent with the diagnosis; however, the extent of the presentation's reversibility and modification with appropriate intervention often distinguish this from autism.

Etiology

Certain medical conditions are associated with autism; tuberous sclerosis, fragile X syndrome, maternal rubella, congenital hypothyroidism, phenylketonuria, Down syndrome, neurofibromatosis, and Angelman's syndrome are some of the conditions that have been identified. In the vast majority of cases (likely greater than 90%), there is no readily identifiable cause for autism.

A growing body of evidence from family, twin, and chromosomal studies supports the genetic basis of autism. First-degree family members of individuals with autism have been shown to have greater-than-expected incidences of anxiety disorders, major depression, and motor tics. Additionally, parents of children with autism have been shown to have higher rates of rigidity, aloofness, anxiety, and limited friendships, part of a constellation of characteristics that has been called the "broad autism phenotype" (Piven et al. 1997).

Course and Prognosis

Although autism is a chronic condition, most individuals demonstrate gradual improvement in their symptoms due to further maturation and understanding a need to modify their behavior. Improvement is consistently maximized when people with autism are provided adequate support, education (which can draw on individual strengths), and management of problematic symptoms or comorbidities. The amount of improvement is closely tied to symptom severity, cognitive and language ability, and the establishment of realistic expectations given the specific areas of difficulty.

Diagnostic Evaluation

Accurate diagnosis is predicated on a complete psychiatric and medical evaluation. Given the rare but recognizable medical conditions associated with autism, close attention to maternal and prenatal histories is necessary. Assessment of the person's early development requires an informed historian. Sensory evaluations (hearing, including brainstem auditory evoked responses [if necessary] and visual screening) are often necessary. The use of standardized diagnostic assessments is not indicated for the clinical diagnosis of autistic disorder but may prove useful along with cognitive and language testing for subsequent treatment decisions. Additional clinically informed laboratory data are often gathered, often based on the age at presentation. Genetic screening for metabolic disorders, chromosome analysis, and genetic counseling in cases of intellectual disability and potentially identifiable syndromes are warranted. Heavy metal screening is appropriate if a possible history of ingestion is identified. Neurological consultation may be warranted secondary to clinical concerns regarding the presence of seizures, and electroencephalograms are often obtained. In most idiopathic cases of autism, neuroimaging is neither warranted nor currently clinically useful.

Treatment

The foundations of effective treatment in autistic disorder comprise parental counseling, child educational interventions that are tailored to an individual student's strengths and difficulties, and behavior (e.g., skill acquisition and practice in a social group) and environmental modification (e.g., the use of schedules, visual cueing, and highly structured settings). Although historically psychotherapy—even for high-functioning individuals—was discouraged, cognitive-behavioral approaches may be beneficial given the level of some individuals' interest and insight as compared with often disparate successes and facility.

There are no pharmacological treatments for autistic disorder. However, psychopharmacological interventions often play a supportive role in the treatment of some individuals. The careful selection and surveillance of appropriate target symptoms are of the utmost importance and demand close contact with families and care providers. Additionally, given the level of rigidity and resistance to change that most individuals with autism demonstrate, the seemingly inconsequential addition of a medication into a morning routine, for example, can be enough to induce significant distress. Thus, extended medication trial durations are often appropriate to ensure that the clinician is measuring a medication effect. Perhaps related to this is the clinical belief that individuals with autism often are responsive to seemingly trivial dosages of psychoactive medication. All of this serves to remind the clinician of the importance of "starting low and going slow" with medications in a population that is often limited or unusual in its ability to report benefit and side effects.

The SSRIs, especially fluoxetine, sertraline, and citalopram, seem to be beneficial in the reduction of compulsive and repetitive behaviors, behavioral rigidity, and aggression (Posey et al. 2006). The atypical antipsychotic risperidone reduces self-injury and aggression (McCracken et al. 2002) and repetitive behaviors (McDougle et al. 2005), but caution is urged, given this drug class's characteristic weight gain and other potential and serious side effects. Other commonly prescribed medications from pediatric formulary include α-agonists targeting impulsivity and hyperactivity, stimulants for hyperactivity and poor concentration, and anticonvulsants for serious aggression.

Despite reports of the benefits of various nutritional and dietary approaches (including the use of "nutriceuticals") in the treatment of autism, the value of these approaches is difficult to assess. Melatonin is often used to facilitate sleep; however, at the present time no specific interventions from these generally unscrutinized reports can be recommended.

Rett's Disorder

Clinical Description and Symptoms

Originally described in 1966, Rett's disorder is characterized by a period of decelerated head growth, loss of purposeful hand movements, midline upper extremity stereotypies (e.g., hand-wringing), severe psychomotor retar-

dation, gait and truncal apraxia, impaired language, and social withdrawal. Typically diagnosed after age 3 years, the disorder exists almost exclusively in females. Associated findings include respiratory symptoms (e.g., breath holding, wakeful apnea, hyperventilation), seizures, spasticity, muscle wasting and dystonia, scoliosis, and growth retardation. Evidence of intrauterine growth retardation, perinatal brain damage, or metabolic or progressive neurological disorder excludes the diagnosis (Table 12–13).

Children with Rett's disorder often also have unusual sleep architecture and increased daytime, decreased nighttime, and increased total sleep. Thyroid problems, increased risk of osteoporosis, and feeding problems due to oropharyngeal abnormalities warrant clinical vigilance.

Table 12–13. DSM-IV-TR diagnostic criteria for Rett's disorder

A. All of the following:
  (1) apparently normal prenatal and perinatal development
  (2) apparently normal psychomotor development through the first 5 months after birth
  (3) normal head circumference at birth

B. Onset of all of the following after the period of normal development:
  (1) deceleration of head growth between ages 5 and 48 months
  (2) loss of previously acquired purposeful hand skills between ages 5 and 30 months with the subsequent development of stereotyped hand movements (e.g., hand-wringing or hand washing)
  (3) loss of social engagement early in the course (although often social interaction develops later)
  (4) appearance of poorly coordinated gait or trunk movements
  (5) severely impaired expressive and receptive language development with severe psychomotor retardation

---

Epidemiology

Estimates of prevalence of Rett's disorder range from 0.44 to 2.10 per 10,000 females. A handful of cases in males have been reported and usually demonstrate an atypical presentation.

Etiology

Multiple different mutations in the gene encoding MECP2 at Xq28 have been identified in a large number of individuals with typical and atypical Rett's disorder (Amir et al. 1999), and nearly all appear to be spontaneous mutations.

Course and Prognosis

A four-stage model of this progressive disorder has been proposed (Hagberg and Witt-Engerström 1986):

1. Early-onset stagnation stage from age 6 months to 1.5 years, with decelerated head growth, hypotonia, and loss of interest in play
2. Rapid developmental regression stage from age 1–2 years and lasting 13–19 months, with the onset of autistic symptoms and often seizures
3. Pseudostationary stage typically occurring at age 3–4 years but may be delayed and persists for years to decades, with the development of characteristic respiratory abnormalities
4. Late motor deterioration stage often occurring during school age or early adolescence, with muscle wasting, weakness, scoliosis, and limb distortion; most individuals with Rett's disorder live well into adulthood (summarized from Tsai 2004)

Diagnostic Evaluation

Clinical diagnosis of Rett's disorder can be supported by molecular analysis of the gene encoding MECP2 at Xq28, although an absence of recognizable gene abnormality at this site does not refute the diagnosis.

Treatment

As is indicated for other PDDs, supportive treatment for families and individuals with Rett's disorder is indicated. Additional education modification is warranted in light of the accompanying intellectual disability. Preparation for the typically worsening physical limitations is appropriate.

Childhood Disintegrative Disorder

Clinical Description

In 1908, Heller described a series of cases of pediatric dementia with onset after age 3–4 years, during which time development had been entirely normal. Originally called *dementia infantilis*, this relatively rare syndrome consists of cognitive decline that usually stabilizes and remains static or improves minimally over time. Additional researchers have described similar presentations and developed the diagnostic term *disintegrative psychosis of childhood*. This has become childhood disintegrative disorder (Table 12–14). The validity of this diagnosis has been well demonstrated (Volkmar and Rutter 1995).

The loss of communication abilities and social functioning in these individuals mimics the presentation in autism. Initial behavioral symptoms (such as tantrums, anxiety, or irritability, sometimes appearing after a neurological illness) are sometimes present, and cognitive symptoms develop abruptly (over days to weeks) or gradually (over weeks to months) and ultimately progress to loss of cognitive ability, speech and language, and social skills. Typically individuals with childhood disintegrative disorder have higher incidences of new-onset seizures (when compared with individuals with intellectual disability alone).

Epidemiology

An incidence of 1 per 100,000 is commonly accepted, with a significant male predominance.

Table 12–14. DSM-IV-TR diagnostic criteria for childhood disintegrative disorder

---

A. Apparently normal development for at least the first 2 years after birth as manifested by the presence of age-appropriate verbal and nonverbal communication, social relationships, play, and adaptive behavior.

B. Clinically significant loss of previously acquired skills (before age 10 years) in at least two of the following areas:
    (1) expressive or receptive language
    (2) social skills or adaptive behavior
    (3) bowel or bladder control
    (4) play
    (5) motor skills

C. Abnormalities of functioning in at least two of the following areas:
    (1) qualitative impairment in social interaction (e.g., impairment in nonverbal behaviors, failure to develop peer relationships, lack of social or emotional reciprocity)
    (2) qualitative impairments in communication (e.g., delay or lack of spoken language, inability to initiate or sustain a conversation, stereotyped and repetitive use of language, lack of varied make-believe play)
    (3) restricted, repetitive, and stereotyped patterns of behavior, interests, and activities, including motor stereotypies and mannerisms

D. The disturbance is not better accounted for by another specific pervasive developmental disorder or by schizophrenia.

Etiology

No underlying cause of childhood disintegrative disorder has been identified.

Course and Prognosis

The progressive loss of abilities over days to months appears to be very consistent, with a minority of individuals experiencing persistent decline and usually death. Most experience stabilization of symptoms (with or without minimal improvement), and the prognosis becomes a product of the person's ultimate level of cognitive ability and adaptive functioning.

Diagnostic Evaluation

The diagnostic workup of childhood disintegrative disorder is similar to that in autistic disorder; however, the extent of neurological evaluation is appropriately intensified.

Treatment

Support for families and adaptation of the psychosocial intervention recommended in autistic disorder are appropriate. A role for medications targeting specific problematic symptoms can be envisioned as being useful; however, there are few data to support this.

Asperger's Disorder

Clinical Description

While Kanner was describing early infantile autism in the United States, Asperger reported on a series of patients in Austria who demonstrated similar presentations. Similar to those with Kanner's infantile autism, these boys demonstrated poor social understanding and skills, intense special interests, and clumsiness but lacked language delay. Asperger referred to these patients as "little professors" (Asperger 1944/1991). The diagnosis of Asperger's disorder came to increased prominence (especially in the United States) during the 1980s. The clinical picture of individuals with Asperger's disorder is notable for the lack of intellectual disability, but as with autistic disorder, variable presentations are common (Table 12–15). The differentiation of Asperger's disorder from autism

---

Table 12–15.   DSM-IV-TR diagnostic criteria for Asperger's disorder

A. Qualitative impairment in social interaction, as manifested by at least two of the following:
   (1) marked impairment in the use of multiple nonverbal behaviors such as eye-to-eye gaze, facial expression, body postures, and gestures to regulate social interaction
   (2) failure to develop peer relationships appropriate to developmental level
   (3) a lack of spontaneous seeking to share enjoyment, interests, or achievements with other people (e.g., by a lack of showing, bringing, or pointing out objects of interest to other people)
   (4) lack of social or emotional reciprocity
B. Restricted repetitive and stereotyped patterns of behavior, interests, and activities, as manifested by at least one of the following:
   (1) encompassing preoccupation with one or more stereotyped and restricted patterns of interest that is abnormal in either intensity or focus
   (2) apparently inflexible adherence to specific, nonfunctional routines or rituals
   (3) stereotyped and repetitive motor mannerisms (e.g., hand or finger flapping or twisting, or complex whole-body movements)
   (4) persistent preoccupation with parts of objects
C. The disturbance causes clinically significant impairment in social, occupational, or other important areas of functioning.
D. There is no clinically significant general delay in language (e.g., single words used by age 2 years, communicative phrases used by age 3 years).
E. There is no clinically significant delay in cognitive development or in the development of age-appropriate self-help skills, adaptive behavior (other than in social interaction), and curiosity about the environment in childhood.
F. Criteria are not met for another specific pervasive developmental disorder or schizophrenia.

(especially in individuals with normal intelligence) can be quite difficult, and controversy exists as to whether Asperger's disorder represents a PDD subtype or the highest-functioning portion of an autistic disorder spectrum (South et al. 2005).

Impairments in social interaction and restricted and repetitive interests and behaviors are hallmarks of the disorder. Unusual communication is common, often characterized by pedantic speech, intense preoccupations, and poor or nonexistent nonverbal communication, although in distinction from autistic disorder, "clinically significant general delay in language" and "cognitive delay" are exclusionary criteria. In addition, it is commonly held that individuals with Asperger's disorder are clumsy.

Epidemiology

Prevalence rates of 0.6–10.0 per 10,000 have been published, although some of these studies lack the application of consistent diagnostic criteria. Investigation of associated psychiatric comorbidities has implicated similar diagnoses to those associated with autistic disorder; affective illness, Tourette's disorder, ADHD, anxiety disorders, and schizophrenia have all been associated with Asperger's disorder.

Etiology

The specific etiology of Asperger's disorder is unknown, although most agree that similarities to autistic disorder imply similar etiologies.

Course and Prognosis

Although the characteristics of Asperger's disorder appear to be lifelong in their duration, more recent research seems to suggest that individuals with the disorder demonstrate higher rates of employment and education and greater levels of self-sufficiency than those with autistic disorder.

Diagnostic Evaluation

The evaluation does not differ significantly from that recommended in autistic disorder. Given the exclusionary criteria of the diagnosis, careful attention to the individual's history of cognitive and language development is necessary.

Treatment

As in autistic disorder, appropriate recognition of the profile of the individual's strengths and difficulties will guide intervention. Cognitive approaches in individual therapy can be beneficial for interested and motivated people. Pharmacological interventions target similar behavioral symptoms to those described for autism.

Attention-Deficit/ Hyperactivity Disorder

Clinical Description

ADHD is defined by three core symptom clusters: inattention, hyperactivity, and impulsivity (Table 12–16). DSM-IV-TR divides ADHD into three types according to the presence or absence of six symptoms in each category. These are primarily inattentive type, primarily hyperactive–impulsive type, and combined type (for those with symptoms in both categories). Some symptoms must be present prior to age 7 years and must occur for at least 6 months in more than one setting. They must cause clinically significant impairment in social, academic, or occupational functioning and be inconsistent for developmental age and intellectual ability (American Psychiatric Association 2000).

Individuals with ADHD have poorer academic performance and higher rates of LDs than other children. They have difficulties in executive functioning as demonstrated by poor planning and deficits in working memory, verbal fluency, and motor sequencing. Additional impairments of executive functioning include an inability to attend, encode, and manipulate information as well as an inability to organize and manage a sequence of actions. These children are often rejected by peers as a result of their impulsive and hyperactive behaviors. This rejection has a strong relationship with poor outcomes such as conduct disturbance, substance abuse, and school failure.

The inattentive subtype shows deficits in focused and selective attention. These children tend to be less active and may have more anxiety and somatic complaints than those with the combined or hyperactive–impulsive type. Children with the combined type have deficits in sustained attention and distractibility. They frequently have more externalizing behaviors, show increased aggression and delinquency, and are more likely to be diagnosed with a comorbid disruptive behavior disorder.

Epidemiology

DSM-IV-TR estimates rates of ADHD to be between 3% and 7% in school-age children, although it has been reported to range from 1.9% to 14.4% (Scahill and Schwab-Stone 2000). Higher IQ can often compensate for the impairments of ADHD and may lead to a later diagnosis. ADHD accounts for 30%–50% of referrals for mental health services for children (Multimodal Treatment of ADHD Cooperative Group 1999).

Teachers identify fewer girls than boys with ADHD symptoms, and the combined type is the most common subtype in both girls and boys. The disorder is more common in males than females, at a ratio of 4:1 (Gershorn 2002), although this decreases to 2:1 for the predominantly inattentive type (Wolraich et al. 1996).

Table 12–16. DSM-IV-TR diagnostic criteria for attention-deficit/hyperactivity disorder

---

A. Either (1) or (2):

(1) six (or more) of the following symptoms of **inattention** have persisted for at least 6 months to a degree that is maladaptive and inconsistent with developmental level:

Inattention

    (a) often fails to give close attention to details or makes careless mistakes in schoolwork, work, or other activities

    (b) often has difficulty sustaining attention in tasks or play activities

    (c) often does not seem to listen when spoken to directly

    (d) often does not follow through on instructions and fails to finish schoolwork, chores, or duties in the workplace (not due to oppositional behavior or failure to understand instructions)

    (e) often has difficulty organizing tasks and activities

    (f) often avoids, dislikes, or is reluctant to engage in tasks that require sustained mental effort (such as schoolwork or homework)

    (g) often loses things necessary for tasks or activities (e.g., toys, school assignments, pencils, books, or tools)

    (h) is often easily distracted by extraneous stimuli

    (i) is often forgetful in daily activities

(2) six (or more) of the following symptoms of **hyperactivity-impulsivity** have persisted for at least 6 months to a degree that is maladaptive and inconsistent with developmental level:

Hyperactivity

    (a) often fidgets with hands or feet or squirms in seat

    (b) often leaves seat in classroom or in other situations in which remaining seated is expected

    (c) often runs about or climbs excessively in situations in which it is inappropriate (in adolescents or adults, may be limited to subjective feelings of restlessness)

    (d) often has difficulty playing or engaging in leisure activities quietly

    (e) is often "on the go" or often acts as if "driven by a motor"

    (f) often talks excessively

Impulsivity

    (g) often blurts out answers before questions have been completed

    (h) often has difficulty awaiting turn

    (i) often interrupts or intrudes on others (e.g., butts into conversations or games)

B. Some hyperactive–impulsive or inattentive symptoms that caused impairment were present before age 7 years.

C. Some impairment from the symptoms is present in two or more settings (e.g., at school [or work] and at home).

D. There must be clear evidence of clinically significant impairment in social, academic, or occupational functioning.

E. The symptoms do not occur exclusively during the course of a pervasive developmental disorder, schizophrenia, or other psychotic disorder and are not better accounted for by another mental disorder (e.g., mood disorder, anxiety disorder, dissociative disorder, or a personality disorder).

Table 12–16.   DSM-IV-TR diagnostic criteria for attention-deficit/hyperactivity disorder *(continued)*

Code based on type:

> **314.01 Attention-deficit/hyperactivity disorder, combined type:**   if both criteria A1 and A2 are met for the past 6 months
>
> **314.00 Attention-deficit/hyperactivity disorder, predominantly inattentive type:**   if criterion A1 is met but criterion A2 is not met for the past 6 months
>
> **314.01 Attention-deficit/hyperactivity disorder, predominantly hyperactive–impulsive type:**   if criterion A2 is met but criterion A1 is not met for the past 6 months

Coding note: For individuals (especially adolescents and adults) who currently have symptoms that no longer meet full criteria, "in partial remission" should be specified.

Approximately 4% of college-age students and adults have ADHD, with a gender ratio of 1:1 (Wilens and Dodson 2004). Anywhere from 4% to 75% of cases persist to adulthood (Fischer 1997; Hechtman 1993). This wide range is likely secondary to methodological differences in the studies. Family history of ADHD, psychosocial adversity, and comorbidity with conduct, mood, and anxiety disorders increase the risk of persistence of ADHD symptoms (Biederman et al. 1996).

ADHD is highly comorbid with other psychiatric disorders. Up to two-thirds of individuals with ADHD have another comorbid psychiatric disorder. Disruptive behavior disorders occur with high frequency. Additionally, 15%–20% of persons with ADHD may have a mood disorder, and another 20%–25% may have a co-occurring anxiety disorder that may affect the overall degree of impairment (Biederman et al. 1991; Jensen et al. 1993; Newcorn and Halperin 1994). LDs may co-occur in 10%–25% of those with ADHD, although, in general, children with ADHD (whether with or without a formal LD) perform more poorly academically than children without ADHD (Faraone et al. 1993). In adolescents, ADHD may also be associated with substance use disorders, CD, and mood and anxiety disorders. Adults with ADHD are most commonly at risk for comorbid depression, anxiety, and substance use disorders (Spencer et al. 1999).

Etiology

ADHD is a heterogeneous behavioral disorder with multiple possible etiologies. A number of biological and environmental factors have been implicated.

Genetics

ADHD is a highly familial disorder, with 25%–50% of cases occurring in families. Among first-degree relatives of children with ADHD, 15%–25% have the disorder, and up to 50% of children whose parents have the disorder also have ADHD (Wilens and Dodson 2004). The specific genes associated with ADHD include the dopamine receptor gene, the dopamine transporter gene, and the dopamine-beta-hydroxylase gene (Wilens and Dodson 2004).

Neuroanatomical and Neurochemical Factors

Although the specific pathophysiology of ADHD remains unclear, recent research on the neural circuits of the prefrontal cortex and striatum, as well as on the brain stem catecholamine systems that innervate these circuits, has advanced our understanding of the possible underlying mechanisms of this disorder. Neuroimaging studies have suggested that impairments in prefrontal-striatal regions play a central role in the pathophysiology of ADHD. Structural imaging studies using magnetic resonance imaging (MRI) have revealed subtle but unique anomalies in the prefrontal cortex and basal ganglia of children with ADHD.

Other Medical Illness

Although an increased risk of ADHD has been reported in a rare genetic disorder of generalized resistance to thyroid hormone (Hauser et al. 1993), the rate of thyroid abnormalities in children with ADHD is very low (Elia et al. 1994). There is no evidence to support routine screening of thyroid function in children with ADHD without other indicators of thyroid disease. There may be increased rates of ADHD in children with a history of recurrent ear infections and acquired sensorineural hearing loss (Elia et al. 1994; Kelly et al. 1993). However, there does not appear to be evidence to support the idea that children with allergies or allergic-type illness such as asthma or eczema have higher rates of ADHD (Biederman et al. 1994; McGee et al. 1993).

Prenatal and Perinatal Factors

Exposure to toxins during pregnancy may contribute to the development of ADHD. Maternal smoking during pregnancy is associated with higher rates of ADHD in offspring, possibly linked to increased fetal testosterone (Rizwan et al. 2007). Children exposed to lead and alcohol during pregnancy can manifest many symptoms of inattention, hyperactivity, and impulsivity. Perinatal complications may also play a role in the development of ADHD.

Diet

The role of preservatives, artificial dyes, or food allergies on hyperactivity and impulsivity remains controversial, with studies both supporting and refuting their importance (Barling and Bullen 1985; Egger et al. 1992; Rowe and Rowe 1994).

Diagnostic Evaluation

The clinical evaluation of ADHD requires multiple sources and types of diagnostic information. Parent and child interviews are supplemented with information from school reports, teacher and parent rating scales, neuropsychological data as indicated, and direct clinical observation. Although there is no simple physical finding or laboratory test that will aid in the diagnosis of ADHD, it is important to rule out other medical causes of inattention and impulsivity.

Interviews and Rating Scales

Diagnosing ADHD in children and adolescents is complicated by the fact that signs may not be directly observable. In a highly structured or novel setting or in a setting with one-to-one supervision or frequent rewards for positive behavior, a child with ADHD may not appear to be inattentive or hyperactive–impulsive. Some children and most adolescents are able to maintain attention in an office setting. Conversely, symptoms of this disorder typically worsen in situations that are unstructured or minimally supervised (American Psychiatric Association 2000). Therefore, multiple sources are necessary for diagnosis. The child interview is best done with a flexible approach that allows for exploration of presenting symptoms. Additional, more structured questioning may be necessary to review symptoms of ADHD and its common comorbidities. Many children lack insight into their behavioral problems or are unable or unwilling to report their symptoms. It is generally held that parents are better reporters of externalizing behaviors, and children are better reporters of internalizing symptoms (American Academy of Child and Adolescent Psychiatry 1997).

The parent interview is the core of the diagnostic assessment, and the diagnosis is more valid when based on parental report (Pelham et al. 1992). Parental report may, however, be influenced by parental psychopathology, the presence of comorbid CD in children, and/or cultural factors (Abikoff et al. 1993; Fergusson et al. 1993). Parent and teacher reports of child behavioral problems and individual child self-report are very different. Although teachers and parents generally agree if a child is at risk, the correlation between their reports is low, likely due to the different environments in which they observe the child. The most commonly used scales are also the best normed and validated. They include the Child Behavior Checklist, the Teacher Report Form of the Child Behavior Checklist, the Conners Parent and Teacher Forms, the Attention Deficit With Hyperactivity Comprehensive Teacher Rating Scale, and the Barkley Home Situations. Identification of behavioral disorders in children is significantly correlated between structured interviews and dimensional scales (Jensen et al. 1993). Structured interviews such as the Diagnostic Interview Schedule for Children continue to be used mainly in research. Although these measures are less useful in identifying ADHD symptoms, they may be helpful in identifying comorbid or alternative diagnoses. Additional scales such as the Conners abbreviated form and the Child Attention Problems Rating Scale are commonly used to assess the patient's response to medication.

Testing

Although there is no specific neuropsychological test for ADHD, testing may provide additional information helpful in establishing a diagnosis and treatment plan. Information from cognitive or educational testing may assist the examiner in providing perspective on level of cognitive or attentional functioning as well as assessing for mental retardation or LDs. This information is essential for developing a treatment plan.

Medical Evaluation

Children with ADHD should have a complete medical evaluation and physical examination. Originally termed *minimal brain dysfunction*, ADHD has been associated with subtle signs of abnormal brain function such as neurological soft signs (asymmetric reflexes, inability to perform rapid alternating movements, minor choreoathetoid movements) and poor motor coordination (Ornoy

et al. 1993; Vitiello et al. 1990). However, these soft neurological signs do not aid in diagnosing ADHD and may be more often associated with anxiety disorders. Although there is evidence both supporting and refuting psychostimulants' effects on growth, height and weight should be measured prior to initiating treatment with a psychostimulant and periodically during the course of treatment (Charach et al. 2006; Spencer et al. 2006; Zachor et al. 2006). These medications may cause a temporary delay in weight gain. Baseline blood pressure and pulse should be obtained, and a family history of sudden cardiac death noted, especially if considering treatment with a psychostimulant (see Chapter 19, "Treatment of Children and Adolescents"). Thyroid function tests are indicated only in the presence of clinical findings of hyperthyroidism or hypothyroidism, goiter, family history of thyroid disease, or decreased growth velocity.

Course and Prognosis

ADHD is a chronic and enduring disorder, with most of those referred for treatment as children experiencing impairment through adolescence. Up to 65% of children continue to have features of ADHD into adulthood (American Academy of Child and Adolescent Psychiatry 1997). Complications of the disorder include lower academic and professional achievement and increased risk of antisocial behaviors and substance abuse (Spencer et al. 1999; Wilens and Dodson 2004).

Treatment

Treatment of ADHD includes both nonpharmacological and pharmacological interventions. The central role of medication for treatment of ADHD was described in the landmark National Institute of Mental Health–funded Multimodal Treatment of ADHD study (Multimodal Treatment of ADHD Cooperative Group 1999). In this study, children ages 7–9 years with ADHD, combined type, were randomly assigned to receive medication (primarily psychostimulants), psychosocial interventions (parent training, intensive summer treatment program, and school consultation), the combined medication and psychosocial treatments, or standard community care. This study suggests that subjects receiving the combination of medication and psychosocial intervention fared only slightly better than those receiving medication alone.

Medication

Psychostimulants. Most hyperactive children improve with psychostimulant medication, although this response is not diagnostic of the disorder. Psychostimulant medication generally remains effective over many years; however, a small subset of patients may develop tolerance to a medication after several months of treatment. These patients who do not have additional psychiatric or medical illness to account for the diminished therapeutic effect of the psychostimulant will frequently respond to an alternate psychostimulant.

Some individuals with ADHD do not respond to psychostimulants. In some cases, symptoms of a comorbid disorder such as an anxiety disorder, bipolar disorder, or psychotic disorder may be exacerbated by these medications. Patients with neurodevelopmental or other neurological disorders may be particularly sensitive to treatment and may have adverse or paradoxical effects even at low dosages.

Methylphenidate is a short-acting agent that generally requires several daily doses. It is approved by the U.S. Food and Drug Administration (FDA) for children to age 6 years, although there are several published reports finding methylphenidate effective in younger children. Dexmethylphenidate hydrochloride (Focalin) is the *d-threo*-enantiomer of short-acting racemic methylphenidate and is currently approved for treatment of ADHD (Wigal et al. 2004). The development of long-acting methylphenidate agents such as Concerta, Metadate CD, and Ritalin LA has allowed for improved benefit from once-daily

dosing and eliminated the need for midday dosing at school. It also seems to have decreased the incidence of rebound—a phenomenon often seen in shorter-acting preparations in which symptom exacerbation occurs prior to administration of the next dose.

Dextroamphetamine and mixed amphetamine salts (Adderall) are additional psychostimulants used in the treatment of ADHD. The short-acting amphetamines have a slightly longer half-life than methylphenidate but still require multiple daily doses. The dextroamphetamine preparations are FDA approved for ADHD treatment in children as young as 3 years. Longer-acting preparations include dextroamphetamine spansules and Adderall XR. Like the longer-acting methylphenidate formulations, these allow for once-daily dosing and a decrease in rebound effects.

The mechanism of action of psychostimulants is not entirely clear but likely augments dopaminergic and adrenergic activity in the central nervous system. Side effects of the psychostimulants are generally mild and may include delayed sleep, decreased appetite, weight loss, stomachache, headache, minor increases in blood pressure and heart rate, tremor, cognitive overfocus, and irritability. In healthy people, the most serious adverse effects of psychostimulants include psychosis and the development or exacerbation of tics. Although psychostimulants have been known to decrease the seizure threshold, there is no evidence to show increased seizure activity with their use. Psychostimulants may cause reduced or slowed height and weight gain, although no long-term adverse effects on final adult height are apparent. The decrease in weight gain is small, and the effects on height may be minimized through the use of "drug holidays" on weekends or school holidays.

Atomoxetine. Atomoxetine (Strattera) is the first nonstimulant medication to be FDA approved for the treatment of ADHD in children and adolescents. It is used as the first line and in treatment-refractory cases. Sometimes it is chosen for treatment of individuals with substance use disorders because of its low potential for abuse. Isolated cases of reversible liver failure have been reported, although these have not affected practice recommendations.

Tricyclic antidepressants.   Tricyclic antidepressants (TCAs) can treat core symptoms of ADHD, although they are less effective than psychostimulants in addressing inattention. However, sudden cardiac death reported in five children and adolescents treated with desipramine (Popper and Elliott 1990; Riddle et al. 1991) has led to concern about use of TCAs.

Alpha-agonists.   α-Adrenergic agonists such as clonidine and guanfacine have some evidence to support their use in the treatment of ADHD. However, they remain third-line agents due to a lack of replicated double-blind, placebo-controlled trials. In general, α-agonists are able to treat the core symptoms of impulsivity and hyperactivity but are typically less effective than psychostimulants in treating inattention. Side effects include drowsiness, hypotension, and bradycardia. Clonidine should be tapered, because sudden discontinuation may cause rebound hypertension and tachycardia.

Other medications.   Bupropion has been helpful in treatment of ADHD in children and adults, although it may worsen tics in children with tic disorders (Spencer et al. 1993). Monoamine oxidase inhibitors have also been effective, although the risk of hypertensive crisis with dietary noncompliance limits their use. Antipsychotics appear to be effective in treating symptoms of ADHD, but the risks of neurological and metabolic side effects make this class of medicines best suited for treatment of patients with severe illness that has been refractory to other interventions. A recent double-blind, placebo-controlled trial found modafinil to be effective and well tolerated in the treatment of ADHD in children (Biederman et al. 2006).

Psychosocial Interventions

For accurate diagnosis and effective treatment, the physician must coordinate all aspects of treatment. Medication; psychoeducation of patients, families, and teachers; and consistent communication with families and schools comprise the core aspects of treatment for ADHD. More intensive psychosocial interventions are commonly used, although their efficacy remains to be validated and their use may be of greater benefit to patients with comorbid disorders or those whose symptoms do not normalize with medication treatment alone. Although medications address the core symptoms of inattention, hyperactivity, and impulsivity, it may be helpful in some cases to include environmental modifications at home and school to treat the behavioral symptoms of the disorder. Disabilities in academic and social spheres may benefit from specific skill development. Adjunctive psychotherapy can address relationship or peer difficulties that are often seen in this population (American Academy of Child and Adolescent Psychiatry 1997; Swanson et al. 1993).

ADHD Summary

ADHD is a common disorder that is well studied, particularly in children. There is strong evidence to support that ADHD has biological underpinnings as well as important environmental influences that affect its presentation and course of illness. Core symptoms of inattention, impulsivity, and hyperactivity often result in poor academic or work performance as well as relational difficulties and low self-esteem. Hyperactivity and impulsivity frequently remit by adulthood, although inattentive symptoms tend to remain. ADHD is highly comorbid and appears to be an enduring condition in some patients. Effective treatments are available with medication as the central component. Psychostimulants are safe and well tolerated in most individuals. In uncomplicated cases, research has shown little benefit of the addition of psychosocial interventions to treatment with psychostimulants. In the future, research will describe the underlying pathophysiology of the disorder and perhaps better define its subtypes.

Disruptive Behavior Disorders

Conduct Disorder

Clinical Description

Conduct disorder is among the most frequently made and probably overused diagnoses in child psychiatry. Despite this, many individuals with this disorder are probably undertreated. *Conduct disorder* describes a pattern of behavior that demonstrates disregard for societal norms and the rights of others (Table 12–17).

The importance of differentiating CD from other delinquent behavior is underappreciated. Recognizing adaptive or subcultural delinquency in specific sociocultural environments is important for accurate diagnosis (Popper et al. 2003). The absence of impulsivity is a hallmark of the diagnosis (Halperin et al. 1995); its presence likely indicates comorbid psychiatric disorder.

Epidemiology

The prevalence of CD has been estimated to be between 1% and 10%, with variable reports attributable to differing detection methods and diagnostic criteria (e.g., clinical interviews vs. arrests) and varying populations. A male predominance is accepted and ranges from 2:1 to 4:1, with the child-onset subtype demonstrating especially greater male predominance.

In most cases CD is comorbid with additional psychiatric disorders, and this contributes to the lack of clear epidemiological evidence for the disorder. ADHD is frequently present and contributes to more severe aggression and antisocial behavior (J.L. Walker et al. 1987). Major and minor mood symp-toms and cognitive difficulties, including LDs and substance use disorders, are frequently comorbid, and prevalence rates in excess of 50% have been reported for all these conditions in individuals with CD.

Etiology

The interplay of biological, psychological, and social factors contributes to the development of the disruptive behavior disorders. It has been suggested that the common co-occurrence of CD, ODD, and ADHD results from shared genetic influences, although each distinct disorder maintains unique genetic factors (Dick et al. 2005).

Neuropsychological associations include relatively low IQ, even in prospective studies, independent of social class. Cognitively, children with conduct problems demonstrate more immature styles of problem solving and social interaction. The importance of parental psychopathology and impoverished home environments is striking, although the linkage is not very clear. The degree of parental discord distinct from actual divorce and separation (Hetherington and Stanley-Hagan 1999), larger family size, absent fathers, and fewer cultural or ethnic interests all correlate with increased risk of behavioral dysfunction.

Course and Prognosis

Younger age at symptom appearance and the presence of aggression are both associated with poorer prognosis. As many as 40% of children with CD become antisocial adults, especially those with drug use prior to age 15 years, those with a history of out-of-home placement, and those who live in extreme poverty (Robins and Ratcliff 1979). "Resilient" children appear to be highly intelligent firstborn children of small, low-discord families (Werner 1989).

Diagnostic Evaluation

Accurate diagnosis of the disruptive behavior disorders requires accurate information. The necessity of accessing multiple sources

Table 12–17. DSM-IV-TR diagnostic criteria for conduct disorder

A. A repetitive and persistent pattern of behavior in which the basic rights of others or major age-appropriate societal norms or rules are violated, as manifested by the presence of three (or more) of the following criteria in the past 12 months, with at least one criterion present in the past 6 months:

Aggression to people and animals

(1) often bullies, threatens, or intimidates others

(2) often initiates physical fights

(3) has used a weapon that can cause serious physical harm to others (e.g., a bat, brick, broken bottle, knife, gun)

(4) has been physically cruel to people

(5) has been physically cruel to animals

(6) has stolen while confronting a victim (e.g., mugging, purse snatching, extortion, armed robbery)

(7) has forced someone into sexual activity

Destruction of property

(8) has deliberately engaged in fire setting with the intention of causing serious damage

(9) has deliberately destroyed others' property (other than by fire setting)

Deceitfulness or theft

(10) has broken into someone else's house, building, or car

(11) often lies to obtain goods or favors or to avoid obligations (i.e., "cons" others)

(12) has stolen items of nontrivial value without confronting a victim (e.g., shoplifting, but without breaking and entering; forgery)

Serious violations of rules

(13) often stays out at night despite parental prohibitions, beginning before age 13 years

(14) has run away from home overnight at least twice while living in parental or parental surrogate home (or once without returning for a lengthy period)

(15) is often truant from school, beginning before age 13 years

B. The disturbance in behavior causes clinically significant impairment in social, academic, or occupational functioning.

C. If the individual is age 18 years or older, criteria are not met for antisocial personality disorder.

Code based on age at onset:

312.81 Conduct disorder, childhood-onset type: onset of at least one criterion characteristic of conduct disorder prior to age 10 years

312.82 Conduct disorder, adolescent-onset type: absence of any criteria characteristic of conduct disorder prior to age 10 years

312.89 Conduct disorder, unspecified onset: age at onset is not known

Specify severity:

Mild: few if any conduct problems in excess of those required to make the diagnosis **and** conduct problems cause only minor harm to others

Moderate: number of conduct problems and effect on others intermediate between "mild" and "severe"

Severe: many conduct problems in excess of those required to make the diagnosis **or** conduct problems cause considerable harm to others of information, often in various agencies, is of paramount importance for making a diagnosis, recommending treatment, and predicting prognosis.

Treatment

Several types of treatment have been shown to be beneficial. It is especially important to recognize and initiate treatment for any comorbid psychiatric disorders. Evidence supports three major types of interventions for CD: parent management training, problem-solving skills training, and multisystemic therapy (Brestan and Eyberg 1998; Farmer et al. 2002).

Parent management training teaches appropriate means of interacting that promote positive and discourage antisocial behaviors. It uses positive reinforcements and negative consequences and teaches negotiation skills. Problem-solving skills training consists of cognitive-based approaches and uses modeling and role-playing to help individuals identify and better handle potentially difficult situations.

Multisystemic therapy is based on making use of available systems within the child's world and maximizing positive interactions and effects. Peers, families, schools, and other communities are all involved. It is then customized for the individual. This strength of the therapy makes it expensive and difficult to replicate, but effective.

Pharmacological interventions for CD are directed at troublesome symptoms and behaviors, but given the lack of specificity of symptoms of this diagnosis, it is not surprising that clear replicable findings are lacking. The most appropriate targets of medication intervention are aggression, impulsivity, hyperactivity, and mood symptoms. Antipsychotics, antidepressants, mood stabilizers, anticonvulsants, stimulants, and adrenergic agents have all been shown to be effective (Tcheremissine and Lieving 2006); however, it remains difficult to differentiate benefit in CD itself from psychiatric comorbidity. (See Chapter 19, "Treatment of Children and Adolescents," for a discussion of treatment.)

Oppositional Defiant Disorder

Clinical Description

ODD recognizes a persistent pathological pattern of interaction, which for briefer periods of time and during well-recognized periods of development is appropriate and typical. Anger and temper management are frequently at the core of the disorder. Authority figures are usually the recipients of often brief tantrums. As in CD, impulsivity is usually absent, and the arguments take on an importance all their own. Many children with ODD would rather win the battle and lose the war. Recognition of societal rules and personal rights distinguishes children with ODD from those with CD. Most children with ODD do not progress to CD; those with earlier onset of symptoms, physical aggression, low socioeconomic status, and parental substance abuse are more likely to develop CD (Loeber et al. 1995; Table 12–18).

Epidemiology

Prevalence estimates for ODD range from 2% to 12%, with a male predominance of approximately 2:1 (American Psychiatric Association 2000). Comorbid psychiatric diagnoses are similar to those for CD and include ADHD and anxiety and mood disorders.

Etiology

The etiology of ODD is unknown, although it appears to be multifactorial. Familial factors are often cited and include inadequate parenting, violence, and attachment issues. (See discussion in "Conduct Disorder" section earlier in this chapter.)

Course and Prognosis

Although the diagnosis has been shown to persist for at least 4 years, most children with ODD do not go on to demonstrate antisocial behaviors as adults.

Diagnostic Evaluation

Given the high incidence of comorbidity and potential etiologies of oppositional behavior,

Table 12–18.   DSM-IV-TR diagnostic criteria for oppositional defiant disorder

A.   A pattern of negativistic, hostile, and defiant behavior lasting at least 6 months, during which four (or more) of the following are present:
   (1)   often loses temper
   (2)   often argues with adults
   (3)   often actively defies or refuses to comply with adults' requests or rules
   (4)   often deliberately annoys people
   (5)   often blames others for his or her mistakes or misbehavior
   (6)   is often touchy or easily annoyed by others
   (7)   is often angry and resentful
   (8)   is often spiteful or vindictive

   Note: Consider a criterion met only if the behavior occurs more frequently than is typically observed in individuals of comparable age and developmental level.

B.   The disturbance in behavior causes clinically significant impairment in social, academic, or occupational functioning.

C.   The behaviors do not occur exclusively during the course of a psychotic or mood disorder.

D.   Criteria are not met for conduct disorder, and, if the individual is age 18 years or older, criteria are not met for antisocial personality disorder.

careful interviewing of the individual and family is necessary. Special attention to common sources of family conflict and individual frustration is worthwhile.

Treatment

Treatment typically consists of psychotherapeutic interventions, including individual behaviorally focused therapy and family work. Parent training involvement appears key for successful intervention. Pharmacotherapy is typically not indicated.

Feeding and Eating Disorders of Infancy or Early Childhood

Pica

Clinical Description

Pica is the persistent eating of nonnutritive substances that is inappropriate to the developmental level of the individual (Table 12–19). The mouthing and eating of nonnutritive substances are commonly observed and developmentally appropriate in a significant number of typically developing 12- to 36-month-old children. Such eating may also be seen in pregnant women and individuals with severe or profound mental retardation. In some cultures, the eating of nonnutritive substances such as clay is thought to be of value.

Epidemiology

Prevalence of pica is not clearly established, although it is estimated that 10%–20% of children display pica-like behavior. Spontaneous remission, often after just a few months, is common. The prevalence of pica in pregnant women has been reported to be from 0% to 70%.

Etiology

Many children with pica have parents who demonstrated the disorder, and a multifactorial etiology is likely. Psychosocial stress, deprivation, family psychopathology, and disruption to parent–child nurturance can be involved in the etiology. Many children with pica also exhibit other excessive oral activities (e.g., thumb sucking, nail biting). In intellectual disability, self-stimulation is the likely etiology. Eating of ice in pregnant women has been associated with iron deficiency.

Table 12–19. DSM-IV-TR diagnostic criteria for pica

A. Persistent eating of nonnutritive substances for a period of at least 1 month.
B. The eating of nonnutritive substances is inappropriate to the developmental level.
C. The eating behavior is not part of a culturally sanctioned practice.
D. If the eating behavior occurs exclusively during the course of another mental disorder (e.g., mental retardation, pervasive developmental disorder, schizophrenia), it is sufficiently severe to warrant independent clinical attention.

Table 12–20. DSM-IV-TR diagnostic criteria for rumination disorder

A Repeated regurgitation and rechewing of food for a period of at least 1 month following a period of normal functioning.
B. The behavior is not due to an associated gastrointestinal or other general medical condition (e.g., esophageal reflux).
C. The behavior does not occur exclusively during the course of anorexia nervosa or bulimia nervosa. If the symptoms occur exclusively during the course of mental retardation or a pervasive developmental disorder, they are sufficiently severe to warrant independent clinical attention.

Course and Prognosis

Pica usually starts in the second year of life and remits prior to age 6 years; however, in intellectual disability, pica may be lifelong.

Diagnostic Evaluation

Evaluation of the child should include detailed developmental and parental histories and an assessment of the home environment, including the parent–child relationship. Children with pica should have a zinc protoporphyrin and lead level taken to assess possibility of lead intoxication.

Treatment

Behavioral therapies that reward appropriate eating or negatively reinforce nonfood ingestion have been successful, notably in individuals with intellectual disability. Reducing the availability of potentially ingestible nonfood items in the home can be beneficial.

Rumination Disorder

Clinical Description

Rumination disorder is the repeated regurgitation and rechewing of food (Table 12–20). It is commonly seen in infants and is frequently accompanied by rhythmic movements and relaxation. Other self-soothing behaviors are often observed in children with rumination disorder, such as thumb sucking, head banging, and body rocking. The behaviors are particularly prominent when the infant is alone.

Epidemiology

No prevalence rates for rumination disorder exist, but it appears to be rare and declining in populations of individuals without intellectual disability.

Etiology

Both environmental and biological causes have been suggested. Genetic factors in the disorder are unknown.

Course and Prognosis

Typically appearing between the ages of 3 and 12 months, rumination disorder frequently spontaneously remits by age 3 years. Individuals with intellectual disability frequently demonstrate longer duration or chronicity.

Diagnostic Evaluation

Evaluation for rumination disorder should include a full psychiatric and behavioral assessment of parent and child. Observation of parent–child interactions is also informative.

Evaluation of potential medical etiologies or resultant effects of rumination may be necessary, including workup for gastroesophageal reflux or physiological abnormalities.

Treatment

No specific treatments for rumination disorder have been developed, although behavioral interventions that attempt to reward nonrumination with parental attention and negatively reinforce further rumination have been shown to be effective (Lavigne et al. 1981).

Feeding Disorder of Infancy or Early Childhood

Clinical Description

Approximately 80% of cases of failure to thrive are attributed to nonorganic causes. The diagnosis of feeding disorder of infancy or early childhood attempts to describe these cases and is characterized by the failure to eat and gain or maintain weight in the presence of adequate food (Table 12–21). Infants may refuse to eat or eat inadequately. Young children's consumption may be limited by behavioral or developmental problems, or they may restrict themselves to excessively nar-

---

Table 12–21. DSM-IV-TR diagnostic criteria for feeding disorder of infancy or early childhood

A. Feeding disturbance as manifested by persistent failure to eat adequately with significant failure to gain weight or significant loss of weight over at least 1 month.

B. The disturbance is not due to an associated gastrointestinal or other general medical condition (e.g., esophageal reflux).

C. The disturbance is not better accounted for by another mental disorder (e.g., rumination disorder) or by lack of available food.

D. The onset is before age 6 years.

---

row choices. Further subtyping is likely appropriate, and additional diagnoses such as feeding disorder of state regulation, feeding disorder of caregiver–infant reciprocity, infantile anorexia, sensory food aversions, posttraumatic feeding disorder, and feeding disorder associated with concurrent medical illness may better clarify potential etiologies and guide treatment (Chatoor 2004).

Epidemiology

Community-based estimates of nonorganic failure to thrive are 1%–4%. These cases represent 1%–5% of pediatric hospital admissions (Popper et al. 2003).

Etiology

Various specific and combined factors are typically involved. Chatoor's (2004) diagnostic subdivisions make clear some of the more common etiologies.

Course and Prognosis

Onset is typically within the first year of life, although it may be somewhat later in individuals with intellectual disability. A full range of outcomes is possible, from spontaneous remission to severe malnutrition and death.

Diagnostic Evaluation

Careful elimination of medical causes of failure to thrive; attention to parental and developmental history and the parent–child relationship, including temperament; evaluation of the home or feeding environment; and elements of behavioral analysis are necessary to clarify the diagnosis.

Treatment

Appropriate treatment targets the specific or suspected etiology of the disorder. At the time of diagnosis, hospitalization is frequently encouraged to completely evaluate the child, control the environment, and alleviate some of the stress incumbent on the parent. Parent education and training are typically important. Specific interventions are then clarified based on the characteristic and supposed etiology.

Tic Disorders

Clinical Description

A *tic* is a rapid, involuntary, and apparently meaningless movement or vocalization. Most simple tics go unnoticed or fail to reach a level of conscious awareness. Many children are not bothered by their motor tics and frequently display some indifference toward them. Vocal tics are frequently disruptive and distressing. Often these are inaccurately described as disruptive habits. In general, tics are sensitive to stress and fatigue. They wax and wane in severity, but for most children, they are not progressive (Walkup et al. 2006; Table 12–22).

Tic disorders are differentiated by the duration, frequency, severity, and anatomical location of the abnormal movements or vocalization. All tic disorders share the common features of a waxing and waning course, an exacerbation by stress and fatigue, and an increased risk of mood-related symptoms. Tourette's disorder is further distinguished by the development of more complex tics over time and the presence of prodromal sensations or urges to perform the tic (Robertson 2000).

Epidemiology

Tics are exceedingly common. Transient tics occur in 10%–25% of early school-age males and in somewhat fewer similarly aged females. Most often tics disappear over a period of weeks to months. Tic disorders demonstrate a greater male predominance than transient tics, with males presenting with tics two to four times more frequently than females.

Tic disorders are frequently associated with additional psychiatric disorders such as ADHD, OCD, mood and anxiety disorders, ODD, or CD. The presence of these disorders has a profound influence on the clinical presentation and course of the tic disorder. LDs, including disorders of written expression, and speech and language disorders, such as stuttering and other forms of speech dysfluency, are additional comorbidities (Robertson 2000; Saint-Cyr et al. 1995).

Etiology

Tic disorders represent dysfunction within a complex network involving the limbic system, prefrontal cortex, and basal ganglia. Analogously, the neurobehavioral symptoms associated with tic disorders involve circuits related to attention, sensory gating, impulse control, capacity for automatization of motor skills (written language), and prepotent inhibition of automatic repetitive be-

Table 12–22. Some common tics

Simple motor tics	Simple vocal tics
Eye blinking	Throat clearing
Shoulder shrugging	Grunting
Mouth opening	Yelling/screaming
Flicking hair out of one's eyes	Sniffing
Arm extending	Barking
Facial grimacing	Snorting
Lip licking	Coughing
Eye rolling	Spitting
Squinting/opening eyes	Humming

Source. Eapen et al. 2003.

haviors (Leckman et al. 2003; Potenza and Hollander 2002; Robertson 2000).

A great deal of effort has gone into determining and defining the genetic risk for tic disorders. There are several promising approaches, although a definitive marker gene remains elusive. Pedigree studies suggest familial clusters of affected probands. These same studies also reveal significant diversity of phenotypic expression. Monozygotic twins yield markedly elevated rates of concordance and similar types and severity of tics when compared with dizygotic twins. It is also apparent that not only are monozygotic twins more likely to have Tourette's disorder (greater than 50% versus 20% for dizygotic twins), but this gap widens when the presence of obsessive-compulsive symptoms is included in the comparison (Leckman et al. 2003).

The precise mode of transmission is unknown. It has been postulated that Tourette's disorder is an autosomal dominant disorder with variable penetrance and phenotypic variability resulting from environmental influences. Other evidence suggests polygenic influences or even a single gene with multiple effects. Most comorbid conditions appear to be inherited independently. Variation in dimensions such as tic type, severity, and course may be secondary to environmental factors such as exposure to neurotoxins, prenatal complications (e.g., hyperemesis gravidarum), or the product of medication side effects (Walkup et al. 2006).

Course and Prognosis

The severity and intensity of tics tend to wax and wane over time. Many resolve spontaneously and, although being worrisome to many parents, rarely result in a referral for treatment. The short duration of transient tic disorders suggests that duration may be related to maturational vulnerabilities and environmental factors. It is likely that transient tics represent a lower genetic loading for movement disorders and more likely that they represent a mild developmental delay in the normal maturation of inhibitory mechanisms. The emergence of commonly co-occurring conditions among preschoolers and early elementary school–age children (e.g., nightmares, parasomnias, migraine headaches, and symptoms associated with ADHD) supports a developmental model (King et al. 2003; Robertson 2000).

Over a period of months, simple tics may develop into persistent motor or phonic tics. By definition, chronic motor tic disorder, phonic tic disorder, and Tourette's disorder persist longer than 1 year. For children with chronic tic disorder, the appearance of either vocalizations or movements tends to remain stable. In contrast, Tourette's disorder often begins with a simple motor tic (e.g., blinking) and progresses over a period of months to years into more complex motor and (often later) phonic tics.

Tic disorders follow a similar trajectory as other nonprogressive hyperkinetic movement disorders. For some, tics reach their peak intensity 4–5 years after onset and then begin to decline in severity. Others experience an increase in severity during the surge in androgen activity present in early puberty. Of course, tics beginning at age 7 years are reaching a natural peak in intensity during early puberty, and the associated androgen surge may be less relevant than previously thought (Bruun and Budman 1994). By late adolescence, most children with tics will experience a gradual decline in tic frequency. Other patients experience increasingly severe tics and repetitive motion injury, self-injury, or complications from long-term treatment (e.g., tardive dyskinesia) (Robertson 2000).

Diagnostic Evaluation

Tics are differentiated from chorea, athetosis, dystonia, myoclonus, and tremors through careful assessment of the age of the patient at symptom onset, distribution, duration, capacity for suppression, provocative agents or events, and the natural course of movements and vocalizations (which can be well characterized through video recording).

The purpose of a detailed neurological examination of children with tic disorders is to characterize the nature of the movement disorder and eliminate more serious developmental neuropsychiatric disorders. In general, tics are not accompanied by lateralizing neurological symptoms such as hemiparesis, severe rigidity, akinesia, or seizures. Many children with tics do have nonspecific developmental soft signs that are also present in ADHD, LDs, and PDDs. Findings such as unilateral rigidity, movement dysfluency, or overflow/synkinesias suggest lateralization within the basal ganglia, whereas perceptual motor skills and executive deficits suggest a more complex brain region relationship. In general, most of these findings may have greater educational than neurological significance (Walkup et al. 2006).

In many settings, an MRI or computed tomography scan is routinely ordered, although lacking other abnormal physical findings or laboratory evidence, the yield from these studies is typically low. An electroencephalogram may show nonspecific findings in the absence of clear-cut myoclonic or paroxysmal events (either nocturnal or daytime). For example, hyperekplexia (excessive startle response) and physiological symptoms associated with acute stress can be confused with tics. The persistence of abnormal movements during sleep or in relation to specific stimuli is helpful in clarifying the differential diagnosis (Jankovic and DeLeon 2002).

Treatment

It is essential to assess the impact of the tic disorder on the person's quality of life and overall psychological adjustment. For most children, the decision to treat tic disorders is not related to tic severity. Treatment is more often related to psychosocial disruptions, peer reactions, or the emotional sensitivity of the affected child. For adults with persistent tics, treatment decisions are often based on the severity of the persistent tics, psychiatric comorbidity, and the degree of interference

with work or social interaction (King et al. 2003). It is essential to evaluate the level of discomfort and distress experienced by the patient and the family.

The treatment of tics proceeds algorithmically in most situations. For simple tics with few indicators of significant distress, a watch-and-wait strategy is often appropriate. On the other hand, individuals with severe tics and highly disruptive comorbid symptoms can require more immediate treatment. Many children with severe tics are resistant to or intolerant of standard treatments outlined in evidence-based protocols. Treatment of these severe cases may require appropriation of neuropharmacological treatments of non-tic-related movement disorders such as dystonia or myoclonic disorders (Walkup et al. 2006).

For most children, tics are stable, generally mild, nonprogressive, and rarely treated. However, watchful waiting may not be an appropriate strategy when severe ADHD or obsessive-compulsive symptoms are present. Because rates of ADHD exceed 40% in many children with tics, the chance of a child having both disorders is quite likely. The presence of ADHD raises several questions. Until relatively recently, the stimulant drugs were considered a causative factor in the development of tic disorders, and this class of drugs was contraindicated in children with abnormal movements. Although there are children for whom stimulants play a key role in the onset and evolution of their tic disorder, subsequent research has failed to support a categorical assumption. In most children, stimulant drugs have minimal or no impact on the course of tics. In some severe tic disorders, both direct and indirect dopamine agonists have palliative effects (Walkup et al. 2006). The severity of the core symptoms of ADHD, coupled with family attitudes, often determines the role of stimulants in treatment. For those disinclined to use stimulants, clonidine, guanfacine, TCAs, modafinil, atomoxetine, SSRIs, SNRIs, and mecamylamine (Inversine) are available as treatments for tics and

ADHD-related symptoms. If nonstimulant treatments of comorbid tic disorder and ADHD are not useful, stimulants should be considered after careful review of the potential risks and benefits with the family and child (King et al. 2003). α-Agonists (e.g., clonidine, guanfacine) may be helpful for tics, ADHD, and explosive behaviors.

Comorbid obsessive-compulsive symptoms can also pose significant diagnostic and treatment difficulties. It can be difficult to differentiate OCD from complex tics and repetitive behaviors common to tic disorders (e.g., arranging, need for symmetry, arithmomania, and "just right" sensations). One approach may be to address phenomenological differences in core symptoms. A second may involve a pharmacological dissection of treatment response (Eapen et al. 2003; Santangelo et al. 1994).

Many patients with obsessive-compulsive spectrum disorders are less responsive to SSRIs. In addition, some exhibit a form of behavioral disinhibition. For these children, compulsive behaviors in the context of significant impulsivity, fewer anxiety-related complaints, and the presence of a growing urge can predict a less complete response to SSRIs and cognitive and behavioral therapies. In these circumstances, the addition of a low dosage of a second-generation antipsychotic drug, anticonvulsant, or naltrexone can be helpful (Potenza and Hollander 2002).

Tic Disorders Summary

Tic disorders, like other hyperkinetic movement disorders, are frequently comorbid with disorders such as OCD, ADHD, LDs (often of written expression), and deficits in executive function. These comorbidities also implicate the basal ganglia and pre-motor pathways, limbic system, and prefrontal regions in the pathophysiology of the disorder. Development affects the course of illness.

Although tic disorders can intensify as they evolve in some individuals, there is no evidence of neurodegenerative changes in cognition or motor skills. Clinicians need to be aware of the differences between transient, primary, and secondary tics as well as causes of abnormal movements acquired later in life.

The appearance of tics and co-occurring conditions early in life can affect subsequent psychological or cognitive development, especially the acquisition of specific skills. Most children with tic disorders have few adverse consequences, but some, especially those with severe tics, comorbid neuropsychiatric symptoms, or psychiatric disorders, have problems that affect a broad range of psychosocial dimensions. Treatment attempts to minimize (and often not completely eliminate) tics and should include both pharmacotherapy and psychotherapy.

Elimination Disorders

Encopresis

Clinical Description

Encopresis is defined by DSM-IV-TR as the repeated involuntary or intentional passage of feces into inappropriate places by children at least 4 years old or with an equivalent developmental level (Table 12–23). It is subdivided into primary and secondary types. In primary encopresis, a period of fecal continence has never developed and is typically associated with developmental delay or fixation. Secondary encopresis, found in slightly more than one-half of cases, follows at least 1 year of fecal continence and is associated with conduct problems. Behavioral problems, found in approximately one-third of individuals afflicted, often resolve with the improvement of encopresis.

Epidemiology

Encopresis is likely individually underreported. Prevalences of 1.5%–7.5% have been reported, with a 3:1 to 4:1 male predominance (C.E. Walker et al. 1988). Some studies have suggested an association with lower socioeconomic status. Psychiatric comorbidity accompanies 35% of children with encopresis (Popper et al. 2003). Associated disorders

---

Table 12–23. DSM-IV-TR diagnostic criteria for encopresis

A. Repeated passage of feces into inappropriate places (e.g., clothing or floor) whether involuntary or intentional.

B. At least one such event a month for at least 3 months.

C. Chronological age is at least 4 years (or equivalent developmental level).

D. The behavior is not due exclusively to the direct physiological effects of a substance (e.g., laxatives) or a general medical condition except through a mechanism involving constipation.

Code as follows:

    787.6 **With constipation and overflow incontinence**

    307.7 **Without constipation and overflow incontinence**

---

include mental retardation, CD, ODD, psychotic disorders, and mood disorders.

Etiology

The diagnosis of encopresis should exclude any medically explained causes of fecal incontinence, such as hypercalcemia, hypothyroidism, lactase deficiency, anal fissure or malformation, aganglionic megacolon, rectal stenosis, and trauma. Altered motility and abnormal secretion of gastrointestinal hormones may also cause encopresis. Encopresis with constipation and overflow incontinence can be due to any nonmedical cause of chronic constipation, inadequate training, or avoidance of toileting. The causes of nonretentive encopresis can include diminished sensory appreciation or lack of appropriate planning, training, or interest.

Course and Prognosis

Most individuals with encopresis get better. Treatment results in recovery rates of 30%–50% after 1 year and 48%–75% after 5 years (Loening-Baucke 2002). Poor prognostic indicators include soiling at night or as an expression of anger, a nonchalant attitude, and conduct problems (Landman and Rappaport 1985).

Diagnostic Evaluation

It is important to rule out medical reasons for fecal incontinence, such as endocrinological sequelae, aganglionic megacolon (Hirschs-

prung's disease), and anal fissure, although extensive workup is not often necessary (Loening-Baucke 2002). An abdominal roentgenogram can aid diagnosis and management of encopresis (Rockney et al. 1995). Careful attention to developmental history, history of toilet training. and observation of family interactions is important to fully assess this often unpleasant and distressing problem.

Treatment

Treatment typically consists of a combination of medical, behavioral, and psychotherapeutic interventions. Education of the patient and family about the disorder, workup, and etiologies can help to alleviate the stresses associated with this problem. For individuals with impaction, laxatives or enemas are frequently required. Subsequently, high-fiber diets and increased water consumption are recommended. A "sitting schedule" is established and compliance is rewarded; sometimes aversive consequences, such as bathing and washing soiled linens, are useful for noncompliance. Psychotherapeutic intervention can target self-esteem in individuals or utilize family work focusing on possible etiologies or results of the disorder.

Enuresis

Clinical Description

Although the term is frequently used to describe urinary incontinence regardless of its cause, more accurately, *enuresis* is the persistence of medically unexplained urinary incontinence after the typical age of bladder control. Subtyping occurs according to the time of day it occurs (Table 12–24). Nocturnal enuresis is more common, and children with diurnal enuresis usually have nocturnal symptoms as well. Approximately 80% of children have primary enuresis, where bladder control has never been attained. The remaining children have previously achieved bladder control, and the term *secondary enuresis* is often used. The relationship between primary and secondary distinction and the incidence and severity of associated psychopathology are not clear.

Epidemiology

Reported prevalence rates vary wildly, with estimates as high as 25% for occasional nocturnal enuresis. More significant enuresis in children older than 5 years is 7%–10% for males and 3% of females.

Etiology

No clear etiology for enuresis is known, although genetic transmission appears likely. Sleep stages do not appear to be related to the occurrence of enuresis. The role of individual diurnal variations of endogenous antidiuretic hormone is not clear. Abnormalities of bladder anatomy, function, and size have been implicated in a minority of cases. Secondary enuresis in young children has been associated with stressful environments or events.

Course and Prognosis

Left untreated, enuresis abates at a rate of about 10%–20% per year. Approximately 1% of adults have enuresis. Adolescent-onset enuresis appears to have more associated psychopathology and poorer prognosis. Individuals with enuresis often feel embarrassment and anger. The secondary effects include punishment from caregivers, teasing from peers, and social withdrawal.

Diagnostic Evaluation

The elimination of possible medical etiologies may require urological evaluation, because approximately 20% of children with nocturnal enuresis are found to have urological abnormalities. Urinary infections and seizure disorders are often suspected, and urinary analysis is warranted, but electroencephalograms are likely to have a low yield.

Treatment

Behavioral and pharmacological interventions are both effective in treating enuresis; however, behavioral interventions likely have greater safety. The most successful and commonly used behavioral interventions are the bell and pad or a simple alarm clock set to the time of night when bladders are typically full. These awaken the child upon, or at the time

---

Table 12–24. DSM-IV-TR diagnostic criteria for enuresis

A. Repeated voiding of urine into bed or clothes (whether involuntary or intentional).

B. The behavior is clinically significant as manifested by either a frequency of twice a week for at least 3 consecutive months or the presence of clinically significant distress or impairment in social, academic (occupational), or other important areas of functioning.

C. Chronological age is at least 5 years (or equivalent developmental level).

D. The behavior is not due exclusively to the direct physiological effect of a substance (e.g., a diuretic) or a general medical condition (e.g., diabetes, spina bifida, a seizure disorder).

Specify type:
   Nocturnal only
   Diurnal only
   Nocturnal and diurnal

most likely for, enuresis. Both of these methods show success rates of approximately 75%.

Imipramine initiated at 25 mg and titrated every 4–7 days to a maximum of 5 mg/kg is effective for enuresis. Most children respond in the 75–125 mg range, and electrocardiograms should be obtained and followed at dosages above 3.5 mg/kg (Mikkelsen and Rapoport 1980). Desmopressin acetate is widely used and approximately as effective as the bell and pad method. Reductions in frequency of enuresis ranging from 10%–91% have been reported; however, continued use of desmopressin acetate is required for continuing bladder control (Moffat et al. 1993). Given the high rate of spontaneous remission in enuresis, long-term continuous treatment with medication is inappropriate (see Chapter 19, "Treatment of Children and Adolescents").

Other Disorders of Infancy, Childhood, or Adolescence

Separation Anxiety Disorder

Clinical Description

Separation anxiety is a normal developmental phenomenon typically beginning around 6 or 7 months, peaking around 18 months, and decreasing after 30 months. Some features of separation anxiety may persist subclinically into childhood and early adolescence. Separation anxiety disorder, however, is characterized by an overwhelming fear of separation or loss of an attachment figure, typically a parent or caregiver. This anxiety response may include cognitive distortions, affective arousal, and behavioral and somatic symptoms. Associated with intense sympathetic arousal, separation distress produces exaggerated proximity-seeking (clinging) and is subject to a rapid expansion of anticipatory triggers and generalization that include enhanced sensitivity to future separations, fears of catastrophic separation, dis-

ruption of sleep initiation, and increased frequency of anxiety dreams (nightmares; Table 12–25). As expected, fear conditioning to both specific (separation) and context-dependent (setting) conditions can become paired with anticipatory experiences (e.g., the ride to school triggers the anxiety response) (Swedo and Pine 2005).

Epidemiology

DSM-IV-TR reports a prevalence of about 4%; however, a large-scale study of children ages 9–13 years found an overall rate of 1% for males and females (Costello et al. 2003). The prevalence of separation anxiety disorder declines with increasing age (American Psychiatric Association 2000). The disorder may be slightly more prevalent in females. It is more common in first-degree relatives and occurs relatively frequently in children of mothers with panic disorder. Separation anxiety frequently accompanies generalized anxiety disorder, although the former often has its onset at an earlier age. Individuals with separation anxiety disorder may be at increased risk for the development of other anxiety disorders, including panic disorder with agoraphobia and depressive disorders.

Etiology

A complicated interaction among genetic factors, temperament, attachment, parental anxiety, parenting style, and life experiences is the generally accepted etiology of anxiety in children. Increased risk factors include high reactivity in novel situations, insecure attachment patterns, parents with anxiety disorders, and parents who are more intrusive and controlling of their children.

Course and Prognosis

Separation anxiety disorder may develop after some life stress, loss, or trauma. Onset may be as young as preschool and may occur any time prior to age 18 years; however, adolescent onset is rare and can have ominous overtones, because it can be an early expression of severe mood disorder or schizophre-

Table 12–25.   DSM-IV-TR diagnostic criteria for separation anxiety disorder

A.   Developmentally inappropriate and excessive anxiety concerning separation from home or from those to whom the individual is attached, as evidenced by three (or more) of the following:

    (1)   recurrent excessive distress when separation from home or major attachment figures occurs or is anticipated

    (2)   persistent and excessive worry about losing, or about possible harm befalling, major attachment figures

    (3)   persistent and excessive worry that an untoward event will lead to separation from a major attachment figure (e.g., getting lost or being kidnapped)

    (4)   persistent reluctance or refusal to go to school or elsewhere because of fear of separation

    (5)   persistently and excessively fearful or reluctant to be alone or without major attachment figures at home or without significant adults in other settings

    (6)   persistent reluctance or refusal to go to sleep without being near a major attachment figure or to sleep away from home

    (7)   repeated nightmares involving the theme of separation

    (8)   repeated complaints of physical symptoms (such as headaches, stomachaches, nausea, or vomiting) when separation from major attachment figures occurs or is anticipated

B.   The duration of the disturbance is at least 4 weeks.

C.   The onset is before age 18 years.

D.   The disturbance causes clinically significant distress or impairment in social, academic (occupational), or other important areas of functioning.

E.   The disturbance does not occur exclusively during the course of a pervasive developmental disorder, schizophrenia, or other psychotic disorder and, in adolescents and adults, is not better accounted for by panic disorder with agoraphobia.

Specify if:

    Early onset: if onset occurs before age 6 years

nia. Left untreated, as many as 80%–95% of children with separation anxiety disorder experience remission; however, continued exposure may intensify the severity of affective response (sensitization) or refusal behaviors (avoiding separation) and expand from specific foci (e.g., the mother) to anticipatory triggers (e.g., school).

Diagnostic Evaluation

Evaluation of separation anxiety disorder requires interviewing the child and parents together and individually. In addition, it should include a systematic review of the classroom environment, the context of the emergence of symptoms, previous interventions, family reactions to these behaviors,

and functions of the behavior within the existing structure of the family system. The age at onset of school refusal should be considered. Transient separation anxiety is not uncommon in preschool or day-care settings. Onset among school-age children may represent true separation anxiety disorder or emerging mood or panic disorders (Labellarte and Ginsburg 2003).

Treatment

The treatment of childhood separation anxiety includes cognitive-behavioral therapy. There is some evidence to support adjunctive parent therapy and parental anxiety management for children (Cobham et al. 1998; Mendlowitz et al. 1999). In conjunction with these therapies, pharmacological interventions include SSRIs, TCAs, and, in some circumstances, short trials of high-potency benzodiazepines (i.e., clonazepam or alprazolam) (Barnett and Riddle 2003; see Chapter 19, "Treatment of Children and Adolescents").

Selective Mutism

Clinical Description

Selective mutism is not classified as either a primary communication or anxiety disorder. Although current diagnostic criteria require exclusion of communication and other psychiatric disorders, it is apparent that there is a considerable overlap between these conditions. As such, selective mutism includes a spectrum of potential communication problems that range from articulation and dysfluency (stuttering) issues and expressive language weakness to concerns about communicating in a second language. However, the key component to the disorder is a form of avoidant behavior: the refusal to speak in public settings despite speaking with minimal difficulty in other situations such as with family, close associates, or members of the primary language community (Table 12–26). Typically, these individuals refuse to speak in certain social settings, although they may use gestures, nods, whispers, or written words to communicate. Associated features include excessive shyness, clinging, compulsive traits, fear of embarrassment, social isolation, controlling behaviors, and temper tantrums (American Psychiatric Association 2000).

Epidemiology

Prevalence estimates range from 0.03% to 2.00%, with the variability likely secondary to differences in ages and threshold for diagnosis. There is a slight female predominance. Comorbid disorders may include language or speech disorders, neurological disorders, and mental retardation. Studies have found high prevalence of comorbid avoidant personality disorder or social phobia. Other anxiety disorders are also often present in these patients (Black and Uhde 1995).

Table 12–26. DSM-IV-TR diagnostic criteria for selective mutism

A. Consistent failure to speak in specific social situations (in which there is an expectation for speaking, e.g., at school) despite speaking in other situations.

B. The disturbance interferes with educational or occupational achievement or with social communication.

C. The duration of the disturbance is at least 1 month (not limited to the first month of school).

D. The failure to speak is not due to a lack of knowledge of, or comfort with, the spoken language required in the social situation.

E. The disturbance is not better accounted for by a communication disorder (e.g., stuttering) and does not occur exclusively during the course of a pervasive developmental disorder, schizophrenia, or other psychotic disorder.

Etiology

Originally selective mutism was understood psychodynamically as a primitive assertion of autonomy. More recently, a posttraumatic etiology is thought to be possible in light of the high prevalence of physical and sexual abuse in these children.

Course and Prognosis

Selective mutism may present between the ages of 3 and 5 years, although diagnosis is often delayed until elementary school. The disorder may persist for a few weeks or months or for several years. Some cases do not emerge until adolescence, although these individuals often show passive-aggressive or antisocial features and generally have a poorer prognosis. Complications include academic difficulties and poor peer relationships.

Diagnostic Evaluation

Diagnostic evaluations generally focus on ruling out comorbid psychiatric disorders such as mood and anxiety disorders as well as other causes of decreased language use such as PDD, autism spectrum disorder, mental retardation, expressive language disorder, or deafness. It is helpful to rule out a primary neurological disorder. It is important to evaluate the familial patterns of communication as well as look at the possibility of physical or sexual abuse.

Treatment

Treatment of selective mutism includes both pharmacological and psychotherapeutic interventions. SSRIs have been shown to improve selective mutism and general level of functioning (Black and Uhde 1994). Fluoxetine specifically has been shown beneficial in case studies, one open trial, and one double-blind, placebo-controlled trial. Anxiolytics and atypical antipsychotics may be used adjunctively. Psychotherapeutic treatment of selective mutism focuses mainly on desensitization procedures. The patient is paired with both an "outsider" and a family member (whom the patient is comfortable speaking around). Decreasing the presence of the family member ideally leads to secondary generalization in which the patient can talk with the "outsider." Contingency management, exposure-based techniques, and self-modeling are also frequently used. The pairing of this behavioral protocol with antianxiety medication serves to desensitize and reduce high levels of anxiety. Medications are eventually tapered and discontinued if possible (Koda et al. 2003). Individual psychodynamically oriented psychotherapy, play therapy, and family therapy are commonly used, although there is limited evidence to support these treatments.

Reactive Attachment Disorder of Infancy or Early Childhood

Clinical Description

Attachment is a central component of social and emotional development, and disordered attachment is defined by specific patterns of abnormal behavior in the context of pathogenic care beginning before age 5 years (American Academy of Child and Adolescent Psychiatry 2005). *Reactive attachment disorder* (RAD) encompasses manifestations of two outcomes of prolonged neglect or physical or emotional abuse: children who are hypervigilant and aloof (inhibited subtype) or children who are indiscriminant in their attachments (disinhibited subtype) (Table 12–27). Inhibited children maintain a degree of wariness and may appear hypoactive or lethargic. As infants, they have little interaction with their environment and often resist being held. Conversely, disinhibited children demonstrate exaggerated, although emotionally empty, attachments and may show inappropriate clinging or hugging. These children fail to discriminate between attachment figures and often seek and are apparently willing to accept comfort from anyone, even strangers. In both types of RAD, disturbances in relatedness, emotional reactivity, and cognition are thought to arise from disordered development of early interpersonal attachment.

Epidemiology

In the few available studies of high-risk children in foster care or institutional settings, 30%–40% had signs of RAD (Smyke et al. 2002; Zeanah et al. 2002, 2005). Associated disorders include mental retardation, developmental delay, language disorder, and posttraumatic stress disorder.

Etiology

By definition, RAD results from pathogenic care that includes a persistent disregard for the basic emotional or physical needs of a child or multiple changes in caregivers that do not allow for the development of a stable attachment. However, our understanding of its etiology has evolved from one of faulty parenting to a transactional model in which a developmental deficit in attachment signaling or behavior may play a role (Zeanah et al. 2002). Infants who have chronic illness or

---

Table 12–27. DSM-IV-TR diagnostic criteria for reactive attachment disorder

A. Markedly disturbed and developmentally inappropriate social relatedness in most contexts, beginning before age 5 years, as evidenced by either (1) or (2):

   (1) persistent failure to initiate or respond in a developmentally appropriate fashion to most social interactions, as manifest by excessively inhibited, hypervigilant, or highly ambivalent and contradictory responses (e.g., the child may respond to caregivers with a mixture of approach, avoidance, and resistance to comforting, or may exhibit frozen watchfulness)

   (2) diffuse attachments as manifest by indiscriminate sociability with marked inability to exhibit appropriate selective attachments (e.g., excessive familiarity with relative strangers or lack of selectivity in choice of attachment figures)

B. The disturbance in criterion A is not accounted for solely by developmental delay (as in mental retardation) and does not meet criteria for a pervasive developmental disorder.

C. Pathogenic care as evidenced by at least one of the following:

   (1) persistent disregard of the child's basic emotional needs for comfort, stimulation, and affection

   (2) persistent disregard of the child's basic physical needs

   (3) repeated changes of primary caregiver that prevent formation of stable attachments (e.g., frequent changes in foster care)

D. There is a presumption that the care in criterion C is responsible for the disturbed behavior in criterion A (e.g., the disturbances in criterion A began following the pathogenic care in criterion C).

Specify type:

   Inhibited type: if criterion A1 predominates in the clinical presentation

   Disinhibited type: if criterion A2 predominates in the clinical presentation

---

handicaps or those who are unwanted may be unable to elicit attachment behaviors from early caregivers. Many parental factors contribute to a disrupted attachment and may include depression, psychosis, mental retardation, or substance abuse as well as poverty, poor education, or chaotic life. Although PDD is excluded from the differential diagnosis of RAD, a study of the core features of autism may provide clues to the origins of detachment and unusual or aberrant forms of attachment behaviors, because children with autism form attachments but do so in an idiosyncratic or peculiar fashion (Sund and Wichstrom 2002). RAD is not the universal outcome of neglectful and abusive parenting. The factors that contribute to resiliency are unknown.

Course and Prognosis

The course and prognosis of untreated RAD range from spontaneous remission to death

and other sequelae of pathological parenting. Children from deprived backgrounds may go on to have low IQ, short stature, and hyperactivity. The persistence of the inhibited type of RAD is exceedingly rare in children adopted out of institutions into more normal environments, although the quality of subsequent attachments may still be compromised. Some children with RAD, disinhibited type, retain a pattern of indiscriminate sociability even after adoption. The quality of the new setting is a significant factor in determining the extent of subsequent behavioral and emotional problems (Zeanah 2000).

Diagnostic Evaluation

In addition to a full psychiatric examination of the child, observation of mother–child interactions and a psychiatric examination of the parents are essential to the diagnosis of RAD. A home visit, if the parents are willing, may provide a more complete picture of the relationship with parents. Physical examination may reveal growth delay, neurological disorder, evidence of physical abuse, vitamin deficiencies, malnutrition, or infectious diseases.

Treatment

The primary intervention in the treatment of RAD is to provide a safe environment and basic medical care. One of the most important interventions for children with RAD who lack an attachment to a discriminated caregiver is for the clinician to advocate for an emotionally available attachment figure for the child (American Academy of Child and Adolescent Psychiatry 2005). This caregiver must be sensitive to and invested in the child. Once the child is in a secure and stable placement, initial therapy should focus on fostering positive interactions with the caregiver. Sometimes, individual treatment for the parent is in order. Dyadic interactive therapy can help promote positive interactions, greater mutual understanding, and a rebuilding of trust. Individual therapy with the child may also be helpful. Therapy designed to improve the quality of attachment through a process of regression and corrective reexperiencing ("therapeutic holding" or "rebirthing therapy") has no empirical support and has been associated with serious injury and death.

No psychopharmacological intervention trials for RAD have been conducted. We can treat comorbid psychiatric disorders, but successful behavioral or pharmacological interventions directed at the core features of disordered attachment may prove more challenging (Zeanah et al. 2002). Recent research indicates that during social contact, reward pathways are activated and communicate with regions processing social, facial, and affective information. These findings suggest that several peptide neuromodulators (endorphins, oxytocin, neuropeptide Y) and neurotransmitters are involved in attachment behaviors and may be the foci of future treatment interventions (Davidson 2003).

Stereotypic Movement Disorder

Clinical Description

The diagnostic criteria for stereotypic movement disorder (SMD) include repetitive and purposeless behaviors, such as hand flapping and body rocking, as well as many forms of self-injury, such as head banging (Table 12–28). The combination of both stereotypy and SIB creates a heterogeneous condition that encompasses a range of repetitive behaviors in which there is considerable variability of typology, severity, motivational or functional states, and treatment approaches (Rapp and Vollmer 2005a). Additional diversity is the result of the changing nature of SMD during child development, the co-occurrence of intellectual disability, and the relationship of symptom severity to other childhood neuropsychiatric disorders (De Raeymaecker 2006).

In the general population, SMD mainly affects infants, toddlers, and young children. Persistence beyond this age group suggests other factors such as intellectual disability, PDD, sensory deficit (deafness, blindness), or possibly psychosis. When compared with typically developing children and adults, persistent stereotypies and SIB are far more common in those with severe intellectual disability. Several stereotypies may occur at once, and their frequency may increase with stress, frustration, and boredom.

Epidemiology

Transient stereotypies during early development occur in 15%–20% of the general population. These are thought to affect men and women equally, although there are indications that head banging is more prevalent in males, with a 3:1 ratio, and self-biting may be more common in women (American Psychiatric Association 2000). The prevalence of SIB is higher in children and adults living in large residential treatment facilities (Barnhill 2003; Symons et al. 2005). SIB resulting in tissue damage affects 15%–20% of adults with severe intellectual disability.

Table 12–28. DSM-IV-TR diagnostic criteria for stereotypic movement disorder

A. Repetitive, seemingly driven, and nonfunctional motor behavior (e.g., hand shaking or waving, body rocking, head banging, mouthing of objects, self-biting, hitting own body).

B. The behavior markedly interferes with normal activities or results in self-inflicted bodily injury that requires medical treatment (or would result in an injury if preventive measures were not used).

C. If mental retardation is present, the stereotypic or self-injurious behavior is of sufficient severity to become a focus of treatment.

D. The behavior is not better accounted for by a compulsion (as in obsessive-compulsive disorder), a tic (as in tic disorder), a stereotypy that is part of a pervasive developmental disorder, or hair pulling (as in trichotillomania).

E. The behavior is not due to the direct physiological effects of a substance or a general medical condition.

F. The behavior persists for 4 weeks or longer.

Specify if:

With self-injurious behavior: if the behavior results in bodily damage that requires specific treatment (or that would result in bodily damage if protective measures were not used)

Etiology

SMD serves multiple functions and is maintained by many different forms of reinforcement (Kennedy et al. 2000). The most common presentations of SMD in those referred for assessment are behavioral responses to significant overarousal or distress. Stereotypies that emerge during periods of increased environmental demands or uncomfortable affect are frequently anxiety reducing and allow the individual to temporarily escape the stressful circumstances (De Raeymaecker 2006). This may lead to an increased frequency of these behaviors and ultimately may interfere with school performance, occupational functioning, and social interaction. This is more likely to occur with intellectual disability, neurodevelopmental disorders, autism, and behavioral phenotypes such as fragile X syndrome (Symons et al. 2005; Troster 1994).

Some repetitive behaviors appear enjoyable and are thought to be intrinsically reinforcing. This self-stimulation often occurs during boredom or isolation. Other behaviors emerge in understimulating environments (vacuous behaviors) but seem to provide little evidence of intrinsic reinforcement or relief from observable distress (Barnhill 2003, 2006). Some individuals experience a compulsive need to self-injure regardless of pain or other adverse consequences. The forces driving these progressive forms of SIB are unknown but share features with compulsive behaviors and addiction (Barnhill 2003).

In the past, a relative dopamine excess and serotonin deficiency were seen as the major factors in repetitive behaviors and SIBs. More recently, γ-aminobutyric acid, glutamate, endorphins, vasopressin, oxytocin, corticotropin-releasing hormone, neurosteroids, and other neuropeptides have been thought to play a role. Other factors include phenotypic differences in enzyme systems, transporter proteins, second messenger systems, differences in stress responses, and pain sensitivity (Edwards et al. 2004; Rapp and Vollmer 2005b).

Course and Prognosis

Once diagnosed, children with SMD follow a variable developmental course. For some, SIBs or repetitive behaviors appear during early childhood but then abate with age. For others, SMD progresses from low-intensity stereotypic behaviors (rocking or nail biting) to more severe behaviors (SIBs). This developmental transformation toward self-injury during childhood is accompanied by changes in typology and severity or a shift from intrinsically motivated repetitive behavior toward escape-motivated SMD (Rapp and Vollmer 2005b; Symons et al. 2005).

Diagnostic Evaluation

In the diagnostic evaluation for SMD, the clinician must acquire a detailed description and behavioral analysis of the behaviors and evaluate for genetic, neurological, psychiatric, and psychosocial variables (Rapp and Vollmer 2005b). In early childhood SMD, one must rule out intellectual disability or PDD. Later-onset SMD requires further evaluation for anxiety, mood, or psychotic disorders. Additionally, the clinician must look carefully for medication side effects that may cause or confound these repetitive movements, particularly with dopamine agonists such as stimulants.

Many stereotypic or repetitive behaviors associated with SMD are also observed in patients with tics, OCD, and autistic spectrum disorders. It can be difficult to distinguish SMD from these disorders (Owley et al. 2005). Additionally, with increasingly severe intellectual disability, many children present with persistent repetitive behaviors that defy easy classification (Troster 1994).

Treatment

SMD is often treatment resistant. Behavioral interventions as well as pharmacotherapy may be indicated. Although typically part of behavioral treatments, positive reinforcement has generally not been effective when used alone in SMD. Overcorrection has the most empirical support, although efforts to reduce anxiety and block the pleasurable effects of self-stimulation can also be useful. In non-SIB, ignoring behaviors can be an effective part of a treatment plan, whereas mildly aversive stimuli in SIB can be helpful.

Behaviors that meet criteria for OCD or comorbid tic disorders may require psychotherapy and, depending on severity, perhaps pharmacotherapy. SSRIs can be helpful but should be used in conjunction with cognitive-behavioral therapy or response prevention therapies (Rapp and Vollmer 2005a, 2005b). Patients with genetic syndromes or specific behavioral phenotypes may require a more comprehensive assessment and referral to clinicians familiar with these syndromes. For patients with SMD and intellectual disability, SSRIs, mood-stabilizing antiepileptic agents, opiate blockers such as naltrexone, and second-generation antipsychotic drugs can be helpful, but the clinician needs to be aware that adverse drug reactions can contribute to an escalation in SMD and SIB (Rapp and Vollmer 2005a; see Chapter 19, "Treatment of Children and Adolescents").

Stereotypic Movement Disorder Summary

SMD is a developmental disorder characterized by repetitive behaviors and, in some situations, SIBs. The clinician must distinguish between normal developmental repetitive behaviors and those that represent significant risk for psychopathology. Although excluded from the diagnosis, tic disorders, OCD, and autistic spectrum disorders may overlap with SMD, and their exclusion can be difficult. Because intellectual disability is also a risk factor for persistent or progressive forms of SMD, the clinician may need to request help from individuals skilled in working with this population. The hasty and injudicious use of medication protocols can become counterproductive and expose children to risks that might be avoided by careful assessment and behavioral interventions.

Conclusion

Many psychiatric disorders have their onset in childhood or adolescence. These disorders can influence development and continue into adulthood, exerting significant and long-lasting effects on a person's self-esteem and sense of satisfaction with relationships or jobs. Variations in presentation may depend on the individual's developmental level. Research in child psychiatric disorders is continuing to increase, and effective treatments are now available for many childhood psychiatric disorders.

Key Points

- Pervasive developmental disorders are neuropsychiatric disorders of development characterized by social, communication, and behavioral symptoms that vary in presentation and severity among individuals.

- Conduct disorder and oppositional defiant disorder are heterogeneous, nonspecific diagnoses with likely multifactorial etiologies. Comorbid psychiatric diagnoses are common and require attention. Effective treatments incorporate cognitive skill development, parental training, and involvement of appropriate community systems.

- Attention-deficit/hyperactivity disorder is a highly comorbid disorder and appears to be an enduring condition in some patients.

- A complete psychiatric examination of a child should include a complete medical evaluation and physical examination to assess for organic etiologies of presenting symptoms.

Suggested Readings

Dulcan MK: Helping Parents, Youth, and Teachers Understand Medications for Behavioral and Emotional Problems: A Resource Book of Medication Information Handouts. Washington, DC, American Psychiatric Publishing, 2007

Dulcan MK, Wiener JM (eds): Essentials of Child and Adolescent Psychiatry. Washington, DC, American Psychiatric Publishing, 2006

Dulcan MK, Martini R, Lake M: Concise Guide to Child and Adolescent Psychiatry, 3rd Edition. Washington, DC, American Psychiatric Publishing, 2003

Gemelli R: Normal Child and Adolescent Development. Washington, DC, American Psychiatric Publishing, 1996

Green WH: Child and Adolescent Clinical Psychopharmacology. Philadelphia, PA, Lippincott Williams & Wilkins, 2006

Lewis M: Child and Adolescent Psychiatry: A Comprehensive Textbook, 3rd Edition. Philadelphia, PA, Lippincott Williams & Wilkins, 2002

Online Resources

American Academy of Child and Adolescent Psychiatry (www.aacap.org)

Children and Adults with Attention Deficit/Hyperactivity Disorder (www.chadd.org)

Learning Disabilities Association of America (www. ldaamerica.org)

Mental Health America (formerly National Mental Health Association) (www.mentalhealthamerica.net; www.nmha.org)

National Institute of Mental Health (www. nimh.nih.gov)

Online Mendelian Inheritance in Man (www. ncbi.nlm.nih. gov/sites/entrez?db=OMIM)

Tourette Syndrome Association (www.tsa-usa.org)

References

Abikoff H, Courtney M, Pelham WEJ, et al: Teacher's ratings of disruptive behaviors: the influence of halo effects. J Abnorm Child Psychol 21:519–533, 1993

Aman MG, Lindsay RL, Nash PL, et al: Individuals with mental retardation, in Pediatric Psychopharmacology. Edited by Martin A, Scahill L, Charney DS, et al. New York, Oxford University Press, 2003, pp 617–630

American Academy of Child and Adolescent Psychiatry: Practice parameters for the assessment and treatment of children, adolescents, and adults with attention deficit/hyperactivity disorder. J Am Acad Child Adolesc Psychiatry 36 (suppl):85S–121S, 1997

American Academy of Child and Adolescent Psychiatry: Practice parameters for the assessment and treatment of children and adolescents with language and learning disorders. J Am Acad Child Adolesc Psychiatry 37:46S–62S, 1998

American Academy of Child and Adolescent Psychiatry: Practice parameters for the assessment and treatment of children and adolescents with reactive attachment disorder of infancy and early childhood. J Am Acad Child Adolesc Psychiatry 44:1206–1219, 2005

American Psychiatric Association: Diagnostic and Statistical Manual of Mental Disorders, 3rd Edition. Washington, DC, American Psychiatric Association, 1980

American Psychiatric Association: Diagnostic and Statistical Manual of Mental Disorders, 4th Edition. Washington, DC, American Psychiatric Association, 1994

American Psychiatric Association: Diagnostic and Statistical Manual of Mental Disorders, 4th Edition, Text Revision. Washington, DC, American Psychiatric Association, 2000

Amir RE, Van den Veyver IB, Wan M, et al: Rett syndrome is caused by mutation in X-linked MECP2, encoding methyl-CpG-binding protein 2. Nat Genet 23:185–188, 1999

Asperger H: "Autistic psychopathy" in childhood (1944), in Autism and Asperger Syndrome. Translated and annotated by Frith U. Cambridge, England, Cambridge University Press, 1991, pp 37–92

Barling J, Bullen G: Dietary factors and hyperactivity: a failure to replicate. J Genet Psychol 146:117–123, 1985

Barnett SR, Riddle MA: Anxiolytics, buspirone, and others, in Pediatric Psychopharmacology. Edited by Martin A, Scahill L, Charney DS, et al. New York, Oxford University Press, 2003, pp 341–352

Barnhill LJ: Neurobiology of self-injurious behavior: is there a relationship to addictions? Nat Assoc Dual Diag Bull 6:29–37, 2003

Barnhill LJ: Stereotypic movement disorder. Nat Assoc Dual Diag Bull 9:23–26, 2006

Biederman J, Newcorn J, Sprich S: Comorbidity of attention deficit hyperactivity disorder with conduct, depressive, anxiety, and other disorders. Am J Psychiatry 148:564–577, 1991

Biederman J, Milberger S, Faraone SV, et al: Associations between childhood asthma and ADHD: issues of psychiatric comorbidity and familiality. J Am Acad Child Adolesc Psychiatry 33:842–848, 1994

Biederman J, Faraone SV, Milberger S, et al: Predictors of persistence and remission of ADHD into adolescence: results from a four-year prospective follow-up study. J Am Acad Child Adolesc Psychiatry 35:343–351, 1996

Biederman J, Swanson JM, Wigal SB, et al: A comparison of once-daily and divided doses of modafinil in children with attention-deficit/hyperactivity disorder: a randomized, double blind, and placebo-controlled study. J Clin Psychiatry 67:727–735, 2006

Black B, Uhde TW: Treatment of elective mutism with fluoxetine: a double blind, placebo-controlled study. J Am Acad Child Adolesc Psychiatry 33:1000–1106, 1994

Black B, Uhde TW: Psychiatric characteristics of children with selective mutism: a pilot study. J Acad Child Adolesc Psychiatry 34:847–856, 1995

Brestan EV, Eyberg SM: Effective psychosocial treatment of conduct-disordered children and adolescents: 29 years, 82 studies, 5275 children. J Clin Child Psychol 27:180–189, 1998

Bruun RD, Budman CL: Natural history of Gilles de la Tourette's syndrome, in Handbook of Tourette's Syndrome and Related

Tic Behavioral Disorders. Edited by Kurlan R. New York, Marcel-Dekker, 1994, pp 27–43

Charach A, Figueroa M, Chen S, et al: Stimulant treatment over 5 years: effects on growth. J Am Acad Child Adolesc Psychiatry 45:415–421, 2006

Chatoor I: Feeding and eating disorders of infancy and early childhood, in The American Psychiatric Publishing Textbook of Child and Adolescent Psychiatry. Edited by Wiener JM, Dulcan MK. Washington, DC, American Psychiatric Publishing, 2004, pp 639–657

Cobham VE, Dadds MR, Spence SH: The role of parental anxiety in the treatment of childhood anxiety. J Consult Clin Psychol 66:893–905, 1998

Connors CK, Schulte AC: Learning disorders, in Neuropsychopharmacology: The Fifth Generation of Progress. Edited by Davis KL, Charney D, Coyle JT, et al. Baltimore, MD, Lippincott Williams & Wilkins, 2002, pp 597–610

Costello EJ, Mustillo S, Erkanli A, et al: Prevalence and development of psychiatric disorders in childhood and adolescence. Arch Gen Psychiatry 60:837–844, 2003

Davidson RJ: Emotion and disorders of emotion: perspectives from affective neuroscience, in Neuropsychiatry, 2nd Edition. Edited by Schiffer RB, Rao SM, Fogel BS. Baltimore, MD, Lippincott Williams & Wilkins, 2003, pp 467–480

De Raeymaecker DM: Psychomotor development and psychopathology in childhood. Int Rev Neurobiology 72:83–101, 2006

Denckla MB, Roeltgen DP: Disorders of motor function and control, in Handbook of Neuropsychology, Vol 6. Edited by Rapin I, Segalowitz SJ. Amsterdam, The Netherlands, Elsevier, 1992, pp 455–476

Dick DM, Viken RJ, Kaprio J, et al: Understanding the covariation among childhood externalizing symptoms: genetic and environmental influences on conduct disorder, attention deficit hyperactivity disorder, and oppositional defiant disorder symptoms. J Abnorm Child Psychol 33:219–229, 2005

Eapen V, Yakeley JW, Robertson MM: Gilles de la Tourette's syndrome and obsessive-compulsive disorder, in Neuropsychiatry, 2nd Edition. Edited by Schiffer RL, Rao SM, Fogel BS. Baltimore, MD, Lippincott Williams & Wilkins, 2002, pp 947–990

Edwards MJ, Dale RC, Church AJ, et al: Adult-onset tic disorders, motor stereotypies, and behavioral disturbances associated with antibasal ganglia antibodies. Mov Disord 19:1190–1196, 2004

Egger J, Stolla A, McEwen LM: Controlled trial of hyposensitization in children with food-induced hyperkinetic syndrome. Lancet 339:1150–1153, 1992

Einfield SL, Aman M: Issues in the taxonomy of psychopathology in mental retardation. J Autism Dev Disord 25:143–167, 1995

Elia J, Gulotta C, Rose SR, et al: Thyroid function and attention deficit hyperactivity disorder. J Am Acad Child Adolesc Psychiatry 33:169–172, 1994

Farmer EM, Compton SN, Bums BJ, et al: Review of the evidence base for treatment of childhood psychopathology: externalizing disorders. J Consult Clin Psychol 70:1267–1302, 2002

Faraone SV, Biederman J, Lehman BK, et al: Intellectual performance and school failure in children with attention deficit hyperactivity disorder and their siblings. J Abnorm Psychol 102:616–623, 1993

Fergusson DM, Lynskey MT, Horwood LJ: The effect of maternal depression on maternal ratings of child behavior. J Abnorm Child Psychol 21:245–269, 1993

Fischer M: Persistence of ADHD into adulthood: it depends on whom you ask. ADHD Rep 5:8–10, 1997

Fletcher JM: Predicting math outcomes: reading predictors and comorbidity. J Learn Disabil 38:308–312, 2005

Fombonne E, Zakarian R, Bennett A, et al: Pervasive developmental disorders in Montreal, Quebec, Canada: prevalence and links with immunizations. Pediatrics 118:e139–e150, 2006

Gershorn J: A meta-analytic review of gender differences in ADHD. J Atten Disord 5:143–154, 2002

Gillberg C, Wing L: Autism: not an extremely rare disorder. Acta Psychiatr Scand 99:399–406, 1999

Goldstein S, Reynolds CR: Handbook of Neurodevelopmental and Genetic Disorders in Children. New York, Guilford, 1999

Griffiths DM, Gardner WI, Nugent JA: Behavioral Supports and Community Living. Kingston, NY, NADD Press, 1998

Guthrie E, Mast J, Engel M: Diagnosing genetic anomalies by inspection. Child Adolesc Psychiatr Clin N Am 8:777–790, 1999

Hagberg BA, Witt-Engerström I: Rett syndrome: a suggested staging system for describing impairment profile with increasing age toward adolescence. Am J Med Genet 24:47–59, 1986

Halperin JM, Newcorn JH, Matier K, et al: Impulsivity and the initiation of fights in children with disruptive behavior disorders. J Child Psychol Psychiatry 36:1199–1211, 1995

Harris JC: Behavioral phenotypes of neurodevelopmental disorders: portals into the developing brain, in Neuropsychopharmacology: Fifth Generation of Progress. Edited by Davis KL, Charney D, Coyle JT, et al. Baltimore, MD, Lippincott Williams & Wilkins, 2002, pp 625–638

Harris JC: Intellectual Disability: Understanding Its Development, Causes, Classification, Evaluation and Treatment. New York, Oxford University Press, 2006

Hauser P, Zametkin AJ, Martinez P, et al: Attention deficit hyperactivity disorder in people with generalized resistance to thyroid hormone. N Engl J Med 328:997–1001, 1993

Hechtman L: Long-term outcome in attention-deficit hyperactivity disorder. Psychiatr Clin North Am 1:553–565, 1993

Hetherington EM, Stanley-Hagan M: The adjustment of children with divorced parents: a risk and resiliency perspective. J Child Psychol Psychiatry 40:129–140, 1999

Jankovic J, DeLeon ML: Basal ganglia and behavioral disorders, in Neuropsychiatry, 2nd Edition. Edited by Schiffer RB, Rao SM, Fogel BS. Baltimore, MD, Lippincott Williams & Wilkins, 2002, pp 934–945

Jensen PS, Shervette RE, Xenakis SN, et al: Anxiety and depressive disorders in attention deficit disorder with hyperactivity: new findings. Am J Psychiatry 150:1203–1209, 1993

Joy SP, Lord JS, Green L, et al: Mental retardation and developmental disabilities, in Neuropsychiatry, 2nd Edition. Edited by Schiffer RB, Rao SM, Fogel BS. Baltimore, MD, Lippincott Williams & Wilkins, 2003, pp 552–604

Kanner L: Autistic disturbances of affective contact. Nervous Child 2:217–250, 1943

Kelly DP, Kelly BJ, Jones MI, et al: Attention deficits in children and adolescents with hearing loss: a survey. Am J Dis Child 147:737–741, 1993

Kennedy CH, Meyer KA, Knowles T, et al: Analyzing the multiple functions of stereotypical behavior for students with autism: implications for assessment and treatment. J Appl Behav Anal 33:559–571, 2000

King RA, Scahill L, Lombroso P, et al: Tourette's syndrome and other tic disorders, in Pediatric Psychopharmacology. Edited by Martin A, Scahill L, Charney DS, et al. New York, Oxford University Press, 2003, pp 526–542

Klein RG, Mannuzza S: Children with uncomplicated reading disorders grown up: a prospective follow-up into adulthood, in Learning Disabilities: Implications for Psychiatric Treatment (Review of Psychiatry Series, Vol 19, No 5; Oldham JO and Riba MB, series eds.). Edited by Greenhill LL. Washington, DC, American Psychiatric Press, 2000, pp 1–31

Koda V, Charney DS, Pine D: Neurobiology of early onset anxiety disorders, in Pediatric Psychopharmacology. Edited by Martin A, Scahill L, Charney DS, et al. New York, Oxford University Press, 2003, pp 138–149

Labellarte M, Ginsburg G: Anxiety disorders, in Pediatric Psychopharmacology. Edited by Martin A, Scahill L, Charney DS, et al. New York, Oxford University Press, 2003, pp 497–510

Lachiewicz AM, Dawson DV, Spirigidiollozzi GA, et al: Arithmetic difficulties in females with the fragile X premutation. Am J Med Genet 140:665–672, 2006

Landman GB, Rappaport L: Pediatric management of severe treatment-resistant encopresis. J Dev Behav Pediatr 6:349–351, 1985

Lavigne JV, Burns WJ, Cotter PD: Rumination in infancy: recent behavioral approaches. Int J Eat Disord 1:70–82, 1981

Leckman JF, Yeh C-B, Lombroso PJ: Neurobiology of tic disorders, in Pediatric Psychopharmacology. Edited by Martin A, Scahill L, Charney DS, et al. New York, Oxford University Press, 2003, pp 164–174

Litt J, Taylor HG, Klein N, et al: Learning disabilities in children with very low birthweight: prevalence, neuropsychological correlations, educational interventions. J Learn Disabil 38:13–41, 2005

Loeber R, Green SM, Keenan K, et al: Which boys will fare worse? Early predictors for the onset of conduct disorder in a six-year longitudinal study. J Am Acad Child Adolesc Psychiatry 34:499–509, 1995

Loening-Baucke V: Encopresis. Curr Opin Pediatr 14:570–575, 2002

McCracken JT, McGough J, Shah B, et al: Risperidone in children with autism and serious behavioral problems. N Engl J Med 347:314–321, 2002

McDougle CJ, Scahill L, Aman MG, et al: Risperidone for the core symptom domains of autism: results from the study by the Autism Network of the Research Units on Pediatric Psychopharmacology. Am J Psychiatry 162:1142–1148, 2005

McGee R, Stanton WR, Sears MR: Allergic disorders and attention deficit disorder in children. J Abnorm Child Psychol 21:79–88, 1993

Mendlowitz SL, Manassis K, Bradley S, et al: Cognitive-behavioral group treatments in childhood anxiety disorders: the role of parental involvement. J Am Acad Child Adolesc Psychiatry 38:1223–1229, 1999

Mikkelsen EJ, Rapoport JL: Enuresis: psychopathology, sleep stage and drug response. Urol Clin North Am 7:361–377, 1980

Moffat ME, Harlos S, Kirshen AJ, et al: Desmopressin acetate and nocturnal enuresis: how much do we know? Pediatrics 92:420–425, 1993

Moldavsky M, Lev D, Lerman-Sagie T: Behavioral phenotypes of genetic syndromes: a reference guide for psychiatrists. J Am Acad Child Adolesc Psychiatry 40:749–760, 2001

Multimodal Treatment of ADHD Cooperative Group: A 14-month randomized clinical trial of treatment strategies for attention-deficit/hyperactivity disorder. The Multimodal Treatment of ADHD Cooperative Group: Multimodal Treatment Study of Children With ADHD. Arch Gen Psychiatry 56:1073–1086, 1999

Newcorn JH, Halperin JM: Comorbidity among disruptive behavior disorders: impact on severity, impairment, and response to treatment. Child Adolesc Psychiatr Clin N Am 3:227–252, 1994

Ornoy A, Uriel L, Tennenbaum A: Inattention, hyperactivity and speech delay at 2–4 years of age as a predictor for ADD-ADHD syndrome. Isr J Psychiatry Relat Sci 30:155–163, 1993

Owley T, Leventhal B, Cook E: EPS or stereotypies? J Child Adolesc Psychopharmacol 15:150–151, 2005

Paul R: Language Disorders From Infancy Through Adolescence: Assessment and Intervention, 2nd Edition. St. Louis, MO, Mosby, 2001

Pelham WEJ, Gnagy EM, Greenslade KE, et al: Teacher ratings of DSM-III-R symptoms for the disruptive behavior disorders. J Am Acad Child Adolesc Psychiatry 31:210–218, 1992

Peters JM, Barnett AL, Henderson SE: Clumsiness, dyspraxia, and developmental coordination disorder. Child Care Health Dev 27:399–412, 2001

Piven J, Palmer P, Landa R, et al: Personality and language characteristics in parents from multiple-incidence autism families. Am J Med Genet 74:398–411, 1997

Popper CW, Elliott GR: Sudden death and tricyclic antidepressants: clinical considerations for children. J Child Adolesc Psychopharmacol 1:125–132, 1990

Popper CW, Gammon GD, West SA, et al: Disorders usually first diagnosed in infancy, childhood, or adolescence, in The American Psychiatric Publishing Textbook of Clinical Psychiatry. Edited by Hales RE, Yudofsky SC. Washington, DC, American Psychiatric Publishing, 2003, pp 833–974

Posey DJ, Erickson CA, Stigler KA, et al: The use of selective serotonin reuptake inhibitors in autism and related disorders. J Child Adolesc Psychopharmacol 16:181–186, 2006

Potenza MN, Hollander E: Pathological gambling and impulse control disorders, in Neuropsychopharmacology: Fifth Generation of Progress. Edited by Davis KL, Charney DS, Coyle JT, et al. Baltimore, MD, Lippincott Williams & Wilkins, 2002, pp 1725–1742

Ramus F, Rosen S, Dakin SC, et al: Theories of developmental dyslexia: insights from multiple case study of dyslexic adults. Brain 126:841–865, 2003

Rapp JT, Vollmer TR: Stereotypy I: a review of behavioral assessment and treatment. Res Dev Disabil 26:527–547, 2005a

Rapp JT, Vollmer TR: Stereotypy II: a review of the neurobiological interpretations and suggestions for integration with behavioral methods. Res Dev Disabil 26:548–564, 2005b

Riddle MA, Nelson JC, Kleinman CS, et al: Sudden death in children receiving Norpramin: a review of three reported cases and commentary. J Am Acad Child Adolesc Psychiatry 30:104–108, 1991

Rizwan S, Manning JT, Brabin BJ: Maternal smoking during pregnancy and possible effects of in utero testosterone: evidence from the 2D:4D finger length ratio. Early Hum Dev 83:87–90, 2007

Robertson MM: Tourette's syndrome, associated conditions, and the complexities of treatment. Brain 23:425–463, 2000

Robins LN, Ratcliff KS: Risk factors in the continuation of childhood antisocial behavior into adulthood. Int J Ment Health 7:96–111, 1979

Rockney RM, McQuade WH, Days AL: The plain abdominal roentgenogram in the management of encopresis. Arch Pediatr Adolesc Med 149:623–627, 1995

Rourke BP, Hayman-Abello BA, Collins DW: Learning disabilities: a neuropsychological perspective, in Neuropsychiatry, 2nd Edition. Edited by Schiffer RB, Rao SM, Fogel BS. Baltimore, MD, Lippincott Williams & Wilkins, 2003, pp 630–659

Rowe KS, Rowe KJ: Synthetic food coloring and behavior: a dose response effect in a double-blind, placebo-controlled, repeated-measures study. J Pediatr 125:691–698, 1994

Rutter M: Concepts of autism: a review of research. J Child Psychol Psychiatry 9:1–25, 1968

Rutter M: Assessment objectives and principles, in Language Development and Disor-

ders. Edited by Yule W, Rutter M. Philadelphia, PA, JB Lippincott, 1987, pp 295–311

Saint-Cyr JA, Taylor AE, Nicholson K: Behavior and the basal ganglia. Adv Neurol 28:273–281, 1995

Santangelo SI, Pauls DL, Goldstein JM, et al: Tourette's syndrome: what are the influences of gender and comorbid obsessive-compulsive disorders? J Am Acad Child Adolesc Psychiatry 33:785–804, 1994

Scahill L, Schwab-Stone M: Epidemiology of ADHD in school-age children. Child Adolesc Psychiatr Clin N Am 9:541–555, 2000

Shaywitz BA, Pugh KR, Fletcher JM, et al: What cognitive and neurobiological studies have taught us about dyslexia, in Learning Disabilities: Implications for Psychiatric Treatment (Review of Psychiatry Series, Vol 19, No 5; Oldham JM and Riba MB, series eds.). Edited by Greenhill LL. Washington, DC, American Psychiatric Press, 2000, pp 59–96

Smyke AT, Dumitrescu A, Zeanah CH: Attachment disturbances in young children, I: the continuum of caretaking casualty. J Am Acad Child Adolesc Psychiatry 41:972–982, 2002

South M, Ozonoff S, McMahon WM: Repetitive behavioral profile in Asperger's syndrome and high functioning autism. J Autism Dev Disord 35:145–158, 2005

Spencer TJ, Biederman J, Steingard R, et al: Bupropion exacerbates tics in children with attention-deficit hyperactivity disorder and Tourette's syndrome. J Am Acad Child Adolesc Psychiatry 32:211–214, 1993

Spencer TJ, Biederman J, Wilens TE: Attention-deficit/hyperactivity disorder and comorbidity. Pediatr Clin North Am 46:915–927, 1999

Spencer TJ, Faraone SV, Biederman J, et al: Does prolonged therapy with a long-acting stimulant suppress growth in children with ADHD? J Am Acad Child Adolesc Psychiatry 45:527–537, 2006

Sund AM, Wichstrom L: Insecure attachment as a risk factor for future depressive symptoms in early adolescence. J Am Acad Child Adolesc Psychiatry 41:1478–1485, 2002

Swanson JM, McBurnett K, Wigal T, et al: Effect of stimulant medication on children with attention deficit disorder: "a review of reviews." Except Child 60:154–162, 1993

Swedo SE, Pine DS (eds): Anxiety disorders. Child Adolesc Psychiatr Clin N Am 14:xv–xviii, 2005

Symons FJ, Sperry LA, Dropik PL, et al: The early development of stereotypy and self-injury: a review of research methods. J Intel Disabil Res 49:144–158, 2005

Tcheremissine OV, Lieving LM: Pharmacological aspects of the treatment of conduct disorder in children and adolescents. CNS Drugs 20:549–565, 2006

Troster H: Prevalence and functions of stereotyped behaviors in nonhandicapped children in residential care. J Abnorm Child Psychol 22:79–97, 1994

Tsai LY: Autistic disorder, in The American Psychiatric Publishing Textbook of Child and Adolescent Psychiatry, 3rd Edition. Edited by Weiner JM, Dulcan MK. Washington, DC, American Psychiatric Publishing, 2004, pp 261–315

U.S. Department of Education: Twenty-Fourth Annual Report to Congress on the Implementation of the Individuals With Disabilities Education Act. Washington, DC, U.S. Office of Special Education Programs, 2002

Vitiello B, Stoff D, Atkins M, et al: Soft neurological signs and impulsivity in children. J Dev Behav Pediatr 11:112–115, 1990

Volkmar FR, Rutter M: Childhood disintegrative disorder: results of the DSM-IV field trial. J Am Acad Child Adolesc Psychiatry 34:1092–1095, 1995

Volkmar FR, Klin A, Siegel B, et al: Field trial for autistic disorder in DSM-IV. Am J Psychiatry 151:1361–1367, 1994

Walker CE, Miller L, Bonner B: Incontinence disorders: enuresis and encopresis, in Handbook of Pediatric Psychology. Edited by Routh D. New York, Guilford, 1988, pp 263–298

Walker JL, Lahey BB, Hynd GW, et al: Comparison of specific patterns of antisocial behavior in children with conduct disorder with or without coexisting hyperactivity. J Consult Clin Psychol 55:910–913, 1987

Walkup JT, Mink JW, Hollenbeck PJ: Advances in Neurology, Vol 99. Baltimore, MD, Lippincott Williams & Wilkins, 2006

Weinberg WA, McLean A: A diagnostic approach to developmental specific learning disorders. J Child Neurol 2:158–172, 1986

Werner EE: High risk children in young adulthood: a longitudinal study from birth to 32 years. Am J Orthopsychiatry 59:72–81, 1989

Wigal S, Swanson JM, Feifel D, et al: A double-blind, placebo-controlled trial of dexmethylphenidate hydrochloride and D,L-threo-methylphenidate hydrochloride in children with attention-deficit/hyperactivity disorder. J Am Acad Child Adolesc Psychiatry 43:1406–1414, 2004

Wilens TE, Dodson W: A clinical perspective of attention-deficit/hyperactivity disorder into adulthood. J Clin Psychiatry 65:1301–1313, 2004

Wolraich M, Hannah J, Pinnock T, et al: Comparison of diagnostic criteria for attention-deficit/hyperactivity disorder in a country-wide sample. J Am Acad Child Adolesc Psychiatry 35:319–324, 1996

Zachor DA, Roberts AW, Hodgens JB, et al: Effects of long-term psychostimulant medication on growth of children with ADHD. Res Dev Disabil 27:162–174, 2006

Zeanah CH: Disturbances of attachment in young children adopted from institutions. J Dev Behav Pediatr 21:230–236, 2000

Zeanah CH, Smyke AT, Dumitrescu A: Attachment disturbances in young children, II: indiscriminant behavior and institutional care. J Am Acad Child Adolesc Psychiatry 41:983–989, 2002

Zeanah CH, Smyke AT, Koga S, et al: Attachment in institutionalized and noninstitutionalized Romanian children. Child Development 75:1015–1028, 2005

13

SLEEP DISORDERS

Daniel J. Buysse, M.D.
Patrick J. Strollo Jr., M.D.
Jed E. Black, M.D.
Phyllis G. Zee, M.D., Ph.D.
John W. Winkelman, M.D., Ph.D.

Sleep and wakefulness are fundamental behavioral-neurobiological states present in all animals, including human beings. Although the function of sleep and sleep–wake rhythms has long been debated, it is unlikely that such a fundamental process will ever be equated with a single function. Theories of the function of sleep focus on several possibilities, including ecological or environmental advantage, physical restoration, optimization of waking neurocognitive and emotional function, learning, and even health and survival.

Sleep and its disorders are particularly relevant to psychiatric practice. Virtually every psychiatric disorder can be associated with disturbances of sleep–wake function or circadian rhythms. Sleep disturbances are associated with increased risk of subsequent psychiatric disorders, and persistent sleep symptoms adversely affect the outcome of psychiatric disorders. Primary sleep disorders often include neuropsychiatric symptoms, which can make differential diagnoses challenging. Finally, many of the treatments used for sleep disorders, including behavioral and pharmacological treatments, fall within the purview of psychiatric practice. Detailed information on the topics in this chapter can be found in more specialized references (Chokroverty 2009; Kryger et al. 2005). Information on pediatric sleep disorders is not presented in this chapter but can be found elsewhere (Sheldon et al. 2005).

Neurobiology of Circadian Rhythms and Sleep

Most physiological and psychological functions in humans demonstrate endogenous rhythms. These rhythms differ in *period*, or the time to complete one cycle, ranging from very short (e.g., electroencephalographic and cardiac rhythms) to very long (e.g., menstrual cycle). *Circadian rhythms* are those with a period length of approximately 24 hours. Humans have a circadian rhythm period of just over 24 hours (Czeisler et al. 1999). Physiological systems that show circadian variation include the sleep–wake cycle, hormone secretion (e.g., cortisol, melatonin), core body temperature, cardiovascular function, sleepiness/alertness, and cognitive and psychomotor function (Czeisler et al. 2005). The *amplitude* of a rhythm is a measure of the "size" of oscillation from peak to trough, and *phase* refers to the timing of a rhythm.

Circadian rhythms are *endogenous* and not the result of the environmental light–dark cycle. Although circadian rhythms can be synchronized *(entrained)* to external time cues, they are expressed even in temporal and environmental isolation. Environmental time cues are also called *zeitgebers*, or "time givers." In humans and most animals, bright light is the strongest zeitgeber for entraining circadian rhythms,. Light-induced phase shifts are most sensitive to short wavelength light of approximately 460 nanometers (nm; blue-green range) (Lockley et al. 2003). The effect of zeitgebers on the timing of rhythms is time dependent. For instance, bright light given toward the end of the usual sleep period causes circadian rhythms to move to an earlier time ("phase advance"), whereas light given near usual bedtime causes circadian rhythms to move to a later time ("phase delay"). Melatonin, a pineal hormone secreted during hours of darkness, is an important endogenous modulator of circadian rhythms and sleep. *Exogenous* melatonin administration in the early evening produces phase advances, and administration in the early morning produces phase delays (Cajochen et al. 2003).

Circadian rhythms are generated and controlled within the central nervous system (CNS). The major pacemakers of the circadian system are the paired suprachiasmatic nuclei (SCN) of the hypothalamus (Moore 1997). Specialized melanopsin-containing retinal ganglion cells project through the retino-hypothalamic tract to the SCN, providing light input independent of vision (Bellingham and Foster 2002). The SCN has efferent pathways to the hypothalamus and thalamus through which it transmits timing information to the rest of the CNS, including sleep–wake systems (Czeisler et al. 2005; Pace-Schott and Hobson 2002). Rhythmic activity of the SCN in turn results from a transcription–translation feedback loop involving a set of circadian rhythm genes (King and Takahashi 2000). Mutations in these genes are associated with lengthening or shortening of the circadian period.

Sleep is a rapidly reversible neurobehavioral state characterized by almost simultaneous change in the activity patterns and mode of firing of CNS neurons and circuits. Sleep onset is an involuntary process that occurs only when neurobiological and environmental circumstances permit.

In humans, the electrophysiological characteristics of sleep can be characterized by polysomnography, which typically includes electroencephalography to measure brain electrical activity, electro-oculography to measure eye movements, and submental surface electromyography to measure muscle tone. Patterns of electroencephalographic activity, eye movements, and muscle tone reveal clear differences between wakefulness and sleep, which is further divided into two states, rapid eye movement (REM) sleep and non–rapid eye movement (NREM) sleep (Carskadon and Rechtschaffen 2005). These three states are distinguished by characteristic patterns of environmental responsiveness, systemic physiology, electroencephalographic waveforms, muscle tone, and mental activity (Table 13–1). NREM sleep is subdivided into three or four stages of increasing "depth," which correlate with decreasing arousability (American Academy of Sleep Medicine 2005; Rechtschaffen and Kales 1968). NREM and REM sleep cycle periodically across the night (Figure 13–1). Most deep NREM sleep occurs in the first half of the night. NREM and REM sleep alternate approximately every 90–100 minutes during the sleep period. REM sleep episodes become longer and more intense toward the morning hours, as measured by the number of eye movements and complexity of dream mentation.

Sleep stages are affected by a number of individual and environmental factors. Age is the most important of these (Ohayon et al. 2004). Newborns spend nearly 50% of sleep in a form of sleep resembling REM, but this decreases rapidly in the first year of life. Sleep duration also dramatically decreases from infancy through childhood and then increases slightly in adolescence. Across the adult life span, deep NREM sleep gradually diminishes from its peak in late adolescence. In later adulthood, the number and duration of awakenings and the amount of Stage 1 sleep increase, whereas Stage 2 NREM and REM sleep are relatively consistent (Ohayon et al. 2004). In addition, the entire sleep period tends to phase delay during adolescence and then phase advance during later adulthood.

Physiologically, human sleep is regulated by two processes, a homeostatic factor and a circadian factor (Figure 13–2). The homeostatic factor represents an increase in sleep "drive" as a function of prior wakefulness and is reflected in electroencephalographic slow-wave activity. Homeostatic sleep drive builds up during waking hours and then decreases during subsequent sleep. The second regulatory factor is the circadian rhythm of sleep and wakefulness. In humans, the circadian drive for sleep is highest in the second half of the usual sleep period.

Sleep and wakefulness are controlled by a number of widely distributed brain systems (B.E. Jones 2005; Pace-Schott and Hobson 2002; Szymusiak and McGinty 2008). Brain regions critical for normal wakefulness include the histaminergic nuclei of the posterior hypothalamus, the cholinergic nuclei of the basal forebrain, and the noradrenergic and serotonergic nuclei of the ascending reticular activating system and the midbrain and pontine tegmentum. The hypocretin system of the lateral hypothalamus stabilizes wakefulness through its innervation of cholinergic, aminergic, and histaminergic brain systems. Regions critical for the generation of NREM sleep include the solitary tract, which projects ventrally through the basal forebrain and dorsally through the thalamus to the cortex. Progressive hyperpolarization of corticothalamic circuits during NREM sleep underlies the characteristic rhythmic waveforms of this state. The ventrolateral and medial preoptic areas of the hypothalamus become more active during sleep than wakefulness, acting as a "sleep switch" through reciprocal interactions with wake-promoting centers described earlier. In addition, homeostatic sleep regulation may involve activity of extracellular adenosine in the basal forebrain. REM sleep results from reciprocal interactions between brain stem cholinergic "REM on" nuclei and noradrenergic/serotonergic "REM off" nuclei in the pontine tegmentum.

Although numerous neurotransmitters are involved in sleep–wake state regulation, their activities are complicated and often apparently contradictory (B.E. Jones 2005). In general, the neurotransmitters acetylcholine, histamine, serotonin, norepinephrine, and hypocretin promote wakefulness. The inhibitory neurotransmitters γ-aminobutyric acid (GABA) and galanin are associated with inhibitory influences that promote NREM sleep. Other substances including cytokines, prostaglandins, and various hormones also influence sleep–wake states.

Table 13–1. Physiological characteristics of sleep–wake states

	Wake	NREM	REM
Electroencephalogram	Fast, low voltage	Slow, high voltage	Fast, low voltage
Eye movement	Vision-related	Slow, irregular	Rapid
Muscle tone	++	+	0
Heart rate, blood pressure, respiratory rate	Variable	Slow/low, regular	Variable, higher than NREM
Responses to hypoxia and hypercarbia	Active	Reduced responsiveness	Lowest responsiveness
Thermoregulation	Behavioral and physiological regulation	Physiological regulation only	Reduced physiological regulation
Mental activity	Full	None or limited	Story-like dreams

Note. += activity level; 0=inactive; NREM=non-rapid eye movement sleep; REM=rapid eye movement sleep.
Source. Adapted from Saper et al. 2001.

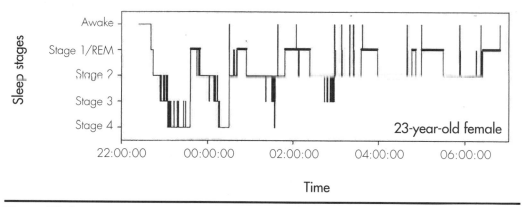

Figure 13–1. Hypnogram of sleep stages in a healthy subject.

Each 20- to 30-second epoch of sleep for an entire night is assigned a sleep stage by a human scorer. These epoch scores can then be displayed graphically in a hypnogram, to display the progression of sleep stages across the night. Sleep stages are indicated by increasing depth on the vertical axis, with rapid eye movement (REM) sleep represented by heavy horizontal lines. Time is indicated on the horizontal axis. Note that most Stage 3–4 non–rapid eye movement (NREM) sleep occurs in the early part of the night, and REM periods get longer toward the end of the night.

Clinical Assessment of Sleep and Sleep Disorders

Clinical Evaluation

The diagnosis and management of patients with sleep complaints rest on an accurate clinical history. Important elements of the history include the nature, severity, and frequency of the symptoms; duration of the complaint; associated impairments; and exacerbating and alleviating factors. The following aspects of the clinical evaluation are particularly relevant to sleep and circadian rhythm disorders:

- *24-hour history.* Following the chronology of a "typical" night and day is essential for assessing sleep problems and daytime sleepiness.
- *Regularity of sleep–wake patterns.* Many patients with sleep disorders develop highly irregular schedules.
- *Bed partner history.* Certain symptoms, including snoring and sleep-related behav-

iors, may not be evident to the person with the disorder itself.
- *Medical, neurological, and psychiatric disorders.* Sleep problems are associated with a wide variety of other disorders that may exacerbate symptoms.
- *Medications and substances.* All drugs affecting control of nervous system function, and many used for medical disorders, can affect sleep.
- *Physical examination.* It is useful to evaluate the following minimal features associated with sleep apnea: height, weight, and body mass index; neck circumference; patency of oral and nasal airways; and craniofacial abnormalities, including retrognathia.
- *Questionnaires.* Sleep–wake diaries may give a more complete picture of the individual's sleep patterns and day-to-day variability and may even help the individual identify patterns that are contributing to sleep problems (Figure 13–3). The Epworth Sleepiness Scale (Johns 1991) assesses daytime sleepiness by asking the likelihood of falling asleep in specific behavioral situations. The Pittsburgh Sleep Quality Index is a 19-item self-rated scale that assesses global sleep quality.

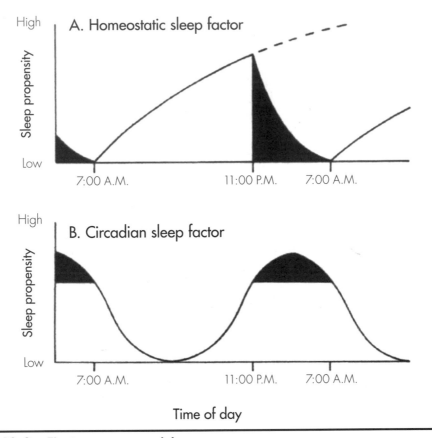

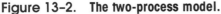

Figure 13–2.   The two-process model.

Alertness and sleepiness are determined by the interaction of two processes. The *homeostatic sleep drive* increases as a function of wake duration, reaches a maximum near the usual sleep time, and dissipates during sleep. The *circadian sleep drive* (technically, the reverse of circadian wake drive) is low during usual waking hours and peaks in the early morning hours to promote consolidated sleep. The *dark* portions of the figure correspond to the usual time of sleep.

Source.   Adapted from Borbély 1982.

- *Actigraphy.* Actigraphy measures body movement patterns during sleep through a small accelerometer worn on the wrist.
- *Polysomnography.* Polysomnography is indicated for the evaluation of patients with suspected sleep apnea and narcolepsy and may be useful to correctly diagnose parasomnias. It is not routinely indicated for the assessment of insomnia, circadian rhythm sleep disorders (CRSDs), or restless legs syndrome (RLS) but is reserved for atypical or treatment-resistant cases (Kushida et al. 2005). Objective daytime sleepiness is assessed with a variant of

polysomnography called the multiple sleep latency test (MSLT).

Classification of Sleep–Wake Disorders

Sleep disorders involve a variety of conditions with physiological, neurological, or behavioral origins. Classification systems for sleep disorders include DSM-IV-TR (American Psychiatric Association 2000), *The International Classification of Sleep Disorders*, 2nd Edition (ICSD-2; American Academy of Sleep Medicine 2005), and ICD-10 (World

A. Graphic sleep diary

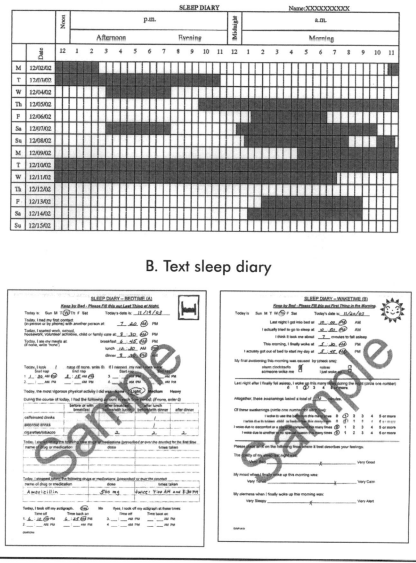

B. Text sleep diary

Figure 13–3. Sleep–wake diaries.

A, In a graphic sleep diary, the subject "blocks out" the times he or she was actually asleep. In this example, the subject had very irregular sleep timing with some very long sleep episodes. **B,** In a text sleep diary, the subject writes in the times of going to bed, waking up, napping, and so on.

Source. Reprinted from Buysse DJ (ed): *Sleep Disorders and Psychiatry* (Review of Psychiatry Series, Volume 24, Number 2; Oldham JM and Riba MB, series editors). Washington, DC, American Psychiatric Publishing, 2005, p. 16. Copyright 2005, American Psychiatric Publishing. Used with permission.

Health Organization 1992). DSM-IV-TR classifies sleep disorders into dyssomnias (insomnias, hypersomnias, and CRSDs), parasomnias, and secondary sleep disorders. This classification may change in the fifth edition of DSM (DSM-V), which is likely to be published in 2012–2013. ICSD-2 categorizes sleep disorders into six groups, as indicated in Table 13–2. The remainder of this chapter follows the ICSD-2 classification.

Table 13-2. ICSD-2 sleep disorder categories

I. Insomnias
Examples: adjustment insomnia, psychophysiological insomnia, paradoxical insomnia, idiopathic insomnia

II. Sleep-related breathing disorders
Examples: central sleep apnea syndromes, obstructive sleep apnea syndromes

III. Hypersomnias of central origin
Examples: narcolepsy with/without cataplexy, idiopathic hypersomnia with/without long sleep time

IV. Circadian rhythm sleep disorders
Examples: delayed sleep phase type, advanced sleep phase type, shift work disorder

V. Parasomnias
Examples: confusional arousals, sleepwalking, sleep terrors, REM sleep behavior disorder, nightmare disorder

VI. Sleep-related movement disorders
Examples: restless legs syndrome, periodic limb movement sleep disorder

Note. ICSD-2= International Classification of Sleep Disorders, 2nd Edition (American Academy of Sleep Medicine 2005); REM=rapid eye movement.

Insomnia Disorders

Definition and Description

Insomnia refers to the complaint of difficulty falling asleep, frequent or prolonged awakenings, or inadequate sleep quality. Insomnia is not defined by polysomnography or a specific sleep duration. Because insomnia occurs only when there is adequate opportunity for sleep, it must be distinguished from sleep deprivation, in which the individual has relatively normal sleep ability but inadequate opportunity for sleep. An *insomnia disorder* is a syndrome consisting of the insomnia complaint together with significant impairment or distress. Common daytime impairments associated with insomnia include mood disturbances (irritability, mild dysphoria, or difficulty tolerating stress), impaired cognitive function (difficulty concentrating, completing tasks, or performing complex, abstract, or creative tasks), and daytime fatigue (Moul et al. 2002). Clinicians are often taught that insomnia is almost always "secondary" to some other condition. However, based on consistencies in clinical features, course, and response to treatment, a 2005 conference suggested that "comorbid" insomnia may be a more appropriate term than "secondary" (National Institutes of Health 2005).

Epidemiology and Consequences

The 1-year prevalence of insomnia symptoms is approximately 30%–40% in the general population and up to 66% in primary care and psychiatric settings. The prevalence of primary insomnia as a specific disorder is in the range of 5%–10% of the general population (Ohayon 2002). Established risk factors for insomnia include older age, female sex, being divorced or separated, unemployment, and comorbid medical and psychiatric illness. Factors that commonly initiate or maintain insomnia include psychosocial stresses such as moves, relationship difficulties, occupational and financial problems, and caregiving responsibilities. Longitudinal studies of clinical patients and population samples indicate that insomnia is a chronic or recurring condition in approximately 40%–85% of affected individuals (Morin et al. 2009).

The consequences of insomnia include increased risk for the later development of depressive, anxiety, and substance use disorders and increased risk of recurrence (Breslau et al. 1996; Riemann and Voderholzer 2003). Insomnia is also associated with increased health care utilization, absenteeism, direct and indirect medical costs, motor vehicle and other accidents, falls in the elderly, and reduced quality of life (reviewed in Buysse 2005).

Pathophysiology and Etiology

Insomnia is often thought to result from increased arousal. Hyperarousal in insomnia is suggested by evidence from psychophysiological, metabolic, electrophysiological, neuroendocrine, and functional neuroanatomical evidence (reviewed in Perlis et al. 2005). Functional imaging studies demonstrate increased glucose metabolic rates during wakefulness and sleep and attenuation of the usual NREM sleep–related decline in metabolism in brain-stem arousal centers in subjects with insomnia compared with healthy control subjects. Self-reported wakefulness during sleep is related to increased metabolic activity in the same regions (Nofzinger 2006; Nofzinger et al. 2004).

Psychological and behavioral theories may also help to explain the development and persistence of insomnia. These theories focus on predisposing, precipitating, and perpetuating factors (Spielman et al. 1987); on the role of ruminative, sleep-focused thoughts (Morin 1993); on conditioned cortical arousal (Perlis et al. 1997); and on cognitive factors such as selective attention (Espie et al. 2001; Harvey 2002).

Assessment and Diagnosis

The assessment of patients with insomnia rests on a detailed clinical history focusing on specific symptoms, chronology, exacerbating and alleviating factors, and response to previous treatments. Symptoms of RLS, snoring or breathing pauses, and other sleep disorders should be investigated. Polysomnography is not routinely recommended for the evaluation of chronic insomnia (Saleia et al. 2000).

Behavioral and Psychological Treatment

Behavioral and psychological treatments aim to reduce sleep latency and improve sleep consolidation by changing behaviors, habits, and cognitions that interfere with sleep. Table 13–3 summarizes the major components of behavioral and psychological treatments for insomnia, which can be administered in individual or group format.

Meta-analyses have demonstrated that behavioral interventions for insomnia significantly reduce sleep-onset latency, reduce wake time after sleep onset, and improve total sleep time (Irwin et al. 2006; Morin et al. 2006). These effects are comparable in magnitude to those achieved with hypnotic medications (Smith et al. 2002). Approximately 70%–80% of insomnia patients benefit from behavioral interventions, and improvements are maintained or enhanced at follow-up. Stimulus control, sleep restriction, and multicomponent cognitive-behavioral interventions show the most robust effects. In general, behavioral interventions have somewhat smaller effects in older adults than in middle-aged subjects. Cognitive-behavioral interventions for insomnia are also effective at improving sleep quality in patients with comorbid medical and psychiatric illnesses and specific conditions such as cancer and chronic pain (Lichstein et al. 2005). A growing number of studies also show that cognitive-behavioral treatments delivered in the primary and psychiatric care settings are also efficacious (Edinger and Sampson 2003; Espie et al. 2001). New treatment modalities such as home-based treatment (Espie et al. 2001), telephone interventions, Internet-based interventions (Ritterband et al. 2009), and self-help material (Mimeault and Morin 1999) are being investigated to disseminate these treatments and reduce patient burden and costs. Most behavioral treatments share basic principles that can be used effectively in a variety of clinical settings (Germain et al. 2006). These specific interventions are reasonably straightforward and rely on principles of the two-process model of sleep regulation described earlier. They include restricting time in bed to match actual sleep time; setting a regular wakeup time, regardless of sleep duration the night before; not go-

Table 13–3. Cognitive-behavioral interventions for insomnia

Intervention	General description
Stimulus control	A set of behaviors that promote associative conditioning between the sleep environment and sleepiness
Sleep restriction therapy	Sleep practices that increase "sleep drive" and facilitate the ability to sleep
Relaxation training	Training in techniques that decrease waking arousal and facilitate sleep at night (muscular tension and cognitive arousal are incompatible with sleep).
Cognitive restructuring of irrational sleep-related beliefs	Identification, challenge, and replacement of dysfunctional beliefs and attitudes regarding sleep and sleep loss. These beliefs increase arousal and tension, which in turn impede sleep and reinforce the dysfunctional beliefs.
Sleep hygiene	Promoting behaviors that improve sleep; limiting behaviors that harm sleep

ing to bed unless sleepy; and not staying in bed during prolonged awakenings.

Pharmacological Treatment

Drugs approved for the treatment of insomnia include benzodiazepine receptor agonists (BzRAs) and a melatonin receptor agonist (Walsh et al. 2005b). However, physicians frequently use other off-label medications for insomnia, despite the lack of systematic efficacy and safety data (Buysse et al. 2005; Walsh 2004).

Benzodiazepine Receptor Agonists

BzRAs are indicated for the treatment of acute insomnia and chronic primary insomnia. They are useful as adjunctive therapies for secondary insomnia related to certain medical conditions, psychiatric disorders, and other primary sleep disorders such as RLS and CRSDs. These agents bind at specific recognition sites on the $GABA_A$ receptor. Some of these drugs, such as zolpidem and zaleplon, bind relatively selectively at $GABA_A$ receptors containing α_1 subunits. The clinical significance of this selectivity is not clear, although such agents may be relatively more specific for hypnotic effects and have lower abuse liability. $GABA_A$ receptors with α_1 subunits mediate the sedative, amnestic, and an-

ticonvulsant effects of BzRAs, whereas those containing α_2 and α_3 subunits mediate anxiolytic and myorelaxant effects (Mohler et al. 2002). The BzRAs have different clinical effects primarily as a result of their different pharmacokinetic properties, including rate of absorption, extent of distribution, and terminal elimination half-life (Table 13–4).

As a class, BzRAs decrease sleep latency; those with longer duration of action also decrease the number and duration of awakenings from sleep and increase sleep duration. Most decrease Stage 3–4 NREM sleep and REM sleep by small amounts, but the clinical significance of these changes is unclear. Meta-analyses have demonstrated these agents to be efficacious in the treatment of chronic insomnia (Holbrook et al. 2000; Nowell et al. 1997; Soldatos et al. 1999) on self-reported outcomes of sleep latency, sleep duration, number of awakenings, and sleep quality. Effects are comparable in magnitude with those of cognitive-behavioral therapies (Smith et al. 2002).

Most studies of BzRAs have been conducted for short durations. More recent data demonstrate the efficacy of nightly BzRA use for 6–12 months (Krystal et al. 2003; Roth et al. 2005). These agents are also efficacious when used intermittently (i.e., 3–5 times per week) (Krystal et al. 2008; Perlis et al. 2004).

Table 13–4. Benzodiazepine receptor agonists: pharmacokinetics

Drug	Onset of action, min	Elimination half-life, h	Typical adult dosage, mg
Zaleplon	10–20	1.0	5–20
Zolpidem	10–20	1.5–2.4	5–10 (IR) 5–10 (MR)
Eszopiclone	10–30	5–6	1–3
Triazolam	10–20	1.5–5	0.125–0.25
Temazepam	45–60	8–20	7.5–30
Estazolam*	15–30	20–30	0.5–2
Quazepam*	15–30	15–120	7.5–15
Flurazepam*	15–30	36–120	15–30

Note. IR = immediate release; MR = modified release.
*Has active metabolite.

BzRAs have similar side effects that differ according to their pharmacokinetic properties. Effects include sedation, impaired psychomotor performance (Vermeeren 2004), falls and hip fractures in the elderly (Cumming and Le Couteur 2003), motor vehicle accidents (Thomas 1998), and respiratory depression of minimal clinical significance in most patients (Camacho and Morin 1995).

Although tolerance has long been a concern with BzRAs, evidence presented here shows no general loss of efficacy with nightly or intermittent treatment. Epidemiological studies show that up to two-thirds of patients taking hypnotics chronically report substantial ongoing benefit (Ohayon and Guilleminault 1999). Discontinuance effects include *rebound insomnia*, defined as an increase in sleep problems to a level greater than the baseline level upon discontinuation of the drug. A meta-analysis suggests that rebound insomnia is a short-lived, dosage-dependent phenomenon (Soldatos et al. 1999). Nevertheless, abrupt discontinuation of BzRAs does lead to worsening of symptoms compared with the treatment period. BzRAs have marginal tendency for self-administration in animals, which is often used as a model of abuse potential in humans (Woods and Winger 1995), and they are infrequently the drug of choice in humans who abuse drugs. Nevertheless, individuals with a past history of

substance abuse, particularly of sedatives or alcohol, should be treated cautiously (Griffiths and Weerts 1997).

Limited evidence suggests that BzRAs are an efficacious adjunctive treatment in patients with insomnia comorbid with medical and psychiatric disorders. For instance, zolpidem and eszopiclone improve sleep time and wakefulness after sleep onset in depressed and anxious patients treated with selective serotonin reuptake inhibitors (SSRIs; Fava et al. 2006, 2009).

Melatonin and Melatonin Receptor Agonists

Melatonin is a pineal hormone secreted exclusively at night in a strong circadian rhythm. Exogenous melatonin has been studied as a hypnotic. It is rapidly absorbed, with peak levels occurring in 20–30 minutes, and has an elimination half-life of 40–60 minutes. Studies of subjective effects in healthy young adults given melatonin during the daytime, when activity of the SCN is greatest, support its hypnotic efficacy (Cajochen et al. 2003). When given at night, melatonin can decrease subjective sleep latency, although other effects are less consistent (Brzezinski et al. 2005), and its efficacy on polysomnographic measures is not well documented. Ramelteon is a synthetic agonist of melatonin MT_1 and MT_2 receptors, with much higher affinity than endogenous melatonin. Controlled clinical trials have demonstrated its efficacy for reducing sleep latency, but with variable effects on sleep duration (Erman et al. 2006; Zammit et al. 2007).

Other Agents

Other drugs and compounds are often used to treat insomnia, despite the lack of a U.S. Food and Drug Administration indication and the small amount of efficacy and safety data supporting their use (reviewed in Buysse et al. 2005). The use of sedating antidepressants may be related to their lack of abuse potential as well as the perception that they may help subsyndromal depression. Small placebo-controlled clinical trials in primary insomnia support the efficacy of trazodone and trimipramine. Doxepin in doses of 1–6 mg has been evaluated for the treatment of chronic primary insomnia (Buysse et al. 2005; Roth et al. 2007). Effects of sedating antidepressants are summarized in Table 13–5.

Other drugs used to treat insomnia include antihistamines, alcohol, valerian, gabapentin and pregabalin, and sedating antipsychotic drugs. As stated earlier, there is generally very little empirical evidence supporting the efficacy and safety of these drugs specifically for treating insomnia. In some cases, potential adverse effects are substantial.

Sleep-Related Breathing Disorders

Sleep-related breathing disorders include central sleep apnea syndromes, obstructive sleep apnea (OSA) syndromes, and sleep-related hypoventilation/hypoxemic syndromes (American Academy of Sleep Medicine 2005). This chapter focuses on OSA syndrome in adults, which is the most prevalent and best studied of these conditions.

Obstructive Sleep Apnea

Definition and Description

OSA is characterized by repetitive episodes of complete (apnea) or partial (hypopnea) upper airway obstruction during sleep that often result in oxygen desaturation and terminate with brief arousals. By definition, apnea and hypopnea events last for 10 seconds or longer and are accompanied by continued efforts to breathe. Obstructive hypopneas are typically defined by a decrease in airflow of 30% or more with desaturation of 4% or more (Strollo and Rogers 1996; Figure 13–4). Because the neurocognitive and cardiovascular outcomes are similar for apneas and hypopneas, these events are typically counted together in an overall index of severity, the apnea–hypopnea index (AHI; number of apneas and hypopneas per hour of sleep) (Gottlieb et al. 1999). Mild OSA is defined as an AHI between 5 and 15, moderate OSA as an AHI of 15–30, and severe OSA as an AHI of greater than 30. In addition to apneas and hypopneas, the OSA syndrome includes a complaint of daytime sleepiness or insomnia, loud snoring, and/or episodes of breath holding, gasping, or choking during sleep. Other findings include complaints of fatigue, memory and cognitive difficulty, obesity, and hypertension or other cardiovascular disease. The clinical symptoms of OSA show considerable overlap with those of depression.

Epidemiology and Consequences

The prevalence of OSA (defined as AHI of 10 or greater with daytime sleepiness and/or hypertension) is approximately 5% (Young et al. 2002). In a longitudinal family study, the 5-year incidence of mild OSA (AHI 5–15) was 7.5% and of moderate to severe OSA (AHI ≥ 15) was 16% (Tishler et al. 2003). Clinical studies indicate an increased risk in men, with a male-to-female prevalence ratio of 3.3 to 1 (Bixler et al. 2001; Young et al. 1993). Increased weight and age also increase the risk of OSA (Young et al. 2002), although the age effect plateaus after age 65 years (Young et al. 1993). Menopause increases risk in women; OSA prevalence is 2.7% in postmenopausal women without hormone replacement therapy versus 0.6% in the premenopausal population (Bixler et al. 2001). The prevalence of OSA appears to be higher among African

Table 13–5. Summary of other drugs used to treat insomnia[a]

Drug	Sleep latency	Sleep continuity[b]	Stage 3–4 NREM sleep amount, %	REM sleep	Other
Trazodone	↓	↔ to ↑	↑	↔ Amount, % (↓ to ↑ in individual studies)	Infrequent side effect of priapism
Doxepin	↓	↑	↔	↓ Amount, % of REM; ↑ phasic eye movements (REM density)	↓ Sleep apnea (minor effect); ↔ or ↑ periodic limb movements;
Amitriptyline	↓	↑	↔	↓ Amount, % of REM; ↑ phasic eye movements (REM density)	↑ restless legs symptoms; may induce eye movements during NREM sleep; anticholinergic effects
Trimipramine	↓	↔ to ↑	↔	↔ Amount, %	
Mirtazapine	↓	↔ to ↑	↔	↔	May cause weight gain
Melatonin	↓	↔ to ↑	↔	↔	
Diphenhydramine	↓	↔ to ↑	↔ to ↑	↓	Anticholinergic effects
Valerian	↓	↔ to ↑	↔ to ↑	↔ to ↑	Inconsistent effects on sleep continuity, Stage 3–4
Gabapentin	↔	↔ to ↑	↑	↔	↓ Periodic limb movements
Tiagabine	↔	↔ to ↑	↑	↔	Infrequent side effect of seizures
Olanzapine, quetiapine	↔ to ↓	↑	↑	↔ to ↓	Reports of increased periodic limb movements, sleep-related eating
γ-Hydroxybutyrate	↔ to ↓	↑	↑	↔ to ↓	Side effects of sleepwalking, enuresis; abuse potential
Chloral hydrate	↓	↑	↔	↔ to ↓	Rapid tolerance; hepatotoxicity

Note. NREM=non-rapid eye movement; REM=rapid eye movement.

[a]Reported effects are based on preponderance of evidence from published studies (see text for details). Many effects are inconsistent between individual studies. "↑" indicates increase from pretreatment baseline; "↓" indicates decrease from pretreatment baseline; "↔" indicates no change from pretreatment baseline.

[b]*Sleep continuity* refers to the proportion of sleep relative to wakefulness after sleep onset as reflected by measures such as sleep efficiency. Other indicators of sleep continuity, such as wakefulness after sleep onset or number of awakenings, would have opposite signs. Thus, "↑" indicates improvement in overall sleep continuity.

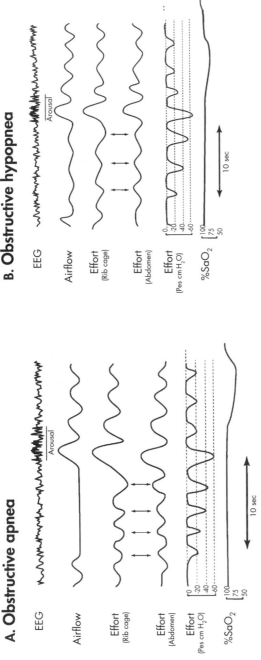

Figure 13–4. Obstructive apnea and obstructive hypopnea.

A, Diagrammatic representation of obstructive apnea. Increasing ventilatory effort is seen in the rib cage, the abdomen, and the level of esophageal pressure (measured with an esophageal balloon), despite lack of oronasal airflow. Arousal on the electroencephalogram (EEG) is associated with increasing ventilatory effort, as indicated by the esophageal pressure. Oxyhemoglobin desaturation follows the termination of apnea. Note that during apnea, the movements of the rib cage and the abdomen (Effort) are in opposite directions (*arrows*) as a result of attempts to breathe against a closed airway. Once the airway opens in response to arousal, rib-cage and abdominal movements become synchronous. B, Diagrammatic representation of obstructive hypopnea. Decreased airflow is associated with increasing ventilatory effort (reflected by the esophageal pressure) and subsequent arousal on the EEG. Rib-cage and abdominal movements are in opposite directions during hypopnea (*arrows*), reflecting increasingly difficult breathing against a partially closed airway. Rib-cage and abdominal movements become synchronous after arousal produces airway opening. Oxyhemoglobin desaturation follows the termination of hypopnea.

Source. Adapted from Strollo PJ, Rogers RM: "Obstructive Sleep Apnea." *New England Journal of Medicine* 334:99–104, 1996.

Americans compared with European Americans (Ancoli-Israel et al. 1995).

OSA is associated with significant cardiovascular, metabolic, and neurocognitive consequences (Table 13–6). AHI is related in a dosage-dependent manner with cardiovascular complications (Shahar et al. 2001) including nocturnal and diurnal systemic hypertension, diurnal pulmonary hypertension, atrial dysrhythmias, heart failure, myocardial infarction, stroke, pulmonary hypertension, and right-sided heart failure (Bady et al. 2000). Treatment of OSA with continuous positive airway pressure (CPAP) is associated with improvement in pulmonary hypertension and right heart failure (Sajkov et al. 2002). AHI is also related in a dosage-dependent manner with biomarkers of the metabolic syndrome (e.g., serum glucose and insulin sensitivity), even after controlling for concomitant obesity (Punjabi et al. 2003). Leptin, an adipokine that regulates metabolic and ventilatory control, is elevated in patients with OSA compared with matched obese control subjects (Ip et al. 2000).

OSA also shows dose–response relationships with neurocognitive consequences, including daytime sleepiness (Gottlieb et al. 1999) and motor vehicle and occupational accidents (Lindberg et al. 2001; Teran-Santos et al. 1999). Untreated OSA is also associated with significant deficits in neuropsychological functions such as vigilance, executive functioning, and coordination (Beebe et al. 2003). Analysis of a large managed-care database identified a significant increase in the odds ratio for OSA in patients prescribed antidepressant medication (Farney et al. 2004). OSA and its consequences ultimately affect quality of life, as measured by both generic and disease-specific measures. Conversely, treatment of OSA improves sleepiness, cognitive function, and quality of life (Engleman and Douglas 2004).

Pathophysiology

During inspiration, negative intrathoracic pressure results in a suction force applied to this small, compliant upper airway, and vibration (snoring), narrowing (hypopnea), or closure (apnea) may occur. Craniofacial structure and function and obesity are the major determinants of small airway diameter in adults. During the transition from wakefulness to sleep, muscle tone decreases and snoring and airway narrowing occur in vulnerable individuals. Arousal from sleep, precipitated by increased airway resistance, hypopnea, or apnea, stimulates resumption of breathing (Gleeson et al. 1990).

Attempting to breathe against a partially or completely obstructed airway leads to increased intrathoracic pressure, hypoventilation, and increased vagal tone; subsequent arousals are accompanied by increased sympathetic tone. Repeated episodes of bradycar-

Table 13–6. Comorbidities and consequences associated with obstructive sleep apnea syndrome

Cardiovascular complications	Metabolic complications	Neurocognitive complications
Nocturnal dysrhythmias	Leptin resistance	Daytime sleepiness
Bradydysrhythmias	Insulin resistance	Motor vehicle accidents
Atrial fibrillation		Work-related accidents
Nocturnal hypertension		Impaired neuropsychological function
Diurnal hypertension		
Pulmonary hypertension		Impaired quality of life
Congestive heart failure		
Myocardial infarction		
Stroke		

dia-tachycardia and increased sympathetic tone (Somers et al. 1995) lead to the cardiovascular effects of OSA. The ischemia–reperfusion associated with intermittent hypoxemia also results in oxidative stress and subsequent endothelial dysfunction (Lavie 2003). Biomarkers of oxidative stress such as C-reactive protein and interleukin 6 increase the risk for, and progression of, cardiovascular and metabolic disease.

Assessment and Diagnosis

History and physical examination can identify patients at high risk for OSA. Nightly loud snoring, breathing pauses during sleep, snorting, choking, and subjective daytime sleepiness all suggest the diagnosis of OSA. Obesity (particularly upper-body obesity) and systemic hypertension are often present. In some individuals, craniofacial abnormalities (retrognathia or micrognathia) and/or soft tissue abnormalities, such as enlarged tonsils, lateral narrowing of the airway, or an elongated soft palate, place the patient at risk for OSA (Schellenberg et al. 2000; Zonato et al. 2003). However, clinical findings alone are not sufficiently precise to confirm a diagnosis of OSA (Schellenberg et al. 2000). Objective measurement and quantification of sleep and breathing with polysomnography are the current standard for diagnosing OSA.

Treatment

Behavioral treatments play a minor role in treatment of OSA. Because obesity is a major risk factor for OSA, weight loss improves both sleep and breathing (Peppard et al. 2000). Sleep deprivation increases the severity of daytime sleepiness and decreases upper airway muscle tone and should therefore be avoided. Alcohol and BzRA hypnotics also reduce upper airway muscle tone. If the patient clearly has positional OSA (typically worse in the supine position), lateral sleep position or elevation of the head of bed may be helpful.

Positive pressure delivered via nasal or nasal–oral mask reliably treats airway closure during sleep and is the first-line treatment for OSA. Positive pressure therapy works by pneumatically "splinting" the airway open during sleep (Figure 13–5). Positive pressure can be applied as CPAP or as bilevel positive airway pressure (BPAP). With BPAP, the pressure setting is higher during inspiration than expiration. Placebo-controlled, randomized clinical trials of positive pressure therapy have documented a favorable effect on quality of life, objective daytime function, and blood pressure. Emerging data indicate that CPAP also improves insulin sensitivity, left ventricular function, pulmonary hypertension, endothelial function, and cardiovascular and overall mortality (Punjabi and Beamer 2005; Strollo et al. 2005; Weaver and George 2005).

Acceptance of and adherence to positive pressure therapy can be improved with patient education and attention to patient–machine interface problems. Proper fit of the nasal or full-face mask is essential. Patients with OSA frequently report nasal congestion prior to treatment, which can be exacerbated by positive pressure therapy and compounded by nasal dryness. Heated humidifiers for the CPAP/BPAP unit frequently improve nasal dryness and subsequent congestion. Occasionally, a mask that covers both the nose and mouth can be helpful. In patients who are claustrophobic, desensitization may be helpful.

Oral appliance therapy (OAP) modifies the position of the mandible and tongue to increase the upper airway size and reduce collapsibility. OAP is regarded as second-line therapy for OSA because it requires multiple adjustments over weeks to months, it is not 100% effective, and objective adherence is difficult to measure. Patients who respond best have mild supine positional OSA and snoring (Marklund et al. 2004). OAP favorably affects subjective sleepiness, sleep-disordered breathing, and blood pressure compared with control interventions (Gotsopoulos et al. 2004).

Surgical therapy has a small but important role in the management of adult OSA and can be broadly divided into two categories: tra-

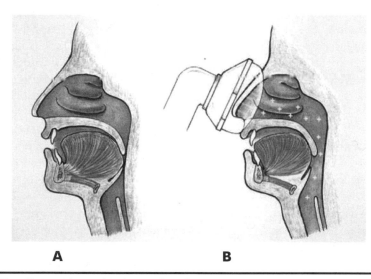

A   **B**

Figure 13–5. **Upper airway in obstructive sleep apnea, without treatment and with CPAP treatment.**

Cross-sectional view of the upper airway, illustrating closure at the level of the palate and base of tongue typically seen in obstructive sleep apnea **(A)** and when the airway is pneumatically splinted open with continuous positive airway pressure (CPAP) **(B)**.

Source.   Reprinted from Buysse DJ (ed): *Sleep Disorders and Psychiatry* (Review of Psychiatry Series, Vol 24, No 2; Oldham JM and Riba MB, series editors). Washington, DC, American Psychiatric Publishing, 2005, p. 93. Copyright 2005, American Psychiatric Publishing. Used with permission.

cheostomy (bypass of the upper airway) and reconstruction of the upper airway, which can involve multiple sites from the nasopharynx to the epiglottis. The most common procedure is uvulopalatopharyngoplasty, which involves altering the size and the stiffness of the soft palate. This procedure is highly effective in treating loud snoring, but its impact on OSA is less certain, with reported success ranging from 7% to 60% (Sher 1995).

Medication plays no role in the treatment of obstructed breathing, per se, but may be important for treating concomitant depression and residual daytime sleepiness after adequate treatment. Residual daytime sleepiness in OSA may be related to the disorder itself (Pack et al. 2001), which is associated with gray matter loss in the frontal, parietal, and temporal cortex, anterior cingulate, hippocampus, and cerebellum (Macey et al. 2002). Long-term intermittent hypoxia may lead to significant oxidative injuries in the wake-promoting regions of the basal forebrain and brain stem and lead to sleepiness

(Veasey et al. 2004). Modafinil is an efficacious adjunctive therapy for OSA patients with residual daytime sleepiness despite adequate treatment with CPAP (Pack et al. 2001). Insomnia can also be encountered in OSA, with prevalences as high as 50% reported (Benetó et al. 2009). Some reports have suggested improvement of insomnia with positive pressure treatment (Guilleminault et al. 2002a, 2002b). BzRAs should generally be avoided in patients with OSA or suspected OSA unless they have been diagnosed and treated.

Hypersomnias of Central Origin

Hypersomnias are sleep disorders characterized by severe sleepiness due to dysfunction of CNS mechanisms regulating sleep–wake states. This distinguishes the hypersomnias from other sleep disorders marked by sleepiness, such as OSA and circadian rhythm disorders, whose etiology relates instead to sleep disruption or abnormal timing of the alertness–sleepiness rhythm. This chapter will focus on four of the most important forms of hypersomnia.

Narcolepsy

Definition and Description

Narcolepsy is a syndrome characterized by profound excessive daytime sleepiness (EDS), which often occurs in association with cataplexy, hypnagogic or hypnopompic hallucinations, sleep paralysis, automatic behavior, and disrupted nocturnal sleep (American Academy of Sleep Medicine 2005). It is subdivided into two types: narcolepsy with cataplexy and narcolepsy without cataplexy. EDS is manifest as an increased propensity to fall asleep in relaxed or sedentary situations or a struggle to avoid sleeping in these situations. Brief naps temporarily relieve the sleepiness in many patients. EDS can lead to related symptoms, including "automatic behavior" (behavior that the individual does not recall), irritability, and poor memory, concentration, and attention. Many patients report fragmented nocturnal sleep, suggesting that the underlying disorder is an inability to maintain any stable sleep–wake state (Guilleminault and Fromherz 2005).

Cataplexy is the partial or complete loss of voluntary muscle tone in response to strong emotion and occurs in 60%–100% of patients with narcolepsy. The atonia may be minimal, occurring in a few muscle groups and causing subtle symptoms (ptosis, head drooping, slurred speech, dropping objects) or severe, resulting in complete collapse. Cataplectic episodes usually last from a few seconds to a minute or two (Honda 1988). The patient is awake and oriented during these episodes, thus distinguishing cataplexy from sleep episodes. Cataplexy is most often triggered by positive emotional experiences, such as laughter, but can be triggered by other strong emotions, such as fear or anger (Gelb et al. 1994), and is exacerbated by stress, fatigue, or sleepiness. *Hypnagogic* and *hypnopompic hal-*

lucinations are visual, tactile, auditory, or multisensory events lasting up to a few minutes during the transition from wakefulness to sleep (hypnagogic) or from sleep to wakefulness (hypnopompic). Hallucinations may combine elements of dream sleep and consciousness and are often bizarre or disturbing to patients. *Sleep paralysis* is the inability to move for a few seconds to a few minutes during wake–sleep or sleep–wake transitions. Sleep paralysis can be frightening, particularly when accompanied by hallucinations or the sensation of being unable to breathe. Hypnagogic hallucinations, sleep paralysis, and automatic behavior are not specific to narcolepsy and may occur in healthy individuals. However, their co-occurrence with EDS strongly suggests narcolepsy.

Epidemiology

The prevalence of narcolepsy in the United States, Western Europe, the Middle East, and Japan is approximately 0.05%, with a range of 0.002%–0.160% (Mignot 1998). Symptoms of narcolepsy most often begin during adolescence or young adulthood but can occur at any age. The usual course of symptoms is stable in the absence of treatment. Narcolepsy is associated with complications including depression, motor vehicle and other accidents, and significant occupational impairment due to sleepiness.

Pathophysiology

Narcolepsy results from dysfunction of the hypothalamic peptide neuromodulator hypocretin (orexin). Narcolepsy was identified in mice with a knockout of the preprohypocretin gene (Chemelli et al. 1999), and canine narcolepsy was associated with mutations in the hypocretin receptor 2 gene (Lin et al. 1999). The majority (85%–90%) of patients with narcolepsy–cataplexy have low or undetectable levels of hypocretin-1 in their cerebrospinal fluid (Nishino et al. 2000), a sensitive and specific finding for this disorder (Mignot 2005). Postmortem studies in narcoleptic patients have confirmed deficiency of the hypocretin-1 and -2 ligand (Thannickal et al. 2000). Human narcolepsy demonstrates familial aggregation but no simple genetic mechanism. Narcolepsy shows a strong association with specific human leukocyte antigen (HLA) haplotypes, particularly DQB1*0602, which is present in approximately 90% of individuals with unequivocal cataplexy (Mignot 2005). Hypocretin deficiency is tightly associated with occurrence of cataplexy and the DQB1*0602 haplotype. The strong association between HLA type and narcolepsy with cataplexy raises the possibility that narcolepsy is an autoimmune disease, but there is no convincing evidence of typical autoimmune markers in narcolepsy (Fredrikson et al. 1990; Matsuki et al. 1988; Mignot 2005).

Assessment and Diagnosis

Clinical assessment of individuals presenting with EDS should focus on the severity, frequency, and situations in which sleepiness occurs. The relationship between EDS and nighttime sleep is also important; individuals with narcolepsy frequently report no strong relationship, which distinguishes narcolepsy from sleep deprivation. A clinical history of severe EDS coupled with cataplexy and/or sleep-related hallucinations or sleep paralysis is virtually diagnostic of narcolepsy. Polysomnography is also an important part of the evaluation and differential diagnosis. It can identify OSA, periodic limb movement disorder (PLMD), and REM sleep behavior disorder that may contribute to EDS and nocturnal sleep disruption (Overeem et al. 2001). The MSLT demonstrates reduced sleep latency (≤8 minutes) coupled with two or more sleep-onset REM periods. However, *sleep-onset REM periods* are not specific for narcolepsy and may also be due to sleep deprivation, rebound from REM-suppressing medication, altered sleep schedules, OSA, and delayed sleep phase syndrome.

Treatment

The effective treatment of EDS requires regular, structured nocturnal sleep and planned daytime naps. A nocturnal sleep period of 8 hours or more should be encouraged, with consistent bedtimes and awakening times. Shift work in any form is usually problematic for individuals with narcolepsy. Scheduling two or more brief naps at regular times during the day is almost always necessary to further enhance daytime function in patients with narcolepsy.

Stimulants are indicated for the treatment of EDS in narcolepsy (Guilleminault and Fromherz 2005; Mitler et al. 1994; Table 13–7). These drugs produce substantial improvement but do not restore daytime alertness to normal levels. Traditional stimulants include methylphenidate, dextroamphetamine, and methamphetamine, which are available as immediate-release and delayed-release preparations. Patients may experience negative effects with any alerting agent, including nervousness, anorexia, weight loss, and sleep disruption. Some patients report rebound hypersomnia (exacerbation of sleepiness) as the dose wears off. Tolerance to the alerting effect may occur with time in some patients. In cases of tolerance, switching to a different class of medication or providing a "drug holiday" can be useful. Dosages of 20–80 mg/day are typical for most stimulants (10–40 mg for methamphetamine).

Modafinil and its *R*-enantiomer, armodafinil, are wake-promoting agents that are somewhat less potent than traditional agents, but with greater tolerability. The mechanism of action of these drugs appears to be mediated through inhibition of the dopamine transporter (Wisor and Eriksson 2005). The duration of effect of modafinil is relatively long as a result of its half-life of 12–15 hours. The efficacy of modafinil has been evaluated extensively in EDS due to narcolepsy, idiopathic hypersomnia, and sleep apnea (U.S. Modafinil in Narcolepsy Multicenter Study Group 1998).

Sodium oxybate (γ-hydroxybutyrate) is an agent unrelated to the traditional stimulants that also enhances alertness in narcolepsy (Mamelak et al. 2004). The mechanism

Table 13–7. Common alerting agents for the treatment of excessive daytime sleepiness

Agent	Receptor	Elimination half-life (h)	Time to maximal plasma concentration (h)	Usual dosage	Side effects
Modafinil	Unknown	15	2–4	100–400 mg + once daily or divided	Headache, nausea, anxiety, irritability
Armodafinil	Dopamine transporter, others (?)	15	2–4	150–250 mg/day	Headache, nausea, anxiety, irritability
Amphetamines	Dopamine agonist	10 (SR: 15+)	2 (SR: 8–10)	5–60 mg divided	Both amphetamines and methylphenidate: headache, anxiety/irritability, increased blood pressure, palpitation, appetite suppression, tremor, insomnia
Methylphenidate	Dopamine agonist	4 (SR: 8–10)	2 (SR: 5)	5–60 mg divided	
Pemoline*	Dopamine agonist	12	2–4	18.75–112.5 mg once daily or divided	Similar to amphetamines and methylphenidate but milder
γ-Hydroxybutyrate	Inadequately characterized	2	1	6–9 g + liquid solution divided nightly	Sedation, nausea, confusional arousals, sleepwalking

Note.   SR = sustained-release.

*Potentially hepatotoxic—frequent liver function monitoring required.

of action of this agent is unknown. Sodium oxybate has similar efficacy as other agents, and its effect may be additive with other stimulants (U.S. Xyrem Multicenter Study Group 2002). Combining two alerting agents of different chemical classes may be necessary when a single agent is insufficient.

Medications used to treat cataplexy also improve hallucinations and sleep paralysis. In addition to its effect on EDS, sodium oxybate reduces cataplexy, reduces nocturnal sleep disruptions, and consolidates sleep (U.S. Xyrem Multicenter Study Group 2002). Low dosages of tricyclic antidepressants and typical antidepressant dosages of SSRIs and serotonin–norepinephrine reuptake inhibitors are also useful in treating cataplexy (Guilleminault and Fromherz 2005). Tolerance to cataplexy medications can occur, requiring a medication switch or drug holiday.

Idiopathic Hypersomnia

Idiopathic hypersomnia is characterized by EDS without the specific features of narcolepsy or other sleep disorders. It occurs in two variants, one with long nocturnal sleep time and difficulty awakening and one without long nocturnal sleep time (Bassetti et al. 2005). Its precise prevalence is uncertain due to the lack of strict diagnostic criteria and specific biological markers. Onset typically occurs in adolescence or early adulthood, and symptoms generally persist throughout adulthood. Distinguishing idiopathic hypersomnia from narcolepsy can be difficult, but patients with idiopathic hypersomnia do not have cataplexy or significant nocturnal sleep disruption. In the subtype with long nighttime sleep, patients are usually difficult to awaken in the morning. Patients often take long naps, which, in contrast to naps in narcolepsy, do not improve alertness. "Microsleeps," with or without automatic behavior, may occur throughout the day. Polysomnography in idiopathic hypersomnia usually reveals short sleep latency, increased total sleep time, and normal sleep continuity. Sleep latency on MSLT is usually short (8 minutes or less), but in contrast to narcolepsy, sleep-onset REM periods are not seen. The etiology and pathophysiology of idiopathic hypersomnia are unknown, but viral illnesses, including Guillain-Barré syndrome, hepatitis, mononucleosis, and atypical viral pneumonia, may precipitate sleepiness in a subset of patients. Some of these patients have associated symptoms suggesting autonomic nervous system dysfunction, including orthostatic hypotension, syncope, vascular headaches, and peripheral vascular complaints. Neurochemical studies using cerebrospinal fluid have suggested that patients with idiopathic hypersomnia may have altered noradrenergic system function (Bassetti et al. 2005). Treatment includes adequate nocturnal sleep time, scheduled daytime naps, and stimulant medications as described earlier for narcolepsy, but these interventions are less consistently helpful in this condition.

Behaviorally Induced Insufficient Sleep Syndrome (Sleep Deprivation)

Sleep deprivation and sleep restriction are endemic in Western societies. Recent data show that American adults on average get approximately 6.5 hours of sleep at night, which represents a decrease in sleep time over the past 100 years (Walsh et al. 2005a). Insufficient sleep syndrome is characterized by complaints of EDS, sometimes quite severe, which is related to curtailed sleep duration at night. Other symptoms of sleep restriction include mood lability, poor concentration, and impaired interpersonal function. When their schedule permits, affected individuals sleep longer and report reduced daytime symptoms (American Academy of Sleep Medicine 2005). However, recovery from sleep restriction does not occur immediately and may require several days to a week for full recovery. A careful history and sleep diary are usually adequate to identify insufficient sleep. However, "treatment" may be quite difficult, because it requires a commitment to behavioral change and acceptance of fewer waking hours.

Hypersomnia Due to Other Conditions

EDS can be a symptom of many medical and psychiatric conditions as well as an effect of medications and/or substances. EDS is often associated with neurological disorders, including structural, vascular, traumatic, toxic, infectious, and metabolic encephalopathic processes. EDS may result either from direct involvement of discrete brain regions (especially the brain-stem reticular formation or midline diencephalic structures) or from the effects of disrupted sleep continuity. Patients with neuromuscular disorders or peripheral neuropathies may also develop EDS because of associated central or obstructive sleep apnea, pain, or PLMD (George 2000). Patients with myotonic dystrophy often have EDS, even in the absence of sleep-disordered breathing (Gibbs et al. 2002). Sleepiness may occur with acute infectious illness even without direct CNS involvement and may be mediated by cytokines, including interferon, interleukins, and tumor necrosis factor (Toth and Opp 2002). Psychiatric disorders, especially depression, are often accompanied by complaints of EDS. Indeed, tiredness, fatigue, and lack of energy are reported by a large majority of patients with major depression. However, rating scales and MSLT findings suggest that actual EDS is much less common than complaints of fatigue or lack of energy (Nofzinger et al. 1991).

Circadian Rhythm Sleep Disorders

Alterations in the regulation of the circadian timing system, or a misalignment between the endogenous circadian rhythm and the external physical or social environment, can affect the timing or duration of sleep and give rise to CRSD (Reid and Zee 2005). Several distinct subtypes of CRSD have been described (Figure 13–6). This chapter will focus on three of the most important CRSDs: delayed and advanced sleep phase disorders and shift work disorder. The approach to assessment and diagnosis is described first, because this is similar across all subtypes.

Assessment and Diagnosis

The diagnosis of CRSD rests on clinical history. CRSDs are distinguished from simple circadian preferences by impairment in social, occupational, or other areas of functioning. Sleep–wake diaries are useful for confirming abnormalities of sleep–wake timing, and actigraphy provides objective verification of rest–activity patterns. Sleep diaries and actigraphy should be obtained for 1–2 weeks in order to capture the individual's typical schedule variations, such as work and nonwork days. Physiological markers of circadian phase, such as melatonin or core body temperature rhythms, can confirm abnormal circadian phase but are rarely used in clinical practice. Although polysomnography is not required for the diagnosis of CRSD, it may be useful to exclude other sleep disorders such as OSA or RLS. When objective evaluation of sleepiness is needed, such as in shift work disorder, the MSLT should be conducted during usual work hours.

Medical history is an important aspect of assessment in CRSD. Shift work disorder is associated with increased prevalence of cardiovascular and gastrointestinal disorders, sleep apnea, obesity, and miscarriage (Scott 2000; Wagner 1996). Neurological disorders affecting the structure of the circadian pacemaker, its afferents, or its efferents (e.g., visual impairment, tumors, dementia, stroke) should be considered in individuals with CRSDs.

Evaluation of CRSD should routinely include screening for psychiatric disorders and psychoactive medications. The prevalence of affective and personality disorders is high in patients with CRSDs (Dagan 2002). Affective and personality disorders may contribute to social withdrawal, which can lead to a de-

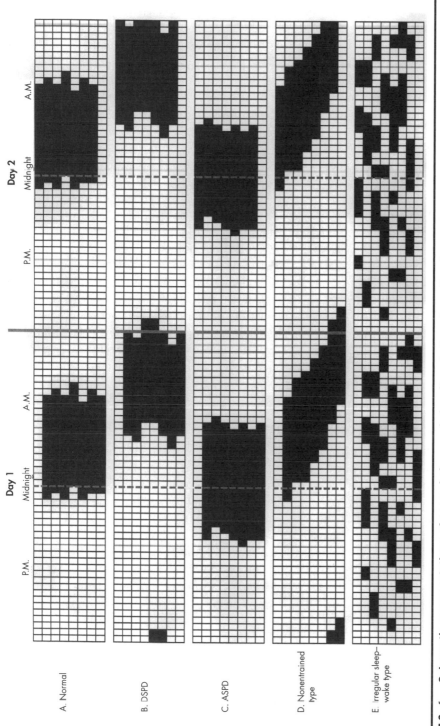

Figure 13–6.   Schematic representations of normal sleep and circadian rhythm sleep disorders.

Data are shown for 7 days and nights for each condition. *Black bars:* Sleep; *Open rectangles:* Wakefulness. For each hypothetical condition, sleep–wake data are "double plotted" (i.e., each day's data are shown both to the right of and below the previous day) to facilitate viewing the pattern across days. Each *horizontal line* shows 2 days; the *heavy vertical line* separates successive days. The *dashed vertical line* indicates midnight. For comparative purposes, each condition is shown with a total sleep time of approximately 8 hours. **A,** Normal sleep. Sleep hours across successive days fall at about midnight to 7:00 A.M. **B,** Delayed sleep phase disorder (DSPD). Sleep hours are consistently delayed, with average sleep times of approximately 4:00 A.M. to noon. **C,** Advanced sleep phase disorder (ASPD). Sleep hours are consistently advanced, with average sleep times of approximately 8:00 P.M. to 4:00 A.M. **D,** Nonentrained type. Sleep hours are progressively later each day, following an underlying circadian rhythm period closer to 25 hours than 24. **E,** Irregular sleep–wake type. Sleep–wake hours occur irregularly over the 24-hour day, with no discernible circadian pattern.

crease in light exposure, physical activity, and social cues, thereby perpetuating abnormal sleep timing. Because depressed patients often complain of early-morning awakening, it is important to distinguish advanced sleep phase disorder (ASPD) from major depression and other affective disorders (Wagner 1996). Individuals with CRSD may use alcohol, sedative-hypnotics, and stimulants to alleviate symptoms, which may lead to substance dependence.

The role of voluntary behavior often poses a problem in the evaluation of CRSD. For instance, some adolescents and young adults prefer delayed sleep–wake schedules and are not strongly motivated to change this pattern. In such cases, altered timing of light exposure can lead to a self-perpetuating cycle of sleep–wake disturbance.

Delayed Sleep Phase Disorder

Definition and Description

Delayed sleep phase disorder (DSPD) is characterized by habitual sleep–wake times that are substantially later than societal norms, resulting in complaints of difficulty falling asleep at night and difficulty waking up in the morning (Regestein and Monk 1995). Individuals with DSPD typically fall asleep between 2:00 and 6:00 A.M. and wake up between 10:00 A.M. and 1:00 P.M. (Weitzman et al. 1981). When allowed to sleep at their preferred sleep–wake times, DSPD patients have relatively normal sleep architecture and quality. The preference for delayed sleep–wake times remains stable over a long period of time, is not the result of external time demands, and is accompanied by greater than usual difficulty adjusting sleep–wake times (Dagan 2002).

Epidemiology and Consequences

The prevalence of DSPD in the general population has been estimated to be less than 1% (Wagner 1996). However, DSPD is more common among adolescents, with a reported prevalence of 7%–16% (Pelayo et al. 1988). Approximately 7% of patients with chronic insomnia presenting to a sleep clinic may have DSPD (Weitzman et al. 1981).

Pathophysiology

Evidence for genetic contributions to DSPD comes from studies of family history (Ancoli-Israel et al. 2001) and polymorphisms in circadian rhythm genes (*Per3, Arylalkylamine N-acetyltransferase, HLA,* and *Clock*) and circadian gene polymorphisms in affected kindreds (Archer et al. 2003; Hohjoh et al. 2003). Circadian physiological dysregulation may also contribute to DSPD through factors including 1) long endogenous circadian period (Regestein and Monk 1995); 2) alteration of circadian entrainment by light, as might result from decreased phase advances to morning light or increased delays to evening light (Weitzman et al. 1981); 3) alteration in light sensitivity, and in particular, increased sensitivity to nighttime light (Aoki et al. 2001); and 4) behavioral factors, such as increased exposure to evening light and decreased exposure to morning light, that may help to perpetuate the phase delay (Ozaki et al. 1996).

Treatment

Treatment success depends on many variables including severity of the disorder, comorbid psychopathology, ability and willingness of the patient to comply with treatment, school or work schedules, and social pressures (Regestein and Monk 1995; Thorpy et al. 1988). Chronotherapy is a behavioral treatment in which bedtime is delayed (i.e., moved to a later clock time) by approximately 3 hours every 2 days until the desired sleep time is achieved (Weitzman et al. 1981). Patients need to adhere to a strict sleep–wake schedule. In addition, light exposure needs to be carefully controlled to avoid inadvertent phase advances. The strict protocol and length of treatment may limit its acceptability for some patients. Bright-light exposure during the early morning hours is an accepted and effective treatment for DSPD

(Chesson et al. 1999). Although the optimal timing, intensity, and duration of light treatment are not well defined, typical regimens include exposure to broad-spectrum light of 2,000–10,000 lux for approximately 1–2 hours shortly after awakening. Compliance with daily or chronic intermittent exposure to light may be difficult. One important factor that affects compliance is the inability of patients to wake up in the morning for light exposure (Thorpy et al. 1988). Blue wavelength light may enhance compliance by permitting shorter-duration, lower-intensity light exposure. Melatonin has both circadian phase shifting effects and mild hypnotic effects. Melatonin, 1–5 mg administered in the evening, advances both sleep onset and wake times and improves quality of life of DSPD patients (Dahlitz et al. 1991; Mundey et al. 2005). Hypnotic medications and stimulants are commonly prescribed for patients with DSPD, but there is little evidence documenting their efficacy.

Advanced Sleep Phase Disorder

Definition and Description

ASPD is characterized by habitual sleep–wake times that are substantially earlier than societal norms, resulting in complaints of sleepiness in the late afternoon and evening and sleep maintenance insomnia or waking up too early in the morning. Individuals with ASPD typically report sleep onset between 6:00 and 9:00 P.M. and wake times between 2:00 and 5:00 A.M. (Kamei et al. 1998). When allowed to follow their usual schedule, ASPD patients have normal sleep architecture and quality for age.

Epidemiology

The actual prevalence of ASPD in the general population is unknown, but it has been estimated to be about 1% in middle-aged and older adults. Because circadian rhythms tend to advance with age, only a few case reports

have described ASPD *not* associated with aging (C. R. Jones et al. 1999; Reid et al. 2001).

Pathophysiology

Genetic factors appear to play an important role in the pathogenesis of ASPD. Several families with ASPD have been identified (C. R. Jones et al. 1999; Reid et al. 2001), and the phenotype segregates with an autosomal dominant mode of inheritance. Mutations in the circadian clock *hPer2* and *CK1 delta* genes have been linked to ASPD, indicating genetic heterogeneity (Toh et al. 2001; Xu et al. 2005). As with DSPD, physiological dysregulation may also play a role. Specifically, ASPD may be related to an unusually short endogenous circadian period or alterations in the entrainment process of the circadian system (C. R. Jones et al. 1999). Similar to DSPD, the interaction between circadian timing and sleep homeostatic regulation may be altered in individuals with ASPD and in older adults with nonpathologically advanced sleep phase (Duffy and Czeisler 2002).

Treatment

Treatment principles for ASPD are similar to those for DSPD, except for the timing of interventions. Chronotherapy for ASPD requires progressively advancing sleep time (i.e., moving it to an earlier clock time) by 2 hours every 2 days until the desired sleep time is achieved (Moldofsky et al. 1986). Exposure to evening bright light (7:00–9:00 P.M.) delays circadian rhythms and improves sleep efficiency, but patients may have difficulty maintaining the treatment regimen (Suhner et al. 2002). Concurrently, patients should avoid bright light in the early morning hours, because exposure to early morning light further advances circadian rhythms. Theoretically, melatonin given in the morning could delay circadian rhythms in ASPD, but there are few empirical data documenting its efficacy, and residual sedating effects may limit its utility. As with DSPD, the appropriate role of hypnotic and stimulant medications in ASPD is uncertain.

Shift Work Type (Shift Work Disorder)

Definition and Description

Shift work disorder is characterized by excessive sleepiness during work hours that are scheduled during the usual sleep period (when circadian alertness is low) and insomnia when attempting to sleep during the usual wake period (when circadian alertness is high). Shift work disorder is most commonly seen in association with night and early-morning shift schedules. Patients report decreased total sleep time, poor sleep quality, and impaired performance at work (Akerstedt 2003; Knauth et al. 1980). Safety at work and during the morning commute is a major concern due to decreased alertness.

Epidemiology

Shift work disorder is likely to be very common, but the actual prevalence is unknown. Approximately 20% of the workforce in industrialized countries has nonstandard work schedules (Presser 1999). Based on data available for night shift workers, approximately 5% of the population is likely to be affected by shift work disorder (Akerstedt 2003). As discussed earlier, shift work disorder is associated with medical and psychiatric morbidity. Mood symptoms and disorders are associated with current and former shift work (Scott 2000). Because irregular schedules and sleep deprivation can exacerbate mania, patients with bipolar disorder may be at particular risk for adverse consequences of shift work.

Pathophysiology

Shift work disorder results from misalignment between scheduled work and sleep times and the endogenous circadian rhythm of alertness and sleep propensity. Even among permanent night workers, internal circadian rhythms are usually out of phase with the desired sleep–wake times (Dumont et al. 2001). Chronic cumulative sleep loss may also contribute to excessive sleepiness.

Treatment

Ideally, the goal of clinical management is to align the circadian propensity for sleep and wakefulness with the work schedule. Because such alignment is difficult to achieve in real work and life environments, it is also important to employ behavioral approaches to improve sleep quality and work performance. For rotating shifts, a clockwise rotation, in which the schedule is delayed from day to evening to night is recommended. Because disturbances in sleep and wakefulness are most common among night shift workers, most treatment strategies have focused on this group. Family, social, and environmental factors are critical in the management of shift work disorder. Adherence to good sleep habits and practices is important and includes protecting sleep time, decreasing daytime noise, and providing a dark and comfortable room. Educating the individual, family members, and employers is essential for effective management.

Timed bright light (1,200–10,000 lux for 3–6 hours) and melatonin accelerate circadian adaptation to night shift (Burgess et al. 2002; Sharkey et al. 2001). A regimen of intermittent exposure to bright light (20-minute blocks per hour) during the night shift may also improve adaptation (Boivin and James 2002). Intermittent or continuous light exposure should begin early in the shift and terminate approximately 2 hours before the end of the shift to avoid the potential advancing effects of early-morning bright light (Crowley et al. 2003). Bright-light exposure during the morning commute may also prevent the desired phase delay and should be avoided (Boivin and James 2002; Crowley et al. 2003). Melatonin given at bedtime after a night shift may increase sleep duration but has limited effects on alertness (Burgess et al. 2002) and questionable additive benefit when combined with intermittent bright-light therapy and morning light avoidance (Crowley et al. 2003).

Pharmacological treatment may target both sleep and alertness. Hypnotics treat insomnia but do not necessarily address circadian misalignment and therefore are often insufficient therapy by themselves. Caffeine alleviates sleepiness, one of the most debilitating symptoms of this disorder (Babkoff et al. 2002). Modafinil and armodafinil are approved for the treatment of excessive sleepiness and neurobehavioral deficits associated with shift work disorder (Walsh et al. 2004).

Parasomnias

Parasomnias are undesirable physical or experiential events that accompany sleep (American Academy of Sleep Medicine 2005) and are generally divided into those arising from NREM sleep and those arising from REM sleep. These types of parasomnias can often be distinguished by their clinical features, time of occurrence, and associated autonomic activation (Table 13–8).

NREM Parasomnias

Clinical Features, Epidemiology, and Pathophysiology

Arousal from sleep is not an all-or-none phenomenon, but rather a continuum of reestablishing alertness, judgment, and control over behavior (Mahowald and Schenck 2001). Behaviors or mood states can be expressed during such partial arousals, which may be partially or completely divorced from awareness. Most commonly, such behaviors involve dissociated motor activities (walking, eating, sexual activity) or emotional responses (fear, anger, sexual excitement) (Schenck and Mahowald 2000). They are distinguished from waking behavior by the absence of complex mentation and sound judgment and by reduced response to environmental feedback. NREM parasomnias show clear familial aggregation (Mahowald and Cramer Bornemann 2005). Several subtypes, defined by clinical features, have been described.

Confusional arousals are brief, simple motor behaviors that usually occur without strong affective expression during partial arousals from NREM sleep. Mental confusion with automatic behavior, indistinct speech, and relative unresponsiveness to the environment are hallmarks (Mahowald and Cramer Bornemann 2005). Amnesia for events is dense. Individuals do not report dreams upon achieving full alertness, but rather simple mentation. Electroencephalographic recordings at the time of confusional arousals may show delta waves (characteristic of slow-wave sleep), theta or alpha activity, or alternation between sleep and waking activity (Gaudreau et al. 2000). Roughly 10%–20% of children and 2%–5% of adults report a history of confusional arousals (Ohayon et al. 1999). The expression of confusional arousals depends on a genetic predisposition combined with a precipitating event, which may be endogenous (e.g., OSA, pain, leg movements) or exogenous (e.g., forced awakening or environmental disruption) (Hublin et al. 2001). In predisposed individuals, sleep deprivation, medications, sleep disorders, stress, and circadian misalignment may aggravate or precipitate NREM parasomnias.

Variants of confusional arousals include sleep inertia ("sleep drunkenness"; Mahowald and Cramer Bornemann 2005), sleep-related abnormal sexual behavior ("sexsomnia"; Shapiro et al. 2003), and sleep-related violence (Cartwright 2004). Unlike confusional arousals, sleep drunkenness arises from final awakenings in the morning, but in other respects it is similar to confusional episodes arising from slow-wave sleep. Sleep-related abnormal sexual behavior is usually distinct from the individual's typical behavior in terms of partner or sexual act. Sleep-related violence is also generally distinct from the individual's waking behavior and occurs with anger or fear as the dominant emotion, agitated resistance to the environment, a slow return to normal levels of alertness following the event, and subsequent amnesia. The majority of cases occur in young or middle-aged males with a prior history of sleepwalking (Bonkalo 1974).

Table 13–8. Overview of parasomnias

	NREM parasomnias			REM parasomnias	
	Confusional arousals	Sleepwalking	Sleep terrors	REM sleep behavior disorder	Nightmare disorder
Stage of arousal	NREM 2–4	NREM 3–4	NREM 3–4	REM	REM
Time of night	Anytime	First 2 hours	First 2 hours	Anytime	Anytime
EEG with event	NA	Mixed	Mixed	Characteristic of REM	NA
EMG with event	Low	Low	Low	High, variable	NA
Relative unresponsiveness during event	Yes	Yes	Yes	Yes	Yes
Autonomic activity	Low	Low	High	High	High
Amnesia	Yes	Yes	Yes	No	No
Confusion following episode	Yes	Yes	Yes	No	No
Family history of parasomnias	Yes	Yes	Yes	No	No

Note. EEG=electroencephalogram; EMG=electromyogram; NA=not available; NREM=non–rapid eye movement; REM=rapid eye movement.

Sleepwalking also occurs within the first 1 or 2 hours of sleep without substantial affective activity, but it involves more elaborate behavior than confusional arousals. Actions are typically simple, such as attempts to use the bathroom, go to the kitchen, or leave the home. Although the sleepwalker's eyes are open, behavior is often clumsy (Crisp 1996). Dreaming is usually not present or consists of only simple mentation (e.g., "had to find my ring"). If the episode is interrupted, responses may be absent, incomplete, or inappropriate. If left alone, sleepwalkers usually return to sleep, at times in unusual places; if attempts are made to arouse them, they may take a prolonged period of time to become fully alert. Individuals may become violent or agitated if sleepwalking episodes are interrupted. As in other NREM parasomnias, full or partial amnesia is typical.

Sleepwalking occurs in 10%–20% of children and 1%–4% of adults (Ohayon et al. 1999). It is most common in children between 5 and 10 years of age and becomes less and less prevalent with increasing age. Genetic factors account for approximately 60%–80% of the variance in sleepwalking, as evidenced by epidemiological and twin studies (Hublin et al. 2001). Risk of sleepwalking roughly doubles when one parent has a positive history and triples when both parents have a history.

Approximately 80% of adults with sleepwalking report a continuous history from childhood, although many will not come to medical attention until their 20s or 30s as a result of bed partner concerns. The frequency of sleepwalking is quite variable, but it usually occurs once or twice a month.

The relationship between psychiatric disorders and sleepwalking is controversial (Schenck and Mahowald 2000). Although childhood sleepwalking does not appear to be associated with psychiatric disorder, a variety of psychiatric disorders may increase the risk of sleepwalking persisting into adulthood (Ohayon et al. 1999). Sleepwalk

ing is not thought to represent latent psychopathology or the underlying "true" motivations of the sufferer (Hartman et al. 2001). Stress, sleep deprivation (Joncas et al. 2002), and chaotic sleep schedules may also increase the risk of sleepwalking.

Polysomnography studies may demonstrate an increase in brief arousals from slow-wave sleep, with preservation of a sleeping electroencephalogram accompanied by autonomic activation (increased heart rate and respiration) following the arousal (Gaudreau et al. 2000). Polysomnography may be useful to identify precipitants to the episodes, such as OSA, periodic leg movements, or nocturnal seizures.

Sleep terrors share many features with sleepwalking but are characterized by more intense motor, autonomic, and affective activity and experience. Sleepwalking and sleep terrors may occur in the same individual and may even co-occur during the same episode. In children, sleep terrors are heralded by a piercing scream, with apparent extreme fear, crying, and inconsolability (Mahowald and Cramer Bornemann 2005). In adults, agitation is common, with the perception of an imminent threat requiring escape or defense (Schenck et al. 1997). For this reason, persons with sleep terrors may cause injury to themselves, others, or property. Dreams are usually not reported, but simple thoughts are sometimes present ("The room is on fire," or "I am being attacked") that can be difficult to dispel, even after awakening. Recollection of the event afterward is limited.

Sleep terrors are less common than sleepwalking, with roughly 5% of children and 1%–2% of adults reporting a history of such events (Ohayon et al. 1999). As with sleepwalking, genetic factors appear to increase susceptibility to sleep terrors, and precipitating factors can be either endogenous or exogenous. Multiple brief arousals from slow-wave sleep with heightened autonomic activity may be observed during polysomnography recordings (Gaudreau et al. 2000).

Assessment and Diagnosis

The differential diagnosis of sleep-related motor or affective behaviors includes nocturnal panic attacks, nocturnal dissociative episodes, frontal lobe seizures, delirium associated with medical or neurological disorders, and REM sleep behavior disorder. A daytime history of behaviors similar to the nocturnal behaviors (e.g., panic or dissociative episode) suggests a diagnosis other than NREM parasomnia. Similarly, overnight polysomnographic monitoring may confirm REM sleep behavior disorder or a seizure disorder.

Treatment

The decision to treat NREM parasomnias is based on the frequency of events, risk of injury to self or others, and distress the behaviors cause the patient or family members (Schenck and Mahowald 2000). Parasomnias typically occur infrequently but unpredictably, raising the question of whether chronic treatment of episodic events is warranted.

For most children, parasomnias do not require treatment, because there is little risk of harm and the child is unaware of the events. Regulating the sleep–wake schedule and avoiding sleep deprivation can reduce the frequency of events. For sleepwalking, the sleeping environment must be made safe by locking doors and windows and keeping hallways and stairs well lit.

Treatment of sleepwalking or sleep terrors in adults involves three steps: modification of predisposing and precipitating factors; enhancing safety of the sleeping environment; and when these are not successful, pharmacotherapy. Sleep disorders, medical disorders (pain, nocturia, dyspnea), and sleep-disrupting medications should be addressed when possible. If the parasomnia occurs within the first half of the sleep period, short-acting BzRAs such as triazolam (0.125–0.25 mg hs) or zolpidem (5–10 mg hs) are recommended. Clonazepam (0.5–1.0 mg qhs) is the most commonly used BzRA for parasomnias and has been used successfully for extended periods without the development of tolerance

(Schenck and Mahowald 1996). These medications may suppress arousals or decrease slow-wave sleep. However, no controlled efficacy trials have been performed for NREM parasomnias.

Sleep-Related Eating Disorder

Sleep-related eating disorder is a recently described disorder, and information regarding its description, course, prevalence, and treatment is more limited. It combines features of a sleep disorder (sleepwalking) with that of an eating disorder (binge-eating disorder) (Schenck et al. 1991; Winkelman 2006). The behavior consists of repeated partial arousals from sleep with eating in a compulsive or driven manner. Preferred foods are typically high in carbohydrates. In distinction to sleepwalking, sleep-related eating disorder usually occurs every night or multiple times per night. Level of awareness varies, but recollection of events is usually incomplete. Individuals are often ashamed of the behavior, gain weight, and alter daytime food consumption in order to limit 24-hour calorie consumption.

The prevalence of this disorder is estimated at 1%–5% of adults and is two to four times more common in women. It most often begins in late adolescence or early adulthood and runs a chronic course without treatment (Winkelman et al. 1999). Eating disorders increase the risk of sleep-related eating disorder, but only a minority of those with the disorder have anorexia, bulimia, or daytime binge-eating disorder (Schenck et al. 1993). A history of sleepwalking is also common. RLS is also commonly observed in those with sleep-related eating disorder, and treatment of the former can eliminate the latter. BzRAs may also be associated with the disorder (Morgenthaler and Silber 2002). Roughly one-third of patients have a first-degree family member with sleep-related eating disorder as well, consistent with the familial patterns observed in both sleepwalking (Hublin et al. 2001) and daytime eating disorders.

In distinction to the other NREM parasomnias, eating episodes in sleep-related eating disorder can occur at any time of the night and from all stages of NREM sleep (Winkelman 2006). Polysomnographic features characteristic of sleepwalking, such as frequent arousals from slow-wave sleep, are commonly observed (Schenck et al. 1991). The underlying pathophysiology is unclear.

The major differential diagnosis for sleep-related eating disorder is nocturnal eating syndrome. In the latter, the individual eats an excessive amount of food either before bed or during nocturnal awakenings while maintaining full consciousness (Schenck et al. 1993). Thus, these two diagnoses represent opposite ends of a continuum of related nocturnal eating disorders distinguished by level of awareness.

Treatment of sleep-related eating disorder is targeted at the underlying causes of abnormal arousals and/or disordered eating. As with other NREM parasomnias, behavioral measures are essential and include ensuring the safety of the sleeping environment, avoiding sleep deprivation and irregular sleep schedules, and normalizing the daytime eating schedule. Individuals with a history of sleepwalking can be treated with short- to intermediate-acting BzRAs or other sedating medications such as trazodone. However, such medications can also aggravate the dissociated eating and amnesia. Agents that suppress or normalize eating disorders, such as SSRIs or topiramate, have been effective in some case series (Winkelman 2003). Dopamine agonists may also be useful, particularly for patients with RLS (Schenck et al. 1993).

REM-Related Parasomnias

REM Sleep Behavior Disorder

In REM sleep behavior disorder (RBD), the usual atonia of REM sleep is absent, allowing the sleeper to enact dreams that, when agitated or violent, can result in injury to the sleeper or bed partner (Mahowald and Schenck 2005). During such episodes, the sleeper has his or her eyes closed and is completely unresponsive to the environment until awakened, at which point he or she will achieve rapid and full alertness and report a dream that usually corresponds to the exhibited behavior. Reported dream content and associated actions often relate to violent themes but may also involve pleasant or nonthreatening themes (Oudiette et al. 2009). Fully expressed episodes of the disorder are intermittent, but talking, shouting, and fragmentary motor activity often occur between such events.

RBD is chronic and usually observed in males older than 50 years. It is strongly associated with neurological disorders characterized by accumulation of α-synuclein protein (Parkinson's disease, dementia with Lewy bodies, and multiple system atrophy) and may serve as an early marker of these disorders (Boeve et al. 2007). Up to two-thirds of patients followed for 10 years developed Parkinson's disease (Postuma et al. 2009; Schenck et al. 1996). Although the site of pathology in RBD is not clear, dopamine transporter abnormalities in the nigrostriatal system and a reduction in peri-locus coeruleus neurons have been reported (Turner et al. 2000). Antidepressants, including SSRIs and monoamine oxidase inhibitors, are an important risk factor for RBD (Mahowald and Schenck 2005). Acute and chronic administration of serotonergic antidepressants can produce subclinical illness, in which motor tone disinhibited during REM has been demonstrated with both acute and chronic administration of serotonergic antidepressants (Winkelman and James 2004).

The diagnosis of RBD is made by polysomnography, which demonstrates elevated muscle tone or excessive phasic muscle activity during REM sleep (American Academy of Sleep Medicine 2005). Large body movements and REM-related behaviors may also appear during the polysomnogram. Periodic limb movements of sleep may be observed during both REM and NREM sleep.

First-line treatment consists of BzRAs. The most commonly used agent is clonazepam (0.5–1.0 mg), which decreases the number and extent of pathological dream-enacting behaviors (Mahowald and Schenck 2005). Although clonazepam is generally well tolerated, its long half-life and the age of most patients with the disorder may lead to daytime sleepiness and/or cognitive impairment. In this case, shorter-acting benzodiazepines (e.g., lorazepam 1–2 mg) may be preferable. Melatonin (3–15 mg qhs) and pramipexole (0.5–1.0 mg qhs) have also been used with some success. Discontinuing medications such as antidepressants should be attempted if clinically possible. As with the NREM parasomnias, ensuring the safety of the sleeping environment for both the patient and bed partner is essential (Mahowald and Schenck 2005).

Nightmare Disorder

Nightmare disorder is characterized by recurrent distressing dreams that usually arise from REM sleep and are followed by an awakening, with full recall. The dominant emotion is usually fear, although anger, sadness, and embarrassment may also be present. Nightmares may occur at any time of night but are more common in the final third of the night when REM is most prominent (American Academy of Sleep Medicine 2005; Nielsen and Zadra 2005). In distinction to sleep terrors, return to sleep after a nightmare is usually delayed, and frequent nightmares may lead to a fear of going to sleep. Nightmares are not associated with complex acting out of dreams as in RBD.

Occasional nightmares are common in both children and adults (Nielsen and Zadra 2005). Approximately 5% of adults report frequent nightmares (Ohayon et al. 1997). The prevalence is higher in women than men. Nightmare distress is associated with psychiatric illness and psychopathology (Nielsen and Zadra 2005). Polysomnography is generally of little diagnostic value for frequent nightmares, except to rule out RBD or NREM parasomnias.

Nightmares occur in more than 50% of individuals with posttraumatic stress disorder (Neylan et al. 1998). In posttraumatic stress disorder the nightmare often has a thematic or literal association with the traumatic event (Harvey et al. 2003). Such nightmares may arise from both REM and NREM sleep.

Nightmare treatment includes pharmacological and behavioral/psychological approaches. Prazosin (4–12 mg qhs; Raskind et al. 2003), cyproheptadine (Gupta et al. 1998), anticonvulsants (Berlant and Van Kammen 2002), and antipsychotic medications (Labbate and Douglas 2000) have all been efficacious in placebo-controlled trials and/or uncontrolled case series. Imagery rehearsal, in which new versions (with better outcomes) of nightmares are rehearsed during the day, has demonstrated consistent benefit for trauma-related and non-trauma-related nightmares (Krakow et al. 2001).

Sleep-Related Movement Disorders: Restless Legs Syndrome and Periodic Limb Movement Disorder

The most prevalent and clinically significant sleep-related movement disorder is RLS. Because this disorder is frequently accompanied by PLMD, the two are described together.

Definition and Description

RLS is a sensory-motor disorder characterized by an urge to move the legs, accompanied by uncomfortable or unpleasant sensations (Allen et al. 2003; Montplaisir et al. 2005; Walters 1995). The restlessness and dysesthesias of RLS are variously described as "achy," "creepy-crawly," "electric," "like a coiled spring," "something running down my veins," "itchy," and "painful." The urge to move and unpleasant leg sensations worsen during periods of rest or inactivity such as lying, sitting, and attempting to sleep. Symptoms are temporarily relieved by movement, such as walking or stretching. Persons with RLS often move excessively in bed or interrupt activities requiring immobility in order to relieve the sensations. Such movement has both voluntary and involuntary aspects. The movement is described as irrepressible but can be delayed or avoided by distraction. While the person is asleep, characteristic periodic movements of the legs appear, with a distinctive pattern and distribution. Finally, the urge to move or unpleasant sensations are typically worse, or occur exclusively, in the evening or night between 8 P.M. and 4 A.M. RLS symptoms demonstrate a true circadian rhythm, in phase with body temperature and melatonin rhythms (Michaud et al. 2004).

The majority of individuals with RLS have symptoms infrequently (up to four times per month), but approximately 25% describe daily or near-daily symptoms. RLS is strongly associated with sleep-onset and sleep-maintenance insomnia. Due to the circadian rhythm of RLS symptoms, some patients adopt atypical sleep–wake schedules. Despite the sleep disruption caused by RLS, excessive daytime sleepiness is not typical, and the ability to nap is often impaired by RLS symptoms.

Approximately 80% of RLS patients have periodic limb movements of sleep (PLMS), which are brief (0.5–5.0 seconds) repetitive, stereotyped movements of the foot and leg appearing at roughly 20-second intervals (Montplaisir et al. 2005). The magnitude of these movements may vary from barely discernible to very large. They can be associated with arousal from sleep and elevated heart rate and blood pressure (Winkelman 1999). More than 5 such movements with arousal per hour of sleep is considered abnormal; however, given the high prevalence of PLMS in the general population, polysomnographic findings are not specific for PLMS (Montplaisir et al. 2005).

Epidemiology and Consequences

The prevalence of RLS is approximately 3%–5% in adult populations of northern European descent, rising roughly linearly with age to 10% of those older than 65 years (Montplaisir et al. 2005; Ohayon and Roth 2002). Preva-lence rates appear to be lower in other ethnic groups and are approximately 50% higher in women than men. RLS is more common in individuals with certain medical disorders, including end-stage renal disease (15%–30%; Unruh et al. 2004; Winkelman et al. 1996), iron deficiency anemia (Berger et al. 2002), and rheumatoid arthritis (Reynolds et al. 1986). It is also common in pregnant women, affecting up to 33% of those in the third trimester (Suzuki et al. 2003). RLS is associated with impaired quality of life (Hening et al. 2004) and with a substantial risk of depression, even when controlling for confounding disorders (Ulfberg et al. 2001). Emerging evidence suggests that RLS/PLMS are also related to hypertension and cardiovascular and cerebrovascular disease (Walters and Rye 2009) through mechanisms including sympathetic hyperactivity and medical comorbidities.

The onset of RLS can occur at any age: 10%–20% of patients reported onset before the age of 10 years and 40% by the age of 20 years (Montplaisir et al. 2005). Early onset is associated with a family history of RLS (Winkelmann et al. 2000), whereas late-onset RLS suggests secondary causes. The longitudinal course of RLS is not well defined, although it has been traditionally thought that the severity progresses over time.

Pathophysiology

Approximately 30%–50% of individuals with RLS report an affected first-degree family member (Winkelmann et al. 2000). In genome-wide association studies, three distinct sequence variants were identified in patients with RLS (Stefansson et al. 2007; Winkelmann et al. 2007). The variant found in both of the studies—a sequence variant in an intron on chromosome 6p—predicted the presence of both PLMS and iron deficiency in patients with RLS and their families. Significant linkages to chromosomes 14q, 12q, and 9p have also been reported (Montplaisir et al. 2005).

Several lines of evidence suggest a role for abnormal CNS iron transport and/or utilization in RLS. The prevalence of iron deficiency is increased in RLS, and iron repletion can relieve RLS (O'Keeffe et al. 1994). Likewise, reductions in cerebrospinal fluid ferritin (the protein storage form of iron) have been observed, even when serum iron is normal (Connor et al. 2003). Iron is also required for dopamine synthesis and dopamine receptor regulation (Allen 2004). Successful treatment of RLS with dopaminergic precursors and agonists has also focused attention on the dopaminergic system. However, studies examining dopamine system structure and function have yielded inconsistent findings, including D_2 dopamine receptor density, response to dopaminergic antagonists, and physiological responses to L-dopa challenge at different times of day (Montplaisir et al. 2005). The A11 dopaminergic system, which originates in the thalamus and descends to the spinal cord, may also be relevant to RLS, as suggested by abnormal responses to tibial nerve stimulation (Bara-Jimenez et al. 2000) and the presence of PLMS in patients with cord transections (de Mello et al. 1996).

Assessment and Diagnosis

RLS is a clinical diagnosis based on the presence of consistent symptoms. Physical examination yields no specific findings for idiopathic RLS, but individuals with comorbid disorders will have findings consistent with that disorder. Polysomnography may be useful to rule out other sleep disorders, including sleep apnea, and for documenting the presence and severity of PLMS. The dysesthesias of RLS are often difficult to distinguish from those of peripheral neuropathies, particularly when RLS is described as "painful." Given the age distribution of neuropathies and RLS, these two disorders commonly co-occur. However, neuropathic symptoms generally do not improve with movement. Nocturnal leg cramps, which occur at night and improve with movement, may also be difficult to distinguish from RLS. However, leg cramps arise precipitously from sleep and are not associated with feelings of motor restlessness.

The distinction between RLS and akathisia related to antipsychotic or serotonergic antidepressant drugs can be difficult to make. It is particularly difficult to determine whether symptoms represent akathisia or medication-related RLS. Both are clinical diagnoses, and both may produce PLMS. A history of RLS prior to antidepressant administration, the presence of a sensory component, nocturnal worsening of symptoms, and a therapeutic response to dopaminergic agonists all suggest a diagnosis of RLS. Anxiety associated with bedtime and sleep onset can also manifest with "an inability to get comfortable," restlessness, and vague sensory complaints. However, the lack of localization to the legs, the strict localization of the experience to the bed, and the anxiety regarding sleeplessness all suggest anxiety rather than RLS.

Treatment

Patients should first be evaluated and treated for reversible causes of RLS, such as iron deficiency, antidepressant use, or opiate withdrawal (Montplaisir et al. 2005; Silber et al. 2004). Behavioral measures include avoidance of caffeine, alcohol, and sleep deprivation. Individuals with RLS should also avoid unnecessary immobility. In individuals with intermittent symptoms, medications may be used on an as-needed basis.

Dopaminergic agents are considered first-line treatments for RLS (Montplaisir et al. 2005; Silber et al. 2004). L-dopa, the first dopaminergic agent used for RLS, can dramatically improve RLS symptoms and sleep latency (Trenkwalder et al. 1995). Its short duration of action is often associated with "rebound" RLS symptoms several hours later, which can be mitigated with use of longer-acting preparations (Collado-Seidel et al. 1999). Two additional problems are often seen with L-dopa: augmentation and tolerance. *Augmentation,* the appearance of RLS symptoms progressively earlier during the day, is observed in roughly two-thirds of individuals treated with L-dopa (Allen and

Earley 1996). Treatment with additional doses of the drug earlier in the day only exacerbates this problem and may lead to severe symptoms throughout the day. Other manifestations of augmentation include extension of RLS symptoms to other body parts and shorter duration of treatment effectiveness after a dose. *Tolerance* to L-dopa is manifested by reduced effectiveness of the medication over time (Allen and Earley 1996).

The long-acting dopamine receptor agonists pramipexole and ropinirole are now considered first-line therapy for RLS and are approved by the U.S. Food and Drug Administration for this indication. The binding profiles of these dopaminergic agonists to dopamine receptor subtypes (D_1–D_5) remain in dispute, but it appears that pramipexole has a higher affinity for the D_3 receptor than ropinirole (Piercey 1998). The efficacy of both pramipexole and ropinirole in RLS has been demonstrated in numerous double-blind, placebo-controlled trials with durations ranging from 3 to 12 weeks (Trenkwalder et al. 2004; Winkelman et al. 2006). Both agents dramatically reduce the number of PLMS and improve subjective sleep quality. Long-term placebo-controlled trials of these agents have not been performed. However, longitudinal naturalistic studies suggest that one-third of patients develop augmentation (i.e., the appearance of RLS symptoms progressively earlier during the day) after 8–12 months on dopaminergic agents (Winkelman and Johnston 2004). Augmentation developing with dopamine agonists can usually be managed by earlier dosing of medication. No randomized studies have examined the comparative efficacy of different dopaminergic agents.

More severely afflicted individuals may require adjunctive treatment. Second-line agents for RLS include short acting opiates such as oxycodone and codeine. Caution is warranted when prescribing opiates, given their potential for abuse and respiratory suppression.

Anticonvulsants are also considered second-line agents for RLS and may be used as adjuncts to dopaminergic agonists or as alternatives for patients who cannot tolerate these drugs or have contraindications to these drugs. Controlled trials have demonstrated efficacy for both gabapentin (Garcia Borreguero et al. 2002) and carbamazepine (Telstad et al. 1984) compared with placebo. Short- to intermediate-acting benzodiazepines can treat mild RLS and persistent sleep disturbance (Silber et al. 2004). Approximately 33%–60% of patients taking pramipexole for RLS also take hypnotics such as benzodiazepines, sedating antidepressants, or anticonvulsants to assist with sleep (Winkelman and Johnston 2004).

Conclusion

Sleep and wakefulness are fundamental neurobiological states that promote physical and mental health and functioning. Sleep disturbances are commonly seen in patients with psychiatric disorders. Conversely, psychiatric symptoms and disorders are common among patients with sleep disorders. Sleep disorders represent a heterogeneous group of conditions characterized by dysfunction in neurobiological and systemic physiological systems. Major categories of sleep disorders include insomnias, sleep-related breathing disorders, hypersomnias, circadian rhythm sleep disorders, parasomnias, and sleep-related movement disorders. Evaluation of sleep disorders rests on an accurate history of sleep and wake symptoms, comorbid psychiatric and medical conditions, and medication and substance use in some cases supplemented by polysomnographic sleep studies and other specialized techniques. Treatments of sleep disorders vary considerably among the specific categories of disorders, and may include psychological and behavioral interventions, medications, somatic treatments, and surgery. Mental health practitioners are well positioned to contribute to the evaluation and management of sleep disorder patients within the multidisciplinary field of sleep medicine.

Key Points

- Human sleep is regulated physiologically by the interaction of homeostatic sleep drive and the circadian timing system. Dysregulation of these factors can contribute to insomnia, hypersomnia, and circadian rhythm sleep disorders. Behavioral treatments of sleep disorders work in part by reinforcing the activity of these regulatory processes.

- Insomnia is a complaint of poor sleep and impaired daytime function in an individual with adequate sleep opportunity. Efficacy has been well demonstrated for behavioral treatments and BzRAs.

- OSA should be suspected in overweight patients with daytime sleepiness, loud snoring, and neurocognitive symptoms including depression. Continuous positive pressure applied via nasal mask is an efficacious first-line treatment.

- Narcolepsy, a disorder characterized by extreme sleepiness, cataplexy, and sleep-related hallucinations and paralysis, is caused by dysfunction of hypocretin-containing neurons in the hypothalamus. Treatment includes stimulants for improving daytime sleepiness and agents such as antidepressants or sodium oxybate to control cataplexy.

- CRSDs result from misalignment of the individual's circadian timing system with the light–dark cycle of the work, social, or physical environment. Behavioral interventions, appropriately timed exposure to light and darkness, and exogenous melatonin may all improve circadian alignment.

- Parasomnias are abnormal behavioral or affective events that occur in association with sleep or arousals from sleep. Distinctive clinical features characterize those occurring in association with NREM sleep and those occurring in association with REM sleep.

- RLS is characterized by unpleasant feelings in the legs and an urge to move, which are temporarily relieved by movement. Efficacious treatments include dopamine receptor agonists, BzRAs, antiepileptic drugs, and opiate analgesics.

Suggested Readings

American Academy of Sleep Medicine: The International Classification of Sleep Disorders, 2nd Edition (ICSD-2): Diagnostic and Coding Manual. Westchester, IL, American Academy of Sleep Medicine, 2005

Buysse DJ (ed): Sleep Disorders and Psychiatry (Review of Psychiatry Series Vol 24, No 2; Oldham JM and Riba MB, series eds). Washington, DC, American Psychiatric Publishing, 2005

Chokroverty S: Sleep Disorders Medicine, 3rd Edition. Boston, MA, Butterworth Heinemann, 2007

Kryger MH, Roth T, Dement W (eds): Principles and Practice of Sleep Medicine, 4th Edition. Philadelphia, PA, Elsevier, 2005

Sheldon SH, Kryger MH, Ferber R: Principles and Practice of Pediatric Sleep Medicine. Philadelphia, PA, Elsevier, 2005

Online Resources

American Academy of Sleep Medicine: aasmnet.org

National Center on Sleep Disorders Research: www.nhlbi.nih.gov/about/ncsdr/index.htm

National Sleep Foundation: www.sleepfoundation.org

Sleep Research Society: www.sleepresearchsociety.org

References

Akerstedt T: Shift work and disturbed sleep/wakefulness. Occup Med 53:88–94, 2003

Allen R: Dopamine and iron in the pathophysiology of restless legs syndrome (RLS). Sleep Med 5:385–391, 2004

Allen R, Earley CJ: Augmentation of the restless legs syndrome with carbidopa/levodopa. Sleep 19:205–213, 1996

Allen R, Picchietti D, Hening WA, et al: Restless legs syndrome: diagnostic criteria, special considerations, and epidemiology: a report from the restless legs syndrome diagnosis and epidemiology workshop at the National Institutes of Health. Sleep Med 4:101–119, 2003

American Academy of Sleep Medicine: The International Classification of Sleep Disorders, 2nd Edition (ICSD-2): Diagnostic and Coding Manual. Westchester, IL, American Academy of Sleep Medicine, 2005

American Psychiatric Association: Diagnostic and Statistical Manual of Mental Disorders, 4th Edition, Text Revision. Washington, DC, American Psychiatric Association, 2000

Ancoli-Israel S, Klauber MR, Stepnowsky C, et al: Sleep-disordered breathing in African-American elderly. Am J Respir Crit Care Med 152:1946–1949, 1995

Ancoli-Israel S, Schnierow B, Kelsoe J, et al: A pedigree of one family with delayed sleep phase syndrome. Chronobiol Int 18:831–840, 2001

Aoki H, Ozeki Y, Yamada N: Hypersensitivity of melatonin suppression in response to light in patients with delayed sleep phase syndrome. Chronobiol Int 18:263–271, 2001

Archer SN, Robilliard DL, Skene DJ, et al: A length polymorphism in the circadian clock gene Per3 is linked to delayed sleep phase syndrome and extreme diurnal preference. Sleep 26:413–415, 2003

Babkoff H, French J, Whitmore J, et al: Single-dose bright light and/or caffeine effect on nocturnal performance. Aviat Space Environ Med 73:341–350, 2002

Bady E, Achkar A, Pascal S, et al: Pulmonary arterial hypertension in patients with sleep apnea syndrome. Thorax 55:934–939, 2000

Bara-Jimenez W, Aksu M, Graham B, et al: Periodic limb movements in sleep: state-dependent excitability of the spinal flexor reflex. Neurology 54:1609–1616, 2000

Bassetti C, Pelayo R, Guilleminault C: Idiopathic hypersomnia, in Principles and Practice of Sleep Medicine, 4th Edition. Edited by Kryger MH, Roth T, Dement WC. Philadelphia, PA, Elsevier, 2005, pp 791–800

Beebe DW, Groesz L, Wells C, et al: The neuropsychological effects of obstructive sleep apnea: a meta-analysis of norm-referenced and case-controlled data. Sleep 26:298–307, 2003

Bellingham J, Foster RG: Opsins and mammalian photoentrainment. Cell Tissue Res 309:57–71, 2002

Benetó A, Gomez-Siurana E, Rubio-Sanchez P: Comorbidity between sleep apnea and insomnia. Sleep Med Rev 13(4):287–293, 2009

Berger K, von Eckardstein A, Trenkwalder C, et al: Iron metabolism and the risk of restless legs syndrome in an elderly general population: the MEMO-Study. J Neurol 249:1195–1199, 2002

Berlant J, Van Kammen DP: Open-label topiramate as primary or adjunctive therapy in chronic civilian posttraumatic stress disorder: a preliminary report. J Clin Psychiatry 63:15–20, 2002

Bixler EO, Vgontzas AN, Lin HM, et al: Prevalence of sleep-disordered breathing in women: effects of gender. Am J Respir Crit Care Med 163:608–613, 2001

Boeve BF, Silber MH, Saper CB, et al: Pathophysiology of REM sleep behaviour disorder and relevance to neurodegenerative disease. Brain 130(Pt 11):2770–2788, 2007

Boivin DB, James FO: Circadian adaptation to night-shift work by judicious light and darkness exposure. J Biol Rhythms 17:556–567, 2002

Bonkalo A: Impulsive acts and confusional states during incomplete arousal from sleep: criminological and forensic implications. Psychiatr Q 48:400–409, 1974

Borbély AA: A two process model of sleep regulation. Hum Neurobiol 1:195–204, 1982

Breslau N, Roth T, Rosenthal L, et al: Sleep disturbance and psychiatric disorders: a longitudinal epidemiological study of young adults. Biol Psychiatry 39:411–418, 1996

Brzezinski A, Vangel MG, Wurtman RJ, et al: Effects of exogenous melatonin on sleep: a meta-analysis. Sleep Med Rev 9:41–50, 2005

Burgess HJ, Sharkey KM, Eastman CI: Bright light, dark and melatonin can promote circadian adaptation in night shift workers. Sleep Med Rev 6:407–420, 2002

Buysse DJ (ed): Sleep Disorders and Psychiatry (Review of Psychiatry Series Vol 24, No 2; Oldham JM and Riba MB, series eds). Washington, DC, American Psychiatric Publishing, 2005

Buysse DJ, Schweitzer PK, Moul DE: Clinical pharmacology of other drugs used as hypnotics, in Principles and Practice of Sleep Medicine, 4th Edition. Edited by Kryger MH, Roth T, Dement WC. Philadelphia, PA, Elsevier, 2005, pp 452–467

Cajochen C, Kräuchi K, Wirz-Justice A: Role of melatonin in the regulation of human circadian rhythms and sleep. J Neuroendocrinol 15:432–437, 2003

Camacho ME, Morin CM: The effect of temazepam on respiration in elderly insomniacs with mild sleep apnea. Sleep 18:644–645, 1995

Carskadon MA, Rechtschaffen A: Monitoring and staging human sleep, in Principles and Practice of Sleep Medicine, 4th Edition. Edited by Kryger MH, Roth T, Dement WC. Philadelphia, PA, Elsevier, 2005, pp 1359–1377

Cartwright R: Sleepwalking violence: a sleep disorder, a legal dilemma, and a psychological challenge. Am J Psychiatry 161:1149–1158, 2004

Chemelli RM, Willie JT, Sinton CM, et al: Narcolepsy in orexin knockout mice: molecular genetics of sleep regulation. Cell 98:437–451, 1999

Chesson AL, Littner M, Davila D, et al: Practice parameters for the use of light therapy in the treatment of sleep disorders. Standards of Practice Committee, American Academy of Sleep Medicine. Sleep 22:641–660, 1999

Chokroverty S: Sleep Disorders Medicine: Basic Science, Technical Considerations, and Clinical Aspects, 3rd Edition. Philadelphia, PA, Saunders Elsevier, 2009

Collado-Seidel V, Kazenwadel J, Wetter TC, et al: A controlled study of additional sustained-release L-dopa in L-dopa-responsive restless legs syndrome with late-night symptoms. Neurology 52:285–290, 1999

Connor JR, Boyer PJ, Menzies SL, et al: Neuropathological examination suggests impaired brain iron acquisition in restless legs syndrome. Neurology 61:304–309, 2003

Crisp AH: The sleepwalking/night terrors syndrome in adults. Postgrad Med J 72:599–604, 1996

Crowley SJ, Lee C, Tseng CY, et al: Combinations of bright light, scheduled dark, sunglasses, and melatonin to facilitate circadian entrainment to night shift work. J Biol Rhythms 18:513–523, 2003

Cumming RG, Le Couteur DG: Benzodiazepines and risk of hip fractures in older people: a review of the evidence. CNS Drugs 17:825–837, 2003

Czeisler CA, Duffy JF, Shanahan TL, et al: Stability, precision, and near-24-hour period of the human circadian pacemaker. Science 284:2177–2181, 1999

Czeisler CA, Buxton OM, Sinngh Khasla SB: Human circadian timing system and sleep–wake regulation, in Principles and Practice of Sleep Medicine, 4th Edition. Edited by Kryger MH, Roth T, Dement WC. Philadelphia, PA, Elsevier, 2005, pp 375–394

Dagan Y: Circadian rhythm sleep disorders (CRSD). Sleep Med Rev 6:45–54, 2002

Dahlitz M, Alvarez B, Vignau J, et al: Delayed sleep phase syndrome response to melatonin. Lancet 337:1121–1124, 1991

de Mello MT, Lauro FA, Silva AC, et al: Incidence of periodic leg movements and of the restless legs syndrome during sleep following acute physical activity in spinal cord injury subjects. Spinal Cord 34:294–296, 1996

Duffy JF, Czeisler CA: Age-related change in the relationship between circadian period, circadian phase, and diurnal preference in humans. Neurosci Lett 318:117–120, 2002

Dumont M, Benhaberou-Brun D, Paquet J: Profile of 24-h light exposure and circadian phase of melatonin secretion in night workers. J Biol Rhythms 16:502–511, 2001

Edinger JD, Sampson WS: A primary care "friendly" cognitive behavior insomnia therapy. Sleep 26:177–182, 2003

Engleman HM, Douglas NJ: Sleep, 4: sleepiness, cognitive function, and quality of life in obstructive sleep apnea/hypopnea syndrome. Thorax 59:618–622, 2004

Erman M, Seiden D, Zammit G, et al: An efficacy, safety, and dose-response study of ramelteon in patients with chronic primary insomnia. Sleep Med 7:17–24, 2006

Espie CA, Inglis SJ, Tessier S: The clinical effectiveness of cognitive behaviour therapy for chronic insomnia: implementation and evaluation of a sleep clinic in general medical practice. Behav Res Ther 39:60, 2001

Farney RJ, Lugo A, Jensen RL, et al: Simultaneous use of antidepressant and antihypertensive medications increases likelihood of diagnosis of obstructive sleep apnea syndrome. Chest, 125:1279–1285, 2004

Fava M, McCall WV, Krystal A, et al: Eszopiclone co-administered with fluoxetine in patients with insomnia coexisting with major depressive disorder. Biol Psychiatry 59:1052–1060, 2006

Fava M, Asnis GM, Shrivastava R, et al: Zolpidem extended-release improves sleep and next-day symptoms in comorbid insomnia and generalized anxiety disorder. J Clin Psychopharmacol 29:222–230, 2009

Fredrikson S, Carlander B, Billiard M, et al: CSF immune variables in patients with narcolepsy. Acta Neurol Scand 81:253–254, 1990

Garcia-Borreguero D, Larrosa O, de la Llave Y, et al: Treatment of restless legs syndrome with gabapentin: a double-blind, cross-over study. Neurology 59:1573–1579, 2002

Gaudreau H, Joncas S, Zadra A, et al: Dynamics of slow-wave activity during the NREM sleep of sleepwalkers and control subjects. Sleep 23:755–760, 2000

Gelb M, Guilleminault C, Kraemer H, et al: Stability of cataplexy over several months: information for the design of therapeutic trials. Sleep 17:265–273, 1994

George CFP: Neuromuscular disorders, in Principles and Practice of Sleep Medicine, 3rd Edition. Edited by Kryger MH, Roth T, Dement WC. Philadelphia, PA, WB Saunders, 2000, pp 1087–1092

Germain A, Moul DE, Franzen PL, et al: Effects of a brief behavioral treatment for late-life insomnia: preliminary findings. J Clin Sleep Med 2:403–406, 2006

Gibbs JW, III, Ciafaloni E, Radtke RA: Excessive daytime somnolence and increased rapid eye movement pressure in myotonic dystrophy. Sleep 25:662–665, 2002

Gleeson K, Zwillich CW, White DP: The influence of increasing ventilatory effort on arousal from sleep. Am Rev Respir Dis 142:295–300, 1990

Gotsopoulos H, Kelly JJ, Cistulli PA: Oral appliance therapy reduces blood pressure in obstructive sleep apnea: a randomized, controlled trial. Sleep 27:934–941, 2004

Gottlieb DJ, Whitney CW, Bonekat WH, et al: Relation of sleepiness to respiratory disturbance index: the Sleep Heart Health Study. Am J Respir Crit Care Med 159:502–507, 1999

Griffiths RR, Weerts EM: Benzodiazepine self-administration in humans and laboratory animals: implications for problems of long-term use and abuse. Psychopharmacology 134:1–37, 1997

Guilleminault C, Fromherz S: Narcolepsy: diagnosis and management, in Principles and Practice of Sleep Medicine, 4th Edition. Edited by Kryger MH, Roth T, Dement WC. Philadelphia, PA, Elsevier, 2005, pp 780–790

Guilleminault C, Palombini L, Poyares D, et al: Chronic insomnia, premenopausal women and sleep disordered breathing: part 1. J Psychosom Res 53:611–615, 2002a

Guilleminault C, Palombini L, Poyares D, et al: Chronic insomnia, premenopausal women and sleep disordered breathing: part 2. J Psychosom Res 53:617–623, 2002b

Gupta S, Popli A, Bathurst E, et al: Efficacy of cyproheptadine for nightmares associated with posttraumatic stress disorder. Compr Psychiatry 39:160–164, 1998

Hartman D, Crisp AH, Sedgwick P: Is there a dissociative process in sleepwalking and night terrors? Postgrad Med J 77:244–249, 2001

Harvey AG: A cognitive model of insomnia. Behav Res Ther 40:869–893, 2002

Harvey AG, Jones C, Schmidt DA: Sleep and posttraumatic stress disorder: a review. Clin Psychol Rev 23:377–407, 2003

Hening W, Walters AS, Allen RP, et al: Impact, diagnosis and treatment of restless legs syndrome (RLS) in a primary care population: the REST (RLS epidemiology, symptoms, and treatment) primary care study. Sleep Med 5:237–246, 2004

Hohjoh H, Takasu M, Shishikura K, et al: Significant association of the arylalkylamine N-acetyltransferase (AA-NAT) gene with delayed sleep phase syndrome. Neurogenetics 4:151–153, 2003

Holbrook AM, Crowther R, Lotter A, et al: Meta-analysis of benzodiazepine use in the treatment of insomnia. Can Med Assoc J 162:225–233, 2000

Honda Y: Clinical features of narcolepsy: Japanese experiences, in HLA in Narcolepsy. Edited by Honda Y, Juti T. Berlin, Germany, Springer-Verlag, 1988, pp 24–57

Hublin C, Kaprio J, Partinen M, et al: Parasomnias: co-occurrence and genetics. Psychiatr Genet 11:65–70, 2001

Ip MS, Lam KS, Ho C, et al: Serum leptin and vascular risk factors in obstructive sleep apnea. Chest 118:580–586, 2000

Irwin MR, Cole JC, Nicassio PM: Comparative meta-analysis of behavioral interventions for insomnia and their efficacy in middle-aged adults and in older adults 55+ years of age. Health Psychol 25:3–14, 2006

Johns MW: A new method for measuring daytime sleepiness: the Epworth Sleepiness Scale. Sleep 14:540–545, 1991

Joncas S, Zadra A, Paquet J, et al: The value of sleep deprivation as a diagnostic tool in adult sleepwalkers. Neurology 58:936–940, 2002

Jones BE: Basic mechanisms of sleep-wake states, in Principles and Practice of Sleep Medicine, 4th Edition. Edited by Kryger MH, Roth T, Dement WC. Philadelphia, PA, Elsevier Saunders, 2005, pp 136–153

Jones CR, Campbell SS, Zone SE, et al: Familial advanced sleep-phase syndrome: a short-period circadian rhythm variant in humans. Nat Med 5:1062–1065, 1999

Kamei Y, Urata J, Uchiyaya M, et al: Clinical characteristics of circadian rhythm sleep disorders. Psychiatry Clin Neurosci 52:234–235, 1998

King DP, Takahashi JS: Molecular genetics of circadian rhythms in mammals. Annu Rev Neurosci 23:713–742, 2000

Knauth P, Landau K, Droge C, et al: Duration of sleep depending on the type of shift work. Int Arch Occup Environ Health 46:167–177, 1980

Krakow B, Hollifield M, Johnston L, et al: Imagery rehearsal therapy for chronic nightmares in sexual assault survivors with posttraumatic stress disorder: a randomized controlled trial. JAMA 286:537–545, 2001

Kryger MH, Roth T, Dement WC (eds): Principles and Practice of Sleep Medicine, 4th Edition. Philadelphia, PA, Elsevier, 2005

Krystal AD, Walsh JK, Laska E, et al: Sustained efficacy of eszopiclone over 6 months of nightly treatment: results of a randomized, double-blind, placebo-controlled study in adults with chronic insomnia. Sleep 26:793–799, 2003

Krystal AD, Erman M, Zammit GK, et al: Long-term efficacy and safety of zolpidem extended-release 12.5 mg, administered 3 to 7 nights per week for 24 weeks, in patients with chronic primary insomnia: a 6-month, randomized, double-blind, placebo-controlled, parallel-group, multicenter study. Sleep 31:79–90, 2008

Kushida CA, Littner MR, Morgenthaler T, et al: Practice parameters for the indications for polysomnography and related procedures: an update for 2005. Sleep 28:499–521, 2005

Labbate LA, Douglas S: Olanzapine for nightmares and sleep disturbance in posttraumatic stress disorder (PTSD). Can J Psychiatry 45:667–668, 2000

Lavie L: Obstructive sleep apnea syndrome: an oxidative stress disorder. Sleep Med Rev 7:35–51, 2003

Lichstein KL, Nau SD, McCrae CS, et al: Psychological and behavioral treatments for secondary insomnias, in Principles and Practice of Sleep Medicine, 4th Edition. Edited by Kryger MH, Roth T, Dement WC. Philadelphia, PA, Elsevier, 2005, pp 738–748

Lin L, Faraco J, Li R, et al: The sleep disorder canine narcolepsy is caused by a mutation in the hypocrotin (orexin) receptor 2 gene. Cell 98:365–376, 1999

Lindberg E, Carter N, Gislason T, et al: Role of snoring and daytime sleepiness in occupational accidents. Am J Respir Crit Care Med 164:2031–2035, 2001

Lockley SW, Brainard GC, Czeisler CA: High sensitivity of the human circadian melatonin rhythm to resetting by short wavelength light. J Clin Endocrinol Metab 88:4502–4505, 2003

Macey PM, Henderson LA, Macey KE, et al: Brain morphology associated with obstructive sleep apnea. Am J Respir Crit Care Med 166:1382–1387, 2002

Mahowald MW, Cramer Bornemann MA: NREM sleep-arousal parasomnias, in Principles and Practice of Sleep Medicine, 4th Edition. Edited by Kryger MH, Roth T, Dement WC. Philadelphia, PA, Elsevier, 2005, pp 889–896

Mahowald MW, Schenck CH: Evolving concepts of human state dissociation. Arch Ital Biol 139:269–300, 2001

Mahowald MW, Schenck CH: REM sleep parasomnias, in Principles and Practice of Sleep Medicine, 4th Edition. Edited by Kryger MH, Roth T, Dement WC. Philadelphia, PA, Elsevier, 2005, pp 897–916

Mamelak M, Black J, Montplaisir J, et al: A pilot study on the effects of sodium oxybate on sleep architecture and daytime alertness in narcolepsy. Sleep 27:1327–1334, 2004

Marklund M, Stenlund H, Franklin KA: Mandibular advancement devices in 630 men and women with obstructive sleep apnea and snoring: tolerability and predictors of treatment success. Chest 125:1270–1278, 2004

Matsuki K, Juji T, Honda Y: Immunological features of narcolepsy in Japan, in HLA in Narcolepsy. Edited by Honda Y, Juti T. Berlin, Germany, Springer-Verlag, 1988, pp 150–157

Michaud M, Dumont M, Selmaoui B, et al: Circadian rhythm of restless legs syndrome: relationship with biological markers. Ann Neurol 55:372–380, 2004

Mignot E: Genetic and familial aspects of narcolepsy. Neurology 50:S16–S22, 1998

Mignot E: Narcolepsy: Pharmacology, pathophysiology, and genetics, in Principles and Practice of Sleep Medicine, 4th Edition. Edited by Kryger MH, Roth T, Dement WC. Philadelphia, PA, Elsevier, 2005, pp 761–779

Mimeault V, Morin CM: Self-help treatment for insomnia: bibliotherapy with and without professional guidance. J Consult Clin Psychol 67:511–519, 1999

Mitler MM, Aldrich MS, Koob GF, et al: Narcolepsy and its treatment with stimulants: ASDA standards of practice. Sleep 17:352–371, 1994

Mohler H, Fritschy J, Rudolph U: A new benzodiazepine pharmacology. J Pharmacol Exp Ther 300:2–8, 2002

Moldofsky H, Musisi S, Phillipson EA: Treatment of a case of advanced sleep phase syndrome by phase advance chronotherapy. Sleep 9:61–65, 1986

Montplaisir J, Allen RP, Walters AS, et al: Restless legs syndrome and periodic limb movements during sleep, in Principles and Practice of Sleep Medicine, 4th Edition. Edited by Kryger MH, Roth T, Dement WC. Philadelphia, PA, Elsevier, 2005, pp 839–852

Moore RY: Circadian rhythms: basic neurobiology and clinical applications. Annu Rev Med 48:253–266, 1997

Morgenthaler TI, Silber MH: Amnestic sleep-related eating disorder associated with zolpidem. Sleep Med 3:323–327, 2002

Morin CM: Insomnia: Psychological Assessment and Management, 17th Edition. New York, Guilford, 1993

Morin CM, Bootzin RR, Buysse DJ, et al: Psychological and behavioral treatment of insomnia: an update of recent evidence (1998–2004). Sleep 29:1398–1414, 2006

Morin CM, Belanger L, LeBlanc M, et al: The natural history of insomnia: a population-based 3-year longitudinal study. Arch Intern Med 169:447–453, 2009

Moul DE, Buysse DJ, Nofzinger EA, et al: Symptoms reports in severe chronic insomnia. Sleep 25:553–563, 2002

Mundey K, Benloucif S, Harsanyi K, et al: Phase-dependent treatment of delayed sleep phase syndrome with melatonin. Sleep 28:1271–1278, 2005

National Institutes of Health: NIH State-of-the-Science Conference Statement on Manifestations and Management of Chronic Insomnia in Adults. Bethesda, MD, National Institutes of Health, 2005

Neylan TC, Marmar CR, Metzler TJ, et al: Sleep disturbances in the Vietnam generation: findings from a nationally representative sample of male Vietnam veterans. Am J Psychiatry 155:929–933, 1998

Nielsen TA, Zadra A: Nightmares and other common dream disturbances, in Principles and Practice of Sleep Medicine, 4th Edition. Edited by Kryger MH, Roth T, Dement WC. Philadelphia, PA, Elsevier, 2005, pp 926–935

Nishino S, Ripley B, Overeem S, et al: Hypocretin (orexin) deficiency in human narcolepsy. Lancet 355:39–40, 2000

Nofzinger EA: Neuroimaging of sleep and sleep disorders. Curr Neurol Neurosci Rep 6:149–155, 2006

Nofzinger EA, Thase ME, Reynolds CF, et al: Hypersomnia in bipolar depression: a comparison with narcolepsy using the multiple sleep latency test. Am J Psychiatry 148:1177–1181, 1991

Nofzinger EA, Buysse DJ, Germain A, et al: Functional neuroimaging evidence for hyperarousal in insomnia. Am J Psychiatry 161:2126–2131, 2004

Nowell PD, Mazumdar S, Buysse DJ, et al: Benzodiazepines and zolpidem for chronic insomnia: a meta-analysis of treatment efficacy. JAMA 278:2170–2177, 1997

Ohayon MM: Epidemiology of insomnia: What we know and what we still need to learn. Sleep Med Rev 6:97–111, 2002

Ohayon MM, Guilleminault C: Epidemiology of sleep disorders, in Sleep Disorders Medicine: Basic Science, Technical Considerations and Clinical Aspects. Edited by Chokroverty S. Boston, MA, Butterworth-Heinemann, 1999, pp 301–316

Ohayon MM, Roth T: Prevalence of restless legs syndrome and periodic limb movement disorder in the general population. J Psychosom Res 53:547–554, 2002

Ohayon MM, Morselli PL, Guilleminault C: Prevalence of nightmares and their relationship to psychopathology and daytime functioning in insomnia subjects. Sleep 20:340–348, 1997

Ohayon MM, Guilleminault C, Priest RG: Night terrors, sleepwalking, and confusional arousals in the general population: their frequency and relationship to other sleep and mental disorders. J Clin Psychiatry 60:268–276, 1999

Ohayon MM, Carskadon MA, Guilleminault C, et al: Meta-analysis of quantitative sleep parameters from childhood to old age in healthy individuals: developing normative sleep values across the human life span. Sleep 27:1255–1273, 2004

O'Keeffe ST, Gavin K, Lavan JN: Iron status and restless legs syndrome in the elderly. Age Ageing 23:200–203, 1994

Oudiette D, De Cock VC, Lavault S, et al: Nonviolent elaborate behaviors may also occur in REM sleep behavior disorder. Neurology 72(6):551–557, 2009

Overeem S, Mignot E, Van Dijk JG, et al: Clinical features, new pathophysiological insights, and future perspectives. J Clin Neurophysiol 18:78–105, 2001

Ozaki S, Uchiyama M, Shirakawa S, et al: Prolonged interval from body temperature nadir to sleep offset in patients with delayed sleep phase syndrome. Sleep 19:36–40, 1996

Pace-Schott EF, Hobson JA: The neurobiology of sleep: genetics, cellular physiology and subcortical networks. Nat Rev Neurosci 3:591–605, 2002

Pack AI, Black JE, Schwartz JR, et al: Modafinil as adjunct therapy for daytime sleepiness in obstructive sleep apnea. Am J Respir Crit Care Med 164:1675–1681, 2001

Pelayo R, Thorpy MJ, Glovinsky P: Prevalence of delayed sleep phase syndrome among adolescents. Sleep Res 17:392, 1988

Peppard PE, Young T, Palta M, et al: Longitudinal study of moderate weight change and sleep-disordered breathing. JAMA 284:3015–3021, 2000

Perlis ML, Giles DE, Mendelson WB, et al: Psychophysiological insomnia: the behavioural model and a neurocognitive perspective. J Sleep Res 6:179–188, 1997

Perlis ML, McCall WV, Krystal AD, et al: Long-term, nonnightly administration of zolpidem in the treatment of patients with primary insomnia. J Clin Psychiatry 65:1128–1137, 2004

Perlis ML, Smith MT, Pigeon WR: Etiology and pathophysiology of insomnia, in Principles and Practice of Sleep Medicine, 4th Edition. Edited by Kryger MH, Roth T, Dement WC. Philadelphia, PA, Elsevier, 2005, pp 714–725

Piercey MF: Pharmacology of pramipexole, a dopamine D3-preferring agonist useful in treating Parkinson's disease. Clin Neuropharmacol 21:141–151, 1998

Postuma RB, Gagnon JF, Vendette M, et al: Quantifying the risk of neurodegenerative disease in idiopathic REM sleep behavior disorder. Neurology 72(15):1296–1300, 2009

Presser HB: Towards a 24 hour economy. Science 284:1778–1779, 1999

Punjabi NM, Beamer BA: Sleep apnea and metabolic dysfunction, in Principles and Practice of Sleep Medicine, 4th Edition. Edited by Kryger MH, Roth T, Dement WC. Philadelphia, PA, Elsevier, 2005, pp 1034–1042

Punjabi NM, Ahmed MM, Polotsky VY, et al: Sleep-disordered breathing, glucose intolerance, and insulin resistance. Respir Physiol Neurobiol 136:167–178, 2003

Raskind MA, Peskind ER, Kanter ED, et al: Reduction of nightmares and other PTSD symptoms in combat veterans by prazosin: a placebo-controlled study. Am J Psychiatry 160:371–373, 2003

Rechtschaffen A, Kales A: A Manual of Standardized Terminology, Techniques and Scoring System for Sleep Stages of Human Subjects (NIH Publ 204). Washington, DC, U.S. Government Printing Office, Department of Health Education and Welfare, 1968

Regestein QR, Monk TH: Delayed sleep phase syndrome: a review of its clinical aspects. Am J Psychiatry 152:602–608, 1995

Reid KJ, Zee PC: Circadian disorders of the sleep–wake cycle, in Principles and Practice of Sleep Medicine, 4th Edition. Edited by Kryger MH, Roth T, Dement WC. Philadelphia, PA, Elsevier, 2005, pp 691–701

Reid KJ, Chang AM, Dubocovich ML, et al: Familial advanced sleep phase syndrome. Arch Neurol 58:1089–1094, 2001

Reynolds G, Blake DR, Pall HS, et al: Restless leg syndrome and rheumatoid arthritis. Br Med J 292:659–660, 1986

Riemann D, Voderholzer U: Primary insomnia: a risk factor to develop depression? J Affect Disord 76:255–259, 2003

Ritterband LM, Thorndike FP, Gonder-Frederick LA, et al: Efficacy of an Internet-based behavioral intervention for adults with insomnia. Arch Gen Psychiatry 66:692–698, 2009

Roth T, Walsh JK, Krystal A, et al: An evaluation of the efficacy and safety of eszopiclone over 12 months in patients with chronic primary insomnia. Sleep Medicine 6:487–495, 2005

Roth T, Rogowski R, Hull S, et al: Efficacy and safety of doxepin 1 mg, 3 mg, and 6 mg in adults with primary insomnia. Sleep 30:1555–1561, 2007

Sajkov D, Wang T, Saunders NA, et al: Continuous positive airway pressure treatment improves pulmonary hemodynamics in patients with obstructive sleep apnea. Am J Respir Crit Care Med 165:152–158, 2002

Saper CB, Chou TC, Scammell TE: The sleep switch: hypothalamic control of sleep and wakefulness. Trends Neurosci 24:726–731, 2001

Sateia MJ, Doghramji K, Hauri PJ, et al: Evaluation of chronic insomnia: an American Academy of Sleep Medicine review. Sleep 23:243–308, 2000

Schellenberg JB, Maislin G, Schwab RJ: Physical findings and the risk for obstructive sleep apnea: the importance of oropharyngeal structures. Am J Respir Crit Care Med 162:740–748, 2000

Schenck CH, Mahowald MW: Long-term, nightly benzodiazepine treatment of injurious parasomnias and other disorders of disrupted nocturnal sleep in 170 adults. Am J Med 100:333–337, 1996

Schenck CH, Mahowald MW: Parasomnias: managing bizarre sleep-related behavior disorders. Postgrad Med 107:145–156, 2000

Schenck CH, Hurwitz TD, Bundlie SR, et al: Sleep-related eating disorders: polysomnographic correlates of a heterogeneous syndrome distinct from daytime eating disorders. Sleep 14:419–431, 1991

Schenck CH, Hurwitz TD, O'Connor KA, et al: Additional categories of sleep-related eating disorders and the current status of treatment. Sleep 16:457–466, 1993

Schenck CH, Bundlie SR, Mahowald MW: Delayed emergence of a parkinsonian disorder in 38% of 29 older men initially diagnosed with idiopathic rapid eye movement sleep behaviour disorder. Neurology 46:388–393, 1996

Schenck CH, Boyd JL, Mahowald MW: A parasomnia overlap disorder involving sleepwalking, sleep terrors, and REM sleep behavior disorder in 33 polysomnographically confirmed cases. Sleep 20:972–981, 1997

Scott AJ: Shift work and health. Prim Care 27:1057–1079, 2000

Shahar DR, Schulz R, Shahar A, et al: The effect of widowhood on weight change, dietary intake and eating behavior in the elderly population. J Aging Health 13:186–199, 2001

Shapiro CM, Trajanovic NN, Fedoroff JP: Sexsomnia: a new parasomnia? Can J Psychiatry 48:311–317, 2003

Sharkey KM, Fogg LF, Eastman CI: Effects of melatonin administration on daytime sleep after simulated night shift work. J Sleep Res 10:181–192, 2001

Sheldon SH, Kryger MH, Ferber R: Principles and Practice of Pediatric Sleep Medicine. Philadelphia, PA, Elsevier, 2005

Sher AE: Update on upper airway surgery for obstructive sleep apnea. Curr Opin Pulm Med 1:504–511, 1995

Silber MH, Ehrenberg BL, Allen RP, et al: An algorithm for the management of restless legs syndrome. Mayo Clin Proc 79:916–922, 2004

Smith MT, Perlis ML, Park A, et al: Comparative meta-analysis of pharmacotherapy and behavior therapy for persistent insomnia. Am J Psychiatry 159:5–11, 2002

Soldatos CR, Dikeos DG, Whitehead A: Tolerance and rebound insomnia with rapidly eliminated hypnotics: a meta-analysis of sleep laboratory studies. Int Clin Psychopharmacol 14:287–303, 1999

Somers VK, Dyken ME, Clary MP, et al: Sympathetic neural mechanisms in obstructive sleep apnea. J Clin Invest 96:1897–1904, 1995

Spielman AJ, Caruso LS, Glovinsky PB: A behavioral perspective on insomnia treatment. Psychiatr Clin North Am 10:541–553, 1987

Stefansson H, Rye DB, Hicks A, et al: A genetic risk factor for periodic limb movements in sleep. N Engl J Med 357:639–647, 2007

Strollo PJ, Rogers RM: Obstructive sleep apnea. N Engl J Med 334:99–104, 1996

Strollo PJ, Atwood CW, Sanders MH: Medical therapy for obstructive sleep apnea-hypopnea syndrome, in Principles and Practice of Sleep Medicine, 4th Edition. Edited by Kryger MH, Roth T, Dement WC. Philadelphia, PA, Elsevier, 2005, pp 1053–1065

Suhner AG, Murphy PJ, Campbell SS: Failure of timed bright light exposure to alleviate age-related sleep maintenance insomnia. J Am Geriatr Soc 50:617–623, 2002

Suzuki K, Ohida T, Sone T, et al: The prevalence of restless legs syndrome among pregnant women in Japan and the relationship between restless legs syndrome and sleep problems. Sleep 26:673–677, 2003

Szymusiak R, McGinty D: Hypothalamic regulation of sleep and arousal. Ann N Y Acad Sci 1129:275–286, 2008

Telstad W, Sorensen O, Larsen S, et al: Treatment of the restless legs syndrome with carbamazepine: a double blind study. Br Med J 288:444–446, 1984

Teran-Santos J, Jimenez-Gomez A, Cordero-Guevara J: The association between sleep apnea and the risk of traffic accidents. N Engl J Med 340:847–851, 1999

Thannickal TC, Moore RY, Nienhuis R, et al: Reduced number of hypocretin neurons in human narcolepsy. Neuron 27:469–474, 2000

Thomas RE: Benzodiazepine use and motor vehicle accidents: systematic review of reported association. Can Fam Physician 44:799–808, 1998

Thorpy MJ, Korman E, Spielman AJ, et al: Delayed sleep phase syndrome in adolescents. J Adolesc Health 9:22–27, 1988

Tishler PV, Larkin EK, Schluchter MD, et al: Incidence of sleep-disordered breathing in an urban adult population: the relative importance of risk factors in the development of sleep-disordered breathing. JAMA 289:2230–2237, 2003

Toh KL, Jones CR, He Y, et al: An hPer2 phosphorylation site mutation in familial advanced sleep phase syndrome. Science 291:1040–1043, 2001

Toth LA, Opp MR: Sleep and infection, in Sleep Medicine. Edited by Lee-Chiong TL, Sateia MJ, Carskadon MA. Philadelphia, PA, Hanley & Belfus, 2002, pp 77–83

Trenkwalder C, Stiasny K, Pollmacher T, et al: L-dopa therapy of uremic and idiopathic restless legs syndrome: a double-blind, crossover trial. Sleep 18:681–688, 1995

Trenkwalder C, Garcia-Borreguero D, Montagna P, et al: Ropinirole in the treatment of restless legs syndrome: results from the TREAT RLS 1 study, a 12 week, randomised, placebo controlled study in 10 European countries. J Neurol Neurosurg Psychiatry 75:92–97, 2004

Turner RS, D'Amato CJ, Chervin RD, et al: The pathology of REM sleep behavior disorder with comorbid Lewy body dementia. Neurology 55:1730–1732, 2000

Ulfberg J, Nystrom B, Carter N, et al: Prevalence of restless legs syndrome among men aged 18 to 64 years: an association with somatic disease and neuropsychiatric symptoms. Mov Disord 16:1159–1163, 2001

Unruh ML, Levey AS, D'Ambrosio C, et al: Restless legs symptoms among incident dialysis patients: association with lower quality of life and shorter survival. Am J Kidney Dis 43:900–909, 2004

U.S. Modafinil in Narcolepsy Multicenter Study Group: Randomized trial of modafinil for the treatment of pathological somnolence in narcolepsy. Ann Neurol 43:88–97, 1998

U.S. Xyrem Multicenter Study Group: A randomized, double-blind, placebo-controlled multicenter trial comparing effects of three doses of orally administered sodium oxybate with placebo for the treatment of narcolepsy. Sleep 25:42–49, 2002

Veasey SC, Davis CW, Fenik P, et al: Long-term intermittent hypoxia in mice: protracted hypersomnolence with oxidative injury to sleep-wake brain regions. Sleep 27:194–201, 2004

Vermeeren A: Residual effects of hypnotics: epidemiology and clinical implications. CNS Drugs 18:297–328, 2004

Wagner DR: Disorders of the circadian sleep–wake cycle. Neurol Clin 14:651–670, 1996

Walsh JK: Pharmacological management of insomnia. J Clin Psychiatry 65 (suppl):41–45, 2004

Walsh JK, Randazzo AC, Stone KL, et al: Modafinil improves alertness, vigilance, and executive function during simulated night shifts. Sleep 27:434–439, 2004

Walsh JK, Dement WC, Dinges DF: Sleep medicine, public policy, and public health, in Principles and Practice of Sleep Medicine, 4th Edition. Edited by Kryger MH, Roth T, Dement WC. Philadelphia, PA, Elsevier, 2005a, pp 648–656

Walsh JK, Roehrs T, Roth T: Pharmacological treatment of primary insomnia, in Principles and Practice of Sleep Medicine, 4th Edition. Edited by Kryger MH, Roth T, Dement WC. Philadelphia, PA, Elsevier, 2005b, pp 749–760

Walters AS: Toward a better definition of the restless legs syndrome. The International Restless Legs Syndrome Study Group. Mov Disord 10:634–642, 1995

Walters AS, Rye DB: Review of the relationship of restless legs syndrome and periodic limb movements in sleep to hypertension, heart disease, and stroke. Sleep 32(5):589–597, 2009

Weaver TE, George CFP: Cognition and performance in patients with obstructive sleep apnea, in Principles and Practice of Sleep Medicine, 4th Edition. Edited by Kryger MH, Roth T, Dement WC. Philadelphia, PA, Elsevier, 2005, pp 1023–1033

Weitzman ED, Czeisler CA, Coleman RM, et al: Delayed sleep phase syndrome: a chronobiological disorder with sleep-onset insomnia. Arch Gen Psychiatry 38:737–746, 1981

Winkelman JW: The evoked heart rate response to periodic leg movements of sleep. Sleep 22:575–580, 1999

Winkelman JW: Treatment of nocturnal eating syndrome and sleep-related eating disorder with topiramate. Sleep Med 4:243–246, 2003

Winkelman JW: Efficacy and tolerability of topiramate in the treatment of sleep-related eating disorder: a retrospective case series. J Clin Psychiatry 67:1729–1734, 2006

Winkelman JW, James L: Serotonergic antidepressants are associated with REM sleep without atonia. Sleep 27:317–321, 2004

Winkelman JW, Johnston L: Augmentation and tolerance with long-term pramipexole treatment of restless legs syndrome (RLS). Sleep Med 5:9–14, 2004

Winkelman JW, Chertow GM, Lazarus JM: Restless legs syndrome in end-stage renal disease. Am J Kidney Dis 28:372–378, 1996

Winkelman JW, Herzog DB, Fava M: The prevalence of sleep-related eating disorder in psychiatric and non-psychiatric populations. Psychol Med 29:1461–1466, 1999

Winkelman JW, Sethi KD, Kushida CA, et al: Efficacy and safety of pramipexole in restless legs syndrome. Neurology 67:1034–1039, 2006

Winkelmann J, Wetter TC, Collado-Seidel V, et al: Clinical characteristics and frequency of the hereditary restless legs syndrome in a population of 300 patients. Sleep 23:597–602, 2000

Winkelmann J, Schormair B, Lichtner P, et al: Genome-wide association study of restless legs syndrome identifies common variants in three genomic regions. Nat Genet 39:1000–1006, 2007

Wisor JP, Eriksson KS: Dopaminergic-adrenergic interactions in the wake-promoting mechanism of modafinil. Neuroscience 132:1027–1034, 2005

Woods J, Winger G: Current benzodiazepine issues. Psychopharmacology 118:107–115; discussion 118, 1995

World Health Organization: International Statistical Classification of Diseases and Related Health Problems, 10th Revision. Geneva, Switzerland, World Health Organization, 1992

Xu Y, Padiath QS, Shapiro RE, et al: Functional consequences of a CKIdelta mutation causing familial advanced sleep phase syndrome. Nature 434:640–644, 2005

Young T, Palta M, Dempsey J, et al: The occurrence of sleep-disordered breathing among middle-aged adults. N Engl J Med 328:1230–1235, 1993

Young T, Peppard PE, Gottlieb DJ: Epidemiology of obstructive sleep apnea: a population health perspective. Am J Respir Crit Care Med 165:1217–1239, 2002

Zammit G, Erman M, Wang-Weigand S, et al: Evaluation of the efficacy and safety of ramelteon in subjects with chronic insomnia. J Clin Sleep Med 3:495–504, 2007

Zonato AI, Bittencourt LR, Martinho FL, et al: Association of systematic head and neck physical examination with severity of obstructive sleep apnea-hypopnea syndrome. Laryngoscope 113:973–980, 2003

14

EATING DISORDERS

Anorexia Nervosa, Bulimia Nervosa, and Obesity

Katherine A. Halmi, M.D.

The eating disorders *anorexia nervosa* and *bulimia nervosa* and the condition of *obesity* have been known since earliest times in Western civilization. Well-documented case reports of anorexia nervosa are found in literature describing early Christian saints, and binge eating and purging behavior are certainly described in Roman civilization.

The eating disorders are best conceptualized as syndromes and are therefore classified on the basis of the clusters of symptoms they present.

Physiology and Behavioral Pharmacology of Eating
A Systems Conceptualization

Eating behavior is now known to reflect an interaction between an organism's physiological state and environmental conditions. Salient physiological variables include the balance of various neuropeptides and neurotransmitters, metabolic state, metabolic rate, condition of the gastrointestinal tract, amount of storage tissue, and sensory receptors for taste and smell. Environmental conditions include features of the food such as taste, texture, novelty, accessibility, and nutritional composition as well as other external conditions such as ambient temperature, presence of other people, and stress (Blundell and Hill 1986).

Neurotransmitters

Biogenic Amines

Underweight anorexia nervosa patients and persons without eating disorders in times of dieting have reduced central and peripheral norepinephrine activity (Pirke 1996). This is confirmed by hypothermia, bradycardia, and hypotension.

Serotonin, an indoleamine, has been shown to facilitate satiety (Hoebel 1977). The serotonin type 2A (5-HT$_{2A}$) receptor is a G protein–coupled receptor that controls signal transduction by activating phospholipase C (Eison and Mullins 1996). Properties of the 5-HT$_{2A}$ receptor such as ligand affinity receptor downregulation or signal transduction could be affected by any disturbance or alteration in a genetic coding variant for this receptor. Such an aberration may contribute to the disturbed and disordered eating behavior in anorexia nervosa and bulimia nervosa.

Dopamine seems to play a more complicated role in eating behavior. There is evidence of increased hypothalamic dopamine turnover during feeding. This finding suggests that central dopamine mechanisms mediate the rewarding effects of food as they mediate the rewarding effects of intracranial self-stimulation and the self-stimulation of psychoactive drugs.

Peptides and Opioids

Corticotropin-releasing factor (CRF) acts within the paraventricular nucleus (PVN) to inhibit feeding. Norepinephrine seems to inhibit the CRF inhibitory feeding effect. The pancreatic polypeptide neuropeptide Y increases both food and water intake when injected into the PVN. Another pancreatic polypeptide, peptide YY, is a more potent stimulator of feeding than neuropeptide Y (Morley and Levine 1985).

Opioid antagonism decreases feeding in many species but has no effect in reducing food intake in other species. Under some physiological conditions, such as starving or insulin-induced hypoglycemia, naloxone fails to inhibit feeding. Stress-induced eating is probably driven by activation of the opioid system. Dynorphin, an endogenous κ opioid receptor ligand, enhances feeding.

Peripheral Satiety Network

Leptin is a protein hormone secreted by adipose tissue cells and believed to act as an afferent signal and regulator of body fat stores (Zhang et al. 1994). Leptin is positively correlated with fat mass in humans in all weight ranges (Considine et al. 1996). Underweight patients with anorexia nervosa have significantly reduced plasma and cerebrospinal fluid (CSF) leptin concentrations compared with normal-weight control subjects (Mantzoros et al. 1997). These levels reach normal values with weight restoration. Because acute fasting-induced weight loss provokes a decline in leptin concentration that is disproportionate to the amount of fat loss (Boden et al. 1996), it has been hypothesized that leptin is a protecting regulator against starvation.

Ghrelin is a gastrointestinal peptide secreted in the stomach that indirectly stimulates hunger. Ghrelin levels increase with food restriction (Gualillo et al. 2002). Levels peak prior to mealtime and decline with feeding and thus seem to have a role in short-term feeding (Cummings et al. 2001). Ghrelin levels are elevated in underweight anorexia nervosa patients and decrease with weight gain; levels are negatively correlated with body mass index (BMI) (Le Roux et al. 2005).

Anorexia Nervosa

Definition

Anorexia nervosa is a disorder characterized by preoccupation with body weight and food, behavior directed toward losing weight, peculiar patterns of handling food, weight loss, intense fear of gaining weight,

---

Table 14–1. DSM-IV-TR diagnostic criteria for anorexia nervosa

---

A. Refusal to maintain body weight at or above a minimally normal weight for age and height (e.g., weight loss leading to maintenance of body weight less than 85% of that expected; or failure to make expected weight gain during period of growth, leading to body weight less than 85% of that expected).

B. Intense fear of gaining weight or becoming fat, even though underweight.

C. Disturbance in the way in which one's body weight or shape is experienced, undue influence of body weight or shape on self-evaluation, or denial of the seriousness of the current low body weight.

D. In postmenarcheal females, amenorrhea, i.e., the absence of at least three consecutive menstrual cycles. (A woman is considered to have amenorrhea if her periods occur only following hormone, e.g., estrogen, administration.)

Specify type:

Restricting type: during the current episode of anorexia nervosa, the person has not regularly engaged in binge-eating or purging behavior (i.e., self-induced vomiting or the misuse of laxatives, diuretics, or enemas)

Binge-eating/purging type: during the current episode of anorexia nervosa, the person has regularly engaged in binge-eating or purging behavior (i.e., self-induced vomiting or the misuse of laxatives, diuretics, or enemas)

---

disturbance of body image, and amenorrhea. DSM-IV-TR (American Psychiatric Association 2000) criteria for anorexia nervosa are included in Table 14–1.

Clinical Features

Individuals with anorexia nervosa typically express an intense fear of gaining weight, tend to be preoccupied with thoughts of food, and worry irrationally about fatness. Denial of their own clearly observable symptoms is characteristic of anorexic patients.

Anorexic patients' fear that they are gaining weight exists even in the face of increasing cachexia, and they characteristically show disinterest in and even resistance to treatment. Some individuals with anorexia will develop rigorous exercise programs. Self-induced vomiting and laxative and diuretic abuse are other purging behaviors by which anorexic persons attempt to lose weight. Weight loss and a refusal to maintain body weight over a minimal normal weight for age and height are the most characteristic features of this disorder. Anorexic individuals have a disturbance in the way in which they experience their body weight and

shape. They often fail to recognize that their degree of emaciation is dangerous.

Amenorrhea can appear before noticeable weight loss has occurred. Poor sexual adjustment is frequently present in patients with anorexia.

Patients with anorexia nervosa can be divided into two groups: those who binge eat and purge and those who merely restrict food intake to lose weight. There is a relatively frequent association with impulsive behavior such as suicide attempts, self-mutilation, stealing, and substance abuse (including alcohol abuse) among bulimic anorexic individuals, who are also less likely to be regressed in their sexual activity and may in fact be promiscuous. Bulimic anorexic patients are more likely to have discrete personality disorder diagnoses (Halmi 1987).

Medical Complications

Most of the physiological and metabolic changes in anorexia nervosa are secondary to the starvation state or purging behavior and are reversed with nutritional rehabilitation (Table 14–2). Individuals with anorexia nervosa who engage in self-induced vomiting or

Table 14-2. Medical complications of anorexia nervosa

Cardiovascular
    Bradycardia
    Orthostatic hypotension
    Arrhythmias
    Electrocardiogram changes—QTc
        prolongation
    ST–T wave abnormalities

Central nervous system
    Peripheral neuropathy
    Enlarged ventricles
    Decreased gray and white matter
    Cognitive impairment

Endocrine/metabolic
    Hypothermia
    Amenorrhea
    Hypokalemia
    Electrolyte abnormalities
    Hypercholesterolemia

Gastrointestinal
    Vomiting
    Constipation
    Diarrhea
    Parotid hyperplasia
    Increased serum amylase
    Abnormal liver function tests

Renal
    Hypokalemic nephropathy

Hematological
    Anemia
    Leukopenia with relative lymphocytosis

Integument
    Lanugo
    Carotenoderma

Muscular
    Muscle wasting
    Creatine kinase abnormalities

Pulmonary
    Decreased pulmonary capacity

Reproductive
    Amenorrhea, secondary or primary
    Decreased serum estrogen in females
    Decreased serum testosterone in males
    Loss of libido

Table 14-2. Medical complications of anorexia nervosa *(continued)*

Skeletal
    Osteopenia
    Osteoporosis
    Pathological stress fractures

who abuse laxatives and diuretics are liable to develop hypokalemic alkalosis. These patients often have elevated serum bicarbonate levels, hypochloremia, and hypokalemia. Patients with electrolyte disturbances have physical symptoms of weakness and lethargy and, at times, have cardiac arrhythmias. The latter condition may threaten sudden cardiac arrest, a frequent cause of death in patients who purge.

Elevation of serum enzymes reflects fatty degeneration of the liver and is observed both in the emaciated anorexic phase and during refeeding. Elevated serum cholesterol levels tend to occur more frequently in younger patients. Carotenemia is often observed in malnourished anorexic patients. All of these physiological changes reverse themselves with nutritional rehabilitation (Halmi and Falk 1981).

Epidemiology, Course, and Prognosis

An incidence study conducted in northeastern Scotland (Eagles et al. 1995) reported that between 1965 and 1991, the incidence of anorexia nervosa increased nearly sixfold (from 3 per 100,000 to 17 cases per 100,000 population). These studies probably underestimate the true incidence, because not all cases come to the attention of health care providers. Rooney et al. (1995) surveyed patients recruited for study from the level of primary care in England. The prevalence among female patients ages 15–29 years was 115.4 cases per 100,000 population (0.1%). A more recent U.S. survey that followed high school students to age 24 years found the incidence of eating disorders to be 2.8% by age 18 years.

The lifetime prevalence of anorexia nervosa was 0.6% (Lewinsohn et al. 2000). Only 4%–6% of the anorexic population is male (Halmi 1974).

In a community epidemiological survey in Canada, Woodside et al. (2001) found that men with eating disorders were very similar to women with the same diagnoses.

Generally speaking, poor outcome in the studies mentioned earlier was associated with longer duration of illness, older age at onset, previous admissions to psychiatric hospitals, poor childhood social adjustment, premorbid personality difficulties, and disturbed relationships between patients and other family members.

Etiology and Pathogenesis

A specific etiology and pathogenesis leading to the development of anorexia nervosa are unknown. Anorexia nervosa begins after a period of severe food deprivation (Table 14–3).

The psychological theories concerning the causes of anorexia have centered mostly on phobic mechanisms and cognitive formulations. Crisp (1976) postulated that anorexia nervosa constitutes a phobic avoidance response to food resulting from the sexual and social tension generated by the physical changes associated with puberty. A cognitive and perceptual developmental defect was postulated by Bruch (1962) as the cause of anorexia nervosa. She described the disturbances of body image (denial of emaciation), disturbances in perception (lack of recognition or denial of fatigue, weakness, hunger), and a sense of ineffectiveness as being caused by untoward learning experiences.

Because central neurotransmitters such as dopamine, serotonin, and norepinephrine all influence appetite, satiety (Table 14–4), and eating behavior, it is reasonable to postulate that a dysregulation of these neurotransmitters is present in patients with anorexia (Table 14–5). The serotonin 1A (5-HT$_{1A}$) receptor is associated with anxiety and feeding behavior. A study using positron emission tomography (PET) imaging and a specific 5-

Table 14–3. Common reasons for severe food deprivation

Willful dieting for the purpose of being more attractive

Willful dieting for the purpose of being more professionally competent (e.g., ballet dancers, gymnasts, jockeys)

Food restriction secondary to severe stress

Food restriction secondary to severe illness and/or surgery

Involuntary starvation

HT$_{1A}$ receptor antagonist, [carbonyl-^{11}C] WAY-100635, found that women who had recovered from the bulimic type of anorexia nervosa had significantly increased binding potential in the cingulate, lateral mesial temporal, lateral medial orbital frontal, parietal, and prefrontal cortical regions and in the dorsal raphe compared with control subjects. No differences were found for women recovered from restricting-type anorexia nervosa relative to control subjects. In women with the restricting type of anorexia, the 5-HT$_{1A}$ postsynaptic receptor binding in the mesial temporal and subgenual cingulate regions was positively correlated with harm avoidance (Bailer et al. 2005). This altered serotonergic function may be related to the anxiety symptoms that persist after recovery from anorexia nervosa. Another study using PET

Table 14–4. Satiety peptides

Hypothalamic neuropeptides
    Corticotropin-releasing hormone
    Thyrotropin-releasing hormone
    α-Melanocyte-stimulating hormone
    Neurotensin
    Somatostatin
    Leptin
Gut-related peptides
    Cholecystokinin
    Peptide YY
    Bombesin
    Gastrin-releasing peptide

Table 14–5. Neurotransmitters and neuropeptides in anorexia nervosa

Hormone	Effect on eating behavior	Functional status in anorexia nervosa	Clinical manifestations
Norepinephrine	Inhibits the CRF-inhibiting feeding effect	↓	Decreased food intake
Serotonin	Facilitates satiety	↑	Feeling full after a minimal intake of food
Dopamine	Mediates rewarding effects of food	↓	?
Corticotropin-releasing factor (CRF)	Inhibits feeding; stimulates motor activity	↑	Decreased food intake; increased motor activity
Neuropeptide Y	Increases food intake	↑	Should stimulate feeding, but ineffective in anorexia nervosa
Cholecystokinin	Attenuates feeding	↑	Decreased meal size

Note. This table is, of course, oversimplified; actual phenomena are more complex.

showed that women recovered from anorexia nervosa had significantly higher [^{11}C] raclopride binding potential in the anteroventral striatum compared with control subjects. The binding potential was positively related to harm avoidance in the dorsal raphe and dorsal putamen. The authors postulated that individuals with anorexia nervosa may have a dopamine-related disturbance of reward mechanisms contributing to their altered hedonics of eating and their ascetic, anhedonic temperament (Frank et al. 2005).

There is increasing evidence for genetic influences in the development of anorexia nervosa. Family studies have shown significantly increased prevalence of eating disorders in relatives of patients with anorexia nervosa compared with relatives of control subjects (Lilenfeld et al. 1998; Strober et al. 1985). The first genomewide linkage analysis of families in which at least two affected relatives had the diagnosis of restricting anorexia nervosa without binge eating or purging behavior showed a peak multipoint nonparametric linkage score of 3.45, suggesting evidence for the presence of an anorexia nervosa susceptibility locus on chromosome 1p (Grice et al. 2002). Finding suggestive linkage sites is of interest because these regions may harbor excellent candidate genes for liability for eating disorders. A subsequent study in this same eating disorder population showed serotonin 1D (5-HT$_{1D}$) and delta opioid receptor loci in the first chromosome linkage region described earlier to exhibit significant association to anorexia nervosa (Bergen et al. 2003). Dopaminergic neuronal function modulates feeding behavior, motor activity, and reward-motivated behavior. For this reason the authors of this study examined in the same eating disorder population the presence of functional polymorphisms or changes at the dopamine D$_2$ receptor. Polymorphisms or changes in the D$_2$ receptor were significantly associated (exhibited significant linkage and association) to the anorexia nervosa diagnosis.

Treatment

A multifaceted treatment endeavor with medical management and behavioral, individual, cognitive, and family therapy is necessary to treat anorexia nervosa (Table 14–6). The first step in treatment is to obtain the anorexic patient's cooperation in a treatment program.

The immediate aim of treatment should be to restore the patient's nutritional state to normal. Mere emaciation or the state of being mildly underweight (15%–25% below normal weight) can cause irritability, depression, preoccupation with food, and sleep disturbance. It is exceedingly difficult to achieve behavioral change with psychotherapy in a patient who is experiencing the psychological effects of emaciation.

The more severely ill patient with anorexia may present an extremely difficult medical-management challenge and should be hospitalized and undergo daily monitoring of weight, food and calorie intake, and urine output. In the patient who is vomiting, frequent assessment of serum electrolytes is necessary. Behavior therapy is most effective in the medical management and nutritional rehabilitation of the patient with anorexia, although there are times when other target behaviors can be changed with this approach. Behavior therapy can be used in both outpatient and inpatient settings.

A family analysis should be done on all patients with anorexia who are living with their families. On the basis of this analysis, a clinical judgment should be made regarding what type of family therapy or counseling is clinically advisable. In some cases, family therapy will not be possible. However, in those cases, issues of family relationships must be dealt with in individual therapy and, in some cases, in brief counseling sessions with immediate family members. A controlled family therapy study by Russell et al. (1987) showed that patients with anorexia younger than 18 years benefited from family therapy and patients older than 18 years did worse in family therapy compared with the

Table 14–6. Treatment of anorexia nervosa

Type of treatment	Key elements	Measurements	Indications
Medical management	Weight restoration	Weight (outpatient—weekly; inpatient—daily)	Below normal weight for age and height by ≥10%
	Rehydration and correction of serum electrolytes	Serum electrolytes	History of vomiting, laxative abuse, severe restriction of food and fluids
Behavior therapy	Positive reinforcements for weight gain	Weight (outpatient—weekly; inpatient—daily)	Underweight
	Response prevention for binge eating and purging	Serum electrolytes and serum amylase	Weakness, puffy cheeks—parotid enlargement, scars on dorsum of hands, fainting spells
Cognitive therapy	Operationalizing beliefs, evaluating automatic thoughts, prospective hypothesis testing, examination of underlying assumptions	Assessment of distorted cognitions (e.g., all-or-none/black-or-white thinking), feeling fat, self-worth measured solely by body image, pervasive sense of ineffectiveness except in losing weight	Disturbance in way one's body weight or shape is experienced; denial of seriousness of low body weight; relentless pursuit of thinness for control of environment
Family therapy	Family counseling or therapy format based on needs of specific family	Analysis of family functioning, roles, and interactions	If patient is living with family, some type of family counseling or therapy is essential
Pharmacotherapy Chlorpromazine	Liquid form, start low doses, such as 10 mg tid, and gradually increase	Complete blood count, lying and standing blood pressure	Severely delusional, overactive, hospitalized patients
Cyproheptadine	Liquid form, start 4 mg bid and increase to 8 mg tid if necessary	Complete blood count with platelets	Severely overactive anorexic patient who does not binge and purge
Fluoxetine	Preferable to use after weight restoration because of tendency to induce arousal	Complete blood count, observation of total sleep and activity	Severely obsessive-compulsive behaviors related or unrelated to eating disorders, severe depression

Table 14–6. Treatment of anorexia nervosa *(continued)*

Type of treatment	Key elements	Measurements	Indications
Clomipramine	Necessary to start in very low doses because of hypotension side effects; preferable to use after weight restoration	Complete blood count, lying and standing blood pressure, electrocardiogram	Severely obsessive-compulsive behaviors
Tricyclic antidepressants	Necessary to start in very low doses because of hypotension side effects; preferable to use after weight restoration	Complete blood count, lying and standing blood pressure, electrocardiogram	Severe depression

control therapy. A subsequent study by LeGrange et al. (1992) compared conjoint family therapy in which the whole family was treated together and a family counseling in which parents were treated separately from their daughter. Both treatments were brief, with an average of nine sessions over a 6-month period. The patients were adolescents, ages 12–17 years. A 32-week assessment showed that the two groups did not differ in their weight, which was in the normal range. A subsequent study with 40 patients replicated these results (Dare and Eisler 2002).

Drugs can be useful adjuncts in the treatment of anorexia nervosa. The first drug used in treating anorexia was chlorpromazine. This medication is especially effective in patients with anorexia who are severely obsessive-compulsive. No controlled, double-blind study has been done to prove definitely the efficacy of chlorpromazine in inducing weight gain in persons with anorexia. This is surprising, given that it was the first drug used and was the preferred drug for most severely ill anorexic patients for many years, especially in Europe.

More recently, atypical antipsychotics have been studied in acutely ill anorexia nervosa patients. A 10-week open-label trial evaluated olanzapine (10 mg/day) in 18 patients with anorexia nervosa. Four of the 18 patients dropped out, and 10 of the 14 patients who completed the study gained an average of 8.75 pounds; the other 4 lost a mean of 2.25 pounds. Olanzapine plasma levels showed that compliance seemed to affect outcome of weight gain. Those patients who lost weight had negligible levels of olanzapine (Powers et al. 2002). Case reports for risperidone show a positive outcome on weight gain.

Another category of drugs frequently used in the treatment of anorexia nervosa is the antidepressants. A double-blind study in which 72 patients with anorexia were randomly assigned to amitriptyline, cyproheptadine (an antihistaminic drug), and placebo therapy showed that both cyproheptadine

and amitriptyline had a marginal effect in decreasing the number of days necessary to achieve a normal weight. Cyproheptadine had an unexpected antidepressant effect demonstrated by a significant decrease in scores on the Hamilton Rating Scale for Depression (Halmi et al. 1986). In the bulimic subgroups of patients with anorexia, cyproheptadine had a negative effect compared with both placebo and amitriptyline. This differential effect within the bulimic anorexic subgroups indicates a real medical distinction and appears to justify this subgrouping. Cyproheptadine has the advantage of not having the tricyclic antidepressant side effects of reducing blood pressure and increasing heart rate. This makes it especially attractive for use in emaciated individuals with anorexia.

Acceptance of treatment and relatively high dropout rates pose a major problem for research in the treatment of anorexia nervosa. In a study of 122 anorexia nervosa patients randomly assigned to cognitive-behavioral therapy (CBT), fluoxetine, or their combination for a 1-year treatment, the overall dropout rate was 46%. Treatment acceptance (defined as staying in treatment for at least 5 weeks) occurred in 73% of the randomized cases. Of the 41 patients assigned to medication alone, acceptance occurred in 56% and in the other two groups the acceptance rate was 81%. This study showed that anorexia nervosa patients will not accept medication unless it is combined with psychotherapy. Among patients who accepted treatment, those with high self-esteem were more likely than those with low self-esteem to complete treatment (Halmi et al. 2005).

A multifaceted treatment approach is necessary for effective care of patients with anorexia nervosa. As medical rehabilitation proceeds, an associated improvement in psychological state occurs. Behavioral contingencies are useful for inducing weight gain and changing the medical condition of the patient. Cyproheptadine may be helpful in facilitating weight gain and decreasing depressive symptomatology in the restricting anorexic patient. If an anorexic patient has a predominance of depressive symptoms and is within 80% of a normal weight range, fluoxetine should be useful for treating the depression.

Severely obsessive-compulsive, anxious, and agitated anorexic patients are likely to require chlorpromazine or an atypical antipsychotic medication such as risperidone or olanzapine. All patients need individual cognitive psychotherapy. Family therapy is essential for children younger than 18 years of age and is equally effective in conjoint or separated format. Effectively treating adolescents before the age of 18 years is the best way to prevent chronic anorexia nervosa.

Bulimia Nervosa

Definition

Bulimia is a term that means "binge eating." This behavior has become a common practice among female students in universities and,

more recently, in high schools. Not all persons who engage in binge eating require a psychiatric diagnosis. Bulimia can occur in anorexia nervosa; when this happens, the patient, under the DSM-IV-TR system, should have a diagnosis of *anorexia nervosa, binge-eating/purging type*. Bulimia also can occur in a normal-weight condition associated with psychological symptomatology. In that case, a diagnosis of *bulimia nervosa* applies (Table 14–7). Normal-weight bingeing and purging patients can fall into two categories: 1) normal-weight bulimic patients who have never had a history of anorexia nervosa and 2) those who have had a history of anorexia nervosa. Unfortunately, the DSM-IV-TR classification system does not separate these two subgroups of bulimic patients. The term *bulimia nervosa* implies a psychiatric impairment and therefore is a better label than simply *bulimia*.

Bulimia is also encountered in DSM-IV-TR *binge-eating disorder* (BED), which did not exist in DSM-III-R (American Psychiatric Association 1987). This disorder is listed as an example under the category "Eating Disorder

---

Table 14–7. DSM-IV-TR diagnostic criteria for bulimia nervosa

A. Recurrent episodes of binge eating. An episode of binge eating is characterized by both of the following:
  (1) eating, in a discrete period of time (e.g., within any 2-hour period), an amount of food that is definitely larger than most people would eat during a similar period of time and under similar circumstances
  (2) a sense of lack of control over eating during the episode (e.g., a feeling that one cannot stop eating or control what or how much one is eating)

B. Recurrent inappropriate compensatory behavior in order to prevent weight gain, such as self-induced vomiting; misuse of laxatives, diuretics, enemas, or other medications; fasting; or excessive exercise.

C. The binge eating and inappropriate compensatory behaviors both occur, on average, at least twice a week for 3 months.

D. Self-evaluation is unduly influenced by body shape and weight.

E. The disturbance does not occur exclusively during episodes of anorexia nervosa.

Specify type:

Purging type: during the current episode of bulimia nervosa, the person has regularly engaged in self-induced vomiting or the misuse of laxatives, diuretics, or enemas

Nonpurging type: during the current episode of bulimia nervosa, the person has used other inappropriate compensatory behaviors, such as fasting or excessive exercise, but has not regularly engaged in self-induced vomiting or the misuse of laxatives, diuretics, or enemas

---

Table 14–8. DSM-IV-TR diagnostic criteria for eating disorder not otherwise specified

---

The eating disorder not otherwise specified category is for disorders of eating that do not meet the criteria for any specific eating disorder. Examples include

1. For females, all of the criteria for anorexia nervosa are met except that the individual has regular menses.
2. All of the criteria for anorexia nervosa are met except that, despite significant weight loss, the individual's current weight is in the normal range.
3. All of the criteria for bulimia nervosa are met except that the binge eating and inappropriate compensatory mechanisms occur at a frequency of less than twice a week or for a duration of less than 3 months.
4. The regular use of inappropriate compensatory behavior by an individual of normal body weight after eating small amounts of food (e.g., self-induced vomiting after the consumption of two cookies).
5. Repeatedly chewing and spitting out, but not swallowing, large amounts of food.
6. Binge-eating disorder: recurrent episodes of binge eating in the absence of the regular use of inappropriate compensatory behaviors characteristic of bulimia nervosa (see Table 14–9 for suggested research criteria).

Not Otherwise Specified" (Tables 14–8 and 14–9). Insufficient data are currently available to make BED a distinct Axis I diagnosis. Preliminary field studies show that most persons who meet criteria for BED are obese. In the next few years, epidemiological studies will determine whether BED is a distinct disorder or merely the nonpurging type of bulimia.

Clinical Features

Bulimia nervosa usually begins after a period of dieting of a few weeks to a year or longer. The dieting may or may not have been successful in achieving weight loss. Most binge-eating episodes are followed by self-induced vomiting. Episodes are less frequently followed by use of laxatives. A minority of bulimic patients use diuretics for weight control.

Most bulimic patients have depressive signs and symptoms. They have problems with interpersonal relationships, self-concept, and impulsive behaviors and show high levels of anxiety and compulsivity. Chemical dependency is not unusual in this disorder, alcohol abuse being the most common. Bulimic persons will abuse amphetamines to reduce their appetite and to lose weight. Impulsive stealing usually occurs af-

ter the onset of binge eating; however, about one-fourth of patients actually begin stealing before the onset of bulimia. Food, clothing, and jewelry are the items most commonly stolen.

Medical Complications

Patients with bulimia nervosa who engage in self-induced vomiting and abuse purgatives or diuretics are susceptible to hypokalemic alkalosis. These patients have electrolyte abnormalities, including elevated serum bicarbonate levels, hypochloremia, hypokalemia, and, in a few cases, low serum bicarbonate levels indicating a metabolic acidosis. The latter is particularly true among individuals who abuse laxatives. It is important to remember that fasting can promote dehydration, which results in volume depletion. This can promote generation of aldosterone, which promotes further potassium excretion from the kidneys. Thus, there can be an indirect renal loss of potassium as well as a direct loss through self-induced vomiting. Patients with electrolyte disturbances have physical symptoms of weakness and lethargy and at times have cardiac arrhythmias. The latter, of course, can lead to a sudden cardiac arrest. Patients with bulimia nervosa can have se-

---

Table 14–9. **DSM-IV-TR research criteria for binge-eating disorder**

A. Recurrent episodes of binge eating. An episode of binge eating is characterized by both of the following:
   (1) eating, in a discrete period of time (e.g., within any 2-hour period), an amount of food that is definitely larger than most people would eat in a similar period of time under similar circumstances
   (2) a sense of lack of control over eating during the episode (e.g., a feeling that one cannot stop eating or control what or how much one is eating)
B. The binge-eating episodes are associated with three (or more) of the following:
   (1) eating much more rapidly than normal
   (2) eating until feeling uncomfortably full
   (3) eating large amounts of food when not feeling physically hungry
   (4) eating alone because of being embarrassed by how much one is eating
   (5) feeling disgusted with oneself, depressed, or very guilty after overeating
C. Marked distress regarding binge eating is present.
D. The binge eating occurs, on average, at least 2 days a week for 6 months.
Note: The method of determining frequency differs from that used for bulimia nervosa; future research should address whether the preferred method of setting a frequency threshold is counting the number of days on which binges occur or counting the number of episodes of binge eating.
E. The binge eating is not associated with the regular use of inappropriate compensatory behaviors (e.g., purging, fasting, excessive exercise) and does not occur exclusively during the course of anorexia nervosa or bulimia nervosa.

---

vere attrition and erosion of the teeth, causing an irritating sensitivity, pathological pulp exposures, loss of integrity of the dental arches, diminished masticatory ability, and an unaesthetic appearance.

Cardiac failure caused by cardiomyopathy from ipecac intoxication is a medical emergency that is being reported more frequently and that usually results in death. Symptoms of precardial pain, dyspnea, and generalized muscle weakness associated with hypotension, tachycardia, and abnormalities on the electrocardiogram should alert one to possible ipecac intoxication. Other laboratory findings may include elevated liver enzymes and an increased erythrocyte sedimentation rate. Obviously, at this point the patient should be under a cardiologist's care. An echocardiogram will show a cardiomyopathy contraction pattern associated with congestive heart failure.

A summary of medical complications of bulimia nervosa is presented in Table 14–10.

Epidemiology, Course, and Prognosis

There have been only a few incidence studies of bulimia nervosa. This is not surprising, given the fact that this disorder emerged only in 1980 as the distinct diagnostic entity presented in DSM-III (American Psychiatric Association 1980). The bulimia nervosa diagnostic criteria have been revised every few years, and this may account for the disparity in reported prevalence rates for this disorder. Studies that used strict criteria found prevalence rates between 1 and 3.8 per 100 females (Hart and Ollendick 1985; Schotte and Stunkard 1987). In a study combining surveys and interviews of women in the first year of college, Kurth et al. (1995) found the prevalence of bulimia nervosa to be 2%. In a Canadian community sample in which a structured interview was used, prevalence rates of this disorder were 1% (Garfinkel et al. 1995). The percentage of males in the bulimia nervosa

Table 14-10. Medical complications of bulimia nervosa

Behavioral and physical aberrations	Physiological disturbances
Binge eating	Acute dilatation of stomach—shock
Self-induced vomiting	Esophageal tears—shock; dehydration
	Metabolic alkalosis—hypochloremia, hypokalemia, weakness, lethargy
	Cardiac arrhythmias—cardiac arrest
	Erosion of dental enamel—caries, exposure of pulp
Parotid gland enlargement (self-induced vomiting or excessive gum chewing)	Elevated serum amylase
Ipecac use	Hypotension, tachycardia, electrocardiographic abnormalities, elevated liver enzymes

population varies between 10% and 15%. In most studies, the average age at onset of bulimia nervosa is 18 years (range: 12–35 years).

Combining the results of meta-analyses by Keel and Mitchell (1997) and Nielsen (2001) yields a corrected mortality rate for bulimia nervosa of 0.4% (11 deaths in 2,692 patients), which indicates that persons with bulimia nervosa have a 1.5 increase in mortality risk. Little information is available on the natural course of this disorder and on outcome predictors.

Etiology and Pathogenesis

Fairburn and Cooper (1984) found that a rigid diet was the most commonly reported precipitant of binge-eating behavior and that a gross bingeing bout was the most common precipitant for vomiting behavior. This finding may shed some light on the physiological mechanisms involved in binge eating and purging. For example, the period of strict dieting may influence peptide and neurotransmitter secretion, which may in turn affect appetite and satiety mechanisms. Studies of satiety responses in patients with eating disorders have shown that the perceptions of hunger and satiety are disturbed in patients who binge and purge (Halmi and Sunday 1991).

Studies of recovered bulimia nervosa women (Kaye et al. 2001), using PET [^{18}F] altanserin, a specific 5-HT$_{2A}$ receptor antago-

nist, found a significant reduction in bilateral medial orbital frontal cortex 5-HT$_{2A}$ binding. These data provide further evidence for serotonergic dysregulation in bulimia nervosa.

In a study of clinical features, Hatsukami et al. (1984) found that 43.5% of a sample of 108 women with bulimia nervosa had an affective disorder at some time in their lives, and 18.5% had a history of alcohol or drug abuse.

The percentage of individuals with DSM-III-R bulimia (including bulimic anorexic individuals) who have at least one personality disorder has been reported to be 77% (Powers et al. 1988), 69% (Wonderlich et al. 1990), 62% (Gartner et al. 1989), 61% (Schmidt and Telch 1990), 33% (Ames-Frankel et al. 1992), and 23% (Herzog et al. 1992). All of these studies used established diagnostic interviews, but the findings are not in agreement. This is probably a result of several factors: 1) some of the studies with very small numbers of patients may represent a biased sample; 2) studies used different criteria, ranging from DSM-III to DSM-III-R, for both eating disorders and personality disorders; and 3) some of the Axis II interviewers lacked information about the patients' Axis I diagnosis, which may have led to false-positive personality disorder diagnoses. Nonetheless, substantial evidence indicates that personality disorders are commonly associated with bulimia nervosa.

There is substantial literature that shows bulimia nervosa is strongly familial (Lilenfeld et al. 1998; Strober et al. 2000) and that this familiality is due largely to the additive effects of genes (Bulik et al. 2000). A linkage study of multiplex families with eating disorders that were identified through a proband with bulimia nervosa showed the highest multipoint logarithm of odds score observed (3.39) was on chromosome 10. This is evidence of the presence of a susceptibility locus for bulimia nervosa on chromosome 10p (Bulik et al. 2002). The next stage of research indicated will be to explore likely candidate genes under the observed linkage peak.

Treatment

Treatment studies of bulimia nervosa have proliferated in the last few decades, in contrast to the relatively few treatment studies of anorexia nervosa. This is probably because of the greater prevalence of bulimia nervosa and the fact that this disorder usually can be treated on an outpatient basis. Specific therapy techniques such as behavior therapy, cognitive therapy, psychodynamic therapy, and "psychoeducation therapy" have been conducted in both individual and group formats (Table 14–11).

Cognitive-Behavioral Therapy

Fourteen published controlled studies have examined the efficacy of CBT in bulimia nervosa. All of the subjects in these 14 studies were outpatients, with the exception of one study of the effectiveness of CBT in individual therapy that involved inpatients. Nearly all of the studies used a psychoeducational component that included information on the social-cultural emphasis on thinness; the physical effects and medical complications of bingeing, purging, and abuse of laxatives and diuretics; and how dieting and fasting precipitate binge–purge cycles. Self-monitoring was an important part of all of these studies and usually consisted of a daily record of the times and durations of meals and a

record of binge-eating and purging episodes as well as descriptions of moods and circumstances surrounding binge–purge episodes. The studies stressed the importance of eating regular meals.

Cognitive restructuring is the basis of all the CBT programs. The first step in cognitive therapy is the assessment of cognition. Patients are asked to write their thoughts on an assessment form so that cognitions can be examined for systematic distortions in the processing and interpretation of events.

Behavior therapy is used specifically to stop the binge-eating/purging behaviors. Behavioral approaches include restricting exposure to cues that trigger a binge–purge episode, developing a strategy of alternative behaviors, and delaying the vomiting response to eating. Response prevention is a technique used specifically to prevent vomiting.

The combined effects of CBT and antidepressant medication for bulimia nervosa were examined in three studies. Mitchell et al. (1990) found that group CBT was superior to imipramine therapy for decreasing binge eating and purging, and the combined treatment showed no additive effects for those treated with group CBT alone. Agras et al. (1992) had similar results comparing individual CBT, desipramine therapy, and the combination at 16 weeks. However, at 32 weeks, only the combined treatment given for 24 weeks was superior to medication given for 16 weeks. In a third study, CBT plus medication (desipramine, followed by fluoxetine in nonresponders) was superior to medication alone, but supportive psychotherapy plus medication was not. CBT plus medication was superior to CBT alone.

A study of interpersonal therapy (IPT), which targets interpersonal functioning, showed that IPT was equivalent to CBT in reducing bulimic symptoms and psychopathology; at follow-up, it was actually superior to CBT (Fairburn et al. 1992b). This was the first study to show that bulimia nervosa may be treated successfully without focusing directly on the patient's eating habits and attitudes to-

Table 14–11. Treatment of bulimia nervosa

Type of treatment	Indications	Measurements	Key elements
Cognitive-behavioral therapy (CBT)			
Group	Outpatients—young adults	Psychiatric and medical evaluations before entering therapy	Psychoeducational component on all aspects of the bulimic disorder
Individual	Inpatients; outpatients—adolescents and adults with severe character disorders	Self-recording of medical consultations available throughout treatment	Self-monitoring, cognitive restructuring
Behavior therapy	Usually used in conjunction with computed tomography	Same as for CBT	Restricting exposure to cues, developing alternative behaviors, response prevention to stop vomiting
Interpersonal therapy	Outpatients—young adults	Psychiatric and medical evaluations before entering therapy and consultation available during treatment	Focuses on interpersonal relationships
Pharmacotherapy			
Antidepressants Fluoxetine Desipramine Imipramine Nortriptyline	Binge-eating behavior, depression, unwillingness to enter CBT	Initial evaluation: complete blood count, serum electrolytes and amylase, electrocardiogram, blood pressure; repeat after 1 week and then as often as clinically indicated	Antidepressant drugs affect catecholamine and indoleamine function, which modulates eating behavior

ward shape and weight. In a multisite study comparing CBT with IPT, bulimic patients received 19 sessions of treatment over a 20-week period and were evaluated for 1 year following treatment. CBT was significantly superior to IPT at the end of treatment for the number of participants recovered (29% vs. 6%). At the 1-year follow-up, no significant difference was found between the two treatments. However, CBT was significantly more rapid in initiating improvement in patients with bulimia nervosa compared with IPT. Accordingly, the authors suggested that CBT should be considered the preferred psychotherapeutic treatment for bulimia nervosa (Agras et al. 2000).

Drug Therapy

Studies of antidepressant medications have consistently shown some efficacy in the treatment of bulimia nervosa. These studies were prompted by observations that patients with bulimia nervosa also had significant mood disturbances. Since 1980, more than a dozen double-blind, placebo-controlled trials of various antidepressants were conducted in normal-weight outpatients with bulimia nervosa. (For a review of these studies, see Fairburn et al. 1992a.) All of these trials found a significantly greater reduction in binge eating when antidepressant medication was administered than when placebo was given. Antidepressants improved mood and reduced psychopathological symptoms such as preoccupation with shape and weight. These studies provide evidence for the short-term efficacy of antidepressant medication, but long-term efficacy remains unknown. The average rate of abstinence from bingeing and purging in these studies was 22%, indicating that most patients remain symptomatic at the end of treatment with antidepressants. Topiramate, an antiepileptic agent, was shown in a placebo-controlled, double-blind trial to be effective in reducing binge–purge behavior in BED (McElroy et al. 2003), and more recently studies have been under way with topiramate in treating bulimia nervosa.

The current data suggest that the treatment of choice for bulimia nervosa should be CBT and that a single antidepressant administered in the absence of psychotherapy cannot be considered an adequate treatment.

Obesity

Definition

In contrast to anorexia nervosa and bulimia nervosa, obesity is classified not as a psychiatric disorder but as a medical disorder. Obesity is an excessive accumulation of body fat and operationally is defined as overweight. The BMI, defined as weight (kg)/height (m^2), has the highest correlation, 0.8, with body fat measured by other, more precise laboratory methods. *Mild overweight* is defined as a BMI of 25–30 or body weight between the upper limit of normal and 20% above that limit on standard height–weight charts. *Obesity* is defined as a BMI greater than 30 or body weight greater than 20% above the upper limit for height (Bray 1978; see Figure 14–1).

Clinical Features

The most obvious clinical features of obesity are physical; these features are discussed in the section on "Medical Complications" that follows. The psychological and behavioral aspects of obesity are best considered grouped in two categories: *eating behavior* and *emotional disturbance*. There is considerable heterogeneity in eating patterns. Most commonly, obese persons complain that they cannot restrain their eating and that they have difficulty achieving satiety. Some obese persons cannot distinguish hunger from other dysphoric states and will eat when they are emotionally upset.

The most methodologically satisfying studies have shown that there is no distinct or excess psychopathology in obesity. In one study of severely obese patients who had gastric bypass surgery, the most prevalent

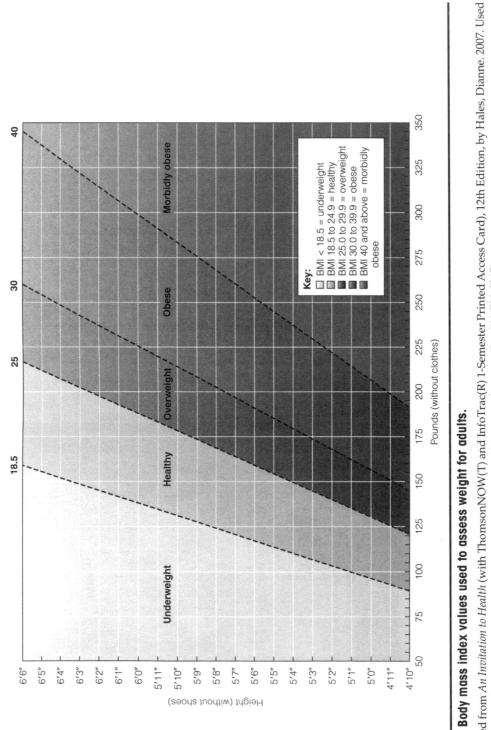

Figure 14–1.   Body mass index values used to assess weight for adults.

Source.   Reprinted from *An Invitation to Health* (with ThomsonNOW(T) and InfoTrac(R) 1-Semester Printed Access Card), 12th Edition, by Hales, Dianne. 2007. Used with permission of Brooks/Cole, a division of Thomson Learning; www.thomsonrights.com. Fax 800-730-2215.

psychiatric diagnosis was major depressive disorder. However, this diagnosis was no more prevalent in the obese patients than in the general population. Self-disparagement of body image is especially prevalent in those who have been obese since childhood. This may be due to the continual bombardment of social prejudice against obese people. The stigmatization and prejudice against obese types are well documented in studies of educational disadvantages and of employment prejudices against obese persons. Many obese individuals develop anxiety and depression when they attempt to diet (Halmi et al. 1980). Because health risks and mortality vary with degree of adiposity, Bray (1986) proposed a classification into low-risk (BMI = 25–30), moderate-risk (BMI = 31–40), and high-risk (BMI > 40) individuals.

Medical Complications

Obesity affects a great variety of physiological functions (Table 14–12). Blood circulation may be overtaxed as body weight increases, and congestive heart failure may occur in grossly obese individuals. Hypertension is strongly associated with obesity, and the prevalence of carbohydrate intolerance in grossly obese subjects is approximately 50%. Increased body fat in the upper region of the body as opposed to the lower region is more likely to be associated with the onset of diabetes mellitus. The impairment of pulmonary function becomes extreme in severe obesity and involves hypoventilation, hypercapnia, hypoxia, and somnolence (i.e., pickwickian syndrome). The latter syndrome has a high mortality rate. Obesity may accelerate the development of osteoarthritis and of dermatological problems from stretching of the skin, intertrigo, and acanthosis nigricans. Obese women are an obstetrical risk, being susceptible to toxemia and hypertension.

Obesity has been associated with several types of cancer. Obese males have a higher rate of prostate and colorectal cancer, and obese females have increased incidences of gallbladder, breast, cervical, endometrial,

Table 14–12. Medical complications of obesity

Insulin resistance
Glucose intolerance
Type 2 diabetes
Low high-density lipoprotein cholesterol
High triglycerides
Elevated blood pressure
Inflammation
Endothelial dysfunction
Susceptibility to thrombosis
Increased incidence of cardiovascular disease
Increased mortality

uterine, and ovarian cancer. Most studies on the topic suggest that obesity influences the development and progression of both endometrial and breast cancer through influences on estrogen production. Low-density lipoprotein levels are increased in obesity, and levels of high-density lipoproteins (high-density lipoprotein cholesterol) are reduced. The low levels of high-density lipoproteins may be one mechanism by which obesity is associated with an increased risk for cardiovascular disease.

Epidemiology, Course, and Prognosis

If obesity is defined as the state of being 20% above ideal weight, then nearly a quarter of the U.S. population would be considered obese (VanItallie 1985). Socioeconomic status is highly correlated with obesity: the condition is much more common among women (less so among men) of low status. This relationship is also present in obese children. Increasing age and obesity are associated until age 50 years. The prevalence of obesity is higher in women compared with men; in those older than 50 years, this may be due to the increased mortality rate among obese men with advancing age.

Unfortunately, life expectancy and obesity studies are restricted to life insurance studies and therefore do not represent a random American population. Despite these limitations, studies have shown a progressive increase in "excess mortality" as BMI increased (Society of Actuaries 1992). Another study of grossly obese persons showed that excess mortality was greatly increased in younger men (ages 25–34 years) and gradually declined with age (Stevens et al. 1998).

Etiology and Pathogenesis

It is unlikely that obesity has a single etiology. In the first section of this chapter, the complex neural mechanisms involved in the control of feeding behavior were discussed. Lipid, amino acid, and glucose metabolism all seem to affect, in some way, central neural regulatory mechanisms that influence eating behavior. Obesity is regarded today by most investigators as a disorder of energy balance, a disorder with a strong genetic component that is modulated by cultural and environmental influences (Flegal et al. 2002).

Obesity has a definite familial aspect. Eighty percent of the offspring of two obese parents are obese, compared with 40% of the offspring of one obese parent and only 10% of the offspring of lean parents. Findings of twin and adoption studies suggest that genetic factors play a strong role in the development of obesity.

The cloning and sequencing of the mouse obese (*Ob*) gene and its human homologue in 1994 (Zhang et al. 1994) provided the basis for further research into the pathways that regulate adiposity and body weight. Leptin, the gene product of the *Ob* gene, was shown to be a 16-kd protein that is present in mouse and human plasma (Halaas et al. 1995). Intraperitoneal injections of recombinant leptin decrease food intake and increase energy expenditure in wild-type mice. Leptin reduces body fat in mice, and its absence in mice with the *Ob* gene leads to a massive increase in body fat. In both humans and rodents, leptin is highly correlated with BMI and amount of body fat (Maffei et al. 1995). Weight loss due to food restriction was associated with a de-

crease in plasma leptin concentrations in mice and obese humans. These data suggest that leptin serves an endocrine function, regulating body weight and stores of body fat.

Obese persons have larger and more numerous fat cells. Cellular proliferation tends to occur early in life but also will occur in adult life when the existing fat cells are greatly enlarged. The regulation of fat cell proliferation and size is not well understood. The relation of physical activity to obesity is complex. It is known that obese people are less active than people of normal weight. The increase in caloric expenditure by physical activity is small. Animal studies show that physical activity actually decreases food intake and may prevent the decline in metabolic rate that usually accompanies dieting.

Treatment

For mild obesity (20%–40% overweight), the most efficient treatment to date is behavioral modification in groups, a balanced diet, and exercise. This is usually done by both commercial and nonprofit large organizations. For moderate obesity (41%–100% overweight), a medically supervised protein-sparing modified fast (400–700 calories per day) is often necessary. This diet may or may not be combined with behavioral modification techniques. A behavior analysis is necessary to set up a sensible behavioral modification program. Antecedents of eating behavior, the eating behavior itself, the consequences of the behavior, and the acceptable rewards for carrying out various prescribed behaviors are all analyzed. Behavioral treatment programs include self-monitoring, nutrition education, physical activity, and cognitive restructuring.

The use of medication such as phenylpropanolamine or fenfluramine was popular in the past. The problem with these drugs is that on withdrawal, a rebound ballooning up of weight occurs; some patients have concomitant lethargy and depression. In 1997, fenfluramine was removed from the market by the U.S. Food and Drug Administration for treatment of obesity because of the adverse effects of pulmonary hypertension and mitral valve impairment.

Severe obesity (more than 100% above a normal weight) is the least common form of obesity and is most effectively treated by surgical procedures that reduce the size of the stomach. These procedures produce a large weight loss and show a good record of weight loss maintenance.

Behavioral modification is the treatment of choice for overweight children and should include involvement of the parents and the schools. Psychotherapy is not recommended as a treatment per se for obesity, although some patients may have particular problems that may be effectively treated or helped with psychotherapy. For excellent discussions on the treatment of obesity, see Brownell (1984), Lasagna (1987), and Stunkard (1984).

Conclusion

The eating disorders are complex syndromes in which the interactions among environmental, psychological, and physiological factors both create and maintain the disturbed eating behavior. The more precise an understanding we obtain of the connectedness of basic physiological changes, psychological changes, and eating behavior, the better we will be able to design effective treatment interventions.

Many questions remain to be asked about our current treatment interventions. For example, how long should the bulimic patient be treated with antidepressants? Would periodic follow-up behavioral sessions prevent relapse in bulimic patients treated with behavior therapy? How can we identify the most likely effective treatment for a patient?

Continued prospective longitudinal studies are necessary for bulimia nervosa, because no information is available on what happens to this addictive-like bingeing–purging behavior over the course of a lifetime. Although disturbed eating behavior has been present throughout the history of humankind, it has been systematically studied with scientific methodology only in the past few decades. There is a continued need for further study of eating disorders.

Key Points

- Chronic anorexia nervosa is best prevented by early diagnosis and early intensive treatment.

- Adolescents with anorexia nervosa are most effectively treated with family therapy, either conjoint or with separate parental counseling.

- CBT specific for bulimia is the most effective treatment for bulimia nervosa.

- Serotonin reuptake inhibitors are effective in reducing bingeing episodes and have a more benign side-effect profile compared with tricyclic antidepressants.

- Obesity is a complex medical disorder with no single etiology. There is no guaranteed effective treatment over time. Behavioral modification is the treatment of choice for overweight children.

Suggested Readings

Bailer UF, Kaye WH: A review of neuropeptide and neuroendocrine dysregulation in anorexia and bulimia nervosa. Curr Drug Targets CNS Neurol Disord 2:53–59, 2003

Bensimhon DR, Kraus WE, Donahue MP: Obesity and physical activity: a review. Am Heart J 151:598–603, 2006

Halmi KA, Agras S, Crow S, et al: Predictors of treatment acceptance and completion in anorexia nervosa. Arch Gen Psychiatry 62:1–6, 2005

Kaye W, Strober M, Jimmerson D: The neurobiology of eating disorders, in The Neurobiology of Mental Illness. Edited by Charney DF, Nestler EJ. New York, Oxford University Press, 2004, pp 1112–1128

Maj M, Halmi K, Lopez-Ibor JJ, et al (eds): Eating Disorders. Chichester, England, Wiley, 2003

References

Agras WS, Rossiter EM, Arnow B, et al: Pharmacological and cognitive-behavioral treatment for bulimia nervosa: a controlled comparison. Am J Psychiatry 149:82–87, 1992

Agras WS, Walsh BT, Fairburn CG: A multicenter comparison of cognitive-behavioral therapy and interpersonal psychotherapy for bulimia nervosa. Arch Gen Psychiatry 57:459–466, 2000

American Psychiatric Association: Diagnostic and Statistical Manual of Mental Disorders, 3rd Edition. Washington, DC, American Psychiatric Association, 1980

American Psychiatric Association: Diagnostic and Statistical Manual of Mental Disorders, 3rd Edition, Revised. Washington, DC, American Psychiatric Association, 1987

American Psychiatric Association: Diagnostic and Statistical Manual of Mental Disorders, 4th Edition, Text Revision. Washington, DC, American Psychiatric Association, 2000

Ames-Frankel J, Devlin MJ, Walsh BT, et al: Personality disorders and eating disorders. J Clin Psychiatry 53:90–96, 1992

Bailer U, Frank G, Henry S, et al: Altered brain serotonin $5HT_{1A}$ receptor binding after recovery from anorexia nervosa measured by positron emission tomography and [carbonyl^{11}C] WAY-100635. Arch Gen Psychiatry 62:1032–1041, 2005

Bergen AW, van Den Bree M, Yeager M, et al: Candidate genes for anorexia nervosa in the 1p33–36 linkage region: serotonin 1D and delta opioid receptor loci exhibit significant association to anorexia nervosa. Mol Psychiatry 8:397–406, 2003

Blundell JE, Hill A: Behavioral pharmacology of feeding: relevance of animal experiments for studies in man, in Pharmacology of Eating Disorders. Edited by Carruba M, Blundell J. New York, Raven, 1986, pp 51–70

Boden G, Chen X, Mazzoli M, et al: Effect of fasting on serum leptin in normal subjects. J Clin Endocrinol Metab 81:3419–3423, 1996

Bray GA: Definition, measurement and classification of the syndromes of obesity. Int J Obesity 2:99–112, 1978

Bray GA: Effects of obesity on health and happiness, in Handbook of Eating Disorders: Physiology, Psychology, and Treatment. Edited by Brownell KD, Foreyt JP. New York, Basic Books, 1986, pp 3–44

Brownell KD: New developments in the treatment of obese children and adolescents, in Eating and Its Disorders. Edited by Stunkard AJ, Stellar E. New York, Raven, 1984, pp 175–184

Bruch H: Perceptual and conceptual disturbance in anorexia nervosa. Psychosom Med 24:187–195, 1962

Bulik C, Sullivan PE, Wade T: Twin studies of eating disorders: a review. Int J Eat Disord 27:1–20, 2000

Bulik C, Devlin B, Bacanu S, et al: Significant linkage on chromosome 10p in families with bulimia nervosa. Am J Hum Genet 72:200–207, 2002

Considine RV, Sinha MK, Heiman ML, et al: Serum immunoreactive-leptin concentrations in normal-weight and obese humans. N Engl J Med 334:292–295, 1996

Crisp AH: The possible significance of some behavioral correlates of weight and carbohydrate intake. J Psychosom Res 11:117–123, 1976

Cummings DE, Purnell JQ, Frayo RS, et al: A preprandial rise in plasma ghrelin levels suggests a role in meal initiation in humans. Diabetes 50:1714–1719, 2001

Dare C, Eisler I: Family therapy and eating disorders, in Eating Disorders and Obesity, 2nd Edition. A Comprehensive Textbook. Edited by Fairburn CG, Brownell KD. New York, Guilford, 2002, pp 314–319

Eagles T, Johnston M, Hunter D, et al: Increasing incidence of anorexia nervosa in the female population of northeast Scotland. Am J Psychiatry 152:1266–1271, 1995

Eison AS, Mullins UL: Regulation of central 5-HT$_{2A}$ receptors: a review of in vivo studies. Behav Brain Res 73:177–181, 1996

Fairburn CG, Cooper PJ: The clinical features of bulimia nervosa. Br J Psychiatry 144:238–246, 1984

Fairburn CG, Agra WS, Wilson GT: The research on the treatment of bulimia nervosa: practical and theoretical implications, in Biology of Feast and Famine: Relevance to Eating Disorders. Edited by Anderson GH, Kennedy SH. New York, Academic Press, 1992a, pp 318–340

Fairburn CG, Jones R, Pevelar RC, et al: Three psychological treatments for bulimia nervosa: a comparative trial. Arch Gen Psychiatry 48:463–469, 1992b

Flegal KM, Carroll MD, Ogden CL, et al: Prevalence and trends in obesity among U.S. adults. JAMA 288:1723–1727, 2002

Frank G, Bailer U, Henry S, et al: Increased dopamine D2/D3 receptor binding after recovery from anorexia nervosa measured by positron emission tomography and [11C] raclopride. Biol Psychiatry 5:1–5, 2005

Garfinkel P, Goering L, Spegg C, et al: Bulimia nervosa in a Canadian community sample: prevalence and comparison of subgroups. Am J Psychiatry 52:1052–1058, 1995

Gartner AF, Marcus RN, Halmi KA, et al: DSM-III-R personality disorders in patients with eating disorders. Am J Psychiatry 146:1585–1591, 1989

Grice D, Halmi KA, Fichter MM, et al: Evidence for a susceptibility gene for anorexia nervosa on chromosome 1. Am J Hum Gent 70:787–792, 2002

Gualillo O, Caminos JE, Nogueiras R, et al: Effective food restriction on ghrelin in normal-cycling female rats and in pregnancy. Obes Res 10:682–687, 2002

Halaas J, Gajiwala K, Maffei M, et al: Weight-reducing effects of the protein encoded by the obese gene. Science 269:543–546, 1995

Halmi KA: Anorexia nervosa: demographic and clinical features in 94 cases. Psychosom Med 36:18–26, 1974

Halmi KA: Anorexia nervosa and bulimia, in Handbook of Adolescent Psychology. Edited by Hersen M, Van Hasselt T. New York, Pergamon, 1987, pp 265–287

Halmi KA, Falk JR: Common physiological changes in anorexia nervosa. Int J Eat Disord 1:16–27, 1981

Halmi KA, Sunday SR: Temporal patterns of hunger and satiety ratings and related cognitions in anorexia and bulimia. Appetite 16:219–237, 1991

Halmi KA, Stunkard AJ, Mason EE: Emotional responses to weight reduction by three methods: gastric bypass, jejunoileal bypass, diet. Am J Clin Nutr 33:446–451, 1980

Halmi KA, Eckert E, LaDu T, et al: Anorexia nervosa: treatment efficacy of cyproheptadine and amitriptyline. Arch Gen Psychiatry 43:177–181, 1986

Halmi KA, Agras S, Crow S, et al: Predictors of treatment acceptance and completion in anorexia nervosa. Arch Gen Psychiatry 62:1–6, 2005

Hart K, Ollendick TH: Prevalence of bulimia in working and university women. Am J Psychiatry 142:851–854, 1985

Hatsukami J, Mitchell J, Eckert E, et al: Affective disorder and substance abuse in women with bulimia. Psychol Med 14:704–710, 1984

Herzog DB, Keller MB, Lavori PW, et al: The prevalence of personality disorders in 210 women with eating disorders. J Clin Psychiatry 53:147–152, 1992

Hoebel BG: Pharmacological control of feeding. Annu Rev Pharmacol Toxicol 17:605–621, 1977

Kaye WH, Nagata T, Weltzin T, et al: Double-blind placebo-controlled administration of fluoxetine in restricting and restricting-purging type anorexia nervosa. Biol Psychiatry 49:644–652, 2001

Keel PK, Mitchell JE: Outcome in bulimia nervosa. Am J Psychiatry 154:313–321, 1997

Kurth C, Krahn D, Nairn K, et al: The severity of dieting and bingeing behaviors in college women: interview validation of survey data. J Psychiatry Res 29:211–225, 1995

Lasagna L: The pharmacotherapy of obesity, in Psychopharmacology: The Third Generation of Progress. Edited by Meltzer HY. New York, Raven, 1987, pp 1281–1284

LeGrange D, Eisler I, Dare C, et al: Evaluation of family treatment in adolescent anorexia nervosa: a pilot study. Int J Eat Disord 12:347–358, 1992

Le Roux CW, Patterson M, Vincent RP, et al: Postprandial plasma ghrelin is suppressed proportional to meal calorie content in normal-weight but not obese subjects. J Clin Endocrinol Metab 90:1068–1071, 2005

Lewinsohn PM, Striegel-Moore RH, Seeley JR: Epidemiology and natural course of eating disorders in young women from adolescence to young adulthood. J Am Acad Child Adolesc Psychiatry 39:1284–1292, 2000

Lilenfeld LR, Kaye WH, Greeno CG, et al: A controlled family study of anorexia nervosa and bulimia nervosa: psychiatric disorders in first-degree relatives and effects of proband comorbidity. Arch Gen Psychiatry 55:603–610, 1998

Maffei M, Halaas J, Ravussin E, et al: Leptin levels in human and rodent: measurement of plasma leptin and OB RNA in obese and weight-reduced subjects. Nat Med 1:1155–1161, 1995

Mantzoros C, Flier JS, Lesem MD, et al: Cerebrospinal fluid leptin in anorexia nervosa: correlation with nutritional status and potential role in resistance to weight gain. J Clin Endocrinol Metab 82:1845–1851, 1997

McElroy SL, Arnold LM, Shapira N: Topiramate in the treatment of binge eating disorder associated with obesity: a randomized, placebo-controlled trial. Am J Psychiatry 160:255–261, 2003

Mitchell JE, Pyle RL, Eckert ED, et al: A comparison study of antidepressants and structured intensive group therapy in the treatment of bulimia nervosa. Arch Gen Psychiatry 47:149–157, 1990

Morley J, Levine AS: Pharmacology of eating behavior. Annu Rev Pharmacol Toxicol 25:127–146, 1985

Nielsen S: Epidemiology and mortality of eating disorders. Psychiatr Clin North Am 24:201–214, 2001

Pirke KM: Central and peripheral noradrenaline regulation in eating disorders. Psychiatry Res 62:43–49, 1996

Powers PS, Covert DL, Brightwell DR, et al: Other psychiatric disorders among bulimic patients. Compr Psychiatry 29:503–508, 1988

Powers PS, Santana CA, Bannon YS: Olanzapine in the treatment of anorexia nervosa: an open label trial. Int J Eat Disord 32:146–154, 2002

Rooney B, McClelland L, Crisp AH, et al: The incidence and prevalence of anorexia nervosa in three suburban health districts in southwest London, UK. Int J Eat Disord 18:299–307, 1995

Russell GFM, Szmukler JI, Dare C, et al: An evaluation of family therapy in anorexia nervosa and bulimia nervosa. Arch Gen Psychiatry 44:1047–1056, 1987

Schmidt ND, Telch MJ: Prevalence of personality disorders among bulimics, non-bulimic binge eaters and normal controls. J Psychopathol Behav Assess 12:170–185, 1990

Schotte D, Stunkard A: Bulimia vs. bulimic behaviors on a college campus. JAMA 9:1213–1215, 1987

Society of Actuaries: Life Tables for the United States Social Security Area 1900–2080: Actuarial Study No 107, August 1992 (SSA Publ No 11-11536). Washington, DC, U.S. Department of Health and Human Services, 1992

Stevens J, Ooi J, Pamuk E, et al: The effect of age on the association between body mass index and mortality. N Engl J Med 338:1–7, 1998

Strober M, Morell W, Burroughs J, et al: A controlled family study of anorexia nervosa. Psychiatry Res 19:329–346, 1985

Strober M, Freeman R, Lampert C, et al: Control family study of anorexia nervosa and bulimia nervosa: evidence of shared liability and transmission of partial syndromes. Am J Psychiatry 157:393–401, 2000

Stunkard AJ: The current status of treatment for obesity in adults, in Eating and Its Disorders. Edited by Stunkard AJ, Stellar E. New York, Raven, 1984, pp 157–174

VanItallie TB: Health implications of overweight and obesity in the United States. Ann Intern Med 103:983–988, 1985

Wonderlich SA, Swift WJ, Slotnick HB, et al: DSM-III-R personality disorders and eating disorder subtypes. Int J Eat Disord 9:607–616, 1990

Woodside DB, Garfinkel PE, Lin E, et al: Comparisons of men with full or partial eating disorders, men without eating disorders, and women with eating disorders in the community. Am J Psychiatry 158:570–574, 2001

Zhang Y, Prenca R, Maffei M, et al: Positional cloning of the mouse obese gene and its human homologue. Nature 372:425–432, 1994

15

PSYCHOPHARMACOLOGY

Melissa Martinez, M.D.
Lauren B. Marangell, M.D.
James M. Martinez, M.D.

This chapter was designed to provide clinicians with an overview of major psychotropic medications. This chapter is not an exhaustive review; we begin with an overview of some general principles that are relevant to the safe and effective prescribing of psychotropic medications, followed by specific discussions of major classes of psychotropic medication classes, including antidepressants, anxiolytics, antipsychotics, and mood stabilizers. Stimulants and cognitive enhancers are discussed elsewhere in this volume.

General Principles

Initial Evaluation

The art and skillful practice of psychopharmacology have multiple facets, including establishing proper diagnoses, identifying medication-responsive target symptoms, ruling out nonpsychiatric causes of a patient's symptomatology, noting the presence of other medical problems that will influence drug selection, evaluating concomitant med-

The text, tables, and figures in this chapter were derived, in part, from Marangell LB, Martinez JM: *Concise Guide to Psychopharmacology*, 2nd Edition, which had its genesis in the previous edition of this chapter.

The authors wish to express sincere gratitude and acknowledgment to Stuart C. Yudofsky, M.D., Donald C. Goff, M.D., and Jonathan M. Silver, M.D., who were coauthors on the previous version of this chapter, and to Dr. Yudofsky and Dr. Silver, who also were coauthors on the first edition of the *Concise Guide to Psychopharmacology*. The "Drug Interactions" sections contain material developed over many years by Lauren B. Marangell, M.D., in collaboration with Ann Callahan, M.D., and Terence Ketter, M.D.

ications that may cause drug–drug interactions, and evaluating personal and family histories of medication response.

Target Symptoms

A key component in arriving at a well-informed treatment decision is the identification of target symptoms. Once the physician determines the proper diagnosis, he or she should identify the specific symptoms that are targets for treatment and monitor the response of these symptoms during the course of treatment. Standard rating scales are useful for monitoring target symptom changes with treatment. In the absence of formal rating scales, target symptoms can be rated on a clinician-determined scale that can be tracked over time. It is also important for the clinician to monitor the patient's functional status because major goals of treatment include both symptomatic and functional recovery.

Use of Multiple Medications

A frequent clinical error is to treat specific symptoms of a disorder with multiple drugs rather than to treat the underlying disorder itself. For example, one may see a patient who has been prescribed two different benzodiazepines (one for anxiety and one for insomnia), an analgesic for pain complaints, a stimulant medication for lethargy and impaired concentration, and a subtherapeutic dose of an antidepressant for other depressive symptoms. In some instances, the cluster of symptoms described in this example may be components of an underlying depression, which may be aggravated by the polypharmaceutical approach inherent in symptomatic treatment. Additionally, this polypharmacy approach may expose the patient to a greater side-effect burden and the potential for significant drug–drug interactions.

Medication Selection

Fortunately, clinicians today are practicing psychiatry in an era that affords them numerous medication options. Because so many medication options exist, a clinician must consider numerous factors when selecting a specific psychotropic medication for a given patient. These factors include the presence of comorbid medical conditions (which may preclude the use of certain medications); the presence of comorbid psychiatric disorders (which may be exacerbated by certain medications but effectively treated by others); the use of concomitant psychotropic and nonpsychotropic medications (which may pose a risk for significant drug–drug interactions); history of response and tolerability to medication; family history of medication responses; patient-specific life circumstances that may be affected by particular side effects; patient concerns regarding the avoidance of particular side effects; and treatment costs.

Generic Substitution

Generic drugs are less expensive alternatives to original proprietary (brand-name) formulations. Some patients may favor the use of a generic medication, if available, so that they may benefit from the cost savings. However, some caution is warranted with respect to generic drugs because generic "equivalents" are not always truly equivalent. The current U.S. Food and Drug Administration (FDA) requirements center around the concept of *bioequivalence*. Products are bioequivalent if they have no significant difference in the rate at which or extent to which the active ingredient becomes available at the site of action, given the same dose and conditions. In some cases, even small differences between a proprietary formulation and a generic preparation may have clinically meaningful consequences. For example, a patient may have an allergic reaction to one generic preparation but not another of the same drug because of differences in the dye used to color the pills.

Drug Interactions

The three main types of drug interactions are *pharmacokinetic interactions, pharmacodynamic interactions,* and *idiosyncratic interactions.*

Pharmacokinetic interactions occur when one medication alters the pharmacokinetics (absorption, distribution, metabolism, or excretion) of another drug. Pharmacodynamic interactions occur when the action of a drug changes at a receptor or biologically active site, which alters the pharmacological effect of a given plasma concentration of the drug. Idiosyncratic interactions occur unpredictably in a small number of patients; they are unexpected, given the known pharmacological actions of the individual drugs.

Cytochrome P450 Enzymes

Most psychotropic medications, except for lithium, are metabolized by cytochrome P450 enzymes. These enzymes are classified by families and subfamilies on the basis of similarities in amino acid sequence. Enzymes within subfamilies have relatively specific affinities for various drugs and other substances. The enzymes primarily involved in drug metabolism include CYP1A2, CYP2C9, CYP2C10, CYP2C19, CYP2D6, CYP3A3, and CYP3A4.

One important drug interaction that may involve cytochrome P450 enzymes is *enzyme inhibition*. Some medications, including several psychotropic medications, can cause clinically meaningful inhibition of one or more cytochrome P450 enzymes. If a cytochrome P450 enzyme is inhibited by a medication, then the plasma levels of concurrently administered drugs that rely on that enzyme for metabolism may increase.

The effects of inhibitors occur relatively rapidly (in minutes to hours) and are reversible within a time frame that depends on the half-life of the inhibitor. Additionally, there is a large amount of interindividual variation in drug metabolism and the propensity for enzyme inhibition to alter metabolism. Part of this variation is the result of genetic polymorphism, which is a heritable alteration of the enzyme. Persons who have a genetic polymorphism that causes a large reduction in the amount of active enzyme are referred to as *poor metabolizers* and are at risk for increased

drug levels, which may lead to toxicity. In contrast, some people have increased amounts of an enzyme. These individuals, referred to as *ultrarapid metabolizers*, may have reduced levels of drugs that are metabolized by the enzyme, resulting in decreased efficacy.

Another important interaction that may occur with cytochrome P450 enzymes is *enzyme induction*. Induction occurs when the liver produces a greater amount of the enzyme. This increase in enzyme availability can increase elimination and reduce plasma levels of a drug (or metabolite) that is a substrate for that enzyme. One risk inherent with this interaction is a potential loss of efficacy for drugs metabolized by the induced enzyme. Indeed, if a drug's clinical effectiveness is diminished as a result of this interaction, the dose of the affected drug should be increased to achieve the same serum concentration that was previously therapeutically effective.

Protein Binding

Another potential drug–drug interaction may occur when drugs compete for protein-binding sites. In short, medications are distributed to their various sites of action through the circulatory system. In the bloodstream, most psychotropic medications (except lithium) are bound to plasma proteins to different degrees. For drugs that are protein bound, the unbound fraction of the drug is pharmacologically active, whereas the bound fraction is not. When two drugs that bind to plasma proteins are present in plasma simultaneously, competition for protein-binding sites occurs. This competition for protein-binding sites can cause displacement of a previously protein-bound drug, which in the free state becomes pharmacologically active. These interactions are often referred to as *protein-binding interactions*. This type of interaction may be clinically significant if the drugs involved are highly protein bound (which results in a large change in plasma concentration of free drug from a small amount of drug displacement) and have a low therapeutic index or narrow therapeutic window (in which case small changes in plasma levels can result in toxicity or loss of efficacy) (Callahan et al. 1996).

Absorption and Excretion

Changes in plasma levels as a result of alterations in absorption or excretion are less common with psychiatric medications. Changes in plasma concentrations as a result of changes in excretion are most frequent with lithium, which is dependent on renal excretion (see "Mood Stabilizers" section later in this chapter).

Pharmacodynamic Interactions

In *pharmacodynamic interactions,* the pharmacological effect of a drug is changed by the action of a second drug at a common receptor or bioactive site. For example, the concomitant administration of two medications with anticholinergic and antihistaminergic actions can result in additive sedation, constipation, and other anticholinergic effects. To avoid these interactions to the extent possible, the clinician must be aware of all medications that a patient is taking, including over-the-counter medications, and be knowledgeable about each medication's various mechanisms of action and receptor effects.

Antidepressant Medications

Overview

One of the most rapidly expanding areas in psychopharmacology is the development of antidepressant medications. Indeed, the antidepressant class contains several different types of medications, categorized largely by their actions on neurotransmission. To date, all antidepressants appear to be similarly effective for treating major depression, but individual patients may respond preferentially to one agent or another. In addition, these medications are significantly different from one another with regard to side effects, lethality in

overdose, pharmacokinetics, drug–drug interaction potential, and the ability to treat comorbid disorders. In this section, we review the pharmacological properties of the various medications within the antidepressant class and discuss some of their clinical uses.

Mechanisms of Action

All currently available antidepressant drugs affect serotonergic and/or noradrenergic neurotransmission. The effects of antidepressants on monoamine availability are immediate, but the clinical response is typically delayed for several weeks. Downregulation of receptors more closely parallels the time course of clinical response. This downregulation can be conceptualized as a marker of antidepressant-induced neuronal adaptation. Therapeutic effects are most likely related to modulation of G proteins, second-messenger systems, and gene expression, particularly genes involved in neuronal growth and regeneration (for a review, see Nestler et al. 2002). As the understanding of the neurobiology of depression progresses, we may gain a better understanding of the mechanisms of action of available antidepressants, as well as identify new targets for drug development.

Indications and Efficacy

All antidepressants are effective in the treatment of major depression. Additionally, some antidepressants are effective in obsessive-compulsive disorder (OCD; selective serotonin reuptake inhibitors [SSRIs] and clomipramine), panic disorder (tricyclic antidepressants [TCAs] and SSRIs), generalized anxiety disorder (venlafaxine and SSRIs), bulimia (TCAs, SSRIs, and monoamine oxidase inhibitors [MAOIs]), dysthymia (SSRIs), bipolar depression (with treatment with a mood stabilizer), social phobia (SSRIs, venlafaxine, MAOIs), posttraumatic stress disorder (SSRIs), irritable bowel syndrome (TCAs), enuresis (TCAs), neuropathic pain (TCAs, duloxetine), migraine headaches (TCAs), attention-deficit/hyperactivity disorder (bupropion), autism (SSRIs), late luteal phase dysphoric disorder (SSRIs), borderline personality disorder (SSRIs), and smoking cessation (bupropion). However, the FDA has not evaluated or approved the use of antidepressants to treat many of these conditions. We refer the reader to current product labeling to determine the indications for use approved by the FDA for a specific medication.

Clinical Use

In the following subsections, clinically relevant information is presented for each commonly used class of antidepressant individually. The pharmacological treatment of depression is also discussed. Information on doses and half-lives is summarized in Table 15–1.

Antidepressants and Suicide

Patients with depression and other psychiatric disorders have an increased risk for suicide and suicidal behavior. Long-term pharmacological treatment is associated with a decreased suicide rate (Angst et al. 2002), but the acute phases of treatment with antidepressants have been associated with increased risks of suicidal thoughts and behaviors. This is of particular concern in children and adolescents. A pooled analysis conducted by the U.S. Food and Drug Administration (2004) of 24 short-term placebo-controlled clinical trials among children and adolescents taking antidepressants found a risk of suicidal thinking or behavior in 4% of the patients who received antidepressants, compared with 2% of the patients who received placebo. Fortunately, no suicides were completed in these studies.

Selective Serotonin Reuptake Inhibitors

Background

SSRIs inhibit serotonin reuptake and are largely devoid of four other major pharmacological properties inherent to other antide-

pressants (e.g., TCAs)—namely, muscarinic receptor blockade, histamine type 1 (H_1) receptor blockade, α_1-adrenergic receptor blockade, and norepinephrine reuptake inhibition. This pharmacological selectivity has several advantages, including a reduction in dangerous side effects. SSRIs are unlikely to affect the seizure threshold or cardiac conduction, and they are relatively safe in overdose. Despite their highly selective pharmacological activity, SSRIs have a broad spectrum of action. They are efficacious in the treatment of depression and of many other psychiatric disorders, including many major anxiety disorders.

Clinical Use

Although all patients with depression should undergo a thorough medical evaluation, no specific tests are required before SSRI therapy is initiated. The usual starting doses of SSRIs are summarized in Table 15–1. These standard doses generally should be decreased by 50% in patients with hepatic disease and in elderly persons (see current product labeling for specific information about dosage adjustments in special populations). In addition, patients with significant anxiety symptoms, or those who are generally sensitive to medication side effects, may experience better tolerability if lower initial doses are used; however, it is important to titrate the dose to a potentially effective dose once tolerability is achieved.

In patients with depression, SSRIs have a flat dose–response curve, meaning that higher doses tend not to be more effective than standard doses, although some patients may respond better to higher doses. Premature escalation of the SSRI dose may result in increased side effects without necessarily improving antidepressant efficacy. Therefore, we recommend maintaining the usual therapeutic dose for at least 4 weeks. If no improvement is seen after 4 weeks, a trial of a higher dose may be warranted. If a partial response is evident after 4 weeks of therapy, the dose should remain constant for an addi-

Table 15–1. Antidepressant medications: dosing and half-life information

Generic drug name	Proprietary drug name	Usual starting dose (mg)[a]	Usual daily dose (mg)	Available oral doses (mg)	Mean half-life, hours (active metabolites)[b]
Monoamine oxidase inhibitors					
Irreversible, nonselective monoamine oxidase inhibitors					
Isocarboxazid	Marplan	10	20–60	10	2
Phenelzine	Nardil	15	15–90	15	2
Tranylcypromine	Parnate	10	30–60	10	2
Transdermal monoamine oxidase inhibitors					
Transdermal selegiline	EMSAM	6	6	None Transdermal doses: 6 mg/24 hours 9 mg/24 hours 12 mg/24 hours	18–25
Reversible inhibitors of monoamine oxidase A					
Moclobemide[c]	Aurorix, Manerix	150	300–600	100, 150	2
Tricyclic antidepressants					
Tertiary-amine tricyclic antidepressants					
Amitriptyline	Elavil	25–50	100–300	10, 25, 50, 75, 100, 150	16 (27)
Clomipramine	Anafranil	25	100–250	25, 50, 75	32 (69)
Doxepin	Sinequan	25–50	100–300	10, 25, 50, 75, 100, 150, L	17
Imipramine	Tofranil	25–50	100–300	10, 25, 50, 75, 100, 125, 150	8 (17)
Trimipramine	Surmontil	25–50	100–300	25, 50, 100	24
Secondary-amine tricyclic antidepressants					
Desipramine	Norpramin	25–50	100–300	10, 25, 50, 75, 100, 150	17
Nortriptyline	Pamelor, Aventyl	25	50–150	10, 25, 50, 75, L	27
Protriptyline	Vivactil	10	15–60	5, 10	79
Tetracyclic antidepressants					
Amoxapine	Asendin	50	100–400	25, 50, 100, 150	8
Maprotiline	Ludiomil	50	100–225	25, 50, 75	43

Table 15–1. Antidepressant medications: dosing and half-life information *(continued)*

Generic drug name	Proprietary drug name	Usual starting dose (mg)[a]	Usual daily dose (mg)	Available oral doses (mg)	Mean half-life, hours (active metabolites)[b]
Selective serotonin reuptake inhibitors					
Citalopram	Celexa	20	20–40[d]	10, 20, 40, L	35
Escitalopram	Lexapro	10	10–20	5, 10, 20, L	27–32
Fluoxetine	Prozac	20	20–60[d]	10, 20, 40, L	72 (216)
Fluoxetine Weekly	Prozac Weekly	90	NA	90	—
Fluvoxamine[e]	Luvox	50	50–300[d]	25, 50, 100	15
Paroxetine	Paxil	20	20–60[d]	10, 20, 30, 40, L	20
Paroxetine CR	Paxil CR	25	25–62.5	12.5, 25, 37.5	15–20
Sertraline	Zoloft	50	50–200[d]	25, 50, 100	26 (66)
Serotonin–norepinephrine reuptake inhibitors					
Duloxetine	Cymbalta	30	60–90	20, 30, 60	12
Venlafaxine	Effexor	37.5	75–225	25, 37.5, 50, 75, 100	5 (11)
Venlafaxine XR	Effexor XR	37.5	75–225	37.5, 75, 150	5 (11)
Serotonin modulators					
Nefazodone[e]	Serzone	50	150–300	100, 150, 200, 250	4
Trazodone	Desyrel	50	75–300	50, 100, 150, 300	7
Norepinephrine–serotonin modulators					
Mirtazapine	Remeron	15	15–45	7.5, 15, 30, 45, soltab	20
Norepinephrine–dopamine reuptake inhibitors					
Bupropion	Wellbutrin	150	300	75, 100	14
Bupropion SR	Wellbutrin SR	150	300	100, 150	21
Bupropion XL	Wellbutrin XL	300	300	100, 150	21

Note. L=liquid; NA=not applicable; CR=controlled release; XL or XR=extended release; soltab=orally disintegrating tablets; SR=sustained release.
[a]Lower starting doses are recommended for elderly patients and patients with panic disorder, significant anxiety, or hepatic disease.
[b]Mean half-lives of active metabolites are given in parentheses.
[c]Not available in the United States.
[d]Dose varies with diagnosis. See text for specific guidelines.
[e]Generic only.

Source. Dosing information from American Psychiatric Association 2000. Half-life data from *Physicians' Desk Reference* 2005. Dosing and half-life information for transdermal selegiline system from EMSAM 2006. Adapted from Marangell LB, Martinez JM: *Concise Guide to Psychopharmacology,* 2nd Edition. Washington, DC, American Psychiatric Publishing, 2006, pp. 13–16. Used with permission.

tional 2 weeks because further improvement at the initial dose may occur.

Treatment of OCD requires a longer duration and higher doses to assess efficacy. A therapeutic trial for OCD should last 8–12 weeks. Late luteal phase dysphoric disorder is more responsive to serotonergic agents than to noradrenergic agents. Interestingly, late luteal phase dysphoric disorder can be treated with medication administered only during the symptomatic period before menses or on a continuous basis (Pearlstein et al. 2000; Wikander et al. 1998; Yonkers et al. 1997).

Risks, Side Effects, and Their Management

Common side effects.   Nausea, loose bowel movements, anxiety, headache, insomnia, and increased sweating are frequent initial side effects of SSRIs. They are usually dose related and may be minimized with low initial dosing and gradual titration. These early adverse effects almost always attenuate after the first few weeks of treatment. Sexual dysfunction (see "Sexual dysfunction" below) is a common long-term side effect of SSRIs.

Gastrointestinal symptoms.   Nausea is a common early, and typically transient, side effect of SSRIs. Some patients report less nausea if they take the medication with food.

Sexual dysfunction.   Decreased libido, anorgasmia, and delayed ejaculation are common side effects of SSRIs. When significant sexual dysfunction persists despite a positive response to treatment, a reduction in the dose may be considered. However, the clinician must balance efficacy and tolerability; for some patients, a lower dose may improve tolerability without compromising the therapeutic benefits, whereas others may not have an adequate therapeutic response to the medication at lower doses. Importantly, some patients may experience sexual side effects throughout the medication dose range. If sexual side effects remain problematic, two main strategies are available: the antidepressant can be replaced with an alternative, or other drugs can be prescribed concomitantly to counteract the side effects. In our experience, switching from one SSRI to another does not tend to decrease sexual side effects. Antidepressants that do not commonly cause sexual dysfunction include bupropion and mirtazapine.

Stimulation and insomnia.   Some patients taking an SSRI may experience jitteriness, restlessness, muscle tension, and disturbed sleep, particularly during the early course of treatment. Patients should be informed of the possibility of the emergence of these side effects and be reassured that if they develop, they tend to be transient. In patients with prominent anxiety, SSRI therapy should be started at low doses, with subsequent titration as tolerated. Additionally, the short-term use of a benzodiazepine (if otherwise safe) may help the patient cope with overstimulation in the early stages of treatment. Despite these transient stimulating effects, SSRIs are effective in patients with anxiety or agitated depression. Similarly, insomnia may occur early in treatment, and short-term, symptomatic treatment with a hypnotic at bedtime is reasonable if necessary.

Bleeding.   SSRIs affect serotonin systems throughout the body, including serotonin in platelets. Because platelets cannot synthesize serotonin, this effect tends to decrease platelet aggregation, which may lead to abnormal bleeding. Two large studies have reported an association between use of SSRIs and increased risk of upper gastrointestinal bleeding or other abnormal bleeding (Dalton et al. 2003; de Abajo et al. 1999). This is most commonly manifested as bruising. Therefore, it is prudent for clinicians to be cautious about prescribing SSRIs for patients with other risk factors for bleeding and to educate patients to inform them if they notice any abnormal bleeding or bruising.

Neurological effects.   Headaches are common early in treatment and usually can be managed with over-the-counter pain relief preparations. SSRIs may initially worsen migraine headaches but are often effective in reducing the severity and frequency of these headaches.

Weight change.   All SSRIs have the potential to cause weight gain in some individuals. In a controlled study, Fava et al. (2000) found that paroxetine was associated with greater weight gain than were fluoxetine and sertraline.

Apathy syndrome.   We and others have noted an apathy syndrome in some patients after months or years of successful treatment with SSRIs. The syndrome is characterized by a loss of motivation, increased passivity, and feelings of lethargy and "flatness." However, sadness, tearfulness, emotional angst, decreased concentration, feelings of hopelessness or worthlessness, and thoughts of suicide are not associated with this syndrome. If specifically asked, patients often remark that the symptoms are not experientially similar to their original depressive symptoms.

Serotonin syndrome.   The serotonin syndrome results from excess serotonergic stimulation and can range in severity from mild to life threatening. The most common symptoms are confusion, flushing, diaphoresis, tremor, and myoclonic jerks. The patient may have symptoms of the serotonin syndrome in the context of monotherapy with a serotonergic medication, but this scenario is less common than symptoms resulting from use of two or more serotonergic drugs simultaneously. Discontinuation of the serotonergic medications is the first step in treatment, followed by emergency medical treatment.

Discontinuation syndrome.   Some patients may experience a series of symptoms after discontinuation or dose reduction of serotonergic antidepressant medications, including dizziness, headache, paresthesia, nausea, diarrhea, insomnia, and irritability. These symptoms also may be seen when a patient misses doses of a serotonergic antidepressant. A prospective double-blind, placebo substitution study confirmed that discontin-

uation symptoms are most common with short-half-life antidepressants, such as paroxetine (Rosenbaum et al. 1998). To avoid a discontinuation syndrome, clinicians should slowly taper antidepressant medications on discontinuation of the drug, particularly medications with short half-lives.

Teratogenicity

Managing major depression, or any psychiatric disorder, in the context of pregnancy is challenging. Although minimizing the risk to the fetus is a clear goal, many patients, families, and even some practitioners need to be reminded that the illness of depression can have adverse effects on the fetus and neonate. Each woman who is facing pregnancy and related psychiatric treatment decisions needs to be approached and advised in the context of her unique circumstances. Some data indicate that the incidence of congenital abnormalities associated with the SSRIs is comparable to that associated with placebo, but other reports note an increased risk of congenital abnormalities, including septal heart defects, with first-trimester exposure and that this risk may be greater with paroxetine and clomipramine (Källén et al. 2006). These data have resulted in a new FDA Category D pregnancy classification for paroxetine.

Drug Interactions

Several deaths have been reported among patients taking a combination of serotonergic antidepressants and MAOIs (Hodgman et al. 1997; Kolecki 1997). Because of the potential lethality of this interaction, a patient who needs to switch from an SSRI to an MAOI must not begin taking the MAOI until the SSRI has been fully eliminated from his or her body. Thus, a period equivalent to at least five times the half-life of the SSRI is required after stopping the SSRI before an MAOI can be initiated. For example, a waiting period of at least 5 weeks is required between discontinuation of fluoxetine and institution of MAOI therapy. A 2-week waiting period is required after stopping an MAOI before an

SSRI can be initiated to allow resynthesis of the monoamine oxidase (MAO) enzyme in the absence of the MAOI.

Serotonin–Norepinephrine Reuptake Inhibitors

Background

Serotonin–norepinephrine reuptake inhibitors (SNRIs) are dual reuptake inhibitors that affect serotonin and norepinephrine but have little effect on muscarinic, H_1, or α_1-adrenergic receptors. Thus, these medications share many of the tolerability and safety benefits of the SSRIs but add an additional pharmacological action compared with SSRIs— namely, norepinephrine reuptake inhibition. Two SNRIs are currently available in the United States: venlafaxine and duloxetine.

Venlafaxine

Background.   Venlafaxine is a dual reuptake inhibitor for both serotonin and norepinephrine; serotonin reuptake inhibition is prominent at lower doses, whereas norepinephrine reuptake inhibition becomes more significant at higher doses.

Clinical use.   The recommended dosage range of venlafaxine is 75–225 mg/day. The extended-release (XL) preparation, which allows for once-daily dosing in most patients, is preferred over the short-acting preparation. The usual starting dosage is 37.5–75 mg/day. Dosages up to 375 mg/day have been used in patients who were otherwise nonresponsive to treatment. Blood pressure monitoring during therapy is recommended because of a dose-dependent risk of increases in mean diastolic blood pressure in some patients.

Risks, side effects, and their management. The side-effect profile of venlafaxine is similar to that of SSRIs and includes gastrointestinal symptoms, sexual dysfunction, and transient discontinuation symptoms. Like the SSRIs, venlafaxine does not affect cardiac conduction or lower the seizure threshold. In most patients, venlafaxine is not associated with sedation or weight gain. Side effects that differ from those of SSRIs are hypothesized to be related to the increased noradrenergic activity of this drug at higher doses; these side effects include dose-dependent anxiety (in some patients) and dose-dependent hypertension. A meta-analysis found that the magnitude of change in blood pressure associated with venlafaxine use is statistically significant but is unlikely to be of clinical significance at dosages less than 300 mg/day. However, the incidence of hypertension is 13% at dosages greater than 300 mg/day.

Overdose.   Few data are available regarding venlafaxine in overdose, but the drug's pharmacological profile suggests that it is safer than TCAs. In most of the reported cases to date, symptoms were not present.

Drug interactions.   Venlafaxine does not appear to inhibit cytochrome P450 enzymes significantly and is not highly protein bound; thus, venlafaxine is less likely to contribute to protein-binding interactions than most other antidepressants. However, venlafaxine should not be combined with MAOIs because of the risk for serotonin syndrome.

Duloxetine

Background.   Duloxetine hydrochloride is an SNRI that is approved by the FDA for the treatment of both major depression and the pain associated with diabetic peripheral neuropathy. Interestingly, it does not appear to induce sustained treatment-emergent hypertension compared with placebo, although rare cases are possible. Its half-life is approximately 12 hours, and it is highly protein bound. The most frequent side effect is early nausea, which is dose dependent and typically transient. Like venlafaxine, duloxetine typically is not associated with significant changes in weight.

Clinical use.   The recommended dosage for the treatment of major depression is 60 mg/day, whereas in diabetic neuropathy, a dosage of up to 120 mg/day is recommended.

Nausea in the early phases of treatment is dose dependent, so treatment-naive patients might benefit from starting at 30 mg/day for the first week and then increasing to the target dosage of 60 mg/day. At present, duloxetine is not recommended for use in patients with end-stage renal disease, severe renal impairment, or any hepatic insufficiency (Cymbalta 2006).

Risks, side effects, and their management. The side-effect profile of duloxetine is similar to that of SSRIs. Like the SSRIs, duloxetine does not affect cardiac conduction or lower the seizure threshold. In most patients, duloxetine is not associated with sedation. Nausea may occur during treatment initiation, but it is generally transient.

Duloxetine has been associated with increases in serum transaminase levels. In controlled trials in major depressive disorder, elevations of alanine aminotransferase (ALT) to greater than three times the upper limit of normal occurred in 0.9% (8 of 930) of the duloxetine-treated patients and in 0.3% (2 of 652) of the placebo-treated patients (Cymbalta 2006). Additionally, postmarketing reports have indicated occurrences of hepatitis, hepatomegaly with liver enzyme elevation, severe hepatic enzyme elevation, and cholestatic jaundice (Cymbalta 2006).

Duloxetine use is associated with an increased risk of mydriasis; therefore, it should not be used in patients with uncontrolled narrow-angle glaucoma.

The controlled clinical trials of duloxetine in the treatment of major depression used a rating scale to assess prospectively treatment-emergent sexual dysfunction. As with SSRIs and venlafaxine, males who received duloxetine experienced more difficulty with ability to reach orgasm than did males who received placebo. However, females taking duloxetine did not experience more sexual dysfunction than did those taking placebo (Cymbalta 2006).

Overdose. Few data are available regarding duloxetine in overdose. Recommended treatment includes general supportive and symptomatic measures. Dialysis is not recommended because the drug is highly protein bound.

Drug interactions. Duloxetine is a moderate inhibitor of the CYP2D6 enzyme and may increase the levels of other medications that use this enzyme. Because of the risk of serotonin syndrome, duloxetine should not be combined with MAOIs. Because duloxetine is highly bound to plasma protein, combination with another drug that is highly protein bound may cause increased free concentrations of the other drug, potentially resulting in adverse events.

Bupropion

Background

Bupropion facilitates dopamine transmission; thus, many clinicians preferentially use this agent for depressed patients with Parkinson's disease. The fact that dopamine is integrally related to the brain's reward mechanisms, which are stimulated by nicotine and other addictive substances, has provided the theoretical underpinning for recent research indicating that bupropion is an effective aid in smoking cessation.

Overall, bupropion has a favorable side-effect profile. The drug is associated with little or no weight gain, has few effects on cardiac conduction, and has minimal sexual side effects. Disadvantages include an increased risk of medication-induced seizures at higher-than-recommended doses.

Clinical Use

Use of the XL preparation is preferred because of increased tolerability, decreased seizure risk, and the convenience of once-daily dosing. Treatment with the sustained-release (SR) or XL preparation is initiated at a dose of 150 mg, preferably taken in the morning. After 4 days, the dosage may be increased to 150 mg twice a day (SR) or 300 mg once daily in the morning (XL).

Contraindications

Patients with seizure disorders should not take bupropion. Similarly, an alternative treatment should be considered in patients with a history of significant head trauma, a central nervous system (CNS) tumor, or an active eating disorder.

Risks, Side Effects, and Their Management

The most common side effects of bupropion are initial headache, anxiety, insomnia, increased sweating, and gastrointestinal upset. Tremor and akathisia also may occur. Management is the same as for SSRI side effects.

Seizures. The incidence of seizures with the immediate-release preparation is 0.4% at dosages less than 450 mg/day, provided no single dose of the short-acting preparation exceeds 150 mg. The incidence increases to 5% at dosages between 450 and 600 mg/day.

Psychosis. Reports of delusions, hallucinations, and paranoia are consistent with bupropion-mediated increases in central dopamine. Bupropion should be used with caution in patients with psychotic disorders.

Overdose

Much more is known about overdose with the immediate-release formulation of bupropion than with the newer SR and XL formulations. Reported reactions to overdose with the immediate-release form include seizures, hallucinations, loss of consciousness, and sinus tachycardia.

One danger associated with bupropion overdose is a risk of seizures. However, seizures are seldom life threatening unless they result in motor vehicle accidents, falls, or other trauma-related events.

Drug Interactions

The combination of bupropion with an MAOI is potentially dangerous but less so than the combination of serotonergic drugs and MAOIs. Although the practice is not recommended, MAOIs and bupropion have been combined in some patients with refractory depression.

Data to date suggest that bupropion is metabolized by CYP2B6 (Faucette et al. 2000). Bupropion inhibits CYP2D6. Because of the risk of dose-dependent seizures, caution is warranted when bupropion is combined with other medications that might inhibit its metabolism.

Nefazodone

Nefazodone is primarily a postsynaptic 5-hydroxytryptamine (serotonin) type 2 (5-HT$_2$) antagonist. The branded product was removed from the market in 2003 after reports of hepatotoxicity. The reported rate of liver failure resulting in death or transplant in the United States is approximately 1 case per 250,000–300,000 patient-years of exposure (Serzone 2002). Nefazodone is available in generic formulations, mostly for patients who have been stabilized previously while taking this medication and need ongoing treatment. Individuals who develop increased serum transaminase levels of three times the upper limits of the normal range or higher should be withdrawn from nefazodone and not be considered for nefazodone rechallenge.

Trazodone

Background

Trazodone is an antidepressant that is associated with significant sedation. Currently, trazodone is not recommended as a first-line antidepressant because of an increased risk of orthostatic hypotension, arrhythmias, and priapism. However, trazodone may be useful in some patients with insomnia (although the use of trazodone specifically for insomnia is not approved by the FDA).

Clinical Use

The recommended dosage range for trazodone is 200–400 mg/day in divided doses. Initial dosing should begin at 50 mg/day. For many patients, even low doses of trazodone may be associated with significant sedation;

thus, most of the daily dose should be administered at night.

Risks, Side Effects, and Their Management

Excessive sedation is the most commonly encountered side effect of trazodone. Although trazodone has virtually no anticholinergic side effects, dry mouth and blurred vision occur more frequently with trazodone treatment than with placebo.

Trazodone can cause orthostatic hypotension and dizziness. Additionally, there have been reports of increased ventricular irritability among patients with conduction defects and preexisting ventricular arrhythmias (Aronson and Hafez 1986; Jankowsky et al. 1983; Vitullo et al. 1990).

Trazodone has been associated with priapism (Scher et al. 1983), which may be irreversible and require surgical intervention.

Overdose

Trazodone overdose carries a risk of myocardial irritation in patients with preexisting ventricular conduction abnormalities.

Mirtazapine

Background

Mirtazapine has been shown to reduce anxiety symptoms and sleep disturbances associated with depression as early as 1 week after the start of treatment. Other advantages are minimal sexual dysfunction, minimal nausea, and once-daily dosing. In addition, mirtazapine is unlikely to be associated with cytochrome P450–mediated drug interactions.

Mechanism of Action

Mirtazapine facilitates central serotonergic and noradrenergic transmission by antagonizing α_2-noradrenergic autoreceptors and heteroreceptors (De Boer 1996). In addition, mirtazapine antagonizes postsynaptic 5-HT$_{2A}$, 5-HT$_3$, and H$_1$ receptors and has moderate activity at α_1-adrenergic and muscarinic receptors.

Clinical Use

Mirtazapine treatment is initiated at a dosage of 15 mg at bedtime. The maximum recommended daily dose is 45 mg. Elderly patients and individuals with renal or hepatic disease may require lower doses.

Risks, Side Effects, and Their Management

Common side effects. The most common side effects associated with mirtazapine are sedation, weight gain, and dizziness. Somnolence occurs in more than 50% of the patients taking mirtazapine (Bremner 1995; Smith et al. 1990). Tolerance to this side effect generally develops after the first few weeks of treatment. Weight gain also may be associated with mirtazapine treatment.

Anticholinergic effects. Mirtazapine is associated with modest anticholinergic side effects, including dry mouth and constipation. Anticholinergic side effects and their management are discussed in the "Tricyclic and Heterocyclic Antidepressants" subsection later in this chapter.

Overdose

Little is known about mirtazapine overdose. To date, patients who have overdosed have fully recovered.

Drug Interactions

Mirtazapine does not significantly inhibit hepatic cytochrome P450 enzymes. Mirtazapine should not be used in combination with an MAOI or within 14 days of discontinuing treatment with an MAOI.

Tricyclic and Heterocyclic Antidepressants

Background

All TCAs have a three-ring nucleus. Most clinicians do not use TCAs as first-line antidepressants because, relative to the newer antidepressants, TCAs tend to have more side effects, require gradual titration, and can be lethal in overdose. Some data suggest that TCAs may be more effective than SSRIs in the treatment of major depression with melancholic features (Danish University Antidepressant Group 1990). However, many clinicians prefer the newer antidepressants because of their safety and tolerability compared with TCAs.

Imipramine, amitriptyline, clomipramine, trimipramine, and doxepin are tertiary-amine TCAs. Desipramine, nortriptyline, and protriptyline are secondary-amine TCAs. Tertiary-amine tricyclics have more potent serotonin reuptake inhibition, and secondary-amine tricyclics have more potent noradrenergic reuptake inhibition. Tertiary-amine TCAs tend to have more side effects than do secondary-amine TCAs. Desipramine and protriptyline tend to be activating. Among the TCAs, nortriptyline is the least likely to produce orthostatic hypotension. Because amoxapine has an active metabolite that antagonizes dopamine type 2 (D_2) receptors, it can cause treatment-emergent extrapyramidal side effects (EPS).

Mechanism of Action

TCAs inhibit norepinephrine, serotonin, and (to a lesser degree) dopamine reuptake. Additionally, they exert inhibitory effects on H_1, muscarinic, and α_1-adrenergic receptors.

Clinical Use

Because of potential cardiovascular effects and risks associated with TCAs, the clinician should obtain a cardiovascular history before initiating TCA therapy. In patients with preexisting heart disease and patients older than 40 years, an electrocardiogram (ECG) should be obtained before TCA treatment. TCAs should not be used in patients with bundle branch block unless all other options have failed. Additionally, other treatment options should be considered for patients with ischemic heart disease. Because orthostatic hypotension can occur with TCA treatment, other potential risk factors for hypotension should be explored.

Imipramine, amitriptyline, doxepin, desipramine, clomipramine, and trimipramine

therapy can be initiated at 25–50 mg/day. Divided dosing may be used at first to minimize side effects, but eventually the entire dose can be given at bedtime. The dosage can be increased to 150 mg/day the second week, 225 mg/day the third week, and 300 mg/day the fourth week. The clomipramine dosage should not exceed 250 mg/day because of an increased risk of seizures at higher doses.

Nortriptyline therapy should be initiated at 25 mg/day, and the dosage should be increased to 75 mg/day over 1–2 weeks depending on tolerability and clinical response. Some patients require dosages of up to 150 mg/day. Amoxapine should be started at 50 mg/day, and the dosage should be titrated to 400 mg/day. Amoxapine has a short half-life and should be given in divided doses. Treatment with protriptyline can be started at 10 mg/day, and the dosage can be increased to 60 mg/day. Maprotiline therapy should be started at 50 mg/day, and that dosage should be maintained for 2 weeks; the risk of seizure increases if the dosage is raised too quickly. The dosage can be increased over 4 weeks to 225 mg/day.

TCA Plasma Levels and Therapeutic Monitoring

Clinically meaningful plasma levels are available for imipramine, desipramine, and nortriptyline. For imipramine, the sum of the plasma levels of imipramine and the desmethyl metabolite (desipramine) should be greater than 200 ng/mL. Desipramine levels should be greater than 125 ng/mL. A therapeutic window has been noted for nortriptyline, with optimal response between 50 and 150 ng/mL. These therapeutic levels are based on steady-state concentrations, which are reached after 5–7 days of administration of these medications. Blood should be drawn approximately 10–14 hours after the last dose of medication.

Risks, Side Effects, and Their Management

Anticholinergic effects. Common anticholinergic side effects include dry mouth, constipation, urinary retention, blurred vision, and tachycardia. Additionally, anticholinergic medications may cause cognitive impairment and confusion. Because the tertiary amine TCAs and protriptyline have a particularly high affinity for muscarinic receptors, these medications are more likely than others within the TCA class to have anticholinergic side effects.

Sedation. Many TCAs can be associated with sedation. The sedative properties of TCAs appear to parallel their respective histamine receptor binding affinities.

Cardiovascular effects. Cardiovascular effects include orthostatic hypotension, tachycardia, and cardiac conduction delays. These side effects may be clinically significant for many patients, particularly those with preexisting heart disease. Although TCAs at toxic levels can cause life-threatening arrhythmias, TCAs are potent antiarrhythmic agents, possessing quinidine-like properties. Because prolongation of PR and QRS intervals can occur with TCA use, these drugs should not be used in patients with preexisting heart block (especially right bundle branch block and left bundle branch block). In such patients, treatment with TCAs may lead to second- or third-degree heart block, both life-threatening conditions (Roose et al. 1987).

Weight gain. Weight gain is a common side effect of TCA treatment.

Seizures. A dose-related risk of seizures has been found with clomipramine, which has led to the recommendation that the total daily dose of this drug not exceed 250 mg. Overdoses of TCAs, particularly amoxapine and desipramine, also are associated with seizures.

Extrapyramidal side effects (amoxapine only). Amoxapine, which has a mild neuroleptic effect, can cause EPS, akathisia, and even tardive dyskinesias.

Overdose

Complications of TCA overdose may include neuropsychiatric impairment, hypotension, cardiac arrhythmias, and seizures. Anticholinergic delirium may occur, as well as other complications of anticholinergic overdose, including agitation, supraventricular arrhythmias, hallucinations, severe hypertension, and seizures. Patients with anticholinergic delirium have hot, dry skin; tachycardia; dilated pupils; dry mucous membranes; and absent bowel sounds. Anticholinergic delirium is a medical emergency and requires emergent care.

Hypotension, which may result from norepinephrine depletion or have other causes related to peripheral and central effects of TCAs, should be treated with vigorous fluid replacement. Seizures and cardiac complications also may occur with TCA overdose. When the QRS interval is less than 0.10 second, the likelihood of seizures or ventricular arrhythmias decreases. Ventricular arrhythmias that occur secondary to overdose are typical of arrhythmias resulting from high doses of quinidine-like agents and begin within the first 24 hours after hospital admission. Ventricular arrhythmias should be treated with lidocaine, propranolol, or phenytoin. Prophylactic treatment with phenytoin and insertion of a temporary pacemaker should be considered in patients with prolonged QRS intervals (i.e., longer than 120 msec).

Drug Interactions

Drugs that induce hepatic microsomal enzymes or inhibit hepatic enzymes (particularly CYP2D6 inhibitors) may alter plasma tricyclic levels. The coadministration of a TCA and a potent CYP2D6 inhibitor may result in dangerously high levels of the TCA.

Monoamine Oxidase Inhibitors

Background

Oral MAOIs are not currently used as first-line agents in the treatment of major depression, largely because newer antidepressants are generally safer and better tolerated. However, these medications remain excellent medications for patients who do not respond to the newer antidepressant drugs. Patients with atypical depression, characterized by oversleeping and overeating, show a preferential response to MAOI therapy (Quitkin et al. 1979).

Mechanism of Action

The enzyme monoamine oxidase A (MAO-A) acts selectively on norepinephrine and serotonin, whereas monoamine oxidase B (MAO-B) preferentially affects phenylethylamine. Both MAO-A and MAO-B oxidize dopamine and tyramine. MAO-A inhibition appears to be most relevant to the antidepressant effects of these drugs. Drugs that inhibit both MAO-A and MAO-B are called *nonselective*. Because tyramine can be metabolized by either MAO-A or MAO-B, drugs that selectively inhibit one of these enzymes but not the other do not require dietary restrictions. MAO-A–selective drugs, such as moclobemide, are available in other countries (e.g., Canada) for the treatment of depression. MAO-B–selective drugs, such as pargyline, are marketed for other indications. Selegiline is an irreversible MAOI that is selective for MAO-B at lower doses—namely, those doses typically used in the treatment of Parkinson's disease, but selegiline inhibits both MAO-A and MAO-B at antidepressant doses.

In addition to potential selectivity for MAO-A or MAO-B, MAOIs may produce either reversible or irreversible enzyme inhibition. An *irreversible inhibitor* permanently disables the enzyme, and the enzyme must be resynthesized in the absence of the drug before the activity of the enzyme can be reestablished. MAO enzyme resynthesis may take up to 2 weeks in the absence of an MAOI; thus, an interval of approximately 14 days is required after discontinuing an irreversible MAOI before instituting treatment with other antidepressants, permitting the use of contraindicated drugs, or permitting the consumption of contraindicated foods. On the other hand, a *reversible inhibitor* can move away from the active site of the enzyme, making the enzyme available to metabolize other substances.

Clinical Use

The physician should discuss the risks associated with MAOI use with the patient and should review and discuss the need to adhere to the appropriate dietary restrictions and avoid medications that may lead to potentially dangerous interactions (Table 15–2). Patients should be advised not to start any new medications without first informing their physician. Indeed, many patients assume that over-the-counter medications and herbal supplements are safe and pose no risk; thus, patients may hastily begin taking one of these agents without discussing it with their physician, potentially putting themselves at risk for serious drug interactions.

Phenelzine therapy is initiated at a dose of 15 mg in the morning, and the dose is increased by 15 mg every other day until a total daily dose of 60 mg is reached. If no response occurs within 2 weeks, the dose may be increased in 15-mg increments to a usual maximum of 90 mg/day. Higher doses are sometimes used, if tolerated, in patients with severe refractory depression. Treatment with tranylcypromine is initiated at a dose of 10 mg, and the dose is then increased every other day to 30 mg/day. As with phenelzine, higher doses may be necessary when the condition is refractory to treatment (Amsterdam and Berwish 1989). After tolerance to the hypotensive side effects has developed, usually after 1 or 2 weeks, the patient may take the medication in a single daily dose in the morning. Morning dosing is preferred because these medications tend to be activating; this is especially true of tranylcypromine, which is related to amphetamine.

Selegiline is an irreversible MAOI that is selective for MAO-B at lower doses and, when administered orally, undergoes extensive first-pass metabolism to amphetamine and methamphetamine metabolites (Karoum et al. 1982). Transdermal selegiline (EMSAM),

Table 15–2. Dietary and medication restrictions for patients taking nonselective monoamine oxidase inhibitors (MAOIs)

Foods to avoid while taking an MAOI and for 2 weeks after discontinuing the medication[a]

Aged cheeses	Meat extracts (e.g., Bovril)
Aged or fermented meats (e.g., sausage, salami, pepperoni)	Sauerkraut
All foods that may be spoiled	Soy sauce
Fava beans and broad bean pods	Tap beer, including nonalcoholic tap beer
	Yeast extracts (e.g., Marmite)

Safe foods

Alcohol (but not tap beer), in moderation	Fresh yogurt
Fresh cheeses (e.g., cream cheese, cottage cheese, ricotta cheese,	Smoked salmon and whitefish
American cheese, moderate amounts of mozzarella)	Yeast and baked goods containing yeast

Drugs to avoid while taking an MAOI and for 2 weeks after discontinuing the medication[b]

All sympathomimetic and stimulant drugs

Amphetamines	Local anesthetic drugs containing epinephrine or cocaine
Buspirone	Meperidine
Diet medications	Methylphenidate
Ephedrine	Other antidepressant medications
Fenfluramine and dexfenfluramine	Phenylephrine
Isoproterenol	Phenylpropanolamine
Levodopa and dopamine	

Over-the-counter nasal decongestants; cold, sinus, and allergy medications containing pseudoephedrine, phenylephrine, or phenylpropanolamine; and supplements

Actifed	NyQuil
Alka-Seltzer Plus	Robitussin PE, DM, CF, Night Relief
Allerest	Sine-Aid
Contac	Sine-Off
Coricidin D	Sinex
CoTylenol	St. John's wort
Dristan	Triaminic
L-Tryptophan	Tylenol
Neo-Synephrine	Vicks 44M, 44D

Table 15–2. Dietary and medication restrictions for patients taking nonselective monoamine oxidase inhibitors (MAOIs) *(continued)*

Other medications

    Carbamazepine

    Oxcarbazepine

Safe cold and allergy medications

    Alka-Seltzer (plain)

    Chlor-Trimeton Allergy (without decongestant)

    Robitussin (plain)

    Tylenol (plain)

Other safe medications

    Antibiotics

    Codeine

    Laxatives and stool softeners

    Local anesthetics without epinephrine or cocaine

    Morphine

    Nonsteroidal anti-inflammatory drugs

[a]Food restrictions based on tyramine content data from Walker et al. 1996.

[b]It is strongly advised that the reader consult the current *Physicians' Desk Reference* before prescribing any medication in combination with an MAOI.

Source. EMSAM 2006; Feinberg and Holzer 1997, 2000; Gardner et al. 1996; *Physicians' Desk Reference* 2006; Shulman and Walker 1999, 2000; Shulman et al. 1997; Walker et al. 1996, 1997; Wing and Chen 1997. Adapted from Marangell LB, Martinez JM: *Concise Guide to Psychopharmacology,* 2nd Edition. Washington, DC, American Psychiatric Publishing, 2006, pp. 48–50. Used with permission.

which allows selegiline to be absorbed directly into the bloodstream, avoids first-pass metabolism (Rohatagi et al. 1997) and selectively targets MAO-A and MAO-B enzymes in the brain relative to those in the gastrointestinal tract (Wecker et al. 2003). Transdermal selegiline has been shown to be effective in the short-term treatment of depression in controlled trials (Amsterdam 2003; Bodkin and Amsterdam 2002). Transdermal selegiline is applied to dry skin on the upper torso, upper thigh, or outer surface of the upper arm once every 24 hours and not applied to the same site on consecutive days (EMSAM 2006). Patients should be advised to wash their hands after applying the transdermal system and also to avoid exposing the transdermal selegiline patch to external sources of heat.

Currently, transdermal selegiline is available in three dosages: 6 mg/24 hours (20 mg/20 cm^2), 9 mg/24 hours (30 mg/30 cm^2), and 12 mg/24 hours (40 mg/40 cm^2). The recommended starting and target dose is 6 mg/24 hours, and dose increases in increments of 3 mg/24 hours should occur at intervals of at least 2 weeks. The maximum recommended daily dosage is 12 mg/24 hours. Additionally, current product labeling does not require dietary restrictions for the 6-mg/24-hour dosing but does require dietary restrictions for the 9-mg/24-hour and 12-mg/24-hour dosing (EMSAM 2006). However, the concomitant medication warnings and restrictions apply across all transdermal selegiline dosages.

Risks, Side Effects, and Their Management

The following side effects apply to the irreversible, nonselective MAOI antidepressants (phenelzine and tranylcypromine). The most common side effects are orthostatic hypotension, headache, insomnia, weight gain, sexual dysfunction, peripheral edema, and afternoon somnolence.

Transdermal selegiline was generally well tolerated in controlled trials; common adverse events included headache, insomnia, diarrhea, dry mouth, dyspepsia, and rash (EMSAM 2006).

Hypertensive crisis Inactivation of intestinal MAO impairs the metabolism of tyramine. Tyramine can act as a false transmitter and displace norepinephrine from presynaptic storage granules. Therefore, large amounts of dietary tyramine can result in a hypertensive crisis in patients taking MAOIs because increased amounts of norepinephrine are displaced from adrenergic terminals, resulting in profound α-adrenergic activation. This reaction has also been called the "cheese reaction" because tyramine is present in relatively high concentrations in aged cheeses.

Tyramine is formed in foods by the decarboxylation of tyrosine during the aging, ripening, or decaying process of foods. Patients receiving MAOIs should be instructed to avoid the foods listed in Table 15–2.

Patients taking MAOIs are advised to carry identification cards that indicate that they are taking MAOIs. Before accepting any medication or anesthetic, patients should notify their physicians that they are taking MAOIs. When patients undergo dental procedures, local anesthetics without vasoconstrictors (e.g., epinephrine) must be used. Additionally, patients may want to have a home blood pressure cuff.

Serotonin syndrome. The combination of serotonergic drugs, such as SSRIs, with MAOIs can result in a potentially fatal hypermetabolic reaction, often referred to as the *serotonin syndrome*. Affected individuals may experience lethargy, restlessness, confusion, flushing, diaphoresis, tremor, and myoclonic jerks. As the condition progresses, hyperthermia, hypertonicity, myoclonus, and death may occur. The syndrome must be identified as rapidly as possible. Discontinuation of the serotonergic medications is the first step in treatment, followed by emergency medical treatment as required.

The combination of MAOIs with meperidine, and perhaps with other phenylpiperidine analgesics, also has been implicated in fatal reactions attributed to the serotonin syndrome.

Cardiovascular effects.   The MAOIs cause significant hypotension, which is often their dose-limiting side effect. Expansion of intravascular volume through administration of salt tablets or fludrocortisone may be an effective treatment.

Weight gain.   MAOIs are associated with a risk of significant weight gain during treatment.

Sexual dysfunction.   MAOIs are commonly associated with treatment-emergent sexual dysfunction, including decreased libido, delayed ejaculation, anorgasmia, and impotence.

CNS effects.   Headache and insomnia are common initial side effects that usually disappear after the first few weeks of treatment. A brief nap may help restore alertness.

Overdose

Most complications related to MAOI overdose arise from the drugs' stimulation of the sympathetic nervous system. MAOIs are most dangerous when patients experience hypertensive crises as the result of ingesting foods with high tyramine content.

Drug Interactions

Inhibition of MAO can cause severe interactions with other drugs, as detailed in the "Hypertensive Crisis" and "Serotonin Syndrome" subsections earlier in this section. A list of some drugs that interact with the nonselective MAOIs is provided in Table 15–2.

Discontinuation of Antidepressants

Discontinuation of antidepressant medication should be concordant with the guidelines for treatment duration. It is advisable to taper the dose while monitoring for signs and symptoms of relapse. Abrupt discontinuation is also more likely to lead to antidepressant discontinuation symptoms, often referred to as *withdrawal symptoms.* The occurrence of these symptoms after medication discontinuation does not imply that antidepressants are addictive.

Discontinuation symptoms appear to occur most commonly after discontinuation of short-half-life serotonergic drugs (Coupland et al. 1996), such as fluvoxamine, paroxetine, and venlafaxine. Patients describe symptoms as "flulike," including nausea, diarrhea, insomnia, malaise, muscle aches, anxiety, irritability, dizziness, vertigo, and vivid dreams (Coupland et al. 1996).

Discontinuation symptoms usually occur within 1–2 days after abrupt discontinuation of a medication and subside within 7–10 days. In some instances, symptoms also may occur during tapering and dose reduction, and they may persist for up to 3 weeks. Restarting treatment with the medication and then tapering more slowly may be necessary, although it is often possible to attenuate withdrawal symptoms produced by short-half-life SSRIs by administering one dose of fluoxetine (which has a longer half-life).

Abrupt discontinuation of TCAs commonly results in diarrhea, increased sweating, anxiety, and dizziness. These symptoms were previously attributed to cholinergic rebound, but the occurrence of similar symptoms after the discontinuation of many of the newer serotonergic antidepressants suggests that the pathophysiology may be more closely related to changes in serotonin.

Anxiolytics, Sedatives, and Hypnotics

Overview

Anxiety and insomnia are prevalent symptoms with multiple etiologies. Effective treatments are available, but they vary by diagnosis. In most instances, the best course of action is to treat the underlying disorder rather than reflexively instituting treatment with a nonspecific anxiolytic.

In some cases, anxiolytics serve a transitional purpose. For example, for a patient with acute-onset panic disorder, severe anticipatory anxiety, and a family history of depression, administration of an antidepressant medication that also has antipanic effects may be the optimal treatment, but this will not help the patient for several weeks, during which time there is a risk of progression to agoraphobia. For this patient, starting antidepressant therapy and also attempting to obtain acute symptom relief with a benzodiazepine may be helpful. After 4 weeks, the benzodiazepine dose should be slowly tapered so that the patient's condition is controlled with the antidepressant alone.

In this section, we review the pharmacology of medications that are primarily classified as anxiolytic, sedative, or hypnotic agents. Common anxiolytics and hypnotics are shown in Table 15–3.

Benzodiazepines

Mechanisms of Action

Benzodiazepines facilitate inhibition by γ-aminobutyric acid (GABA), a major inhibitory neurotransmitter in the brain (reviewed by Tallman et al. 1980). The benzodiazepine receptor is a subtype of the $GABA_A$ receptor. Activation of the benzodiazepine receptor facilitates the action of endogenous GABA, which results in the opening of chloride ion channels and a decrease in neuronal excitability.

Indications and Efficacy

Benzodiazepines are highly effective anxiolytics and sedatives. They also have muscle relaxant, amnestic, and anticonvulsant properties. Benzodiazepines effectively treat acute and chronic generalized anxiety and panic disorder. The high-potency benzodiazepines alprazolam and clonazepam have received more attention as antipanic agents, but double-blind studies also have confirmed the efficacy of diazepam and lorazepam in the treatment of panic disorder. Although only a few benzodiazepines are specifically ap-

proved by the FDA for the treatment of insomnia, almost all benzodiazepines may be used for this purpose. Benzodiazepines are most clearly valuable as hypnotics in the hospital setting, where high levels of sensory stimulation, pain, and acute stress may interfere with sleep. The safe, effective, and time-limited use of benzodiazepine hypnotics may, in fact, prevent chronic sleep difficulties (NIMH/NIH Consensus Development Conference Statement 1985). Benzodiazepines are also used to treat akathisia and catatonia and as adjuncts in the treatment of acute mania.

Because alcohol and barbiturates also act, in part, via the $GABA_A$ receptor–mediated chloride ion channel, benzodiazepines show cross-tolerance with these substances. Thus, benzodiazepines are used frequently for treating alcohol or barbiturate withdrawal and detoxification. Alcohol and barbiturates are more dangerous than benzodiazepines because they can act directly at the chloride ion channel at higher doses. In contrast, benzodiazepines have no direct effect on the ion channel; the effects of benzodiazepines are limited by the amount of endogenous GABA.

Benzodiazepine Selection

At equipotent doses, all benzodiazepines have similar effects. The choice of benzodiazepine is generally based on half-life, rapidity of onset, metabolism, and potency. In patients with moderate to severe hepatic dysfunction, it may be useful to avoid benzodiazepines. All benzodiazepines are metabolized at various levels by the liver, which leads to an increased risk of sedation and confusion in patients with hepatic failure. If it is necessary to prescribe this class of medication, lorazepam and oxazepam are reasonable choices because their elimination will not be significantly affected (Abernethy et al. 1984).

Risks, Side Effects, and Their Management

Sedation and impairment of performance. Benzodiazepine-induced sedation may be considered either a therapeutic action or a

Table 15–3. Commonly used anxiolytic and hypnotic agents

Generic drug	Proprietary name	Dose equivalence (mg)	Typical starting dose in adults[a] (mg)	Typical daily dosage range in adults[a] (mg/day)
Anxiolytic medications				
Benzodiazepines used as anxiolytics				
Alprazolam	Xanax	0.5	0.25–0.5 tid (0.5 tid for panic)	0.75–4 (divided) (1–6 for panic)
Alprazolam extended-release	Xanax XR	NA	0.5–1	3–6
Chlordiazepoxide	Librium	10	5–25 tid or qid	15–100 (divided tid or qid)
Clonazepam	Klonopin	0.25	0.25 bid	1–4
Clorazepate	Tranxene	7.5	15 (T-tab)	T-tab: 15–60 (divided) SD: 22.5 qd to replace T-tab 7.5 tid
Diazepam	Valium	5	2–10 bid–qid	4–40 (divided)
Lorazepam	Ativan	1	0.5–2 tid–qid	2–4 (divided)
Oxazepam	Serax	15	10–30 tid–qid	30–120 (divided)
Nonbenzodiazepines used as anxiolytics				
Buspirone	BuSpar	NA	10–30 (divided)	30–60 (divided)
Hypnotic medications				
Benzodiazepines used as anxiolytics				
Estazolam	ProSom	—	1	1–2
Flurazepam	Dalmane	—	15–30	15–30
Quazepam	Doral	—	7.5–15	7.5–15
Temazepam	Restoril	—	15	15–30
Triazolam	Halcion	—	0.125	0.125–0.25
Nonbenzodiazepine GABA–benzodiazepine receptor agonists used as hypnotics				
Eszopiclone	Lunesta	NA	2	2–3
Zaleplon	Sonata	NA	5–10	5–10
Zolpidem	Ambien	NA	5–10	5–10
Zolpidem extended-release	Ambien CR	NA	12.5	6.25–12.5

Table 15–3. Commonly used anxiolytic and hypnotic agents *(continued)*

Generic drug	Proprietary name	Dose equivalence (mg)	Typical starting dose in adults[a] (mg)	Typical daily dosage range in adults[a] (mg/day)
Nonbenzodiazepine melatonin MT₁ and MT₂ receptor agonists used as hypnotics				
Ramelteon	Rozerem	NA	8	8

Note. td=three-times-per-day dosing; NA=not applicable; qid=four-times-per-day dosing; bid=twice-daily dosing; qd=once-daily dosing; CR=extended release; SD=single dose; T-tab=T-shaped tablet; GABA=γ-aminobutyric acid.

[a]The typical starting doses are for healthy adults. Special populations, such as the elderly, debilitated, or hepatically or renally impaired, may require lower doses or may preclude the use of certain agents.

Source. Drug Facts and Comparisons 2002; Fuller and Sajatovic 2004; Jenkins et al. 2001; Nishino et al. 2004; *Physicians' Desk Reference* 2006; Pies 1998; Shader and Greenblatt 2003.

side effect. When a patient takes a benzodiazepine at night, particularly an agent with a
long half-life, residual sedation may be present on awakening. Additionally, any benzodiazepine has the potential to cause sedation.

Impairment of performance on sensitive
psychomotor tests has been well documented
after the administration of benzodiazepines.
Patients must be warned that driving, engaging in dangerous physical activities, and using hazardous machinery should be avoided
during treatment with benzodiazepines, particularly during the early course of treatment.

*Dependence, withdrawal, and rebound ef-
fects.* Many patients and clinicians are concerned about the abuse and dependence potential of benzodiazepines. Most benzodiazepines have a low abuse potential when they
are properly prescribed and their use is supervised (American Psychiatric Association
1990). However, physical dependence often
occurs when benzodiazepines are taken at
higher-than-usual doses or for prolonged periods.

If benzodiazepines are discontinued precipitously, withdrawal effects (including hy-
perpyrexia, seizures, psychosis, and even
death) may occur. Signs and symptoms of
withdrawal may include tachycardia, increased blood pressure, muscle cramps, anxiety, insomnia, panic attacks, impairment of
memory and concentration, perceptual disturbances, and delirium. In addition, with-
drawal-related derealization, hallucinations,
and other psychotic symptoms may occur.
These withdrawal symptoms may begin as
early as the day after discontinuation of the
benzodiazepine, and they may continue for
weeks to months. Evidence indicates that
withdrawal reactions associated with
shorter-half-life benzodiazepines peak more
rapidly and more intensely. These withdrawal symptoms may be alleviated by rein-
troducing the withdrawn benzodiazepine.

Rebound anxiety and insomnia also may
occur when benzodiazepines are abruptly
discontinued. As a general rule, most psychoactive medications should be discontinued

gradually, not abruptly. For patients who have
been taking benzodiazepines for longer than
2–3 months, the benzodiazepine dose should
be decreased by approximately 10% per week.
Therefore, in the case of a patient receiving alprazolam 4 mg/day, the dose should be tapered by 0.5 mg/week for 8 weeks.

Memory impairment. Benzodiazepines are
associated with anterograde amnesia, especially when they are administered intravenously and in high doses (Dixon et al. 1984;
Lucki et al. 1986; Reitan et al. 1986). Amnesia
may be a desirable effect of benzodiazepines
when they are used for surgical procedures,
but memory impairment in other instances
may be a serious liability. Clinicians should
warn patients about the potential risk for amnesia when prescribing all benzodiazepines.

Disinhibition and dyscontrol. Anecdotal
reports suggest that benzodiazepines may
occasionally cause paradoxical anger and behavioral disinhibition (see review by Rothschild 1992). A history of hostility, impulsivity, or borderline or antisocial personality
disorder is a potential predictor of this reaction. Some caution should be exercised when
benzodiazepines are prescribed to patients
with a history of poor impulse control and
aggression.

Overdose

Benzodiazepines are remarkably safe in
overdose when taken alone. Dangerous effects occur when the overdose includes several sedative drugs, especially alcohol, because of synergistic effects at the chloride ion
site and resultant membrane hyperpolarization.

Drug Interactions

Most sedative drugs, including narcotics and
alcohol, potentiate the sedative effects of
benzodiazepines. In addition, medications
that inhibit hepatic CYP3A3/4 increase
blood levels and hence side effects of clonazepam, alprazolam, midazolam, and triazolam. Lorazepam, oxazepam, and temazepam

are not dependent on hepatic enzymes for metabolism; thus, cytochrome P450 enzyme inhibition should not significantly affect these particular benzodiazepines.

Use in Pregnancy

Anxiolytics, like most medications, should be avoided during pregnancy and breast-feeding when possible. There have been concerns that benzodiazepines, when administered during the first trimester of pregnancy, may increase the risk of malformations, particularly cleft palate. Pooled data from cohort studies do not support an increased risk, but data from case–control studies do suggest a risk (Rosenberg et al. 1983).

Buspirone

Background

Buspirone is a partial agonist at $5\text{-}HT_{1A}$ receptors. It is important to note that buspirone does not interact with the GABA receptor or chloride ion channels. Therefore, it does not produce sedation, interact with alcohol, impair psychomotor performance, or pose a risk of abuse. Importantly, there is no cross-tolerance between benzodiazepines and buspirone, so benzodiazepines cannot be abruptly replaced with buspirone. Likewise, buspirone cannot be used to treat alcohol or barbiturate withdrawal and detoxification. Like the antidepressants, buspirone has a relatively slow onset of action.

Indications and Efficacy

Buspirone is effective in the treatment of generalized anxiety. Although the onset of therapeutic action is less rapid, buspirone's efficacy is not statistically different from that of benzodiazepines (Cohn and Wilcox 1986; Goldberg and Finnerty 1979). Despite its success in the treatment of generalized anxiety disorder, buspirone does not appear to be effective against panic disorder (Sheehan et al. 1990). Buspirone is also used as an augmenting agent in the treatment of OCD (Harvey and Balon 1995; Laird 1996) and depression (Sramek et al.

1996; Trivedi et al. 2006), and some evidence suggests that buspirone therapy may be an effective treatment for social phobia (Munjack et al. 1991; Schneier et al. 1992).

Clinical Use

Buspirone is available for oral administration in a variety of dosage forms. The usual initial dosage is 7.5 mg twice a day, increased after 1 week to 15 mg twice a day. The dose may then be increased as needed to achieve optimal therapeutic response. The usual recommended maximum daily dose is 60 mg. Because buspirone is metabolized by the liver and excreted by the kidneys, it should not be administered to patients with severe hepatic or renal impairment.

Side Effects

The side effects that are more common with buspirone therapy than with benzodiazepine therapy are nausea, headache, nervousness, insomnia, dizziness, and light-headedness (Rakel 1990). Restlessness also has been reported.

Overdose

No fatal outcomes of buspirone overdose have been reported. However, overdose of buspirone with other drugs may result in more serious outcomes.

Drug Interactions

Buspirone is metabolized by CYP3A3/4. Therefore, the initial dose should be lower in patients who are also taking medications known to inhibit this enzyme. Additionally, buspirone should not be administered in combination with an MAOI.

Zolpidem and Zaleplon

Zolpidem and zaleplon are hypnotics that act at the omega-1 receptor of the central $GABA_A$ receptor complex. This selectivity is hypothesized to be associated with a lower risk of dependence. Unlike benzodiazepines, zolpidem and zaleplon do not appear to have significant anxiolytic, muscle relaxant, or anticonvulsant properties. However, amnestic effects may occur.

Indications and Efficacy

Zolpidem is a short-acting hypnotic with established efficacy in inducing and maintaining sleep. Because of the short half-life of this drug, most patients taking zolpidem report minimal daytime sedation. Zaleplon is an ultra-short-acting hypnotic; minimal residual sedative effects are seen after 4 hours of administration.

Clinical Use

Both zolpidem and zaleplon are available in 5- and 10-mg tablets for oral administration. The maximum recommended dosages for adults are 10 mg/day and 20 mg/day, respectively, administered at night. The initial dose for elderly persons should not exceed 5 mg. Caution is advised in patients with hepatic dysfunction. In general, hypnotics should be limited to short-term use, with reevaluation for more extended therapy. Zolpidem XL is available in 6.25- and 12.5-mg tablets. The recommended dose for adults is 12.5 mg before sleep (6.25 mg for elderly patients).

Side Effects

In general, side effects of zolpidem and zaleplon are similar to those of short-acting benzodiazepines. These agents should not be considered free of abuse potential.

Overdose

Both zolpidem and zaleplon appear to be nonfatal in overdose. However, overdoses in combination with other CNS depressant agents pose a greater risk. Recommended treatment consists of general symptomatic and supportive measures, including gastric lavage. Use of flumazenil may be helpful.

Drug Interactions

Research on drug interactions is limited, but any drug with CNS depressant effects could potentially enhance the CNS depressant effects of zolpidem and zaleplon through phar-

macodynamic interactions. In addition, zolpidem is primarily metabolized by CYP3A3/4, and zaleplon is partially metabolized by CYP3A3/4. Thus, inhibitors of these enzymes may increase blood levels and the toxicity of zolpidem.

Ramelteon

Ramelteon is a hypnotic medication with melatonin receptor agonist activity targeting melatonin MT_1 and MT_2 receptors. It has not been proved to induce dependence. No appreciable activity on serotonin, dopamine, GABA, or acetylcholine occurs with the parent compound, but in vitro studies report that ramelteon's primary metabolite, M-II, has weak $5\text{-}HT_{2B}$ receptor agonist activity.

Indications and Efficacy

Ramelteon is indicated for the treatment of insomnia. Because its half-life is 1–2.6 hours, this medication is not thought to be associated with daytime sedation.

Clinical Use

Ramelteon is available in 8-mg tablets for oral administration. The current maximum dosage is 8 mg administered at night. Ramelteon should be used with caution in elderly patients because plasma levels were twice those in healthy nonelderly adults in clinical trials. Ramelteon should not be used by patients with severe hepatic impairment. This medication has been evaluated in moderate sleep apnea and chronic obstructive pulmonary disease but not in subjects with severe sleep apnea or severe chronic obstructive pulmonary disease and is not recommended for use in these patients.

Side Effects

Common side effects include somnolence, dizziness, and fatigue. Additionally, ramelteon has been associated with decreased testosterone levels and increased prolactin levels. To date, trials of ramelteon have not indicated high abuse potential with this medication.

Overdose

Supportive measures are recommended if overdose occurs. Gastric lavage also should be considered.

Drug Interactions

Ramelteon is metabolized by hepatic metabolism; CYP1A2 is the major isoenzyme involved. Caution is recommended with other inhibitory agents such as fluvoxamine. Ramelteon is also metabolized, to a lesser extent, by CYP2C9 and CYP3A4; thus, additional caution is warranted with medications that affect these cytochrome P450 enzymes.

Eszopiclone

Eszopiclone is a hypnotic agent that is thought to act on GABA receptor complexes close to benzodiazepine receptors.

Indications and Efficacy

Eszopiclone has a half-life of approximately 6 hours and is indicated for the treatment of insomnia.

Clinical Use

Eszopiclone is available in 1-, 2-, and 3-mg tablets for oral administration. The maximum recommended dose is 3 mg/night. In the elderly, this dose is reduced to a maximum of 2 mg. No evidence of tolerance or dependence has been reported, but long-term use should be approached with caution. In addition, eszopiclone should be used cautiously in patients with substance abuse because clinical trials have shown euphoric effects at high doses.

Side Effects

Eszopiclone has side effects similar to those of short-acting benzodiazepines. Dizziness, headache, and unpleasant taste were the most commonly reported side effects in patients taking eszopiclone in clinical trials (Lunesta 2005).

Overdose

Limited information on overdose with eszopiclone is available at this time. No fatali-

ties have been reported with up to 36 mg being taken in overdose. Overdose symptoms include impairment in consciousness, including somnolence or coma. Treatment is symptom-driven and supportive. Flumazenil may be beneficial.

Drug Interactions

Eszopiclone is metabolized in the liver by CYP3A4. Eszopiclone should not be used in patients with severe hepatic impairment. Dose adjustment and caution are recommended when prescribing eszopiclone to patients taking enzyme inhibitors such as ketoconazole, ciprofloxacin, erythromycin, isoniazid, and nefazodone. The use of other sedative-hypnotics is not recommended with administration of this medication.

Antipsychotic Medications

Background

Antipsychotic medications, previously referred to as *major tranquilizers* or *neuroleptics,* are effective for the treatment of a variety of psychotic symptoms. Antipsychotics can be classified in several ways. One classification system is based on chemical structure; for example, phenothiazines and butyrophenones make up two chemical classes. We use the term *conventional* to signify older or first-generation antipsychotic drugs—to differentiate them from newer *atypical* or second-generation antipsychotics. Among the conventional antipsychotics, we distinguish between high- and low-potency agents because the level of potency predicts side effects. Although the term *atypical antipsychotic* lacks a single consistent definition, it generally refers to the newer antipsychotic medications that affect both 5-HT_2 and D_2 receptors. Atypical antipsychotics available in the United States include clozapine, olanzapine, risperidone, quetiapine, ziprasidone, aripiprazole, and paliperidone.

The favorable neurological side-effect profile of atypical antipsychotics led to their use as first-line agents for the treatment of psychosis. Additionally, atypical antipsychotics as a class were often considered to be more effective than conventional antipsychotics. As discussed later in this section, superior efficacy has clearly been documented for clozapine but not necessarily for all agents in the class (Lieberman et al. 2005). Although neurological side effects are less frequent with atypical antipsychotics compared with conventional agents, atypical antipsychotics may place some patients at risk for medical morbidity resulting from weight gain and adverse metabolic effects. Therefore, medication choices must be individualized. In this section, we first discuss properties common to most of the antipsychotic medications and then describe each of the atypical antipsychotics and treatment recommendations.

Mechanisms of Action

All available antipsychotics antagonize D_2 receptors in vitro. However, the theory that psychosis results from hyperdopaminergia is overly simplistic. Underactivity of dopamine in mesocortical pathways, specifically those projecting to the frontal lobes, may account for the negative symptoms of schizophrenia (e.g., anergia, apathy, lack of spontaneity) (K.L. Davis et al. 1991; Goff and Evins 1998). In addition, this underactivity in the frontal lobes may serve to disinhibit mesolimbic dopamine activity via a corticolimbic feedback loop. Overactivity of mesolimbic dopamine is the result, which manifests as the positive symptoms of schizophrenia (e.g., hallucinations, delusions).

The atypical antipsychotics have other physiological properties as well, some of which appear to relate to antagonism of the $5\text{-}HT_2$ receptor, which may modify dopamine activity in a regionally specific manner. This dual $5\text{-}HT_2/D_2$ antagonism is believed to account, at least in part, for the unique properties of this group of medications. An additional hypothesis is that the atypical antipsychotic medications have a lower liability for EPS because they have looser binding to the D_2 receptor (Kapur and Seeman 2001).

Indications and Efficacy

The most common indications for antipsychotic drugs are the treatment of acute psychosis and the maintenance of psychotic symptom remission in patients with schizophrenia. All conventional antipsychotics have comparable efficacy in schizophrenia when given in equivalent doses (Table 15–4) but differ somewhat in their propensity for some side effects. The atypical antipsychotics appear to be at least as effective as the conventional antipsychotics in the treatment of schizophrenia (Glick and Marder 2005; Goff et al. 1998), but they differ with respect to their tolerability profiles. Clozapine has shown efficacy in patients with schizophrenia after nonresponse to one or more antipsychotic medication trials, including other atypical antipsychotics (Kane 1996; Lewis et al. 2006; McEvoy et al. 2006).

Atypical antipsychotics also have become a key part of the pharmacological armamentarium to treat bipolar disorder. Indeed, all atypical antipsychotics (except clozapine) are approved by the FDA for the treatment of acute mania. Additionally, olanzapine and aripiprazole are approved as maintenance treatments for bipolar disorder. Olanzapine–fluoxetine combination therapy (marketed in the United States under the trade name Symbyax) and quetiapine are approved by the FDA for the treatment of acute bipolar depressive episodes. The potential use of other atypical antipsychotics in acute bipolar depression is an area of current research interest.

Antipsychotic drugs also effectively target psychotic symptoms associated with drug intoxications, delusional disorders, and nonspecific agitation, although the data supporting their use in these conditions are limited. In addition, low doses of antipsychotics may be effective in some patients with borderline or schizotypal personality disorders, particularly when psychotic ideation is targeted (Oldham 2005). In patients with severe OCD, antipsychotics have been used to augment treatment with antiobsessional agents. Antipsychotics and other drugs with dopamine receptor–blocking action (e.g., metoclopramide) are also used for their antiemetic effect. Gilles de la Tourette's syndrome also may be controlled with antipsychotic agents.

Because of the sedating properties of some antipsychotics, these agents may be misused in certain clinical situations, such as for their use solely as hypnotic agents for patients with insomnia or as anxiolytics for patients with anxiety. Because of both short- and long-term adverse event risks associated with antipsychotic medications (such as neuroleptic malignant syndrome [NMS] and tardive dyskinesias, which are reviewed later in this section), antipsychotic medications should not be used solely as hypnotic or anxiolytic agents.

Clinical Use

Medication Selection

The choice of antipsychotic medication is often determined, in part, by their safety and tolerability profiles. The prescribing clinician should engage the patient in a discussion of available treatment options and their potential for both short- and long-term side effects. Clozapine is generally reserved for patients with refractory illness, particularly for patients whose symptoms have failed to respond to two or more antipsychotic medication trials (Lewis et al. 2006), because of the risk of agranulocytosis.

A useful construct for conceptualizing differences in side-effect profiles for the conventional antipsychotics is the concept of "high potency" versus "low potency." Drug potency refers to the milligram equivalence of drugs. For example, although haloperidol is more potent than chlorpromazine (haloperidol 2 mg = chlorpromazine 100 mg), therapeutically equivalent doses are equally effective (haloperidol 12 mg = chlorproma-

zine 600 mg). As a rule, for conventional antipsychotics only, the high-potency antipsychotic drugs have an equivalent dose of less than 5 mg (see Table 15–4). Compared with low-potency conventional antipsychotics, the high-potency agents generally have a higher degree of EPS but less sedation, fewer anticholinergic side effects, and less hypotension. Low-potency conventional antipsychotic drugs have an equivalent dose of greater than 40 mg. These drugs have a high level of sedation, anticholinergic side effects, and hypotension but a lower degree of acute EPS. Importantly, tardive dyskinesia rates do not differ between high- and low-potency conventional antipsychotics. Antipsychotic drugs with intermediate potency (i.e., equivalent dose between 5 and 40 mg) have a side-effect profile that lies between the profiles of these two groups.

The atypical antipsychotics produce fewer EPS than do conventional antipsychotics, particularly clozapine and quetiapine. Additionally, evidence to date suggests that the atypical agents are associated with lower rates of tardive dyskinesia than are the conventional agents. With the exception of risperidone, the atypical antipsychotics also produce substantially less hyperprolactinemia than do the conventional agents. However, several safety and tolerability issues are associated with atypical antipsychotic medications, including the potential for weight gain and metabolic abnormalities. Weight gain is an important side effect associated to varying degrees with all atypical agents, with less weight gain propensity associated with ziprasidone and aripiprazole.

Optimal Dosages

An optimal dosage or therapeutic range of blood levels has not been identified for most of the antipsychotics. High-dosage strategies are no longer recommended because controlled studies found that modest dosages of conventional antipsychotic drugs are as effective as higher dosages and are better tolerated. Several reviews of controlled trials of

Table 15–4. Commonly used atypical and conventional antipsychotic drugs

Generic drug name	Trade name	Usual adult daily dose (mg)	Formulations for administration	Available oral doses (mg)	Approximate oral dose equivalents (mg)
Atypical antipsychotics					
Aripiprazole	Abilify	15–30	po, L, ODT	5, 10, 15, 20, 30; 1 mg/mL	4
Clozapine	Clozaril	250–500	po, ODT	25, 100	100
Olanzapine	Zyprexa	10–20	po, ODT, im	2.5, 5, 7.5, 10, 15, 20	4
Paliperidone	Invega	3–12	po	3, 6, 9	—
Quetiapine	Seroquel	300–600	po	25, 100, 200, 300	125
Quetiapine extended-release	Seroquel XR	400–800	po	200, 300, 400	125
Risperidone	Risperdal	4–6	po, L, ODT, D	0.25, 0.5, 1, 2, 3, 4; 1 mg/mL	1
Ziprasidone	Geodon	80–160	po, im	20, 40, 60, 80	40
Conventional antipsychotics					
Butyrophenones					
Droperidol	Inapsine	2.5–10	im	2.5 mg/mL	—
Haloperidol	Haldol	5–15	po, im, D	0.5, 1, 2, 5, 10, 20	2
Dibenzoxazepines					
Loxapine	Loxitane	45–90	po	5, 10, 25, 50	10
Dihydroindolones					
Molindone	Moban	30–60	po	5, 10, 25, 50	15
Phenothiazines					
Aliphatics					
Chlorpromazine	Thorazine	300–600	po, L, im	10, 25, 50, 100, 200; 100 mg/mL	100
Piperazines					
Fluphenazine	Prolixin	5–15	po, L, im, D	1, 2.5, 5, 10	2
Perphenazine	Trilafon, Etrafon	32–64	po, L	2, 4, 8, 16; 16 mg/mL	10
Trifluoperazine	Stelazine	15–30	po	1, 2, 5, 10	5

Table 15–4. Commonly used atypical and conventional antipsychotic drugs *(continued)*

Generic drug name	Trade name	Usual adult daily dose (mg)	Formulations for administration	Available oral doses (mg)	Approximate oral dose equivalents (mg)
Piperidines					
Mesoridazine	Serentil	150–300	po	10, 25, 50, 100	50
Thioridazine	Mellaril	300–600	po, im	10, 15, 25, 50, 100	100
Diphenylbutylpiperidine					
Pimozide	Orap	2–6	po	1, 2	2
Thioxanthenes					
Thiothixene	Navane	15–30	po, L	1, 2, 5, 10, 20; 5 mg/mL	4

Note.   po=oral tablets or capsules; L=liquid; ODT=oral disintegrating tablets; im=intramuscular injections; D=decanoate.
Source.   Equivalent doses from Fuller and Sajatovic 2004. Adapted from Marangell LB, Martinez JM: *Concise Guide to Psychopharmacology*, 2nd Edition. Washington, DC, American Psychiatric Publishing, 2006, pp. 92–93. Used with permission.

conventional antipsychotics concluded that the optimal dosage for most patients is between 300 and 600 mg/day of chlorpromazine equivalents, with some patients responding to lower doses and with little benefit at doses greater than 700 mg/day (Appleton and Davis 1980; Baldessarini et al. 1988; J.M. Davis 1985).

It is important to note that reversal of psychosis is generally not an immediate effect of antipsychotic treatment; instead, improvement in psychosis is often gradual and may occur over several weeks to several months. Thus, clinicians should avoid premature antipsychotic dose escalations during the early phase of treatment if psychotic symptoms do not immediately respond to treatment. Typical dosing for antipsychotic medications is outlined in Table 15–4.

Risks, Side Effects, and Their Management

Many side effects of antipsychotic drugs can be understood in terms of the drugs' receptor-blocking properties. When antipsychotics reduce dopamine activity in the nigrostriatal pathway (via dopamine receptor blockade), extrapyramidal signs and symptoms similar to those of Parkinson's disease result. Another locus of dopamine receptors is in the pituitary and hypothalamus (the tuberoinfundibular system), where dopamine is synonymous with prolactin-inhibiting factor. Blockade of dopamine in this system results in hyperprolactinemia. Similarly, antagonism of acetylcholine receptors produces symptoms such as dry mouth, blurred vision, and constipation. Antagonism of α_1-adrenergic receptors results in hypotension, and antagonism of histamine receptors is associated with sedation.

Extrapyramidal Side Effects

EPS include acute dystonic reactions, parkinsonian syndrome, akathisia, tardive dyskinesia, and NMS. Although high-potency conventional antipsychotics are more likely than low-potency conventional antipsychotics to cause EPS, all first-generation antipsychotic drugs are equally likely to cause tardive dyskinesia. The atypical antipsychotics cause substantially fewer EPS, although careful titration of risperidone is necessary to avoid neurological side effects. Although the use of anticholinergic agents or amantadine may prevent or ameliorate EPS, the use of atypical agents is increasingly recommended to avoid these side effects without introducing additional medications. Clozapine appears to be the only agent that does not cause tardive dyskinesia, and data suggest that a reduced risk with the atypical agents is possible (Correll et al. 2004; Jeste et al. 1999; Margolese et al. 2005; Tarsy and Baldessarini 2006; Tollefson et al. 1997).

Acute dystonic reactions are among the most disturbing and acutely disabling adverse reactions that can occur with the administration of antipsychotic drugs. These reactions occur within hours or days of initiation of treatment with a high-potency conventional antipsychotic medication. The uncontrollable tightening of muscles typically involves spasms of the neck, back (opisthotonos), tongue, or muscles that control lateral eye movement (oculogyric crisis). Laryngeal involvement may compromise the airway and result in ventilatory difficulties (stridor). These reactions are often terrifying to the patient and may seriously jeopardize compliance with medications. Intravenous or intramuscular administration of anticholinergic medication is a rapid and effective treatment for acute dystonia. The drugs and dosages used to treat dystonic reactions are listed in Table 15–5. The effects of the anticholinergic drug given to reverse the dystonia wear off after several hours. Because antipsychotic drugs have long half-lives and durations of action, additional oral anticholinergic drugs should be prescribed for several days after an acute dystonic reaction or longer if treatment with the antipsychotic drug is continued unchanged. Amantadine, 100 mg twice a day, should be considered for treatment of EPS in elderly patients who are highly sensitive to anticholinergic activity, particularly if a switch to an atypical agent is not appropriate.

Acute dystonic reactions may be treated prophylactically with anticholinergic medications, such as benztropine 1–2 mg twice a day. Young patients taking high-potency antipsychotic drugs are at particularly high risk for the development of acute dystonia. We suggest that prophylactic treatment be considered for patients for whom the risk of developing extrapyramidal reactions is high, especially patients younger than 40 years starting high-potency conventional agents. Anticholinergic medication can be tapered and stopped after 10 days.

Parkinsonian syndrome has many of the features of classic idiopathic Parkinson's disease, including a diminished range of facial expression, cogwheel rigidity, slowed movements, drooling, small handwriting (micrographia), and pill-rolling tremor. This side effect may appear weeks after the initiation of the antipsychotic medication. The most common treatments for idiopathic Parkinson's disease restore the dopamine–acetylcholine balance by increasing dopamine availability. The treatment of antipsychotic medication-related parkinsonism most often involves decreasing the level of acetylcholine (although amantadine, a dopaminergic drug, often effectively attenuates parkinsonian side effects without exacerbating the underlying psychotic illness). Drugs used in the treatment of the parkinsonian side effects of antipsychotic agents are listed in Table 15–5.

The rabbit syndrome, consisting of fine, rapid movements of the lips that resemble the chewing movements of a rabbit, is often considered a subset of parkinsonian side effects. This side effect occurs after more prolonged treatment and may be confused with buccolingual tardive dyskinesia. It has been found in approximately 4% of patients receiving antipsychotics without concomitant anticholinergics (Yassa and Lal 1986). Like parkinsonian side effects, the rabbit syndrome is treated effectively with anticholinergic drugs.

Akinesia is a behavioral state of diminished spontaneity characterized by decreased gestures, unspontaneous speech, apathy, and difficulty with initiating usual activities. Akinesia may appear after several weeks of therapy and is often an element of the parkinsonism syndrome. This drug-induced syndrome may be mistaken for depression or for negative symptoms of schizophrenia.

Akathisia is an extrapyramidal disorder consisting of a subjective feeling of restlessness in the lower extremities, often manifested as an inability to sit still. It is a common reaction that most often occurs shortly after initiation of treatment with a conventional antipsychotic medication or aripiprazole. After a single oral dose of 5 mg of haloperidol, 40% of patients in one study experienced akathisia; this rate increased to 75% after receiving a 10-mg nighttime dose for 1 week (van Putten et al. 1984).

Akathisia is among the most treatment resistant of the acute EPS. Benzodiazepines are helpful in some cases. The current treatment of choice for akathisia is either a switch to an atypical agent (with the exception of aripiprazole) or the addition of a β-adrenergic–blocking drug, particularly propranolol. Several well-controlled studies have documented that propranolol, in dosages up to 120 mg/day, is an effective treatment for akathisia (Adler et al. 1985, 1989; Lipinski et al. 1984). In general, the lipophilic β-blockers are more effective in treating akathisia than the hydrophilic ones. At present, controversy remains as to whether β-selective drugs effectively treat akathisia, with some negative findings (Zubenko et al. 1984b) and some positive reports (Dumon et al. 1992; Dupuis et al. 1987).

Tardive Disorders

Tardive dyskinesia is a disorder characterized by involuntary choreoathetoid movements of the face, trunk, or extremities. The syndrome is usually associated with prolonged exposure to dopamine receptor–blocking agents—most frequently, antipsychotic drugs. However, the antidepressant

Table 15–5. Drugs used to treat extrapyramidal side effects

Generic drug name	Trade name	Drug type (mechanism)	Usual adult dosage	Indications for extrapyramidal side effects
Amantadine	Symmetrel	Dopaminergic agent	100 mg po bid	Parkinsonian syndrome
Benztropine	Cogentin	Anticholinergic agent	1–2 mg po bid 2 mg iv[a]	Dystonia, parkinsonian syndrome Acute dystonia
Diphenhydramine	Benadryl	Anticholinergic agent	25–50 mg po tid 25 mg im or iv[a]	Dystonia, parkinsonian syndrome Acute dystonia
Propranolol	Inderal	β-Blocker	20 mg po tid 1 mg iv	Akathisia
Trihexyphenidyl	Artane	Anticholinergic agent	5–10 mg po bid	Dystonia, parkinsonian syndrome

Note. po=oral administration of tablets or capsules; bid=twice daily; iv=intravenous; tid=three times a day; im=intramuscular.
[a]Follow with oral medication.
Source. Adapted from Marangell LB, Martinez JM: *Concise Guide to Psychopharmacology,* 2nd Edition. Washington, DC, American Psychiatric Publishing, 2006, p. 98. Used with permission.

amoxapine and the antiemetic agents meto-clopramide and prochlorperazine can also cause tardive dyskinesia. The American Psychiatric Association Task Force on Tardive Dyskinesia estimated a cumulative incidence of 5% per year of exposure among young adults and a prevalence of 30% after 1 year of treatment with conventional antipsychotics among elderly patients (American Psychiatric Association 1992). Clozapine seems to carry little or no risk of inducing tardive dyskinesia. The incidence of tardive dyskinesia associated with other atypical antipsychotics is higher than that associated with clozapine and lower than that associated with conventional antipsychotics (Correll et al. 2004; Jeste et al. 1999; Tollefson et al. 1997). Elderly patients taking antipsychotics are at increased risk for tardive dyskinesia.

Clinicians can use the Abnormal Involuntary Movement Scale (AIMS) to examine patients for the presence or emergence of tardive dyskinesia (Guy 1976). An evaluation for abnormal movements should be conducted before treatment begins and every 6 or 12 months thereafter. In typical cases, the patient is unaware of mild involuntary movements. Severe dyskinetic movements are less common, which can be disfiguring or even disabling as a result of affecting the muscles involved in the production of speech or swallowing. Although the most common form of tardive disorder is the dyskinetic variety (nonrhythmic, quick choreiform movements), other types have been identified. These include tardive akathisia, tardive dystonia, and tardive tics.

The most commonly accepted hypothesis of the mechanism for the development of tardive dyskinesia is that postsynaptic dopamine receptors develop supersensitivity to dopamine after prolonged dopamine receptor blockade. This model does not account for the time course of tardive dyskinesia onset or for the persistence of tardive dyskinesia after medication has been discontinued. Research has implicated an interaction between oxidative load (free radicals) and glu-

tamatergic neurotoxicity in the disorder (Tsai et al. 1998).

The most significant and consistently documented risk factor for the development of tardive dyskinesia is increasing age of the patient (Branchey and Branchey 1984; Jeste and Wyatt 1982; Kane and Smith 1982). The duration of exposure to a conventional antipsychotic is also an important factor because the cumulative incidence has been shown to remain constant at about 5% for the first 8 years in nonelderly patients. Women have been found to be at greater risk for severe tardive dyskinesia, although the evidence suggests that this finding is limited to geriatric populations (Kennedy et al. 1971; Seide and Muller 1967). Other risk factors may include EPS early in the course of treatment, a history of drug holidays (a greater number of drug-free periods is associated with an increased risk), the presence of brain damage, diabetes mellitus, and a diagnosis of a mood disorder.

Because antipsychotic medications are the most effective treatment for most patients with schizophrenia, the situation often arises in which a patient develops tardive dyskinesia but still requires an antipsychotic medication to function. If discontinuation of the antipsychotic drug is clinically possible, tardive dyskinesia may gradually diminish; however, involuntary movements often worsen initially with tapering of the antipsychotic dose, a phenomenon referred to as *withdrawal-emergent dyskinesia* (Glazer et al. 1984). Withdrawal-emergent dyskinesia also may occur when a conventional antipsychotic is replaced with an atypical antipsychotic.

Withdrawal-emergent dyskinesia typically resolves within 6 weeks; however, suppressed or latent tardive dyskinesia that has been suppressed by D_2 receptor blockade may not resolve once it has appeared. Conversely, movements may be masked temporarily by increasing the dosage of the antipsychotic medication, but the symptoms eventually reemerge, often in a more severe form. Anticholinergic drugs may reversibly worsen dyskinetic movements (Reunanen et al. 1982; Yassa 1985), whereas anticholinergic drugs in high doses may improve tardive dystonia (Burke et al. 1982; Fahn 1985).

No definitive treatment for tardive dyskinesias has been identified to date. Clozapine may be useful for certain patients with tardive dyskinesia who need an antipsychotic medication.

Neuroleptic Malignant Syndrome

In rare instances, patients taking antipsychotic medications develop a potentially life-threatening disorder known as NMS. Although it occurs most frequently with the use of high-potency conventional antipsychotic drugs, this condition may appear during treatment with any antipsychotic agent, including atypical antipsychotics. Patients with NMS typically have marked muscle rigidity, although this feature may be absent in patients taking atypical antipsychotics. Other features include fever, autonomic instability, increased white blood cell (WBC) counts (>15,000/mm^3), increased creatine kinase levels (>300 U/mL), and delirium. The increased creatine kinase concentrations are the result of muscle breakdown, which can lead to myoglobinuria and acute renal failure.

Treatment of NMS includes discontinuation of the antipsychotic medication, a thorough medical evaluation, administration of intravenous fluids and antipyretic agents, and the use of cooling blankets.

Anticholinergic Side Effects

Anticholinergic side effects are categorized as peripheral effects or central effects. The most common peripheral side effects are dry mouth, decreased sweating, decreased bronchial secretions, blurred vision, difficulty with urination, constipation, and tachycardia. Central side effects of anticholinergic drugs include impairment in concentration, attention, and memory. In cases of toxicity, anticholinergic delirium—which includes hot and dry skin, dry mucous membranes, dilated pupils, absent bowel sounds, tachycardia, and confusion—may occur. Anticho-linergic delirium is a medical emergency, and full supportive medical care is required.

Adrenergic Side Effects

Antipsychotics block α_1-adrenergic receptors, which can result in orthostatic hypotension and dizziness. Orthostatic hypotension is commonly associated with low-potency conventional agents. Among the atypical agents, clozapine, quetiapine, risperidone, and ziprasidone require initial dose titration, particularly in the elderly, to avoid orthostatic hypotension. Administration of epinephrine, which stimulates both α- and β-adrenergic receptors, will result in a paradoxical drop in blood pressure as a result of the stimulation of β-adrenergic receptors in the presence of α-receptor blockade. In asthmatic patients who require treatment with antipsychotics as well as episodic treatment with β-adrenergic drugs, specific warnings are necessary regarding the dangers associated with the use of epinephrine in the treatment of an acute asthmatic attack.

Endocrine Effects

Numerous studies have suggested a relation between the use of atypical antipsychotic medications and the development of hyperglycemia, dyslipidemia, and metabolic syndrome (American Diabetes Association et al. 2004; review by Citrome et al. 2005). The metabolic syndrome comprises several metabolic risk factors that may be associated with an increased cardiovascular risk. One definition of the metabolic syndrome specifies the presence of three or more of the following five clinical or laboratory features: 1) elevated plasma triglyceride levels (≥150 mg/dL); 2) decreased plasma high-density lipoprotein levels (<50 mg/dL in women or <40 mg/dL in men); 3) elevated fasting glucose levels (≥110 mg/dL); 4) waist circumference greater than 35 inches in women or greater than 40 inches in men; 5) elevated blood pressure (≥130/85 mm Hg) (Citrome et al. 2005; Expert Panel on the Detection, Evaluation, and Treatment of High Blood Cholesterol in Adults 2001).

Hyperglycemia can develop independent of or secondary to weight gain and, in some cases, resolves after discontinuation of the medication. Patients taking clozapine and olanzapine have a higher risk of developing diabetes compared with patients taking other conventional and atypical antipsychotics (see American Diabetes Association et al. 2004). Data indicate that alterations in serum lipids are concordant with changes in body weight. Clozapine and olanzapine are associated with the greatest increases in total cholesterol, low-density lipoprotein, and triglycerides, as well as decreases in high-density lipoprotein. Aripiprazole and ziprasidone do not appear to be associated with dyslipidemia. However, monitoring should be considered for all patients taking an antipsychotic medication.

At present, it appears appropriate to monitor all patients taking atypical antipsychotics for metabolic changes. Published guidelines recommend monitoring patients taking atypical antipsychotics for several metabolic risk factors, including personal and family history of metabolic risks (baseline and annually), waist circumference (baseline and annually), body mass index (baseline, week 4, week 8, week 12, and quarterly), blood pressure and fasting glucose levels (baseline, week 12, and annually), and lipid panel (baseline, week 12, and every 5 years) (American Diabetes Association et al. 2004).

All conventional antipsychotic medications and risperidone may cause hyperprolactinemia. Clinical signs and symptoms of hyperprolactinemia may include gynecomastia, galactorrhea, amenorrhea, and decreased libido. Although such side effects were frequently associated with hyperprolactinemia resulting from conventional antipsychotics, a review of clinical experience with risperidone found relatively low rates of side effects despite markedly elevated prolactin levels (Kleinberg et al. 1997). Hyperprolactinemia secondarily can lower estrogen levels, resulting in amenorrhea and theoretically placing patients at risk for osteoporosis and pathological fractures (Klibanski et al. 1981).

Weight Gain

Both conventional and atypical antipsychotic medications can be associated with weight gain. Antipsychotics associated with weight gain include risperidone, quetiapine, chlorpromazine, thioridazine, olanzapine, and clozapine (Allison et al. 1999; American Diabetes Association et al. 2004); however, all patients taking an antipsychotic medication should be monitored for weight gain throughout treatment.

Sexual Effects

A combination of anticholinergic effects, α-adrenergic receptor blockade, and hormonal effects may lead to several types of sexual difficulty. In men, inability to achieve or maintain erections, decreased ability to achieve orgasm, and changes in the pleasurable quality of orgasm have been reported with conventional agents (Ghadirian et al. 1982).

Ocular Effects

Antipsychotics may cause pigmentary changes in the lens and retina, especially if the drugs are administered for long periods. Pigment deposition in the lens of the eye does not affect vision; however, pigmentary retinopathy, which can lead to irreversible blindness, has been associated specifically with the use of thioridazine.

Quetiapine was associated with cataracts in preclinical safety studies conducted in beagles (Seroquel 2001). Subsequent studies involving nonhuman primates did not detect an increased risk of cataracts; postmarketing surveys have not detected an increased risk of cataracts in patients taking quetiapine compared with patients taking other antipsychotics (Laties et al. 2000).

Dermatological Effects

Patients taking antipsychotics, especially the aliphatic phenothiazines (e.g., chlorpromazine), may become more sensitive to sunlight, which can lead to severe sunburn.

Cardiac Effects

In materials submitted to the Psychopharmacological Drugs Advisory Committee of the FDA, Pfizer, Inc., reported results from a trial designed to examine the ECG effects of atypical agents and thioridazine at maximum therapeutic serum concentrations and at the potentially higher concentrations that might occur in clinical practice if these agents were co-prescribed with metabolic inhibitors. After correcting the QT interval for heart rate, thioridazine produced the greatest mean delay in QTc (35.6 msec), followed by ziprasidone (20.6 msec), quetiapine (9.1 msec), olanzapine (6.8 msec), and haloperidol (4.7 msec). Quetiapine produced the greatest increase in heart rate (11 beats/minute).

Hepatic Effects

Increased levels on liver function tests have been associated with antipsychotic treatment. If abnormalities suggest obstructive liver disease, with increases in bilirubin and alkaline phosphatase, the drug must be immediately discontinued. This reaction appears to be more common with low-potency conventional antipsychotics. Transient elevations in hepatic enzymes have been observed with olanzapine and quetiapine, but these laboratory findings have not been linked to liver injury.

Hematological Effects

Transient leukopenia and, in rare cases, agranulocytosis have been associated with neuroleptic treatment. Although agranulocytosis is strictly defined as a complete absence of all granulocytes in the blood, it also may refer to severe neutropenia, with a neutrophil count of less than 500/mL. This idiosyncratic reaction usually occurs within the first 3–4 weeks after the initiation of treatment with an antipsychotic drug. However, this risk continues for 2–3 months during therapy. A higher risk of agranulocytosis is

associated with low-potency conventional antipsychotic drugs and, most significantly, clozapine.

Lowered Seizure Threshold

Most conventional antipsychotics are associated with a dose-dependent risk of a lowered seizure threshold, although the incidence of seizures with most of these drugs is quite small. Of all the conventional antipsychotics, molindone and fluphenazine have been shown most consistently to have the lowest potential for this side effect (Itil and Soldatos 1980; Oliver et al. 1982). The atypical antipsychotic clozapine is associated with a dose-dependent risk of seizure and has been estimated to produce seizures in as many 10% of the patients receiving the drug for 3.8 years.

Suppressed Temperature Regulation

Antipsychotic drugs directly affect the hypothalamus and suppress temperature regulation. In combination with the α-adrenergic receptor antagonism and cholinergic receptor antagonism of antipsychotics, this effect becomes particularly serious in hot, humid weather. Severe hyperthermia, rhabdomyolysis, renal failure, and death may result. This potentially life-threatening condition requires immediate medical intervention and supportive treatment. A cool environment and adequate amounts of fluids are mandatory for patients taking antipsychotic agents.

Risks in Elderly Patients With Dementia

Treatment with atypical antipsychotics recently has been associated with an almost twofold increased mortality rate when used in elderly patients with dementia. It is important to note that these medications are often used in clinical practice, but they are not approved by the FDA for the treatment of dementia-related psychosis (Herrmann and Lanctot 2005). The risk associated with atypical antipsychotics is not statistically different from the risk associated with treatment with conventional antipsychotics (Gill et al. 2005).

Use in Pregnancy

Like most other drugs, antipsychotic agents should be avoided, if possible, during pregnancy and during lactation periods for breast-feeding mothers. The use of low-potency phenothiazine antipsychotics during the first trimester of pregnancy may increase the baseline risk of congenital anomalies by 0.4%, or 4 cases per 1,000 pregnancies (Altshuler et al. 1996). Infants born to mothers who were first exposed to antipsychotic drugs during the sixth to tenth week of gestation may have an increase in birth defects (Edlund and Craig 1984).

Less is known about the risks for teratogenicity, perinatal complications, and neurobehavioral problems associated with atypical antipsychotic medications. Data from a prospective comparative study indicated that treatment with olanzapine, risperidone, quetiapine, and clozapine was not associated with a significantly higher risk of major malformations; however, treatment with these agents was associated with a lower birthrate ($P=0.05$) and higher rate of therapeutic abortions ($P=0.003$) (McKenna et al. 2005).

Drug Interactions

Antipsychotic drugs have profound effects on multiple CNS receptors, and these effects are compounded when other medications are added. For example, the α-adrenergic receptor blockade of antipsychotics may affect the efficacy of the antihypertensive drug guanethidine. The sedative and anticholinergic effects of antipsychotic drugs are increased with the addition of other sedating or anticholinergic drugs. As mentioned previously, patients taking drugs with potentially serious adverse effects should be monitored through plasma level determinations when other medications are used concurrently.

Pharmacokinetic interactions with antipsychotic drugs are common and have been reviewed elsewhere (Goff and Baldessarini 1995). Most antipsychotics are metabolized by the hepatic CYP2D6 isoenzyme. Exceptions include ziprasidone and quetiapine, which are metabolized mainly by the CYP3A4 enzyme. The activity of the CYP2D6 enzyme varies greatly (on the basis of genetic polymorphisms) among individuals and can be inhibited by certain drugs, such as SSRIs. For example, the addition of fluoxetine increased serum haloperidol concentrations by 20% and serum fluphenazine concentrations by 65% in one study (Goff et al. 1995). Two categories of potential drug–drug interactions are of particular concern. The first includes interactions that can increase serum concentrations of antipsychotics to dangerous levels. For example, clozapine is metabolized by the CYP2D6, CYP3A4, and CYP1A2 isoenzymes. When taken with CYP3A4 and CYP1A2 inhibitors, such as erythromycin and fluvoxamine, serum clozapine concentrations can rise to toxic levels (L.G. Cohen et al. 1996; Wetzel et al. 1998). The other category of potentially serious interactions includes those that induce metabolism of antipsychotic agents, thereby lowering serum concentrations below a therapeutic threshold. Large reductions in serum clozapine and haloperidol concentrations have been reported with the addition of carbamazepine, phenobarbital, and phenytoin (Arana et al. 1986; Byerly and DeVane 1996). Notably, cigarette smoking can affect antipsychotic metabolism; serum concentrations of clozapine in particular are reduced with smoking and increased after smoking cessation (Byerly and DeVane 1996; Haring et al. 1989).

Atypical Antipsychotics

The atypical antipsychotics are referred to as *atypical* (compared with conventional antipsychotics) for several reasons, including their receptor binding profiles, improved side-effect profile, and spectrum of efficacy in patients with schizophrenia. In general, the atypical antipsychotic drugs provide superior efficacy for the treatment of negative symptoms, produce fewer acute motor side effects, and may reduce the risk of tardive dyskinesia compared with conventional antipsychotic drugs. These drugs also may improve cognitive function in patients with schizophrenia (Green et al. 1997; Hagger et al. 1993; Purdon et al. 2000; Rossi et al. 1997). In this subsection, we review the atypical antipsychotic medications currently available in the United States: clozapine, olanzapine, risperidone, quetiapine, ziprasidone, aripiprazole, and paliperidone.

Clozapine

Clozapine, the first of the class of atypical antipsychotic drugs, was a landmark in the treatment of schizophrenia for several reasons. It was the first medication shown to be efficacious in otherwise nonresponsive patients. In addition, clozapine was the first agent to attenuate significantly the negative symptoms of schizophrenia, such as marked social withdrawal and apathy, thereby helping many patients return to meaningful and productive lives. Also, clozapine rarely produces EPS, and to date it is the only antipsychotic drug that is not associated with treatment-emergent tardive dyskinesia. This important clinical property is concordant with the observation that chronic administration of clozapine results in selective inhibition of dopamine neurons in the mesolimbic pathways, with little functional effect on striatal dopamine tracts. Finally, clozapine has minimal effects on the tuberoinfundibular system, and therefore it does not cause hyperprolactinemia.

Clozapine is the prototype for the atypical antipsychotic medication class. However, because it is associated with a risk for agranulocytosis, clozapine use is restricted to patients who have not adequately responded to or tolerated treatment with two other antipsychotics (Lewis et al. 2006).

Mechanism of action. Clozapine has a wide range of physiological actions. A great deal of research has focused on clozapine's relatively greater 5-HT$_2$ than D$_2$ antagonism,

and this property has been the predominant focus of new drug development in the atypical antipsychotic medication class.

Clinical use. Because of prominent sedation and orthostatic hypotension, clozapine therapy is initiated at a dosage of 12.5 mg/day, with a rapid increase to 12.5 mg twice a day. The dose is then increased as tolerated, generally in 25- or 50-mg increments every day or every other day. Clozapine is usually added to the previous antipsychotic agent in a cross-titration in which the dose of the previous drug is tapered once a clozapine dosage of approximately 100 mg/day has been achieved. This strategy should be used with caution if the existing medication is a low-potency conventional antipsychotic because of the possibility of additive α-adrenergic and anticholinergic side effects. Clozapine doses can be increased much more rapidly in an inpatient setting, with monitoring of vital signs, than in an outpatient setting. The typical target dose is 300–500 mg/day in divided doses.

Risks, side effects, and their management.

Agranulocytosis. Agranulocytosis was previously estimated to occur in 0.8% of the patients receiving clozapine during the first year of treatment, with a peak incidence at 3 months. However, a system of hematological monitoring has reduced agranulocytosis-related fatalities to extremely low levels (Honigfeld et al. 1998). The dispensing of clozapine in the United States is linked to weekly WBC counts during the first 6 months of treatment and biweekly counts thereafter.

If agranulocytosis develops, prompt consultation with a hematologist is indicated. Although lithium often causes leukocytosis, it does not appear to treat or prevent clozapine-induced agranulocytosis. Once a patient has developed agranulocytosis while taking clozapine, he or she should not be rechallenged with this medication.

Extrapyramidal side effects. EPS are uncommon with any dose of clozapine, although some patients experience akathisia or hand tremors. Note that a risk for NMS exists; indeed, NMS has been reported in patients medicated with clozapine alone (Anderson and Powers 1991; DasGupta and Young 1991; Miller et al. 1991).

Sedation. Sedation is the most common side effect of clozapine, and it is particularly prominent early in treatment. Sedation generally attenuates when the dose is reduced, when tolerance to this side effect develops, or when a disproportionate amount is given at bedtime.

Cardiovascular effects. Hypotension and tachycardia occur in most patients taking clozapine.

Weight gain. Weight gain is a common side effect of clozapine. Body weight increases by 10% or more in many patients.

Endocrine effects. As noted earlier, numerous studies suggested a relation between the use of atypical antipsychotic medications and the development of hyperglycemia, dyslipidemia, and metabolic syndrome (American Diabetes Association et al. 2004; review by Citrome et al. 2005). Patients should receive nutritional counseling at the initiation of treatment with clozapine, and weight and other metabolic parameters should be monitored, as noted earlier in this section.

Hypersalivation. Hypersalivation occurs in one-third of the patients taking clozapine. However, because clozapine has potent anticholinergic properties, addition of an anticholinergic agent is not recommended for control of hypersalivation.

Fever. Clozapine is associated with benign, transient temperature increases, generally within the first 3 weeks of treatment. Patients taking clozapine who develop fevers should be evaluated for infections, agranulocytosis, and NMS.

Seizures. Clozapine is associated with a dose-dependent risk of seizures. The vast majority of clozapine-induced seizures are tonic-clonic, but myoclonic seizures also occur.

Doses less than 300 mg/day are associated with a 1%–3% risk of seizures. Doses of 300–600 mg/day carry a 2.7% risk, and doses greater than 600 mg/day are associated with a 4.4% risk (Devinsky et al. 1991).

Anticholinergic side effects. Anticholinergic effects, such as dry mouth, blurred vision, constipation, and urinary retention, are common early side effects.

Drug interactions. Clozapine should not be combined with any drugs that have the potential to suppress bone marrow function, such as carbamazepine. There have been isolated reports of respiratory arrest in patients taking both clozapine and a high-potency benzodiazepine. Thus, benzodiazepines (particularly in high doses) should not be administered to patients taking clozapine.

Clozapine is metabolized by hepatic CYP1A2 and, to a lesser degree, CYP3A3/4; therefore, the drug is subject to changes in serum concentration when combined with medications that inhibit or induce these enzymes. Serum clozapine levels increase with coadministration of fluvoxamine or erythromycin and decrease with coadministration of phenobarbital or phenytoin and with cigarette smoking (Byerly and DeVane 1996). These pharmacokinetic interactions are particularly important because of the dose-dependent risk of seizures.

Olanzapine

Olanzapine represents a modification of the clozapine molecule. Like risperidone, olanzapine is a monoaminergic antagonist with high-affinity binding at the 5-HT$_2$ and D$_1$, D$_2$, D$_3$, and D$_4$ receptors. Compared with clozapine, olanzapine has greater D$_2$ and weaker D$_4$ and α-adrenergic affinity. Despite its structural similarity to clozapine, olanzapine is not associated with higher-than-expected rates of agranulocytosis.

Acute dystonia is uncommon. Akathisia may occur, but it is significantly less common than with the conventional antipsychotic drugs. Olanzapine is associated with modest dose-dependent elevations in serum prolactin levels, but most often these elevations are transient and within the normal reference range (Tollefson et al. 1997).

Clinical use.   The recommended starting dosage of olanzapine is 10 mg at bedtime for patients with schizophrenia and 10–15 mg at bedtime for acutely manic patients. The clinically effective dosage range is 7.5–20 mg/day (5–20 mg/day in mania). Olanzapine can be administered in a single daily dose at bedtime. It is important to note that meaningful improvement may not be evident for the first several weeks after initiation of treatment. Usual dosages for maintenance treatment in patients with bipolar disorder range from 5 to 20 mg/day.

Olanzapine is available in a short-acting intramuscular injectable form, providing clinicians with another option for treating acute agitation associated with psychosis or mania.

Risks, side effects, and their management.

Somnolence.   Somnolence is a common, dose-dependent side effect of olanzapine. Patients often become tolerant to this side effect over time.

Anticholinergic side effects.   Anticholinergic side effects are clinically less significant than would be predicted on the basis of in vitro muscarinic receptor–binding affinity. However, dry mouth has been reported in association with olanzapine treatment (Beasley et al. 1996).

Seizures.   Treatment-emergent seizures are rare in the absence of concomitant medical disorders.

Hepatic effects.   Transaminase levels were increased in approximately 2% of the patients taking olanzapine in premarketing evaluation. In many cases, these levels normalized without medication discontinuation. Routine laboratory monitoring is not recommended, but olanzapine should be used with caution in patients with hepatic disease or with additional risk factors for hepatic toxicity.

Weight gain.   Treatment-emergent weight gain is common with olanzapine therapy and averages about 4.15 kg after 10 weeks of treatment (Allison et al. 1999). By 39 weeks, weight gain tends to plateau (Kinon et al. 2001), and approximately 20% of patients may not gain weight. Patients with higher body mass indices ($>27.6 \text{ kg/m}^2$) tend to gain less weight than do those with lower body mass indices. Weight gain is independent of dose (Kinon et al. 2001).

Drug interactions.   Olanzapine is metabolized by several pathways and is unlikely to be affected by concurrent administration of other medications. Additionally, olanzapine does not appear to inhibit any cytochrome P450 enzymes.

Risperidone

Risperidone is an atypical antipsychotic medication that combines D_2 receptor antagonism with potent 5-HT_2 receptor antagonism. Risperidone has a higher affinity for D_2 receptors than does clozapine. Risperidone also antagonizes D_1 and D_4 receptors, α_1- and α_2-adrenergic receptors, and H_1 receptors. The optimal dosage of risperidone in the North American trials was 6 mg/day, but subsequent clinical experience has indicated that most patients do well on lower dosages of 3–6 mg/day, and the elderly may require dosages as low as 0.5 mg/day. Clinicians should titrate the dose of risperidone to avoid EPS. Unlike the other atypical agents, risperidone elevates prolactin levels.

Clinical use.   Risperidone is most effective at total daily doses of 4–6 mg. For initial treatment, we recommend using divided doses, starting at 1 mg twice a day and quickly increasing to 2 mg twice a day. For elderly persons, the initial dose should be much lower (0.25–0.5 mg/day). After the first week of treatment, the entire dose can be given at bedtime. This approach usually helps the patient sleep and reduces daytime side effects. However, we do not suggest this practice for elderly persons because of an increased risk of falling.

Risperidone is available in a long-acting injectable form (Risperdal Consta).

Risks, side effects, and their management. Insomnia, hypotension, agitation, headache, and rhinitis are the most common side effects of risperidone. These tend to lessen with time. Overall, the drug tends to be well tolerated. Risperidone does not have significant anticholinergic side effects. Hyperprolactinemia is common.

Extrapyramidal side effects. In comparison with relatively high dosages of haloperidol (20 mg/day), risperidone is associated with a lower prevalence of acute extrapyramidal effects and akathisia. EPS occurs in a dose-dependent manner, with more frequent occurrence when the dosage is greater than 6 mg/day. Thus, clinicians are advised to titrate the dose of risperidone in a manner that maximizes its clinical benefits and minimizes EPS.

Cardiovascular effects. Brief hypotension may occur, as may be expected with α-adrenergic receptor blockade. Tachycardia is also common.

Tardive disorders. Risperidone at low doses produces few parkinsonian side effects. The incidence of risperidone-induced tardive dyskinesia is not known, but it is assumed to be between that of clozapine and the conventional antipsychotics. In one 9-month study of elderly patients, risperidone produced very low rates of tardive dyskinesia compared with haloperidol (Jeste et al. 1999).

Weight gain. Weight gain associated with risperidone treatment is quite variable and is generally less than weight gain associated with olanzapine and clozapine (Allison et al. 1999). The mean weight gain after 10 weeks of exposure to risperidone is approximately 2.1 kg. All patients taking atypical antipsychotics should be monitored for weight gain, particularly during the early course of treatment.

Drug interactions. Risperidone is metabolized primarily by CYP2D6 (Byerly and DeVane 1996). Medications that inhibit this enzyme, such as many of the SSRIs, cause increases in plasma risperidone levels. However, there does not appear to be an increase in side effects resulting from such an interaction, possibly because the primary metabolite of risperidone, 9-OH risperidone, is fully active and is excreted unchanged by the kidneys (Shelton and Stahl 2004).

Quetiapine

Quetiapine is a dibenzothiazepine derivative with weak affinity for $5-HT_{1A}$, $5-HT_2$, D_1, D_2, H_1, α_1, and α_2 receptors. Quetiapine has very "loose" binding to D_2 receptors. Quetiapine's relatively high $5-HT_2$-to-D_2 ratio is consistent with the hypothesized advantageous properties of the atypical antipsychotics. Antagonism of H_1 receptors is associated with sedative side effects, and α_1 antagonism is associated with orthostatic hypotension.

Clinical use. Quetiapine is indicated for the treatment of schizophrenia, acute mania, and bipolar depression. Quetiapine therapy is initiated at a dose of 25 mg twice a day for patients with schizophrenia, with increases to 50 mg twice a day on day 2, 100 mg twice a day on day 3, and 100 mg in the morning and 200 mg in the evening on day 4. The optimal dosage for most patients appears to range between 400 and 600 mg/day, although the drug is safe and efficacious for some patients within a dose range of 150–750 mg. Slower titration and lower daily doses may be warranted in patients with hepatic disease and in elderly patients. Because of its relatively short half-life of 6–8 hours, quetiapine is usually administered twice daily. A new formulation of quetiapine, quetiapine XR (extended-release tablets), is administered once daily, usually in the evening. The recommended initial dosage is 300 mg/day, and the effective dosage range is 400–800 mg/day. The dose can be increased by up to 300 mg/day, and increases can occur at 1-day intervals.

For patients who have acute mania, treatment should be initiated with twice-daily doses totaling 100 mg on day 1, 200 mg on day 2, 300 mg on day 3, and 400 mg on day 4. Additional adjustments up to 800 mg/day by day 6 can be made. Doses should not be increased by more than 200 mg/day on days 5 and 6. Most patients respond to dosages between 400 and 800 mg/day. Some clinicians use lower starting doses and slower titrations for less ill outpatients; however, this practice is not supported by controlled data.

For patients struggling with bipolar depression, the recommended starting dosage for quetiapine is 50 mg/day. This dosage can be increased to 100 mg on day 2, 200 mg on day 3, and 300 mg on day 4. Although no additional benefit has been observed for dosages higher than 300 mg/day, the dosage can be titrated upward to 400 mg on day 5 and 600 mg on day 8.

Risks, side effects, and their management. Quetiapine was no different from placebo in dosages to 750 mg/day regarding EPS and changes in serum prolactin levels (Arvanitis and Miller 1997).

Somnolence. Somnolence is one of the most common side effects of quetiapine. Somnolence and psychomotor slowing are dose dependent, and patients often become tolerant to these side effects over time.

Ocular changes. As noted earlier, the development of cataracts was observed in association with quetiapine treatment in preclinical studies of beagles, but a causal relation has not been established in humans.

Cardiovascular effects. Given α_1-adrenergic receptor antagonism, quetiapine may induce orthostatic hypotension and concomitant symptoms of dizziness, tachycardia, and syncope. The risk of symptomatic hypotension is particularly pronounced during initial dose titration. Quetiapine should be used with caution in patients with cardiovascular disease, cerebrovascular disease, or other illnesses predisposing to hypotension.

Hepatic effects. In premarketing trials, increased transaminase levels were noted in 6% of the patients taking quetiapine. These changes usually occur during the first weeks of treatment. Routine laboratory monitoring currently is not recommended, but quetiapine should be used with caution in patients with hepatic disease or with additional risk factors for hepatic toxicity.

Weight gain. Quetiapine is associated with weight gain. In premarketing placebo-controlled studies, a weight gain of at least 7% of body weight was observed in 23% of the quetiapine-treated patients with schizophrenia, compared with 6% of the control subjects given placebo. Thus, patients should be educated about the potential risk for weight gain, and weight should be monitored periodically throughout treatment.

Drug interactions. Quetiapine is metabolized by hepatic CYP3A3/4. Concurrent administration of cytochrome P450–inducing drugs, such as carbamazepine, decreases blood levels of quetiapine. In such circumstances, increased doses of quetiapine are appropriate. Quetiapine does not appreciably affect the pharmacokinetics of other medications. Pharmacodynamic effects are expected if quetiapine is combined with medications that also have antihistaminic or α-adrenergic side effects. Because of its potential for inducing hypotension, quetiapine also may enhance the effects of certain antihypertensive agents.

Ziprasidone

Ziprasidone is the only atypical antipsychotic available in capsule form. This medication combines a high affinity for 5-HT$_2$ receptors with an intermediate affinity for D$_2$, resulting in a very high 5-HT$_2$-to-D$_2$ affinity ratio.

Clinical use. Ziprasidone is approved for the treatment of schizophrenia and acute mania. For patients with schizophrenia, ziprasidone is usually started at a dosage of 20–40 mg twice a day. In medically healthy noneld-erly patients, the dose can be rapidly titrated over 2–4 days to a typical therapeutic dosage of 60–80 mg twice a day. For patients with acute mania, treatment should be initiated at 40 mg twice a day. This dosage should be in-creased to 60 or 80 mg twice a day on day 2 and subsequently adjusted on the basis of in-dividual tolerance and symptoms to be-tween 40 and 80 mg twice a day. Ziprasidone has a half-life of 5–10 hours and is usually ad-ministered twice daily with meals. Food in-creases absorption by approximately 100%.

Ziprasidone is also available for intra-muscular administration. The recommended dose for intramuscular injection (for the treatment of acute agitation associated with schizophrenia) is 10–20 mg, with a maximum dosage of 40 mg/day. The 10-mg doses can be administered every 2 hours, whereas the 20-mg doses can be administered every 4 hours. Peak plasma concentrations are achieved by 60 minutes.

Risks, side effects, and their management. In general, ziprasidone is well tolerated. The most common side effects are headache, dys-pepsia, nausea, constipation, abdominal pain, somnolence, and EPS. Ratings of par-kinsonism and akathisia with ziprasidone, 120 mg/day, did not differ from those with placebo. Although dizziness has been re-ported, rates of orthostatic hypotension have not differed from rates associated with pla-cebo in controlled clinical trials. Ziprasidone produces transient hyperprolactinemia, which returns to predrug baseline levels af-ter 12 hours; prolactin levels are significantly lower with ziprasidone than with haloperi-dol (Goff et al. 1998).

Cardiovascular effects. The FDA delayed approval of ziprasidone until additional safety data could be obtained regarding ef-fects on cardiac conduction. Ziprasidone de-lays the QTc interval at maximum therapeu-tic blood levels by approximately 20 msec, on average, which is a larger effect than with other atypical agents but less than with thior-idazine. Although monitoring of ECGs is not routinely required, clinicians should consider the relative risk of cardiac conduction delay compared with the benefits of ziprasidone (which include tolerability and minimal weight gain) when selecting a medication.

Weight gain. Ziprasidone is associated with less weight gain than are other atypical antipsychotic agents. Allison et al. (1999) cal-culated a mean weight gain of less than 1 kg after 10 weeks of ziprasidone treatment.

Drug interactions. Drugs that inhibit CYP3A4 reduce metabolism of ziprasidone: concurrent treatment with ketoconazole in-creased blood levels of ziprasidone by ap-proximately 40%. Carbamazepine (and pos-sibly other enzyme inducers) may decrease ziprasidone levels by approximately 35%. Ef-fects of ziprasidone on metabolism of other drugs have not been reported. Ziprasidone is contraindicated for use in patients taking other medications that can prolong the QT interval.

Aripiprazole

Aripiprazole has a high affinity for D_2 and D_3 receptors, as well as 5-HT$_{1A}$ and 5-HT$_{2A}$ re-ceptors. Aripiprazole has partial agonist ac-tivity at the D_2 and 5-HT$_{1A}$ receptors and an-tagonist activity at the 5-HT$_{2A}$ receptor.

Clinical use. Aripiprazole has been ap-proved for treatment of schizophrenia, treat-ment of acute manic or mixed episodes in bi-polar disorder, and maintenance treatment of bipolar disorder. The recommended start-ing and target dosage for aripiprazole in pa-tients with schizophrenia is 10 or 15 mg/day. The recommended starting dose for treat-ment of an acute manic or mixed episode is 30 mg; the recommended dosage for mainte-nance treatment in stable patients is 15 mg/day. The elimination half-life is 75 hours, and steady-state concentrations are reached within 2 weeks. Therefore, dosage adjust-ments are recommended every 2 weeks, to allow time for clinical assessments of the medication's effects to be observed at steady-state concentrations.

Risks, side effects, and their management.
The most common side effects associated with aripiprazole include headache, nausea, dyspepsia, agitation, anxiety, insomnia, somnolence, and akathisia. Aripiprazole is not associated with significant sedation, anticholinergic side effects, weight gain, or cardiovascular side effects. As with most other antipsychotic medications, aripiprazole is associated with a risk for NMS and tardive dyskinesias.

As noted earlier, elderly patients with dementia-related psychosis treated with atypical antipsychotics are at an increased risk for death compared with those receiving placebo. This warning applies across all atypical antipsychotic medications. Additionally, in controlled trials of dementia-related psychosis, aripiprazole-treated patients had an increased incidence of cerebrovascular adverse events, including deaths, with one study showing a dose-dependent relationship for these adverse events (Abilify 2005).

Drug interactions.   Aripiprazole is hepatically metabolized, mainly by two cytochrome P450 enzymes: CYP2D6 and CYP3A4. Therefore, dosage adjustments are necessary when this medication is given with other medications that either inhibit or induce these enzymes. For example, the dose of aripiprazole should be halved when this medication is given with ketoconazole, a CYP3A4 inhibitor, or at least decreased when given with fluoxetine, a CYP2D6 inhibitor. When aripiprazole is given with CYP3A4 inducers such as carbamazepine, the dose should be doubled.

Paliperidone

Paliperidone, a benzisoxazole derivative, is the major active metabolite of risperidone. This medication functions as an antagonist at the D_2, $5\text{-}HT_{2A}$, α_1, α_2, and H_1 receptors. Whereas risperidone reaches peak plasma concentrations approximately 1 hour following a single oral dose, paliperidone reaches peak plasma concentrations 24 hours following a single oral dose, allowing for once-daily dosing rather than twice-daily dosing.

Clinical use.   Paliperidone is approved for the acute and maintenance treatment of schizophrenia. Clinical efficacy for acute treatment was established in several randomized, controlled trials (Davidson et al. 2007; Kane et al. 2007; Marder et al. 2007). Effective dosages, as measured by a significant decrease in Positive and Negative Syndrome Scale scores compared with placebo, included 3–12 mg/day. In a randomized, double-blind, placebo-controlled trial, Kramer et al. (2007) found that treatment with paliperidone (3–15 mg/day) significantly delayed time to relapse compared with placebo. At dosages of 3 and 6 mg/day, the rate of adverse events was similar for paliperidone and placebo. In some studies, at dosages greater than 6 mg/day, the rate of adverse events was significantly higher in the paliperidone group.

The recommended dosage for paliperidone is 6 mg/day. No initial titration is necessary. If a dosage greater than 6 mg/day is required, increases in 3-mg increments every 5 days are recommended. The minimum and maximum dosages are 3 mg/day and 6 mg/day, respectively.

Risks, side effects, and their management.
The risks associated with paliperidone use are similar to those for other atypical antipsychotics. The most common adverse events, which were reported significantly more often with paliperidone than with placebo, included tachycardia (12%–14%), headache (11%–14%), somnolence (6%–11%), and anxiety (6%–9%). Extrapyramidal symptoms, including parkinsonism (3%–14%), akathisia (4%–9%), dyskinesias (3%–9%), and tremor (3%–5%), also occurred.

Drug interactions.   Paliperidone is not expected to interact significantly with drugs metabolized by cytochrome P450 enzymes. However, an additive effect may occur when this medication is administered with other agents that cause orthostatic hypotension.

Long-Acting Injectable Antipsychotics

For patients with chronic psychotic symptoms who are not compliant with antipsychotic medication, a long-acting depot preparation should be considered after stabilization with oral medication.

Conversion to a decanoate preparation is complicated by the highly variable individual pharmacokinetics of the oral and long-term depot agents. Most patients respond to a fluphenazine decanoate dose of 10–30 mg given every 2 weeks. A loading dose strategy has been established for haloperidol decanoate, in which patients receive an initial dose that is 20 times the oral maintenance dose (Ereshefsky et al. 1993). Steady-state serum concentrations are achieved after approximately 10 weeks (five injection intervals) with fluphenazine decanoate and after approximately 20 weeks with haloperidol decanoate. Side effects may take months to subside, and withdrawal dyskinesia may not appear for months after discontinuation of the decanoate formulation.

The recommended starting dose for the risperidone long-acting injection is 25 mg. Although an initial release of medication occurs, the amount released is small, and the main release of the drug begins 3 weeks after the injection. This release is maintained from 4 to 6 weeks and subsides by 7 weeks. Because not much drug is released for the first 3 weeks after the injection, oral antipsychotic supplementation is recommended. Injections are given every 2 weeks, and steady-state plasma concentrations are achieved after four injections. Dosing adjustments should not be made more often than once a month; the maximum dose is 50 mg every 2 weeks. Doses of 25, 37.5, and 50 mg are available, and different dosage strengths should not be combined. Dose titration depends on clinical symptoms. If the patient has not taken risperidone before, a trial of oral risperidone is recommended to determine whether the patient has a hypersensitivity reaction to the medication.

Mood Stabilizers

The term *mood stabilizer* is used to refer to a group of medications that are effective in the treatment of bipolar disorder. These treatments serve as the foundation for the psychopharmacological treatment of bipolar illnesses. Currently, lithium, valproate, carbamazepine, lamotrigine, and most of the atypical antipsychotic medications are approved by the FDA for the treatment of one or more phases of bipolar disorder.

Lithium

Mechanism of Action

Lithium is a cation that inhibits several steps in phosphoinositide metabolism, as well as many second and third messengers, including G proteins and protein kinases (Bitran et al. 1995; Lenox et al. 1992; Manji et al. 1993, 1995, 1999). Recent evidence suggests that lithium ultimately stimulates neurite growth, regeneration, and neurogenesis, which is likely related to its therapeutic effect (Coyle and Duman 2003; Kim et al. 2004).

Indications and Efficacy

Lithium has been proved effective for acute and prophylactic treatment of both manic and depressive episodes in patients with bipolar disorder (American Psychiatric Association 2002), although patients with rapid-cycling bipolar disorder have been reported to respond less well to lithium treatment (Dunner and Fieve 1974). Lithium is also effective in prevention of future depressive episodes in patients with recurrent unipolar depressive disorder (American Psychiatric Association 2002) and as an adjunct to antidepressant therapy in depressed patients whose illness is partially refractory to treatment with antidepressants alone. Furthermore, lithium may be useful in maintaining remission of depressive disorders after electroconvulsive therapy (Sackeim et al. 2001), as well as in the management of some cases of aggression and behavioral dyscontrol.

Clinical Use

Lithium carbonate is completely absorbed by the gastrointestinal tract and reaches peak plasma levels in 1–2 hours. The elimination half-life is approximately 24 hours. Steady-state lithium levels are achieved in approximately 5 days. Therapeutic plasma levels for the treatment of bipolar disorder range from 0.5 to 1.2 mEq/L. Although lower plasma levels are associated with less troubling side effects, many clinicians target lithium levels of 0.8 mEq/L or more when treating acute manic episodes. Therefore, treatment of acute mania with lithium should not be considered a failure until the treatment has been tried throughout the therapeutic plasma level range (provided that the treatment is tolerated). Additionally, more severely or acutely ill patients may require combination treatment.

Lithium dosing is based on achieving therapeutic blood levels, targeting clinical response, and minimizing side effects if possible. Lithium can be administered either as a single daily dose or in divided doses. Divided daily dosing with lithium carbonate results in several peak lithium levels a day, whereas a single daily dose is associated with a single, but higher, peak level. Some clinicians prefer evening dosing because some side effects are associated with peak blood levels. Lithium levels should be determined 12 hours after the last lithium dose. After therapeutic lithium levels have been established, levels should be measured every month for the first 3 months and every 3 months thereafter. In patients who have remained stable and who are aware of early signs of both relapse and lithium toxicity, lithium levels may be measured less frequently. In addition, serum urea nitrogen and creatinine levels should be measured before lithium therapy has commenced and every 3–6 months during therapy, with more frequent testing if there are specific complaints or signs of renal dysfunction. As with any treatment, patients should be informed of the potential benefits and risks of lithium treatment and also should be educated about other treatment alternatives.

Contraindications and Pretreatment Medical Evaluation

Lithium should not be administered to patients with unstable renal function. Because lithium may affect functioning of the cardiac sinus node, patients with sinus node dysfunction (e.g., sick sinus syndrome) should not receive lithium. Although lithium also has acute and chronic effects on the thyroid, patients with hypothyroidism may receive lithium if the thyroid disease is adequately treated and monitored. Laboratory tests that should be performed before initiation of lithium treatment are listed in Table 15–6.

Lithium treatment during pregnancy has been associated with teratogenic effects. The risk of Ebstein's anomaly in infants exposed to lithium in utero is 0.1%–0.7%, compared with 0.01% in the general population. The overall risk of major congenital anomalies associated with lithium exposure is 4%–12%, compared with 2%–4% in comparison groups (L.S. Cohen et al. 1994). The increased risk of malformations must be weighed against the risk of harm to both mother and fetus if lithium discontinuation results in a manic relapse.

Risks, Side Effects, and Their Management

Renal effects.   In the absence of toxicity, most of the effects of lithium on the kidneys are largely reversible after discontinuation of the drug (although permanent morphological changes in renal structure may occur in some patients). However, lithium inhibits vasopressin and may result in an impairment in renal concentrating ability, called *nephrogenic diabetes insipidus* (NDI). This condition results in polyuria for up to 60% of patients taking lithium. NDI may result in serious complications, including dehydration, lithium toxicity, and electrolyte imbalance. Clinically significant polyuria usually reverses itself after discontinuation of lithium therapy, but it may persist for many months. However, less serious increases in urine volume may persist indefinitely, an effect that some investigators believe is a consequence of renal tubular atrophy (Hetmar et al. 1991).

Preventive and management strategies for NDI include increasing the patient's fluid intake and decreasing the amount of lithium given to the lowest effective dosage. Once-daily dosing also results in lower urinary output than the multiple-dosing schedule (Hetmar et al. 1991; Plenge et al. 1982). For some patients, potassium supplementation, 10–20 mEq/day, may be effective. The nonthiazide diuretic amiloride also may treat lithium-induced NDI. For lithium-induced NDI, amiloride is prescribed in a dosage of 5 mg twice a day and increased to 10 mg twice a day if necessary. Even though amiloride does not appear to increase plasma lithium levels, it is prudent to continue to monitor serum lithium levels with greater frequency (at least every 2 months) when amiloride is combined with lithium.

Interstitial nephritis has been reported to be a consequence of long-term lithium therapy. Proteinuria has been reported as a rare side effect and is thought to be the consequence of either glomerular leakage or the inhibition of tubular resorption.

Thyroid dysfunction. Reversible hypothyroidism may occur in as many as 20% of the patients receiving lithium. Therefore, thyroid function should be evaluated every 6–12 months during lithium treatment or if symptoms develop that might be attributable to thyroid dysfunction, including depression or rapid cycling. If laboratory studies indicate the development of hypothyroidism, the patient should be referred to an endocrinologist for further evaluation and management. The psychiatrist and endocrinologist can also collaborate on the appropriate treatment for the patient's bipolar illness, including whether to continue lithium treatment or switch to another medication.

Parathyroid dysfunction. The effects of lithium on calcium metabolism may be re-

lated to lithium-induced hyperparathyroidism (Anath and Dubin 1983; Mallette and Eichhorn 1986). Clinically significant effects of hypercalcemia associated with lithium have been reported, including back pain, kyphoscoliosis, osteoporosis, hypertension, cardiomegaly, and impaired renal function. Potential neuropsychiatric sequelae include affective changes, anxiety, aggressiveness, sleep disturbance, apathy, psychosis, delirium, dementia, and seizures. Symptoms of hyperparathyroidism may be misdiagnosed as lithium toxicity or the effects of the underlying mood disorder. When signs or symptoms that might be related to hyperparathyroidism develop, serum calcium ion levels should be checked, and if they are abnormal, parathyroid hormone levels should be measured and an endocrinologist consulted.

Neurotoxicity. Several types of neurological adverse events may occur with lithium treatment. A fine resting tremor is a common side effect of lithium. β-Blockers, such as propranolol (<80 mg/day in divided doses), may effectively treat this tremor (Zubenko et al. 1984a). Additionally, subjective memory impairment commonly occurs (Goodwin and Jamison 1990).

Cardiac effects. Benign flattening of the T wave on the ECG occurs in 20%–30% of patients taking lithium (Bucht et al. 1984). In addition, lithium may suppress the function of the sinus node and result in sinoatrial block. Thus, an ECG should be obtained before initiating lithium treatment in patients older than 40 years or in those with a history or symptoms of cardiac disease.

Weight gain. Weight gain is a frequent side effect of lithium treatment. Indeed, weight gain can be problematic with numerous psychotropic medications and is a potential cause for treatment noncompliance. Therefore, patients should be informed of the risk for weight gain before initiating lithium therapy and counseled regarding weight management strategies, such as dietary habits and regular exercise. If weight gain occurs

Table 15–6. Key characteristics of mood stabilizers[a]

	Lithium	Valproate	Carbamazepine	Lamotrigine
Available preparations	Lithium carbonate (Eskalith, Lithonate, Lithotabs; 150-, 300-, 600-mg tablets, capsules) Lithium citrate liquid (8 mEq/5 mL) Extended-release lithium (Eskalith CR, 450 mg; Lithobid, 300 mg)	Divalproex sodium (Depakote, 125-, 250-, 500-mg tablets; 125-mg sprinkle capsules) Valproate sodium injection (Depacon) Valproic acid (Depakene, 250-mg capsules; 250 mg/5 mL syrup) Extended-release divalproex sodium (Depakote ER, 250, 500 mg)	Carbamazepine (Tegretol; 100-mg chewable tablets; 200-mg tablets) Extended-release carbamazepine capsules (Equetro, 100, 200, 300 mg; Carbatrol, 200, 300 mg) Carbamazepine suspension (100 mg/5 mL) Extended-release carbamazepine tablets (Tegretol XR, 100, 200, 400 mg)	Lamotrigine (Lamictal, 25-, 100-, 150-, 200-mg tablets; Lamictal CD [chewable dispersible], 2-, 5-, 25-mg tablets)
Half-life (hours)	24	96	Initially, 25–65; decreases to 12–17 because of autoinduction	25–33[b]
Starting dosage	300 mg bid	250 mg tid or 20 mg/kg[c]	Tablets/capsules: 200 mg bid[d]; suspension: 100 mg qid	25 mg/day[b]
Blood level	0.8–1.2 mEq/L	45–125 µg/mL	Not helpful; monitor for signs or symptoms of toxicity	Not monitored; target dose of lamotrigine is 200 mg/day
Metabolism	Renal	Hepatic	Hepatic	Hepatic
Contraindications[e]	Unstable renal function	Hepatic dysfunction	Hepatic dysfunction, bone marrow suppression	Previous hypersensitivity to lamotrigine

Table 15–6. Key characteristics of mood stabilizers[a] *(continued)*

	Lithium	Valproate	Carbamazepine	Lamotrigine
Key side effects, risks, and features	Nephrogenic diabetes insipidus Reversible hypothyroidism Tremor Benign leukocytosis Weight gain Narrow therapeutic index Potentially fatal toxicity Risk of Ebstein's anomaly with first-trimester exposure	Titration or loading dose strategies Rare hepatotoxicity Rare pancreatitis Polycystic ovarian syndrome Weight gain Tremor Alopecia Rare blood cell dyscrasias Risk of neural tube defects with first-trimester exposure	Cytochrome P450 inducer (oral contraceptive failure) Autoinduction Rare blood cell dyscrasias: aplastic anemia, agranulocytosis Hepatotoxicity Rash risk, including Stevens-Johnson syndrome Risk for SIADH Teratogenicity risk: neural tube defects, craniofacial defects	Rash risk in 5%–10% Rarely, life-threatening rash (including Stevens-Johnson syndrome) Risk minimized by low starting dose and slow titration Metabolism inhibited by valproate Metabolism induced by carbamazepine
Pretreatment laboratory evaluation	Chem 20,[f] CBC, TSH level determination, ECG (if patient is 40 years of age or older or has cardiac disease), pregnancy test	AST and ALT level determination, pregnancy test	AST, ALT, CBC, sodium level; pregnancy test	None; might consider a pregnancy test

Note. bid=twice daily; iv=intravenous; qid=four times a day; tid=three times a day; SIADH=syndrome of inappropriate secretion of antidiuretic hormone; CBC=complete blood count; TSH=thyroid-stimulating hormone; ECG=electrocardiogram; AST=aspartate aminotransaminase; ALT=alanine aminotransaminase.

[a]The atypical antipsychotics are not included in this table. Please refer to the antipsychotics section of this chapter for information about their characteristics.

[b]The effective half-life of lamotrigine approximately doubles with valproate and decreases by approximately half with carbamazepine, primidone, phenytoin, phenobarbital, and rifampin; therefore, initial doses may vary depending on concomitant medications. The reader should refer to current product labeling for specific information regarding drug–drug interactions, their effects on lamotrigine, and lamotrigine dosing guidelines.

[c]Increase close by 10%–20% when converting from valproate, divalproex, or valproic acid to the extended-release formulation of divalproex sodium.

[d]100 mg bid if given in combination with a neuroleptic or lithium.

[e]Lithium, valproate, and carbamazepine should be avoided in pregnancy, if possible; see text for discussion. Recent reports also have noted cases of oral clefts with lamotrigine use; see text for discussion.

[f]Especially serum urea nitrogen, creatinine, sodium, and calcium levels.

Source. Adapted from Marangell LB, Martinez JM: *Concise Guide to Psychopharmacology*, 2nd Edition. Washington, DC, American Psychiatric Publishing, 2006, pp. 138–141. Used with permission.

during treatment and weight management interventions fail, the clinician should discuss further treatment options with the patient.

Dermatological effects. Dermatological reactions to lithium include acne, follicular eruptions, and psoriasis. Hair loss and thinning also have been reported. Except for cases of exacerbation of psoriasis, these reactions are usually benign. Lithium-induced acne responds to topical treatment with retinoid acid, such as tretinoin (Retin-A).

Gastrointestinal symptoms. Gastrointestinal side effects, particularly nausea and diarrhea, are common and occur early during treatment. These side effects may be alleviated by decreasing the lithium dose (must balance this strategy against the risk for reduced efficacy) or instructing the patient to take lithium with meals. In general, the slow-release formulations of lithium are more often associated with nausea, whereas the immediate-release preparations are more commonly associated with diarrhea.

Hematological effects. The most frequent hematological change associated with lithium therapy is leukocytosis (approximately 15,000 WBCs/mm^3). This change is generally benign and typically reversible on lithium discontinuation.

Overdose and Toxicity

There is a narrow margin between therapeutic and toxic plasma lithium levels. Thus, the physician should educate the patient about the risks for lithium toxicity, the signs and symptoms of lithium toxicity, and the importance of preventing lithium toxicity by ensuring adequate salt and water intake, taking the lithium as prescribed, and following through with recommended laboratory monitoring.

Drug Interactions

Because lithium treatment is associated with a narrow therapeutic range, it is crucial that clinicians have good knowledge about the potential drug–drug interactions that may be associated with the concomitant administration of lithium and other drugs. Because lithium is excreted by the kidneys, any medication that alters renal function can affect lithium levels. Thiazide diuretics and nonsteroidal anti-inflammatory agents may increase lithium levels by decreasing renal clearance of lithium. Other medications that may increase lithium levels include angiotensin-converting enzyme inhibitors and cyclooxygenase-2 inhibitors (e.g., celecoxib, rofecoxib). Drugs that may decrease lithium levels include theophylline and aminophylline. Lithium may potentiate the effects of succinylcholine-like muscle relaxants.

Valproate

Valproate is approved by the FDA for the treatment of acute mania. It is commonly used for all phases of bipolar disorder, but its major body of evidence in bipolar disorder to date is in its efficacy in acute mania.

Mechanism of Action

Although many mechanisms of action have been proposed, the basis for the mood-stabilizing effects of valproate is most likely concordant with lithium's mechanism of action—specifically, attenuation of the activity of protein kinase C and other steps in the signal transduction pathway, leading to neuronal adaptation and changes in gene expression (Chen et al. 1994; Manji et al. 1996), including neurotrophic effects (Coyle and Duman 2003).

Clinical Use

Before starting treatment with valproate, patients should be told that they might experience nausea, sedation, and a fine hand tremor. These effects are often transient, but in some patients they persist. Several valproate preparations are available in the United States, including valproic acid, sodium valproate, divalproex sodium, and an XL preparation of divalproex sodium. Divalproex sodium is a dimer of sodium valproate and valproic acid with an enteric coating, and it is much better tolerated than other oral valproate preparations. The half-life of valproate is 9–16 hours.

Most clinicians use two general dosing strategies when treating acute mania: 1) a gradual dose titration or 2) a more rapid loading-dose strategy. Most commonly, treatment with valproate is initiated with a gradual titration strategy in which it is started at a dosage of 250 mg three times a day, with subsequent increases of 250 mg every 3 days. Most patients require a daily dose of 1,250–2,000 mg. Although valproate has a relatively short half-life, moderate doses may be given once a day at bedtime to reduce daytime sedation in patients with bipolar disorder (this strategy should not be used when the drug is being used to treat seizure disorders).

When an acutely manic patient requires rapid stabilization, valproate treatment can be initiated at a dose of 20 mg per kilogram of body weight (Keck et al. 1993). Plasma levels of 45–100 µg/mL are recommended for the treatment of acute mania (Bowden et al. 1996); however, dosing should be based on the balance between clinical response and side effects rather than on absolute blood level alone. Patients with less severe disorders, such as bipolar II disorder or cyclothymia, often respond at lower doses and blood levels (Jacobsen 1993). The XL preparation of divalproex sodium has 80%–90% of the bioavailability of the initial divalproex sodium, so doses may need to be slightly higher when this preparation is used.

Contraindications

Valproate is relatively contraindicated in patients with hepatitis or liver disease. If a patient has significant liver disease, alternative medications to treat his or her bipolar illness should be considered. Valproate should be used in such cases only as a last resort and only with the approval and continuous involvement of a gastroenterologist. Valproate has been linked to spina bifida and other neural tube defects in the offspring of pa-

tients exposed to this medication in the first trimester of pregnancy (Lammer et al. 1987; Robert and Guibaud 1982). Thus, the risks of continuing valproate therapy during pregnancy must be balanced against the risk of relapse. Abrupt discontinuation of medication in a woman with severe illness who is otherwise stable while taking valproate in the second or third trimester of pregnancy may be more harmful than helpful.

Risks, Side Effects, and Their Management

Hepatotoxicity. Although it is estimated that 1 in 118,000 patients dies from non-dose-related hepatic failure, no cases have occurred in patients older than 10 years who were receiving valproate monotherapy. Nonetheless, baseline liver function tests are indicated. If baseline test results are normal, monitoring for clinical signs of hepatotoxicity is more important than routine monitoring of liver enzyme levels, which has little predictive value and may be less effective than clinical monitoring (Pellock and Willmore 1991).

Transient mild increases in liver enzyme levels, up to three times the upper limit of normal, do not necessitate discontinuation of valproate. Although γ-glutamyltransferase levels are often checked by clinicians, these levels are often increased, without clinical significance, in patients receiving valproate and carbamazepine (Dean and Penry 1992). Likewise, plasma ammonia levels are often increased transiently during valproate treatment, but this finding does not necessitate interruption of treatment (Jaeken et al. 1980). Increases in transaminase levels are often dose dependent. If no suitable alternative treatment is available, dose reduction (with careful monitoring) may be attempted.

Hematological effects. Valproate has been associated with changes in platelet counts, but clinically significant thrombocytopenia has rarely been documented (Dean and Penry 1992). Coagulation defects also have been reported. Overall, the risk of inducing a coagulation disturbance in an otherwise healthy adult is extremely low. However, in patients in whom anticoagulation is strictly contraindicated and in patients who are already receiving anticoagulation therapy, monitoring of the coagulation profile is required at baseline, after 1 month of therapy, and then at least every 3 months.

Gastrointestinal symptoms. Multiple gastrointestinal side effects may be associated with valproate, including indigestion, nausea, and heartburn. Use of the divalproex sodium preparation and administration of the medication with food may alleviate these effects. Pancreatitis is a rare occurrence in patients receiving relatively high doses of valproate (Murphy et al. 1981). If vomiting and severe abdominal pain develop during valproate therapy, serum amylase levels should be determined immediately.

Weight gain. Weight gain is a common side effect of valproate treatment that does not appear to be dose dependent. Isojarvi et al. (1996) reported significant weight gain with associated hyperinsulinemia in approximately 50% of a cohort of women taking valproate. Given the risk of weight gain, diet and exercise should be recommended early in treatment.

Neurological effects. A benign essential tremor is a common side effect of valproate therapy. Drowsiness is another common side effect, but tolerance often develops once a steady-state level of the drug is reached.

Alopecia. Both transient and persistent hair loss have been associated with valproate use. Patients with valproate-induced alopecia may benefit from zinc supplementation, at a dosage of 22.5 mg/day (Hurd et al. 1984).

Polycystic ovarian syndrome. Polycystic ovarian syndrome is characterized by menstrual irregularity, hyperandrogenism, and the exclusion of other etiologies. Isojarvi et al. (1993) reported an association between polycystic ovarian syndrome and valproate in women receiving long-term valproate

treatment for epilepsy, especially those who were younger than 20 years.

Overdose

Valproate overdose results in increasing sedation, confusion, and ultimately coma. The patient also may manifest hyperreflexia or hyporeflexia, seizures, respiratory suppression, and supraventricular tachycardia. Treatment should include gastric lavage, electrocardiographic monitoring, treatment of emergent seizures, and respiratory support.

Drug Interactions

Valproate can inhibit hepatic enzymes, resulting in increased levels of other medications. Valproate is also highly bound to plasma proteins and may displace other highly bound drugs from protein-binding sites. Therefore, coadministered drugs that are either highly protein bound or reliant on hepatic metabolism may require dose adjustment. Drugs that may increase valproate levels include cimetidine, macrolide antibiotics (e.g., erythromycin), and felbamate. Valproate may increase concentrations of phenobarbital, ethosuximide, and the active 10,11-epoxide metabolite of carbamazepine, increasing the risk of toxicity. Valproate also may raise lamotrigine levels, increasing the risk of rash (current lamotrigine product labeling provides specific lamotrigine dosing guidelines for patients who are taking valproate). Valproate metabolism may be induced by other anticonvulsants, including carbamazepine, phenytoin, primidone, and phenobarbital, resulting in an increased total clearance of valproate and perhaps decreased efficacy.

Carbamazepine

Carbamazepine is effective in both acute and prophylactic treatment of mania (Gerner and Stanton 1992; Keck et al. 1992; Weisler et al. 2004, 2005). An XL formulation of carbamazepine, marketed in the United States under the brand name Equetro, is approved by the FDA for the treatment of acute mania. XL preparations of carbamazepine are preferred because the simplified dosage schedules may facilitate patient adherence. Other XL carbamazepine preparations include Tegretol XR and Carbatrol, although neither has been specifically indicated for the treatment of bipolar disorder.

Clinical Use

Carbamazepine should be initiated at a dosage of 200 mg twice a day, with increments of 200 mg/day every 3–5 days. Cited plasma levels of 8–12 μg/mL are based on clinical use in patients with seizure disorders and do not correlate with clinical response in patients with psychiatric disorders. We recommend a dose titration strategy that emphasizes achievement of a clinical response and minimizes side effects. During the titration phase, patients may be particularly prone to side effects such as sedation, dizziness, and ataxia; if these occur, titration should be continued more gradually (the dosage might be 100 mg twice a day, for example). Because carbamazepine induces its own metabolism (autoinduction), dosage adjustments may be required for weeks or months after initiation of treatment to maintain therapeutic plasma levels.

Contraindications

Because of the potential for hematological and hepatic toxicity, carbamazepine should not be administered to patients with liver disease or thrombocytopenia or to those at risk for agranulocytosis. For this reason, carbamazepine is strictly contraindicated in patients receiving clozapine. Because of reports of teratogenicity, including increased risks of spina bifida (Rosa 1991), microcephaly (Bertollini et al. 1987), and craniofacial defects (Jones et al. 1989), carbamazepine is relatively contraindicated in pregnant women. Additionally, because carbamazepine has a tricyclic structure, there are concerns about concomitant use of carbamazepine and MAOIs.

Pretreatment evaluation should include a complete blood count and determination of ALT and aspartate aminotransferase (AST)

levels. Because of the risk for teratogenicity, a pregnancy test also should be obtained in women of childbearing potential (see Table 15–6).

Risks, Side Effects, and Their Management

Hematological effects. The most serious toxic hematological side effects of carbamazepine are agranulocytosis and aplastic anemia, which can be fatal. Whereas carbamazepine-induced agranulocytosis or aplastic anemia is extremely rare (Pellock 1987), other hematological effects, such as leukopenia (total WBC count<3,000 cells/mm^3), thrombocytopenia, and mild anemia, may occur more frequently. Although it is important to assess hematological function and risk factors before initiating treatment, there appears to be no benefit to ongoing monitoring in the absence of clinical indicators. When carbamazepine-induced agranulocytosis occurs, the onset is rapid. Thus, a normal complete blood count one day does not mean that agranulocytosis will not develop the next day. Therefore, it is more important to educate the patient regarding early signs and symptoms of agranulocytosis and thrombocytopenia and to urge the patient to inform the psychiatrist immediately if these signs and symptoms develop.

If significant leukopenia develops, such as an absolute neutrophil count of less than 1,000, carbamazepine therapy should be discontinued, and a hematologist should be consulted.

Hepatotoxicity. Carbamazepine therapy is occasionally associated with hepatic toxicity (Gram and Bentsen 1983), usually a hypersensitivity hepatitis that appears after a latency period of several weeks and involves increases in ALT, AST, and lactate dehydrogenase levels. Cholestasis is also possible, with increases in bilirubin and alkaline phosphatase concentrations. Mild transient increases in transaminase levels generally do not necessitate discontinuation of carbamazepine. If ALT or AST levels increase more than three times the upper limit of normal, carbamazepine should be discontinued.

Dermatological effects.   Rash is a common side effect of carbamazepine, occurring in 3%–17% of patients (Warnock and Knesevich 1988) and typically occurring within 2–20 weeks after treatment initiation. Carbamazepine is generally discontinued if a rash develops because of the risk of progression to an exfoliative dermatitis or Stevens-Johnson syndrome, a severe bullous form of erythema multiforme (Patterson 1985).

Endocrine disorders.   Carbamazepine may cause reductions in circulating thyroid hormones (Bentsen et al. 1983; Yeo et al. 1978). syndrome of inappropriate secretion of antidiuretic hormone (SIADH), with resultant hyponatremia, may be induced by carbamazepine treatment. Alcoholic patients may be at greater risk for hyponatremia. Patients taking carbamazepine who develop signs or symptoms of hyponatremia should have their serum sodium level measured.

Gastrointestinal symptoms.   Nausea and occasional vomiting are common side effects of carbamazepine.

Neurological effects.   Patients taking carbamazepine may develop dizziness, drowsiness, or ataxia, particularly during the early phases of treatment. If this occurs, the carbamazepine dose should be reduced and a slower titration schedule implemented.

Overdose

Carbamazepine overdose may initially present with neuromuscular disturbances, such as nystagmus, myoclonus, and hyperreflexia, which may then progress to seizures and coma. Cardiac conduction changes, nausea, vomiting, and urinary retention also may occur. Treatment of carbamazepine overdose should include induction of vomiting, gastric lavage, and supportive care. After a serious overdose, blood pressure and respiratory and kidney function should be monitored for several days.

Drug Interactions

Carbamazepine induces hepatic cytochrome P450 enzymes, which may reduce levels of other medications. Importantly, carbamazepine therapy can lead to oral contraceptive failure (Coulam and Annegers 1979). Therefore, women who are planning to initiate therapy with carbamazepine should be advised to consider alternative forms of birth control while taking carbamazepine. Use of medications or substances that inhibit CYP3A3/4 may result in significant increases in plasma carbamazepine levels (Brodie and MacPhee 1986; Cozza et al. 2003; Ketter et al. 1995).

Lamotrigine

Lamotrigine is an anticonvulsant medication that decreases sustained high-frequency repetitive firing of the voltage-dependent sodium channel, which may then decrease glutamate release (Leach et al. 1991; Macdonald and Kelly 1995). Lamotrigine is approved by the FDA for the prevention of mania and depression in patients with bipolar disorder. Two randomized, controlled trials showed a greater time to intervention for any mood episode for both lamotrigine and lithium compared with placebo (Bowden et al. 2003; Calabrese et al. 2003). However, lamotrigine has not shown efficacy as a monotherapy treatment for acute mania. Lamotrigine has shown efficacy in a double-blind, placebo-controlled trial for the treatment of bipolar depression (Calabrese et al. 1999). Although lamotrigine is frequently used for the acute and longer-term control of the depressed phase of bipolar disorder (American Psychiatric Association 2002; Marangell et al. 2004), its use as a treatment for acute bipolar depression has not been approved by the FDA.

Clinical Use

Lamotrigine treatment is usually initiated at 25 mg once a day. Because the risk of a serious rash increases with rapid titration, it is essential to follow the recommended titration schedule. After 2 weeks, the dosage is increased to 50 mg/day for another 2 weeks. At week 5, the dosage can be increased to 100 mg/day and at week 6 to 200 mg/day. In patients who are taking valproate or other medications that decrease the clearance of lamotrigine, the dosing schedule and target dose are halved. Conversely, the titration schedule and dose are increased in those taking carbamazepine. In the absence of carbamazepine or other enzyme inducers, doses higher than 200 mg are typically not recommended in the treatment of bipolar disorder.

Risks, Side Effects, and Their Management

Lamotrigine is well tolerated and is not associated with hepatotoxicity, weight gain, or significant sedation. Common early side effects include headache, dizziness, gastrointestinal distress, and blurred or double vision.

Rash. Lamotrigine has been associated with both benign and severe rashes. A maculopapular rash develops in 5%–10% of patients taking lamotrigine, usually in the first 8 weeks of treatment. Lamotrigine also has been associated with serious rashes requiring hospitalization and discontinuation of treatment. The incidence of these rashes, which have included Stevens-Johnson syndrome, is approximately 0.3% in adults receiving adjunctive treatment for epilepsy, 0.13% in adults receiving adjunctive therapy in mood disorders clinical trials, and 0.08% in adults receiving lamotrigine as initial monotherapy in mood disorders clinical trials (Lamictal 2005).

To minimize the risk of a rash, the clinician must prescribe lamotrigine in accordance with the current product labeling's recommended starting dose and titration schedule (noting that the titration schedules vary depending on the presence or absence of concomitant medications, particularly valproate). Additionally, Ketter et al. (2005) reported a decreased incidence of treatment-emergent rash by advising patients who are starting lamotrigine to avoid other new medicines and new foods, cosmetics, condition-

ers, deodorants, detergents, and fabric softeners, as well as sunburn and exposure to poison ivy and poison oak.

Teratogenicity. Data published from the North American Antiepileptic Drug Registry reported 3 cases of cleft palate and 2 cases of cleft lip in infants from a total of 564 infants exposed in the first trimester to lamotrigine monotherapy (8.9 cases per 1,000) (Holmes et al. 2006). At present, clinicians should discuss the possibility of these risks with their patients and consider treatment alternatives for patients who are contemplating pregnancy.

Drug Interactions

Several important potential drug–drug interactions may occur with lamotrigine. Of particular importance to patients with bipolar disorders, valproate will increase lamotrigine levels, and carbamazepine will decrease lamotrigine levels. These two interactions are of particular importance to psychiatrists because both drugs are commonly prescribed as mood stabilizers for patients with bipolar disorder. Many other anticonvulsants interact with lamotrigine as well. Oral contraceptives can result in decreases in lamotrigine concentrations, but lamotrigine does not affect the availability of oral contraceptives.

Oxcarbazepine

Oxcarbazepine is a keto derivative of carbamazepine but offers several advantages over carbamazepine. Specifically, oxcarbazepine does not require blood cell count, hepatic, or serum drug level monitoring; causes less cytochrome P450 enzyme induction than does carbamazepine (but may decrease effectiveness of oral contraceptives containing ethinyl estradiol and levonorgestrel); and does not induce its own metabolism. These properties, combined with its similarity to carbamazepine, led many clinicians to use this medication for the treatment of bipolar disorder. However, it is important to note that oxcarbazepine has not been approved by the FDA for the acute or long-term treatment of bipolar disorder. To date, small controlled trials have suggested efficacy in the treatment of acute mania compared with lithium and haloperidol (Emrich 1990).

Oxcarbazepine has been associated with hyponatremia (Pendlebury et al. 1989; Trileptal 2006); thus, serum sodium levels should be monitored in patients at risk. Additionally, Stevens-Johnson syndrome and toxic epidermal necrolysis may occur at rates 3- to 10-fold higher than background incidence rates (Trileptal 2006).

Other Anticonvulsants

There is considerable interest in the potential usefulness of newer anticonvulsants for the treatment of bipolar disorder. However, positive data from well-designed controlled monotherapy trials to date are lacking for these agents.

Atypical Antipsychotics

All of the atypical antipsychotic medications (olanzapine, risperidone, quetiapine, ziprasidone, and aripiprazole) except clozapine are approved by the FDA for the treatment of acute mania. Across randomized, controlled trials, atypical antipsychotics have shown efficacy in treating the core symptoms of mania. General dosing guidelines for acute mania are shown in Table 15–7. It is common clinical practice to use lower starting dosages for patients who are less ill, particularly those patients receiving treatment in outpatient settings, but this practice has not been studied in randomized, controlled trials. At present, only two of the atypical antipsychotics—olanzapine and aripiprazole—have been approved by the FDA as maintenance-phase treatments for bipolar disorder, although studies are under way with the other agents. The use of these agents for the depressed phase of bipolar disorder is an area of active clinical investigation. Clozapine has not received FDA approval for use in bipolar disorder, but it is a valuable option for patients whose symptoms are otherwise resistant to treatment (Suppes et al. 1999).

Olanzapine–Fluoxetine Combination

The olanzapine–fluoxetine combination is currently the only medication approved by the FDA specifically for the treatment of depression in patients with bipolar disorder. This indication was based on data from a double-blind, randomized study in which the combination was superior to both olanzapine monotherapy and placebo (Tohen et al. 2003). Treatment-emergent mania or hypomania did not occur more frequently in the olanzapine–fluoxetine combination group than in the placebo group during the acute trial.

Clinical Use

The olanzapine–fluoxetine combination is available in four dosing preparations (6 mg/25 mg, 12 mg/25 mg, 6 mg/50 mg, 12 mg/50 mg) that allow clinicians to tailor treatment individually to provide greater or lesser amounts of each medication component. The typical starting dose for most patients is 6 mg/25 mg. Common side effects include somnolence, weight gain, increased appetite, asthenia, peripheral edema, and tremor. As one might expect, warnings and precautions that apply to either olanzapine or fluoxetine also apply to this combination treatment. For example, concomitant use of MAOIs is contraindicated given the fluoxetine component. Similarly, warnings and precautions regarding the potential association between olanzapine and hyperglycemia also apply. Additionally, clinicians should be aware of the potential drug–drug interactions that apply to either olanzapine or fluoxetine alone, such as the potential for clinically relevant CYP2D6 isoenzyme inhibition by the fluoxetine component.

Conclusion

The pharmacological armamentarium for treatment of psychiatric illnesses continues to expand. Results from multisite effective-

Table 15–7. Atypical antipsychotic dosing in the treatment of acute mania

| Generic drug | Trade name | Dosing in acute mania (mg/day)[a] | | |
		Starting dose	Dose titration	Target dose
Olanzapine	Zyprexa	10–15	5 mg/day increments	5–20
Risperidone	Risperdal	2–3	1 mg/day increments	1–6
Aripiprazole	Abilify	15–30	15 mg increments	30
Quetiapine	Seroquel	100	50–100 mg/day increments	600
Ziprasidone	Geodon	80 (divided twice daily)	40–80 mg/day increments	120–160

[a]Lower doses and slower dose titrations are indicated for the elderly. The reader is referred to current product labeling for specific information regarding approved indications for use and dosing in special populations.

Source.   Adapted from Marangell LB, Martinez JM: *Concise Guide to Psychopharmacology,* 2nd Edition. Washington, DC, American Psychiatric Publishing, 2006, p. 161. Used with permission.

ness and efficacy trials, such as Clinical Antipsychotic Trials of Intervention Effectiveness (CATIE) and Sequenced Treatment Alternatives to Relieve Depression (STAR*D), inform treatment and help define areas where improvement is needed. Current medications often have limited efficacy, and side effects decrease tolerability and compliance. More research is needed to address these hurdles that interfere with achieving remission.

Key Points

- Accurate diagnosis is the key to a well-informed treatment decision; whenever possible, treat the primary diagnosis and not the symptoms.

- Several factors are important when selecting an appropriate medication, including identifying medication-responsive target symptoms, ruling out nonpsychiatric causes of a patient's symptomatology, noting the presence of other medical problems that will influence drug selection, evaluating concomitant medications that may cause drug–drug interactions, and evaluating personal and family histories of medication response.

- Whenever possible, the clinician should involve the patient in medication decisions and educate the patient and significant others about the illness and potential benefits, risks, and side effects of any medication being prescribed.

- Patients must be educated about the typical time to response for the medication being prescribed and the need for strict adherence to the treatment regimen to ensure an optimal chance for treatment success.

- In addition to pharmacotherapy, other interventions such as disease-specific psychotherapies should be considered.

- When evaluating a patient with a history of treatment failures, a detailed treatment history should include a review of the dose, duration, tolerability, adherence, and reason for discontinuation for each prior treatment; many prior medication failures may be a result of inadequate dosing, inadequate treatment duration, noncompliance, or poor tolerability.

- Ongoing psychiatric and medical monitoring during treatment should be individualized to each patient according to several factors, including the severity of the illness, the current clinical status of the patient (e.g., acutely ill, partially remitted), and the specific medication(s) being prescribed.

- The clinician should evaluate response to each prescribed treatment by monitoring symptomatic and functional improvement and strive for complete symptomatic and functional recovery.

- Clinicians should be mindful of the response to each medication and consider discontinuing any treatment that has provided no benefit despite an adequate dose and duration of treatment.

Suggested Readings

Books

Marangoll LB, Martinez JM. Concise Guide to Psychopharmacology, 2nd Edition. Washington, DC, American Psychiatric Publishing, 2006

Schatzberg AF, Nemeroff CB: The American Psychiatric Publishing Textbook of Psychopharmacology, 4th Edition. Washington, DC, American Psychiatric Publishing, 2009

Wynn GH, Oesterheld JR, Cozza KL, Armstrong SC: Clinical Manual of Drug Interaction for Medical Practice. Washington, DC, American Psychiatric Publishing, 2009

Articles

Lieberman JA, Stroup TS, McEvoy JP, et al: Effectiveness of antipsychotic drugs in patients with chronic schizophrenia. N Engl J Med 353:1209–1223, 2005

McEvoy JP, Lieberman JA, Stroup TS, et al: Effectiveness of clozapine versus olanzapine, quetiapine, and risperidone in patients with chronic schizophrenia who did not respond to prior atypical antipsychotic treatment. Am J Psychiatry 163:600–610, 2006

Rush AJ, Trivedi MH, Wisniewski SR, et al: Bupropion-SR, sertraline, or venlafaxine-XR after failure of SSRIs for depression. N Engl J Med 354:1231–1242, 2006

Stroup TS, Lieberman JA, McEvoy JP, et al: Effectiveness of olanzapine, quetiapine, risperidone, and ziprasidone in patients with chronic schizophrenia following discontinuation of a previous atypical antipsychotic. Am J Psychiatry 163:611–622, 2006

Trivedi MH, Fava M, Wisniewski SR, et al: Medication augmentation after the failure of SSRIs for depression. N Engl J Med 354:1243–1252, 2006

Trivedi MH, Rush AJ, Wisniewski SR, et al: Evaluation of outcomes with citalopram for depression using measurement-based care in STAR*D: implications for clinical practice. Am J Psychiatry 163:28–40, 2006

Online Resources

American Psychiatric Association: www.psych.org

MedScape Psychiatry & Mental Health: www.medscape.com/psychiatry

References

Abernethy DR, Greenblatt DJ, Ochs HR, et al: Benzodiazepine drug-drug interactions commonly occurring in clinical practice. Curr Med Res Opin 8 (suppl 4):80–93, 1984

Abilify (product information). Princeton, NJ, Bristol-Myers Squibb, 2005

Adler LA, Angrist B, Peselow E, et al: Efficacy of propranolol in neuroleptic-induced akathisia. J Clin Psychopharmacol 5:164–166, 1985

Adler LA, Angrist B, Reiter S, et al: Neuroleptic-induced akathisia: a review. Psychopharmacology (Berl) 97:1–11, 1989

Allison DB, Mentore JL, Heo M, et al: Antipsychotic-induced weight gain: a comprehensive research synthesis. Am J Psychiatry 156:1686–1696, 1999

Altshuler LL, Cohen L, Szuba MP, et al: Pharmacological management of psychiatric illness during pregnancy: dilemmas and guidelines. Am J Psychiatry 153:592–606, 1996

American Diabetes Association, American Psychiatric Association, American Association of Clinical Endocrinologists, North American Association for the Study of Obesity: Consensus development conference on antipsychotic drugs and obesity and diabetes. Diabetes Care 27:596–601, 2004

American Psychiatric Association: Benzodiazepine Dependence, Toxicity, and Abuse: A Task Force Report of the American Psychiatric Association. Washington, DC, American Psychiatric Association, 1990

American Psychiatric Association: Tardive Dyskinesia: A Task Force Report of the American Psychiatric Association. Washington, DC, American Psychiatric Association, 1992

American Psychiatric Association: Practice Guideline for the Treatment of Patients With Major Depressive Disorder, 2nd Edition. Washington, DC, American Psychiatric Association, 2000

American Psychiatric Association: Practice guideline for the treatment of patients with bipolar disorder (revision). Am J Psychiatry 159 (4 suppl):1–50, 2002

Amsterdam J: A double-blind, placebo-controlled trial of the safety and efficacy of selegiline transdermal system without dietary restrictions in patients with major depressive disorder. J Clin Psychiatry 64:208–214, 2003

Amsterdam J, Berwish NJ: High dose tranylcypromine therapy for refractory depression. Pharmacopsychiatry 22:21–25, 1989

Anath J, Dubin SE: Lithium and symptomatic hyperparathyroidism. J R Soc Med 96:1026–1029, 1983

Anderson ES, Powers PS: Neuroleptic malignant syndrome associated with clozapine use. J Clin Psychiatry 52:102–104, 1991

Angst F, Stassen HH, Clayton PJ, et al: Mortality of patients with mood disorders: follow-up over 34–38 years. J Affect Disord 68:167–181, 2002

Appleton WS, Davis JM: Practical Clinical Psychopharmacology, 2nd Edition. Baltimore, MD, Williams & Wilkins, 1980

Arana GW, Goff DC, Friedman H, et al: Does carbamazepine-induced reduction of plasma haloperidol levels worsen psychotic symptoms? Am J Psychiatry 143:650–651, 1986

Aronson MD, Hafez H: A case of trazodone-induced ventricular tachycardia. J Clin Psychiatry 47:388–389, 1986

Arvanitis LA, Miller BG: Multiple fixed doses of "Seroquel" (quetiapine) in patients with acute exacerbation of schizophrenia: a comparison with haloperidol and placebo. The Seroquel Trial 13 Study Group. Biol Psychiatry 42:233–246, 1997

Baldessarini RJ, Cohen BM, Teicher MH: Significance of neuroleptic dose and plasma level in the pharmacological treatment of psychoses. Arch Gen Psychiatry 45:79–91, 1988

Beasley CM, Tollefson G, Tran P, et al: Olanzapine versus placebo and haloperidol: acute phase results of the Northern American double-blind olanzapine trial. Neuropsychopharmacology 14:111–123, 1996

Bentsen KD, Gram L, Veje A: Serum thyroid hormones and blood folic acid during mono-therapy with carbamazepine or valproate: a controlled study. Acta Neurol Scand 67:235–241, 1983

Bertollini R, Kallen B, Mastroiacovo P, et al: Anticonvulsant drugs in monotherapy: effect on fetus. Eur J Epidemiol 3:164–171, 1987

Bitran JA, Manji HK, Potter WZ, et al: Down-regulation of PKC alpha by lithium in vitro. Psychopharmacol Bull 31:449–452, 1995

Bodkin J, Amsterdam JD: Transdermal selegiline in major depression: a double-blind, placebo-controlled, parallel-group study in outpatients. Am J Psychiatry 159:1869–1875, 2002

Bowden CL, Janicak PG, Orsulak P, et al: Relation of serum valproate concentration to response in mania. Am J Psychiatry 153:765–770, 1996

Bowden CL, Calabrese JR, Sachs G, et al: A placebo-controlled 18-month trial of lamotrigine and lithium maintenance treatment in recently manic or hypomanic patients with bipolar I disorder. Lamictal 606 Study Group. Arch Gen Psychiatry 60:392–400, 2003

Branchey M, Branchey L: Patterns of psychotropic drug use and tardive dyskinesia. J Clin Psychopharmacol 4:41–45, 1984

Bremner JD: A double-blind comparison of Org 3770, amitriptyline, and placebo in major depression. J Clin Psychiatry 56:519–525, 1995

Brodie MJ, MacPhee GJ: Carbamazepine neurotoxicity precipitated by diltiazem. BMJ 292:1170–1171, 1986

Bucht G, Smigan L, Wahlin A, et al: ECG changes during lithium therapy: a prospective study. Acta Med Scand 216:101–104, 1984

Burke RE, Fahn S, Jankovic J, et al: Tardive dyskinesia: late-onset and persistent dystonia caused by antipsychotic drugs. Neurology 32:1335–1346, 1982

Byerly MJ, DeVane CL: Pharmacokinetics of clozapine and risperidone: a review of recent literature. J Clin Psychopharmacol 16:177–187, 1996

Calabrese JR, Bowden CL, Sachs GS, et al: A double-blind placebo-controlled study of lamotrigine monotherapy in outpatients with bipolar I depression. Lamictal 602 Study Group. J Clin Psychiatry 60:79–88, 1999

Calabrese JR, Bowden CL, Sachs GS, et al: A placebo-controlled 18-month trial of lamotrigine and lithium maintenance treatment in recently depressed patients with bipolar I disorder. Lamictal 605 Study Group. J Clin Psychiatry 64:1013–1024, 2003

Callahan AM, Marangell LB, Ketter TA: Evaluating the clinical significance of drug interactions: a systematic approach. Harv Rev Psychiatry 4:153–158, 1996

Chen G, Manji HK, Hawver DB, et al: Chronic sodium valproate selectively decreases protein kinase C alpha and epsilon in vitro. J Neurochem 63:2361–2364, 1994

Citrome L, Blonde L, Damatarca C: Metabolic issues in patients with severe mental illness. South Med J 98:714–720, 2005

Cohen LG, Chesley S, Eugenio L, et al: Erythromycin-induced clozapine toxic reaction. Arch Intern Med 156:675–677, 1996

Cohen LS, Friedman JM, Jefferson JW, et al: A reevaluation of risk of in utero exposure to lithium [published erratum appears in JAMA 271:1485, 1994]. JAMA 271:146–150, 1994

Cohn JB, Wilcox CS: Low-sedation potential of buspirone compared with alprazolam and lorazepam in the treatment of anxious patients: a double-blind study. J Clin Psychiatry 47:409–412, 1986

Correll CU, Leucht S, Kane JM: Lower risk for tardive dyskinesia associated with second generation antipsychotics: a systematic review of 1-year studies. Am J Psychiatry 161:414–425, 2004

Coulam CB, Annegers JF: Do anticonvulsants reduce the efficacy of oral contraceptives? Epilepsia 20:519–525, 1979

Coupland NJ, Bell CJ, Potokar JP: Serotonin reuptake inhibitor withdrawal. J Clin Psychopharmacol 16:356–362, 1996

Coyle JT, Duman RS: Finding the intracellular signaling pathways affected by mood disorder treatments. Neuron 38:157–160, 2003

Cozza KL, Armstrong SC, Oesterheld JR: Concise Guide to Drug Interaction Principles for Medical Practice: Cytochrome P450s, UGTs, P-Glycoproteins, 2nd Edition. Washington, DC, American Psychiatric Publishing, 2003

Cymbalta (package insert). Indianapolis, IN, Eli Lilly & Co, 2006

Dalton SO, Johansen C, Mellemkjaer L, et al: Use of selective serotonin reuptake inhibi-

tors and risk of upper gastrointestinal tract bleeding: a population-based cohort study. Arch Intern Med 163:59–64, 2003

Danish University Antidepressant Group: Paroxetine: a selective serotonin reuptake inhibitor showing better tolerance, but weaker antidepressant effect than clomipramine in a controlled multicenter study. J Affect Disord 18:289–299, 1990

DasGupta K, Young A: Clozapine-induced neuroleptic malignant syndrome. J Clin Psychiatry 52:105–107, 1991

Davidson M, Emsley R, Kramer M, et al: Efficacy, safety and early response of paliperidone extended-release tablets (paliperidone ER): results of a 6-week, randomized, placebo-controlled study. Schizophr Res 93:117–130, 2007

Davis JM: Maintenance therapy and the natural course of schizophrenia. J Clin Psychiatry 46:18–21, 1985

Davis KL, Kahn RS, Ko G, et al: Dopamine in schizophrenia: a review and reconceptualization. Am J Psychiatry 148:1474–1486, 1991

de Abajo FJ, Rodriguez LA, Montero D: Association between selective serotonin reuptake inhibitors and upper gastrointestinal bleeding: population based case-control study. BMJ 319:1106–1109, 1999

Dean JC, Penry JK: Valproate, in The Medical Treatment of Epilepsy. Edited by Resor SR Jr, Kutt H. New York, Marcel Dekker, 1992, pp 265–278

De Boer T: The pharmacological profile of mirtazapine. J Clin Psychiatry 57 (suppl 4):19–25, 1996

Devinsky O, Honigfeld G, Patin J: Clozapine-related seizures. Neurology 41:369–371, 1991

Dixon J, Power SJ, Grundy EM, et al: Sedation for local anaesthesia: comparison of intravenous midazolam and diazepam. Anaesthesia 39:372–378, 1984

Drug Facts and Comparisons, 56th Edition. St. Louis, MO, Facts & Comparisons, A Wolters Kluwer Company, 2002, pp 915–921, 1012–1014

Dumon J-P, Catteau J, Lanvin F, et al: Randomized, double-blind, crossover, placebo-controlled comparison of propranolol and betaxolol in the treatment of neuroleptic-induced akathisia. Am J Psychiatry 149:647–650, 1992

Dunner DL, Fieve RR: Clinical factors in lithium carbonate prophylaxis failure. Arch Gen Psychiatry 30:229–233, 1974

Dupuis B, Catteau J, Dumon J-P, et al: Comparison of propranolol, sotalol, and betaxolol in the treatment of neuroleptic-induced akathisia. Am J Psychiatry 144:802–805, 1987

Edlund MJ, Craig TJ: Antipsychotic drug use and birth defects: an epidemiologic reassessment. Compr Psychiatry 25:32–37, 1984

Emrich HM: Studies with oxcarbazepine (Trileptal) in acute mania. Int Clin Psychopharmacol 5:83–88, 1990

EMSAM (product information). Princeton, NJ, Bristol-Myers Squibb, 2006

Ereshefsky L, Toney G, Saklad SR, et al: A loading-dose strategy for converting from oral to depot haloperidol. Hosp Community Psychiatry 44:1155–1161, 1993

Expert Panel on the Detection, Evaluation, and Treatment of High Blood Cholesterol in Adults: Executive summary of the third report of the National Cholesterol Education Program (NCEP) expert panel on detection, evaluation, and treatment of high blood cholesterol in adults (Adult Treatment Panel III). JAMA 285:2486–2497, 2001

Fahn S: A therapeutic approach to tardive dyskinesia. J Clin Psychiatry 46:19–24, 1985

Faucette SR, Hawke RL, Lecluyse EL, et al: Validation of bupropion hydroxylation as a selective marker for human cytochrome P450 2B6 catalytic activity. Drug Metab Dispos 28:1222–1230, 2000

Fava M, Judge R, Hoog SL, et al: Fluoxetine versus sertraline and paroxetine in major depressive disorder: changes in weight with long-term treatment. J Clin Psychiatry 61:863–867, 2000

Feinberg SS, Holzer B: The monoamine oxidase inhibitor (MAOI) diet and kosher pizza (letter). J Clin Psychopharmacol 17:227–228, 1997

Feinberg SS, Holzer B: Clarifying the safety of the MAOI diet and pizza (letter). J Clin Psychiatry 61:145, 2000

Fuller MA, Sajatovic M: Lexi-Comp's Drug Information Handbook for Psychiatry, 4th Edition. Hudson, OH, Lexi-Comp, 2004, pp 1420, 1440–1441

Gardner DM, Shulman KI, Walker SE, et al: The making of a user friendly MAOI diet. J Clin Psychiatry 57:99–104, 1996

Gerner RH, Stanton A: Algorithm for patient management of acute manic states: lithium, valproate, or carbamazepine? J Clin Psychopharmacol 12 (suppl):57S–63S, 1992

Ghadirian AM, Chouinard G, Annable L: Sexual dysfunction and plasma prolactin levels in neuroleptic-treated schizophrenic outpatients. J Nerv Ment Dis 170:463–467, 1982

Gill SS, Rochon PA, Herrmann N, et al: Atypical antipsychotic drugs and risk of ischaemic stroke: population based retrospective cohort study. BMJ 330:445, 2005

Glazer WM, Moore DC, Schooler NR, et al: Tardive dyskinesia: a discontinuation study. Arch Gen Psychiatry 41:623–627, 1984

Glick ID, Marder SR: Long term maintenance therapy with quetiapine versus haloperidol decanoate in patients with schizophrenia or schizoaffective disorder. J Clin Psychiatry 66:638–641, 2005

Goff DC, Baldessarini R: Antipsychotics, in Drug Interactions in Psychiatry, 2nd Edition. Edited by Ciraulo D, Shader R, Greenblatt D, et al. Baltimore, MD, Williams & Wilkins, 1995, pp 129–174

Goff DC, Evins AE: Negative symptoms in schizophrenia: neurobiological models and treatment response. Harv Rev Psychiatry 6:59–77, 1998

Goff DC, Midha KK, Sarid-Segal O, et al: A placebo-controlled trial of fluoxetine added to neuroleptic in patients with schizophrenia. Psychopharmacology (Berl) 117:417–423, 1995

Goff D, Posever T, Herz L, et al: An exploratory haloperidol-controlled dose-finding study of ziprasidone in hospitalized patients with schizophrenia or schizoaffective disorder. J Clin Psychopharmacol 18:296–304, 1998

Goldberg HL, Finnerty RJ: The comparative efficacy of buspirone and diazepam in the treatment of anxiety. Am J Psychiatry 136:1184–1187, 1979

Goodwin FK, Jamison R: Manic-Depressive Illness. New York, Oxford University Press, 1990

Gram LM, Bentsen KD: Hepatic toxicity of antiepileptic drugs: a review. Acta Neurol Scand Suppl 97:81–90, 1983

Green MF, Marshall BD Jr, Wirshing WC, et al: Does risperidone improve verbal working memory in treatment-resistant schizophrenia? Am J Psychiatry 154:799–804, 1997

Guy W: Abnormal Involuntary Movement Scale (AIMS), in ECDEU Assessment Manual for Psychopharmacology, Revised. Washington, DC, U.S. Department of Health, Welfare, and Education, 1976, pp 534–537

Hagger C, Buckley P, Kenny JT, et al: Improvement in cognitive functions and psychiatric symptoms in treatment-refractory schizophrenic patients receiving clozapine. Biol Psychiatry 34:702–712, 1993

Haring C, Barnas C, Saria A, et al: Dose-related plasma levels of clozapine. J Clin Psychopharmacol 9:71–72, 1989

Harvey KV, Balon R: Augmentation with buspirone: a review. Ann Clin Psychiatry 7:143–147, 1995

Herrmann N, Lanctot KL: Do atypical antipsychotics cause stroke? CNS Drugs 19:91–103, 2005

Hetmar O, Poulsen UJ, Ladefoged J, et al: Lithium: long-term effects on the kidney: a prospective follow-up study ten years after kidney biopsy. Br J Psychiatry 158:53–58, 1991

Hodgman MJ, Martin TG, Krenzelok EP: Serotonin syndrome due to venlafaxine and maintenance tranylcypromine therapy. Hum Exp Toxicol 16:14–17, 1997

Holmes LB, Wyszynski DF, Baldwin EJ, et al: Increased risk for non-syndromic cleft palate among infants exposed to lamotrigine during pregnancy (abstract). Birth Defects Res A Clin Mol Teratol 76:318, 2006

Honigfeld G, Arellano F, Sethi J, et al: Reducing clozapine-related morbidity and mortality: 5 years of experience with the Clozaril National Registry. J Clin Psychiatry 59 (suppl 3): 3–7, 1998

Hurd RW, Van Rinsvelt HA, Wilder BJ, et al: Selenium, zinc, and copper changes with valproic acid: possible relation to drug side effects. Neurology 34:1393–1395, 1984

Isojarvi JIT, Laatikainen TJ, Pakarinen AJ, et al: Polycystic ovaries and hyperandrogenism in women taking valproate for epilepsy. N Engl J Med 39:579–584, 1993

Isojarvi JI, Laatikainen TJ, Knip M, et al: Obesity and endocrine disorders in women taking valproate for epilepsy. Ann Neurol 39:579–584, 1996

Itil TM, Soldatos C: Epileptogenic side effects of psychotropic drugs: practical recommendations. JAMA 244:1460–1463, 1980

Jacobsen FM: Low-dose valproate: a new treatment for cyclothymia, mild rapid cycling disorders, and premenstrual syndrome. J Clin Psychiatry 54:229–234, 1993

Jaeken J, Casaer P, Corbeel L: Valproate, hyperammonaemia, and hyperglycinaemia (letter). Lancet 2(8188):260, 1980

Jankowsky D, Curtis G, Zisook S, et al: Trazodone-aggravated ventricular arrhythmias. J Clin Psychopharmacol 3:372–376, 1983

Jenkins SC, Tinsley JA, Van Loon JA: A Pocket Reference for Psychiatrists, 3rd Edition. Washington, DC, American Psychiatric Publishing, 2001, pp 133–134

Jeste DV, Wyatt RJ: Understanding and Treating Tardive Dyskinesia. New York, Guilford, 1982

Jeste DV, Lacro JP, Bailey A, et al: Lower incidence of tardive dyskinesia with risperidone compared to haloperidol in older patients. J Am Geriatr Soc 47:716–719, 1999

Jones KL, Lacro RV, Johnson KA, et al: Pattern of malformations in the children of women treated with carbamazepine during pregnancy. N Engl J Med 320:1661–1666, 1989

Källén B, Otterblad Olausson P: Antidepressant drugs during pregnancy and infant congenital heart defect. Reprod Toxicol 21:221–222, 2006

Kane JM: Treatment-resistant schizophrenic patients. J Clin Psychiatry 57:35–40, 1996

Kane JM, Smith JM: Tardive dyskinesia: prevalence and risk factors, 1959 to 1979. Arch Gen Psychiatry 39:473–481, 1982

Kane J, Canas F, Kramer M, et al: Treatment of schizophrenia with paliperidone extended-release tablets: a 6-week placebo-controlled trial. Schizophr Res 90:147–161, 2007

Kapur S, Seeman P: Does fast dissociation from the dopamine D2 receptor explain the action of atypical antipsychotics? A new hypothesis. Am J Psychiatry 158:360–369, 2001

Karoum F, Chuang LW, Eisler T, et al: Metabolism of (-)deprenyl to amphetamine and methamphetamine may be responsible for deprenyl's therapeutic benefit: a biochemical assessment. Neurology 32:503–509, 1982

Keck PE Jr, McElroy SL, Nemeroff CB: Anticonvulsants in the treatment of bipolar disorder. J Neuropsychiatry Clin Neurosci 4:395–405, 1992

Keck PE Jr, McElroy SL, Tugrul KC, et al: Valproate oral loading in the treatment of acute mania. J Clin Psychiatry 54:305–308, 1993

Kennedy PF, Hershon HI, McGuire RJ: Extrapyramidal disorders after prolonged phenothiazine therapy. Br J Psychiatry 118:509–518, 1971

Ketter TA, Flockhart DA, Post RM, et al: The emerging role of cytochrome P450 3A in psychopharmacology. J Clin Psychopharmacol 15:387–398, 1995

Ketter TA, Wang PW, Chandler RA, et al: Dermatology precautions and slower titration yield low incidence of lamotrigine treatment-emergent rash. J Clin Psychiatry 66:642–645, 2005

Kim JS, Chang MY, Yu IT, et al: Lithium selectivity increases neuronal differentiation of hippocampal neural progenitor cells both in vitro and in vivo. J Neurochem 89:324–336, 2004

Kinon BJ, Basson BR, Gilmore JA, et al: Long-term olanzapine treatment: weight change and weight-related health factors in schizophrenia. J Clin Psychiatry 62:92–100, 2001

Kleinberg D, Brecher M, Davis J: Prolactin levels and adverse events in patients treated with risperidone. Paper presented at the 150th annual meeting of the American Psychiatric Association, San Diego, CA, May 17–22, 1997

Klibanski A, Neer R, Beitins I: Decreased bone density in hyperprolactinemic women. N Engl J Med 303:1511–1514, 1981

Kolecki P: Venlafaxine induced serotonin syndrome occurring after abstinence from phenelzine for more than two weeks (letter). J Toxicol Clin Toxicol 35:211–212, 1997

Kramer M, Simpson G, Maciulis V, et al: Paliperidone extended-release tablets for prevention of symptom recurrence in patients with schizophrenia: a randomized, double-blind, placebo-controlled study. J Clin Psychopharmacol 27:6–14, 2007

Laird LK: Issues in the monopharmacotherapy and polypharmacotherapy of obsessive-compulsive disorder. Psychopharmacol Bull 32:569–578, 1996

Lamictal (product information). Research Triangle Park, NC, GlaxoSmithKline, 2005

Lammer EJ, Sever LE, Oakley GP Jr: Teratogen update: valproic acid. Teratology 35:465–473, 1987

Laties AM, Dev V, Geller W, et al: Safety update on lenticular opacities: benign experience with 620,000 US patient exposures to quetiapine (p 354), in Abstracts of the 39th Annual Meeting of the American College of Neuropharmacology. Nashville, TN, American College of Neuropharmacology, 2000

Leach MJ, Baxter MG, Critchley MA: Neurochemical and behavioral aspects of lamotrigine. Epilepsia 32 (suppl 2): S4–S8, 1991

Lenox RH, Watson DG, Patel J, et al: Chronic lithium administration alters a prominent PKC substrate in rat hippocampus. Brain Res 570:333–340, 1992

Lewis SW, Barnes TR, Davies L, et al: Randomized controlled trial of effect of prescription of clozapine versus other second-generation antipsychotic drugs in resistant schizophrenia. Schizophr Bull 32:715–723, 2006

Lieberman JA, Stroup TS, McEvoy JP, et al: Effectiveness of antipsychotic drugs in patients with chronic schizophrenia. N Engl J Med 353:1209–1223, 2005

Lipinski JF, Zubenko GS, Cohen BM, et al: Propranolol in the treatment of neuroleptic induced akathisia. Am J Psychiatry 141:412–415, 1984

Lucki I, Rickels K, Geller AM: Chronic use of benzodiazepines and psychomotor and cognitive test performance. Psychopharmacology (Berl) 88:426–433, 1986

Lunesta (product information). Marlborough, MA, Sepracor, 2005

Macdonald RL, Kelly KM: Antiepileptic drug mechanisms of action. Epilepsia 36:S2–S12, 1995

Mallette LE, Eichhorn E: Effects of lithium carbonate on human calcium metabolism. Arch Intern Med 146:770–776, 1986

Manji HK, Bebchuk JM, Moore GJ, et al: Modulation of CNS signal transduction pathways and gene expression by mood-stabilizing agents: therapeutic implications. J Clin Psychiatry 60 (suppl 2):27–39, 1993

Manji HK, Chen G, Shimon H, et al: Guanine nucleotide-binding proteins in bipolar affective disorder: effects of long-term lithium treatment. Arch Gen Psychiatry 52:135–144, 1995

Manji HK, Chen G, Hsiao JK, et al: Regulation of signal transduction pathways by mood-stabilizing agents: implications for the delayed onset of therapeutic efficacy. J Clin Psychiatry 57 (suppl 13):34–46, 1996

Manji HK, Chen G, Hsiao JK, et al: Regulation of signal transduction pathways by mood-stabilizing agents: implications for the delayed onset of therapeutic efficacy. J Clin Psychiatry 57:34–46, 1999

Marangell LB, Martinez JM, Ketter TA, et al: Lamotrigine treatment of bipolar disorder: data from the first 500 patients in STEP-BD. Bipolar Disord 6:139–143, 2004

Marder SR, Kramer M, Ford L, et al: Efficacy and safety of paliperidone extended-release tablets: results of a 6-week, randomized, placebo-controlled study. Biol Psychiatry 62:1363–1370, 2007

Margolese HC, Chouinard G, Kolivakis TT, et al: Tardive dyskinesia in the era of typical and atypical antipsychotics, part 2: incidence and management strategies in patients with schizophrenia. Can J Psychiatry 50:703–714, 2005

McEvoy JP, Lieberman JA, Stroup TS, et al: Effectiveness of clozapine versus olanzapine, quetiapine, and risperidone in patients with chronic schizophrenia who did not respond to prior atypical antipsychotic treatment. Am J Psychiatry 163:600–610, 2006

McKenna K, Koren G, Tetelbaum M, et al: Pregnancy outcome of women using atypical antipsychotic drugs: a prospective comparative study. J Clin Psychiatry 66:444–449, 2005

Miller DD, Sharafuddin MJ, Kathol RG: A case of clozapine-induced neuroleptic malignant syndrome. J Clin Psychiatry 52:99–101, 1991

Munjack DJ, Bruns J, Baltazar PL, et al: A pilot study of buspirone in the treatment of social phobia. J Anxiety Disord 5:87–98, 1991

Murphy MJ, Lyon IW, Taylor JW, et al: Valproic acid associated pancreatitis in an adult (letter). Lancet 1(8210):41–42, 1981

Nestler EJ, Barrot M, DiLeone RJ, et al: Neurobiology of depression. Neuron 34:13–25, 2002

NIMH/NIH Consensus Development Conference Statement: Mood disorders: pharmacological prevention of recurrences. Consensus Development Panel. Am J Psychiatry 142:469–476, 1985

Nishino S, Mishima K, Mignot E, et al: Sedative-hypnotics, in The American Psychiatric Publishing Textbook of Psychopharmacology, 3rd Edition. Edited by Schatzberg AF, Nemeroff CB. Washington, DC, American Psychiatric Publishing, 2004, pp 651–670

Oldham JM: Guideline Watch: Practice Guidelines for the Treatment of Patients With Borderline Personality Disorder. Arlington, VA, American Psychiatric Association, 2005

Oliver AP, Luchins DJ, Wyatt RJ: Neuroleptic-induced seizures: an in vitro technique for assessing relative risk. Arch Gen Psychiatry 39:206–209, 1982

Patterson JF: Stevens-Johnson syndrome associated with carbamazepine therapy. J Clin Psychopharmacol 5:185, 1985

Pearlstein TB, Halbreich U, Batzar ED, et al: Psychosocial functioning in women with premenstrual dysphoric disorder before and after treatment with sertraline or placebo. J Clin Psychiatry 61:101–109, 2000

Pellock JM: Carbamazepine side effects in children and adults. Epilepsia 28:S64–S70, 1987

Pellock JM, Willmore LJ: A rational guide to routine blood monitoring in patients receiving antiepileptic drugs. Neurology 41:961–964, 1991

Pendlebury SC, Moses DK, Eadie MJ: Hyponatremia during oxcarbazepine therapy. Hum Toxicol 8:337–344, 1989

Physicians' Desk Reference, 59th Edition. Montvale, NJ, Thompson PDR, 2005

Physicians' Desk Reference, 60th Edition. Montvale, NJ, Thompson PDR, 2006

Pies RW: Handbook of Essential Psychopharmacology. Washington, DC, American Psychiatric Press, 1998

Plenge P, Mellerup ET, Bolwig C, et al: Lithium treatment: does the kidney prefer one daily dose instead of two? Acta Psychiatr Scand 66:121–128, 1982

Purdon SE, Jones BDW, Stip E, et al: Neuropsychological change in early phase schizophrenia during 12 months of treatment with olanzapine, risperidone, or haloperidol. Arch Gen Psychiatry 57:249–258, 2000

Quitkin FM, Rifkin A, Klein DF: Monoamine oxidase inhibitors: a review of antidepressant effectiveness. Arch Gen Psychiatry 36:749–760, 1979

Rakel RE: Long-term buspirone therapy for chronic anxiety: a multicenter international study to determine safety. South Med J 83:194–198, 1990

Reitan JA, Porter W, Braunstein M: Comparison of psychomotor skills and amnesia after induction of anesthesia with midazolam or thiopental. Anesth Analg 65:933–937, 1986

Reunanen M, Kaarnen P, Vaisanen E: The influence of anticholinergic treatment on tardive dyskinesia caused by neuroleptic drugs. Acta Neurol Scand 65 (suppl 90): 278–279, 1982

Robert E, Guibaud P: Maternal valproic acid and congenital neural tube defects (letter). Lancet 2(8304):937, 1982

Rohatagi S, Barrett JS, DeWitt KE, et al: Integrated pharmacokinetic and metabolic modeling of selegiline and metabolites after transdermal administration. Biopharm Drug Dispos 18:567–584, 1997

Roose SP, Glassman AH, Giardina EGV, et al: Tricyclic antidepressants in depressed patients with cardiac conduction disease. Arch Gen Psychiatry 44:273–275, 1987

Rosa FW: Spina bifida in infants of women treated with carbamazepine during pregnancy. N Engl J Med 324:674–677, 1991

Rosenbaum JF, Fava M, Hoog SL, et al: Selective serotonin reuptake inhibitor discontinuation syndrome: a randomized clinical trial. Biol Psychiatry 44:77–87, 1998

Rosenberg L, Mitchell AA, Parsells JL, et al: Lack of relation of oral clefts to diazepam use during pregnancy. N Engl J Med 309:1282–1285, 1983

Rossi A, Mancini F, Stratta P, et al: Risperidone, negative symptoms, and cognitive deficit in schizophrenia: an open study. Acta Psychiatr Scand 95:40–43, 1997

Rothschild AJ: Disinhibition, amnestic reactions, and other adverse reactions secondary to triazolam: a review of the literature. J Clin Psychiatry 53 (suppl):69–79, 1992

Sackeim HA, Haskett RF, Mulsant BH, et al: Continuation pharmacotherapy in the prevention of relapse following electroconvulsive therapy: a randomized controlled trial. JAMA 285:1299–1307, 2001

Scher M, Krieger JN, Juergens S: Trazodone and priapism. Am J Psychiatry 140:1362–1363, 1983

Schneier FR, Saoud JB, Campeas RC, et al: Buspirone in social phobia. J Clin Psychopharmacol 13:251–256, 1992

Seide H, Muller HR: Choreiform movements as side effects of phenothiazine medication in elderly patients. J Am Geriatr Soc 15:517–522, 1967

Seroquel (package insert). Wilmington, DE, Zeneca Pharmaceuticals, 2001

Serzone (package insert). Princeton, NJ, Bristol-Myers Squibb Co, 2002

Shader RI, Greenblatt DJ: Approaches to the treatment of anxiety states, in Manual of Psychiatric Therapeutics, 3rd Edition. Edited by Shader RI. Philadelphia, PA, Lippincott Williams & Wilkins, 2003, pp 199–200

Sheehan DV, Raj AB, Sheehan KH, et al: Is buspirone effective for panic disorder? J Clin Psychopharmacol 10:3–11, 1990

Shelton RC, Stahl SM: Risperidone and paroxetine given singly and in combination for bipolar depression. J Clin Psychiatry 65:1715–1719, 2004

Shulman KI, Walker SE: Refining the MAOI diet: tyramine content of pizzas and soy products. J Clin Psychiatry 60:191–193, 1999

Shulman KI, Walker SE: Reply: clarifying the safety of the MAOI diet and pizza (letter). J Clin Psychiatry 61:145–146, 2000

Shulman KI, Tailor SA, Walker SE, et al: Tap (draft) beer and monoamine oxidase inhibitor dietary restrictions. Can J Psychiatry 42:310–312, 1997

Smith WT, Glaudin V, Panagides J, et al: Mirtazapine vs. amitriptyline vs. placebo in the treatment of major depressive disorder. Psychopharmacol Bull 26:191–196, 1990

Sramek JJ, Tansman M, Suri A, et al: Efficacy of buspirone in generalized anxiety disorder with coexisting mild depressive symptoms. J Clin Psychiatry 57:287–291, 1996

Suppes T, Webb A, Paul B, et al: Clinical outcome in a randomized 1-year trial of clozapine versus treatment as usual for patients with treatment-resistant illness and a history of mania. Am J Psychiatry 156:1164–1169, 1999

Tallman JF, Paul SM, Skolnick P, et al: Receptors for the age of anxiety: pharmacology of the benzodiazepines. Science 207:274–281, 1980

Tarsy D, Baldessarini RJ: Epidemiology of tardive dyskinesia: is risk declining with modern antipsychotics? Mov Disord 21:589–598, 2006

Tohen M, Vieta E, Calabrese J, et al: Efficacy of olanzapine-fluoxetine combination in the treatment of bipolar I depression. Arch Gen Psychiatry 60:1079–1088, 2003

Tollefson GD, Beasley CM Jr, Tamura RN: Blind, controlled long-term study of the comparative incidence of treatment-emergent tardive dyskinesia with olanzapine or haloperidol. Am J Psychiatry 154:1248–1254, 1997

Trileptal (product information). East Hanover, NJ, Novartis Pharmaceuticals, 2006

Trivedi MH, Fava M, Wisniewski SR, et al: Medication augmentation after the failure of SSRIs for depression. N Engl J Med 354:1243–1252, 2006

Tsai G, Goff D, Chang R, et al: Markers of glutamatergic neurotransmission and oxidative stress associated with tardive dyskinesia. Am J Psychiatry 9:1207–1213, 1998

U.S. Food and Drug Administration Public Health Advisory: Suicidality in children and adolescents being treated with antidepressant medications, October 15, 2004. Available at: http://www.fda.gov/cder/drug/antidepressants/SSRIPHA200410.htm. Accessed December 7, 2005

van Putten T, May PRA, Marder SR: Akathisia with haloperidol and thiothixene. Arch Gen Psychiatry 31:67–72, 1984

Vitullo RN, Wharton JM, Allen NB, et al: Trazodone-related exercise-induced nonsustained ventricular tachycardia. Chest 98:247–248, 1990

Walker SE, Shulman KI, Tailor SAN, et al: Tyramine content of previously restricted foods in monoamine oxidase inhibitor diets. J Clin Psychopharmacol 16:383–388, 1996

Walker SE, Shulman KE, Tailor SAN: Reply: tyramine content in Chinese food. J Clin Psychopharmacol 17:227–228, 1997

Warnock JK, Knesevich J: Adverse cutaneous reactions to antidepressants. Am J Psychiatry 145:425–430, 1988

Wecker L, James S, Copeland N, et al: Transdermal selegiline: targeted effects on monoamine oxidases in the brain. Biol Psychiatry 54:1099–1104, 2003

Weisler RH, Kalali AH, Ketter TA, et al: A multicenter, randomized, double-blind, placebo-controlled trial of extended-release carbamazepine capsules as monotherapy for bipolar disorder patients with manic or mixed episodes. J Clin Psychiatry 65:478–484, 2004

Weisler RH, Keck PE Jr, Swann AC, et al: Extended-release carbamazepine capsules as monotherapy for acute mania in bipolar disorder: a multicenter, randomized, double-blind, placebo-controlled trial. J Clin Psychiatry 66:323–330, 2005

Wetzel H, Anghelescu I, Szegedi A, et al: Pharmacokinetic interactions of clozapine with selective serotonin reuptake inhibitors: differential effects of fluvoxamine and paroxetine in a prospective study. J Clin Psychopharmacol 18:2–9, 1998

Wikander I, Sundblad C, Andersch B, et al: Citalopram in premenstrual dysphoria: is intermittent treatment during luteal phases more effective than continuous medication throughout the menstrual cycle? J Clin Psychopharmacol 18:390–398, 1998

Wing YK, Chen CN: Tyramine content in Chinese food (letter). J Clin Psychopharmacol 17:227, 1997

Yassa R: Antiparkinsonian medication withdrawal in the treatment of tardive dyskinesia: a report of three cases. Can J Psychiatry 30:440–442, 1985

Yassa R, Lal S: Prevalence of the rabbit syndrome. Am J Psychiatry 143:656–657, 1986

Yeo PP, Bates D, Howe JG, et al: Anticonvulsants and thyroid function. BMJ 1:1581–1583, 1978

Yonkers KA, Halbreich U, Freeman E, et al: Symptomatic improvement of premenstrual dysphoric disorder with sertraline treatment: a randomized controlled trial. Sertraline Premenstrual Dysphoric Collaborative Study Group. JAMA 278:983–988, 1997

Zubenko GS, Cohen BM, Lipinski JF: Comparison of metoprolol and propranolol in the treatment of lithium tremor. Psychiatry Res 11:163–164, 1984a

Zubenko GS, Lipinski JF, Cohen M, et al: Comparison of metoprolol and propranolol in the treatment of akathisia. Psychiatry Res 11:143–149, 1984b

16

BRIEF PSYCHOTHERAPIES

Mantosh J. Dewan, M.D.
Brett N. Steenbarger, Ph.D.
Roger P. Greenberg, Ph.D.

Brief therapy refers to time-limited psychotherapies that seek to accelerate change through the active, focused interventions of therapists and enhanced patient involvement in treatment. Descriptions of brief psychotherapies date back to Freud's own cases and to subsequent purposeful attempts to abbreviate the duration of psychoanalytic treatments (Breuer and Freud 1893–1895/1955; Fisher and Greenberg 1985). More recently, various brief approaches to therapy have evolved, ranging from single-session treatments and strategic interventions of several sessions to short-term psychodynamic modalities that frequently exceed 20 sessions.

As rising health care costs brought attempts to manage health care in the 1980s, brief therapy found an economic and a practice rationale. Research suggesting that brief therapy could be time-effective (Budman and Gurman 1988) and clinically effective for a variety of patients and problems (Steen-

barger 1992) supported the adoption of short-term work among clinicians and managed health care organizations. The movement toward evidence-based medicine spurred the development of manualized psychotherapeutic treatments, which, by their very nature, are highly structured and limited in duration. Despite concerns about the limitations of such treatments, especially for severe and persistent emotional disorders and conditions with high relapse rates, it is fair to say that by the twenty-first century, brief therapies had become the practice rule rather than the exception among psychotherapists.

Current Models of Brief Psychotherapy

The various brief therapies make different assumptions about the causes of presenting problems and the procedures necessary to alter them. These approaches cluster within three broad models: relational, learning, and contextual (Steenbarger 2002). Because of their distinctive assumptions and practice patterns, each of these models defines brevity differently. As we emphasize later in this chapter, however, many features are common to the models, several of which are central to their efficacy.

Relational Therapies

Relational modalities include short-term psychodynamic treatments and interpersonal therapy (IPT). The key assumption of these approaches is that the presenting problems of patients reflect difficulties in significant relationships. Several important differences are evident between short-term dynamic therapies and IPT, chief among them being the focus on the therapeutic relationship as a vehicle for change.

Psychodynamic Therapy

Psychodynamic brief therapies share the premise of all psychodynamic therapies that the presenting problems of patients result from an internalization of conflicts from earlier significant relationships. The anxiety from these conflicts is controlled through defenses that aid short-term coping but forestall the conscious assimilation and working through of core relational issues. As a result, these issues resurface in future relationships whenever similar anxiety and conflict are experienced, triggering old patterns of defense. These coping efforts are no longer appropriate to present-day relationship contexts, yielding secondary conflict and the consequences that typically bring people to therapy. Thus, the psychodynamic therapist views presenting problems as more than symptoms of an underlying disorder; they are the result of outmoded, currently maladaptive (defensive) efforts in the face of repeated interpersonal conflict.

Several features of short-term psychodynamic therapy enable it to accelerate this change curve:

Circumscribed, here-and-now focus—Brief dynamic work focuses on "core conflictual relationship themes" (Luborsky and Mark 1991) that represent "cyclical maladaptive patterns" (Binder and Strupp 1991) linking current, past, and therapeutic relationships. Although an understanding of the role of the past in the genesis of these themes is relevant, it is not the primary focus of short-term dynamic therapy. Rather, brief dynamic work actively focuses on highly salient present-day manifestations of the cyclical patterns.

Patient selection criteria—Most short-term psychodynamic practitioners acknowledge that brief treatment is not appropriate for all patients and disorders. By limiting such work to patients who are experiencing emotional discomfort, able to readily form a trusting relationship, and willing to view problems in an interpersonal context, therapists help ensure that treatment will progress quickly.

Active provision of positive relationship experiences within the therapy—Following Alexander and French's (1946) early formulations, brief dynamic therapists do not rely primarily on interpretation as a source of change. Rather, change is catalyzed by the involvement of the therapist. When a core conflict (e.g., hostility toward the parent [therapist]) is repeated in therapy, the therapist purposefully provides responses different (e.g., acceptance, inquiry) from those anticipated by patients (e.g., rejection, silence) (Levenson 1995). Moreover, countertransference is not viewed merely as something for the therapist to guard against but as an inevitable and potentially useful experience that allows therapists to detect and counteract the emotional pulls of their patients.

Creation of heightened emotional contexts for change—Sifneos (1972) and Davanloo (1980) suggested that change can be accelerated by fostering an enhanced state of experiencing among patients. Such anxiety-provoking therapies seek to challenge and break through patterns of defense and resistance rather than relying solely on interpretation. Under these emotionally charged conditions, patients can more readily gain access to memories, impulses, and feelings associated with core conflictual patterns, facilitating an accelerated working through of these experiences within therapy.

In short, brief dynamic therapists, unlike their traditional counterparts who conduct long-term therapy (including psychoanalysis), take an active role in the helping process, fostering and sustaining a treatment focus and initiating interventions within this focus to challenge maladaptive defensive patterns and provide new, corrective relationship experiences (Table 16–1). Although such short-term work may not be brief by managed care standards, extending to 20 or more sessions, it significantly abbreviates the traditional treatment course of psychoanalytically oriented psychotherapy. The idea that an abbreviated form of psychoanalytic therapy can achieve good results for many patients (Shedler 2010) has been bolstered by research observations that (even in traditional psychoanalysis) relationship factors, persuasion, suggestion, catharsis, and the therapist as a model are much more pivotal to the change process than was previously recognized (Fisher and Greenberg 1996).

Interpersonal Therapy

IPT also sustains a focus on relationship issues but abbreviates treatment even further by not making the therapeutic relationship a primary focus. Indeed, unlike short-term psychodynamic therapy, IPT began in 1984 as a brief manualized treatment that has been successfully applied to a variety of presenting problems and interpersonal concerns (Stuart 2004).

Central to IPT and its brevity is the establishment of a treatment focus on difficulties and changes that patients are experiencing in relationships. Much of the work of IPT emphasizes changing patterns of communication, altering expectations within relationships, and using social supports to help patients deal with interpersonal crises. Because this focus stresses current relationship

concerns and how these can be handled, lengthy explorations of past relationship conflicts are not a core ingredient of IPT. Similarly, the IPT therapist does not focus on transference relationships with patients and a reenactment of past interpersonal patterns. As a result, IPT tends to be briefer than most short-term psychodynamic therapies, with treatment for depression ranging from 12 to 20 sessions (Stuart 2004).

Specific targets for IPT work include grief, interpersonal disputes, role transitions (e.g., from a professional woman to a mother), and interpersonal sensitivity. Within these areas, more specific targets for change involve patterns of communication and patterns of attachment. The therapist takes an active role in treatment, sustaining the focus on these issues. As in short-term dynamic work, IPT achieves brevity in part by limiting its application to patients who meet specific assessment criteria. In general, IPT has been found to be efficacious for patients with mood and anxiety disorders and may not be appropriate for patients with personality disorders who have difficulty forming and sustaining therapeutic alliances (Stuart 2004).

After a period of assessment and establishment of a focus through a therapeutic contract, IPT explores current interpersonal concerns and brainstorms ways of handling them (Table 16–2). These potential solutions form the basis for between-session efforts by patients, securing their active involvement in treatment. Subsequent sessions review and refine these efforts, casting the therapist in the role of collaborative problem solver. Resistances to change are dealt with in a straightforward manner by the therapist, not as pattern reenactments to be interpreted and worked through. The goal of therapy is to promote independent functioning on the part of the patient, as well as symptom relief. IPT, unlike other therapies, does not presume a complete termination of therapy at the end of treatment. Rather, therapists assume that future sessions may be necessary to maintain gains and prevent relapse.

Table 16–1. Differences between short-term psychodynamic and traditional therapies

	Short-term dynamic therapies	Traditional dynamic therapies
Therapeutic focus	Focal relationship patterns	Personality change
Therapist role	Active significant other	Blank screen
Emphasized change mechanism	Corrective relationship experiences	Insight
Mechanism for dealing with resistances	Challenge and confrontation	Interpretation

Table 16–2. Differences between interpersonal therapy and short-term psychodynamic therapy

	Interpersonal therapy	Short-term psychodynamic therapy
Therapeutic focus	Current patterns in interpersonal communications and attachments	Patterns repeated in past, present, and therapeutic relationships
Therapist role	Problem solver	Transference object
Emphasized change mechanism	Attempting new patterns of communication and altered expectations in extratherapeutic relationships	Corrective relationship experiences within therapy
Structure	Brief; manualized	Time-effective; open-ended

Comparison and Summary

In summary, the relational model of therapy achieves brevity by creating a circumscribed focus on the patient's interpersonal patterns and by limiting treatment to patient groups able to sustain this focus. Whereas the role of the therapist is different in short-term dynamic therapy (a significant other) compared with IPT (a collaborative problem solver), the ultimate goal is similar: altering problem patterns by generating new, constructive relational experiences.

Learning Therapies

The learning model of treatment, which includes a wide range of cognitive-behavioral therapies, starts from a different set of premises from those in the relational model. The presenting concerns of patients are viewed as learned maladaptive patterns that can be unlearned. Moreover, patients are seen as capable of acquiring new, adaptive patterns of thought and action through skill development. As a result, the learning therapies feature the therapist in an active, directive teaching mode and the patient as a student. This structuring of the helping relationship lends itself to active skill rehearsal within sessions and directed homework between meetings. The combination of tight learning focus and active practice of techniques ensures that most learning therapies are short term by their very nature.

For purposes of exposition, it is helpful to distinguish between primarily *behavioral treatments* that emphasize exposure as a central therapeutic ingredient and *cognitive approaches* that more broadly target dysfunctional patterns of information processing for restructuring. Although these approaches have elements that overlap (e.g., patients exposed to traumatic cues may rehearse thoughts that emphasize self-control), the relative degree of emphasis is different, which affects the conduct and brevity of treatment.

Behavior Therapy

Learning therapies that use *exposure* as a core therapeutic ingredient include the work of

Edna Foa and colleagues (Hembree et al. 2004) in the treatment of posttraumatic stress disorder and obsessive-compulsive disorder and David Barlow's (2002) work on panic disorder. Treatment typically begins with a period of assessment and psychosocial education. During this time, patients may keep detailed logs that track the appearance of symptoms and the circumstances surrounding these. Examination of these logs during the early sessions helps to generate a focus on the specific triggers for symptom appearance. Concurrently, therapists educate patients about the learning model, explaining how and why symptoms appear. This can be highly reassuring for patients with disorders such as panic, who may be bewildered by their symptoms.

Also early in treatment, exposure-based learning therapies introduce specific skills designed to help control symptoms. These can include efforts at relaxation, thought stopping, self-reassurance, and seeking social support. The skills are typically introduced one at a time, explained in detail as part of the aforementioned psychosocial education, modeled in session by the therapist, and rehearsed in session by patients. Only after patients understand and master skills in session do they rehearse the skills as part of between-session homework.

An important component of the brevity of these therapies stems from the subsequent employment of these skills. Once triggers for presenting symptoms have been identified, they are deliberately introduced into therapy sessions via imagery and in vivo exercises. Patients are thus required to actively use their coping skills while they are exposed to the very stimuli that have provoked symptoms. For example, a patient with a handwashing compulsion might be exposed to dirt and then prevented from washing his hands (i.e., response prevention). A patient experiencing panic might simulate panic experiences by spinning in a chair and then using cognitive and relaxation skills to maintain composure. This in vivo exposure provides patients with firsthand emotional experiences of mastery, which appear to accelerate the pace of symptom resolution. Once initial gains are achieved, efforts at generalization commence, and the skills are used across a variety of symptom-related cues (Table 16–3). Variations in technique—and the specific needs of patients—dictate whether the exposure is attempted in a gradual way or in a more rapid, intensive fashion. Interestingly, research suggests that a significant immersion into anxiety-arousing situations often may be therapeutic because patients benefit from extended sessions of exposure. Exposure appears to be effective because of the opportunity it affords patients to reprocess cues associated with distress.

Cognitive Therapy

Whereas the exposure therapies have found their greatest application in the treatment of anxiety disorders, *cognitive reprocessing therapies* have been applied to depression, anxiety, eating disorders, and child and adolescent disorders (Hollon and Beck 2004). Symptoms, according to this approach, can be traced to automatic thought patterns that distort information processing about self, others, and the future. The goal of therapy is to identify these thought patterns, challenge them, and replace them with more constructive alternatives. The combination of in-session rehearsal and out-of-session homework targeting core patterns of automatic thought ensures that the cognitive work is time efficient.

Like the exposure-based learning therapies, cognitive restructuring treatments begin with a period of assessment and psychosocial education. The education in the cognitive model helps patients understand the relation between thoughts and feelings and the ways in which automatic thought patterns can sustain unwanted patterns of emotion and action. Throughout cognitive therapy, therapists engage patients in a highly collaborative manner, minimizing resistances and sustaining the helping alliance.

This collaboration continues with the maintenance of a dysfunctional thought record in which patients track events, reactions to those events, and mediating beliefs.

Most of these beliefs pertain to the sense of being helpless or unlovable (Beck and Bieling 2004); patients then form schemas that filter and color future perception, which creates cognitive distortions. The dysfunctional thought record enables therapists to create cognitive conceptualizations of patients, linking core beliefs to automatic thoughts, emotions, and behaviors. The record also helps patients observe their distortions as they are occurring and realize their role in maintaining presenting symptoms. From the observations of patients and therapists, a focus for intervention emerges that targets specific cognitive distortions.

Central to the cognitive restructuring therapies is a Socratic process of guided discovery between therapist and patient that questions these distortions and encourages a consideration of alternative explanations. This process also occurs between sessions because therapists encourage patients to use thought records to evaluate their own degree of belief in the distortions. Each dysfunctional thought pattern is viewed by therapist and patient as a hypothesis to be questioned and tested. Behavioral experiments devised during sessions are carried out between meetings to provide direct experiential tests of patient assumptions. The goal of this "collaborative empiricism" is to create vivid experiences of disconfirmation for patients, which aid the building of new, accurate schemas (Table 16–4).

Comparison and Summary

Whereas the exposure therapies target specific conditioned responses for extinction, the cognitive restructuring therapies entail a comprehensive collaborative relationship between therapists and patients that evaluates and restructures a range of cognitive patterns. For this reason, as well as the differences between the therapies in the range of problems that they typically address, the exposure treatments tend to be briefer than the restructuring therapies, with the former frequently lasting fewer than 10 sessions and the latter typically ranging between 10 and 20 visits. Despite the

Table 16–3. Comparison of learning and relational models of brief therapy

	Learning models	Relational models
View of presenting problems	Learned maladaptive patterns of behavior and thought	Internalized relationship conflicts and patterns
Goal of therapy	Unlearning old dysfunctional patterns; acquiring new constructive ones	Novel interpersonal experiences that can be internalized
Therapist role	Directive teacher	Facilitator of exploration
Emphasized change mechanism	Rehearsal of skills and experiences of mastery during problematic situations	Changing interpersonal patterns in current relationships
Structure	Brief, often manualized or highly structured	Sometimes brief and manualized (interpersonal therapy); sometimes not (short-term dynamic)

Table 16–4. Differences between exposure and cognitive restructuring brief therapies

	Exposure therapies	Cognitive restructuring therapies
View of presenting problems	Conditioned patterns of emotion and behavior triggered by internal and environmental cues	The result of information processing distortions arising from dysfunctional schemas
Goal of therapy	Deconditioning of patterns through skill enactment during exposure to symptom triggers	Challenging and replacing cognitive distortions with realistic, constructive alternatives
Therapist role	Directive teacher	Collaborative empiricist
Emphasized change mechanism	Firsthand experiences of mastery	Altered cognitive schemas
Structure	Brief, with circumscribed symptom focus; often manualized or highly structured	More extended, with broader focus; often manualized or highly structured

differences in their specific methods, many similarities link these learning therapies. They are highly structured and focused, with active assignments during and between sessions. They seek to challenge directly and undercut the patterns that bring patients to therapy, achieving brevity by replacing verbal exploration with experiences of mastery.

Contextual Therapies

The aforementioned relational and learning therapies begin with a common premise—that the presenting concerns of patients are acquired over the life span as the result of problematic experience: faulty relationships or faulty learning. Both, in that sense, place the locus of problems within the patient. Contextual brief therapies, on the other hand, do not view problems as intrinsic to patients. Rather, they are seen as artifacts of person–situation interactions, which, once identified, can be rapidly modified. Short-term couples therapies, for instance, view problem patterns as sustained by the reciprocal contributions of each partner (Baucom et al. 2004). Because difficulties are seen as situational, targeted problem-solving interventions to alter these situations make the contextual therapies among the briefest of therapies.

Strategic Therapy

Strategic therapies, including single-session treatments (Hoyt et al. 1992), view presenting concerns as the result of attempts at solutions that unwittingly reinforce the very problems patients are attempting to address. A person concerned about rejection in relationships, for instance, might interact in guarded ways, leading others to avoid future interaction. The problem, from the vantage point of the strategic therapist, is a function of the patient's construal of the situation. It can be resolved through skillful reframing that opens the door to new action alternatives and the creation of directed tasks that disconfirm existing understandings. The goal of treatment is to catalyze initial change

that patients can then sustain on their own, not to effect fundamental changes of personality. For this reason, strategic therapies are intentionally brief.

The initial interview of strategic therapy is designed to identify current complaints of patients and their attempts at resolution. The therapist's conceptualization is neither a diagnosis nor a formulation of personality, but a description of the current situational factors that help to maintain the patient's presenting concerns. This description includes the people involved in the patient's concerns and the roles they take, the patient's view of the situation, the sequence of behaviors that result in the patient's complaints, and the specific contexts in which these complaints arise. From this conceptualization, therapists gain an appreciation of the ways in which patients feel stuck in their attempts at resolution and can begin to generate ways of becoming unstuck.

The goal of the therapy is not to find a solution for a patient's problem but to create a situation that lends itself to spontaneous goal attainment. Many times, fresh construals and solutions will result simply when patients behave in new and unpredictable ways. The patient who is afraid of social interaction, for instance, will not interact with others if rejection is anticipated. That same patient, however, may view himself to be a kind, sensitive person and will initiate interactions to help others. Such interactions offer the possibility of positive feedback and fresh incentives to seek out further social contact. By changing the patient's context—from being stuck in a pattern to enacting a strength—the therapist allows naturally occurring growth processes to take their own course. In that sense, strategic therapy is a process for removing barriers to change and not a self-contained change process in itself (Table 16–5).

Solution-Focused Therapy

An offshoot of strategic therapy, solution-focused brief therapy (SFBT), provides a somewhat different contextual approach to

Table 16–5. Contextual models of brief therapy

- Presenting complaints are the result of self-reinforcing problem–solution cycles.
- Problems are a function of patients and their context, not internal to patients.
- Goal of therapy is initiating change, not seeing it to completion.
- Role of therapist is to structure experiences that undermine the stuck behavior of patients.
- Therapy is highly abbreviated.

short-term change. Solution-focused brief therapists start from the premise that people are changing all the time, enacting solution patterns as well as problem ones. Indeed, there is an important sense in SFBT in which problems do not exist at all. When patients cannot reach their goals, they at some point identify that they have a problem. This reification becomes self-fulfilling: the more patients focus on their problems, the more troubled they feel and act. Equally important, such a problem focus blinds patients to the occasions in which they do, in fact, reach their goals.

The aim of SFBT is to break this self-fulfilling conceptualization. The therapist accomplishes this by focusing on solution patterns rather than on problems. Thus, the initial assessment in SFBT asks patients to identify positive pre-session changes and occasions during which problems either do not occur or occur less often or less intensely (Walter and Peller 1992). Enacting these exceptions to problem patterns—doing more of what is already working (de Shazer 1988; O'Hanlon and Weiner-Davis 1989)—is the focus of therapy, not an analysis of core conflicts or a teaching of skills to remediate deficits. Because the therapy is not initiating new behavior and thought patterns but instead is building on existing ones, it tends to be highly targeted, lasting several sessions on average (Steenbarger 2004).

Several other factors contribute to the brevity of SFBT, including working within

patient goals to minimize resistance; maintaining a tight solution focus; involving patients in between-session efforts to enact solution patterns; and having a high degree of therapist activity (Steenbarger 2004). The emphasis on patient strength undercuts the cycle of problem-based thinking and stuck emotion and behavior. The focus on constructive change also paves the way for therapists and patients to frame goals in positive, action terms that can be supported by directed homework tasks extending the solution patterns. Such goals can be formulated with minimal historical exploration, which further contributes to brevity.

Comparison and Summary

One way SFBT differs from strategic brief therapies is that SFBT lends itself to manualization (Table 16–6). SFBT manuals (de Shazer 1988; Walter and Peller 1992) view therapy as a series of steps involving the following:

- Identification of pre-session change.
- Formulation of solution-based goals (e.g., "I will reach out to others when I feel depressed").
- Use of the miracle question ("Suppose that one night, while you were asleep, a miracle occurred and this problem was solved. How would you know? What would be different? How would your husband know without your saying a word to him about it?") and of scaling questions (e.g., "On a scale of 1 to 10, where 1 is 'arguing constantly' and 10 is 'getting along perfectly,' on average how would you rate your relationship?") to elicit exceptions to patient complaints ("A 5? What is happening differently when you are arguing less than a 5?").
- Provision of feedback to support change.
- Assignment of tasks to extend solution patterns.

Like strategic therapies, SFBT relies less on verbal exploration and more on direct experience to break circular patterns that interfere

Table 16–6. Differences between strategic and solution-focused brief therapies

	Strategic therapies	Solution-focused therapies
View of presenting problems	Attempted solutions to problems further reinforce those problems	De-emphasis of problems and emphasis on exceptions to problem patterns
Goal of therapy	Interruption of problem cycles and attempts to initiate new action patterns	Creating solution patterns out of exceptions to problem patterns
Therapist role	Facilitator of change through structured tasks and experiences	Facilitator of change through construction of solution patterns
Emphasized change mechanism	Reframing of problems and direct experiences of novel action patterns	Undermining of problem focus through enactment of solutions
Structure	Highly abbreviated, but not highly structured	Highly abbreviated; often manualized or highly structured

with the achievement of patient goals. The goal of both therapies is not so much to resolve a problem as it is to help patients see that what they thought was a problem was in fact a function of their punctuation of experience, their ways of construing themselves and the world.

Research Pertaining to Brief Therapy and Its Effectiveness

An impressive body of research documents the effectiveness of psychotherapy across a variety of presenting problems (Dewan et al. 2004; Gabbard 2009; Roth and Fonagy 2006). This is relevant to brief therapy because most treatments that have been tested for efficacy—including the manualized therapies commonly used in controlled, double-blind outcome studies—are short term. Indeed, it would not be an exaggeration to say that most of the studies on psychotherapy outcomes are investigations of the effectiveness of short-term therapies. This is partly because cognitive and behavioral therapies dominate the outcome literature (Epp et al. 2009; Roth and Fonagy 2006), although a sizable body of studies does support the effectiveness of short-term dynamic therapy (Leichsenring

2009), IPT (Markowitz and Weissman 2009), and SFBT (Steenbarger 2004).

What Works in Brief Therapy?

A large body of research suggests that the ingredients common to the psychotherapies are more important than their specific interventions in generating clinical outcomes (Greenberg 2004; Wampold 2001). These common effective ingredients include the quality of the therapeutic relationship (Lambert and Barley 2002); patient expectations, readiness for change, and capacity for attachment (Greenberg et al. 2006); and therapist ability to engage patients in a constructive manner. Given these findings, the brief therapies likely achieve their results by 1) providing the structure (Table 16–7) to intensify the change ingredients found among all therapies, including longer-term ones (Steenbarger 2002), and 2) limiting application of short-term methods to patient populations most likely to benefit from psychosocial interventions (Table 16–8). Lambert and Archer (2006) reported that patients who benefited from the initial sessions of therapy were most likely to have favorable outcomes by the end of treatment and at follow up periods. This is significant because it suggests that the course and outcome are determined before most of the procedures that distinguish the various therapeutic schools have

---

Table 16–7. Structural elements common to the brief therapies

Engagement
  Rapid formation of a therapeutic alliance and translation of presenting problems into focal goals

Discrepancy
  Provision of novel skills, insights, and experiences that challenge patient patterns and facilitate new understandings and actions

Consolidation
  Rehearsal of new patterns in varied contexts, accompanied by feedback, to ensure internalization and relapse prevention

---

Table 16–8. Patient selection criteria predictive of success in brief therapy (DISCUS)

- Duration of presenting problems: brief
- Interpersonal functioning: good, able to quickly form a trusting relationship
- Severity of presenting problems: mild to moderate
- Complexity of presenting problems: limited, circumscribed, with low relapse potential
- Understanding of the need for change: and ready to take action
- Social supports: strong and easily accessible

been initiated: it has been estimated that techniques specific to particular psychotherapy models account for only 15% of the observed improvements (Asay and Lambert 1999).

Among the brief therapies, therapists' skill factors—their ability to flexibly facilitate and sustain a treatment focus and their ability to provide novel experiences for patients— may be more important than the specific methods they use. Lambert and Archer (2006) observed that therapists who are given feedback about the progress of their poor-prognosis patients early in treatment have more favorable outcomes than do therapists who are not given feedback. A detailed analysis by Wampold (2001) indicated that therapist competence accounts for greater treatment variance than do specific treatments themselves. Indeed, when outcome studies assigned therapists to multiple treatments, competent therapists tended to have significantly better outcomes than did less competent ones, regardless of the treatment modality.

Finally, all this research suggests that the factors that make therapy efficient are not entirely separable from those that make therapy effective. It may not be far wrong to assert that therapy is most likely to be brief when it is performed skillfully with patients most open to, and likely to benefit from, psychosocial intervention. The skills that make for successful treatment—the ability to foster novel experiences of self and others in an emotionally charged context via the medium of a supportive alliance—appear to be equally essential to brevity.

Conclusion

Seeking to make psychotherapy treatment more efficient, innovative psychoanalysts originally presented the key components of brief therapy. They stressed narrowed patient inclusion criteria, narrowed treatment focus, an active therapist, a limit on time and/or number of sessions, and facilitation of corrective emotional experiences. Building on dynamic tradition, behaviorists, cognitive therapists, and strategic therapists went on to develop three broad models of brief therapy based on their understanding about the causes of presenting problems and the techniques necessary to alter them. *Relational therapies,* which assume that presenting symptoms are a result of problems with significant relationships, include brief psychodynamic therapies and interpersonal therapy. *Learning therapies,* such as behavior therapies and cognitive therapy, view symptoms as arising from maladaptive learned behavior patterns that can be unlearned. *Contextual therapies* place the emphasis on ways in which presenting problems are situated within—and sustained by—their psychosocial contexts. Strategic therapies and solution-focused therapy are major models of contextual therapy.

Brief therapies vary from single-session approaches and very brief strategic treatments to dynamic interventions that often exceed 20 sessions. Behavioral and cognitive therapies are of intermediate duration. Treatment manuals have made it easier to practice these techniques with fidelity and to conduct research. Indeed, most psychotherapy research is focused on brief therapy and clearly supports the efficacy of brief therapy approaches for a broad range of patients. As a result of the growth of brief therapy models, manuals, and research evidence, in association with fiscal constraints and demonstrated positive patient outcomes, brief therapy has become the norm for the majority of today's patients.

Key Points

- Brief therapy consists of a group of approaches to psychotherapy that include short-term psychodynamic, interpersonal, behavioral, cognitive, strategic, and solution focused modalities.

- The various brief therapies differ in their average treatment duration, their targets for change, and their assumptions regarding change processes.

- Several common ingredients link the brief therapies, including a circumscribed treatment focus, increased therapist and patient activity, an emphasis on generating novel experiences, and patient inclusion criteria.

- Brief therapies overall are effective but are most likely to benefit patients who are ready for change and who present concerns that are recent, nonsevere, and simple, not patients with severe, chronic disorders.

- Although a sizable proportion of patients can benefit from short-term treatment, the relation between time and change is complex, mediated by the nature of the outcomes measured, the time at which progress is assessed, and the degree of patient impairment.

- Brief therapies appear to be effective to the degree that they intensify the common factors that account for change across all therapies.

Suggested Readings

Barlow DH: Clinical Handbook of Psychological Disorders, 3rd Edition. New York, Guilford, 2001

Beck JS: Cognitive Therapy: Basics and Beyond. New York, Guilford, 1995

Dewan MJ, Steenbarger BN, Greenberg RP (eds): The Art and Science of Brief Psychotherapies: A Practitioner's Guide. Washington, DC, American Psychiatric Publishing, 2004

Levenson H: Time-Limited Dynamic Psychotherapy: A Guide to Clinical Practice. New York, Basic Books, 1995

Stuart S, Robertson M: Interpersonal Psychotherapy: A Clinician's Guide. London, Edward Arnold, 2003

Walter JL, Peller JE: Becoming Solution-Focused in Brief Therapy. New York, Brunner/Mazel, 1992

Online Resources

Academy of Cognitive Therapy: www.academyofct.org

Association of Advancement of Behavior Therapy (AABT)/Association for Behavioral and Cognitive Therapies (ABCT): www.aabt.org

International Society for Interpersonal Psychotherapy: www.interpersonalpsychotherapy.org

Society for Psychotherapy Research: www.psychotherapyresearch.org

Solution-Focused Brief Therapy Association: www.sfbta.org

References

Alexander F, French TM: Psychoanalytic Therapy: Principles and Applications. New York, Ronald Press, 1946

Asay TP, Lambert MJ: The empirical case for the common factors in therapy: quantitative findings, in The Heart and Soul of Change: What Works in Therapy. Edited by Hubble MA, Duncan BL, Miller SD. Washington, DC, American Psychological Association, 1999, pp 33-56

Barlow D: Anxiety and Its Disorders: The Nature and Treatment of Anxiety and Panic, 2nd Edition. New York, Guilford, 2002

Baucom DH, Epstein NB, Sullivan LJ: Brief couple therapy, in The Art and Science of Brief Psychotherapies: A Practitioner's Guide. Edited by Dewan MJ, Steenbarger BN, Greenberg RP. Washington, DC, American Psychiatric Publishing, 2004, pp 189–230

Beck JS, Bieling PJ: Cognitive therapy: introduction to theory and practice, in The Art and Science of Brief Psychotherapies: A Practitioner's Guide. Edited by Dewan MJ, Steenbarger BN, Greenberg RP. Washington, DC, American Psychiatric Publishing, 2004, pp 15–50

Binder JL, Strupp HH: The Vanderbilt approach to time-limited dynamic psychotherapy, in Handbook of Short-Term Dynamic Psychotherapy. Edited by Crits-Christoph P, Barber JP. New York, Basic Books, 1991, pp 137–165

Breuer J, Freud S: Studies in hysteria (1893–1895), in The Standard Edition of the Complete Psychological Works of Sigmund Freud, Vol 2. Translated and edited by Strachey J (in collaboration with Freud A). London, Hogarth Press, 1955, pp 1–311

Budman SH, Gurman AS: Theory and Practice of Brief Therapy. New York, Guilford, 1988

Davanloo H: Short-Term Dynamic Psychotherapy. New York, Jason Aronson, 1980

de Shazer S: Clues: Investigating Solutions in Brief Therapy. New York, WW Norton, 1988

Dewan MJ, Steenbarger BN, Greenberg RP (eds): The Art and Science of Brief Psychotherapies: A Practitioner's Guide. Washington, DC, American Psychiatric Publishing, 2004

Epp A, Dobson K, Cottraux J: Applications of individual cognitive behavioral therapy to specific disorders: efficacy and indications, in Textbook of Psychotherapeutic Treatments. Edited by Gabbard G. Washington, DC, American Psychiatric Publishing, 2009, pp 239–262

Fisher S, Greenberg RP: The Scientific Credibility of Freud's Theories and Therapy. New York, Columbia University Press, 1985

Fisher S, Greenberg RP: Freud Scientifically Reappraised: Testing the Theories and Therapy. New York, Wiley, 1996

Gabbard GO (ed): Textbook of Psychotherapeutic Treatments. Washington, DC, American Psychiatric Publishing, 2009

Greenberg RP: Essential ingredients for successful psychotherapy: effect of common factors, in The Art and Science of Brief Psychotherapies: A Practitioner's Guide. Edited by Dewan MJ, Steenbarger BN, Greenberg RP. Washington, DC, American Psychiatric Publishing, 2004, pp 231–242

Greenberg RP, Constantino MJ, Bruce N: Are patient expectations still relevant for psychotherapy process and outcome? Clin Psychol Rev 26:657–678, 2006

Hembree EA, Roth D, Bux DA Jr, et al: Brief behavior therapy, in The Art and Science of Brief Psychotherapies: A Practitioner's Guide. Edited by Dewan MJ, Steenbarger BN, Greenberg RP. Washington, DC, American Psychiatric Publishing, 2004, pp 51–84

Hollon SD, Beck AT: Cognitive and cognitive-behavioral therapies, in Bergin and Garfield's Handbook of Psychotherapy and Behavior Change, 5th Edition. Edited by Lambert MJ. New York, Wiley, 2004, pp 447–492

Hoyt MF, Rosenbaum R, Talmon M: Planned single-session therapy, in The First Session in Brief Therapy. Edited by Budman SH, Hoyt MF, Friedman S. New York, Guilford, 1992, pp 59–86

Lambert MJ, Archer A: Research findings on the effects of psychotherapy and their implications for practice, in Evidence-Based Psychotherapy: Where Practice and Research Meet. Edited by Goodheart CD, Kazdin AE, Sternberg RJ. Washington, DC, American Psychological Association, 2006, pp 111–130

Lambert MJ, Barley DE: Research summary on the therapeutic relationship and psychotherapy outcome, in Psychotherapy Relationships That Work: Therapist Contributions and Responsiveness to Patients. Edited by Norcross JC. New York, Oxford University Press, 2002, pp 17–36

Leichsenring F: Applications of psychodynamic psychotherapy to specific disorders: efficacy and indications, in Textbook of Psychotherapeutic Treatments. Edited by Gabbard GO. Washington, DC, American Psychiatric Publishing, 2009, pp 97–132

Levenson H: Time-Limited Dynamic Psychotherapy: A Guide to Clinical Practice. New York, Basic Books, 1995

Luborsky L, Mark D: Short-term supportive-expressive psychoanalytic psychotherapy, in Handbook of Short-Term Dynamic Psychotherapy. Edited by Crits-Christoph P, Barber JP. New York, Basic Books, 1991, pp 110–136

Markowitz J, Weissman M: Applications of individual interpersonal psychotherapy to specific disorders: efficacy and indications, in Textbook of Psychotherapeutic Treatments. Edited by Gabbard GO. Washington, DC, American Psychiatric Publishing, 2009, pp 339–364

O'Hanlon W, Weiner-Davis J: In Search of Solution: A New Direction in Psychotherapy. New York, WW Norton, 1989

Roth A, Fonagy P: What Works for Whom? A Critical Review of Psychotherapy Research, 2nd Edition. New York, Guilford, 2006

Shedler J: The efficacy of psychodynamic psychotherapy. Am Psychol 65:98–109, 2010

Sifneos PE: Short-Term Psychotherapy and Emotional Crisis. Cambridge, MA, Harvard University Press, 1972

Steenbarger BN: Toward science-practice integration in brief counseling and therapy. Couns Psychol 20:403–450, 1992

Steenbarger BN: Brief therapy, in Encyclopedia of Psychotherapy, Vol 1. Edited by Hersen M, Sledge W. New York, Elsevier, 2002, pp 349–358

Steenbarger BN: Solution-focused brief therapy: doing what works, in The Art and Science of Brief Psychotherapies: A Practitioner's Guide. Edited by Dewan MJ, Steenbarger BN, Greenberg RP. Washington, DC, American Psychiatric Publishing, 2004, pp 85–118

Stuart S: Brief interpersonal psychotherapy, in The Art and Science of Brief Psychotherapies: A Practitioner's Guide. Edited by Dewan MJ, Steenbarger BN, Greenberg RP. Washington, DC, American Psychiatric Publishing, 2004, pp 119–156

Walter JL, Peller JE: Becoming Solution-Focused in Brief Therapy. New York, Brunner/Mazel, 1992

Wampold BE: The Great Psychotherapy Debate: Models, Methods, and Findings. Mahwah, NJ, Lawrence Erlbaum, 2001

17

PSYCHODYNAMIC PSYCHOTHERAPY

Robert J. Ursano, M.D.

Stephen M. Sonnenberg, M.D.

Susan G. Lazar, M.D.

Psychodynamic psychotherapy may be brief, long-term, or intermittent. The principles and techniques are similar, but each form of therapy has its advantages and limitations. Psychodynamic psychotherapy requires the therapist to recognize patterns of interpersonal interaction and to recognize and understand his or her own reactions as early indicators of events transpiring in the treatment and as potential roadblocks to a successful treatment.

Why Psychotherapy?

Psychotherapy has long been a part of the treatment of psychiatric patients. Clinical experience and empirical research have shown psychotherapy to be both efficacious and cost-effective. The effectiveness of psycho-

therapy can be presented in several ways. A reevaluation of a classic study by Eysenck indicates that psychotherapy accomplishes in 15 sessions what spontaneous remission takes 2 years to do (McNeilly and Howard 1991). Smith et al. (1980) found an average effect size for psychotherapy of 0.68; this means that after treatment, the average treated person was better off than 75% of the untreated sample (Sonnenberg et al. 1996, 2003). The effect size found by Smith and colleagues is larger than the effect sizes for some other medical treatment trials; these trials were stopped before completion because the data indicated the treatment was efficacious enough that it would be unethical to withhold treatment (Rosenthal 1990). Similarly, such effect sizes are the equivalent of a surgeon's saying that with the surgery, 66% will survive, and without it, only 34% will survive (Rosenthal and Rubin 1982). Is there any question about whether to have such a surgery? Similar effect sizes have been found for psychodynamic psychotherapy in particular (Bond and Perry 2004; Crits-Christoph 1992; Leichsenring et al. 2004).

Psychiatric illness is not uncommon. There are psychiatric "common colds" as well as psychiatric "cancers." Often we forget the range of psychiatric illnesses and therefore the range of interventions—including psychotherapy—that are needed when one considers community health needs as a whole.

Psychotherapy is essential to the care of many diagnostic groups of psychiatric patients. It can be crucial for many depressed patients, especially for those who cannot take antidepressant medication, such as pregnant and nursing mothers, some elderly depressed patients, and some depressed patients with concomitant medical illnesses. Approximately 3% of the U.S. population receives psychotherapy each year (Weissman et al. 2006). In 1997, 10.3% of patients had 20 visits or more, compared with 15.7% in 1987. In 1997, nearly 10 million Americans spent $5.7 billion on outpatient psychotherapy (Olfson et al. 2002).

Behavior, which includes thoughts, feelings, fantasies, and actions, has both direct and indirect effects on health. Psychopathology usually limits the individual's ability to see options and exercise choice. Feelings, thoughts, and actions are frequently restricted, painful, and repetitive. Psychotherapy, the "talking cure," is the medical treatment directed to changing behavior through verbal means. Through talk, psychotherapy provides understanding, support, and new experiences that can result in learning. The goal of all psychotherapies is to increase the range of behaviors available to the patient and, in this way, to relieve symptoms and alter patterns that have created increased morbidity and potential mortality. The target organ of psychotherapeutic treatment is the brain. Feelings, thoughts, and behavior are

basic brain functions (Etking et al. 2005; Kandel 1999; Meany 2001).

Behavioral change can be the result of direct biological effects at the brain level (e.g., toxins, tumors), the unfolding of biology in maturation, or the effect of past and present life experiences interacting with biological givens. Psychotherapy itself is a life experience and can become a means by which what is "outside" changes what is "inside."

Our understanding of the basic sciences of this process—how what is outside affects what is inside—is only now emerging (Huttenlocher 2002; McEwen 2001; Ursano and Fullerton 1991).

A wide array of infant systems (activity level, arousal, and brain neurochemistry) are regulated by the mother–infant interaction and can be profoundly affected by it (Hofer 1984; Meany 2001). In adults, as well, the extent of social relatedness has been repeatedly shown to affect behavior as well as morbidity and mortality (House et al. 1988). Our understanding of how the outside world (psychotherapy) can change the inside world (biology) is growing but is still in its infancy. Our basic sciences of psychotherapy have changed the question from *whether* organization, meaning, memory, expectations, and interpersonal contact influence health and behavior to *how* they influence them and to what extent.

The Focus of Psychodynamic Psychotherapy

The different psychotherapies target different aspects of psychological functioning for change. Psychodynamic (psychoanalytically oriented) psychotherapy focuses primarily on the effects of past experience on molding patterns of behavior and expectations through particular cognitions (defenses) and interpersonal styles of interaction and perception (transference) that have become repetitive and that interfere with health (Table 17–1).

Table 17–1. Psychodynamic psychotherapy

Focus

Effects of past experience on present behaviors (cognitions, affects, fantasies and actions)

Goal

Understanding the defense mechanisms and the transference responses of the patient, particularly as they appear in the doctor–patient relationship

Technique

Therapeutic alliance

Free association

Defense and transference interpretation

Frequent meetings

Duration of treatment

Months to years

Expectations—the anticipated present and future—are formed by one's past experiences and biology. Likewise, the way in which language is used metaphorically by a patient may reflect a particular organization (cluster of feelings, thoughts, and behaviors) formed in the past and affecting present perception and behavior. By exploring the past and present meaning of events and their context, the psychodynamic psychotherapist aims to alter the organizers of behavior, restructuring how information and experience are organized.

Psychodynamic psychotherapy (also called *psychoanalytic psychotherapy, exploratory psychotherapy,* or *insight-oriented psychotherapy*) is a method of treatment for psychiatric disorders that uses words exchanged between two people to effect changes in behavior. There are both indications and contraindications to this form of treatment.

Psychodynamic psychotherapy is based on the principles of mental functioning and the psychotherapeutic techniques originally developed by Sigmund Freud. Freud focused on unrecognized (unconscious) conflicts that arose from development and continued into adult life. Such conflicts are patterns of behavior—that is, patterns of feelings, thoughts, and behaviors laid down in the brain during childhood.

Typically, these unconscious conflicts are between libidinal or aggressive desires (wishes) and the fear of loss, the fear of retaliation, the limits imposed by the real world, or the opposition of conflicting desires. *Libidinal wishes* are best thought of as longings for sexual and emotional gratification. *Aggressive wishes,* on the other hand, are destructive wishes that either are primary or are the result of perceived frustration or deprivation (Ursano et al. 1990). The beginning therapist frequently confuses the old terminology of libidinal wishes with the idea of specifically genital feelings. *Sexual gratification* in psychodynamic work refers to the broad concept of bodily pleasure—the states of excitement and pleasure experienced since infancy. The patient talking about happiness, excitement, pleasure, anticipation, love, or longing is describing libidinal wishes. The desire to destroy or the experience of pleasure in anger, hate, and pain is usually the expression of aggressive wishes.

Neurotic conflict (i.e., conflicted feelings/ambivalence derived from past [usually childhood] experiences and usually out of awareness) can result in anxiety, depression, and somatic symptoms; work, social, or sexual inhibitions; or maladaptive interpersonal relations. These unconscious neurotic conflicts are evident as patterns of behavior: feelings, thoughts, fantasies, and actions. These patterns, learned in childhood, may at one time have been appropriate to the patient's childhood view of the world and may have been adaptive or even necessary for survival.

Psychodynamic psychotherapy is more focused than psychoanalysis, per se, and somewhat more oriented to the here and now. However, both these techniques share the goal of understanding the nature of the patient's conflicts—maladaptive patterns of behavior derived from childhood (also called the *infantile neurosis*)—and their effects in adult life.

The Setting of Psychodynamic Psychotherapy

Duration and Frequency

Psychodynamic psychotherapy may be brief (see Chapter 16, "Brief Psychotherapies"), intermittent, or long term. Intermittent psychotherapy is often the norm. This is the result of episodes of brief or time-limited psychodynamic psychotherapy being given to a patient over a longer period of time. Intermittent psychotherapy may also be necessary due to resources of time, money, or the patient's unwillingness to undertake longer-term treatment.

Psychodynamic psychotherapy may extend over months or years. Typically, a longer-term treatment is open ended; no termination date is set in the beginning of treatment. The length of treatment depends on the number of conflict areas to be addressed and the course of the treatment. Psychotherapy sessions are usually held one, two, or three times a week, although in brief treatments once a week is the norm. The frequent meetings permit a more detailed exploration of the patient's inner life and a fuller development of the transference.

Medications

Medications are used as needed with patients in psychodynamic psychotherapy. Medications may relieve biological symptoms or regulation disruptions that evidence shows do not respond to psychotherapy. In addition, medication may alleviate persistent and impairing symptoms, which can allow the patient to participate in psychotherapy to learn new behaviors and avoid old impairing behaviors while experiencing a fuller range of affect. In some disorders, medication may be alleviating a primary disease process so that the psychotherapy can address the illness-onset conditions and facilitate the patient's avoidance of relapse, re-adjustment, recovery, and integration into family and community, thus decreasing the risk of morbidity and mortality. The meaning to the patient of the medication he or she may be taking is an important area for exploration during psychotherapy, particularly when it is time to discontinue use of the medication.

The Technique of Psychodynamic Psychotherapy

Behavioral change occurs in psychodynamic psychotherapy primarily through two processes of treatment: understanding the cognitive and affective patterns derived from childhood (defense mechanisms) and understanding the conflicted relationship(s) one had with one's childhood significant figures as they are reexperienced in the doctor–patient relationship (transference). The recovery and understanding of these feelings and perceptions are the focus of treatment. The treatment setting is designed to facilitate the emergence of these patterns in a way that allows them to be analyzed rather than being confused with the reality of the doctor–patient relationship or being dismissed as trivial. This therapeutic alliance is built on the reality-based elements of the treatment, such as the mutual working together toward a common goal and the consistency and reliability of the therapist (Bruch 1974).

Beginning therapists often think that as soon as they see something, it is time to tell the patient. The timing of when to tell the patient is the essence of the skill of the therapist; careful thought and planning are needed to determine the appropriate time. Although the actual event of interpreting—explaining a piece of behavior in the context of the present and past and in relation to transference elements—is spontaneous, it is "spontaneous" after much preparation. When to tell the patient a new piece of information is determined by when the patient can hear and understand what the therapist has to say.

The patient's free association—that is, speaking without censoring or inhibiting his or her thoughts—is encouraged. This encouragement can be as simple as telling a patient that she is free to talk about whatever she wishes. The therapist's main task is to listen to the undercurrents of the patient's associations. Frequently this involves wondering about the connection between one vignette and the next or listening for how the patient is experiencing a particular person she describes or a particular interaction with the therapist. Often, listening to the ambiguity in a patient's associations may open the door to the unconscious conflict and the person from the past to which it relates.

For example, one patient came into a psychotherapy session shortly after breaking up with his girlfriend, saying, "I want to get her back." If one hears the double meaning in the sentence—to be back with her or to take revenge on her—it will not be surprising to learn that although the patient thought he was only talking about wanting to get back together with his girlfriend, by the end of the session he was describing his particular revenge fantasy. (This patient's fantasy derived from an old movie. He fantasized about "smushing" a grapefruit in his girlfriend's face.) The conflicted feelings—longing for and hating—were foretold in the opening of the session. This long-held pattern of response to rejections matched his early experiences with a mother who would alternately see him as having exactly the same feelings as she did and later chase him with a knife. He was not yet ready to hear this connection, but it was already becoming evident. The pattern could now be watched, and the patient's awareness of it slowly increased.

The transference may be experienced by the therapist as a pressure to act in a certain way toward the patient. The transference is a specific example of the tendency of the brain to see the past in the present, to make use of old patterns of perception and response, and to exclude new information. Exploring the transference is just a special case of the ongoing work of examining the patterns of relationships that the patient experiences. Transference is not unique to the psychotherapeutic setting. It occurs throughout life and in medical treatments of all kinds. What is unique is the attempt to understand the transference and to examine it when it occurs rather than to try to undo it (Gabbard 2000; Luborsky and Crits-Christoph 1998).

The therapist may also experience feelings toward the patient that come from the therapist's past. This is called the *countertransference*. The countertransference is increased during times of stressful events and unresolved conflicts in the life of the therapist. The countertransference can be a friend, guiding one to see subtle aspects of the doctor–patient relationship that may have gone unnoticed. It can also be a block to a successful treatment, causing the therapist to misperceive and mishear the patient.

Evaluation

Assessment, Diagnosis, and Prescription of Brief, Intermittent, or Long-Term Psychodynamic Psychotherapy

Psychiatric evaluation is critical to the assessment of a patient for psychotherapy, just as for the patient who is to be seen for medication management (Ursano and Silberman 1988). The prescription of psychotherapy can be the outcome of the psychiatric evaluation.

Psychodynamic psychotherapy may be short term (brief; see Chapter 16, "Brief Psychotherapies"), long term, or intermittent. The structure of each of these requires consideration and planning of goals and targets of treatment. The choice of brief, intermittent, or long-term treatment is determined by the patient, type of problems (recent precipitant versus character related), degree of social supports to aid treatment responsiveness, extent of the disorder (multifocal versus unifocal conflict), and practical issues of patient availability and preferences.

As part of the evaluation for psychodynamic psychotherapy, the clinician must assess the presence or absence of organic causes for the patient's psychiatric disturbance, the need for medication, the risk of untoward outcomes (suicide, homicide, divorce, work disruption), and the possibility that the patient's condition will worsen. At times, the beginning therapist starting work in a busy outpatient service may neglect to consider the option that the patient assigned for psychotherapy was evaluated incorrectly and that individual psychodynamic psychotherapy is not the appropriate treatment or that no treatment is indicated.

The psychiatric assessment for psychodynamic psychotherapy includes the use of two important techniques: psychodynamic listening (Chessick 2000) and the psychodynamic assessment or evaluation.

Psychodynamic listening (Mohl 2003; Sonnenberg 1995) puts the psychiatrist in an attitude of curious inquiry, listening to the meanings, metaphors, developmental sequencing, and interpersonal nuances of the patient's story and of the doctor–patient interaction (Edelson 1993) (Table 17–2). Particular attention is paid to stories, present and past. The focus areas of the stories reflect the six psychodynamic perspectives on psychopathology: drive theory, ego function, self psychology, object relations, intersubjectivity and relational theory, and attachment theory (Table 17–3).

The *psychodynamic assessment or evaluation* uses the data obtained from questioning and from psychodynamic listening (MacKinnon et al. 2006; Sullivan 1954; Table 17–4). This psychodynamic formulation provides an integrated understanding through the patient's life cycle from the four psychodynamic perspectives on the past and present

---

Table 17–2. Psychodynamic listening

I. Wishes/desires

What is the patient wishing for?

What in the patient's developmental history caused this wish to be prominent?

Are the wishes developmentally appropriate?

II. Defenses

What in the patient's developmental history disrupted his or her wishes and desires?

How does the patient keep wishes out of awareness?

III. Self-esteem

Does the patient like him- or herself?

Does he or she feel valued, admired, recognized by others?

How does the patient respond to events in life that decrease self-esteem or the feeling of being valued?

IV. Interpersonal relations—present and in memory/fantasy

Who are the important people in the patient's past and present?

How are they recalled and spoken of at the different phases of the patient's life and development?

Whom from the past does the patient behave and feel and think like (even if the patient is not aware of it)?

Whom does the patient miss and long for?

Who was lost from the patient's life at an early age (by death, moving, illness, conflict, or absence/neglect)?

Table 17–3. Psychodynamic perspectives

Theory	Focus
Drive theory	Wishes and feelings
Ego function	Defense mechanisms, cognitive style, and areas of health in the personality
Self psychology	Regulation of self-esteem
Object relations	Internalized memories of interpersonal relationships
Intersubjectivity and relational theory	Subjective experience and interpersonal relations
Attachment theory	Infant–caregiver attachment

experiences of the patient, and it makes predictions of potential doctor–patient interactions and the patient's patterns of defense mechanisms and interpersonal interactions.

After a well-conducted evaluation, the patient feels respected and safe, believes that his or her best interests are the primary concern of the clinician, and feels that any topic can be talked about (Levinson et al. 1967). The therapist's asking about medical signs and symptoms and suicidal and homicidal thoughts and actions frequently relieves the patient of the feeling that he or she is the only one worried about these areas.

Beginning the Evaluation

The evaluation begins when the therapist meets the patient (Lazare and Eisenthal 1989; Lazare et al. 1989). In the outpatient setting, it is best for the therapist to introduce him- or herself and explain to the patient what the therapist knows about the patient's problems. One should not assume that a patient knows that a session is an evaluation. Rather, the therapist should set the context of the meeting, explaining that he or she, the therapist, would like to spend some time getting to know the nature of the patient's difficulties and inviting the patient to tell more (Table 17–5).

The number of evaluation sessions usually ranges from one to four, but more sessions may be needed. Usually, the beginning therapist errs on the side of short evaluations and an incomplete assessment.

The clinician uses two methods for data collection during the evaluation: asking questions and listening unobtrusively (Silberman and Certa 2003; Table 17–6). Life-threatening issues must be dealt with early in order to gather the needed diagnostic information. However, other historical information can be collected as part of the patient's story (Horowitz et al. 1995; Perry et al. 1987). Frequently, the skill of the therapist lies in how the history and diagnostic information are collected. The skilled therapist can establish rapport across a wide array of socioeconomic classes and sexual, racial, religious, cultural, and emotional differences.

Table 17–4. Guidelines for psychodynamic assessment

Listen to and explore:
  The precipitants of the symptoms, of the illness, and of seeking help
  The history of significant events from childhood to the present
Identify the significant people in the patient's history from childhood to present
Ask for the patient's earliest memory
Explore any recurrent or recent dreams and the context of when they were dreamed
Observe how the patient relates to the therapist
Discuss the patient's previous treatments and therapists
Give a trial interpretation
Invite collaboration in "understanding"

Table 17–5. The evaluation

Goal

Educate the patient about the evaluation process

Establish an atmosphere of safety and inquiry

Assess for the appropriate treatment

Tasks

Assess for life-threatening behaviors

Assess for organic causes of the patient's illness

Determine the diagnosis

Identify areas of conflict across the life cycle

Duration

Meet for one to four sessions

Techniques

Use questioning and listening

Listen for the patient's fears about starting treatment

Attend to the precipitants of the illness and of seeking treatment

---

In the first session, the therapist should listen for the patient's fears of starting psychotherapy (Table 17–7). These fears should be explored early, as they appear and are articulated by the patient. (In clinic settings, about 50% of patients stop before the fifth session [Malan et al. 1973].)

Indications and Selection Criteria

Psychodynamic psychotherapy has its best outcomes with individuals who have conflicts that are primarily oedipal in nature (e.g., competition, guilt, independence, adult sexuality and intimacy, parental loss and identification) and that are experienced as internal by the patient. Although the diagnoses in DSM-IV-TR (American Psychiatric Association 2000) are not organized by their developmental conflict level (or level of maturity of defenses), some of the disorders are more likely than others to present with a primarily neurotic-level conflict. DSM-IV-TR disorders that frequently involve a primarily neurotic conflict include obsessive-compulsive disorder, anxiety disorders (Bond and Perry 2004), conversion disorder, psychological factors affecting physical disease, dysthymic disorder, mild to moderate mood disorders (Bond 2006), adjustment disorders, and mild to moderate personality disorders (Gabbard et al. 2002; Leichsenring 2005; Leichsenring and Leibing 2003). Patients who are psychologi-

---

Table 17–6. Helpful hints for the evaluation

When the clinician is only doing the evaluation and the patient will be referred to another therapist for treatment, it is most helpful to the evaluation and to its successful termination that the patient know this plan at the beginning.

Infrequently, it may be advantageous and important to have the initial evaluation done by a clinician who will not be the treating therapist. In the case where the patient needs a very firm, direct, confrontational approach to enter a much-needed treatment, the evaluating clinician who is not expecting to treat the patient may feel freer to be blunt, in a tactful manner, with the patient.

Patients must be given the time and space in which to paint a picture of their world without the therapist choosing the colors! Being either too intrusive or too silent can lead to missed information and can needlessly confuse the patient.

All therapists also experience certain therapist–patient differences that they cannot bridge, and in such cases they refer the patient to another clinician.

Early termination may be due to defenses against seeking help, a transference reaction, a decision that this is not the right treatment, or, at times, a relief of symptoms as a result of the evaluation.

Table 17–7. First session

By the end of the first session, the clinician should know the answers to these questions:

What further organic workup is needed?

Is psychosis in the differential diagnosis?

Are there any life-threatening issues, either now or possibly in the future?

How many (if any) more sessions will be taken for the evaluation?

cally minded, who are able to observe feelings without acting on them, and who can obtain symptom relief through understanding may benefit from psychodynamic psychotherapy. The patient who has a supportive environment—family, friends, work—usually does better because he or she is able to use the therapy in a more intensive manner. Such a patient does not need the therapist to be a primary reality support in order to weather the stresses of life or the treatment.

When not in the acute phase of illness and when dealing with rehabilitation, adjustment, and recovery, more seriously disturbed patients—those with major depression, schizophrenia, or borderline personality disorder—can also be treated in psychodynamically informed psychotherapy, with the addition of psychosocial supports and interventions as needed (Blatt and Shahar 2004; Fonagy et al. 2005). For these patients, the treatment is usually directed toward modifying the illness-onset conditions and facilitating readjustment, recovery, and integration into the community. Supportive treatment, derived from many principles of psychodynamic psychotherapy, is the primary treatment in the acute phase of these illnesses. The regressive tendencies of such patients are managed in psychodynamic psychotherapy with the use of medication and with greater support and reality feedback through face-to-face meetings with the therapist (Gabbard 2005).

Patients with severe preoedipal pathology are not good candidates for psychodynamic psychotherapy. This type of pathology is manifested by an inability to form a sup-

portive dyadic relationship, the presence of severely exploitative relationships, a chaotic lifestyle, or substantial (or dangerous) acting-out.

Although psychological mindedness is important, intelligence per se is not a selection criterion; in fact, it can reflect a highly organized obsessional character structure that may be very difficult to treat. Socioeconomic class is also not a good predictor of success in treatment.

Treatment

Psychodynamic psychotherapy is usually not a familiar form of medical treatment to the patient who is about to begin psychotherapy. At the end of the evaluation, the clinician discusses with the patient alternative forms of treatment that might in various ways be of benefit. In addition, the clinician must discuss with the patient how each of these treatments works. Psychodynamic psychotherapy can be explained to the patient as a process for learning a new method of problem solving based on an understanding of the personal life history, the workings of the mind that are outside conscious awareness, and the personal view of the world—one's psychic reality.

Teaching the patient about the goals and process of psychodynamic psychotherapy is very important to the successful beginning of the psychotherapy. One way to conceptualize this phase of treatment is that an atmosphere of safety must be established.

The patient is educated directly, both through teaching and explanation and through example. At times, the clinician should explain very directly and supportively to the patient the process of the treatment. Generally, the new therapist struggles with how much to educate and how much to listen in the opening sessions. Understanding the goals and processes of treatment is important to the patient's feeling safe and comfortable enough to explore and tolerate the anxiety that arises in the treatment setting (Sonnenberg et al. 1996, 2003).

Abstinence, Neutrality, and Free Association

After the patient has begun to understand the process of treatment, the therapist will, over time, become somewhat less verbally active in order to hear more about how the patient organizes his or her psychological world. Technically this is called being abstinent. Again the therapist may need to explain this to the patient if he or she asks about the therapist's silence. The therapist might say, "I am listening to you very closely. I want to be able to best understand how you see the world and not interfere with what you are telling me." The therapist also encourages the patient to speak as freely as possible and to suspend judgment about the accuracy or logic of what is said. This may be explained to the patient in the following manner: "You are free to say whatever you would like. In fact, it is most helpful if you say whatever comes to mind. I know that is difficult to do." The therapist helps the patient say whatever comes to mind—to speak without editing thoughts—even though the patient may say things that he or she fears would be untrue or hurtful to the therapist or to loved ones. This method of communication is known as *free association* (S. Freud 1917/1963).

The ways of thinking that block uncomfortable feelings and conflicts from being experienced are called *defense mechanisms* (discussed later in this chapter). The therapist carefully observes, and at the right time shares with the patient, the patterns the patient shows in his or her thoughts and feelings and the blocks to these thoughts and feelings.

The clinician and patient work together to recognize the patterns of the patient's thoughts and feelings. This collaborative work allows the patient to experience this task as one he or she can eventually assume, rather than as something magical. This task—the analysis of defenses—forms the basis on which the patient can eventually choose alternative behaviors.

What the patient says is met with an effort to understand, not with judgment or criticism. The therapist maintains neutrality. The job of the psychodynamic psychotherapist does not involve managing the patient's life (one reason why patient selection is so important) or judging its worth or the value of the way in which it is conducted (Poland 1984). The therapist's abstinent, neutral demeanor in the therapeutic setting is, in part, a technique, a special form of behavior designed to offer the patient the opportunity to experience his or her own feelings, thoughts, and fantasies. Over time, the therapy becomes a laboratory in which the patient can examine in detail the feelings, thoughts, and fantasies he or she experiences toward another person (the therapist) within the safety of the therapeutic alliance (Bender 2005).

The therapist and the patient develop a working (Greenson 1965) or therapeutic alliance (Curtis 1979; Zetzel 1956). The psychiatrist doing this form of therapy works from the perspective of the concerned physician, with gentleness and an awareness of the patient's pain (Schafer 1983; Stone 1981).

Transference, Defense Mechanisms, and Resistance

Transference

Transference is at the core of how psychodynamic psychotherapy works. All human beings experience others by superimposing their perceptions of figures from the past on new individuals. Today, it is generally felt that memories of the past are activated in all relationships. To some extent, each individual unconsciously plays out in current relationships certain aspects of important past relationships (Table 17–8).

People form transferences in all relationships. This is because we use the past as a pattern for understanding the present and because there seems to be in all people a psychological need to repeat the past in an effort to master that which was difficult or emotionally painful (S. Freud 1912/1958; McLaughlin 1981).

What we see when we observe individuals and talk with them about their present life

Table 17–8. Transference

Transference...

Is part of all relationships

Is a primary focus of psychodynamic psychotherapy

Brings the past alive to the patient in the doctor–patient relationship

Aids in remembering the past

Provides examples of patterns of interpersonal behaviors, fantasies, feelings, and thoughts that influence the patient's present relationships

Can be felt by the therapist as "role pressure"—a pressure to respond in a particular way to the patient

or current relationships is the surface of their psychological life. Beneath that surface are the memories of their important past relationships, which—like the muscles, nerves, and bones beneath the skin—constitute vital parts of the organic whole of their interpersonal world, present as well as past (Goldstein and Goldberg 2003; Sandler et al. 1973).

The development and understanding of the transference is one of the therapist's most important tools. It is the vehicle for bringing alive—in the consulting room—the patient's difficulties and for examining these in depth in an existentially meaningful environment.

Defense Mechanisms, Resistance, and Dreams

Defenses are our cognitive mechanisms of structuring mental and emotional experience to keep psychic pain at a minimum and bring our interpersonal and intrapsychic functioning and relationships into some congruence with external reality. The therapist is hoping to point out the kinds of thoughts and feelings that the patient obscures and the ways they are obscured, defended against, and kept unconscious. Throughout treatment, the patient's defensive ways of thinking are elucidated. In the opening phase, the therapist will have the opportunity to identify patterns of defense and resistance and must orient the

patient to how awareness of these patterns can be used to advance the patient's knowledge of him- or herself (Loewald 1960).

Resistance is a general term referring to all the forces in the patient that oppose the painful work of therapy. There are many different categories of resistance, including general fear of any change, an overly harsh conscience that punishes a patient with the continuation of suffering, and the insistence on the gratification of childish impulses that forms part of an emotional illness. All people, including patients in therapy, employ mechanisms of defense to keep painful feelings and memories outside conscious awareness. These defense mechanisms are specific, discrete maneuvers or ways of thinking that the mind employs to avoid painful emotional material (Nemiah 1961; Shapiro 1965).

Whenever a patient is manifesting resistance, in whatever form, it is because the patient is protecting him- or herself from experiencing, including remembering or reliving, the old dangers and fears associated with the childhood conflicts and developmental difficulties of his or her life. Character (the set of expectable responses from a person in a given setting) is a result of the defense mechanisms each person characteristically uses.

The patient's defense mechanisms are an important source of resistance in psychotherapy. In 1936, Anna Freud, in *The Ego and the Mechanisms of Defense* (A. Freud 1966), outlined the functioning of many of these defense maneuvers. Since that time, the list has grown and been elaborated upon (Table 17–9). More primitive mechanisms of defense, including splitting, projection, projective identification, omnipotence, devaluing, and primitive idealization, are seen in severe personality disorders such as borderline personality disorder and psychotic disorders (Kernberg 1975).

In psychotherapy the therapist strives to help the patient understand the origins and functions of his or her defenses so that the patient can become aware of the feelings, thoughts, and fantasies that the patient fears from the conflicts of long ago.

Table 17–9.   Defense mechanisms

Common defense mechanisms	Primitive defense mechanisms
Repression	Splitting
Denial	Projection
Reaction formation	Projective identification
Displacement	Omnipotence
Identification	Devaluing
Identification with the aggressor	Primitive identification
Intellectualization	
Isolation of affect	
Sublimation	

The therapist also attends to the dream life of the patient (Brenner 1976; S. Freud 1900/1953). Not all patients in psychotherapy work extensively with dreams, but many do, and for those who can, the work is an important tool. Frequently, dreams reported early in treatment are particularly revealing of the core conflicts of the patient. They can also serve to educate the patient about unconscious processes (Sharpe 1961). Dreams can be presented to the patient as thoughts and concerns the patient is having while asleep, although the rules for how these thoughts and concerns are created are different (i.e., primary process thinking) than during waking life (i.e., secondary process thinking) (Reiser 1994).

Countertransference

Countertransference is the emotional reaction of the therapist to the patient. Historically, countertransference was limited in meaning to the therapist's transference onto the patient. This was felt to be a response to the patient's transference. Like all transferences, the therapist's countertransference was the result of unconscious conflicts; however, these unresolved conflicts were those of the therapist rather than those of the patient. This countertransference was thought to obscure the therapist's judgment in conducting the therapy (Gabbard 1995; Gabbard and Wilkinson 2001).

Countertransferences are many and varied. Often they are the result of events occurring in the therapist's life that may make him or her more sensitive to certain themes in the patient's associations. The developmental period of the therapist's life—involving issues of intimacy, achievement, or old age, for example—may also affect how the therapist hears the patient. Intense transferences of all kinds—erotic, aggressive, devaluing, idealizing, and others—are ripe for serving as the stimulus to awaken in the therapist elements of his or her own past (Mitchell and Aron 1999).

There are generally two types of countertransference reactions: concordant and complementary (Racker 1968; Table 17–10).

Termination

Often, psychodynamic psychotherapy is conducted in an open-ended fashion regard-

Table 17–10. Countertransference

Concordant countertransference

The therapist experiences and empathizes with the patient's emotional position (e.g., therapist thinks: "Boy, my patient is right! His boss sounds like a terrible person!").

Complementary countertransference

The therapist experiences and empathizes with the feelings of an important person from the patient's life (e.g., therapist thinks: "My patient is infuriating—I certainly see why his boss gets so angry at him!").

less of whether it is to be short or longer term. There comes a time, however, when the patient and the psychiatrist agree that it is time to end the treatment. At this juncture, the troublesome areas of the patient's personality seem to be separate from the core of the patient's sense of self (Alexander 1941).

The therapist must remember and the patient must come to realize that treatment goals are related to, but different from, the patient's life goals (Ticho 1972). Treatment goals are always dependent to some extent on life's demands and possibilities—what is possible at a given time of life and in a given context. Termination does not mean a patient has realized all of his or her hopes and wishes. Rather, the patient entering the end phase of treatment after a successful treatment has experienced substantial relief of psychological suffering, and this relief is evident to both the patient and the therapist. In addition, the internal conflicts of the patient, as well as the presenting symptoms, have been resolved, and reasonably permanent changes in behavior have occurred.

The patient shows a detailed understanding of the working of his or her mind and is beginning to use self-inquiry as a method of problem solving. Often there have been gains in most of these areas, although not necessarily all. The gains are observed by the therapist and shared with the patient as part of the patient's increasing awareness of new areas of strength and conflict resolution (Table 17–11). The termination phase has its own tasks to consolidate the treatment and facilitate leave-taking while maintaining the therapeutic relationship (Table 17–12).

Table 17–11. Criteria for termination

The patient...
  Experiences relief of symptoms.
  Experiences symptoms as alien.
  Understands his or her characteristic defenses.
  Is able to understand and recognize his or her characteristic transference responses.
  Engages in ongoing self-inquiry as a method of resolving internal conflicts.

Table 17–12. Tasks of the termination phase

Review the treatment.

The patient reviews the treatment, reconsidering his or her history and conflicts and placing in perspective what has been learned. Frequently the patient experiences a feeling of pride, strength, and gratitude to the therapist in this process while refreshing the "table of contents" of the patient's knowledge about him- or herself.

Experience the loss of the psychotherapy and the therapist.

In termination, the patient experiences what is an essential and poignant aspect of the human condition: the experience of separation—the loss of a relationship with a person who has been very helpful and who often is perceived as kind and understanding. This loss may reawaken the conflicts of previous losses.

Reexperience and remaster the transference.

Very often, in the context of termination, there is a recrudescence of the patient's symptoms and a return of old transference patterns and styles of interacting with the therapist.

Increase skills in self-inquiry as a method of problem solving.

The patient now begins to take over the functions of the therapist. The patient increasingly exercises a greater degree of self-inquiry to resolve now well-known and well-understood internal conflicts.

Conclusion

The patterns of early childhood—laid down on the basis of our biological givens, our early familial experiences, and our interpersonal world—form the lenses through which we view the world throughout our lives and give meaning to our adult experiences. Psychodynamic psychotherapy looks to change current maladaptive patterns of behavior through understanding the relationship of present symptomatic behaviors to past experiences that have provided the templates for these behaviors and for adult cognitive and emotional perception. The core concepts of psychodynamic psychotherapy—the role of conflict in our feelings, thoughts, and behaviors; the interaction of our neurobiology with our experiences throughout development and particularly in childhood; and the fact that we have feelings and thoughts outside of our awareness—require study across a wide array of health-related behaviors to identify new psychodynamically informed interventions and treatments.

Key Points

- Transference occurs in all interpersonal relationships.

- Defense mechanisms are cognitive mechanisms to decrease anxiety and other distressing feelings.

- Early childhood development structures brain development and leaves patterns of feelings, thoughts, behaviors, and interpersonal relating.

- Psychotherapy is an effective form of treatment, as effective as many other medical interventions.

- The working, reality-based relationship with the patient is called the therapeutic alliance.

- Psychodynamic psychotherapy may be brief, intermittent, or longer term.

- The principles of psychodynamic psychotherapy are used in many doctor–patient interactions other than psychodynamic psychotherapy.

Suggested Readings

Ellenberger HF: The Discovery of the Unconscious: The History and Evolution of Dynamic Psychiatry. New York, Basic Books, 1970

Foelsch PA, Levy KN, Hull JW, et al: The development of a psychodynamic treatment for patients with borderline personality disorder: a preliminary study of behavioral change. J Personal Disord 15:487–495, 2001

Freud S: The interpretation of dreams (1900), in The Standard Edition of the Complete Psychological Works of Sigmund Freud, Vols 4 and 5. Translated and edited by Strachey J. London, Hogarth Press, 1953

Freud S: The psychopathology of everyday life (1901), in The Standard Edition of the Complete Psychological Works of Sigmund Freud, Vol 6. Translated and edited by Strachey J. London, Hogarth Press, 1960

Gabbard GO: Long-Term Psychodynamic Psychotherapy: A Basic Text. Washington, DC, American Psychiatric Publishing, 2004

Gabbard GO, Gabbard K: Psychiatry and the Cinema. Washington, DC, American Psychiatric Press, 1999

Kohut H: The Analysis of the Self: A Systematic Approach to the Psychoanalytic Treatment of Narcissistic Personality Disorders. New York, International Universities Press, 1971

Meissner WW: Freud and Psychoanalysis. Notre Dame, IN, University of Notre Dame Press, 2000

Stern DN: The Interpersonal World of the Infant: A View From Psychoanalysis and Developmental Psychology. New York, Basic Books, 2000

Ursano RJ, Sonnenberg SM, Lazar SG: Concise Guide to Psychodynamic Psychotherapy: Principles and Techniques of Brief, Intermittent, and Long-Term Psychodynamic Psychotherapy. Washington, DC, American Psychiatric Publishing, 2004

References

Alexander F: The voice of the intellect is soft. Psychoanal Rev 28:12–29, 1941

American Psychiatric Association: Diagnostic and Statistical Manual of Mental Disorders, 4th Edition, Text Revision. Washington, DC, American Psychiatric Association, 2000

Bender DS: The therapeutic alliance in the treatment of personality disorders. J Psychiatr Pract 11:73 87, 2005

Blatt S, Shahar G: Psychoanalysis—with whom, for what and how? Comparisons with psychotherapy. J Am Psychoanal Assoc 52:393–447, 2004

Bond M: Psychodynamic psychotherapy in the treatment of mood disorders. Curr Opin Psychiatry 19:40–43, 2006

Bond M, Perry C: Long-term changes in defense styles with psychodynamic psychotherapy for depressive, anxiety and personality disorders. Am J Psychiatry 161:1665–1671, 2004

Brenner C: Psychoanalytic Technique and Psychic Conflicts. New York, International Universities Press, 1976

Bruch H: Learning Psychotherapy: Rationale and Ground Rules. Cambridge, MA, Harvard University Press, 1974

Chessick RD: Psychoanalysis: clinical and theoretical. Am J Psychiatry 157:846–848, 2000

Crits-Christoph P: The efficacy of brief dynamic psychotherapy: a meta-analysis. Am J Psychiatry 149:151–158, 1992

Curtis HC: The concept of therapeutic alliance: implications for the "widening scope." J Am Psychoanal Assoc 27 (suppl):159–192, 1979

Edelson M: Telling and enacting stories in psychoanalysis and psychodynamic psychotherapy. Psychoanal Study Child 48:293–325, 1993

Etking A, Pittenger, C, Polan HJ, et al: Toward a neurobiology of psychotherapy: basic research and clinical applications. J Neuropsychiatry Clin Neurosci 17:145–158, 2005

Fonagy P, Roth A, Higgitt A: Psychodynamic psychotherapies: evidence-based practice and clinical wisdom. Bull Menninger Clin 69:1–58, 2005

Freud A: The Ego and the Mechanisms of Defense, Revised Edition. New York, International Universities Press, 1966

Freud S: The interpretation of dreams (1900), in The Standard Edition of the Complete Psychological Works of Sigmund Freud, Vols 4 and 5. Translated and edited by Strachey J. London, Hogarth Press, 1953

Freud S: The dynamics of transference (1912), in The Standard Edition of the Complete Psychological Works of Sigmund Freud, Vol 12. Translated and edited by Strachey J. London, Hogarth Press, 1958, pp 97–108

Freud S: Resistance and repression (1917), in The Standard Edition of the Complete Psychological Works of Sigmund Freud, Vol 16. Translated and edited by Strachey J. London, Hogarth Press, 1963, pp 286–302

Gabbard GO: Countertransference: the emerging common ground. Int J Psychoanal 76:475–485, 1995

Gabbard GO: Psychodynamic Psychiatry in Clinical Practice, 3rd Edition. Washington, DC, American Psychiatric Press, 2000

Gabbard GO: Psychodynamic Psychiatry in Clinical Practice, 4th Edition. Washington, DC, American Psychiatric Publishing, 2005

Gabbard GO, Wilkinson SM: Management of Countertransference With Borderline Patients. Washington, DC, American Psychiatric Publishing, 2001

Gabbard GO, Gunderson JG, Fonagy P: The place of psychoanalytic treatments within psychiatry. Arch Gen Psychiatry 59:505–510, 2002

Goldstein WN, Goldberg ST: The Transference in Psychotherapy. Northvale, NJ, Jason Aronson, 2003

Greenson RR: The working alliance and the transference neurosis. Psychoanal Q 34:155–181, 1965

Hofer MA: Relationships as regulators: psychobiological perspective on bereavement. Psychosom Med 46:183–197, 1984

Horowitz MJ, Eells T, Singer J, et al: Role-relationship models for case formulation. Arch Gen Psychiatry 52:625–633, 1995

House JS, Landis KR, Umberson D: Social relationships and health. Science 241:540–545, 1988

Huttenlocher PR: Neural Plasticity. Cambridge, MA, Harvard University Press, 2002

Kandel ER: Biology and the future of psychoanalysis: a new framework for psychiatry revisited. Am J Psychiatry 156:505–524, 1999

Kernberg OF: Borderline Conditions and Pathological Narcissism. New York, Jason Aronson, 1975

Lazare A, Eisenthal S: Clinician/patient relations, I: attending to the patient's perspective, in Outpatient Psychiatry. Edited by Lazare A. Baltimore, MD, Williams & Wilkins, 1989, pp 125–136

Lazare A, Eisenthal S, Frank A: Clinician/Patient relations, II: conflict and negotiation, in Outpatient Psychiatry. Edited by Lazare A. Baltimore, MD, Williams & Wilkins, 1989, pp 137–157

Leichsenring F: Are psychodynamic and psychoanalytic therapies effective? A review of empirical data. Int J Psychoanal 86:841–868, 2005

Leichsenring F, Leibing E: The effectiveness of psychodynamic therapy and cognitive behavior therapy in the treatment of personality disorders: a meta analysis. Am J Psychiatry 160:1223–1232, 2003

Leichsenring F, Rabung S, Leibing E: The efficacy of short-term psychodynamic psychotherapy in specific psychiatric disorders: a meta analysis. Arch Gen Psychiatry 61:1208–1216, 2004

Levinson D, Merrifield J, Berg K: Becoming a patient. Arch Gen Psychiatry 17:385–406, 1967

Loewald HW: On the therapeutic action of psycho-analysis. Int J Psychoanal 41:16–33, 1960

Luborsky L, Crits-Christoph P: Understanding Transference: The CCRT Method, 2nd Edition. Washington, DC, American Psychological Association Press, 1998

MacKinnon RA, Michels R, Buckley PJ (eds): The Psychiatric Interview in Clinical Practice, 2nd Edition. Washington, DC, American Psychiatric Publishing, 2006

Malan DH, Heath ES, Baral HA, et al: Psychodynamic changes in untreated neurotic patients, II: apparently genuine improvement. Arch Gen Psychiatry 32:110–126, 1973

McEwen BS: Plasticity of the hippocampus: adaptation to chronic stress and allostatic load. Ann NY Acad Sci 933:265–277, 2001

McLaughlin JT: Transference, psychic reality, and countertransference. Psychoanal Q 50:639–664, 1981

McNeilly CL, Howard KI: The effects of psychotherapy: a reevaluation based on dosage. Psychother Res 1:74–78, 1991

Meany MK: Maternal care, gene expression and the transmission of individual differences in stress reactivity across generations Annu Rev Neurosci 24:1161–1192, 2001

Mitchell S, Aron L (eds): Relational Psychoanalysis: The Emergence of a Tradition. Hillsdale, NJ, Analytic Press, 1999

Mohl PC: Listening to the patient, in Psychiatry, 2nd Edition. Edited by Tasman A, Kaye J, Lieberman J. New York, Wiley, 2003, pp 3–18

Nemiah JC: Foundations of Psychopathology. New York, Oxford University Press, 1961

Olfson M, Marcus SC, Druss B, et al: National trends in the use of outpatient psychotherapy. Am J Psychiatry 159:1914–1920, 2002

Perry S, Cooper AM, Michels R: The psychodynamic formulation: its purpose, structure and clinical application. Am J Psychiatry 144:543–550, 1987

Poland WS: On the analyst's neutrality. J Am Psychoanal Assoc 32:283–299, 1984

Racker H: Transference and Countertransference. New York, International Universities Press, 1968

Reiser MF: Memory in Mind and Brain: What Dream Imagery Reveals. New Haven, CT, Yale University Press, 1994

Rosenthal R: How are we doing in soft psychology? Am Psychol 45:775–777, 1990

Rosenthal R, Rubin DB: A simple, general-purpose display of magnitude of experimental effect. J Educ Psychol 74:166–169, 1982

Sandler J, Dare C, Holder A: The Patient and the Analyst: The Basis of the Psychoanalytic Process. New York, International Universities Press, 1973

Schafer R: The atmosphere of safety: Freud's "Papers on Technique" (1911–1915), in The Analytic Attitude. New York, Basic Books, 1983, pp 14–33

Shapiro D: Neurotic Styles. New York, Basic Books, 1965

Sharpe EF: Dream Analysis. London, Hogarth Press, 1961

Silberman EK, Certa K. The psychiatric interview: settings and techniques, in Psychiatry, 2nd Edition. Edited by Tasman A, Kaye J, Lieberman J. New York, Wiley, 2003, pp 30–51

Smith ML, Glass GV, Miller TI: The Benefits of Psychotherapy. Baltimore, MD, Johns Hopkins University Press, 1980

Sonnenberg SM: Analytic listening and the analyst's self-analysis. Int J Psychoanal 76:335–342, 1995

Sonnenberg SM, Sutton L, Ursano RJ: Physician–patient relationship, in Psychiatry. Edited by Tasman A, Kaye J, Lieberman J. Philadelphia, PA, WB Saunders, 1996, pp 41–49

Sonnenberg SM, Ursano AM, Ursano RJ: Physician–patient relationship, in Psychiatry, 2nd Edition. Edited by Tasman A, Kay J, Lieberman JA. New York, Wiley, 2003, pp 52–63

Stone L: Notes on the noninterpretive elements in the psychoanalytic situation and process. J Am Psychoanal Assoc 29:89–118, 1981

Sullivan HS: The Psychiatric Interview. New York, WW Norton, 1954

Ticho E: Termination of psychoanalysis: treatment goals, life goals. Psychoanal Q 41:315–333, 1972

Ursano RJ, Fullerton CS: Psychotherapy: medical intervention and the concept of normality, in Normality: Context and Theory. Edited by Offer D, Sabshin M. New York, Basic Books, 1991, pp 39–59

Ursano RJ, Silberman EK: Individual psychotherapies, in The American Psychiatric Press Textbook of Psychiatry. Edited by Talbott JA, Hales RE, Yudofsky SC. Washington, DC, American Psychiatric Press, 1988, pp 855–889

Ursano RJ, Silberman EK, Diaz A Jr: The psychotherapies: basic theoretical principles, techniques and indications, in Clinical Psychiatry for Medical Students. Edited by Stoudemire A. Philadelphia, PA, JB Lippincott, 1990, pp 855–890

Weissman MM, Verdell H, Gameroff JM, et al: National survey of psychotherapy training psychiatry, psychology and social work. Arch Gen Psychiatry 63:925–934, 2006

Zetzel ER: Current concepts of transference. Int J Psychoanal 37:369–376, 1956

18

COGNITIVE THERAPY

Jesse H. Wright, M.D., Ph.D.
Michael E. Thase, M.D.
Aaron T. Beck, M.D.

Cognitive therapy (CT) is a system of psychotherapy based on theories of pathological information processing in mental disorders. Treatment is directed primarily at modifying distorted or maladaptive cognitions and related behavioral dysfunction. Therapeutic interventions are usually focused and problem oriented. Although the use of specific techniques is a major feature of this approach, there can be considerable flexibility and creativity in the clinical application of CT.

In this chapter we explain basic theories and detail commonly used CT techniques. The main focus is on the treatment of depression and anxiety disorders in adults. Methods have been developed for using CT with children and adolescents, but these applica-tions are not discussed in this chapter. Readers who wish to learn about CT for younger persons are referred to the excellent books on this topic, including those by Reinecke et al. (2003), Albano and Kearney (2000), and March and Mulle (1998).

Basic Concepts
The Cognitive Model

The cognitive model for psychotherapy is grounded on the theory that there are characteristic errors in information processing in psychiatric disorders, and that these alterations in thought processes are closely linked to emotional reactions and dysfunctional be-

Drs. Wright and Beck receive a portion of profits from sales of the "Good Days Ahead" software for computer-assisted cognitive therapy discussed in this chapter.

havior patterns (A.T. Beck 1976; Wright et al. 2006). For example, Beck and co-workers (A.T. Beck 1976) have proposed that there are three major areas of cognitive distortion in depression (the negative cognitive triad of self, world, and future) and that patients with anxiety disorders habitually overestimate the danger or risk in situations. Cognitive distortions such as misperceptions, errors in logic, or misattributions are thought to lead to dysphoric moods and maladaptive behavior. Furthermore, a vicious cycle is perpetuated when the behavioral response confirms and amplifies negatively distorted cognitions (Wright et al. 2006).

This point is illustrated by the case of Mr. S, a 45-year-old recently divorced, depressed man. After being rebuffed on his first attempt to ask a woman for a date, Mr. S had a series of dysfunctional cognitions, such as, "You should have known better.... You're a loser.... There's no use trying." His subsequent behavioral pattern was consistent with these cognitions—he made no further social contacts and became more lonely and isolated. The negative behavior led to additional maladaptive cognitions (e.g., "No one will want me.... I'll be alone the rest of my life.... What's the use of going on?").

The CT perspective can be summarized in a working model (Figure 18–1) that expands on the well-known stimulus–response paradigm (Wright et al. 2006). Cognitive mediation is given the central role in this model. However, an interactive relationship between environmental influences, cognition, emotion, and behavior is also recognized. It should be emphasized that this working model does not presume that cognitive pathology is the cause of specific syndromes or that other factors such as genetic predisposition, biochemical alterations, or interpersonal conflicts are not involved in the etiology of psychiatric illnesses. Instead, the model is used simply as a guide for the actions of the cognitive therapist in clinical practice. It is assumed that most forms of psychopathology have complex etiologies in-

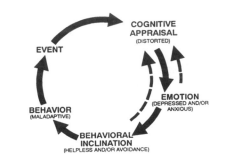

Figure 18–1.   A working model for cognitive therapy.
Source.   Adapted from Wright 1988.

volving cognitive, biological, social, and interpersonal influences, and that there are multiple potentially useful approaches to treatment. In addition, it is assumed that cognitive changes are accomplished through biological processes and that psychopharmacological treatments can alter cognitions (Wright and Thase 1992). This position is consistent with outcome research on CT and pharmacotherapy (Blackburn et al. 1981) and with other studies that have documented neurobiological changes associated with conditioning in animals (Kandel and Schwartz 1982; Mohl 1987) or psychotherapy in humans (Baxter et al. 1992; Goldapple et al. 2004).

The working model in Figure 18–1 posits a close relationship between cognition and emotion. The general thrust of CT is that emotional responses are largely dependent upon cognitive appraisals of the significance of environmental cues. For example, sadness is likely when an event (or memory of an event) is perceived in a negative way (such as a loss, a defeat, or a rejection), and anger is common when it is judged that there are threats to one's self or loved ones.

Levels of Dysfunctional Cognitions

Beck and colleagues (A.T. Beck 1976; A.T. Beck et al. 1979; Dobson and Shaw 1986) have suggested that there are two major levels of

Table 18–1. Cognitive errors

Selective abstraction (sometimes termed "mental filter")	Drawing a conclusion based on only a small portion of the available data
Arbitrary inference	Coming to a conclusion without adequate supporting evidence or despite contradictory evidence
Absolutistic thinking ("all or none" thinking)	Categorizing oneself or personal experiences into rigid dichotomies (e.g., all good or all bad, perfect or completely flawed, success or total failure)
Magnification and minimization	Over- or undervaluing the significance of a personal attribute, a life event, or a future possibility
Personalization	Linking external occurrences to oneself (e.g., taking blame, assuming responsibility, criticizing oneself) when there is little or no basis for making these associations
Catastrophic thinking	Predicting the worst possible outcome while ignoring more likely eventualities

Source.   Adapted from Beck AT, Rush AJ, Shaw BF, Emery G: *Cognitive Therapy of Depression.* New York, Guilford Press, 1979. Used with permission.

dysfunctional information processing: 1) automatic thoughts and 2) basic beliefs incorporated in schemas. Automatic thoughts are the cognitions that occur rapidly while a person is in a situation (or recalling an event). These automatic thoughts usually are not subjected to rational analysis and often are based on erroneous logic. Although the individual may be only subliminally aware of these cognitions, automatic thoughts are accessible through questioning techniques used in CT (A.T. Beck et al. 1979; Wright and Beck 1983). The different types of faulty logic in automatic thinking have been termed *cognitive errors* (A.T. Beck et al. 1979). Descriptions of typical cognitive errors, such as selective abstraction, arbitrary inference, and absolutistic thinking, are provided in Table 18–1.

Schemas are deeper cognitive structures that contain the basic rules for screening, filtering, and coding information from the environment (A.T. Beck et al. 1979; D.A. Clark et al. 1999; Wright and Beck 1983). These organizing constructs are developed through early childhood experiences and subsequent formative influences. Schemas can play a highly adaptive role in allowing rapid assimilation of data and appropriate decision making. However, in psychiatric disorders there are clusters

of maladaptive schemas that perpetuate dysphoric mood and ineffective or self-defeating behavior (A.T. Beck 1976; A.T. Beck and Freeman 1990). Examples of adaptive and maladaptive schemas are presented in Table 18–2.

Cognitive Pathology in Depression and Anxiety Disorders

The role of cognitive functioning in depression and anxiety disorders has been studied extensively. Information processing also has been examined in eating disorders, characterological problems, and other psychiatric conditions. In general, the results of this investigative effort have confirmed Beck's hypotheses (A.T. Beck 1963, 1964, 1976; A.T. Beck et al. 1979; D.A. Clark et al. 1999; Wright and Beck 1983). These findings have played an important role in both confirming and shaping the treatment procedures used in CT.

Reviews of the voluminous research on cognitive processes in depression have found strong evidence for a negative cognitive bias in this disorder (D.A. Clark et al. 1999). For example, distorted automatic thoughts and cognitive errors have been found to be much more frequent in de-

Table 18–2. Adaptive and maladaptive schemas

Adaptive	Maladaptive
No matter what happens, I can manage somehow.	I must be perfect to be accepted.
If I work at something, I can master it.	If I choose to do something, I must succeed.
I'm a survivor.	I'm a fake.
Others can trust me.	Without a woman [man], I'm nothing.
I'm lovable.	I'm stupid.
People respect me.	No matter what I do, I won't succeed.
I can figure things out.	Others can't be trusted.
If I prepare in advance, I usually do better.	I can never be comfortable around others.
I like to be challenged.	If I make one mistake, I'll lose everything.
There's not much that can scare me.	The world is too frightening for me.

pressed persons than in control subjects (Blackburn et al. 1986; Dobson and Shaw 1986), and substantial evidence has been collected to support the concept of the negative cognitive triad (D. A. Clark et al. 1999).

Findings of studies on cognitive pathology in depression and anxiety disorders are summarized in Table 18–3.

Therapeutic Principles

General Procedures

CT is usually a short-term treatment, lasting from 5 to 20 sessions. In some instances, very brief treatment courses are used for patients with mild or circumscribed problems, or longer series of CT sessions are used for those with chronic or especially severe conditions. However, the typical patient with major depression or an anxiety disorder can be treated successfully within the short-term format. After completion of the initial course of treatment, intermittent booster sessions may be useful in some cases, particularly for individuals with a history of recurrent illness or incomplete remission.

The bulk of the therapeutic effort in CT is devoted to working on specific problems or issues in the patient's present life. The problem-oriented approach is emphasized for several reasons. First, directing the patient's attention to current problems stimulates the development of action plans that can help reverse helplessness, hopelessness, avoidance, or other dysfunctional symptoms. Second, data on cognitive responses to recent life events are more readily accessible and verifiable than for events that happened years in the past. Third, practical work on present problems helps to prevent the development of excessive dependency or regression in the therapeutic relationship. Finally, current problems usually provide ample opportunity to understand and explore the impact of past experiences.

The Therapeutic Relationship

The therapeutic relationship in CT is characterized by a high degree of collaboration between patient and therapist and an empirical tone to the work of therapy. The therapist and patient function much like an investigative team. They develop hypotheses about the validity of automatic thoughts and schemas or alternately about the effectiveness of patterns of behavior. A series of exercises or experiments is then designed to test the validity of the hypotheses and, subsequently, to modify cognitions or behavior. A. T. Beck et al. (1979) have termed this form of therapeutic relationship *collaborative empiricism*. Methods of building a collaborative and empirical relationship are listed in Table 18–4.

Table 18–3. Pathological information processing in depression and anxiety disorders

Predominant in depression	Predominant in anxiety disorders	Common to both depression and anxiety disorders
Hopelessness	Fears of harm or danger	Demoralization
Low self-esteem	High sensitivity to information about potential threat	Self-absorption
Negative view of environment		Heightened automatic information processing
Automatic thoughts with negative themes	Automatic thoughts associated with danger, risk, uncontrollability, incapacity	Maladaptive schemas
Misattributions	Overestimates of risk in situations	Reduced cognitive capacity for problem solving
Overestimates of negative feedback	Enhanced recall of memories for threatening situations	
Enhanced recall of negative memories		
Impaired performance on cognitive tasks requiring effort, abstract thinking		

Table 18–4. Methods of enhancing collaborative empiricism

Work together as an investigative team.

Adjust therapist activity level to match the severity of illness and phase of treatment.

Encourage self-monitoring and self-help.

Obtain accurate assessment of validity of cognitions and efficacy of behavior.

Develop coping strategies for real losses and actual deficits.

Promote essential "nonspecific" therapist variables (e.g., kindness, empathy, equanimity, positive general attitude).

Provide and request feedback on regular basis.

Recognize and manage transference.

Customize therapy interventions.

Use gentle humor.

The therapist usually is more active in CT than in most other psychotherapies. The degree of therapist activity varies with the stage of treatment and the severity of the illness. Generally, a more directive and structured approach is emphasized early in treatment, when symptoms are severe. For example, a markedly depressed patient who is beginning treatment may benefit from considerable direction and structure because of symptoms such as helplessness, hopelessness, low energy, and impaired concentration. As the patient improves and understands more about the methods of CT, the therapist can become somewhat less active. By the end of treatment, the patient should be able to use self-monitoring and self-help techniques with little reinforcement from the therapist.

Collaborative empiricism is fostered throughout the therapy, even when directive work is required. Although the therapist may suggest specific strategies or give homework assignments designed to combat severe depression or anxiety, the patient's input is always solicited and the self-help component of CT is emphasized from the outset of treatment. Also, it is made clear that CT is not an attempt to convert all negative thoughts to positive ones. In fact, bad things do occur to people, and some individuals have behaviors that are ineffective or self-defeating. It is emphasized that in CT one seeks to obtain an accurate assessment of 1) the validity of cognitions, and 2) the adaptive versus maladaptive

nature of behavior. If cognitive distortions have occurred, then the patient and therapist will work together to develop a more rational perspective. On the other hand, if actual negative experiences or characteristics are identified, they will attempt to find ways to cope or to change.

The development of a collaborative working relationship is dependent on a number of therapist and patient characteristics. The "nonspecific" therapist variables that are important components of all effective psychotherapies (Davis and Wright 1994; Wright et al. 2006) are equally significant in CT (see Table 18–4).

Additional procedures that cognitive therapists use to encourage collaborative empiricism are 1) providing feedback throughout sessions, 2) recognizing and managing transference, 3) customizing therapy interventions, and 4) using gentle humor. The therapist gives feedback to keep the therapeutic relationship anchored in the "here and now" and to reinforce the working aspect of the therapy process. Comments are made frequently throughout the session to summarize major points, to give direction, and to keep the session on target. Also, questions are asked at several intervals in each session to determine how well the patient has understood a concept or has grasped the essence of a therapeutic intervention. Because CT is highly psychoeducational, the therapist functions to some degree as a teacher. Thus, discreet positive feedback is given to help stimulate and reward the patient's efforts to learn.

Patients also are encouraged to give feedback throughout the sessions. In the beginning of treatment, patients are told that the therapist will want to hear from them regularly about how the sessions are going. What are the patient's reactions to the therapist? What things are going well? What would the patient like to change? What points are clear and make sense? What seems confusing?

Another feature of CT that increases the collaborative nature of the therapeutic relationship is the customization of therapy interventions to meet the level of the patient's cognitive and social functioning. A profoundly depressed or anxious individual of low average intelligence may require a primarily behavioral approach, with limited efforts at understanding concepts such as automatic thoughts and schemas, especially in the beginning of treatment. Conversely, a less symptomatic patient with higher intelligence and ability to grasp abstract concepts may be able to profit from schema assessment early in therapy. If treatment procedures are pitched at a proper level, the patient is more likely to understand the material of therapy and to form a collaborative relationship with the therapist who is directing the treatment.

The therapeutic relationship also can be enhanced by using gentle humor during CT sessions. For example, the therapist may encourage the patient's sense of humor by providing opportunities to laugh together at some improbable situation or humorously distorted cognition. Humor needs to be injected carefully into the therapeutic relationship. However, appropriate use of humor can strengthen the therapeutic relationship in CT if patient and therapist are able to laugh with one another and to use humor to deflate exaggerated or distorted cognitions.

Assessment and Case Conceptualization

Assessment for CT begins with completion of a standard history and mental status exami-

nation. Although special attention is paid to cognitive and behavioral elements, a full biopsychosocial evaluation is completed and used in formulating the treatment plan. The Academy of Cognitive Therapy, a certifying organization for cognitive therapists, has outlined a method for assessment and case conceptualization. This method involves consideration of developmental influences, family history, social and interpersonal issues, genetic and biological contributions, and strengths and assets, in addition to key automatic thoughts, schemas, and behavioral patterns (Figure 18–2). The book *Learning Cognitive-Behavior Therapy: An Illustrated Guide* (Wright et al. 2006) provides detailed methods, worksheets, and examples of use of the Academy of Cognitive Therapy formulation methods. Worksheets from this book can be downloaded from the American Psychiatric Publishing Inc. Web site (www.appi.org). Also, the Academy of Cognitive Therapy Web site (www.academyofct.org) supplies illustrations of how to complete case conceptualizations.

Structuring Therapy

Several of the structuring procedures commonly employed in CT are listed in Table 18–5. One of the most important techniques for CT is the use of a therapy agenda. At the beginning of each session, the therapist and patient work together to derive a short list of topics, usually consisting of two to four items. Generally, it is advisable to shape an agenda that 1) can be managed within the time frame of an individual session, 2) follows up on material from earlier sessions, 3) reviews any homework from the previous session and provides an opportunity for new homework assignments, and 4) contains specific items that are highly relevant to the patient but are not too global or abstract.

Agenda setting helps to counteract hopelessness and helplessness by reducing seemingly overwhelming problems down into workable segments. The agenda-setting process also encourages patients to take a prob-

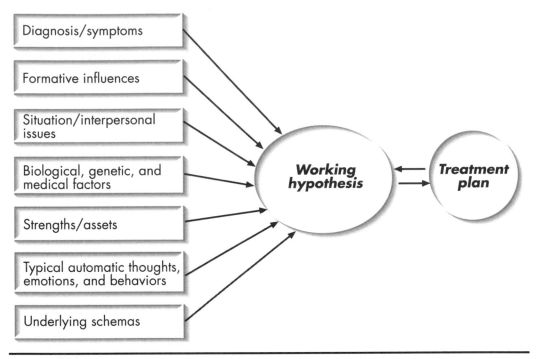

Figure 18–2.   Case conceptualization flow chart.

Source.   Reprinted from Wright JH, Basco MR, Thase ME: *Learning Cognitive-Behavior Therapy: An Illustrated Guide* (Core Competencies in Psychotherapy Series, Glen O. Gabbard, series ed.). Washington, DC, American Psychiatric Publishing, 2006, p. 51. Copyright 2006, American Psychiatric Publishing. Used with permission.

lem-oriented approach to their difficulties. Simply articulating a problem in a specific manner often can initiate the process of change. In addition, the agenda keeps the patient focused on salient issues and encourages efficient use of the therapy time.

Feedback procedures described earlier are also used in structuring CT sessions. For example, the therapist may observe that the patient is drifting from the established agenda or is spending time discussing a topic of questionable relevance. In situations such as these, constructive feedback is given to direct the patient back to a more profitable area of inquiry.

Commonly used CT techniques add an additional structural element to the therapy. Examples include activity scheduling, thought recording, and graded task assignments. Repeated use of procedures such as recording, labeling, and modifying automatic thoughts helps to link sessions together, especially if they are introduced in therapy and then assigned as homework.

Psychoeducation

Psychoeducational procedures are a routine component of CT. One of the major goals of the treatment approach is to teach patients a new way of thinking and behaving that can be applied in resolving their current symptoms and in managing problems that will be

---

Table 18–5.   Structuring procedures for cognitive therapy

Set agenda for therapy sessions.
Give constructive feedback to direct the course of therapy.
Employ common cognitive therapy techniques on a regular basis.
Assign homework to link sessions together.

encountered in the future. The psychoeducational effort usually begins with the process of socializing the patient to therapy. In the opening phase of treatment, the therapist explains the basic concepts of CT and introduces the patient to the format of CT sessions. The therapist also devotes time early in treatment to discussing the therapeutic relationship in CT and the expectations for both patient and therapist. Psychoeducational work during a course of CT often involves brief explanations or illustrations coupled with homework assignments. These activities are woven into treatment sessions in a manner that emphasizes a collaborative, active learning approach. Some cognitive therapists have described the use of "mini-lectures," but a heavily didactic approach is generally avoided.

Psychoeducation can be facilitated with reading assignments and computer programs that reinforce learning, deepen the patient's understanding of CT principles, and promote the use of self-help methods. Table 18–6 contains a list of useful psychoeducational tools, including a pamphlet, books, and a computer

program, that teach the CT model and encourage self-help. Most cognitive therapists liberally use psychoeducational tools as a basic part of the therapy process.

Cognitive Techniques

Identifying Automatic Thoughts

Much of the work of CT is devoted to recognizing and then modifying negatively distorted or illogical automatic thoughts (Table 18–7). The most powerful way of introducing the patient to the effects of automatic thoughts is to find an in vivo example of how automatic thoughts can influence emotional responses. Mood shifts during the therapy session are almost always good places to pause to identify automatic thoughts. The therapist observes that a strong emotion such as sadness, anxiety, or anger has appeared and then asks the patient to describe the thoughts that "went through your head" just prior to the mood shift. This technique is illustrated in the exam-

Table 18–6. Psychoeducational materials and programs for cognitive therapy

Title	Authors	Description
"Coping With Anxiety"	A.T. Beck et al. 1985	Appendix to book
"Coping With Depression"	A.T. Beck et al. 1995	Short booklet
Feeling Good	Burns 1980, 1999	Book with self-help program
Getting Your Life Back: The Complete Guide to Recovery From Depression	Wright and Basco 2002	Book with self-help program; integrates cognitive therapy and biological approaches
Good Days Ahead: The Multimedia Program for Cognitive Therapy	Wright et al. 2004	Computer-assisted therapy and self-help program
Mastery of Your Anxiety and Panic	Barlow and Craske 1999	Self-help workbook for anxiety
Mind Over Mood	Greenberger and Padesky 1995	Self-help workbook
Never Good Enough	Basco 1999	Book on perfectionism
Stop Obsessing! How to Overcome Your Obsessions and Compulsions	Foa and Wilson 2001	Self-help book for obsessive-compulsive disorder

Table 18–7. Methods for identifying and modifying automatic thoughts

Socratic questioning (guided discovery)
Use of mood shifts to demonstrate automatic thoughts in vivo
Imagery exercises
Role-play
Thought recording
Generating alternatives
Examining the evidence
Decatastrophizing
Cognitive rehearsal

ple of Mr. B, a 50-year-old depressed man who had suffered several recent losses and had developed extremely low self-esteem.

Therapist: "How did you react to your wife's criticism?"

Mr. B: (Suddenly appears much more sad and anxious) "It was just too much to take."

Therapist: "I can see this really upsets you. Can you think back to what went through your mind right after I asked you the last question? Just try to tell me all the thoughts that popped into your head."

Mr. B: (Pause, then recounts) "I'm always making mistakes. I can't do anything right. There's no way to please her. I might as well give up."

Therapist: "I can see why you felt so sad. When these kinds of thoughts just automatically pop into your mind, you don't stop to think if they are accurate or not. That's why we call them automatic thoughts."

Mr. B: "I guess you're right. I hardly realized I was having those thoughts until you asked me to say them out loud."

Therapist: "Recognizing that you're having automatic thoughts is one of the first steps in therapy. Now let's see what we can do to help you with your thinking and with the situation with your wife."

One of the most frequently used procedures in CT is Socratic questioning. There is no set format or protocol for this technique. Instead, the therapist must rely on his or her experience and ingenuity to formulate questions that will help patients move from having a "closed mind" to a state of inquisitiveness and curiosity. Socratic questioning stimulates recognition of dysfunctional cognitions and development of a sense of dissonance about the validity of strongly held assumptions.

Socratic questioning usually involves a series of inductive questions that are likely to reveal dysfunctional thought patterns. The use of this technique to identify automatic thoughts is illustrated in the case of Ms. P, a 42-year-old woman with an anxiety disorder.

Therapist: "What things seem to trigger your anxiety?"

Ms. P: "Everything. It seems like no matter what I do, I'm nervous all the time."

Therapist: "I suppose that 'everything' could trigger your anxiety and that you have no control over it. But let's stop for a moment and see if there are any other possibilities. Is that okay?"

Ms. P: "Sure."

Therapist: "Then try to think of a situation where your anxiety is very high and one where it's much lower."

Ms. P: "Well, a high-anxiety time would be whenever I try to go out in public, like to go shopping or to a party. And a low-anxiety time would be sitting at home watching TV."

Therapist: "So there's some variation depending on what you are doing at the time."

Ms. P: "I guess that's right."

Therapist: "Would you like to find out what's behind the variation?"

Ms. P: "I guess. But I suppose it's just because being out with people makes me nervous and being at home feels safe."

Therapist: "That's one explanation. I wonder if there might be any others—ones that would give you some clues on how to get over the problem."

Ms. P: "I'm willing to look."

Therapist: "Well then, let's try to find out something about the different thoughts that you have about these two situations. When you think of going out to a party, what comes to mind?"

Ms. P: "I'll be embarrassed. I won't have any idea what to say or do. I'll probably panic and run out the door."

Imagery and role-play are used as alternate methods of uncovering cognitions when direct questions are unsuccessful in generating suspected automatic thinking (A.T. Beck et al. 1979). Some patients may be able to use imagery procedures with few prompts or directions. In this case, the clinician may only need to ask the patient to imagine himself or herself back in a particularly troubling or emotion-provoking situation and then to describe the thoughts that occurred. However, most patients, particularly in the early phases of therapy, can benefit from "setting the scene" for the use of imagery. The patient is asked to describe the details of the setting. When and where did the incident take place? What happened immediately before the incident? How did the characters in the scene appear?

Role-play is a related technique for evoking automatic thoughts. When this procedure is used, the therapist first asks a series of questions to try to understand a vignette involving an interpersonal relationship or other social interchange that is likely to stimulate dysfunctional automatic thinking. Then, with the permission of the patient, the therapist briefly steps into the role of the individual in the scene and facilitates the playing out of a typical response set.

Thought recording is one of the most frequently used CT procedures for identifying automatic thoughts (J. Beck 1995; Wright et al. 2006). Patients can be asked to log their thoughts in a number of different ways. For example, a three-column exercise could include a description of the situation, a list of automatic thoughts, and a notation of the emotional response. Thought recording helps the patient to recognize the effects of underlying automatic thoughts and to understand how the basic cognitive model (i.e., relationship between situations, thoughts, feelings, and behaviors) applies to his or her own experiences. This procedure also initiates the process of modifying dysfunctional cognitions.

Modifying Automatic Thoughts

There usually is no sharp division in CT between the phases of eliciting and modifying automatic thoughts. In fact, the processes involved in identifying automatic thoughts often are enough to initiate substantive change. As the patient begins to recognize the nature of his or her dysfunctional thinking, there typically is an increased degree of skepticism regarding the validity of automatic thoughts. Although patients can start to revise their cognitive distortions without specific additional therapeutic interventions, modification of automatic thoughts can be accelerated if the therapist applies Socratic questioning and other basic CT procedures to the change process (see Table 18–7).

Techniques used for revising automatic thoughts include 1) generating alternatives, 2) examining the evidence, 3) decatastrophizing, 4) thought recording, and 5) cognitive rehearsal (A.T. Beck et al. 1979; J. Beck 1995; Wright et al. 2006). Socratic questioning is used in all of these procedures.

Generating alternatives is illustrated in the case of Ms. D, a 32-year-old woman with major depression. The therapist's questions were pointed toward helping Ms. D to see a broader range of possibilities than she had originally considered.

Ms. D: "Every time I think of going back to school, I panic."

Therapist: "And when you start to think of going to school, what thoughts come to mind?"

Ms. D: "I'll botch it up. I won't be able to make it. I'll feel so ashamed when I have to drop out."

Therapist: "What else could happen? Anything even worse, or are there any better possibilities?"

Ms. D: "Well, it couldn't get much worse unless I never even tried at all."

Therapist: "How would that be so bad?"

Ms. D: "Then I'd just be the same—stuck in a rut, not going anywhere."

Therapist: "We can take a look at that conclusion later—that not going to school would mean that you would stay in a rut; but for now let's look at the other possibilities if you do try to go to school again."

Ms. D: "Okay. I guess there's some chance that it would go pretty well, but it'll be hard for me to manage school, the house, and all my family responsibilities."

Therapist: "When you try to step back from the situation and not listen to your automatic thoughts, what's the most likely outcome of your going back to school?"

Ms. D: "It will be a difficult adjustment, but it's something I want to do. I have the intelligence to do it if I apply myself."

Examining the evidence is a major component of the collaborative empirical experience in CT. Specific automatic thoughts or clusters of related automatic thoughts are set forth as hypotheses, and the patient and therapist then search for evidence both for and against the hypothesis. In the case of Ms. D, the thought "If I don't go to school, I'd just be the same—stuck in a rut, not going anywhere" was selected for an examining-the-evidence exercise. The therapist believed that returning to school was probably an adaptive action for the patient to take. However, it also was

thought that seeing further education as the only route to change would excessively load this activity with a "make or break" mentality and would promote a disregard for other modifications that might increase self-esteem and self-efficacy.

Decatastrophizing involves efforts to reconceptualize feared outcomes in a manner that encourages coping and problem solving. This technique can be effective even if there is a reasonably high likelihood that a negative prediction will actually occur. For example, a man might correctly judge his marriage to be so troubled that his wife may ask for a divorce. In this instance, the therapist would help the patient to recognize distorted cognitions about his ability to manage a possible breakup of the marriage. The patient might think, "I couldn't make it without her" or "I'd lose everything." The decatastrophizing procedure would involve examining negative automatic thoughts for their validity; looking for previously unrecognized attributes, interests, or coping mechanisms; reviewing the ways that the patient had managed losses in the past; and stimulating the patient to think beyond the immediate situation.

Five-column Thought Change Records (TCRs; A. T. Beck et al. 1979) or other similar thought-recording devices are standard tools used in modification of automatic thoughts. The five-column TCR is used to encourage both identification and change of dysfunctional cognitions. A fourth (rational response) and fifth (outcome) column are added to the three-column thought record (situation, automatic thoughts, and emotions) typically used to identify automatic thoughts. There are a wide variety of procedures that can be used to facilitate the development of rational thoughts for the TCR.

Most patients can learn about cognitive errors and can start to label specific instances of erroneous logic in their automatic thoughts. This is often the first step in generating a more rational pattern of cognitive responses to life events. This process is illustrated in the case of Mr. E, a 58-year-old man with major depression, who completed a TCR during the middle phase of CT (Table 18–8). He had learned how to use the TCR during prior therapy sessions and had been acquainted with the concept of cognitive errors through therapy experiences and from reading self-help materials (see Table 18–6). Mr. E noted the particular cognitive errors involved with each of his automatic thoughts and wrote out a more rational set of cognitions.

Techniques such as generating alternatives and examining the evidence also are used by the patient in a self-help format when the TCR is assigned for homework. In addition, the therapist often is able to help the patient refine or add to the list of rational thoughts when the TCR is reviewed at a subsequent therapy session. Repeated attention to generating rational thoughts on the TCR is usually quite helpful in breaking maladaptive patterns of automatic and negatively distorted thinking.

The fifth column of the TCR, outcome, is used to record any changes that have occurred as a result of revising and modifying automatic thoughts. In the case of Mr. E, there was a significant decrease in dysphoric affect. Although the use of the TCR will usually lead to the development of a more adaptive set of cognitions and a reduction in painful affect, on some occasions the initial automatic thoughts will prove to be accurate. In such situations, the therapist helps the patient take a problem-solving approach, including the development of an action plan, to manage the stressful or upsetting event.

Cognitive rehearsal is used to help uncover potential negative automatic thoughts in advance and to coach the patient in ways of developing more adaptive cognitions. First, the patient is asked to use imagery or role-play to identify possible distorted cognitions that could occur in a stressful situation. Second, the patient and therapist work together to modify the dysfunctional cognitions. Third, imagery or role-play is used again, this time to practice the more adaptive pattern of thinking. Finally, for a homework assign-

ment, the patient is asked to try out the newly acquired cognitive patterns in vivo.

Identifying and Modifying Schemas

The process of identifying and modifying schemas is somewhat more difficult than changing negative automatic thoughts because these core beliefs are more deeply embedded, may be largely out of the patient's awareness, and usually have been reinforced through years of life experience. However, many of the same techniques described for automatic thoughts are employed successfully in therapeutic work at the schema level (A. T. Beck et al. 1979; Wright et al. 2006). Procedures such as Socratic questioning, imagery, role-play, and thought recording are used to uncover maladaptive schemas (Table 18–9).

Modification of schemas may require repeated attention, both in and out of therapy sessions. One commonly used procedure is to ask the patient to keep a list in a therapy notebook of all the schemas that have been identified to date. The schema list can be reviewed before each session. This technique promotes a high level of awareness of schemas and usually encourages the patient to place issues pertaining to schemas on the agenda for therapy.

CT interventions that are particularly helpful in modifying schemas include examining the evidence, listing advantages and disadvantages, generating alternatives, and using cognitive rehearsal. After a schema has been identified, the therapist may ask the patient to do a pro/con analysis (examining the evidence) using a double-column procedure. This technique usually induces the patient to doubt the validity of the schema and to start to think of alternate explanations. An examining-the-evidence intervention is illustrated in the case of Ms. R, a 24-year-old woman with depression and bulimia (Table 18–10). During the course of her CT, Ms. R identified an important schema that was affecting both the depression and the eating disorder ("I must

Table 18–8. Thought Change Record—an example

Situation	Automatic thought(s)	Emotion(s)	Rational response	Outcome
Describe: a. Actual event leading to unpleasant emotion; or b. Stream of thoughts, daydream, or recollection leading to unpleasant emotion; or c. Unpleasant physiological sensations	a. Write automatic thought(s) that preceded emotion(s). b. Rate belief in automatic thought(s), 0%–100%.	a. Specify sad, anxious, angry, etc. b. Rate degree of emotion, 1%–100%.	a. Identify cognitive errors. b. Write rational response to automatic thought(s). c. Rate belief in rational response, 0%–100%.	a. Once again, rate belief in automatic thought(s), 0%–100%. b. Specify and rate subsequent emotion(s), 0%–100%.
Date: 4/15/98 I wake up and I'm immediately troubled. I start to worry about work.	1. I can't face another day. (90%)	Sad: 90% Anxious: 80%	1. Magnification. Even though it has been rough, I have been able to get to work every day. Get a shower and make breakfast—that will get things started. (80%)	Sad: 30% Anxious: 40%
	2. The big project is due in 2 weeks; I'll never get it done. (100%)		2. Catastrophizing, all-or-none thinking. About half of the work is done. Don't panic. Break it down into pieces. Taking one step at a time helps. (95%)	
	3. Everybody knows I'm ready to fall apart. (90%)		3. Overgeneralization, magnification. Some people know I've been in trouble, but they haven't gotten down on me. I'm the one who puts me down. (95%)	
	4. It's hopeless. (85%)		4. Magnification. I know my job well and have a good track record. If I stick with this, I can probably make it. (90%)	

Source. Adapted from Beck AT, Rush AJ, Shaw BF, Emery G: *Cognitive Therapy of Depression.* New York, Guilford Press, 1979. Used with permission.

Table 18–9. Methods for identifying and modifying schemas

Socratic questioning

Imagery and role play

Thought recording

Identifying repetitive patterns of automatic thoughts

Psychoeducation

Listing schemas in therapy notebook

Examining the evidence

Listing advantages and disadvantages

Generating alternatives

Cognitive rehearsal

---

be perfect to be accepted"). By examining the evidence, she was able to see that her schema was based at least in part on faulty logic.

Ms. R also used the listing advantages and disadvantages technique as part of the strategy to modify this maladaptive schema (Table 18–11). Some schemas appear to have few, if any, advantages (e.g., "I'm stupid"; "I'll always lose in the end"), but many schemas have both positive and negative features (e.g., "If I decide to do something, I must succeed"; "I always have to work harder than others or I'll fail"). The latter group of schemas may be maintained even in the face of their dysfunctional aspects because they en-

courage hard work, perseverance, or other behaviors that are adaptive. Yet the absolute and demanding nature of the schemas ultimately leads to excessive stress, failed expectations, low self-esteem, or other deleterious results. Listing advantages and disadvantages helps the patient to examine the full range of effects of the schema and often encourages modifications that can make the schema both more adaptive and less damaging. In Ms. R's case, this exercise set the stage for another step of schema modification, generating alternatives (Table 18–12).

Behavioral Procedures

Behavioral interventions are used in CT to 1) change dysfunctional patterns of behavior (e.g., helplessness, isolation, phobic avoidance, inertia, bingeing and purging); 2) reduce troubling symptoms (e.g., tension, somatic and psychic anxiety, intrusive thoughts); and 3) assist in identifying and modifying maladaptive cognitions. Table 18–13 presents a listing of behavioral techniques.

The Socratic questions used in cognitively oriented procedures have a direct parallel when the emphasis is on behavioral change. The therapist asks a series of questions that help differentiate actual behavioral deficits from negatively distorted accounts of

---

Table 18–10. Schema modification through examining the evidence

Schema: "I must be perfect to be accepted."

Evidence for	Evidence against
The better I do, the more people seem to like me.	Others who aren't "perfect" seem to be to be loved and accepted. Why should I be different?
Women who have a perfect figure are most attractive to men.	You don't have to have a perfect figure. Hardly anybody has one—just the models on television.
My parents have the highest standards; they are always pushing me to do better.	My parents want me to do well. But they'll probably accept me as long as I try to do my best, even if I don't meet all of their expectations. This statement is absolute and sets me up for failure, because no one can be perfect all the time.

Table 18–11. Schema modification through listing advantages and disadvantages

Schema: "I must be perfect to be accepted."

Advantages	Disadvantages
I've tried very hard to be the best.	I never really feel accepted because I've never reached perfection.
I've received top marks in school.	I'm always down on myself. I've developed bulimia. I'm obsessed with my body size.
I'm in lots of activities, and I've won dancing competitions.	I have trouble accepting my successes. I drive myself too hard and can't enjoy ordinary things.

Table 18–12. Schema modification through generating alternatives

Schema: "I must be perfect to be accepted."

Possible alternatives

People who are successful are more likely to be accepted.

If I try to do my best (even if it's not perfect), others are likely to accept me.

I would like to be perfect, but that's an impossible goal. I'll choose certain areas to try to excel (school, work, and career) and not demand perfection everywhere.

You don't need to be perfect to be accepted.

I'm worthy of love and acceptance without trying to be perfect.

Table 18–13. Behavioral procedures used in cognitive therapy

Questioning to identify behavioral patterns

Activity scheduling with mastery and pleasure recording

Self-monitoring

Graded task assignments

Behavioral rehearsal

Exposure and response prevention

Coping cards

Distraction

Relaxation exercises

Respiratory control

Assertiveness training

Modeling

Social skills training

behavior. Depressed and anxious patients usually overreport their symptomatic distress or the difficulties they have in managing situations. Often, well-framed questions can reveal cognitive distortions and also stimulate change as the patient considers the negative impact of dysfunctional behavior. Four specific behavioral techniques—activity scheduling, graded task assignments, exposure, and coping cards—are explained below. A more detailed description of behavioral methods is available in Wright et al. (2006) or Meichenbaum (1977).

Activity scheduling is a structured method of learning about the patient's behavioral patterns, encouraging self-monitoring, increasing positive mood, and designing strategies for change (A. T. Beck et al. 1979; Wright et al. 2006). A daily or weekly activity log is employed in which the patient is asked to record what he or she does during each hour of the day and then to rate each activity for mastery and pleasure on a 0–10 scale. When the activity record is first introduced, the patient usually is asked to make a record of baseline activities without attempting to make any changes. The data are then reviewed in the next therapy session.

Almost invariably, the patient rates some activities higher than others on mastery and/ or pleasure. For example, Mr. G, a 48-year-old depressed man who had told his therapist that "I don't enjoy anything anymore," described several activities on his daily activity log that contradicted this statement. Reading while sitting alone was rated as a 6 on mastery and 8 on pleasure, and attending his son's choir concert was rated as 7 on mastery and 10 on pleasure. Conversely, attempting to work in his home office was rated as a 1 on mastery and a 0 on pleasure. Discussion of the activity scheduling assignment with Mr. G helped him to see that he was still capable of performing reasonably well in certain activities and also that he was able to derive considerable enjoyment from some of his actions. In addition, the schedule was used to target problem areas (e.g., working in his home office) that would require further work in therapy. Finally, the activity schedule provided data that could be used in adjusting Mr. G's daily routine to promote a heightened sense of mastery and greater enjoyment.

Another behavioral procedure, the graded task assignment, can be used when the patient is facing a situation that seems excessively difficult or overwhelming. A challenging behavioral goal is broken down into small steps that can be taken one at a time. The graded task assignment is somewhat similar to the systematic desensitization protocols that are used in traditional behavior therapy (Wolpe 1969). However, a cognitive component is added to the methodology. There is an added emphasis placed on improving self-esteem and self-efficacy, countering hopelessness and helplessness, and using the graded task assignment to disprove maladaptive thoughts and schemas. With depressed individuals, the graded task assignment typically is used as a problem-solving technique. This stepwise approach, coupled with cognitive techniques such as Socratic questioning and thought recording, can reactivate the patient and focus his or her energy in a productive manner.

An example of the use of a graded task assignment can be found in the case of Mr. G, the 48-year-old man described earlier. One of the particularly troublesome items uncovered with activity scheduling was the patient's difficulty in getting to work at his home office. Socratic questioning revealed that Mr. G had been unable to work in his home office for over 6 weeks. Mail, bills, and correspondence

with friends were piled up to the point that he saw the situation as impossible. Cognitions related to this problem included automatic thoughts such as "It's too much....I've procrastinated too long this time....I'm totally swamped....I can't handle it."

The therapist and patient constructed a series of steps that encouraged Mr. G to approach the task and eventually master the problem. The graded task assignment included the following steps: 1) walk into the office and sit down at the desk for at least 15 minutes; 2) spend at least 20 minutes sorting mail into categories; 3) open and discard any junk mail; 4) open and read any personal letters and write list of responses required; 5) open and stack all bills; 6) clean office; 7) respond in writing to at least one letter; 8) balance checkbook; 9) pay all current or overdue bills; 10) respond to additional letters if necessary. Reasonable goals for specific time intervals were discussed, and the therapist used coaching, Socratic questioning, and other cognitive techniques to help Mr. G accomplish the task.

Exposure techniques are a central part of cognitive-behavioral approaches to anxiety disorders. For example, a phobia can be conceptualized as an unrealistic fear of an object or a situation coupled with a conditioned pattern of avoidance. Treatment can proceed along two complementary lines: cognitive restructuring to modify the dysfunctional thoughts and exposure therapy to break the pattern of avoidance. Typically, a hierarchy of feared stimuli is developed with the patient. The hierarchy should contain a number of different stimuli that cause varying degrees of distress. Usually the items are ranked by degree of distress. One commonly used system involves rating each item on a scale from 0 to 100, with 100 representing the maximum distress possible. After the hierarchy is established, the therapist and patient work collaboratively to set goals for gradual exposure, starting with the items that are ranked lower on the distress scale. Breathing training, relaxation exercises, and other be-

> **Situation:** My girlfriend comes in late or does something else that makes me think she doesn't care.
>
> **Coping Strategies:**
> - Spot my extreme thinking, especially when I use words like <u>never</u> or <u>always</u>.
> - Stand back from the situation and check my thinking before I start yelling.
> - Think of the positive parts of our relationship.
> - Take a "time-out" if I start getting into a rage.
> - Tell her that I need to take a break to calm down.
> - Take a brief walk or go to another room.

Figure 18–3.   Mr. W's coping card.

This example shows how Mr. W, a middle-aged man with bipolar disorder, developed an effective coping strategy for managing anger in situations with his girlfriend.
Source.   Wright et al. 2006.

havioral methods (see Table 18–13) may be used to enhance the patient's ability to carry out the exposure protocol.

Coping cards are another commonly used method to achieve behavioral change. The therapist helps the patient to identify specific actions that are likely to help her or him cope with an anticipated problem or put CT skills into action. These ideas are then written down on a small card, which the patient carries with her or him as a reminder and as a tool to help in solving problems. Coping cards often contain both cognitive and behavioral interventions, as illustrated in Figure 18–3.

Selection of Patients for Cognitive Therapy

CT procedures have been described for a large number of diagnostic categories (A.T. Beck 1993). Although there are no contraindications to using this treatment approach, CT is usually not attempted with patients who have marked brain disease. CT can be considered a primary treatment for 1) disorders in which it has been proved to be effective in controlled research (e.g., unipolar depression [nonpsychotic], anxiety disorders, eating disorders, and psychophysiological disorders), and 2) other conditions for which a clearly detailed treatment method has been developed (e.g., personality disorders, substance abuse) and there is some evidence for CT's effectiveness. CT should be considered an adjunctive therapy for disorders such as major depression with psychotic features, bipolar illness, and schizophrenia, in which there is clear evidence for the effectiveness of biological treatments and the effects of CT alone compared with pharmacotherapy have not been studied.

Clinical experience has suggested that patients who do not have severe character pathology (especially borderline or antisocial features), have previously formed trusting relationships with significant others, have a belief in the importance of self-reliance, and have a curious or inquisitive nature are especially suitable for CT (Wright et al. 2006). Above-average intelligence is not associated with better outcome, and CT procedures can be simplified for those with subnormal intellectual skills or impaired learning and memory functioning. Of course, most patients do not have a full combination of the ideal features noted above. A flexible approach can be employed in which CT procedures are customized to match the special characteristics of the patient's social background, intellectual level, personality structure, and clinical disorder (Wright et al. 2006).

Applications of Cognitive Therapy

The basic procedures described in this chapter are used in all CT applications. However, the targets for change, selection of techniques, and timing of interventions may vary depending on the condition being treated and the format for therapy. A full discussion of the multiple applications and formats for CT is beyond the scope of this chapter. The reader is referred to comprehensive books on CT for a more detailed accounting of the modifications of this treatment approach for different clinical disorders (see "Suggested Readings" at end of chapter). CT methods have been outlined for a number of clinical problems not covered here, including conditions such as personality disorders (A. T. Beck and Freeman 1990), substance abuse (Wright et al. 1993), bipolar disorder (Basco and Rush 2005), hypochondriasis (Warwick and Salkovskis 1990), and psychophysiological disorders (Sensky 2004). Group CT techniques have been described by Covi and Primakoff (1988) and Freeman et al. (1992); procedures for marital and family CT have been set forth by A.T. Beck (1988), Epstein et al. (1988), and others. In this portion of the chapter, we briefly examine the distinctive features of CT for four common psychiatric illnesses—depression, anxiety disorders, eating disorders, and psychosis.

Depression

In the opening phase of treatment of depression, the cognitive therapist focuses on establishing a collaborative relationship and introduces the patient to the cognitive model. Agendas, feedback, and psychoeducational procedures are used to structure sessions. The emphasis is placed on two major forms of cognitive dysfunction: negatively distorted thinking and deficits in learning and memory functioning. Early in therapy, a special effort may be placed on relieving hopelessness because of the close link between this element of the negative cognitive triad and suicide risk. Also, reduction in hopelessness can be an important step in reactivating and reenergizing the depressed patient. Behavioral techniques such as activity scheduling and graded task assignments often are a major component of the opening phase of CT for depression.

The middle portion of treatment is usually devoted to eliciting and modifying negatively distorted automatic thoughts. Behavioral techniques continue to be used in most cases. By this point in the therapy, patients should understand the cognitive model and be able to employ thought-monitoring techniques to reverse all three elements of the negative cognitive triad (self, world, and future). Typically, the patient is taught to identify cognitive errors (e.g., selective abstraction, arbitrary inference, absolutistic thinking) and to use procedures such as generating alternatives and examining the evidence to alter negatively distorted thinking.

Work on eliciting and testing automatic thoughts continues during the latter portion of treatment. However, if there have been gains in functioning and the patient has grasped the basic principles of CT, therapy can turn primarily to identifying and altering maladaptive schemas. The concept of schemas usually has been introduced earlier in therapy, but the principal efforts at changing these underlying structures are reserved for the late phase of treatment when the patient is more likely to grasp and retain complex therapeutic initiatives. Before therapy concludes, the therapist helps the patient review what has been learned during the course of treatment and also suggests thinking ahead to possible circumstances that could trigger a return of depression. The potential for relapse is recognized, and problem-solving strategies are developed that can be employed in future stressful situations.

Anxiety Disorders

Although the techniques used in CT for anxiety disorders are similar to those employed in the treatment of depression, treatment efforts are directed toward altering four major types of dysfunctional anxiety-producing cognitions: 1) overestimates of the likelihood of a feared event, 2) exaggerated estimates of the severity of a feared event, 3) underestimation of personal coping abilities, and 4) unrealistically low estimates of the help that others can offer. Most authors have recommended that a mixture of cognitive and behavioral measures be used in patients who have anxiety disorders (Barlow and Cerney 1988; A.T. Beck et al. 1985).

In panic disorder, the emphasis is placed on helping the patient to recognize and change grossly exaggerated estimates of the significance of physiological responses or fears of imminent psychological disaster (A.T. Beck et al. 1985, 1992; D.M. Clark 1986). For example, an individual with panic disorder may begin to perspire or breathe more rapidly, after which cognitions such as "I can't catch my breath....I'll pass out....I'll have a stroke" increase the intensity of the autonomic nervous system activity. The vicious cycle interaction between catastrophic cognitions and physiological arousal can be broken in two complementary ways: 1) altering the dysfunctional cognitions and 2) interrupting the cascading autonomic hyperactivity. Commonly used cognitive interventions include Socratic questioning, imagery, thought recording, generating alternatives, and examining the evidence. Behavioral measures such as relaxation training, positive imagery, and respiratory control are used to dampen the physiological arousal associated with panic (D.M. Clark et al. 1985). Also, when panic attacks are stimulated by specific situations

(e.g., driving, public speaking, crowds), graded exposure may be particularly useful in helping patients to both master a feared task and overcome their panic symptoms.

CT of phobic disorders centers on modifying unrealistic estimates of risk or danger in situations and engaging the patient in a series of graded exposure assignments. Generally, cognitive and behavioral procedures are used simultaneously. For example, a graded task assignment for an individual with agoraphobia might include a stepwise increase in experiences in a social setting accompanied by use of a TCR to record and revise maladaptive automatic thinking.

Behavioral techniques such as exposure and response prevention (ERP) are used together with cognitive restructuring for patients with obsessive-compulsive disorder (OCD) (Salkovskis 1985). Cognitive interventions include challenging the validity of obsessional thoughts, attempting to replace dysfunctional cognitions with positive self-statements, and modifying negative automatic thoughts. Salkovskis and Warwick (1985) have noted that cognitive procedures may be needed in some cases to help the patient engage in ERP. A combined approach of cognitive techniques to modify maladaptive thought patterns and behavioral interventions to counter patterns of avoidance is also used in CT for posttraumatic stress disorder (PTSD) (Harvey et al. 2003).

Eating Disorders

CT is a well-established first-line treatment for bulimia nervosa and binge-eating disorder. CT for both conditions was given a grade A rating by the United Kingdom's National Institute for Clinical Excellence, indicating that there is strong support for efficacy from empirical trials (Wilson and Shafran 2005).

Individuals with eating disorders may have many of the same cognitive distortions that are seen in depression. However, they have an additional cluster of cognitive biases about body image, eating behavior, and weight (D.A. Clark et al. 1989). Patients with eating disorders usually place inordinate value on body shape as a measure of self-worth and as a condition for acceptance (e.g., "I must be thin to be accepted"; "If I'm overweight, nobody will want me"; "Fat people are weak"). They also may believe that any variance from their excessive standards means a total loss of control. CT interventions are used to subject these maladaptive cognitions to empirical testing. Commonly used procedures include eliciting and testing automatic thoughts, examining the evidence, and giving in vivo homework assignments. In addition, behavioral techniques are used to stimulate more adaptive eating behavior and to uncover significant cognitions related to eating.

Psychosis

Psychotic illnesses are one of the indications for adjunctive CT. Although biological treatments are the accepted form of therapy for psychotic patients, several randomized, controlled trials have demonstrated that CT can reduce symptoms in patients who have residual symptomatology after stabilization on medication. It has also been observed that cognitive psychotherapy can help psychotic individuals understand their disorders, adhere to treatment recommendations, and develop more effective psychosocial functioning (Cochran 1986; Kingdon and Turkington 2005).

In CT of patients who have psychotic symptoms, the therapist conveys that maladaptive cognitions and reactions to life stress may interact with biological factors in the expression of the illness. Therefore, attempts to develop more adaptive cognitions or to learn how to cope better with environmental pressures can assist with efforts toward managing the disorder. During the early part of therapy with a psychotic patient, there is a strong emphasis on building a therapeutic alliance (Kingdon and Turkington 2005). The therapist tries to normalize and destigmatize the condition (Kingdon and Turkington 2005), and the rationale for antipsychotic medication in combination with CT is explained. Usually,

work on challenging hallucinations or delusions directly is delayed until a solid therapeutic relationship has been established. However, efforts are made to reverse delusional self-destructive cognitions as early as possible in the treatment process.

Reality testing is performed in a gentle, nonconfrontational manner (Kingdon and Turkington 2005). Usually delusions with lowest level of conviction are targeted first. The therapist uses guided discovery as a major intervention, but also may help the patient to record and change distorted automatic thoughts or perform examining-the-evidence exercises. Behavioral techniques such as activity scheduling, graded task assignments, and social skills training also are used with psychotic patients. These procedures can be used to provide needed structure or to teach adaptive behaviors. Negative symptoms are typically approached slowly in a manner that gives consideration to the difficulty of changing this manifestation of psychotic disorders (Kingdon and Turkington 2005).

Learning Cognitive Therapy

Psychiatry residents are now required to achieve competency in CT before completing their training, and many other mental health disciplines are emphasizing CT training in their educational programs. Also, clinicians who have previously completed their training without special emphasis on CT may be interested in gaining expertise in this approach. Although there are many ways to receive training in CT and to achieve competency, typical programs include at least a year of educational experiences with a series of didactic presentations, readings, video and role-play illustrations, and supervision.

Workshops on CT are offered at annual meetings of the American Psychiatric Association, the American Psychological Association, the Association for the Advancement of Behavioral and Cognitive Therapies, and others.

Basic textbooks used for training in CT include *Learning Cognitive-Behavior Therapy: An Illustrated Guide* (Wright et al. 2006), which includes a DVD with demonstrations of CT methods; *Cognitive Therapy: Basics and Beyond* (J. Beck 1995); and *Cognitive Behavioral Therapy for Clinicians* (Sudak 2006). Other recommended readings and Web sites are provided at the end of this chapter.

Effectiveness of Cognitive Therapy

CT has been investigated in many carefully designed outcome trials that have documented the effectiveness of this treatment approach. The most intensive research has been directed at CT of depression and anxiety disorders. However, there has been a steady increase in investigations of CT for eating disorders, psychosis, bipolar disorder, and other conditions (see, for example, Butler et al. 2006). Our focus here is on providing an overview of outcome research. Representative or especially important studies are discussed briefly to illustrate investigative work on CT.

Depression

Early studies of CT for depression have been the subject of a detailed review by Thase (2001). Meta-analyses of these studies have found that CT compares well with other treatments for depression, including antidepressant medications across 12–16 weeks of treatment (Dobson 1989; Gaffan et al. 1995; Robinson et al. 1990). In one of the most recent trials, a two-center study conducted at the University of Pennsylvania and Vanderbilt University (DeRubeis et al. 2005), CT was as effective as the selective serotonin reuptake inhibitor paroxetine, which in turn was significantly more effective than a double-blind placebo.

Several studies have investigated the durability of treatment effects across 1 and 2 years of follow-up. Results of these studies have generally supported the hypothesis that short-term CT has enduring benefits and that patients who respond to CT have a relatively low risk of subsequent relapse (Blackburn et al. 1981; Evans et al. 1992; Hollon et al. 2005; Kovacs et al. 1981; Simons et al. 1986). The only investigation that did not find clear-cut evidence that CT had an enduring effect was the National Institute of Mental Health Treatment of Depression Collaborative Research Program. However, as CT was not a particularly effective acute-phase therapy in this study (Elkin et al. 1995), it would not be expected to have an enduring effect (Thase 2001). Several other studies have focused on sequential CT treatment of residual symptoms following pharmacotherapy (Fava et al. 1996; Paykel et al. 1999) or longer-term models of CT (Jarrett et al. 2001) to reduce risk of relapse or recurrent depression. Taken together, results of these investigations provide further support for the view that CT can decrease the risk of relapse or recurrence.

Anxiety Disorders

CT also has been found to be an effective therapy for anxiety disorders, with particularly strong evidence emerging for treatment of panic disorder. Two major forms of CT have been tested: 1) panic control treatment (PCT), a combination of relaxation training, cognitive restructuring, and exposure (Barlow and Cerney 1988); and 2) focused cognitive therapy, a more cognitively oriented treatment that uses exposure but places less emphasis on behavioral interventions than does PCT (A.T. Beck et al. 1985). In the largest study of PCT conducted to date, Barlow et al. (2000) found its short-term effects comparable to those of imipramine; both active interventions were significantly more effective than a double-blind pill placebo–clinical management condition. Following termination of treatment, patients treated with PCT had more durable responses than those withdrawn from imipramine. In studies of focused CT, superiority was found in comparison to supportive psychotherapy (A.T. Beck et al. 1992) and relaxation training or imipramine (D.M. Clark et al. 1994).

Several well-executed studies have found evidence for the effectiveness of CT for social phobia (Davidson et al. 2004; Gelernter et al. 1991; Heimberg et al. 1990; Hope et al. 1995). In a large trial of 295 persons with social phobia, no differences in treatment response were found between subjects receiving group CT and those receiving fluoxetine (51.7% vs. 50.9%) (Davidson et al. 2004). In another trial, individual CT was superior to fluoxetine plus self-exposure (D.M. Clark et al. 2003).

ERP, a treatment that is primarily behavioral in focus, has been studied widely for OCD. ERP is typically combined with CT in comprehensive treatment packages (James and Blackburn 1995). Van Oppen et al. (1995) randomly assigned 71 patients with OCD who were not taking antidepressants to either Beck's form of CT or ERP. Both treatments led to statistically significant improvement, but CT was superior to ERP in reducing symptoms of OCD. In contrast, Whittal et al. (2005) found that CT and ERP were equally effective in treating OCD.

PTSD has also been shown to be responsive to CT. One example is the work of Foa et al. (2005), who compared CT with ERP in a large study ($n=171$) of women with chronic PTSD after sexual trauma. Both treatments were significantly better than a wait-list control condition in relieving symptoms of PTSD. Another study compared CT with supportive therapy and a wait-list control group in 78 persons with chronic PTSD symptoms after motor vehicle accidents (Blanchard et al. 2003). Results of this study indicated that CT was more effective than supportive therapy, which in turn was more effective than the wait-list condition.

Eating Disorders

Reviews of controlled studies of CT for bulimia nervosa have concluded that there is convincing evidence for the efficacy of cognitive-behavioral treatment (Mitchell et al. 1996; Ricca et al. 2000; Wilson 1999; Wilson and Shafran 2005). Typically, CT reduces the frequency of binge behaviors by 73%–93%

(Fairburn et al. 1992) and leads to a complete remission of bulimic symptoms in 51%–84% of cases (Carter et al. 2003; Ricca et al. 2000). Although binge-eating disorder has been studied less intensively than has bulimia nervosa, there is growing evidence that CT is also effective for this disorder (Ricca et al. 2000; Wilson 1999).

Psychosis

There has been growing interest in studying the use of CT and related therapies in psychotic disorders. A meta-analysis of 14 investigations completed between 1990 and 2004 found that cognitive-behavioral treatment was significantly better than adjunctive measures in lowering psychotic symptoms (Zimmerman et al. 2005). Although the overall results of studies of CT for nonaffective psychosis document additive effects in combination with medication and routine care, results have varied, and some studies have found only short-term benefit or partial impact on various psychotic symptoms. Possible explanations for such variability include differences in treatment methods or in the experience and skill of therapists.

Outcome Research in Other Disorders

The majority of CT outcome research has been concerned with depression, anxiety disorders, eating disorders, and psychosis. However, a substantial amount of investigative work has been completed on the efficacy of CT for other conditions, such as bipolar disorder, psychophysiological disorders, substance abuse, and personality disorders. Readers interested in this research are referred to a more detailed review of CT outcome studies (Wright et al. 2008).

Conclusion

CT is a recently developed system of psychotherapy that is linked philosophically with a long tradition of viewing cognition as a primary determinant of emotion and behavior. The theoretical constructs of CT are supported by a large body of experimental findings regarding dysfunctional information processing in psychiatric disorders. In clinical practice, CT is usually short term, problem oriented, and highly collaborative. Therapists and patients work together in an empirical style, seeking to identify and modify maladaptive patterns of thinking. Behavioral techniques are used to uncover distorted cognitions and to promote more effective functioning. Also, psychoeducational procedures and homework assignments help reinforce concepts learned in therapy sessions. The goals of CT include both immediate symptom relief and the acquisition of cognitive and behavioral skills that will decrease the risk for relapse.

The efficacy of CT for depression, generalized anxiety disorder, panic disorder, eating disorders, and other conditions has been established in a wide range of outcome studies. Newer applications for CT, such as personality disorders, substance abuse, and psychosis are beginning to receive attention from investigators. Detailed treatment manuals or other guidelines for therapy have been described for most psychiatric illnesses.

CT has rapidly evolved into one of the major psychotherapeutic orientations in modern psychiatric treatment. Future challenges for this therapy model include study of the relative importance of treatment components, detailed examination of predictors for outcome, elucidation of the interface between biological and cognitive processes, and incorporation of new developments in computer-assisted learning. The empirical nature of CT should promote further exploration of the potential uses for this treatment approach.

Key Points

- Studies of information processing in mental disorders have found characteristic patterns of cognitions that are linked with dysphoric emotions and maladaptive behavior.

- Treatment with cognitive therapy involves modification of dysfunctional cognitions and associated behaviors.

- Cognitive therapy is an active treatment characterized by a highly collaborative therapeutic relationship.

- Structure, psychoeducation, and homework are important components of treatment.

- Cognitive therapists help patients identify and change automatic thoughts and core beliefs (schemas).

- Behavioral methods are used to reverse helplessness, anhedonia, avoidance, and other core symptoms of mental disorders.

- Cognitive therapy has been extensively researched. There is strong empirical support for the efficacy of this treatment approach.

- Cognitive therapy methods have been developed for many conditions including mood and anxiety disorders, schizophrenia, eating disorders, substance abuse, and personality disorders.

Suggested Readings

Barlow DH, Cerney JA: Psychological Treatment of Panic. New York, Guilford, 1988

Basco MR, Rush AJ: Cognitive-Behavioral Therapy for Bipolar Disorder. New York, Guilford, 2005

Beck AT, Freeman A: Cognitive Therapy of Personality Disorders. New York, Guilford, 1990

Beck AT, Rush AJ, Shaw BF, et al: Cognitive Therapy of Depression. New York, Guilford, 1979

Beck AT, Emery GD, Greenberg RL: Anxiety Disorders and Phobias: A Cognitive Perspective. New York, Basic Books, 1985

Beck AT, Wright FD, Newman CF, et al: Cognitive Therapy of Substance Abuse. New York, Guilford, 1993

Beck J: Cognitive Therapy: Basics and Beyond. New York, Guilford, 1995

Clark DA, Beck AT, Alford BA: Scientific Foundations of Cognitive Theory and Therapy of Depression. New York, Wiley, 1999

Clark DM, Fairburn CG (eds): Science and Practice of Cognitive Behavior Therapy. New York, Oxford University Press, 1997

Fairburn C, Brownell K (eds): Eating Disorders and Obesity: A Comprehensive Handbook, 2nd Edition. New York, Guilford, 2002

Kingdon D, Turkington D: Cognitive Therapy for Schizophrenia. New York, Guilford, 2005

Leahy RL: Contemporary Cognitive Therapy: Theory, Research, and Practice. New York, Guilford, 2004

Linehan MM: Cognitive-Behavioral Treatment of Borderline Personality Disorder. New York, Guilford, 1993

Mahoney MJ, Freeman A (eds): Cognition and Psychotherapy. New York, Plenum, 1985

Meichenbaum DB: Cognitive-Behavior Modification: An Integrative Approach. New York, Plenum, 1977

Reinecke MA, Dattilio FM, Freeman A (eds): Cognitive Therapy With Children and Adolescents: A Casebook for Clinical Practice, 2nd Edition. New York, Guilford, 2003

Salkovskis PM (ed): Frontiers of Cognitive Therapy. New York, Guilford, 1996

Wilkes TCR, Belsher G, Rush AJ, et al: Cognitive Therapy for Depressed Adolescents. New York, Guilford, 1994

Wright JH, Basco MR, Thase ME: Learning Cognitive-Behavior Therapy: An Illustrated Guide (Core Competencies in Psychotherapy Series, Glen O. Gabbard, series ed). Washington, DC, American Psychiatric Publishing, 2006

Online Resources

Academy of Cognitive Therapy: www.academyofCT.org

American Psychiatric Publishing, Inc. (for downloading of worksheets from *Learning Cognitive-Behavior Therapy: An Illustrated Guide,* by J.H. Wright, M.R. Basco, and M.E. Thase): www.appi.org

Association for Behavioral and Cognitive Therapies: www.aabt.org

Beck Institute for Cognitive Therapy and Research: www.beckinstitute.org

British Association for Behavioural and Cognitive Psychotherapies: www.babcp.com

Good Days Ahead (for computer-assisted CT software): www.mindstreet.com

International Association for Cognitive Psychotherapy: www.the-iacp.com

References

Albano AM, Kearney CA: When Children Refuse School: A Cognitive Behavioral Therapy Approach (Therapist Guide). San Antonio, TX, Psychological Corporation, 2000

Barlow DH, Cerney JA: Psychological Treatment of Panic. New York, Guilford, 1988

Barlow DH, Craske MG: Mastery of Your Anxiety and Panic (MAP3). Boston, MA, Graywind Publications, 1999

Barlow DH, Gorman JM, Shear MK, et al: Cognitive-behavioral therapy, imipramine, or their combination for panic disorder: a randomized controlled trial. JAMA 283:2529–2536, 2000

Basco MR: Never Good Enough. New York, Free Press, 1999

Basco MR, Rush AJ: Cognitive-Behavioral Therapy for Bipolar Disorder. New York, Guilford, 2005

Baxter LR Jr, Schwartz JM, Bergman KS, et al: Caudate glucose metabolic rate changes with both drug and behavior therapy for obsessive-compulsive disorder. Arch Gen Psychiatry 49:681–689, 1992

Beck AT: Thinking and depression. Arch Gen Psychiatry 9:324–333, 1963

Beck AT: Thinking and depression, II: theory and therapy. Arch Gen Psychiatry 10:561–571, 1964

Beck AT: Cognitive Therapy and the Emotional Disorders. New York, International Universities Press, 1976

Beck AT: Love Is Never Enough. New York, Harper & Row, 1988

Beck AT: Cognitive therapy: past, present, and future. J Consult Clin Psychol 61:194–198, 1993

Beck AT, Freeman A: Cognitive Therapy of Personality Disorders. New York, Guilford, 1990

Beck AT, Rush AJ, Shaw BF, et al: Cognitive Therapy of Depression. New York, Guilford, 1979

Beck AT, Emery GD, Greenberg RL: Anxiety Disorders and Phobias: A Cognitive Perspective. New York, Basic Books, 1985

Beck AT, Sokol L, Clark DA, et al: A cross-over study of focused cognitive therapy for panic disorder. Am J Psychiatry 149:778–783, 1992

Beck AT, Greenberg RL, Beck J: Coping with depression (a booklet). Bala Cynwyd, PA, The Beck Institute, 1995

Beck J: Cognitive Therapy: Basics and Beyond. New York, Guilford, 1995

Blackburn IM, Bishop S, Glen AIM, et al: The efficacy of cognitive therapy in depression: a treatment trial using cognitive therapy and pharmacotherapy, each alone and in combination. Br J Psychiatry 139:181–189, 1981

Blackburn IM, Jones S, Lewin RJP: Cognitive style in depression. Br J Clin Psychol 25:241–251, 1986

Blanchard EB, Hickling EJ, Devineni T, et al: A controlled evaluation of cognitive behavioral therapy for posttraumatic stress in motor vehicle accident survivors. Behav Res Ther 41:79–96, 2003

Burns DD: Feeling Good. New York, William Morrow, 1980

Burns DD: Feeling Good: The New Mood Therapy. New York, HarperCollins, 1999

Butler AC, Chapman JE, Forman EM, et al: The empirical status of cognitive-behavioral therapy: a review of meta-analyses. Clin Psychol Rev 26:17–31, 2006

Carter FA, McIntosh VVW, Joyce PR, et al: Role of exposure with response prevention in cognitive-behavioral therapy for bulimia nervosa: three-year follow-up results. Int J Eat Disord 33:127–135, 2003

Clark DA, Feldman J, Channon S: Dysfunctional thinking in anorexia and bulimia nervosa. Cognit Ther Res 13:377–387, 1989

Clark DA, Beck AT, Alford BA: Scientific Foundations of Cognitive Theory and Therapy of Depression. New York, Wiley, 1999

Clark DM: A cognitive approach to panic. Behav Res Ther 24:461–470, 1986

Clark DM, Salkovskis PM, Chalkley AJ: Respiratory control as a treatment for panic attacks. J Behav Ther Exp Psychiatry 16:23–30, 1985

Clark DM, Salkovskis PM, Hackmann A, et al: A comparison of cognitive therapy, applied relaxation and imipramine in the treatment of panic disorder. Br J Psychiatry 164:759–769, 1994

Clark DM, Ehlers A, McManus F, et al: Cognitive therapy versus fluoxetine in generalized social phobia: a randomized placebo-controlled trial. J Consult Clin Psychol 71:1058–1067, 2003

Cochran SD: Compliance with lithium regimens in the outpatient treatment of bipolar affective disorders. J Compliance Health Care 1:151–169, 1986

Covi L, Primakoff L: Cognitive group therapy, in The American Psychiatric Press Review of Psychiatry. Edited by Frances AJ, Hales RE. Washington, DC, American Psychiatric Press, 1988, pp 608–616

Davidson JR, Foa EB, Huppert JD, et al: Fluoxetine, comprehensive cognitive behavioral therapy, and placebo in generalized social phobia. Arch Gen Psychiatry 61:1005–1013, 2004

Davis D, Wright JH: The therapeutic relationship in cognitive-behavioral therapy: patient perceptions and therapist responses. Cogn Behav Pract 1:25–45, 1994

DeRubeis RJ, Hollon SD, Amsterdam JD, et al: Cognitive therapy vs medications in the treatment of moderate to severe depression. Arch Gen Psychiatry 62:409–416, 2005

Dobson KS: A meta-analysis of the efficacy of cognitive therapy for depression. J Consult Clin Psychol 57:414–419, 1989

Dobson KS, Shaw BF: Cognitive assessment with major depressive disorders. Cognit Ther Res 10:13–29, 1986

Elkin I, Gibbons RD, Shea MT, et al: Initial severity and differential treatment outcome in the National Institute of Mental Health Treatment of Depression Collaborative Research Program. J Consult Clin Psychol 63:841–847, 1995

Epstein N, Schlesinger SE, Dryden W: Cognitive-Behavioral Therapy With Families. New York, Brunner/Mazel, 1988

Evans MD, Hollon SD, DeRubeis RJ, et al: Differential relapse following cognitive therapy and pharmacotherapy for depression. Arch Gen Psychiatry 49:802–808, 1992

Fairburn CG, Agras WS, Wilson GT: The research on the treatment of bulimia nervosa: practical and theoretical implications, in The Biology of Feast and Famine: Relevance to Eating Disorders. Edited by Anderson GH, Kennedy SH. San Diego, CA, Academic Press, 1992, pp 318–340

Fava GA, Grandi S, Zielezny M, et al: Four-year outcome for cognitive behavioral treatment of residual symptoms in major depression. Am J Psychiatry 153:945–947, 1996

Foa E, Wilson R: Stop Obsessing! How to Overcome Your Obsessions and Compulsions, Revised Edition. New York, Bantam Books, 2001

Foa EB, Hembree EA, Cahill SP, et al: Randomized trial of prolonged exposure for posttraumatic stress disorder with and without cognitive restructuring: outcome at academic and community clinics. J Consult Clin Psychol 73:953–964, 2005

Freeman A, Schrodt GR, Gilson M, et al: Cognitive group therapy with inpatients, in Cognitive Therapy With Inpatients: Developing a Cognitive Milieu. Edited by Wright JH,

Thase ME, Beck AT, et al. New York, Guilford, 1992, pp 121–153

Gaffan EA, Tsaousis I, Kemp-Wheeler SM: Researcher allegiance and meta-analysis: the case of cognitive therapy for depression. J Consult Clin Psychol 63:966–980, 1995

Gelernter CS, Uhde TW, Cimbolic P, et al: Cognitive-behavioral and pharmacological treatments of social phobia: a controlled study. Arch Gen Psychiatry 48:938–945, 1991

Goldapple K, Segal Z, Garson C, et al: Modulation of cortical-limbic pathways in major depression: treatment-specific effects of cognitive behavior therapy. Arch Gen Psychiatry 61:34–41, 2004

Greenberger D, Padesky CA: Mind Over Mood. New York, Guilford, 1995

Harvey AG, Bryant RA, Tarrier N: Cognitive behaviour therapy for posttraumatic stress disorder. Clin Psychol Rev 23:501–522, 2003

Heimberg RG, Dodge CS, Hope DA, et al: Cognitive behavioral group treatment for social phobia: comparison with a credible placebo control. Cognit Ther Res 14:1–23, 1990

Hollon SD, DeRubeis RJ, Shelton RC, et al: Prevention of relapse following cognitive therapy vs medications in moderate to severe depression. Arch Gen Psychiatry 62:417–422, 2005

Hope DA, Heimberg RG, Bruch MA: Dismantling cognitive-behavioral group therapy for social phobia. Behav Res Ther 33:637–650, 1995

James IA, Blackburn IM: Cognitive therapy with obsessive-compulsive disorder. Br J Psychiatry 166:444–450, 1995

Jarrett RB, Kraft D, Doyle J, et al: Preventing recurrent depression using cognitive therapy with and without a continuation phase: a randomized clinical trial. Arch Gen Psychiatry 58:381–388, 2001

Kandel ER, Schwartz JH: Molecular biology of learning: modulation of transmitter release. Science 218:433–443, 1982

Kingdon D, Turkington D: Cognitive Therapy for Schizophrenia. New York, Guilford, 2005

Kovacs M, Rush AJ, Beck AT, et al: Depressed outpatients treated with cognitive therapy or pharmacotherapy. Arch Gen Psychiatry 38:33–39, 1981

March JS, Mulle K: OCD in Children and Adolescents: A Cognitive-Behavioral Treatment Manual. New York, Guilford, 1998

Meichenbaum DB: Cognitive-Behavior Modification: An Integrative Approach. New York, Plenum, 1977

Mitchell JE, Hoberman HN, Peterson CB, et al: Research on the psychotherapy of bulimia nervosa: half empty or half full. Int J Eat Disord 20:219–229, 1996

Mohl PC: Should psychotherapy be considered a biological treatment? Psychosomatics 28:320–326, 1987

Paykel ES, Scott J, Teasdale JD, et al: Prevention of relapse in residual depression by cognitive therapy. Arch Gen Psychiatry 56:829–835, 1999

Reinecke MA, Dattilio FM, Freeman A (eds): Cognitive Therapy With Children and Adolescents: A Casebook for Clinical Practice, 2nd Edition. New York, Guilford, 2003

Ricca V, Mannucci E, Zucchi T, et al: Cognitive-behavioural therapy for bulimia nervosa and binge eating disorder: a review. Psychother Psychosom 69:287–295, 2000

Robinson LA, Berman JS, Neimeyer RA: Psychotherapy for the treatment of depression: a comprehensive review of controlled outcome research. Psychol Bull 108:30–49, 1990

Salkovskis PM: Obsessional-compulsive problems: a cognitive-behavioral analysis. Behav Res Ther 25:571–583, 1985

Salkovskis PM, Warwick HM: Cognitive therapy of obsessive-compulsive disorder: treating treatment failures. Behavioural Psychotherapy 13:243–255, 1985

Sensky T: Cognitive-behavior therapy for patients with physical illnesses, in Cognitive-Behavior Therapy. Edited by Wright JH. Washington, DC, American Psychiatric Publishing, 2004, pp 83–121

Simons AD, Murphy GE, Levine JE, et al: Cognitive therapy and pharmacotherapy for depression: sustained improvement over one year. Arch Gen Psychiatry 43:43–49, 1986

Sudak D: Cognitive Behavioral Therapy for Clinicians. Baltimore, MD, Lippincott Williams & Wilkins, 2006

Thase ME: Depression-focused psychotherapies, in Treatments of Psychiatric Disorders, 3rd Edition, Vol 2. Edited by Gabbard GO. Washington, DC, American Psychiatric Publishing, 2001, pp 1181–1227

Van Oppen P, De Haan E, Van Balkom AJLM, et al: Cognitive therapy and exposure in vivo in the treatment of obsessive compulsive disorder. Behav Res Ther 33:379–390, 1995

Warwick HM, Salkovskis PM: Hypochondriasis. Behav Res Ther 28:105–117, 1990

Whittal ML, Thordarson DS, McLean PD: Treatment of obsessive-compulsive disorder: cognitive behavior therapy vs. exposure and response prevention. Behav Res Ther 43:1559–1576, 2005

Wilson GT: Cognitive behavior therapy for eating disorders: progress and problems. Behav Res Ther 37:S79–S95, 1999

Wilson GT, Shafran R: Eating disorders guidelines from NICE. Lancet 365:79–81, 2005

Wolpe J: The Practice of Behavior Therapy. New York, Pergamon, 1969

Wright JH: Cognitive therapy of depression, in The American Psychiatric Press Review of Psychiatry, Vol 7. Edited by Frances AJ, Hales RE. Washington, DC, American Psychiatric Press, 1988, pp 554–590

Wright JH, Basco MR: Getting Your Life Back: The Complete Guide to Recovery From Depression (Paperback Edition). New York, Touchstone, 2002

Wright JH, Beck AT: Cognitive therapy of depression: theory and practice. Hosp Community Psychiatry 34:1119–1127, 1983

Wright JH, Thase ME: Cognitive and biological therapies: a synthesis. Psychiatr Ann 22:451–458, 1992

Wright JH, Thase ME, Beck AT, et al (eds): Cognitive Therapy With Inpatients: Developing a Cognitive Milieu. New York, Guilford, 1993

Wright JH, Wright AS, Beck AT: Good Days Ahead: The Multimedia Program for Cognitive Therapy. Louisville, KY, MindStreet, 2004

Wright JH, Basco MR, Thase ME: Learning Cognitive-Behavior Therapy: An Illustrated Guide (Core Competencies in Psychotherapy Series, Glen O. Gabbard, series ed). Washington, DC, American Psychiatric Publishing, 2006

Wright JH, Thase ME, Beck AT: Cognitive therapy, in The American Psychiatric Publishing Textbook of Clinical Psychiatry, 5th Edition. Edited by Hales RE, Yudofsky SC, Gabbard GO. Washington, DC, American Psychiatric Publishing, 2008, pp 1211–1256

Zimmerman G, Favrod J, Trieu VH, et al: The effect of cognitive behavioral treatment on the positive symptoms of schizophrenia spectrum disorders: a meta-analysis. Schizophr Res 77:1–9, 2005

19

TREATMENT OF CHILDREN AND ADOLESCENTS

Glen C. Crawford, M.D.

Stephen J. Cozza, M.D.

Mina K. Dulcan, M.D.

This chapter outlines the basic principles of psychiatric treatment for children and adolescents, with an emphasis on psychopharmacology. Readers seeking a more in-depth treatment of the subject should consult *Dulcan's Textbook of Child and Adolescent Psychiatry* (Dulcan 2010).

Techniques used in the treatment of child psychiatric conditions have developed from two different sources: the traditions of understanding and treating children that were based on developmental uniqueness, and treatments that were originally designed for adults and were then applied to children and adolescents. Increasingly, more rigorous evaluation and diagnostic procedures have allowed greater specificity in the application of treatments to our younger patients. In addition, expanding research on the efficacy of specific therapeutic approaches continues to enlarge our armamentarium of empirically tested interventions.

Evaluation

The American Academy of Child and Adolescent Psychiatry (AACAP) has developed practice parameters as guides to the evaluation and treatment of specific disorders. Completed practice parameters are available on the AACAP Web site (www.aacap.org).

Special considerations for children make evaluation different from that for adult patients. Practitioners must have a clear understanding of normal development and the differences that may exist among children at the same or different ages, in order to distinguish normal from pathological behaviors. Also, practitioners must be able to apply developmental understanding in the diagnostic interview of the child, using approaches like imaginative play with younger children or with those less skilled in verbal communication.

Information from the school is always useful and is essential when there is concern about learning or behavior in school or peer functioning. With parental consent, the clinician talks with the teacher; obtains records of testing, grades, and attendance; and requests completion of a standardized checklist, such as the Teacher Report Form of the Child Behavior Checklist (Achenbach 1991) or the Vanderbilt ADHD Rating Scales (Wolraich et al. 1998). Even better, though less convenient, is a visit to the school to observe the youngster with peers in the classroom and on the playground and to talk with teachers and counselors.

A referral to another provider such as a pediatrician, pediatric neurologist, child psychologist, or speech and language specialist may be necessary to complete the assessment. Psychological evaluation, including an intelligence test and achievement tests, should be obtained when there is any question about learning or IQ, with additional testing as indicated.

Treatment Planning

Treatment planning takes into consideration psychiatric diagnosis, target emotional and behavioral symptoms, and the strengths and weaknesses of the patient and family. Resources and risks in the school, neighborhood, and social support network and any religious group affiliation also influence the selection of treatment strategies. The clinician must decide which treatment is likely to be the most efficient or to have the highest benefit–risk ratio and whether treatments should be administered simultaneously or in sequence. Parents are best included in the choice of treatment strategies, with the strength of the clinician's recommendation depending on the clarity of the indications.

The motivation and ability of the responsible adults to carry out the treatment should be considered because the best treatment has little chance of success without the cooperation of the family. Treatment planning is an ongoing process, with reevaluations done as interventions are attempted and their results observed and as additional information about the child and family comes to light.

Informed Consent

The implementation of any treatment plan requires carefully obtained informed consent from parents before the plan is initiated. The concept of informed consent is more complicated with children because of their lack of legal competency. Although parents provide informed consent for children, clinicians should strive to obtain assent from child patients before initiating any treatment, keeping in mind the cognitive capacities and developmental level of the patient. Such consent should include a general discussion of the selected treatment, its intended purpose, the availability of any alternative treatments (to include a choice of no treatment), and the nature of any adverse reactions that could result. An open discussion of any questions or concerns not only meets the legal obligations of practice, but also can safeguard the therapeutic alliance should undesirable side effects occur. Although not always necessary, parents' written consent may be useful in some situations.

Printed materials to supplement discussion with the physician in educating parents and children regarding a variety of treatments are now available (Dulcan 2007). In addition, the Internet has become an important source of information about medications and treatments for health care consumers. Because the quality of information available on the World Wide Web is inconsistent, patients and their families benefit from guidance as to the best sources of information about mental health issues. Clinicians should also be prepared to respond to questions or concerns about treatments that may arise from a patient's or parent's "surfing" of the Internet. A good Internet resource for child and adolescent psychiatry is the AACAP Web site (www.aacap.org).

Confidentiality

It is essential that the guidelines for confidentiality and for sharing information between parent and child be clear. Adolescents are usually more sensitive to this issue than younger children. As a general rule, either party should be told when information from one party's session will be relayed to the other. When children are engaged in potentially dangerous activities or have serious thoughts of harming themselves or others, parents must be informed. Carefully planned family sessions in which the therapist coaches and supports a parent or child in sharing information may be more useful than secondhand reports. Clinicians should also ensure that they inform children and parents of the possible need to share some information with third-party entities (such as insurance companies) and make prudent choices as to the nature and quantity of information that are appropriate to pass on.

Psychopharmacology

Two important general principles of pediatric psychopharmacology are worth repeating: polypharmacy should be minimized, and medication should virtually never be used as the only treatment. Most disorders of children and adolescents that require medication are either chronic (e.g., attention-deficit/hyperactivity disorder [ADHD], autistic disorder, Tourette's disorder) or likely to have recurrent episodes (e.g., mood disorders), and a long-term relationship with the physician is crucial. It is important to educate the family regarding the disorder, its treatment, and the different needs at each developmental stage. The physician must consider the meaning of the prescription and administration of a med-

ication to the child, the family, the school, and the child's peer group.

Special Issues for Children and Adolescents

Pharmacokinetics, Pharmacodynamics, and Pharmacogenetics

Pharmacokinetics is the study of the movement of drugs into, around, and out of the body by the processes of absorption, distribution, metabolism, and elimination. Although children share some similarities in the physiological processing of medications with adults, developmental differences are clinically relevant, particularly in regard to drug distribution and metabolism.

The distribution of drugs in children is influenced by developmental differences in proportion of extracellular water volume, which decreases substantially from birth through early adolescence. This decrease results in a larger distribution volume for water-soluble drugs in younger children, requiring a relatively higher dose to achieve a comparable plasma concentration (Clein and Riddle 1995).

By late infancy to early childhood, hepatic metabolic activity is at its peak. This substantially greater metabolic rate is related to the proportionally larger liver size of children compared with adults. Relative to body weight, the liver of a toddler is 40%–50% greater and that of a 6-year-old is 30% greater than the liver of an adult. This greater metabolic rate has been postulated as the principal factor contributing to decreased drug plasma concentration levels and decreased drug half-lives in children compared with adults (Clein and Riddle 1995).

An understanding of the cytochrome P450 (CYP) enzyme system is becoming increasingly important. Many medications either are substrates of or inhibit or induce one or more of the CYP isoenzymes. Potentially toxic interactions can result from inappropriate combinations of medications that inhibit

CYP enzymes. An excellent source of information on this topic is the work by Cozza et al. (2003).

Medication dosage also is determined by pharmacodynamics, or how the biological system responds to the drug. For example, interaction with receptors is determined by receptor number, distribution, structure, function, sensitivity, and mechanism of action. Little is known about the influence of growth and development on these variables.

Pharmacogenetics is the study of how genetics influences the physiological effect of and response to drugs. Genetic variations in the CYP2D6 isoenzyme, for example, may enhance the metabolism of medications frequently used in child and adolescent psychiatry. Polymorphisms that have been identified in certain isoenzymes of uridine 5'-diphospho-glucuronosyltransferase (UDP-glucuronosyltransferase) may affect the metabolism of almost all psychotherapeutic agents except lithium. Research is ongoing into genetic variations in drug and neurotransmitter receptor sites important to the field of psychiatry, such as serotonin, norepinephrine, and acetylcholine (Anderson and Cook 2000).

Ideally, medication doses in children should be derived from studies of children rather than adults, but such studies are too rare. Dosage is typically determined empirically or by extrapolation from adults, or, for a few drugs, by weight. Generally, children require a higher weight-adjusted dose to achieve the same blood levels and therapeutic effects as adults. However, clinicians should remain alert to the possibility that such practice occasionally results in toxicity.

Side Effects and Measurement of Outcome

Side effects are common in children being treated with psychiatric medications. Clinicians must actively look for adverse reactions, as children often will not report them and parents may not notice. Children may occasionally develop a paradoxical response to a particular medication. Such a response may be extremely individual in its manifestation, affecting one child but not another.

Effective medication management in children requires the identification of clear target symptoms that are monitored during the course of a medication trial. The physician must obtain emotional, behavioral, and physical data at baseline, periodically during treatment, and posttreatment. Therapeutic effects can be assessed by interviews and rating scales, direct observation, collection of data from outside sources (e.g., teachers), or specific tests evaluating attention or learning.

Developmentally Disabled Patients

Medication effects are even more difficult to assess in children and adolescents with mental retardation or pervasive developmental disorders (PDDs). Their impaired ability to verbalize symptoms is relevant to diagnosis, measurement of efficacy, and detection of side effects. These individuals are prone to physical side effects and are at risk for idiosyncratic behavioral effects or simply less prominent therapeutic effects.

Adherence to Medication Regimen

Taking medication as directed can be particularly problematic for children, because the cooperation of two people, parent and child, and often school personnel as well, is required. In general pediatric practice, adherence to medication regimens is associated with degree of parental concern about the seriousness of the child's illness, the severity of the child's symptoms, and prior adherence to treatment (Lewis 1995). Adherence appears to be inversely related to the complexity of the medication regimen (including the number of medicines used and the frequency of dosing). Although experiences in general pediatrics and adult psychiatry indicate that educational efforts may improve compliance, administration of psychotropic medications in children is more complex. Understanding a child's feelings about taking medication may also help in promoting adherence (Bastiaens 1995).

Stimulants

This category of medications is the most studied and most used in pediatric psychopharmacology and is most often prescribed by non–child psychiatrists such as pediatricians and general practitioners. Methylphenidate and dextroamphetamine, the "gold standard" medications used to treat ADHD in children, have been enhanced over the past few years by the introduction of a racemic salt formulation of amphetamine (Adderall), innovative delivery systems for methylphenidate (Concerta and Daytrana), an isomeric form of methylphenidate (Focalin), and a prodrug of dextroamphetamine (Vyvanse).

Indications and Efficacy

The most established indication for stimulant use is in the treatment of ADHD. There is extensive empirical support of the short-term efficacy and safety of stimulant medications (American Academy of Child and Adolescent Psychiatry 2002; Connor 2002). Side effects of medication in this age group were considered mild and varied with the age of the child. The Preschool ADHD Treatment Study (PATS; Greenhill et al. 2006a) found methylphenidate to be safe and effective in preschool children, although improvement was less, and side effects were somewhat greater, in comparison with school-age children. In addition, a review of studies of stimulant treatment in adolescents (Spencer et al. 1996) concluded that stimulants are just as effective in adolescents as they are in school-age children.

The long-term therapeutic effect of stimulant medication remains unclear, as most studies to date have been of short duration. Analysis of 14-month treatment outcomes in the National Institute of Mental Health Collaborative Multisite Multimodal Treatment Study of Children With ADHD (MTA) has suggested that combined medication and behavioral treatments provide no more clinical benefit in treating core ADHD symptoms than carefully managed medication alone but may offer some added benefit in other ar-

eas of social skills and academic performance (Jensen 2000). The 10-month open-label continuation phase of the PATS study suggested maintenance of improvement of ADHD symptoms in preschool-age children, although there was notable variation in medication dose (Vitiello et al. 2007).

Stimulants have been found to be effective in treating ADHD symptoms in children with mental retardation, although the treatment response is not as robust as it is in children with normal IQ and ADHD (Aman et al. 2003) and, as one might expect, an increase in side effects (such as insomnia and appetite suppression) was noted as the dosage increased (Pearson et al. 2003). Children with fragile X syndrome also have been shown to benefit significantly from stimulant treatment of ADHD symptoms (Hagerman et al. 1988).

The benefit of stimulant medication in the treatment of inattention and hyperactivity in children with PDDs remains unclear. Small studies have described the effective use of these medications in this patient group. A study of children with autism and hyperactivity conducted by the Research Units on Pediatric Psychopharmacology (RUPP) Autism Network (Aman et al. 2005) demonstrated the superiority of methylphenidate over placebo. However, the response observed was less vigorous than that seen in children with ADHD who do not have a PDD, and the incidence of side effects was greater.

Although current U.S. product labeling either contraindicates or cautions against the use of stimulants in patients with tics or Tourette's disorder, a meta-analysis by Bloch et al. (2009) showed no significant exacerbation of tics with therapeutic doses of stimulant medication. Previously, the greatest concern about using stimulants in this population has been precipitating new tics. However, patients with Tourette's disorder are often far more disabled by their ADHD symptoms than by their tics. The Tourette's Syndrome Study Group (2002) trial showed that the frequency of tics was no more increased with methylphenidate than it was with clonidine or placebo. The apparent increase in tics, previously attributed to stimulant treatment in children with ADHD and a tic disorder, may instead be a function of the natural waxing and waning nature of tics. Nevertheless, if stimulants are to be used in patients with ADHD and a tic disorder, monitoring for tics during treatment is advised.

Initiation and Maintenance

The decision to medicate a child or adolescent with a stimulant is based on the presence of persistent target symptoms that are sufficiently severe to cause functional impairment at school and usually also at home and with peers. Parents must be willing to monitor medication and to attend appointments.

Multiple outcome measures, determined by using more than one source, setting, and method of gathering data and including premedication baseline school data on behavior and academic performance, are essential. Education for the child, family, and teacher is helpful before the start of medication (see N.L. Miller and Findling 2010). The physician should explicitly debunk common myths about stimulant treatment—for example, that stimulants have a paradoxical sedative action, that they lead to drug abuse, and that they are not needed or are ineffective after puberty. The physician should work closely with parents on dosage adjustments and obtain annual academic testing and more frequent reports from teachers.

Although methylphenidate is the most commonly used and best studied, no patient characteristics are helpful in suggesting which stimulant drug is best for a particular child.

The current edition of the Texas Children's Medication Algorithm for ADHD (Pliszka et al. 2006) provides useful guidance to clinicians in approaching the pharmacological management of ADHD, as well as the treatment of ADHD with other comorbid disorders. In brief, the algorithm recommends initiating the treatment of ADHD with a stimulant medication. If the treatment response is suboptimal, or if side effects or other circumstances warrant, the next step would be the use of a different stimulant. For example, if methylphenidate (or one of its formulations) is tried first, then the next step would be the use of an amphetamine preparation, or vice versa.

Adderall, a racemic mixture of four amphetamine salts, has been shown in several randomized, controlled studies to be of equal efficacy to methylphenidate in treating the behavioral symptoms of ADHD (Pliszka 2000), with no significant difference in side effects noted. Adderall XR (extended release) incorporates immediate-release and delayed-release formulations of Adderall in a 50:50 ratio within a single capsule to provide a more extended period of action; its efficacy in improving attention and classroom behavior has been demonstrated in controlled trials (McCracken et al. 2003). The long-term effectiveness and tolerability of Adderall XR has been suggested by a 24-month open-label extension study by McGough et al. (2005).

In February 2005, Health Canada suspended the sale of Adderall XR in the Canadian market after it reviewed worldwide reports of 20 instances of sudden death and 12 instances of stroke in patients taking this medication, which included 14 and 2 children, respectively (Health Canada 2005a). After an independent review of the data, Health Canada (2005b) authorized the resumption of the use of Adderall XR in August 2005, contingent upon stronger product labeling warning against the use of Adderall XR in patients with structural heart defects, as well as the potential dangers resulting from the misuse of amphetamines. The current U.S. product labeling contains similar cautions for both Adderall and Adderall XR.

Several long-acting formulations of methylphenidate are currently available. Concerta is a single-daily-dose methylphenidate preparation that provides an immediate dose of methylphenidate followed by gradual release of methylphenidate over several hours by means of an osmotic release system. It has been found comparable to three-times-daily dosing of methylphenidate, and superior to placebo, in several blinded trials (Swanson et al. 2002). No significant increases in side effects were reported in the active treatment groups. An open-label multicenter study of Concerta by Wilens et al. (2005) suggested that Concerta remains effective and well tolerated in long-term treatment, although modest increases in dose may be required. Metadate CD (controlled delivery) is a modified-release preparation of methylphenidate that incorporates immediate-release and extended-release preparations of methylphenidate to extend its length of action. In a blinded, placebo-controlled multicenter study, Greenhill et al. (2002) found Metadate CD to be safe and effective in controlling ADHD symptoms. Ritalin LA (long acting), which uses the proprietary Spheroidal Oral Drug Absorption System (SODAS) to deliver immediate- and delayed-release doses of medication, was also shown to be superior to placebo in a brief (2-week) randomized, controlled multicenter trial (Biederman et al. 2003).

Daytrana is a transdermal patch preparation of methylphenidate that has been shown to be effective in treating the symptoms of ADHD in randomized, controlled trials (McGough et al. 2006). This method of administering methylphenidate is particularly useful for children who have difficulty swallowing tablets or capsules. The patch should be applied 2 hours before medication effect is needed, and it may remain in place for up to 9 hours. If a shorter duration of action is needed, the patch may be removed sooner, with medication effect ending 2-4 hours afterwards (Wilens et al. 2008). Although erythema at the site of application of the patch is common, use of the patch should be discontinued if contact sensitization occurs (Shire U.S. Inc.). Several dosage strengths are available, allowing for titration of dose.

Focalin (dexmethylphenidate), the *d*-enantiomer of racemic *d,l-threo*-methylphenidate, was found to be significantly superior to placebo, and as effective as racemic methylphenidate, on several measures of behavior and performance in a randomized, controlled trial (Wigal et al. 2004). Although a slightly longer duration of action of dexmethylphenidate compared with methylphenidate was observed, further studies are needed to determine whether dexmethylphenidate offers any other distinct clinical advantages over racemic methylphenidate. The efficacy of the extended-release preparation of dexmethylphenidate (Focalin XR) in controlling ADHD symptoms has also been demonstrated in a randomized, controlled trial (Greenhill et al. 2006b).

Vyvanse (lisdexamfetamine dimesylate) is a prodrug of dextroamphetamine. Dosed once a day, lisdexamfetamine was superior to placebo in treating symptoms of ADHD in a randomized, controlled crossover study (Biederman et al. 2007a) and a randomized, controlled, parallel-group study (Biederman et al. 2007b).

Stimulant medication should be initiated with a low dose and titrated within the recommended range every week or two according to response and side effects, with body weight as a rough guide. When children reach 3 years of age, their absorption, distribution, protein binding, and metabolism of stimulants are similar to those of an adult (Coffey et al. 1983), although adults have more side effects than children do at the same mg/kg dose. Giving medication after meals minimizes anorexia. Preschool-age children or patients with ADHD, predominantly inattentive type; mental retardation; or PDDs may benefit from (and have fewer side effects with) doses lower than are used in patients with ADHD with prominent symptoms of hyperactivity or impulsivity. Starting with only a morning dose may be useful in assessing drug effect by comparing morning and afternoon school performance. The need for an after-school dose or medication on weekends should be individually determined. Whereas some children who experience sleep or appetite disturbance but a good clinical response to stimulants may benefit from a suspension of treatment on weekends and school holidays, those who are actively involved in weekend sports or extracurricular activities may require treatment during the weekends. Results from the MTA study suggest that most children continue to benefit from maintenance medication doses that are similar to the initial titration dose. However, adjustments to dose were often required in children, indicating the need for ongoing monitoring of treatment response and active medication management (Vitiello et al. 2001). MTA study results support the superiority of full-day, 7-day-per-week stimulant coverage in children with combined-type ADHD.

Behavioral checklists such as the revised versions of the Conners Teacher and Parent Rating Scales (Conners et al. 1998a, 1998b), and the parent and teacher versions of the Vanderbilt ADHD Rating Scales (Wolraich et al. 1998, 2003) are useful in assessing the severity of inattentive and hyperactive symptoms in a variety of settings prior to initiating treatment, as well as monitoring the efficacy of medication during treatment.

If symptoms are not severe outside of the school setting, children may have an annual drug-free trial in the summer, at least 2 weeks' duration but longer if possible. If school behavior and academic performance are stable, a carefully monitored trial off medication during the school year (but *not* at the beginning) will provide data on whether medication is still needed.

Tolerance is reported anecdotally, but adherence is often irregular and should be the first possibility considered when medication appears ineffective. Children should not be responsible for their medication because youngsters are impulsive and forgetful at best, and most dislike the idea of taking medication, even when they can verbalize its positive effects and cannot identify any side effects. They will often avoid, "forget," or simply refuse medication. Lower efficacy of a generic preparation may be another possibility. Decreased drug effect also may be due to a reaction to a change at home or school.

Greenhill (1995) used the term *pseudotolerance* to define circumstances in which increased symptomatology is inaccurately ascribed to decreased medication efficacy (e.g., when symptoms are exacerbated due to changes in a child's life rather than changes in response to medication). True tolerance may be more likely with the long-acting formulations (Birmaher et al. 1989); if it occurs, another of the stimulants may be substituted.

Table 19–1 lists the currently available stimulant medications, their formulations, and dose ranges.

Risks and Side Effects

Most side effects are similar for all stimulants. Insomnia may be due to drug effect, to rebound, or to a preexisting sleep problem. Stimulants may worsen or improve irritable mood (Gadow 1992). Black male adolescents who take stimulants may be at higher risk for elevated blood pressure (Brown and Sexson 1989).

The issue of stimulant-induced growth retardation remains a significant concern. In their extensive literature review, Faraone et al. (2008) found that the magnitude of growth delay appears to be dose related, and while no significant differences between dextroamphetamine and methylphenidate were noted, more direct comparisons of the two drugs are required. The possible mechanisms of stimulant use on growth interference and the long-term implications for final stature remain to be clearly elucidated. Although some authors have suggested that growth delays in ADHD children may be related to dysmaturity inherent in the disorder itself rather than to medication effects (Spencer et al. 1996), Swanson et al. (2007) found just the opposite: compared with age-matched children without ADHD, medication-naive children with ADHD had greater-than-expected initial height and weight, and those who remained unmedicated throughout the study experienced a greater growth rate. In light of these findings, measurement of height and weight at the initiation of treatment and at regular intervals throughout is recommended.

Rebound effects, consisting of increased excitability, activity, talkativeness, irritability, and insomnia, beginning 4–15 hours after a dose, may be seen as the last dose of the day wears off or for up to several days after sudden withdrawal of high daily doses of stimulants. This effect may resemble a worsening of the original symptoms (Zahn et al. 1980).

Although psychosis is a well-known side effect of all stimulant medications, psychotic symptoms have not been rigorously studied within the child and adolescent population being treated for ADHD. There is no evidence that stimulants produce an increase in seizure activity. Addiction has *not* been found to result from the prescription of stimulants for ADHD.

Alpha₂-Noradrenergic Agonists

Clonidine and guanfacine are α_2-noradrenergic agonists approved for the treatment of hypertension.

Indications and Efficacy

The α_2-noradrenergic agonists clonidine and guanfacine have been shown to be effective in the treatment of ADHD as well as tics. A randomized, controlled trial of 136 children with ADHD and a chronic tic disorder conducted by the Tourette's Syndrome Study Group (2002) noted significant improvements in all treatment groups (clonidine, methylphenidate, and the combination of the two), with the greatest benefit found in the group of children taking both clonidine and methylphenidate. However, a 16-week controlled trial by Palumbo et al. (2008) comparing clonidine with methylphenidate, either alone or in combination, in the treatment of ADHD without a comorbid tic disorder showed a less robust effect of clonidine in the treatment of ADHD compared with methylphenidate.

A meta-analysis of the literature from 1980 to 1999 by Connor et al. (1999) demonstrated an effect size of clonidine on symptoms of ADHD that was intermediate between a higher stimulant medication response and a lower tricyclic antidepressant (TCA) medication response.

Guanfacine has been shown effective in open trials of children with ADHD and comorbid ADHD and Tourette's disorder. The extended-release formulation of guanfacine has been shown to be effective in the treatment of ADHD in blinded, placebo-controlled trials (Biederman et al. 2008; Sallee et al. 2009). A meta-analysis of studies examining the treatment of children with ADHD and a comorbid tic disorder showed significant improvement in tics with the use of either clonidine or guanfacine (Bloch et al. 2009).

Initiation and Maintenance

Because clonidine and guanfacine have similar pharmacological profiles, blood pressure and pulse should be measured before treatment and at regular intervals throughout treatment. An electrocardiogram (ECG) and baseline laboratory blood studies (especially fasting glucose) may be considered.

Clonidine is initiated at a low dose of 0.05 mg (one-half of the smallest manufactured tablet) at bedtime. This low dose converts the side effect of initial sedation into a benefit. An alternate strategy is to begin with 0.025 mg qid. Either way, the dosage is then titrated gradually over several weeks to 0.15–0.30 mg/day (0.003–0.01 mg/kg/day) in three or four divided doses. Young children (ages 5–7 years) may require lower initial and maintenance doses. The transdermal form (skin patch) may be useful to improve compliance and reduce variability in blood levels. It lasts only 5 days in children (compared with 7 days in adults) (Hunt et al. 1990). Once the daily dose has been determined using pills, an equivalent-size patch may be substituted (0.1, 0.2, 0.3 mg/day). Patches should not be cut to adjust the dose, as this may damage the delivery membrane, potentially causing an increase in the delivered dose of clonidine (Broderick-Cantwell

Table 19–1. Clinical use of stimulant medications in pediatric patients

Generic name	Duration of action	Proprietary name	How supplied	Starting dose	Maximum daily dose	Remarks
Methylphenidate	3–4 hours	Methylin	5-, 10-, 20-mg tablets 2.5-, 5-, 10-mg chewable tablets 5 mg/5 mL oral solution 10 mg/5 mL oral solution	5 mg bid	60 mg	Give doses 3–5 hours apart. Consider a smaller starting dose for children <6 years of age.
		Ritalin Generic	5-, 10-, 20-mg tablets 5-, 10-, 20-mg tablets			
Dexmethylphenidate	3–4 hours	Focalin	2.5-, 5-, 10-mg tablets	2.5 mg bid	20 mg	Start with 2.5 mg bid for children not previously treated with racemic methylphenidate. If converting from methylphenidate, start with half of daily dose of methylphenidate (maximum 20 mg/day divided bid).
Dextroamphetamine	≤6 hours	Dexedrine	5-mg tablets	<6 years: 2.5 mg/day	40 mg	Give doses 4–6 hours apart.
		Dextrostat	5-, 10-mg tablets	≥6 years: 5 mg/day		
		Generic	5-, 10- mg tablets			
Mixed amphetamine salts	≤6 hours	Adderall	5-, 7.5-, 10-, 12.5-, 15-, 20-, 30-mg tablets	<6 years: 2.5 mg/day	40 mg	Start with once-daily dosing; may dose twice daily if necessary.
		Generic	5-, 7.5-, 10-, 12.5-, 15-, 20-, 30-mg tablets	≥6 years: 5 mg/day		

Table 19–1. Clinical use of stimulant medications in pediatric patients *(continued)*

Generic name	Duration of action	Proprietary name	How supplied	Starting dose	Maximum daily dose	Remarks
Methylphenidate	≤8 hours	Metadate ER	10-, 20-mg tablets	10 mg/day	60 mg	Do not cut, crush, or chew tablets.
		Metadate CD	10-, 20-, 30-, 40-, 50-, 60-mg capsules	20 mg/day		Capsule may be swallowed whole or opened and sprinkled on applesauce. Do not crush or chew capsules.
		Methylin ER	10-, 20-mg tablets	10 mg/day		Do not cut, crush, or chew tablets.
		Ritalin SR	20-mg tablets	20 mg/day		Do not cut, crush, or chew tablets.
		Ritalin LA	10-, 20-, 30-, 40-mg capsules	20 mg/day		Capsule may be swallowed whole or opened and sprinkled on applesauce. Do not crush or chew capsules.
		Generic	20-mg tablets	20 mg/day		Do not cut, crush, or chew tablets.
Dextroamphetamine	≤8 hours	Dexedrine Spansule	5-, 10-, 15-mg capsules	5 mg/day	40 mg	Start with once-daily dosing; may dose twice daily if necessary.
		Generic	5-, 10-, 15-mg capsules			
Methylphenidate	≤12 hours	Concerta	18-, 27-, 36-, 54-mg tablets	18 mg/day	<13 years: 54 mg/day ≥13 years: 72 mg/day or 2 mg/kg	MUST swallow whole. OROS® tablet is passed in stool.

Table 19–1. Clinical use of stimulant medications in pediatric patients *(continued)*

Generic name	Duration of action	Proprietary name	How supplied	Starting dose	Maximum daily dose	Remarks
Methylphenidate *(continued)*	≤9 hours	Daytrana	10-, 15-, 20-, 30-mg transdermal patches (nominal dose delivered over 9 hours)	10 mg/day	30 mg/day	Start with 10-mg patch applied to the hip; increase dosage weekly as necessary. Apply 2 hours before medication effect is needed. Remove patch after 9 hours' use. Erythema is a common side effect at the site of application. Alternate application site daily. More severe skin reactions may necessitate discontinuation of use.
Dexmethylphenidate	≤12 hours	Focalin XR	5-, 10-, 15-, 20-mg capsules	5 mg/day	20 mg/day	Start with 5 mg/day for children not previously treated with racemic methylphenidate. If converting from methylphenidate, start with half of daily dose of methylphenidate (maximum 20 mg/day divided bid). Capsule may be swallowed whole or opened and sprinkled on applesauce. Do not crush or chew capsule.
Mixed amphetamine salts	≤12 hours	Adderall XR	5-, 10-, 15-, 20-, 25-, 30-mg capsules	10 mg/day	30 mg/day	Capsule may be swallowed whole or opened and sprinkled on applesauce. Do not crush or chew capsule.

Table 19–1. Clinical use of stimulant medications in pediatric patients *(continued)*

Generic name	Duration of action	Proprietary name	How supplied	Starting dose	Maximum daily dose	Remarks
Lisdexamfetamine	≤12 hours	Vyvanse	20-, 30-, 40-, 50-, 60-, 70-mg capsules	30 mg/day	70 mg/day	Capsule may be swallowed whole or opened and dissolved in water. Not studied in children younger than 6 years or older than 12 years of age.

Note. bid=twice-daily dosing. Amphetamine preparations carry a black box warning regarding their potential for abuse and the possibility of sudden death and serious cardiovascular events if misused. They should also be avoided in patients with structural cardiac defects. All of the above medications are Drug Enforcement Administration Schedule II controlled substances and should be used cautiously in patients with a history of substance abuse. Many generic preparations of the above medications are available. Proprietary names are included for informational purposes only and do not imply endorsement of a particular preparation. Please consult chapter text and manufacturers' product inserts for further prescribing information.

Source. Adapted from product labeling and information available from Drugs@FDA (www.fda.gov/cder).

1999). Unfortunately, patches do not adhere well in hot, humid climates.

For guanfacine, dosages range from 0.5 to 4.0 mg/day. A recommended starting regimen for immediate-release guanfacine is 0.5 mg once or twice daily in children and 1 mg once or twice daily in adolescents, to be increased every 3 or 4 days until therapeutic effect is noted (Silver 1999). An extended-release formulation of guanfacine (Intuniv) with 1-, 2-, 3-, and 4-mg tablets is available for the treatment of ADHD. The extended-release preparation of guanfacine is recommended for once-daily dosing in the morning. Because of pharmacokinetic differences between the immediate- and extended-release preparations, the dose of immediate-release guanfacine should not be substituted with an equivalent extended-release dose. Instead, whether changing from the immediate-release preparation or starting treatment de novo with the extended-release formulation, the recommended starting dose is 1 mg daily, in the morning, with dosage increases no more frequent than 1 mg a week. Tablets should not be broken or crushed, nor administered with high-fat foods (Intuniv product labeling). When clonidine or guanfacine is discontinued, it should be tapered gradually over 1–2 weeks to avoid any withdrawal phenomena.

Risks and Side Effects

Sedation and irritability are troublesome side effects of clonidine therapy, although these tend to decrease after several weeks. Dry mouth, nausea, and photophobia have been reported, with hypotension and dizziness possible at high doses. The clonidine skin patch often causes local pruritic dermatitis; daily rotation of the patch site or use of a steroid cream may minimize this. Depression may occur, often in patients with a personal or family history of depressive symptoms (Hunt et al. 1991). Glucose tolerance may decrease, especially in those patients at risk for diabetes. Although guanfacine is less sedating and less hypotensive than cloni-

dine, it shares many of the side effects of this class of medication.

Reports of serious adverse drug reactions (including sudden death) in children treated with clonidine, alone or in combination with methylphenidate, have raised concerns about the safety of this medication in the pediatric population. In several cases, the presence of polypharmacy or other medical conditions made it more difficult to implicate clonidine in these adverse events (Wilens et al. 1999). More recent studies (Hazell and Stuart 2003; Tourette's Syndrome Study Group 2002) have demonstrated the benefits and safety of combination clonidine and methylphenidate therapy in select patient groups. Cardiovascular screening and monitoring of children treated with clonidine or guanfacine are still recommended, however, as well as gradual titration and tapering of dose to reduce cardiovascular side effects.

Atomoxetine

Atomoxetine, a norepinephrine reuptake inhibitor, is a nonstimulant medication approved for the treatment of ADHD in children and adults.

Indications and Efficacy

The efficacy of atomoxetine in the treatment of ADHD in the pediatric age group has been demonstrated in several controlled clinical trials (M. Weiss et al. 2005), with studies in young children showing continued efficacy and tolerability for up to 2 years (Kratochvil et al. 2006). Atomoxetine was shown to be beneficial in children with comorbid ADHD and oppositional defiant disorder in a randomized, controlled trial by Newcorn et al. (2005), and a small controlled pilot trial by Arnold et al. (2006) demonstrated the efficacy and safety of atomoxetine in the treatment of ADHD symptoms in children with a comorbid autism spectrum disorder.

Studies comparing the efficacy of atomoxetine with that of stimulant medications are limited. A retrospective analysis of pooled data from six controlled trials by Newcorn et al. (2009) suggested a bimodal distribution of atomoxetine efficacy, with almost half of children showing a good response, but with about 40% of children considered nonresponders. Unfortunately, the analysis was not able to offer any insights into which children would ultimately respond.

In the meantime, atomoxetine should be considered a second-line treatment for ADHD. The revised Texas Children's Medication Algorithm (Pliszka et al. 2006) recommends the use of atomoxetine only after trials of two different stimulants, unless severe side effects from stimulants or contraindications to their use require that atomoxetine be used preferentially.

Initiation and Maintenance

Based on clinical studies and current drug labeling, atomoxetine may be started at a dose of 0.5 mg/kg/day. The dose can be given once a day, or in equal divided doses in the morning and evening. The dose may then be incrementally increased every few days, as tolerated, to 1.2 mg/kg/day. The total daily dose in children and adolescents weighing less than 70 kg should not exceed 1.4 mg/kg/day or 100 mg, whichever is less. For children and adults who weigh over 70 kg, the maximum daily dose is 100 mg.

Risks and Side Effects

The product labeling of atomoxetine currently includes a black box warning about the possibility of increased suicidal ideation in children and adolescents taking this medication. Similar to the recommendations for the use of antidepressants in the pediatric population, this risk should be discussed with parents before initiating treatment. Patients should be closely monitored for increases in anxiety, irritability, aggressiveness, or mood disturbance or the presence of suicidal thoughts. Atomoxetine should be used with caution in children with a history of bipolar disorder or who have a family history of bipolar disorder or suicide.

Atomoxetine is generally well tolerated. The most common side effects include abdominal pain, headache, irritability or mood lability, dizziness, somnolence or fatigue, decreased appetite, and nausea and vomiting. Modest dose-related increases in pulse and blood pressure have also been noted. Most side effects appear to subside over time and only rarely result in discontinuation of treatment. A meta-analysis of the effect of atomoxetine on growth over a 2-year treatment period by Spencer et al. (2005) showed only minimal effects on height and weight compared with expected growth rates based on extrapolated baseline measurements and comparison to growth charts from the U.S. Centers for Disease Control and Prevention (CDC), with relative decreases of height and weight of less than 0.5 cm and 1 kg, respectively.

Selective Serotonin Reuptake Inhibitors

Six selective serotonin reuptake inhibitors (SSRIs) are currently approved by the FDA for use in the United States. Of these, only four have an indicated use in children. Escitalopram is indicated for the treatment of depression in children ages 12–17 years. Fluoxetine is approved for the treatment of depression in children 8–17 years of age and obsessive-compulsive disorder (OCD) in children ages 7–17 years. Fluvoxamine is approved for the treatment of OCD in children 8 years of age and older, and sertraline is approved for the treatment of OCD in children 6 years of age and older. However, all of the SSRIs have been used to treat a wide variety of disorders in children and adolescents. The use of SSRIs in children has become more controversial over the past few years as the results of clinical trials, some unpublished, called into question the efficacy of this class of medication in the treatment of pediatric depression. More importantly, concerns were raised that antidepressants in general, and the SSRI class of antidepressants in particular, may actually induce suicidal thinking or behavior in susceptible individuals.

A meta-analysis of 24 pediatric drug trials by Hammad et al. (2006) concluded that the use of antidepressant medications in children and adolescents is associated with a "modestly increased risk of suicidality." Of course, one would hasten to add, as did Hammad and colleagues, that association does not necessarily imply cause and effect, and that several possible alternative explanations exist, including an increased rate of reporting of suicidal thoughts and behaviors rather than an increase in the incidence of these phenomena.

After considering the matter carefully, the FDA stopped short of contraindicating the use of antidepressants in this age group but required that a black box warning of the increased risk of suicidality in pediatric patients be added to the labeling of all antidepressants (U.S. Food and Drug Administration 2004a).

The debate over SSRI use in children has not ended. No suicides actually occurred in the more than 4,000 children included in the studies of SSRI use in the pediatric population (U.S. Food and Drug Administration 2004b). The controlled studies analyzed by the FDA excluded children who had suicidal thoughts or behavior. As such, it is possible that SSRIs may reduce suicidality in medicated depressed children more than they induce it in nonsuicidal depressed children who initiate treatment (Riddle 2004). Some studies suggest that suicide rates have decreased in areas of the country where SSRI use has increased (Gibbons et al. 2005). Although the conversation about antidepressant use in children and adolescents continues, many health care providers believe, based on their own experience and the results of clinical studies, that SSRIs can be beneficial for children suffering from depression, anxiety, and other disorders.

Indications and Efficacy

Depressive disorders.   Fluoxetine and escitalopram are currently the only SSRIs with an FDA indication for the treatment of depression in children and adolescents. The efficacy of fluoxetine in treating pediatric de-

pression has been demonstrated in several controlled trials (Emslie et al. 2002, 2004; March et al. 2006).

Obsessive-compulsive disorder.   At present, fluoxetine, fluvoxamine, and sertraline possess FDA indications for their use in pediatric OCD, with several studies demonstrating the efficacy of these agents, along with paroxetine (D. A. Geller et al. 2003; March et al. 2004). A small randomized, controlled trial also supports the use of citalopram (Alaghband-Rad and Hakimshooshtary 2009). A 52-week open follow-up study of 120 children and adolescents diagnosed with OCD suggested that sertraline may be effective in the long-term treatment of OCD symptoms (Cook et al. 2001).

In 2004, the Pediatric OCD Treatment Study (POTS) (March et al. 2004) examined the use of sertraline, cognitive-behavioral therapy (CBT), and the combination of the two in a 12-week randomized, controlled study of 112 children and adolescents with OCD. All treatment modalities were found to be significantly superior to placebo. The combination of CBT and sertraline was superior to either CBT or sertraline monotherapy. Sertraline monotherapy was not superior to CBT monotherapy in treating pediatric OCD.

Other disorders.   SSRIs have been shown to be effective in the treatment of other anxiety disorders, such as social phobia, separation anxiety disorder, and generalized anxiety disorder, in the pediatric age group (Birmaher et al. 2003; Rynn et al. 2001; Wagner et al. 2004; Walkup et al. 2001, 2008).

A double blind, placebo-controlled study examining the effectiveness of fluoxetine in the treatment of elective mutism in a small group of children showed mixed results (Black and Uhde 1994).

Dosage and Administration

All of the SSRIs possess a black box warning about the potential for increased suicidality in patients taking these medications, and patients and parents should be cautioned accordingly. While the FDA recommends weekly monitoring of children during the first 4 weeks of treatment, with additional monitoring at weeks 6, 8, and 12, the American Psychiatric Association and AACAP suggest a monitoring schedule tailored to the individual needs of the patient and his or her family (PhysiciansMedGuide 2010).

The following dosing guidelines should be considered in light of the current evidence regarding the efficacy of SSRIs in pediatric psychiatric disorders. Fluoxetine, citalopram, and paroxetine may be started at dosages of 5–10 mg/day. These dosages may be increased as needed to 20 mg/day. Although most children will obtain an adequate response to 20 mg/day or less of these medications, some children may require dosages in excess of 20 mg/day. All three of these medications are available in a liquid formulation that may facilitate medication administration or dosage titration in small children. Escitalopram is generally dosed at half the usual dose for citalopram.

For sertraline and fluvoxamine, dosages may be started at 25 mg/day, and increased as necessary to a dosage of 100–150 mg/day. Doses may be increased every few days as tolerated. Sertraline is also available in a liquid preparation.

Although children and adolescents as well as adults usually tolerate this class of medication well, children may experience the same constellation of side effects as seen in adults, such as gastrointestinal complaints or headache. In addition, patients may experience a discontinuation syndrome if the medication is stopped abruptly. Symptoms include malaise, myalgias, headache, and anxiety, and these may occur even if only one dose is missed. It is therefore preferable to taper the dose of medication over several days rather than discontinue the medication abruptly. This discontinuation syndrome is not usually noted with fluoxetine, because of its active metabolites and long half-life. In a patient who has a recurrence of symptoms after an initial good response, gentle inquiry

about medication compliance should be made prior to making a change in dose.

Adverse Effects

Several cases of "behavioral activation" and manic symptoms, presumed to be caused by treatment with SSRIs, have been reported in pediatric patients. In many of these cases, the manic symptoms appeared within days to weeks of initiating treatment with an SSRI. Symptoms usually resolved within a few days of the reduction in dose or cessation of medication. In some cases, treatment with a mood stabilizer was necessary. In many of the cases, there was no premorbid or family history of a cyclical mood disorder.

Adolescents, like adults, may experience sexual dysfunction from SSRI therapy. Given the potential for SSRI-induced sexual dysfunction to affect treatment adherence, clinicians should be sensitive to the potential presence of this adverse effect in their adolescent patients. Movement disorders (acute dystonic reactions, akathisia, and tic-like movements) have also been noted in children taking SSRIs (Sokolski et al. 2004).

Serotonin syndrome is a potentially fatal reaction to serotonergic agents. It is more likely to occur when serotonergic agents are used in combination. Several signs characterize this syndrome: mental status changes, fever, tremor, diaphoresis, and agitation. While uncommon, there are several case reports of serotonin syndrome in the pediatric population. The syndrome may arise after only one dose of a serotonergic agent. Clinicians should be alert to the possibility of serotonin syndrome occurring in their pediatric patients and counsel patients and parents as appropriate.

Tricyclic Antidepressants

Until the introduction of the SSRIs into the U.S. market in the late 1980s, TCAs were a mainstay in the pharmacological treatment of a wide variety of disorders in children and adolescents. However, the paucity of clinical studies demonstrating the efficacy of TCAs in children, an increased awareness of the potential cardiac effects of this class of medication, and the availability of alternative medications have resulted in a shift away from using tricyclic agents as first-line treatment (Safer 1997).

Indications and Efficacy

Depression. TCAs have consistently failed to show superiority over placebo in treating pediatric depression (B. Geller et al. 1999). Given the absence of empirical data demonstrating efficacy and the unfavorable side-effect and risk profile, TCAs appear to have no place in the treatment of pediatric depression.

Attention-deficit/hyperactivity disorder. TCAs may be indicated for those patients who do not respond to stimulants. TCAs may also be useful for the treatment of ADHD symptoms in patients with tics or Tourette's disorder (Spencer et al. 2002). Efficacy in improving cognitive symptoms does not appear to be as great as for stimulants. The revised Texas Children's Medication Algorithm (Pliszka et al. 2006) describes TCAs as a fourth-line medication in the treatment of ADHD.

Obsessive-compulsive disorder. Clomipramine, a TCA that inhibits serotonin reuptake, is indicated for the treatment of OCD in children older than 10 years of age. In their meta-analysis of pharmacological treatments for pediatric OCD, D.A. Geller et al. (2003) found clomipramine to be more effective than SSRIs. As in depression, the more favorable side-effect and safety profile of the SSRIs makes clomipramine a second- or third-line treatment of OCD in children.

Enuresis. All of the TCAs have been found to be effective in the treatment of nocturnal enuresis. However, wetting invariably returns when the drug is discontinued. Behavioral treatments that avoid drug side effects and have higher remission rates are the best first choice. Should pharmacological intervention be necessary, desmopressin (1-desamino-8-D-arginine vasopressin [DDAVP]) is a first-line treatment and is preferred over TCAs due to its greater efficacy and more favorable safety profile (Hjalmas et al. 2004). A trial with imipramine may be useful if other interventions are unsuccessful (Gepertz and Nevéus 2004).

Anxiety disorders. The majority of studies have examined the use of TCAs for separation anxiety disorder and school absenteeism. The efficacy of imipramine in patients with anxiety disorders is controversial (Klein et al. 1992), and other medications are now available. Medication may be useful as an adjunct if psychosocial treatment is ineffective. In a randomized, double-blind trial of imipramine plus CBT in the treatment of school refusal, imipramine plus CBT was shown to be more effective than placebo plus CBT in decreasing depressive symptoms and improving school attendance (Bernstein et al. 2000).

Initiation and Maintenance

Pharmacokinetics for TCAs are different in children than in adolescents or adults. The smaller fat-to-muscle ratio in children leads to a decreased volume of distribution, and children are not protected from excessive dosage by a large volume of fat in which the drug can be stored. Children have larger livers relative to body size, leading to faster metabolism (Sallee et al. 1986), more rapid absorption, and lower protein binding than in adults (Winsberg et al. 1974). As a result, children are likely to need a higher weight-corrected dose of TCAs than adults. Prepubertal children are prone to rapid dramatic swings in blood levels from toxic to ineffective and should have divided doses to produce more stable levels (Ryan 1992). Parents must be reminded to supervise closely the administration of medication and to keep pills in a safe place. Wilens et al. (1996) recommended guidelines for monitoring the cardiovascular effects of TCAs. If the patient's history suggests head trauma or seizures, an electroencephalogram (EEG) is indicated before starting treatment.

Attention-deficit/hyperactivity disorder. Imipramine is begun at a dosage of 10 or 25 mg/day and increased weekly. The maximum dosage is 5 mg/kg/day (given in three divided doses in children). Plasma levels do not predict efficacy. Some patients respond to a daily dose as low as 2 mg/kg. Nortriptyline is given at 25–75 mg/day in two divided doses (Saul 1985).

Obsessive-compulsive disorder. Doses of clomipramine used to treat OCD are generally lower than TCA doses used for depression. Response is delayed for 10–14 days, as in the treatment of depression, and is unlike the immediate response seen in the treatment of ADHD or enuresis (Rapoport 1986). Clomipramine is started at 25 mg/day (or every other day) and gradually increased over 2 weeks to a maximum of 100 mg/day or 3 mg/kg/day, whichever is less. If necessary, the dosage in children and adolescents may be gradually increased up to a maximum of 200 mg/day or 3 mg/kg/day, whichever is less. Divided doses are preferable during dosage titration. Chronic treatment may be required.

Enuresis. Daily charting of wet and dry nights is used before starting medication to obtain a baseline and subsequently to monitor progress. Much lower doses are needed than for the treatment of depression. Imipramine is started at 10–25 mg at bedtime and increased by 10- to 25-mg increments weekly to 50 mg (75 mg in preadolescents), if necessary. The maximum dosage is 2.5 mg/kg/day (Ryan 1990). Tolerance may develop, requiring a dose increase. For some children, TCAs lose their effect entirely. If medication is used chronically, the child or adolescent should have a drug-free trial at least every 6 months because enuresis has a high spontaneous remission rate.

Anxiety disorders. In separation anxiety disorder and school nonattendance, psychological interventions such as family therapy, work with school personnel, and desensitization should be used before and along with medication. For children with school phobia,

McDaniel (1986) recommends 125 mg as the maximum dose of imipramine. The starting dosage for children ages 6–8 years is 10 mg at bedtime and for older children, 25 mg at bedtime. The dosage may be increased by 10–50 mg/day, but those with school avoidance require at least 75 mg/day. Some patients require a higher dose for complete response, but if there is no detectable positive response at 125 mg/day, improvement at higher doses is unlikely. After clinical response (6–8 weeks), medication is continued at least another 8 weeks and then gradually withdrawn.

Risks and Side Effects

As with other antidepressants, TCAs are considered to have the potential to induce suicidal thoughts or behavior, regardless of the condition for which they are being used, and consequently carry a black box warning to this effect. Patients and their caregivers should be cautioned about this potential adverse effect and advised on the behavioral signs and symptoms that may indicate developing suicidality. Frequent monitoring of patients by clinicians in the early stages of treatment is essential. TCAs are particularly lethal in overdose.

The quinidine-like effect of TCAs slows cardiac conduction time and repolarization. At dosages of more than 3 mg/kg/day of imipramine, children and adolescents may develop an increased pulse and small but statistically significant ECG changes (intraventricular conduction defects, such as lengthened P-R interval, that may progress to a first-degree atrioventricular heart block and occasional widening of the QRS complex) (Wilens et al. 1996). The tendency of prepubertal children to have wider swings in blood levels may place them at higher risk for serious cardiac conduction changes. A minority of the population has a genetic defect in TCA metabolism, increasing risk for toxicity.

Anticholinergic side effects may occur in children, although less commonly than in adults. Most of these side effects are transient and/or respond to a decrease in dose. Of particular importance for children are dry mouth (which may lead to an increase in dental caries in long-term use [Herskowitz 1987]), drying of bronchial secretions (especially problematic for asthmatic children), sedation, anorexia, constipation, nausea, tachycardia, palpitations, and increased diastolic blood pressure.

Other reported side effects include abdominal pain, chest pain, headache, orthostatic hypotension (rare in young patients), syncope, mild tremors of hands and fingers, weight loss, and tics. The seizure threshold may be lowered, with worsening of preexisting EEG abnormalities and rarely a seizure. Seizures appear to be more common with clomipramine. Side effects with a probable allergic mechanism include rash, worsening of eczema, and rarely thrombocytopenia (Campbell et al. 1985).

Behavioral toxicity may be manifested by irritability, worsening of psychosis, mania, agitation, anger, aggression, forgetfulness, or confusion. Central nervous system (CNS) toxicity may be mistaken for exacerbation of the primary condition. A drug blood level is often required to differentiate the two. As depressed children, especially those who are anergic and withdrawn, improve with TCA treatment, crying and verbalizations of sadness and anger may transiently increase.

Sudden cessation of moderate or higher doses results in flu-like anticholinergic withdrawal syndrome, with nausea, cramps, vomiting, headaches, and muscle pains. Other manifestations may include social withdrawal, hyperactivity, depression, agitation, and insomnia (Ryan 1990). TCAs should therefore be tapered over a 2- to 3-week period. The short half-life of TCAs in prepubertal children often produces daily withdrawal symptoms if medication is given only once a day. These symptoms also may indicate that poor compliance is resulting in missed doses. Because of the predictability of TCA-induced electrocardiographic changes, a rhythm strip is useful in monitoring compliance.

The physician should be alert to the risk of intentional overdose or accidental poisoning, not only by the patient but by other family members, especially young children.

Cautionary note on the use of desipramine. Seven cases of sudden death have been reported in children being treated with desipramine, three of whom died immediately after physical exertion (Varley and McClellan 1997). A causal relationship between the medication and the deaths has not been established. Cardiac etiology is often suspected; however, a review of cardiovascular changes in children treated with TCAs (Wilens et al. 1996) concluded that although changes in blood pressure, heart rate, and ECG parameters are identifiable, they are probably of minor significance.

A study of the effects of desipramine on cardiac function during exercise concluded that desipramine had only minor effects on the cardiovascular response to exercise and that these effects did not appear to be age related (Waslick et al. 1999). A further study by Walsh et al. (1999) showed that desipramine reduced parasympathetic input to the heart as measured by R-R interval variability. While this reduction in parasympathetic tone could, theoretically, increase vulnerability to cardiac arrhythmias, the R-R interval variability did not differ with age in the 42 subjects (ages 7–66 years) who were studied. Nevertheless, because other safe and effective medications are available, the use of desipramine in children is discouraged.

Other Antidepressants

Several other antidepressants are used to treat depression and other psychiatric conditions in the pediatric population, although none have an FDA indication for their use in children. All possess a black box warning because of their perceived potential to induce suicidality. Studies demonstrating efficacy of these agents in the pediatric age group are limited, and in some cases studies have failed to demonstrate efficacy in children. Most of these agents would be considered second- or third-line treatments, if considered at all.

Serotonin–Norepinephrine Reuptake Inhibitors

Few studies have examined the use of serotonin–norepinephrine reuptake inhibitors (SNRIs) in children. In light of the current literature, the use of SNRIs in the treatment of pediatric depression is unsupported.

Bupropion

Small controlled studies have demonstrated the superiority of bupropion to placebo in the treatment of ADHD in children. Bupropion has been reported to exacerbate tics in children with comorbid ADHD and Tourette's disorder and may not be suitable for use in this population (Spencer et al. 1993).

Although bupropion is marketed in the United States as an antidepressant and as an aid in smoking cessation, the literature on its use in treating childhood depression is limited to small open-label studies.

Bupropion is available in regular-, sustained-, and extended-release tablets in addition to the hydrobromide formulation (bupropion HBr; Aplenzin). Regular-release bupropion is administered in two or three daily doses, beginning with a low dose (37.5 or 50 mg bid), with titration over 2 weeks to a usual maximum of 250 mg/day (300–400 mg/day in adolescents). A sustained-release preparation of this medication is available in generic form, allowing for once- or twice-daily dosing. An extended-release preparation of bupropion (Wellbutrin XL) permits once-daily dosing, as does Aplenzin, which comes in 522-mg, 358-mg, and 174-mg tablets (considered to be equivalent to 450 mg, 300 mg, and 150 mg of Wellbutrin XL, respectively). The most serious side effect is a decrease in the seizure threshold, seen most frequently in patients with an eating disorder. Bupropion is contraindicated in this population. Other side effects in children include skin rash, perioral edema, nausea, increased appetite, agitation, and exacerbation of tics.

Monoamine Oxidase Inhibitors

The nonselective monoamine oxidase inhibitors (MAOIs) phenelzine, tranylcypromine, and isocarboxazid are infrequently prescribed in adults nowadays and their use in the pediatric age group is almost unheard of, given the availability of other safe and effective treatments.

Although some studies have suggested a possible role for selegiline in the treatment of children with ADHD (Akhondzadeh et al. 2003; Mohammadi et al. 2004; Rubinstein et al. 2006), further study is needed before its use can be routinely considered in pediatric ADHD. Selegiline, unlike the nonselective MAOIs, selectively inhibits MAO-B in therapeutic doses and is therefore much less likely to induce potentially fatal hypertensive crises due to the ingestion of tyramine-rich foods. Selegiline is metabolized to amphetamine and methamphetamine (Standaert and Young 2006), which may in part account for its usefulness in treating ADHD.

A transdermal formulation of selegiline is available for the treatment of depression. Studies of the safety and efficacy of this preparation in pediatric patients are required. We identified no studies of the use of selegiline in pediatric depressive disorders.

Mood-Stabilizing Agents

Lithium has been approved for use in the treatment of mania in patients 12 years of age and older. The antiepileptic drugs carbamazepine, oxcarbazepine, divalproex sodium, lamotrigine, and clonazepam have been used for a variety of non–FDA approved psychiatric indications. Divalproex sodium has an FDA-approved indication for the treatment of mania in adults, and lamotrigine is approved for maintenance treatment in adult bipolar disorder. The mood-stabilizing efficacy of these agents may be unrelated to their anticonvulsant effects. Wide variations in bioavailability and rate of absorption of generic products have led to recommendations that the brand name (or at least a single generic) product be prescribed. Two second-generation antipsychotics—aripiprazole and risperidone—also have an indication for the treatment of mania in children age 10 years and older; these are discussed in greater detail in the section on antipsychotic medications. Data on children and adolescents are far more limited than on adults, but side-effect patterns appear to be similar. All of the mood stabilizers, particularly the anticonvulsants, have complex interactions with multiple other drugs.

Lithium

Indications and efficacy.   In a controlled study of 25 adolescents with bipolar disorder and a substance dependence disorder, B. Geller et al. (1998) found that lithium significantly improved global functioning and decreased substance use compared with placebo. While a small sample size and lack of a follow-up phase limited this study, it is the first to examine the use of lithium in this particular population.

Lithium may be more useful in the treatment of the depressive phase of pediatric bipolar disorder than in the treatment of unipolar depression in children at risk of developing bipolar disorder because of a strong family history. Lithium is not indicated for prophylaxis in bipolar disorder in children and adolescents unless there is well-documented history of recurrent episodes.

It is not yet clear whether lithium is efficacious for the treatment of behavior disorders without an apparent mood disorder in children of bipolar parents or for children and adolescents who have behavior disorders accompanied by mood swings. Lithium has been shown to be effective in some placebo-controlled studies of children with severe impulsive aggression, while other controlled studies have rendered less encouraging results (Malone et al. 2000). Lithium may be useful in mentally retarded or autistic youths with severe aggression directed toward themselves or others or with symptoms suggestive of bipolar disorder (Campbell et al.

1985; Kerbeshian et al. 1987; Steingard and Biederman 1987).

Initiation and maintenance.   Lithium should not be prescribed unless the family is willing and able to comply with regular multiple daily doses and with blood monitoring of lithium levels. In addition to the usual detailed medical history and physical examination, complete blood count (CBC) with differential, liver function tests, electrolytes, serum thyroxine and thyroid-stimulating hormone (TSH), blood urea nitrogen (BUN), creatinine, and ECG should be determined before starting lithium. Some clinicians recommend determining renal concentrating ability (urine specific gravity or osmolality after overnight fluid deprivation). A patient with a history suggesting increased risk of seizures warrants an EEG. Height, weight, TSH, creatinine, and morning urine specific gravity (or osmolality) should be obtained every 3–6 months.

Lithium levels, drawn 10–12 hours after the last dose, should be obtained twice weekly during initial dose adjustment and monthly thereafter. Three to four days are required to reach steady-state levels after a dose change. Therapeutic levels are the same as for adults, 0.6–1.2 mEq/L. The starting dose is 150–300 mg/day, gradually titrated upward in divided doses according to serum levels and clinical effects. Total daily therapeutic dosing is typically reached between 900 and 1,200 mg. Because lithium excretion occurs primarily through the kidney, and most children have more efficient renal function than adults, they may require higher doses for body weight than do adults (Weller et al. 1986). More steady blood levels may be obtained by using a slow-release formulation. Lithium should be taken with food to minimize gastrointestinal distress. Some difference may be present in pharmacokinetics between lithium carbonate and lithium citrate, and clinicians should not assume equal dosing when shifting between the two forms (Reischer and Pfeffer 1996). Given lithium's teratogenicity, the clinician should address this potential with sexually mature female adolescent patients and consider contraceptive options as appropriate.

Risks and side effects.   The younger the child, the more likely the occurrence of side effects (Campbell et al. 1991). Autistic children have more frequent and severe side effects from lithium than do children with conduct disorder, even at lower doses (Campbell et al. 1991). Children may experience side effects at serum levels that are lower than those in adults: most commonly, weight gain, vomiting, headache, nausea, tremor, enuresis, stomachache, weight loss, sedation, and anorexia (Campbell et al. 1991). Common early-onset side effects, which seem to be related to rapid increase in serum level, include nausea, diarrhea, muscle weakness, thirst, urinary frequency, a dazed feeling, and hand tremor. Polydipsia and polyuria secondary to vasopressin-resistant diabetes insipidus may result in enuresis (Campbell et al. 1985). In growing children, the consequences of hypothyroidism (which could resemble retarded depression) are potentially more severe than in adults. The calcium mobilization from bones that has been noted in adults might cause a significant problem in growing children (Herskowitz 1987). Lithium's tendency to aggravate acne may be especially significant for adolescents. Lithium's effects on glucose are controversial, but both hyperglycemia and exercise-induced hypoglycemia are possible. Rarely, lithium may cause extrapyramidal side effects (EPS) in children (Samuel 1993).

Toxicity is closely related to serum levels, and the therapeutic margin is narrow. Symptoms of lithium toxicity include vomiting, drowsiness, hyperreflexia, sluggishness, slurred speech, ataxia, anorexia, convulsions, stupor, coma, and death. Adequate salt and fluid intake is necessary to prevent levels rising into the toxic range. The family should be instructed in the importance of preventing dehydration from heat or exercise and in the need to stop the lithium and contact the physician if the child or adolescent develops an illness with fever, vomiting, diarrhea, and/or decreased fluid intake. The erratic consumption of large amounts of salty snack foods may cause fluctuations in lithium levels (Herskowitz 1987). Clinicians should also be aware of potential drug–drug interactions, especially with nonsteroidal anti-inflammatory drugs, antipsychotic agents, SSRIs, and antibiotics (Kowatch and Bucci 1998).

Carbamazepine and Oxcarbazepine

The evidence suggesting a potential benefit of carbamazepine in the treatment of juvenile bipolar disorder is limited (Kowatch et al. 2000; Woolston 1999). No controlled studies have been reported. Carbamazepine usage has largely been supplanted by other, more effective treatments.

Oxcarbazepine is the 10-keto analog of carbamazepine, and is approved for use in children and adults as an anticonvulsant. The literature on its use in pediatric bipolar disorder consists of only a few case reports and one multicenter randomized, controlled trial (Wagner et al. 2006) in which oxcarbazepine was not found to be more effective than placebo. Any recommendations regarding its use in pediatric bipolarity must await further controlled trials.

Divalproex Sodium

Indications and efficacy.   Open-label trials of divalproex sodium as monotherapy (Wagner et al. 2002), in comparison with lithium or carbamazepine (Kowatch et al. 2000), and in combination with lithium (Findling et al. 2003b) have found it to be generally well tolerated and beneficial in the treatment of children and adolescents with mania. However, a recent blinded and controlled trial of divalproex extended-release in the treatment of pediatric bipolar disorder did not show the its superiority over placebo (Wagner et al. 2009). Further controlled studies are required to clarify whether divalproex sodium is beneficial in the treatment of pediatric bipolar disorder.

Initiation and maintenance.   Hemoglobin, hematocrit, CBC, platelets, liver function,

BUN, and creatinine should be measured before the patient begins taking valproate. Liver function tests and CBC may be repeated weekly for the first month and then every 4–6 months. For children younger than age 10 years, monthly liver function tests are advisable (Trimble 1990). Divalproex sodium may be initiated at 250 mg once or twice daily, depending on the weight of the child. Trough plasma levels should be drawn after reaching a dosage of 15 mg/kg/day dispensed in three divided doses. Dosages should be titrated to achieve a serum level within the therapeutic range (50–120 μg/mL). Clinicians are cautioned that the use of mg/kg loading doses for divalproex sodium may lead to supratherapeutic levels in overweight children (Good et al. 2001).

Risks and side effects.   The most frequent adverse effects are nausea, vomiting, and gastrointestinal distress (which may be diminished by using enteric-coated divalproex sodium), sedation, weight gain, and tremor (Trimble 1990). Acute hepatic failure is almost always restricted to children younger than age 3 years, especially those who have mental retardation or who are following a regimen of anticonvulsant polytherapy. Other side effects are similar to those seen in adults. Of uncertain significance is the report of menstrual disturbances, polycystic ovaries, and hyperandrogenism in a series of women treated with divalproex sodium for epilepsy (Isojarvi et al. 1993). These findings have been challenged in one review of the literature (Genton et al. 2001).

Lamotrigine

Lamotrigine is an anticonvulsant approved for the treatment of certain seizure disorders and as maintenance therapy for adults with bipolar disorder. Only a handful of reports describe its use in children with psychiatric disorders. Carandang et al. (2003) reported on their observations of a beneficial response in eight of nine adolescents with a mood disorder (predominantly bipolar or unipolar depression) treated with lamotrigine; three of the children received lamotrigine as monotherapy. Similar results in adolescent bipolar depression were described in an open-label trial by Chang et al. (2006).

Lamotrigine has the potential to induce serious, potentially life-threatening rashes in patients. This risk appears to be greater in pediatric patients treated for seizure disorders (0.8%) compared with adults (0.3%) (GlaxoSmithKline 2005). Prompt discontinuation of treatment at the first signs of rash is necessary, although this may not necessarily prevent a more serious rash from developing. Very slow titration of the medication seems to mitigate the potential for rash development. Until controlled trials establish lamotrigine's efficacy in the treatment of pediatric mood disorders, its use should be relegated to second- or third-line status.

Antipsychotic Medications

Indications and Efficacy

In addition to their use in the treatment of schizophrenia and other psychotic disorders, antipsychotic medications have been used in the pediatric population to treat bipolar disorders, conduct and other aggressive disorders, Tourette's disorder, and the behavioral manifestations of PDDs. The introduction of second-generation or "atypical" antipsychotic medications (aripiprazole, clozapine, olanzapine, quetiapine, risperidone, and ziprasidone) has added significantly to the child and adolescent psychiatrist's pharmaceutical armamentarium. Second-generation agents are increasingly being used over first-generation agents due to their more favorable side-effect profile and decreased risk of inducing EPS and tardive dyskinesia.

Psychotic disorders.   Few studies examining the efficacy of first-generation antipsychotic medications in schizophrenic children exist (Findling et al. 2005). Of the second-generation antipsychotics, only aripiprazole and risperidone possess an FDA-approved indication for the treatment of schizophrenia in adolescents, with efficacy demonstrated in randomized, controlled trials (Findling et al. 2008; Sikich et al. 2004). A randomized, controlled trial also showed olanzapine to be effective in this patient population (Kryzhanovskaya et al. 2009), although significant increases in weight and serum triglycerides were noted with olanzapine treatment.

Open trials and double-blind studies examining the efficacy of clozapine in adolescent patients with treatment-resistant childhood-onset schizophrenia have consistently demonstrated clozapine's superiority to standard treatments, specifically haloperidol (Kumra et al. 1996). And in a more recent study, clozapine was shown to be superior to olanzapine (Kumra et al. 2008). Because treatment with clozapine is compounded by possible serious side effects (agranulocytosis, seizures, and significant weight gain), clozapine's use is reserved for treatment of those select pediatric patients who have failed to respond to trials of first-generation or other second-generation antipsychotics.

Mood disorders. Although aripiprazole and risperidone are the only second-generation antipsychotic agents also approved for the treatment of bipolar disorder in patients age 10 years and older, olanzapine, quetiapine, and ziprasidone have also been shown to be superior to placebo in the treatment of pediatric bipolar disorder in clinical trials (McVoy and Findling 2009).

Pervasive developmental disorders. Of the second-generation agents, risperidone is the only one approved for use in treating the irritability associated with autistic disorder in children ages 5–16 years, with efficacy demonstrated in randomized, controlled trials (McCracken et al. 2005; Scahill et al. 2002; Shea et al. 2004; Troost et al. 2005). Risperidone was generally well tolerated in all of these studies, although weight gain was significant.

While the above studies demonstrate the efficacy of risperidone in controlling aggression, self-injurious behavior, and tantrums, risperidone appears to have limited benefit

in treating the primary symptoms of autism (McDougle et al. 2005).

A small randomized, controlled trial suggests that olanzapine may be a safe and effective treatment of core symptoms in children and adolescents with autism spectrum disorders (Hollander et al. 2006). Of all the second-generation antipsychotics, risperidone has the strongest evidence for its beneficial use in the treatment of the disruptive behaviors associated with PDDs, with efficacy being demonstrated in controlled trials. The evidence for the other second-generation agents is limited. Further controlled study of these medications in the treatment of PDDs is clearly needed.

Tourette's disorder. Two 8-week randomized, controlled trials in pediatric and adult patients with Tourette's disorder showed risperidone to be significantly superior to placebo in reducing symptom severity (Dion et al. 2002; Scahill et al. 2003). The mean daily dose of risperidone was comparable in both studies (2.5 mg/day), and risperidone was generally well tolerated. An average weight increase of 2.5 kg was reported in the treatment group of one study (Scahill et al. 2003), with no increase in weight in the placebo group. Although small open trials and pilot studies have been undertaken with other second-generation antipsychotics, controlled studies are needed in order to more clearly establish their safety and efficacy in Tourette's disorder.

Conduct disorder and aggression. Risperidone is the most studied second-generation antipsychotic for the treatment of pediatric aggression, with several double-blind placebo-controlled studies demonstrating efficacy in treating disruptive behavior disorders (Aman et al. 2002; Findling et al. 2000; Snyder et al. 2002). Among the various studies, dosages ranged from 1 to 3 mg/day and were generally well tolerated.

Literature on the use of aripiprazole (Findling et al. 2003a), clozapine (Soderstrom et al. 2002), olanzapine (Handen and Hardan

2006; Soderstrom et al. 2002), and quetiapine (Findling et al. 2007) in the treatment of aggression in pediatric patients is limited to case reports, small case series, or small open trials.

Initiation and Maintenance

Medication should not be used as the sole treatment in the aforementioned complex disorders. Before medication is initiated, a complete physical examination and baseline laboratory workup, including CBC with differential, serum chemistries including fasting glucose and liver-associated enzymes, TSH, lipid studies, and urinalysis, should be done. A baseline EEG is recommended in children being treated with clozapine, and a weekly white blood cell count with differential is mandatory for at least the first 6 months of clozapine therapy. Antipsychotic medication use has been linked to the development of type 2 diabetes mellitus that may or may not be related to weight gain. Patients treated with atypical agents should specifically be monitored for changes in weight, as well as changes in fasting glucose levels. Both first- and second-generation antipsychotic agents have been shown to increase QT intervals on ECG, potentially leading to dysrhythmias and sudden death. Clinicians should consider ECG monitoring, when appropriate.

Doses must be titrated individually, with careful attention to positive and negative effects. Age, weight, and severity of symptoms do not provide clear guidelines. The initial dose should be very low, with gradual increments no more than once or twice a week. Although divided doses are often used during titration, in most cases, once a therapeutic dosage has been reached, a single daily dose (usually at bedtime) can be used. Children metabolize these drugs more rapidly than do adults but also require lower plasma levels for efficacy (Teicher and Glod 1990). Antipsychotic medications can interact with a wide variety of other drugs (Teicher and Glod 1990). Dosing guidelines for the second-generation antipsychotics can be found in Table 19–2.

Schizophrenia.   While data are few, they are suggestive of the benefit and safety of the use of atypical antipsychotics as first-line agents for schizophrenia in this population. Children and younger adolescents generally need lower dosages than adults, whereas older adolescents may require dosages in the adult range. It may require several weeks for full efficacy to be achieved. Due to potential for lethal side effects, clozapine should be used only in cases refractory to treatment with other first- or second-generation agents and should be started at very low dosages—12.5 mg/day or 25 mg/day—and titrated slowly to minimize side effects to an expected dosage range of 250–500 mg/day.

Pervasive developmental disorders. It is important to give a trial of sufficient length to determine if the drug is efficacious in a child with PDD, barring serious side effects requiring immediate discontinuation. Developmentally disturbed children treated with risperidone may benefit from dosages as low as 0.5–1.0 mg/day, with most responding to dosages between 0.5 and 2 mg/day. Therapeutic daily dosages for olanzapine may range from 5 to 20 mg.

Tourette's disorder.   Careful monitoring of patients with Tourette's disorder for several months before starting medication is possible, given that Tourette's is a chronic condition and not usually an emergency. This monitoring permits the clinician to establish a baseline of symptoms and to assess the need for psychological and educational interventions. Risperidone dosages in the range of 0.5–2.5 mg/day appear to be useful. Sallee et al. (2000) initiated ziprasidone at 5 mg/day, titrating as high as 40 mg/day to achieve clinical effect in the Tourette's disorder children they studied. Effective dosages of quetiapine in the two published reports ranged from 50 to 150 mg/day (Mukaddes and Abali 2003; Párraga et al. 2001). For olanzapine, dosages of 10–15 mg/day may be helpful (Stephens et al. 2004).

Table 19–2. Clinical use of second-generation antipsychotics in pediatric patients

Generic name	How supplied	Indications	Target adult dosing	Pediatric dosing	Remarks
Aripiprazole	2-, 5-, 10-, 15-, 20-, 30-mg tablets 10-, 15-mg orally disintegrating tablets 1 mg/mL oral solution	Schizophrenia Acute bipolar mania Maintenance treatment for bipolar disorder Adjunct treatment for major depression[a]	10–15 mg/day 15–30 mg/day 15–30 mg/day 2–15 mg/day	10–30 mg/day[b]	Start with a dose of 2 mg/day in pediatric patients. Maximum dosage is 30 mg/day.
Clozapine	12.5-, 25-, 50-, 100-, 200-mg tablets 12.5-, 25-, 100-mg orally disintegrating tablets	Treatment-resistant schizophrenia[a]	300–600 mg/day	250–500 mg/day[c]	Use only in cases where patients do not adequately respond to first- or second-generation agents. Start treatment with 12.5 mg/day; maximum dosage in adults is 900 mg/day. Patients taking clozapine are at risk of developing agranulocytosis, myocarditis, other cardiac side effects, or seizures. Frequent blood monitoring required.
Olanzapine	2.5-, 5.0-, 7.5-, 10-, 15-, 20-mg tablets 5-, 10-, 15-, 20-mg orally disintegrating tablets	Schizophrenia[a] Bipolar disorder[a]	10 mg/day 10–15 mg/day (range 5–20 mg/day)	5–15 mg/day	Start with a dosage of 2.5 mg/day in children, 5 mg/day in adolescents, and 5–10 mg/day in adults. Dosage changes should be made weekly, due to the medication's long half-life.
	10 mg intramuscular	Acute agitation associated with schizophrenia or bipolar mania[a]	5–20 mg/day		Maximum adult dosage is 20 mg/day. Maximum adult dosage is 30 mg/day.

Table 19–2. Clinical use of second-generation antipsychotics in pediatric patients *(continued)*

Generic name	How supplied	Indications	Target adult dosing	Pediatric dosing	Remarks
Quetiapine	25-, 50-, 100-, 200-, 300-, 400-mg tablets 50-, 150-, 200-, 300-, 400-mg extended-release	Schizophrenia[a] Bipolar disorder, mania[a] Bipolar disorder, depression[a]	150–750 mg/day 400–800 mg/day 300 mg/day	300–800 mg/day[d]	Dosed bid or tid. Start with 25–50 mg/day in divided doses; increase by 25–50 mg every 1–2 days as tolerated. Maximum dosage in adults is 800 mg/day. Ophthalmological examination for cataracts is recommended before starting treatment and at 6-month intervals thereafter.
Risperidone	0.25-, 0.5-, 1-, 2-, 3-, 4-mg tablets 0.5-, 1-, 2-, 3-, 4-mg orally disintegrating tablets 1 mg/mL oral solution 25-mg, 37.5-mg, 50-mg intramuscular depot	Schizophrenia Bipolar disorder, mania Autistic disorder, irritability	4–8 mg/day 1–6 mg/day N/A	1–6 mg/day Maximum 1 mg/day if <20 kg; 2.5 mg/day if 20–40 kg; 3 mg/day if >40 kg	May be dosed qd or bid. Maximum adult dosage is 16 mg/day. Start with 0.25 mg in children, 0.5 mg in adolescents.

Table 19–2. Clinical use of second-generation antipsychotics in pediatric patients *(continued)*

Generic name	How supplied	Indications	Target adult dosing	Pediatric dosing	Remarks
Ziprasidone	20-, 40-, 60-, 80-mg tablets 20 mg intramuscular	Schizophrenia[a] Acute bipolar mania[a]	40–160 mg/day 80–160 mg/day	20–120 mg/day	Dosed bid. Usual adult starting doses are 20 mg bid in schizophrenia, and 40 mg bid in acute mania, increased every 1–2 days as tolerated. Baseline electrocardiogram, with repeat after dose stabilization, is recommended due to potential for QTc prolongation.

Note.   bid=twice-daily dosing; qd=once-daily dosing; tid=three-times-per-day dosing. Pediatric dosing guidelines are derived from available literature and are recommendations only. Dosing of these medications in pediatric patients should be titrated based on tolerability and symptom response. These medications are often used in pediatric patients for conditions other than those for which they are indicated in adults, such as for disruptive behavior disorders, pervasive developmental disorders, and Tourette's disorder. Published reports of the use of second-generation antipsychotics in conditions other than schizophrenia and acute mania are limited, especially in the pediatric age group. Reported dosage ranges vary widely when used for these other conditions and may differ from the dosage ranges used for schizophrenia or acute mania. Please consult chapter text and manufacturers' product inserts for further prescribing information.

[a]Not a U.S. Food and Drug Administration (FDA)-approved pediatric indication.

[b]Dosages in most pediatric studies ranged from 1 to 15 mg/day.

[c]Dosages in most pediatric studies in schizophrenia ranged from 75 to 500 mg/day.

[d]Limited information on pediatric dosing of quetiapine is available. Individual case studies report dosages of 100–600 mg/day, with Tourette's disorder being treated by dosages of 50–150 mg/day. Larger case studies report dosages ranging from 300 to 800 mg/day, predominantly for schizophrenia or acute mania.

Source.   Adapted from product labeling and information available from Drugs@FDA (www.fda.gov/cder).

Risks and Side Effects

An excellent review of second-generation antipsychotic side effects in children can be found in Correll et al. (2006).

Extrapyramidal side effects. Acute EPS, including dystonic reactions, parkinsonian tremor, rigidity and drooling, and akathisia, occur as in adults and may be induced by either first- or second-generation agents. Acute dystonia may be treated with oral or intramuscular diphenhydramine, 25 mg or 50 mg, or benztropine mesylate, 0.5–2.0 mg. Adolescent boys seem to be more vulnerable to acute dystonic reactions than are adult patients, so the physician may be more inclined to use prophylactic antiparkinsonian medication. In children, however, reduction of antipsychotic dose is preferable to the use of antiparkinsonian agents (Campbell et al. 1985).

For treatment or prevention of parkinsonian symptoms, adolescents may be given the anticholinergic drug benztropine mesylate, 1–2 mg/day, in divided doses. Chronic parkinsonian symptoms are often drastically underrecognized by clinicians (Richardson et al. 1991). The neuromuscular consequences may impair the performance of age-appropriate activities, and the subjective effects may lead to noncompliance with medication. Akathisia may be especially difficult to identify in young patients or those with limited verbal abilities.

Tardive and withdrawal dyskinesias. Tardive or withdrawal dyskinesias, some transient but others irreversible, mandate caution regarding the casual use of these drugs. Tardive dyskinesia has been documented in children and adolescents after as brief a period of treatment as 5 months with a first-generation agent (Herskowitz 1987) and may appear even during periods of constant medication dose. Cases of tardive dyskinesia have also been reported in youths treated with second-generation antipsychotics (Kumra et al. 1998), indicating that patients treated with these newer medications may not be immune to this serious adverse reaction. In children

with autism or Tourette's disorder, it may be especially difficult to distinguish medication-induced movements from those characteristic of the disorder. Before patients begin taking an antipsychotic medication, they should be examined carefully for abnormal movements by using a scale such as the Abnormal Involuntary Movement Scale (AIMS 1988) and should be periodically reexamined. Parents and patients (if they are able) should receive regular explanations of the risk of movement disorders.

Cardiovascular side effects. Antipsychotic medications have been associated with prolongation of the QTc interval, torsades de pointes, and sudden death (Glassman and Bigger 2001). Certain antipsychotics may be at greater risk for causing these problems. Thioridazine possesses a black box warning due to its significantly greater risk for causing QTc prolongation and sudden death. Haloperidol has also been associated with torsades de pointes.

Ziprasidone has been shown to have a clear effect on cardiac repolarization, resulting in QTc prolongation that is greater than with most antipsychotic agents, but less than with thioridazine. While no evidence of serious cardiac events occurred during the premarketing testing of ziprasidone, its association with sudden death remains unclear (Glassman and Bigger 2001).

The use of clozapine has been associated with the development of other cardiotoxicities, such as cardiomyopathy, myocarditis, and pericarditis, which have also occurred in the pediatric age group (Wehmeier et al. 2004). Clinicians considering the use of clozapine in pediatric patients should be mindful of the potential development of these cardiac side effects and should monitor patients accordingly.

Metabolic side effects. Weight gain may be problematic with the use of antipsychotics, especially second-generation medications (Martin et al. 2004). The weight gain associated with risperidone, while significant, appears less than that associated with olanzapine (Vieweg et al. 2005). Distinguishing growth-related weight gain from weight gain associated with antipsychotic use can be problematic in children and adolescents, and no specific criteria have been widely adopted (Correll 2005). Measurements of height and weight and calculations of body mass index (BMI) are recommended before initiation of treatment with antipsychotic agents and at regular intervals thereafter.

Reports of children and adolescents developing hyperglycemia or diabetes mellitus after treatment with second-generation agents have been published, although polypharmacy or a family history of diabetes was present in many instances. Until further studies elucidate a clear relationship (or not) between second-generation agents and the development of hyperglycemia or diabetes mellitus in children, prudence would suggest especially cautious use of these agents in children who are already overweight or who have a strong family history of diabetes. Baseline measurement of fasting blood sugar, with occasional measurements thereafter, is recommended for all patients treated with these medications.

Other side effects. Hyperprolactinemia is a potential effect of treatment with antipsychotic agents, due to their effects on tuberoinfundibular pathways within the CNS, although this potential is theoretically lower with the second-generation agents, due to their serotonergic effects that result in decreased stimulation of prolactin secretion (Stahl 2000). Hyperprolactinemia has been associated with galactorrhea, menstrual irregularities, sexual dysfunction, and osteoporosis.

With first-generation agents, another concern is behavioral toxicity, manifested as worsening of preexisting symptoms or development of new symptoms such as hyperactivity or hypoactivity, irritability, apathy, withdrawal, stereotypies, tics, or hallucinations (Campbell et al. 1985). Sedation, which is common with atypical antipsychotics, may

also be experienced with low-potency first-generation antipsychotic drugs such as chlorpromazine and thioridazine and can interfere with the patient's ability to benefit from school. Children may be at greater risk of antipsychotic-induced seizures than adults because of their immature nervous systems and in view of the high prevalence of abnormal EEGs in seriously disturbed children.

Anticholinergic side effects such as hypotension, dry mouth, constipation, nasal congestion, blurred vision, and urinary retention are most commonly experienced with low-potency first-generation antipsychotics and appear to be unusual in children. Potentially fatal neuroleptic malignant syndrome has been reported in children and adolescents (Chungh et al. 2005), with a presentation similar to that seen in adults.

Anxiolytics, Sedatives, and Hypnotics

There are few data on the safety and efficacy of anxiolytics and sedative-hypnotics in children and adolescents, although this population appears to respond similarly to adults (Spencer et al. 1995). In most cases, psychosocial interventions should precede and accompany pharmacotherapy.

Benzodiazepines

Indications and efficacy. Little research has been done on the use of benzodiazepines for pediatric psychiatric conditions. Benzodiazepines may be useful in the short-term treatment of children with severe anticipatory anxiety (Pfefferbaum et al. 1987). Some evidence suggests that clonazepam may be useful in the treatment of panic disorder and neuroleptic-induced akathisia in adolescents (Biederman 1987; Kutcher et al. 1989).

Initiation and maintenance. Infants and children absorb diazepam faster and metabolize it more quickly than do adults (Simeon and Ferguson 1985). Usual daily dose ranges for children and adolescents are as follows: lorazepam, 0.25–6.00 mg; diazepam, 1–20 mg;

and alprazolam, 0.25–4.00 mg. Clonazepam has been used at 0.5–3.0 mg/day. Dosage schedule depends on age (more frequent in children) and the specific drug (Coffey 1990). When the medication is being discontinued, the dose needs to be tapered gradually to avoid withdrawal seizures or rebound anxiety.

Risks and side effects.   In addition to the risks of substance abuse and physical or psychological dependence, side effects include sedation, cognitive dulling, ataxia, confusion, emotional lability, and worsening of psychosis. Paradoxical or disinhibition reactions may occur, manifested by acute excitation, irritability, increased anxiety, hallucinations, increased aggression and hostility, rage reactions, insomnia, euphoria, and/or incoordination.

Naltrexone and Acamprosate

Abnormalities of endogenous opioids have been suggested to occur in persons who have autism and in mentally retarded persons who engage in self-injurious behavior. Published reports are mixed regarding the benefits of naltrexone, a potent opiate antagonist, in these conditions. Several double-blind and placebo-controlled studies have shown naltrexone to be effective in the treatment of hyperactivity in autistic children (Kolmen et al. 1995; Willemsen-Swinkels et al. 1996). Although earlier reports suggested that naltrexone treatment increased social interaction and decreased self-injury in autistic patients, these later controlled studies failed to demonstrate statistical difference from response to placebo in regard to these behaviors (Feldman et al. 1999).

In doses of 0.5–2.0 mg/kg/day, naltrexone appears to be safe, with only mild side effects noted. No changes in any laboratory measures, ECG, or vital signs have been demonstrated in children or adolescents.

Acamprosate is a glutamate receptor modulator recently approved in the United States for the treatment of alcohol dependence in adult patients who are abstinent at the time of initiation of treatment. A small double-blind, placebo-controlled study of adolescents with alcohol dependence by Niederhofer and Staffen (2003) reported that, at the end of the 3-month study, 7 of the 13 adolescents treated with acamprosate remained abstinent, compared with 2 of the 13 adolescents treated with placebo. Larger controlled trials of the use of acamprosate in alcohol-dependent adolescents are needed.

Desmopressin

Desmopressin (DDAVP) is an analog of antidiuretic hormone administered as a nasal spray or oral tablet to treat nocturnal enuresis. DDAVP acts by increasing water absorption in the kidneys, thereby reducing the volume of urine. Onset of action is rapid, and side effects are mild (nasal mucosal dryness or irritation, headache, epistaxis, and nausea) in patients with normal electrolyte regulation. In their review of the literature, Thompson and Rey (1995) concluded that DDAVP is superior to placebo in the treatment of nocturnal enuresis. They further noted that behavioral methods are more effective and that the relapse rate after cessation of DDAVP is high. Most of the studies cited at that time were of brief duration, usually 2 weeks. A year-long open study by Hjalmas et al. (1998) supports the safe and effective longer-term use of DDAVP.

The usual dosage is 0.2–0.6 mg orally at bedtime; use of the intranasal preparation is no longer recommended. Relapse is likely upon discontinuation of treatment. Water intoxication is rare, but children should be encouraged to limit fluid intake in the evenings when taking DDAVP.

Electroconvulsive Therapy

Electroconvulsive therapy (ECT) is currently reserved for the treatment of adolescents with depression, mania, or certain psychotic disorders who have not responded to more conservative interventions (such as several trials of medication) or whose symptoms (such as severe and persistent suicidal intent) require an urgent treatment response. Experience in the use of ECT in adolescents is limited and is extremely rare in prepubertal children. The current AACAP practice parameter on the use of ECT in adolescents (Ghaziuddin et al. 2004) offers a thorough review of the literature and guidelines for the use of this treatment modality in adolescents.

Psychotherapy

While psychotherapy for children has been shown to be effective when performed in a research setting (Kazdin 2000; Weisz 2000), the results are often less favorable when psychotherapy provided in the clinical or office setting is studied (B. Weiss et al. 2000; Weisz and Jensen 2001). Compared with children seen in research environments, children seen in "real world" clinical practice are often more symptomatic, have other comorbid conditions, have more psychosocially stressed families, and receive more eclectic forms of psychotherapy (Borkovec and Miranda 1996; Kazdin 2000; Weisz 2000).

There are currently more than 550 therapeutic techniques used in child and adolescent psychotherapy (Kazdin 2000). More data are emerging regarding the use and efficacy of specific forms of psychotherapy for particular disorders, especially depressive and anxiety disorders. The following sections describe, in very general terms, some of the more common forms of psychotherapy used in children. More thorough explanations of the various techniques of psychotherapy as they are applied to children may be found in therapy-specific reference materials and treatment manuals.

Individual Psychotherapy

All individual therapies have certain common themes (Strupp 1973):

- Relationship with a therapist who is identified as a helping person and who has some degree of control and influence over the patient
- Instillation of hope and improved morale
- Use of attention, encouragement, and suggestion
- Goals of helping the patient to achieve greater control, competence, mastery, and/or autonomy; to improve coping skills; and to abandon or modify unrealistic expectations of himself or herself, others, and the environment

In the treatment of children, it is essential to consider the patients' environment and family dynamics. In most cases, work with parents and school, and often pediatricians, welfare agencies, courts, or recreation leaders, must accompany individual therapy. The cooperation of parents, and often teachers, is required to maintain the child in treatment and to remove any secondary gain resulting from the symptoms. The therapist must be aware of a patient's level of physical, cognitive, and emotional development in order to understand the symptoms, set appropriate goals, and tailor effective interventions.

Communication With Children and Adolescents

Children are less able to use abstract language than are adults. They use play to express feelings, to narrate past events, to work through trauma, and to express wishes and hopes. It is less threatening and anxiety provoking if the therapist uses the metaphor of the play and bases questions and comments on characters in the play rather than on the child (even if the connection is clear to the therapist). Effective communications are tailored to the child's stage of language, cognitive, and affective development. The therapist must be aware that the vocabulary of some bright and precocious children exceeds their emotional understanding of events and concepts.

Dramatic play with dolls or puppets, drawing, painting, or modeling with clay, as well as questions about dreams, wishes, or favorite stories or television shows, can provide access to children's fantasies, emotions, and concerns. Adolescents may prefer creative writing or more complex expressive art techniques.

The Resistant Child or Adolescent

It is not surprising that many children or adolescents do not cooperate in therapy. Most are brought to treatment by adults. These young patients often do not wish to change themselves or their behaviors and view their parents' and teachers' complaints as unreasonable or unfair. In addition, a child or adolescent may refuse to participate in or may attempt to sabotage therapy for a variety of dynamic reasons (Gardner 1979). Effective interventions are tailored to the cause of the resistance.

A child who is feeling anxious or having difficulty separating from a parent may be helped by initially permitting the parent to remain in the therapy room. When a child or adolescent does not talk, whether from anxiety or opposition, the therapist often addresses this reluctance, either directly or through play. Long silences are not generally helpful and tend to increase anxiety or battles for control. Attractive play materials help to make therapy less threatening and to encourage participation while the therapist builds an alliance. However, the therapist must guard against the danger of sessions becoming mere play or recreation instead of therapy. A variety of techniques incorporate therapeutic activities with storytelling, drama, and game boards (Gardner 1979). Using behavioral contingencies in therapy also may improve motivation and cooperation.

Types of Individual Psychotherapy

Psychodynamic psychotherapies. In *psychoanalysis,* a relatively infrequently used treatment modality for children and adolescents, neurotic symptoms are viewed as arising from internalized intrapsychic conflict, nonorganic developmental arrest, or regression. The goal is to remove these symptoms through structural changes in defensive organization and personality. The expense, frequency of sessions, length of treatment, and often lack of immediate symptom relief have contributed to the decreased use of psychoanalysis.

Psychodynamically oriented psychotherapy is grounded in psychoanalytic theory but is more flexible and emphasizes the real relationship with the therapist and the provision of a corrective emotional experience rather than the transference. Frequency is typically once or twice a week, most commonly over a period of 1–2 years, although shorter, time-limited dynamic psychotherapies are also available (Dulcan 1984). Interaction between the parents and the therapist is more active. Goals of therapy include symptom resolution, change in behavior, and return to normal developmental process. Change occurs via transference interpretation and maturation of defenses, catharsis, development of insight, ego strengthening, improved reality testing, and sublimation (Adams 1982). The therapist forms an alliance with the child or adolescent, reassures, promotes controlled regression, identifies feelings, clarifies thoughts and events, makes interpretations, judiciously educates and advises, and acts as an advocate for the patient (Adams 1982).

Supportive therapy. Supportive therapy has less ambitious goals than dynamically oriented psychotherapies and is usually focused on a particular crisis or stressor. The therapist provides support to the patient until a stressor resolves, a developmental crisis has passed, or the patient or environment changes sufficiently so that other adults can take on the supportive role. There is a real relationship with the therapist, who facilitates catharsis and provides understanding and judicious advice.

Time-limited therapy. All of the various models of time-limited therapy have in common a planned, relatively brief duration; a predominant focus on the presenting problem; a high degree of structure and attention to specific, limited goals; and active roles for both therapist and patient. Length of treatment varies among models from several sessions to 6 months. The short duration is used to increase patient motivation, participation, and reliance on resources within the patient's world rather than on the therapist. Theoretical foundations include psychodynamic, crisis, family systems, cognitive, behavioral or social learning and guidance, or educational theories (Dulcan 1984; Dulcan and Piercy 1985).

Interpersonal psychotherapy. A model of interpersonal psychotherapy has been modified for depressed adolescents (IPT-A) (Mufson et al. 2004a). This 12-week treatment focuses on improving interpersonal relationships in the lives of depressed adolescents through role clarification and enhanced communication. This modality has been elaborated in a treatment manual and has demonstrated efficacy in several controlled studies (Mufson et al. 2004b).

Cognitive-behavioral therapy. The CBT techniques developed for the treatment of depression in adults have been adapted for use in children and adolescents. CBT has been shown in numerous controlled trials to be efficacious in the treatment of anxiety and depressive disorders in children and adolescents (Compton et al. 2004) as well as in pediatric posttraumatic stress disorder (Cohen et al. 2005; Smith et al. 2007). Caution is needed to ensure that homework assignments that are an integral part of this therapy are not perceived as aversive when added to homework assigned in school. Studies have also shown that cognitive self-control training may be effective in reducing aggressive behavior in adolescents (Kazdin 2000; Weisz et al. 2004).

Other psychotherapies. Dialectical behavior therapy (DBT) and motivational interviewing are two psychotherapeutic techniques developed for adults that have been adapted for use in adolescents.

Originally developed by Marsha Linehan (1993) for women with borderline personality disorder, DBT combines cognitive-behavioral therapy and Eastern meditation techniques. A.L. Miller et al. (2007) developed a modified 16-week outpatient treatment for use with suicidal adolescents that has been shown to be beneficial in a clinical study (Rathus and Miller 2002). A program for use in adolescent inpatients has also been described (Katz and Cox 2002).

Motivational interviewing is a client-centered directive therapy (W.R. Miller and Rollnick 2002). Commonly used in the treatment of substance abuse and to help decrease negative health behaviors and reinforce positive behaviors, its use has also been reported in the treatment of adolescent depression (Brody 2009). As with DBT, there are no published randomized, controlled trials in the adolescent population, although initial reports are promising.

Parent Counseling

Parent counseling or guidance is primarily a psychoeducational intervention, conducted in a mental health setting. It may be conducted with a single parent or couple, or in groups. In counseling sessions, parents learn about normal child and adolescent development. Efforts are made to help parents better understand their child and his or her problems and to modify practices that may be contributing to the current difficulties (whatever their original cause). The therapist's understanding of the parents' point of view and of the hardships of living with a disturbed child is crucial to the therapist's successful work with the child. For some parents who have serious difficulties of their own, parent counseling may merge into or pave the way for individual treatment of the adult or couple.

Behavior Therapy

In behavior therapy, symptoms are viewed as resulting from bad habits, faulty learning, or inappropriate environmental responses to behavior rather than as stemming from unconscious or intrapsychic motivation. Attention is focused on observable behaviors, psychophysiological responses, and self-report statements. Behavioral approaches are characterized by detailed assessment of problematic responses and the environmental conditions that elicit and maintain them, the development of strategies to produce change in the environment and therefore in the patient's behavior, and repeated assessment to evaluate the success of the intervention.

Indications and Efficacy

Behavior therapy is by far the most thoroughly evaluated psychological treatment for children. Maximally effective programs require home and school cooperation, focus on specific target behaviors, and ensure that contingencies follow behavior quickly and consistently.

Behavior therapy is the most effective treatment for simple phobias, for enuresis and encopresis, and for the noncompliant behaviors seen in oppositional defiant disorder and conduct disorder. For youngsters with ADHD, behavior modification can improve both academic achievement and behavior, if specifically targeted. Both punishment (time-out and response cost) and reward components are required. Behavior modification is more effective than medication in improving peer interactions, but skills may need to be taught first. Many youngsters require programs that are consistent, intensive, and prolonged (months to years). A wide variety of other childhood problems, such as motor and vocal tics, trichotillomania, and sleep problems, are treated by behavior modification, either alone or in combination with pharmacotherapy.

Parent Management Training

Effective training packages, based on social learning theory, have been developed for parents of noncompliant, oppositional, and aggressive children (Barkley 1997; Forehand and Long 2002; McMahon and Forehand 2003) and delinquent adolescents (Kazdin 2005; Patterson and Forgatch 2005). Such behaviors in children have been found to lead to inappropriately harsh or ineffective parental responses. Through training, parents are taught to give clear instructions, to positively reinforce good behavior, and to use punishment effectively. One frequently used negative contingency is the time-out, so called because it puts the child in a quiet, boring area where there is a time-out from accidental or naturally occurring positive reinforcement. The most powerful parent training programs use a combination of written materials, verbal instruction, and videotapes in social learning principles and contingency management, modeling by the therapist, and behavioral rehearsal of skills to be used. Parent management training has been shown to be effective in improving child behavior in meta-analyses conducted by Serketich and Dumas (1996) and Montgomery et al. (2006).

Classroom Behavior Modification

Techniques for behavior modification in schools include token economies, class rules, and attention to positive behavior, as well as response cost programs in which reinforcers are withdrawn in response to undesirable behavior. Reinforcers such as positive recognition or stars on a chart may be dispensed by teachers or more tangible rewards or privileges by parents through the use of daily report cards. Effective programs for use in the classroom environment include the Academic and Behavioral Competencies (ABC) Program (Pelham et al. 2005) and the Positive Behavior Support program (Sugai and Horner 2002).

Behavioral Treatment of Specific Symptoms

Behavioral treatments are useful for treating enuresis, encopresis, and certain anxiety disorders in children. An evaluation for other psychiatric disorders or trauma as well as a medical history and physical examination should precede behavioral treatment.

Enuresis. In younger children, especially those who wet only at night, enuresis is largely a consequence of delayed maturation. While waiting for the child to outgrow it, the most useful strategy is to minimize secondary symptoms by discouraging the parents from punishing or ridiculing the child. Older children can be taught to change their own beds, thus reducing expectable negative reactions from parents. A simple monitoring and reward procedure that includes a chart with stars to be exchanged for rewards may be effective for some children who are motivated to stop wetting the bed.

Two additional programs found to be effective in treating nocturnal enuresis are the urine alarm device and dry-bed training. The urine alarm is a conditioning treatment that results in dryness in 65%–75% of children (Butler and Gasson 2005). The success rate can be increased and relapses minimized by the addition of various behavioral interventions (Houts 1995). Dry-bed training (Azrin et al. 1974) is an equally effective (but somewhat more cumbersome) behavioral program that includes positive practice, contingent response, and the urine alarm in combination.

Combining the urine alarm with a pharmacological treatment is particularly effective in children who are frequent bed-wetters and has been shown to be more effective than the urine alarm alone in one study (Bradbury and Meadow 1995). Butler et al. (2001) have developed a structured withdrawal program to assist in relapse prevention by systematically withdrawing medication (either desmopressin or imipramine) while using a chart to allow children to track dry nights. Almost 75% of children remained dry in the last 2 weeks of the 10-week program (when no medication was administered), with over 70% of those remaining dry at 6 months' posttreatment.

Children who are secondarily enuretic (having previously been dry) and those who have accompanying psychiatric problems are more difficult to treat. Other interventions may be necessary before they are motivated to participate in or be responsive to behavioral techniques.

Encopresis. The treatment of encopresis is somewhat more complex, because encopresis

frequently results from chronic constipation and stool withholding, which create physiological consequences requiring medical treatment. In addition, children with encopresis more commonly have associated psychiatric disorders than do those with enuresis.

Behavioral treatment of encopresis must be integrated into a plan that also includes educational and psychological approaches (Levine 1982). Because encopresis often results in stool retention and impaction, an initial bowel cleanout is sometimes required. This regimen is followed by a bowel "retraining" program using oral mineral oil, a high-roughage diet, ample fluid intake, and a mild suppository. The behavioral program focuses on the development of a regular toileting routine with scheduled positive toilet practicing. Behaviors that progressively approximate the appropriate passing of feces in the toilet are rewarded. Routine pants checks followed by contingent positive or negative response are often included. Administration of enemas by parents is contraindicated, as that alone does not improve bowel function and is toxic to the parent–child relationship.

Anxiety disorders. Desensitization, in vivo or in fantasy, is the treatment of choice for simple phobias, often supplemented by modeling. The principles and techniques are essentially the same as those used with adults, with modification for developmental level. In vivo desensitization, often combined with contingency management and parent guidance, may be effective in the treatment of school avoidance (school phobia) resulting from separation anxiety disorder. Behavioral approaches using exposure and response prevention appear to be effective in the treatment of OCD in children and adolescents (March et al. 2004).

Behavioral Medicine Techniques

Behavioral methods can be used to treat somatic symptoms. These interventions should be carried out in collaboration with the primary physician and any necessary medical specialists. Children are just as sensitive as adults are to implications that their symptoms are not "real," so care must be taken to explain the interaction of psychological processes and physical symptoms and to develop a working alliance.

A variety of techniques, such as hypnotherapy, relaxation training, and pain behavior management, have been used for children in much the same way as for adults, but with adaptations for the children's level of cognitive or emotional development. Especially important is an understanding of any misconceptions youngsters may have about the disease state and its treatment. These notions vary according to a patient's stage of cognitive development and his or her unique experience.

Family Treatment

Attempts to treat children and adolescents without considering the persons with whom they live and the patients' relationships with other significant persons are doomed to failure. Any change in one family member, whether resulting from a psychiatric disorder, psychiatric treatment, a normal developmental process, or an outside event, is likely to produce change in other family members and in their relationships. Family constellations vary widely, ranging from the traditional nuclear family to the single-parent family, a blended family or stepfamily, an adoptive or foster family, or a group home. The term *parents* in this chapter applies to adults filling the parenting role, whatever their actual relationship to the patient.

Evaluation of Families

Data should be gathered on each person living with the patient, as well as on others who may be important or have been so in the past (e.g., noncustodial parents, grandparents, siblings who are no longer living at home). It is often useful to have at least one session that includes all significant family members. For families with young children, techniques such as the use of family drawings or puppet play or the assignment of family tasks to be carried out in the session are often useful. A variety of schemas exist by which to assess a family's structure and dynamic functioning. The family's developmental stage offers a clue to predictable transitional crises as children are born, become adolescents, and are launched from the nuclear family (Carter and McGoldrick 1980).

Family Therapy

Family therapy addresses primarily the interaction *among* family members rather than the processes *within* an individual. In the most general sense, family therapy is psychological treatment conducted with an identified patient and at least one biological or functional (by marriage, adoption, and so forth) family member. Related techniques include therapy with an individual patient that takes a family systems perspective, or therapy sessions with family members other than the identified patient, based on noncompliance with treatment, severity of illness, or other factors. Nowadays it is rare for family therapists to insist that all family members attend sessions.

Family therapy may be particularly useful when there are dysfunctional interactions or impaired communication within the family, especially when these appear to be related to the presenting problem. It also may be useful when symptoms seem to have been precipitated by difficulty with a developmental stage for an individual or the family or by a change in the family such as divorce or remarriage. If more than one family member is symptomatic, family therapy may be both more efficient and more effective than multiple individual treatments. Family therapy should be considered when one family member improves with treatment but another, not in treatment, worsens. In any case, the family must have, or be induced to have, sufficient motivation to participate. When the identified patient is relatively unmotivated to participate or to change, family therapy is likely to be more effective than individual therapy.

Attention to family systems issues also may be useful when progress is blocked in individual therapy or in behavior therapy.

Family therapy is contraindicated as a sole treatment method in cases of clearly organic physical or mental illness or if the family equilibrium is precarious and one or more family members are at serious risk of decompensation. In these situations, family therapy may be useful in combination with other treatments, such as medication or hospitalization. It is counterproductive to include in family therapy sessions a patient who is acutely psychotic, violent, or delusional regarding the family. Family sessions may not be helpful when a parent has severe, intractable, or minimally relevant psychopathology or when the child strongly prefers individual treatment. Children should not be included in sessions in which parents persist (despite redirection) in criticizing the children or in sharing inappropriate information, when the most critical need is marital therapy, or when parents primarily need specific, concrete help with practical affairs.

Group Therapy

Group therapy is particularly appropriate for children, who are often more willing to reveal their thoughts and feelings to peers than to adults. Also, the therapist can observe behavior with peers rather than depending on the reports of others. Establishing rewarding social relationships, a crucial developmental task for children of all ages, is especially difficult for youths with a psychiatric disorder. Group therapy offers unparalleled opportunities for the clinician to model and facilitate practice of important skills and to provide youngsters with companionship and mutual support. Interventions by peers may be far more acute and powerful in their effect than those by an adult therapist. An additional benefit is the larger number of patients who can benefit from limited therapist time.

Target symptoms include absent or conflictual peer relationships, aggression, withdrawal, timidity, difficulty with separation, and deficient social interactive or problem-solving skills. These problems often are not apparent or accessible to intervention in individual therapy sessions. Group therapy can be a powerful modality in the treatment of adolescents with eating disorders or substance abuse.

Group psychotherapy is contraindicated for those who are acutely psychotic, paranoid, or actively suicidal. Adolescents with sociopathic traits or behaviors should not be included in groups with teenagers who might be victimized or intimidated. Severely aggressive or hyperactive children probably should not be included in outpatient groups because of the difficulty in controlling their behavior, the contagion of problem behaviors, and the intimidation of less assertive children. Groups should *not* be used as a repository for unmotivated, nonverbal, difficult patients.

Inpatient and Residential Treatment

Indications

Because children should be treated in the setting that is least restrictive and disruptive to their lives, inpatient or residential treatment is indicated only in emergencies or for youngsters who have not responded to efforts at outpatient treatment because of severity of the disorder, lack of motivation, resistance, or disorganization of patients and/or family. Programs vary widely in their criteria for admission.

Placement in a residential treatment center may be indicated for children and adolescents with chronic behavior problems such as aggression, running away, truancy, substance abuse, school phobia, or self-destructive acts that the family, foster home, and/or community cannot manage or tolerate. Some parents harbor negative attitudes toward their children or adolescents or have severe psychopathology of their own. Children for whom it is not advisable to return home—because of factors in the youngsters, their families, or both—may be referred to a residential treatment center following a hospital stay.

Short-term hospitalization is typically an acute event, stemming from immediate physical danger to self or others, acute psychosis, a crisis in the environment that reduces the ability of the caregiving adults to cope with the child or adolescent, or the need for more intensive, systematic, and detailed evaluation and observation of the patient and family than is possible on an outpatient basis or in a day program. Managed care pressures have forced hospital lengths of stay to decrease significantly, often allowing only clinical stabilization of the patient before his or her discharge from the hospital. Briefer hospitalizations of severely ill child psychiatric patients require well-coordinated transfer to less restrictive levels of care in the clinical continuum (residential, day, and intensive outpatient treatments).

Longer-term hospitalization may be indicated for those patients who do not improve sufficiently in a brief period and who continue to require a secure setting and intensive treatment.

Differences in Settings

Residential treatment centers, compared with hospital units, tend to be longer term, more open to and integrated with the community, and not organized by the medical model. Usually, residential centers have a lower staff-to-patient ratio and less highly trained personnel. These centers are more likely to be based on a family group model and divided into sections or cottages.

Inpatient units for children can be classified according to the usual length of stay on such units. The lengths of stay on brief-stay or crisis intervention units average 1–2 weeks. These units emphasize rapid evaluation, triage, stabilization, and development of a treatment plan that will be implemented on an outpatient basis or in another facility. Stays on intermediate units last several weeks to months, and more definitive treatment can be conducted. Children may stay on long-term units from several months to longer than 1 year. On these units, care for the most severely impaired youth is provided. Increasing financial pressures have resulted in reduced overall lengths of stay in all types of units.

Treatment Planning

Ideally, hospitalization forms part of a comprehensive continuum of care for children. With ever-shorter lengths of stay, rapid and efficient planning and execution of evaluation and treatment strategies are essential. The goal is not to eliminate all psychopathology but to address the "focal problem" that precipitated hospitalization and then to discharge the patient to home, residential treatment, or foster placement, where he or she can receive outpatient or day treatment (Harper 1989).

Partial Hospitalization

Partial hospitalization (day treatment) may be best for the child who requires more intensive intervention than can be provided in outpatient visits but who is able to live at home. Partial hospitalization is less disruptive to the patient and family than inpatient treatment or residential placement and can offer an opportunity for more intensive work with parents, who may attend the program on a regular basis. Partial hospitalization may be used as a transition for a child who has been hospitalized or to avert a hospitalization. It may be implemented in combination with placement in a foster or group home.

Adjunctive Treatments

At times, an intervention that is not a psychiatric treatment may be recommended as part of a treatment plan. These programs may be crucial for the child's well-being and/or the treatment of the psychiatric disorder, or they may be facilitative, speeding progress or improving level of function.

Parent Support Groups

Parents of children with psychiatric disorders, together with mental health professionals and teachers, have established groups that provide education and support for parents, as well as advocacy for services and fundraising for research. National organizations with local chapters include Parents Anonymous, for abusive or potentially abusive parents; the Arc, for people with intellectual and developmental disabilities; the Autism Society of America; Children and Adults with Attention-Deficit/Hyperactivity Disorder (CHADD); and the Learning Disabilities Association of America. Recently, the National Alliance on Mental Illness (NAMI) established a Child and Adolescent Network (NAMI-CAN) as its concerns broadened to include children and adolescents. Local groups focused on a particular disorder or on more generic issues can provide a powerful adjunct to direct clinical services.

Special Education

Modified school programs are indicated for those children who cannot perform satisfactorily in regular classrooms or who need special structure or teaching techniques to reach their academic potential. These programs range in intensity from tutoring or resource classrooms several hours a week, to special classrooms in mainstream schools, to public or private schools that serve only children with special educational needs. Resources differ from community to community, but most communities have programs for mentally retarded youth, for those with learning disabilities (specific developmental disorders), and for those whose emotional and/or behavioral problems require a special setting for learning or for the control of their behavior. Classes are small, with a high teacher-to-student ratio and teachers who are specially trained.

Foster Care

Placement in a foster home may be needed when parents are unwilling or unable to care for a child. Indications are clearest in cases of physical neglect or physical or sexual abuse. Other families may be unable to provide the appropriate emotional or physical environment. Court intervention is required for placement. Although foster placement can be a suitable and effective intervention, children in foster care may have a variety of unmet physical, developmental, and mental health needs, often making foster care less than optimal and clearly unsatisfactory as a long-term solution (Rosenfeld et al. 1997). A study by McMillen et al. (2005) showed that older youths in foster homes have a much higher rate of psychiatric illness, compared with age-matched peers.

Dietary Treatments

Since the mid-1970s, advocates of dietary treatment of behavioral problems have been remarkably persistent, despite the lack of scientific evidence. A variety of food additives and food allergens have been proposed as contributory or even causal in childhood behavior disorders, especially hyperactivity and autism. Reviews of methodologically adequate studies (Rojas and Chan 2005) have consistently failed to demonstrate behavioral or cognitive improvement on the Kaiser Permanente Diet. A thorough meta-analysis by Wolraich et al. (1995) debunked the notion that dietary sugar contributes to hyperactivity. There are no data to support dietary treatments or supplements for autism, although parents may pursue these treatments out of desperation.

Conclusion

The treatment of psychiatric disorders in children and adolescents is both an art and a science. Research on assessment and diagnosis, biological correlates of disorders, and outcome of traditional and newly developed techniques will continue to improve the specificity and outcome of treatment. However, a need always will exist for clinical skills in tailoring and applying psychosomatic techniques to individual patients and their families.

Key Points

- As in adults, treatment of pediatric psychiatric patients requires expertise in psychiatric evaluation and case formulation, effective use of complex treatment strategies, and a respect for the principles of informed consent and confidentiality.

- An understanding of human development is key to the successful treatment of pediatric psychiatric patients, to include an appreciation of the differences between youngsters and adults as well as the developmental differences between children of all ages.

- Ideally, treatments identified specifically for children and adolescents should reflect evidence-based practices. However, many have been developed by applying known effective adult treatments to the pediatric population.

- Pediatric psychopharmacology research remains limited despite escalations in the use of psychiatric medications in children. Caution should be exercised to prescribe medications in a safe and monitored fashion.

- Decisions regarding the use of psychoactive medications in children, as in adults, are best supported through double-blind, placebo-controlled efficacy trials and through the collection of longitudinal data regarding medication safety. Clinicians should avoid the routine use of medication in youngsters that is based solely on case reports or uncontrolled drug trials.

- Parents should be carefully informed of the presence or absence of scientific evidence supporting the use of a specific medication in a child, as well as that medication's possible side effects and adverse effects.

- Psychotherapy remains a mainstay in the effective practice of child and adolescent psychiatry and may be used solely or in combination with other treatments, depending on a patient's treatment needs.

- Further studies are required to demonstrate which types of psychotherapy are most effective for which child psychiatric diagnoses. Such efficacy studies remain methodologically challenging.

- Although each psychotherapy is based on its own theoretical constructs and purported therapeutic principles, all psychotherapies tend to rely on several similar precepts: the importance of the relationship with the therapist, an emphasis on hopefulness, the use of therapist attention and suggestion, and the expectation of change in one or more realms—psychological makeup, cognition, behavior, sense of self, or emotional experience.

Suggested Readings

General

Barkley RA: Attention-Deficit Hyperactivity Disorder: A Handbook for Diagnosis and Treatment, 3rd Edition. New York, Guilford, 2006

Connor DF, Meltzer B: Pediatric Psychopharmacology: Fast Facts. New York, WW Norton, 2006

Dulcan MK, Wiener JM (eds): Essentials of Child and Adolescent Psychiatry. Washington, DC, American Psychiatric Publishing, 2006

Dulcan MK, Martini, DR, Lake MB: Concise Guide to Child and Adolescent Psychiatry,

3rd Edition. Washington, DC, American Psychiatric Publishing, 2003

Mash EJ, Barkley RA (eds): Treatment of Childhood Disorders, 3rd Edition. New York, Guilford, 2006

Rating Scales

Collett B, Ohan J, Myers K: Ten-year review of rating scales, V: scales assessing attention-deficit/hyperactivity disorder. J Am Acad Child Adolesc Psychiatry 42:1015–1037, 2003

Collett B, Ohan J, Myers K: Ten-year review of rating scales, VI: scales assessing externalizing behaviors. J Am Acad Child Adolesc Psychiatry 42:1143–1170, 2003

Myers K, Winters N: Ten-year review of rating scales, I: overview of scale functioning, psychometric properties, and selection. J Am Acad Child Adolesc Psychiatry 41:114–122, 2002

Myers K, Winters N: Ten-year review of rating scales, II: scales for internalizing disorders. J Am Acad Child Adolesc Psychiatry 41:634–659, 2002

Ohan J, Myers K, Collett B: Ten-year review of rating scales, IV: scales assessing trauma and its effects. J Am Acad Child Adolesc Psychiatry 41:1401–1422, 2002

Rush AJ Jr, First MB, Blacker D (eds): Handbook of Psychiatric Measures, 2nd Edition. Washington, DC, American Psychiatric Publishing, 2008

Winters N, Myers K, Proud L: Ten-year review of rating scales, III: scales assessing suicidality, cognitive style, and self-esteem. J Am Acad Child Adolesc Psychiatry 41:1150–1181, 2002

Winters N, Collett B, Myers K: Ten-year review of rating scales, VII: scales assessing functional impairment. J Am Acad Child Adolesc Psychiatry 44:309–338, 2005

References

Abnormal Involuntary Movement Scale (AIMS). Psychopharmacol Bull 24:781–783, 1988

Achenbach TM: Manual for the Teacher's Report Form and 1991 Profile. Burlington, University of Vermont, Department of Psychiatry, 1991

Adams PL: A Primer of Child Psychotherapy, 2nd Edition. Boston, MA, Little, Brown, 1982

Akhondzadeh S, Tavakolian R, Davari-Ashtani R, et al: Selegiline in the treatment of attention deficit hyperactivity disorder in children: a double blind and randomized trial. Prog Neuropsychopharmacol Biol Psychiatry 27:841–845, 2003

Alaghband-Rad J, Hakimshooshtary M: A randomized controlled clinical trial of citalopram versus fluoxetine in children and adolescents with obsessive-compulsive disorder (OCD). Eur Child Adolesc Psychiatry 18:131–135, 2009

Aman MG, De Smedt G, Derivan A, et al: Double-blind, placebo-controlled study of risperidone for the treatment of disruptive behaviors in children with subaverage intelligence. Am J Psychiatry 159:1337–1346, 2002

Aman MG, Buican B, Arnold LE: Methylphenidate treatment in children with borderline IQ and mental retardation: analysis of three aggregated studies. J Child Adolesc Psychopharmacol 13:29–40, 2003

Aman MG, Arnold LE, Ramadan Y, et al (Research Units on Pediatric Psychopharmacology Autism Network): Randomized, controlled, crossover trial of methylphenidate in pervasive developmental disorders with hyperactivity. Arch Gen Psychiatry 62:1266–1274, 2005

American Academy of Child and Adolescent Psychiatry: Practice parameter for the use of stimulant medications in the treatment of children, adolescents, and adults. J Am Acad Child Adolesc Psychiatry 41 (2 suppl):26S–49S, 2002

Anderson GM, Cook EH: Pharmacogenetics: promise and potential in child and adolescent psychiatry. Child Adolesc Psychiatr Clin N Am 9:23–42, 2000

Arnold LE, Aman MG, Cook AM, et al: Atomoxetine for hyperactivity in autism spectrum disorders: placebo-controlled crossover pilot trial. J Am Acad Child Adolesc Psychiatry 45:1196–1205, 2006

Azrin NH, Sneed TJ, Foxx RM: Dry-bed training: rapid elimination of childhood enuresis. Behav Res Ther 12:147–156, 1974

Barkley RA: Defiant Children: A Clinician's Manual for Assessment and Parent Training, 2nd Edition. New York, Guilford, 1997

Bastiaens L: Compliance with pharmacotherapy in adolescents: effects of patients' and parents' knowledge and attitudes toward treatment. J Child Adolesc Psychopharmacol 5:39–48, 1995

Bernstein GA, Borchardt CM, Perwien AR, et al: Imipramine plus cognitive-behavioral therapy in the treatment of school refusal. J Am Acad Child Adolesc Psychiatry 39:276–283, 2000

Biederman J: Clonazepam in the treatment of prepubertal children with panic-like symptoms. J Clin Psychiatry 48 (suppl):38–41, 1987

Biederman J, Quinn D, Weiss M, et al: Efficacy and safety of Ritalin LA, a new, once daily, extended-release dosage form of methylphenidate, in children with attention deficit hyperactivity disorder. Paediatr Drugs 5:833–841, 2003

Biederman J, Boellner SW, Childress A, et al: Lisdexamfetamine dimesylate and mixed amphetamine salts extended-release in children with ADHD: a double-blind, placebo-controlled, crossover analog classroom study. Biol Psychiatry 62:970–976, 2007a

Biederman J, Krishnan S, Zhang Y, et al: Efficacy and tolerability of lisdexamfetamine dimesylate (NRP-104) in children with attention-deficit/hyperactivity disorder: a phase III, multicenter, randomized, double-blind, forced-dose, parallel-group study. Clin Ther 29:450–463, 2007b

Biederman J, Melmed RD, Patel A, et al: A randomized, double-blind, placebo-controlled study of guanfacine extended release in children and adolescents with attention-deficit/hyperactivity disorder. Pediatrics 121:e73–e84, 2008

Birmaher B, Greenhill LL, Cooper TB, et al: Sustained release methylphenidate: pharmacokinetic studies in ADHD males. J Am Acad Child Adolesc Psychiatry 28:768–772, 1989

Birmaher B, Axelson DA, Monk K, et al: Fluoxetine for the treatment of childhood anxiety disorders. J Am Acad Child Adolesc Psychiatry 42:415–423, 2003

Black B, Uhde TW: Treatment of elective mutism with fluoxetine: a double-blind, placebo-controlled study. J Am Acad Child Adolesc Psychiatry 33:1000–1006, 1994

Bloch MH, Panza KE, Landeros-Weisenberger A, et al: Meta-analysis: treatment of attention-deficit/hyperactivity disorder in children with comorbid tic disorders. J Am Acad Child Adolesc Psychiatry 48:884–893, 2009

Borkovec TD, Miranda J: Between-group psychotherapy outcome research and basic science. Psychotherapy and Rehabilitation Research 5:14–20, 1996

Bradbury MG, Meadow SR: Combined treatment with enuresis alarm and desmopressin for nocturnal enuresis. Acta Paediatr 84:1014–1018, 1995

Broderick-Cantwell JJ: Accidental clonidine patch overdose in attention-deficit/hyperactivity disorder patients. J Am Acad Child Adolesc Psychiatry 38:95–98, 1999

Brody AE: Motivational interviewing with a depressed adolescent. J Clin Psychol: In Session 1168–1179, 2009

Brown RT, Sexson SB: Effects of methylphenidate on cardiovascular responses in attention deficit hyperactivity disordered adolescents. J Adolesc Health Care 10:179–183, 1989

Butler RJ, Gasson SL: Enuresis alarm treatment. Scand J Urol Nephrol 39:349–357, 2005

Butler RJ, Holland P, Robinson J: Examination of the structured withdrawal program to prevent relapse of nocturnal enuresis. J Urol 166:2463–2466, 2001

Campbell M, Green WH, Deutsch SI: Child and Adolescent Psychopharmacology. Beverly Hills, CA, Sage, 1985

Campbell M, Silva RR, Kafantaris V, et al: Predictors of side effects associated with lithium administration in children. Psychopharmacol Bull 27:373–380, 1991

Carandang CG, Maxwell DJ, Robbins DR, et al: Lamotrigine in adolescent mood disorders. J Am Acad Child Adolesc Psychiatry 42:750, 2003

Carter E, McGoldrick M (eds): The Family Life Cycle: A Framework for Family Therapy. New York, Gardner, 1980

Chang K, Saxena K, Howe M: An open-label study of lamotrigine adjunct or monotherapy for the treatment of adolescents with bipolar depression. J Am Acad Child Adolesc Psychiatry 45:298–301, 2006

Chungh DS, Kim BN, Cho SC: Neuroleptic malignant syndrome due to three atypical antipsychotics in a child. J Psychopharmacol 19:422–425, 2005

Clein PD, Riddle MA: Pharmacokinetics in children and adolescents. Child Adolesc Psychiatr Clin N Am 4:59–75, 1995

Coffey BJ: Anxiolytics for children and adolescents: traditional and new drugs. J Child Adolesc Psychopharmacol 1:57–83, 1990

Coffey BJ, Shader RI, Greenblatt DJ: Pharmacokinetics of benzodiazepines and psychostimulants in children. J Clin Psychopharmacol 3:217–225, 1983

Cohen JA, Mannarino AP, Knudsen K: Treating sexually abused children: 1 year follow-up of a randomized controlled trial. Child Abuse Negl 29:135–145, 2005

Compton SN, March JS, Brent D, et al: Cognitive-behavioral psychotherapy for anxiety and depressive disorders in children and adolescents: an evidence-based medicine review. J Am Acad Child Adolesc Psychiatry 43:930–959, 2004

Conners C, Sitarenios G, Parker JD, et al: The revised Conners' Parents Rating Scale (CPRS-R): factor structure, reliability, and criterion validity. J Abnorm Child Psychol 26:257–268, 1998a

Conners C, Sitarenios G, Parker JD, et al: Revision and restandardization of the Conners' Teacher Rating Scale (CTRS-R): factor structure, reliability, and criterion validity. J Abnorm Child Psychol 26:279–291, 1998b

Connor DF: Preschool attention deficit hyperactivity disorder: a review of prevalence, diagnosis, neurobiology, and stimulant treatment. J Dev Behav Pediatr 23 (1 suppl):S1–S9, 2002

Connor DF, Fletcher KE, Swanson JM: A meta-analysis of clonidine for symptoms of attention-deficit hyperactivity disorder. J Am Acad Child Adolesc Psychiatry 38:1551–1559, 1999

Cook EH, Wagner KD, March JS, et al: Long-term sertraline treatment of children and adolescents with obsessive-compulsive disorder. J Am Acad Child Adolesc Psychiatry 40:1175–1181, 2001

Correll CU: Metabolic side effects of second-generation antipsychotics in children and adolescents: a different story? J Clin Psychiatry 66:1331–1332, 2005

Correll CU, Penzner JB, Parikh UH, et al: Recognizing and monitoring adverse events of second-generation antipsychotics in children and adolescents. Child Adolesc Psychiatric Clin N Am 15:177–206, 2006

Cozza KL, Armstrong SC, Oesterheld JR: Concise Guide to Drug Interaction Principles for Medical Practice: Cytochrome P450s, UGTs, P-Glycoproteins. Washington, DC, American Psychiatric Publishing, 2003

Dion Y, Annable L, Sandor P, et al: Risperidone in the treatment of Tourette syndrome: a double-blind, placebo-controlled trial. J Clin Psychopharmacol 22:31–39, 2002

Dulcan MK: Brief psychotherapy with children and their families: the state of the art. J Am Acad Child Psychiatry 23:544–551, 1984

Dulcan MK (ed): Helping Parents, Youth, and Teachers Understand Medications for Behavioral and Emotional Problems: A Resource Book of Medication Information Handouts, 3rd Edition. Washington, DC, American Psychiatric Publishing, 2007

Dulcan MK (ed): Dulcan's Textbook of Child and Adolescent Psychiatry. Washington, DC, American Psychiatric Publishing, 2010

Dulcan MK, Piercy PA: A model for teaching and evaluating brief psychotherapy with children and their families. Professional Psychology: Research and Practice 16:689–700, 1985

Emslie GJ, Heiligenstein JH, Wagner KD, et al: Fluoxetine for acute treatment of depression in children and adolescents: a placebo-controlled, randomized clinical trial. J Am Acad Child Adolesc Psychiatry 41:1205–1215, 2002

Emslie GJ, Heiligenstein JH, Hoog SL, et al: Fluoxetine treatment for prevention of relapse of depression in children and adolescents: a double-blind, placebo-controlled study. J Am Acad Child Adolesc Psychiatry 43:1397–1405, 2004

Faraone SV, Biederman J, Morley CP, et al: Effect of stimulants on height and weight: a review of the literature. J Am Acad Child Adolesc Psychiatry 47:994–1009, 2008

Feldman HM, Kolmen BK, Gonzaga AM: Naltrexone and communication skills in young children with autism. J Am Acad Child Adolesc Psychiatry 38:587–593, 1999

Findling RL, McNamara NK, Branicky LA, et al: A double-blind pilot study of risperidone in the treatment of conduct disorder. J Am Acad Child Adolesc Psychiatry 39:509–516, 2000

Findling RL, Blumer JL, Kauffman R, et al: Aripiprazole in pediatric conduct disorder: a pilot study. Eur Neuropsychopharmacol 13 (suppl 4):S335, 2003a

Findling RL, McNamara NK, Gracious BL, et al: Combination lithium and divalproex sodium in pediatric bipolarity. J Am Acad Child Adolesc Psychiatry 42:895–901, 2003b

Findling RL, Steiner H, Weller EB: Use of antipsychotics in children and adolescents. J Clin Psychiatry 66 (suppl 7): 29–40, 2005

Findling RL, Reed MD, O'Riordan MA, et al: A 26-week open-label study of quetiapine in children with conduct disorder. J Child Adolesc Psychopharmacol 17:1–9, 2007

Findling RL, Robb A, Nyilas M, et al: A multiple-center, randomized, double-blind, placebo-controlled study of oral aripiprazole for treatment of adolescents with schizophrenia. Am J Psychiatry 165:1432–1441, 2008

Forehand R, Long N: Parenting the Strong-Willed Child: The Clinically Proven Five-Week Program for Parents of Two- to Six-Year-Olds, Revised and Updated Edition. New York, Contemporary Books, 2002

Gadow KD: Pediatric psychopharmacology: a review of recent research. J Child Psychol Psychiatry 33:153–195, 1992

Gardner RA: Helping children cooperate in therapy, in Basic Handbook of Child Psychiatry, Vol 3: Therapeutic Interventions. Edited by Harrison SI. New York, Basic Books, 1979, pp 414–433

Geller B, Coper TB, Sun K, et al: Double-blind and placebo-controlled study of lithium for adolescent bipolar disorders with secondary substance dependency. J Am Acad Child Adolesc Psychiatry 37:171–178, 1998

Geller B, Reising D, Leonard HL, et al: Critical review of tricyclic antidepressant use in children and adolescents. J Am Acad Child Adolesc Psychiatry 38:513–516, 1999

Geller DA, Biederman J, Steward SE, et al: Which SSRI? A meta-analysis of pharmacotherapy trials in pediatric obsessive-compulsive disorder. Am J Psychiatry 160:1919–1928, 2003

Genton P, Bauer J, Duncan S, et al: On the association between valproate and polycystic ovary syndrome. Epilepsia 42:305–310, 2001

Gepertz S, Nevéus T: Imipramine for therapy resistant enuresis: a retrospective evaluation. J Urol 171:2607–2610, 2004

Ghaziuddin N, Kutcher SP, Knapp P, et al: Practice parameter for use of electroconvulsive therapy with adolescents. Work Group on Quality Issues, AACAP. J Am Acad Child Adolesc Psychiatry 43:1521–1539, 2004

Gibbons RD, Hur K, Bhaumik DK, et al: The relationship between antidepressant medication use and rate of suicide. Arch Gen Psychiatry 62:165–172, 2005

Glassman AH, Bigger JT: Antipsychotic drugs: prolonged QTc interval, torsade de pointes, and sudden death. Am J Psychiatry 158:1774–1782, 2001

GlaxoSmithKline: U.S. product labeling for Lamictal (lamotrigine). August 2005. Available at: http://us.gsk.com/products/assets/us_lamictal.pdf. Accessed June 3, 2006.

Good CR, Feaster CS, Krecko VF: Tolerability of oral loading of divalproex sodium in child psychiatry inpatients. J Child Adolesc Psychopharmacol 11:53–57, 2001

Greenhill LL: Attention-deficit hyperactivity disorder. Child Adolesc Psychiatr Clin N Am 4:123–168, 1995

Greenhill LL, Findling RL, Swanson JM: A double-blind, placebo-controlled study of modified-release methylphenidate in children with attention-deficit/hyperactivity disorder. Pediatrics [serial online] 109:e39, 2002. Available at: http://www.pediatrics.org/cgi/content/full/109/3/e39. Accessed January 16, 2006.

Greenhill LL, Kollins S, Abikoff H, et al: Efficacy and safety of immediate-release methylphenidate treatment for preschoolers with ADHD. J Am Acad Child Adolesc Psychiatry 45:1284–1293, 2006a

Greenhill LL, Muniz R, Ball RR, et al: Efficacy and safety of dexmethylphenidate extended-release capsules in children with attention-deficit hyperactivity disorder. J Am Acad Child Adolesc Psychiatry 45:817–823, 2006b

Hagerman RJ, Murphy MA, Wittenberg MD: A controlled trial of stimulant medication in children with the fragile X syndrome. Am J Med Genet 30:377–392, 1988

Hammad TA, Laughren T, Racoosin J: Suicidality in pediatric patients treated with antidepressant drugs. Arch Gen Psychiatry 63:332–339, 2006

Handen BL, Hardan AY: Open label, prospective trial of olanzapine in adolescents with subaverage intelligence and disruptive behavior disorders. J Am Acad Child Adolesc Psychiatry 45:928–935, 2006

Harper G: Focal inpatient treatment planning. J Am Acad Child Adolesc Psychiatry 28:31–37, 1989

Hazell PL, Stuart JE: A randomized controlled trial of clonidine added to psychostimulant medication for hyperactive and aggressive children. J Am Acad Child Adolesc Psychiatry 42:886–894, 2003

Health Canada (2005a): Health Canada suspends the market authorization of Adderall XR, a drug prescribed for attention deficit hyperactivity disorder (ADHD) in children. February 9, 2005. Available at: http://www.hc-sc. gc.ca/ahc-asc/media/advisories-avis/2005/2005_01_e.html. Accessed June 3, 2006.

Health Canada (2005b): Health Canada allows Adderall XR back on the Canadian Market. August 24, 2005. Available at: http://www.hc-sc.gc.ca/ahc-asc/media/nr-cp/2005/2005_92_e.html. Accessed June 3, 2006.

Herskowitz J: Developmental neurotoxicology, in Psychiatric Pharmacosciences of Children and Adolescents. Edited by Popper C. Washington, DC, American Psychiatric Press, 1987, pp 81–123

Hjalmas KI, Hanson E, Hellstrom AL, et al: Long-term treatment with desmopressin in children with primary monosymptomatic nocturnal enuresis: an open multicentre study. Swedish Enuresis Trial Group (SWEET). Br J Urol 82:704–709, 1998

Hjalmas K, Arnold T, Bower W, et al: Nocturnal enuresis: an international evidence based management strategy. J Urol 171:2545–2561, 2004

Hollander E, Wasserman S, Swanson EN, et al: A double-blind placebo-controlled pilot study of olanzapine in childhood/adolescent pervasive developmental disorder. J Child Adolesc Psychopharmacol 16:541–548, 2006

Houts AC: Behavioural treatment for enuresis. Scand J Urol Nephrol 173 (suppl):83–86, 1995

Hunt RD, Capper S, O'Connell P: Clonidine in child and adolescent psychiatry. J Child Adolesc Psychopharmacol 1:87–102, 1990

Hunt RD, Lau S, Ryu J: Alternative therapies for ADHD, in Ritalin: Theory and Patient Management. Edited by Greenhill LL, Osman BB. New York, Mary Ann Liebert, 1991, pp 75–95

Intuniv (guanfacine) product labeling. Available at: http://www.intuniv.com/documents/INTUNIV-Full_Prescribing_Information.pdf. Accessed September 26, 2009.

Isojarvi JI, Laatikainen TJ, Pakarinen AJ, et al: Polycystic ovaries and hyperandrogenism in women taking valproate for epilepsy. N Engl J Med 329:1383–1388, 1993

Jensen PS: Current concepts and controversies in the diagnosis and treatment of attention deficit hyperactivity disorder. Curr Psychiatry Rep 2:102–109, 2000

Katz LY, Cox BJ: Dialectical behavior therapy for suicidal adolescent inpatients: a case study. Clinical Case Studies 1:81–92, 2002

Kazdin AD: Developing a research agenda for child and adolescent psychotherapy. Arch Gen Psychiatry 57:829–835, 2000

Kazdin AD: Parent Management Training: Treatment for Oppositional, Aggressive, and Antisocial Behavior in Children and Adolescents. New York, Oxford University Press, 2005

Kerbeshian J, Burd L, Fisher W: Lithium carbonate in the treatment of two patients with infantile autism and atypical bipolar symptomatology. J Clin Psychopharmacol 7:401–405, 1987

Klein RG, Koplewicz HS, Kanner A: Imipramine treatment of children with separation anxiety disorder. J Am Acad Child Adolesc Psychiatry 31:21–28, 1992

Kolmen BK, Feldman HM, Handen BL, et al: Naltrexone in young autistic children: a double-blind, placebo-controlled crossover study. J Am Acad Child Adolesc Psychiatry 34:223–231, 1995

Kowatch RA, Bucci JP: Mood stabilizers and anticonvulsants. Pediatr Clin North Am 45:1173–1186, 1998

Kowatch RA, Suppes T, Carmody TJ, et al: Effect size of lithium, divalproex sodium, and carbamazepine in children and adolescents with bipolar disorder. J Am Acad Child Adolesc Psychiatry 39:713–720, 2000

Kratochvil CJ, Wilens TE, Greenhill LL, et al: Effects of long-term atomoxetine treatment for young children with attention-deficit/hyperactivity disorder. J Am Acad Child Adolesc Psychiatry 45:919–927, 2006

Kryzhanovskaya L, Schulz SC, McDougle C, et al: Olanzapine versus placebo in adolescents with schizophrenia: a 6-week, randomized, double-blind, placebo-controlled trial. J Am Acad Child Adolesc Psychiatry 48:60–70, 2009

Kumra S, Frazier JA, Jacobsen LK, et al: Child-onset schizophrenia: a double-blind clozapine-haloperidol comparison. Arch Gen Psychiatry 53:1090–1097, 1996

Kumra S, Jacobsen L, Lenane M, et al: Case series: spectrum of neuroleptic-induced movement disorders and extrapyramidal side effects in childhood-onset schizophrenia. J Am Acad Child Adolesc Psychiatry 37:221–227, 1998

Kumra S, Kranzler H, Gerbino-Rosen G, et al: Clozapine and "high-dose" olanzapine in refractory early-onset schizophrenia: a 12-week randomized and double-blind comparison. Biol Psychiatry 63:524–529, 2008

Kutcher SP, Williamson P, MacKenzie S, et al: Successful clonazepam treatment of neuroleptic-induced akathisia in older adolescents and young adults: a double-blind, placebo-controlled study. J Clin Psychopharmacol 9:403–406, 1989

Levine MD: Encopresis: its potentiation, evaluation and alleviation. Pediatr Clin North Am 29:315–330, 1982

Lewis O: Psychological factors affecting pharmacological compliance. Child Adolesc Psychiatr Clin N Am 4:15–22, 1995

Linehan MM: Cognitive-Behavioral Treatment of Borderline Personality Disorder. New York, Guilford, 1993

Malone RP, Delaney MA, Luebbert JF, et al: A double-blind placebo-controlled study of lithium in hospitalized aggressive children and adolescents with conduct disorder. Arch Gen Psychiatry 57:649–654, 2000

March JS, Foa E, Gammon P, et al: Cognitive-behavior therapy, sertraline, and their combination for children and adolescents with obsessive-compulsive disorder. The Pediatric OCD Treatment Study (POTS) randomized controlled trial. JAMA 292:1969–1976, 2004

March JS, Silva S, Vitiello B: The Treatment for Adolescents with Depression Study: methods and message at 12 weeks. J Am Acad Child Adolesc Psychiatry 45:1393–1403, 2006

Martin A, Scahill L, Anderson G, et al: Weight and leptin changes among risperidone-treated youths with autism: 6-month prospective data. Am J Psychiatry 161:1125–1127, 2004

McCracken JT, Biederman J, Greenhill LL, et al: Analog classroom assessment of a once-daily mixed amphetamine formulation, SLI381 (Adderall XR), in children with ADHD. J Am Acad Child Adolesc Psychiatry 42:673–683, 2003

McCracken JT, Aman MG, McDougle CJ, et al (Research Units on Pediatric Psychopharmacology Autism Network): Risperidone treatment of autistic disorder: longer-term benefits and blinded discontinuation after 6 months. Am J Psychiatry 162:1361–1369, 2005

McDaniel KD: Pharmacological treatment of psychiatric and neurodevelopmental disorders in children and adolescents, I. Clin Pediatr (Phila) 25:65–71, 1986

McDougle CJ, Scahill L, Aman M, et al: Risperidone for the core symptom domains of autism: results from the study by the Autism Network of the Research Units on Pediatric Psychopharmacology. Am J Psychiatry 162:1142–1148, 2005

McGough JJ, Biederman J, Wigal SB, et al: Long-term tolerability and effectiveness of once-daily mixed amphetamine salts (Adderall XR) in children with ADHD. J Am Acad Child Adolesc Psychiatry 44:530–538, 2005

McGough JJ, Wigal SB, Abikoff H, et al: A randomized, double-blind, placebo-controlled, laboratory classroom assessment of methylphenidate transdermal system in children with ADHD. J Atten Disord 9:476–485, 2006

McMahon R, Forehand R: Helping the Noncompliant Child: Family-Based Treatment for Oppositional Behavior, 2nd Edition. New York, Guilford, 2003

McMillen JC, Zima BT, Scott LD, et al: Prevalence of psychiatric disorders among older youths in the foster care system. J Am Acad Child Adolesc Psychiatry 44:88–95, 2005

McVoy M, Findling R: Child and adolescent psychopharmacology update. Psychiatr Clin N Am 32:111–133, 2009

Miller AL, Rathus JH, Linehan MM: Dialectical Behavior Therapy for Childhood Anxiety Disorders. New York, Guilford, 2007

Miller NL, Findling RL: Principles of psychopharmacology, in Dulcan's Textbook of Child and Adolescent Psychiatry. Washington, DC, American Psychiatric Publishing, 2010, pp 667–679

Miller WR, Rollnick S: Motivational Interviewing: Preparing People for Change, 2nd Edition. New York, Guilford, 2002

Mohammadi MR, Ghanizadeh A, Alaghband-rad J, et al: Selegiline in comparison with methylphenidate in attention deficit hyperactivity disorder children and adolescents in a double-blind, randomized clinical trial. J Child Adolesc Psychopharmacol 14:418–425, 2004

Montgomery P, Bjornstad G, Dennis J: Media-based behavioural treatments for behavioural problems in children. Cochrane Database Syst Rev (1):CD002206, 2006

Mufson L, Dorta KP, Moreau D, et al: Interpersonal Psychotherapy for Depressed Adolescents, 2nd Edition. New York, Guilford, 2004a

Mufson L, Dorta KP, Wickramaratne P, et al: A randomized effectiveness trial of interpersonal psychotherapy for depressed adolescents. Arch Gen Psychiatry 61:577–584, 2004b

Mukaddes NM, Abali O: Quetiapine treatment of children and adolescents with Tourette's disorder. J Child Adolesc Psychopharmacol 13:295–299, 2003

Newcorn JH, Spencer TJ, Biederman J, et al: Atomoxetine treatment in children and adolescents with attention-deficit hyperactivity disorder and comorbid oppositional defiant disorder. J Am Acad Child Adolesc Psychiatry 44:240–248, 2005

Newcorn JH, Sutton VK, Weiss MD, et al: Clinical responses to atomoxetine in attention-deficit/hyperactivity disorder: the Integrated Data Exploratory Analysis (IDEA) study. J Am Acad Child Adolesc Psychiatry 48:511–581, 2009

Niederhofer H, Staffen W: Acamprosate and its efficacy in treating alcohol dependent adolescents. Eur Child Adolesc Psychiatry 12:144–148, 2003

Palumbo DR, Sallee FR, Pelham WE, et al: Clonidine for attention-deficit/hyperactivity disorder, I: efficacy and tolerability outcomes. J Am Acad Child Adolesc Psychiatry 47:180–188, 2008

Párraga HC, Párraga MI, Woodward RL, et al: Quetiapine treatment of children with Tourette's syndrome: report of two cases. J Child Adolesc Psychopharmacol 11:187–191, 2001

Patterson GR, Forgatch M: Parents and Adolescents Living Together: The Basics, 2nd Edition. Champaign, IL, Research Press, 2005

Pearson DA, Santos CW, Roache JD, et al: Treatment effects of methylphenidate on behavioral adjustment in children with mental retardation and ADHD. J Am Acad Child Adolesc Psychiatry 42:209–216, 2003

Pelham WE, Massetti GM, Wilson T, et al: Implementation of a comprehensive school-wide behavioral intervention: the ABC Program. J Atten Disord 9:248–260, 2005

Pfefferbaum B, Overall JE, Boron HA, et al: Alprazolam in the treatment of anticipatory and acute situational anxiety in children with cancer. J Am Acad Child Adolesc Psychiatry 26:532–535, 1987

PhysiciansMedGuide: The Use of Medication in Treating Childhood and Adolescent Depression: Information for Physicians. 2010. Available at: http://www.psych.org/ Share/Parents-Med-Guide/HTML-Physician-Depression.aspx. Accessed May 28, 2010.

Pliszka SR: A double-blind, placebo-controlled study of Adderall and methylphenidate in the treatment of attention-deficit/hyperactivity disorder. J Am Acad Child Adolesc Psychiatry 39:619–626, 2000

Pliszka SR, Crismon ML, Hughes CW, et al: The Texas Children's Medication Algorithm Project: revision of the algorithm for pharmacotherapy of attention-deficit/hyperactivity disorder. J Am Acad Child Adolesc Psychiatry 45:642–657, 2006

Rapoport JL: Antidepressants in childhood attention deficit disorder and obsessive-compulsive disorder. Psychosomatics 27 (suppl): 30–36, 1986

Rathus JH, Miller AL: Dialectical behavior therapy adapted for suicidal adolescents. Suicide Life Threat Behav 32:146–157, 2002

Reischer H, Pfeffer CR: Lithium pharmacokinetics. J Am Acad Child Adolesc Psychiatry 35:130–131, 1996

Richardson MA, Haugland G, Craig TJ: Neuroleptic use, parkinsonian symptoms, tardive dyskinesia, and associated factors in child and adolescent psychiatric patients. Am J Psychiatry 148:1322–1328, 1991

Riddle MA: Paroxetine and the FDA. J Am Acad Child Adolesc Psychiatry 43:128–130, 2004

Rojas NL, Chan E: Old and new controversies in the alternative treatment of attention-deficit hyperactivity disorder. Ment Retard Dev Disabil Res Rev 11:116–130, 2005

Rosenfeld AA, Pilowsky DJ, Fine P, et al: Foster care: an update. J Am Acad Child Adolesc Psychiatry 36:448–457, 1997

Rubinstein S, Malone MA, Roberts W, et al: Placebo-controlled study examining effects of selegiline in children with attention-deficit/ hyperactivity disorder. J Child Adolesc Psychopharmacol 16:404–415, 2006

Ryan ND: Heterocyclic antidepressants in children and adolescents. J Child Adolesc Psychopharmacol 1:21–31, 1990

Ryan ND: The pharmacological treatment of child and adolescent depression. Psychiatr Clin North Am 15:29–40, 1992

Rynn MA, Siqueland L, Rickels K: Placebo-controlled trial of sertraline in the treatment of children with generalized anxiety disorder. Am J Psychiatry 158:2008–2014, 2001

Safer DJ: Changing patterns of psychotropic medications prescribed by child psychiatrists in the 1990s. J Child Adolesc Psychopharmacol 7:267–274, 1997

Sallee F, Stiller R, Perel J, et al: Targeting imipramine dose in children with depression. Clin Pharmacol Ther 40:8–13, 1986

Sallee FR, Kurlan R, Goetz CG, et al: Ziprasidone treatment of children and adolescents with Tourette syndrome: a pilot study. J Am Acad Child Adolesc Psychiatry 39:292–299, 2000

Sallee FR, McGough J, Wigal T, et al: Guanfacine extended release in children and adolescents with attention-deficit/hyperactivity disorder: a placebo-controlled trial. J Am Acad Child Adolesc Psychiatry 48:155–165, 2009

Samuel RZ: EPS with lithium (letter). J Am Acad Child Adolesc Psychiatry 32:1078, 1993

Saul RC: Nortriptyline in attention deficit disorder. Clin Neuropharmacol 8:382–384, 1985

Scahill L, McCracken JT, McGough J, et al (Research Units on Pediatric Psychopharmacology Autism Network): Risperidone in children with autism and serious behavioral problems. N Engl J Med 347:314–321, 2002

Scahill L, Leckman JF, Schultz RT, et al: A placebo-controlled trial of risperidone in Tourette syndrome. Neurology 60:1130–1135, 2003

Serketich WJ, Dumas JE: The effectiveness of behavioral parent training to modify antisocial behavior in children: a meta-analysis. Behavioral Therapy 27:171–186, 1996

Shea S, Turgay A, Carroll A, et al: Risperidone in the treatment of disruptive behavioral symptoms in children with autistic and other pervasive developmental disorders. Pediatrics 114:634–641, 2004

Shire U.S. Inc: U.S. product labeling for Daytrana (methylphenidate transdermal system). Available at: http://www.daytrana. com/pdf/pdf1.pdf. Accessed June 25, 2006.

Sikich L, Hamer RM, Bashford RA, et al: A pilot study of risperidone, olanzapine, and haloperidol in psychotic youth: a double-blind, randomized, 8-week trial. Neuropsychopharmacology 29:133–145, 2004

Silver LB: Alternative (nonstimulant) medications in the treatment of attention-deficit/hyperactivity disorder in children. Pediatr Clin North Am 46:965–975, 1999

Simeon JG, Ferguson HB: Recent developments in the use of antidepressant and anxiolytic medications. Psychiatr Clin North Am 8:893–907, 1985

Smith P, Yule W, Perrin S, et al: Cognitive-behavioral therapy for PTSD in children and adolescents: a preliminary randomized controlled trial. J Am Acad Child Adolesc Psychiatry 46:1051–1061, 2007

Snyder R, Turgay A, Aman M, et al: Effects of risperidone on conduct and disruptive behavior disorders in children with subaverage IQs. J Am Acad Child Adolesc Psychiatry 41:1026–1036, 2002

Soderstrom H, Rastam M, Gillberg C: A clinical case series of six extremely aggressive youths treated with olanzapine. Eur Child Adolesc Psychiatry 11:138–141, 2002

Sokolski KN, Chicz-Demet A, Demet EM: Selective serotonin reuptake inhibitor-related extrapyramidal symptoms in autistic children: a case series. J Child Adolesc Psychopharmacol 14:143–147, 2004

Spencer T, Biederman J, Steingard R, et al: Bupropion exacerbates tics in children with attention-deficit hyperactivity disorder and Tourette's syndrome. J Am Acad Child Adolesc Psychiatry 32:211–214, 1993

Spencer T, Wilens T, Biederman J: Psychotropic medication for children and adolescents. Child Adolesc Psychiatr Clin N Am 4:97–121, 1995

Spencer T, Biederman J, Wilens T, et al: Pharmacotherapy of attention-deficit hyperactivity disorder across the life cycle. J Am Acad Child Adoles Psychiatry 35:409–432, 1996

Spencer T, Biederman J, Coffey B, et al: A double-blind comparison of desipramine and placebo in children and adolescents with chronic tic disorder and comorbid attention-deficit/hyperactivity disorder. Arch Gen Psychiatry 59:649–656, 2002

Spencer T, Newcorn JH, Kratochvil CJ, et al: Effects of atomoxetine on growth after 2-year treatment among pediatric patients with attention-deficit/hyperactivity disorder. Pediatrics [serial online] 116:e74–e80, 2005. Available at: http://www.pediatrics/org/cgi/doi/10.1542/peds.2004–0624. Accessed March 17, 2006.

Stahl SM: Essential Pharmacology: Neuroscientific Basis and Practical Applications, 2nd Edition. New York, Cambridge University Press, 2000, pp 246–255

Standaert DG, Young AB: Treatment of central nervous system degenerative disorders (Chapter 20), in Goodman and Gilman's The Pharmacological Basis of Therapeutics, 11th Edition. Edited by Brunton LL. New York, McGraw-Hill, 2006. Available at: http://www.accessmedicine.com. Accessed May 2, 2006.

Steingard R, Biederman J: Lithium responsive manic-like symptoms in two individuals with autism and mental retardation. J Am Acad Child Psychiatry 26:932–935, 1987

Stephens RJ, Bassel C, Sandor P: Olanzapine in the treatment of aggression and tics in children with Tourette's syndrome—a pilot study. J Child Adolesc Psychopharmacol 14:255–266, 2004

Strupp HII: Psychotherapy: Clinical, Research, and Theoretical Issues. New York, Jason Aronson, 1973

Sugai G, Horner RH: Introduction to the special series on positive behavior support in schools. J Emotional Behavioral Disorders 10:130–136, 2002

Swanson JM, Gupta S, Williams L, et al: Efficacy of a new pattern of delivery of methylphenidate for the treatment of ADHD: effects on activity level in the classroom and on the playground. J Am Acad Child Adolesc Psychiatry 41:1306–1314, 2002

Swanson JM, Elliott GR, Greenhill LL, et al: Effects of stimulant medication on growth rates across 3 years in the MTA follow-up. J Am Acad Child Adolesc Psychiatry 46:1015–1027, 2007

Teicher MH, Glod CA: Neuroleptic drugs: indications and guidelines for their rational use in children and adolescents. J Child Adolesc Psychopharmacol 1:33–56, 1990

Thompson S, Rey JM: Functional enuresis: is desmopressin the answer? J Am Acad Child Adolesc Psychiatry 34:266–271, 1995

Tourette's Syndrome Study Group: Treatment of ADHD in children with tics: a randomized controlled trial. Neurology 58:527–536, 2002

Trimble MR: Anticonvulsants in children and adolescents. J Child Adolesc Psychopharmacol 1:33–56, 1990

Troost PW, Lahuis BE, Steenhuis MP, et al: Long-term effects of risperidone in children with autism spectrum disorders: a placebo-discontinuation study. J Am Acad Child Adolesc Psychiatry 44:1137–1144, 2005

U.S. Food and Drug Administration (2004b): Center for Drug Evaluation and Research. Transcript of the joint meeting of the CDER psychopharmacological drugs advisory committee and the FDA pediatric advisory committee. September 14, 2004. Available at: http://www.fda.gov/ohrms/dockets/ac/04/transcripts/2004-4065T2.pdf. Accessed April 30, 2006.

U.S. Food and Drug Administration (2004c): FDA statement on recommendations of the psychopharmacological drugs and pediatric advisory committees. September 16, 2004. Available at: http://www.fda.gov/bbs/topics/news/2004/NEW01116.html. Accessed January 8, 2006.

Varley C, McClellan J: Case study: two additional sudden deaths with tricyclic antidepressants. J Am Acad Child Adolesc Psychiatry 36:390–394, 1997

Vieweg WVR, Sood AB, Pandurangi A, et al: Newer antipsychotic drugs and obesity in children and adolescents. How should we assess drug-associated weight gain? Acta Psychiatr Scand 111:177–184, 2005

Vitiello B, Severe JB, Greenhill LL, et al: Methylphenidate dosage for children with ADHD over time under controlled conditions: lessons from the MTA. J Am Acad Child Adolesc Psychiatry 40:188–196, 2001

Vitiello B, Abikoff HB, Chuang SZ, et al: Effectiveness of methylphenidate in the 10-month continuation phase of the Preschoolers with ADHD Treatment Study (PATS). J Child Adolesc Psychopharmacol 17:593–603, 2007

Wagner KD, Weller EB, Carlson GA, et al: An open-label trial of divalproex in children and adolescents with bipolar disorder. J Am Acad Child Adolesc Psychiatry 41:1224–1230, 2002

Wagner KD, Berard R, Stein MB, et al: A multicenter, randomized, double-blind, placebo-controlled trial of paroxetine in children and adolescents with social anxiety disorder. Arch Gen Psychiatry 61:1153–1162, 2004

Wagner KD, Kowatch RA, Emslie, GJ, et al: A double-blind, randomized, placebo-controlled trial of oxcarbazepine in the treatment of bipolar disorder in children and adolescents. Am J Psychiatry 163:1179–1186, 2006

Wagner KD, Redden L, Kowatch RA, et al: A double-blind, randomized, placebo-controlled trial of divalproex extended-release in the treatment of bipolar disorder in children and adolescents. J Am Acad Child Adolesc Psychiatry 48:519–532, 2009

Walkup JT, Labellarte MJ, Riddle MA, et al: Fluvoxamine for the treatment of anxiety disorders in children and adolescents. N Engl J Med 344:1279–1285, 2001

Walkup JT, Albano AM, Piacentini J, et al: Cognitive behavioral therapy, sertraline, or a combination in childhood anxiety. N Engl J Med 359:2753–2766, 2008

Walsh BT, Greenhill LL, Elsa-Grace V, et al: Effects of desipramine on autonomic input to the heart. J Am Acad Child Adolesc Psychiatry 38:1186–1193, 1999

Waslick BD, Walsh BT, Greenhill LL, et al: Cardiovascular effects of desipramine in children and adults during exercise testing. J Am Acad Child Adolesc Psychiatry 38:179–186, 1999

Wehmeier PM, Schüler-Springorum M, Heiser P, et al: Chart review for potential features of myocarditis, pericarditis, and cardiomyopathy in children and adolescents treated with clozapine. J Child Adolesc Psychopharmacol 14:267–271, 2004

Weiss B, Catron T, Harris V: A 2-year follow-up of the effectiveness of traditional child psychotherapy. J Consult Clin Psychol 68:1094–1101, 2000

Weiss M, Tannock R, Kratochvil C, et al: A randomized, placebo-controlled study of once-daily atomoxetine in the school setting in children with ADHD. J Am Acad Child Adolesc Psychiatry 44:647–655, 2005

Weisz JR: Agenda for child and adolescent psychotherapy research. On the need to put science into practice. Arch Gen Psychiatry 57:837–838, 2000

Weisz JR, Jensen AL: Child and adolescent psychotherapy in research and practice contexts: review of the evidence and suggestions for improving the field. Eur Child Adolesc Psychiatry 10 (suppl 1):I/12–I/18, 2001

Weisz JR, Hawley KM, Doss AJ: Empirically tested psychotherapies for youth internalizing and externalizing problems and disorders. Child Adolesc Psychiatric Clin N Am 13:729–815, 2004

Weller EB, Weller RA, Fristad MA: Lithium dosage guide for prepubertal children: a preliminary report. J Am Acad Child Psychiatry 25:92–95, 1986

Wigal S, Swanson JM, Feifel D, et al: A double-blind, placebo-controlled trial of dexmethylphenidate hydrochloride and d,l-threo-methylphenidate hydrochloride in children with attention-deficit/hyperactivity disorder. J Am Acad Child Adolesc Psychiatry 43:1406–1414, 2004

Wilens TE, Biederman J, Baldessarini RJ, et al: Cardiovascular effects of therapeutic doses of tricyclic antidepressants in children and adolescents. J Am Acad Child Adolesc Psychiatry 35:1491–1501, 1996

Wilens TE, Spencer TJ, Swanson JM, et al: Combining methylphenidate and clonidine: a clinically sound medication option. J Am Acad Child Adolesc Psychiatry 38:614–622, 1999

Wilens T, McBurnett K, Stein M, et al: ADHD treatment with once-daily OROS methylphenidate: final results from a long-term open-label study. J Am Acad Child Adolesc Psychiatry 44:1015–1023, 2005

Wilens TE, Boellner SW, López FA, et al: Varying the wear time of the methylphenidate transdermal system in children with attention-deficit/hyperactivity disorder. J Am Acad Child Adolesc Psychiatry 47:700–708, 2008

Willemsen-Swinkels SH, Buitelaar JK, van Engeland H: The effects of chronic naltrexone treatment in young autistic children: a double-blind placebo-controlled crossover study. Biol Psychiatry 39:1023–1031, 1996

Winsberg BG, Perel JM, Hurwic MJ, et al: Imipramine protein binding and pharmacokinetics in children, in The Phenothiazines and Structurally Related Drugs. Edited by Forrest IS, Carr CJ, Usdin E. New York, Raven, 1974, pp 425–431

Wolraich ML, Wilson DB, White JW: The effect of sugar on behavior or cognition in children: a meta-analysis. JAMA 274:1617–1621, 1995

Wolraich ML, Feurer I, Hannah JN, et al: Obtaining systematic teacher reports of disruptive behavior disorders utilizing DSM-IV. J Abnorm Child Psychol 26:141–152, 1998

Wolraich ML, Lambert W, Doffing MA, et al: Psychometric properties of the Vanderbilt ADHD diagnostic parent rating scale in a referred population. J Pediatr Psychol 28:559–568, 2003

Woolston JL: Case study: carbamazepine treatment of juvenile-onset bipolar disorder. J Am Acad Child Adolesc Psychiatry 38:335–338, 1999

Zahn TP, Rapoport JL, Thompson CL: Autonomic and behavioral effects of dextroamphetamine and placebo in normal and hyperactive prepubertal boys. J Abnorm Child Psychol 8:145–160, 1980

20

TREATMENT OF SENIORS

Dan G. Blazer, M.D., Ph.D.

Psychiatrists who work with older adults encounter diagnostic and therapeutic problems that are more complex than those encountered in young adult and middle-aged patients. Most older patients with psychiatric disorders do not fit easily into the diagnostic categories of DSM-IV-TR (American Psychiatric Association 2000) because they experience multiple symptoms that affect both physical and psychiatric functioning. This is especially true when treating the oldest members of this population (Blazer 2000). Once the problem is formulated by the clinician, usual treatment approaches must be modified both to manage the functional disability that results from the psychiatric problem and to reverse the underlying disorder.

In an era in which specific psychiatric disorders are emphasized, psychiatrists working with older adults can benefit from the syndromal approach to impairment, a paradigm shift developed by geriatricians to structure diagnostic and therapeutic strategies for older patients. In this chapter, I follow this syndromal approach by identifying

seven psychiatric syndromes that are most prevalent among older individuals—acute confusion, memory loss, insomnia, anxiety, suspiciousness and agitation, depression, and hypochondriasis—and describing them within the context of managing the resultant impairment (Table 20–1).

Acute Confusion

Acute confusion, or delirium, is a transient organic brain syndrome characterized by acute onset and global impairment of cognitive function. The older person with acute confusion exhibits a decreased ability to maintain attention to environmental stimuli and has difficulty shifting attention from one set of stimuli to another (Table 20–2). Thinking is disorganized, speech becomes rambling, and a decreased level of consciousness is exhibited. Emotional disturbances often, but not always, accompany acute confusion and may be the presenting problem in late life. These emotional disturbances include

Table 20–1. Geriatric psychiatric syndromes
Acute confusion
Memory loss
Insomnia
Anxiety
Suspiciousness and agitation
Depression
Hypochondriasis

Table 20–2. Characteristics of acute confusion
Acute onset
Decreased ability to maintain attention
Difficulty shifting attention
Disorganized thinking and speech
Memory disturbance
Altered levels of consciousness
Sleep–wake cycle disturbance
Anxiety, fear, irritability, and anger
May appear apathetic and withdrawn
Fluctuating course usually brief in duration

anxiety, fear, irritability, and anger. Some older persons, in contrast, are apathetic and withdrawn during an episode of delirium and thus are much more difficult to diagnose. Acute confusion, by definition, is brief, usually lasting a few hours but possibly lasting weeks, such as in the case of confusion secondary to medications.

Frequency and Origins

The frequency of delirium among the older population is difficult to estimate because many episodes are undetected due to their brevity. Most estimates of incidence range from 15% to 25% on medical and surgical wards (Martin et al. 2000). The incidence is higher on intensive care units and among persons recovering from cardiovascular surgery. When delirium is diagnosed in a hospitalized older patient, the hospitalization is usually prolonged, and both in-hospital and posthospital mortality rates are increased. Mortality at 2-year follow-up approaches 50%.

Acute confusion in late life is the common outcome of a cascade of biological, cognitive, and environmental contributors. Biological brain function declines with age, although functional capacity varies greatly within age groups. Degenerative changes, such as those characteristic of Alzheimer's disease, render the older person more susceptible to physiological changes secondary to aging and disease. These physiological changes include drug intoxication, electrolyte disturbance, infection, dehydration, hypoalbuminemia, and hypoxia. Visual and hearing impairment may also contribute to delirium.

Cognitive contributors to delirium include a predisposition to hallucinations and delusions, such as that in an aging patient with a history of schizophrenia. Environmental contributors include the unfamiliar surroundings of a hospital or long-term-care facility and social isolation. Therefore, the hospital, where the convergence of these contributors is likely, is a high-risk environment for delirium. Additional factors that may contribute to delirium in the hospital include physical restraint and bladder catheter (S. Inouye 2000).

Treatment

General therapy for the confused older individual, to be administered in parallel with specific therapy for the underlying cause of the acute confusion, begins with medical support (Table 20–3). Vital signs and level of consciousness should be closely monitored (S.K. Inouye et al. 1999). All medications that are not critical should be discontinued. Vasopressor agents may be needed to increase blood pressure, and excessive fever should be treated with ice baths and alcohol sponges. When the syndrome of acute confusion is recognized and the precipitant of the confusion is established through history, physical examination, and laboratory studies, the clinician can begin therapy. Laboratory tests should be

Table 20–3. Treatment of acute confusion

Monitor levels of consciousness with brief bedside tests (serial 7s and digit span).

Check vital signs.

Discontinue all nonessential medications.

Establish an adequate airway (if necessary).

Administer 100 mL of 50% dextrose plus 100 mg of thiamine intravenously.

Leave lights on in the room.

Avoid unnecessary stimuli (e.g., keep the room quiet and simply furnished).

Use antipsychotic medications (haloperidol 0.5–1.0 mg po, bid; 0.5–1.0 mg im prn).

Note. po=oral administration; bid=twice daily; prn=as needed; im=intramuscular.

ordered as indicated, including thyroid function tests, measurement of drug levels, toxicology screen, measurement of ammonia or cortisol levels, electrocardiogram (ECG), and neuroimaging (S. Inouye 2006). Acute confusion may present as a psychiatric emergency that threatens permanent brain damage. Severe hypoglycemia, hypoxia, and hyperthermia are examples of critical conditions that may present as acute confusion. Therefore, the initial treatment should include the establishment of an adequate airway to ensure that the patient is breathing and the administration of 100 mL 50% dextrose plus thiamine 100 mg intravenously if hypoglycemia and Wernicke's encephalopathy cannot be ruled out.

The clinician also must pay special attention to reducing the demands that excess and conflicting environmental stimuli make on the patient's cerebral function. Order and simplicity in the environment are critical to the management of the confused older patient, who should be maintained in a quiet, simply furnished, and well-lit room. Lights should be left on at night. Care can best be facilitated by constant attention from familiar persons such as family members, who should frequently orient the patient to time, place, and person. Physicians, nurses, and other hospital personnel should explain all procedures. Restraints should be kept to a minimum. Behavioral ag-

itation generally can be managed by judicious use of antipsychotic medications, such as risperidone, in low doses (administered either intramuscularly or orally).

Memory Loss

The syndrome of memory loss (the dementia syndrome) is one of the more frequent and disabling syndromes experienced by older adults. Late-life memory loss is usually accompanied by a more or less sustained decline in cognitive function from a previously obtained intellectual level, usually with an insidious onset. Other cognitive capacities that decline with memory include language (e.g., aphasia), spatial or temporal orientation, judgment, executive function, and abstract thought. State of consciousness is usually not altered until very late in the memory loss syndrome, which is in contrast with acute confusion.

Frequency and Origins

Disabling memory loss may begin in midlife, but it is much more frequent in persons older than 75 years than in those between 65 and 74 years of age. Alzheimer's disease (AD), the most common disorder contributing to the dementia syndrome, has been estimated to be prevalent in 6%–8% of community-dwelling persons older than 65 years, with more than 30% of persons 85 years or older having AD. Prevalence estimates of AD include both mild and severe cases, so significant memory impairment may be found in only a proportion of persons identified as having the condition in community samples. Until age 75 years, the life expectancy of persons with AD or vascular dementia is reduced by one-half. After 75 years of age, life expectancy is less affected by memory loss. Other causes of memory loss are listed in Table 20–4.

More than 50% of persons with chronic memory loss will, at autopsy, exhibit the changes of AD only. AD is characterized by neurofibrillary tangles, deposition of β-amyloid, and brain atrophy. The next most com-

Table 20–4. Differential diagnosis of memory loss

Dementia of the Alzheimer's type
Vascular dementia
Dementia due to HIV disease
Dementia due to head trauma
Dementia due to Parkinson's disease
Dementia due to Huntington's disease
Dementia due to Pick's disease
Lewy body dementia

mon contributor to the syndrome is vascular dementia, characterized by multiple small infarcts of the brain. Clinically and pathophysiologically, it is difficult to disaggregate the dementias. Vascular dementia frequently is comorbid with AD. In contrast to AD, however, vascular dementia is more common in males than in females. Many patients with Parkinson's disease develop brain changes late in the course of the disease similar to those changes found in AD. Clinically, except for their parkinsonian symptoms, these patients cannot be distinguished from patients with AD. In addition, many patients with AD exhibit changes in the substantia nigra at autopsy. Approximately 5% of older persons experience memory loss as a result of alcohol-induced amnestic disorder. A variant of AD is Lewy body dementia, characterized by synaptophysin-containing cytoplasmic inclusions outside the substantia nigra. In addition to memory impairment, fluctuating cognitive function is characteristic of this disorder.

The primary risk factors for AD are age and family history, with the prevalence of AD, as mentioned previously, being an exponential function of age. Other risk factors for AD include Down syndrome, head trauma, and possibly lack of education. (Use of statins and/or nonsteroidal anti-inflammatory drugs [NSAIDs] may be protective [Breitner and Zandi 2001].) Genetic risk factors have received much attention in recent years, especially the relationship between the disease and the ε4 allele of the apolipoprotein E (*APOE*) gene (Roses 1994). Persons who carry at least one copy of the *APOE* ε4 allele are at increased risk for AD.

Diagnostic Workup

The diagnostic workup of the older adult with memory loss begins with a history (Table 20–5). A history should be obtained from both family members and the patient. The nature and severity of memory loss should be assessed in conjunction with a chronological account of the onset of the older adult's problems and specific behavioral changes. Patient and family should be asked about common problems resulting from memory loss, such as becoming lost in a familiar place, having difficulties with driving, becoming repetitious, and losing objects.

The nature and degree of the cognitive dysfunction should be assessed by both a thorough mental status examination and objective cognitive testing, such as use of the Mini-Mental State Exam (Folstein et al. 1975).

The in-office or hospital-based initial assessment of memory and cognitive functioning is followed by a more in-depth evaluation of cognition with tests of specific functions such as executive functioning (Trail Making Test), language (Boston Naming Test), memory (Wechsler Memory Scale), and spatial ability (tests of constructional praxis).

Routine laboratory examination is essential, with special focus on findings that could contribute to memory loss, such as hypothyroidism, anemia, and (in rarer cases) vitamin deficiencies, such as deficiency of vitamin B_{12}. Magnetic resonance imaging (MRI) or computed tomography scans are now routine in the initial evaluation of memory loss. Genotyping a patient with AD or a patient's family members cannot be justified at this time, despite the emerging evidence of a hereditary predisposition with certain genotypes such as APOE 4/4 (Roses 1997).

Treatment

Most pharmacological therapies are based on the cholinergic hypotheses of memory and include primarily cholinesterase inhibitors

Table 20–5. Diagnostic workup of memory loss

Detailed history from the patient and a family member

A mental status exam, such as the Mini-Mental State Exam

A physical, including a thorough neurological exam

Report of all medications and frequency of use

More complex neuropsychological exams

Routine laboratory exam: complete blood count, electrolytes, liver function tests, thyroid function tests, vitamin B_{12}, and folate

Magnetic resonance imaging or computed tomography scan

Routine genetic testing is not recommended

Table 20–6. Medications for the primary treatment of memory loss

Cholinesterase inhibitors

  Donepezil (begin with 5 mg and increase to target dosage of 10 mg/day)

  Rivastigmine (begin with 1.5 mg bid and increase to at least 3 mg bid)

  Galantamine (begin with 4–8 mg/day and increase to 16–24 mg/day)

NMDA receptor antagonist

  Memantine (begin with 5 mg/day and increase to 20 mg/day)

Note. bid = twice daily; NMDA = *N*-methyl-D-aspartate.

(Table 20–6). Tacrine, donepezil, rivastigmine, and galantamine are available to physicians in office-based practice. These drugs have proved moderately effective in reducing decline in memory up to 6 months after administration, but their long-term ability to retard memory loss is questioned. Studies are now emerging to suggest that cognitive function among subjects using these agents is indistinguishable from that among control subjects after 1–2 years. Memantine, an *N*-methyl-D-aspartate (NMDA) receptor antagonist, has been approved for the treatment of moderate to severe AD (based on the theory that glutamatergic overstimulation may cause excitotoxic neuronal changes).

Psychotropic medications are used extensively in patients with memory loss, primarily because of secondary symptoms such as verbal or physical aggression, anxiety, depression, psychoses, and severe agitation or regressive behavior (see "Suspiciousness and Agitation" section later in chapter) (Katz et al. 1999).

After determining that the emerging behavioral problem cannot be handled through nonpharmacological means and is ongoing, medication can be prescribed with caution.

Agitation and anxiety can be treated with antianxiety agents (e.g., short-acting benzodiazepines), neuroleptics (e.g., risperidone, olanzapine), and occasionally low doses of antidepressant agents (e.g., trazodone) at night.

The antipsychotics are the most effective psychotropic agents for controlling severe agitation, aggressive behavior, and psychoses. Most neuroleptics are effective but produce side effects; therefore, selection of a drug is usually made on the basis of the least adverse side-effect profile for a given patient. The atypical antipsychotic agents, such as olanzapine and risperidone, are the preferred drugs at present, primarily because of their more benign immediate side-effect profile (but see the "Suspiciousness and Agitation" section later in this chapter for black box warning in connection with use of these drugs).

Because depression is frequent among patients with chronic memory loss, the use of an antidepressant agent is often indicated (Reifler et al. 1989). In general, the antidepressant agent will not lead to an improvement in memory. Selective serotonin reuptake inhibitors (SSRIs) with the fewest potential side effects are preferred (e.g., sertraline, escitalopram).

Behavioral management of the patient with memory loss not only is useful to the patient but also provides the patient's family with a sense of accomplishment in the presence of an illness that tends to leave a family feeling helpless and bewildered. The family and the physician should develop behaviors that promote both patient and family security. Familiar routines and consistent repetition of instructions usually enhance security. The family, as much as possible, should provide moments of fun with the patient, even when these brief moments of relief are quickly forgotten by the patient.

Management of memory loss must include a review of the patient's environment for safety. Typical safety problems include behaviors such as becoming lost or wandering into busy traffic, using medicines erratically or accidentally, falling (secondary to poor lighting or slippery surfaces), having accidents while driving, and leaving things unattended (e.g., leaving appliances turned on). Home visits by geriatric nurse specialists are most helpful in reviewing the household for potential problems.

Perhaps the most important long-term component for managing the older adult with memory loss is support of the family through educational materials and support groups. Families are the primary caregivers of elderly persons with memory loss until the memory loss becomes severe enough to lead to institutionalization. With proper support, the older person can remain at home for a longer period of time, and the family can function more effectively in the midst of the devastation of the severe memory loss. Education of the family about the expected progression of memory loss, and the many behaviors that accompany such loss but that may not be intuitively recognized as resulting from the illness, is key to family support.

Insomnia

Insomnia is more frequent in the elderly population than in any other age group; 28% report difficulty falling asleep, and 46% report symptoms of difficulty both falling asleep and staying asleep and use of more sedative-hypnotic medications (Foley et al. 1995). Both the lack of sleep and the subsequent medication use frequently lead to deterioration in daytime alertness and functioning. The most common causes of sleep disturbances include primary insomnia, sleep-disordered breathing, sleep–wake schedule disorder, and secondary insomnia due to conditions such as depression, dementing disorders, and sleep problems secondary to medication use.

Sleep changes characteristic in late life include decreased total sleep time, frequent arousals, increased percentages of Stage 1 and Stage 2 sleep, decreased percentages of Stage 3 and Stage 4 sleep, decreased rapid eye movement (REM) latency, decreased absolute amounts of REM sleep, and a tendency to exhibit a redistribution of sleep across the 24-hour day (e.g., napping during the day). Many of these sleep changes are similar to those that occur in depression and dementing disorders, although not as severe. Older persons are also more likely to phase-advance in the sleep cycle, with a phase tendency toward "morningness."

Frequency

Approximately 5% of all elderly persons who initially report no sleep problems report new symptoms each year (Ancoli-Israel 2000). The proportion of older persons living in long-term care facilities who have sleep problems and take sedative-hypnotic agents is much higher than in the community. Sleep apnea is more prevalent in elderly men than women, with the apnea index (i.e., the number of apneic episodes per hour of sleep) being 5 or greater in 25%–35% of elderly persons in the community.

Diagnostic Workup

The diagnostic workup of an older person with insomnia begins with a recognition of the severity of the sleep disturbance (Table 20–7).

A medication history is essential in determining the etiology of insomnia. Prescribed medications, especially sedative-hypnotics

Table 20–7. Diagnostic workup of insomnia in later life

Screening (satisfaction with sleep, daytime napping, sleep–wake cycle problems, fatigue, and complaints [e.g., snoring] from a bed partner)
Medical history
Psychiatric history
Medication use
Polysomnography
Previous treatments of insomnia

and anxiolytics, as well as alcohol, have significant effects on sleep and also may impair cardiopulmonary function. Symptoms of the major psychiatric disorders affecting older persons, such as dementia, depression, or severe anxiety, may also lead to insomnia. If a sleep–wake cycle dysfunction is suspected, patients may be asked to keep a log of napping, going to sleep, and awakening. Physical and neurological examinations are necessary, especially when sleep apnea is suspected. Heavy snoring requires a thorough examination of the nose and throat, usually by an otolaryngologist.

If referred to a psychiatrist or neurologist, most patients are evaluated by polysomnography. Polysomnographic techniques have been improved in recent years; patients can now be fitted with a portable recording instrument and returned home to sleep for 2 evenings.

Treatment

The cornerstones of effective treatment of insomnia in late life are management of the underlying causes of the sleep disturbance and improved sleep hygiene. For example, a significant portion of older adults experiencing chronic insomnia also experience psychiatric disorders, especially depression and alcohol problems. Both of these conditions are responsive to therapy. Physical problems such as hypothyroidism or arthritis may not be reversed, but the symptoms can be relieved

with medications or other therapeutic interventions. Nocturnal myoclonus or restless legs syndrome may respond to medication such as dopamine agonists (e.g., pergolide), anticonvulsants (e.g., carbamazepine), benzodiazepines (e.g., clonazepam), and opiates in severe and otherwise treatment-resistant cases. Sleep apnea syndrome that does not respond to conservative management (e.g., the use of positive-pressure breathing) may require surgery to improve flow in the nasopharyngeal region.

Institution of good sleep hygiene is the next step in managing insomnia among elderly patients. First, the patient should be encouraged to initiate sleep at the same time every night, preferably at a later rather than an earlier time (to prevent early-morning wakefulness). The bedroom should be used primarily for sleeping and not for napping. Therefore, if the elderly patient has difficulty sleeping at night, the bed should be made up in the morning and the patient should be encouraged not to nap in the bed and to spend as little time as possible in the bedroom during the day. Exercising can facilitate sleep, but exercise should not be initiated after later afternoon. Alcohol and caffeine should be avoided in the evenings, and the evening meal should be moderate and at least 2–3 hours before bedtime. Fluid intake should also be limited during the 2–3 hours before bedtime (to prevent nocturia).

Bedrooms should generally be maintained at a temperature between 65°F and 72°F. To maintain a cool bedroom, many elderly persons who cannot afford air conditioning are forced to leave their windows open at night, possibly exposing them to noises that are likely to disturb sleep. One means for decreasing the potential of noise to disrupt the night's sleep is to institute white noise (e.g., a waterfall or rain sounds) using specially built devices or to run a fan during the night.

A number of medications can be used to facilitate sleep in the elderly population, although these medications should be used with care (Table 20–8). The antidepressant

Table 20–8. Medications and recommended doses for treating late-life insomnia

Trazodone 25–50 mg
Zolpidem (Ambien) 5 mg
Temazepam (Restoril) 15 mg
Zaleplon (Sonata) 10 mg
Eszopiclone (Lunesta) 1–2 mg

agents not only are useful in managing the older adult with insomnia secondary to depression but also can be used as sedative agents, especially if prescribed in low doses. For example, 25–50 mg of trazodone may be preferable to using a long-term benzodiazepine if chronic use of a sedative is indicated. In general, short- to medium-acting benzodiazepines are preferred over those that are more extended in length of action. Therefore, shorter-acting agents such as zolpidem (5 mg) and temazepam (15 mg) are preferred as a sedative-hypnotic. A new benzodiazepine receptor agonist, zaleplon (10 mg), has the shortest half-life among these agents and does not appear to cause rebound insomnia or adversely affect psychomotor function (Ancoli-Israel 2000). Eszopiclone (1–2 mg), although approved for long-term use to improve sleep, should be used with the same caution as other agents. Each of the newer agents has been proved to be safe and effective in older adults (Ancoli-Israel and Ayalon 2006).

Anxiety

Anxiety is a frequent symptom among older persons secondary to physical illness such as hyperthyroidism, comorbid with other psychiatric disorders such as depression, or as the primary symptom of a disorder such as generalized anxiety disorder (Blazer 1997). Many of the anxiety disorders, however, are relatively less frequent in late life. Generalized anxiety disorder is a frequent diagnosis regardless of age, yet generalized anxiety is often comorbid with other psychiatric disorders such as major depression. Panic disor-

der is relatively frequent and severe among younger persons but much less so among older persons (although data documenting a lower prevalence among older persons are sparse). Posttraumatic stress disorder can occur at any age but is found more frequently in younger persons than older persons. Obsessive-compulsive traits are common throughout the life cycle, although the severe manifestations of this disorder are less likely to be observed in older persons. Therefore, the management of anxiety in older persons usually consists of managing the symptoms of generalized anxiety that are the primary problem or comorbid with other disorders.

Frequency and Origins

Community surveys of individuals with anxiety symptoms estimate that approximately 5% of older persons meet DSM-III (American Psychiatric Association 1980) criteria for the diagnosis of generalized anxiety disorder (Blazer et al. 1991). Approximately 20% of older persons report some cognitive or somatic symptoms of anxiety in community surveys, with somatic symptoms being more prevalent than cognitive symptoms. In a survey in North Carolina, DSM-III simple phobia was found in 10% of persons 65 years or older compared with 13% of persons in middle age (Blazer et al. 1985). Yet these phobias are generally not disabling.

Anxiety can result from a number of medical (Table 20–9) and psychiatric conditions.

Table 20–9. Medical causes of anxiety in the elderly

Hyperthyroidism
Cardiac arrhythmia
Pulmonary emboli
Hypoglycemia
Medications
  Caffeine
  Over-the-counter sympathomimetic drugs
  Anticholinergic agents
  Withdrawal from anxiolytic agents

Many psychiatric disorders are manifested, in part, by symptoms of anxiety. Moderate to severe acute confusion is usually associated with anxiety and agitation, especially when the older person is in an unfamiliar place. Anxiety is a common accompaniment of major depression; older patients who experience major depression also meet the criteria for generalized anxiety disorder in more than 50% of the cases. Hypochondriasis is associated with anxiety, especially when dependency needs are not met by family and health care professionals. Dementing disorders, especially in the early and middle stages, are associated with anxiety and agitation. The clinician must not overlook the possibility that the anxiety symptoms may be secondary to appropriate fear. Many older persons must expose themselves daily to situations that threaten their security. Older adults living in inner cities often fear being attacked as they walk the streets. Those with memory loss who live alone may fear that they will get lost driving to the doctor's office. Individuals who have lost the acuteness of their reflexes fear driving on busy, crowded highways.

Treatment

The use of nonpharmacological therapies such as relaxation training, cognitive restructuring, and activity structuring for the treatment of anxiety in older adults has not been studied extensively. Nevertheless, the danger of medication, as well as the successful application of cognitive-behavior therapies to other psychiatric disorders in late life (especially depression), suggests that nonpharmacological therapies may be applicable to anxiety disorders. Older persons who do not have cognitive dysfunction may be good candidates for relaxation training and biofeedback.

The cornerstone of pharmacological therapy for the anxiety disorders is the benzodiazepines (Table 20–10). They are generally well tolerated by persons of all ages but present unique problems when prescribed to older persons. For example, the half-life of the benzodiazepines may be increased dra-

Table 20–10. Medications and typical starting doses for treating anxiety in the elderly

Alprazolam (begin with 0.25 mg bid)
Oxazepam (begin with 15 mg bid)
Lorazepam (begin with 0.5 mg bid)
Buspirone (begin with 5 mg bid and increase to a total of 20–30 mg/day)
Selective serotonin reuptake inhibitors (see Table 20–13 for dosages)
Propranolol (begin with 10 mg bid)

Note. bid = twice daily.

matically in late life. Older persons are also more susceptible to potential side effects of benzodiazepines such as fatigue, drowsiness, motor dysfunction, and memory impairment. Therefore, the shorter-acting benzodiazepines, such as alprazolam (0.25 mg), oxazepam (15 mg), and lorazepam (0.5 mg), given two to three times a day, have been preferred agents in late life. Nevertheless, shortacting drugs in some older patients may lead to brief withdrawal episodes during the day and a rebound of anxiety.

The antidepressant agents are useful in treating anxiety mixed with depression. Nevertheless, in many older persons with a mixed anxiety–depression syndrome, the depressive symptoms improve while the antidepressant is being used, yet the anxiety symptoms persist. Therefore, a combination of a benzodiazepine and an antidepressant is sometimes used. Some have suggested that β-blockers such as propranolol (10 mg twice daily) are valuable in treating anxiety disorders. These drugs must be monitored carefully, given their propensity to slow the heart rate.

Suspiciousness and Agitation

A frequent symptom in older adults, especially older adults experiencing cognitive impairment, is suspiciousness, which may range from increased cautiousness and distrust of family and friends to overt paranoid delusions.

The predominant delusions encountered in older persons are persecutory delusions and somatic delusions. Persecutory delusions often revolve around a single theme or a series of connected themes, such as family and neighbors conspiring against the older person or a delusion of sexual abuse. Somatic delusions often involve the gastrointestinal tract and frequently reflect the older person's fear that he or she is experiencing cancer. Regardless of the etiology of suspiciousness and paranoid delusions, when older persons believe they are threatened from the social environment, often because they do not understand what is happening in that environment, agitation becomes paramount. Agitation in the suspicious older person is an acute symptom that may require emergency management, as described later in this discussion.

Frequency and Origins

Suspiciousness and paranoid behavior were found in 17% of persons in one community survey (Christenson and Blazer 1984; Lowenthal 1964), and a sense of persecution was reported in 4% in another survey (Christenson and Blazer 1984). Fewer than 1% were found to have schizophrenia or a paranoid disorder.

Many different disorders may lead to suspiciousness, delusions, and agitation. Chronic schizophrenic disorder, which has its onset earlier in life and persists into late life, is perhaps the most easily identified cause of late-life suspiciousness (Jeste et al. 2004). Schizophrenia-like illness may have its first onset in late life. These patients are less likely to experience negative symptoms and neuropsychological impairment and often respond to lower doses of antipsychotic medication. Usually, depression and organic mental disorders do not contribute to these late-onset schizophrenia-like states. In contrast, organic mental disorders and late-onset depression are frequently associated with some psychotic symptoms.

Late-onset delusional disorder, with mild to moderate symptoms, is a more frequent cause of suspiciousness in late life. Delusions, often of being persecuted by family and friends, usually center on a single theme or a connection of themes. For example, an older woman may become convinced that her daughter was instrumental in the death of her husband (or that the daughter neglected her father during a chronic illness). That woman, in turn, may not listen to reason regarding the daughter's behavior and may never forgive the daughter for the perceived abuse or neglect. These delusions may lead to a withdrawal of affection, financial support, and social contact with the daughter.

Another common cause of suspiciousness in late life is organic delusional syndrome (or dementia with psychosis). These delusions, in contrast to late-onset delusional disorder, wax and wane over time in severity and in content. In some cases, the older adult functions well and does not appear to be disturbed by the delusional thoughts, though the thoughts are frequently expressed. Imagined infidelity by a marriage partner is a common example. If the delusion does not create subjective stress and/or problems in management, regular evaluation of the patient and family without the use of medications is the preferred intervention. Suspiciousness usually results from the dementing disorders. For some persons with AD, paranoid thoughts may dominate other symptoms of the dementing illness, especially in the early stages. Perhaps the most common encounter psychiatrists have with suspicious older persons is with patients with dementia who have become a management problem because of suspiciousness and agitation. Suspiciousness and agitation are also frequent symptoms of delirium, as described earlier.

A family history of suspiciousness and delusional thought is uncommon among suspicious older persons, and therefore hereditary contributions are probably less important than at earlier stages of the life cycle. Degeneration of subcortical tissues with aging may disrupt neurotransmission and higher brain functions, which in turn contributes to a deficiency in maintaining attention and filtering information, symptoms that have been associated with psychotic thinking. Sensory deprivation also has been identified as a potential risk factor for suspiciousness, regardless of the underlying disorder. Social isolation also may contribute to suspiciousness.

Diagnostic Workup

The key to the diagnostic workup of the suspicious older person is the psychiatric evaluation. Delusional thinking and agitation usually render the patient's history inaccurate, and therefore family members should be interviewed to review the patient's behavior, especially any change in behavior. Previous psychotic or delusional episodes should be documented, as well as previous treatment. Clinicians evaluating the suspicious older person should remember that older adults are occasionally abused by family members and that the seemingly delusional description of family behavior by the older individual may contain some truth.

Treatment

The management of suspiciousness in older adults requires 1) ensuring a safe environment; 2) initiating a therapeutic alliance; 3) considering and, if appropriate, instituting pharmacological therapy (Table 20–11); and 4) managing acute behavioral crises. The clinician must first decide whether hospitalization is necessary. In general, paranoid older persons do not adapt well to the hospital. Change from familiar surroundings and interaction with strange persons tend to exacerbate the suspiciousness. Nevertheless, older patients often are so disabled in their behavior secondary to schizophrenic or delusional disorder that hospitalization is necessary.

It is rarely necessary for clinicians to confront patients regarding suspicious or delusional thinking; therefore, clinician responses

Table 20–11. Medications for the management of suspiciousness and agitation in the elderly

Atypical antipsychotic agents
  Risperidone (Risperdal) 1–3 mg/day
  Olanzapine (Zyprexa) 5–15 mg/day
  Quetiapine (Seroquel) 50–100 mg/day

Older antipsychotic agents
  Haloperidol (Haldol) 0.5–2.0 mg tid

Note. tid=three times a day.

to older patients' answers to questions can be supportive, and clinicians do not need to agree with statements made by the patients that are known to be untrue.

The cornerstone of managing the moderately to severely suspicious older patient is medication, especially antipsychotic agents (see Table 20–11). Medications most frequently used to treat older persons are risperidone (1–3 mg/day), olanzapine (5–15 mg/day), quetiapine (50–100 mg/day), and haloperidol (0.5–2.0 mg orally three times a day). Dosage of these agents is relatively small initially, and one-half of the dose should be given during the evening. Recent reports suggest that older adults taking both the typical and atypical antipsychotic agents for the treatment of dementia-related behavioral disorders may be at some increased risk for mortality, leading to a black box warning from the U.S. Food and Drug Administration. Physicians who prescribe antipsychotic medications for the treatment of suspiciousness in an older adult should carefully monitor the success of these agents and should discuss the potential benefits and potential risks with the patient and family. If the drug is deemed not successful—for example, if the target symptoms do not change with the medication—then it should be discontinued, given the significant side effects that may result. Tardive dyskinesia is five to six times more prevalent in elderly than in younger patients (Jeste 2000).

Table 20–12. Suggestions for preventing aggressive and violent behavior in the older adult

Psychologically disarm the patient by helping him or her to express his or her fears.

Distract the attention of the older patient.

Provide directions to the patient in simple terms.

Avoid threatening body language or gestures.

Remain at a safe distance from the patient until help is available.

Finally, the physician must be prepared to deal with severe agitation and violent behavior (Table 20–12). Medications alone will not control these behaviors. Physicians must work with the nursing staff to prevent such behavior in patients at risk while they are in the hospital and must instruct families on methods of prevention when these patients are at home.

Periods of severe agitation are usually brief and, if managed properly, are soon forgotten by the older patient. Then the physician once more can work toward establishing a sustained therapeutic relationship with the patient.

Depression

Depression is one of the more frequent and the second most disabling geriatric psychiatry syndrome (after memory loss) experienced by older adults (Blazer 2002, 2003). Late-life depression that is not comorbid with physical illness and/or a dementing disorder is characterized by symptoms similar to those experienced at earlier stages of the life cycle, with some significant differences. Depressed mood is usually apparent in the older adult but may not be a spontaneous complaint. Older persons are more likely to experience weight loss (as opposed to weight gain or no change in weight) during a major depressive episode and are less likely to report feelings of worthlessness or guilt. Although older persons experience more difficulty with cognitive performance tests during a depressive episode, they are no more likely than persons in midlife to report cognitive problems subjectively. Complaints of cognitive dysfunction are common in more severe depressive episodes regardless of the person's age. Persistent anhedonia associated with a lack of response to pleasurable stimuli is a common and central symptom of late-life depression. Older persons are also more likely than younger persons to exhibit psychotic symptoms during a depressive episode. Recent studies have suggested that executive function is impaired in older adults with depression and that this impairment may be associated with a higher likelihood of relapse and recurrence of symptoms (Alexopoulos et al. 2000).

Frequency and Origins

In community surveys, older adults are less likely to be diagnosed as having major depression than are persons in young adulthood or middle age. Depressive symptoms, however, are about equally prevalent across the life cycle. Standardized interviews reveal that 1%–3% of persons in the community are diagnosed as having dysthymia (Blazer et al. 1987). Major depression is much more prevalent among older persons in the hospital and in long-term care facilities, ranging from 10% to 20% (Koenig et al. 1988).

Major depression is relatively infrequent among older persons, yet it can be a challenging disorder to manage. Older persons also may experience bipolar disorder, with a first-onset manic episode after age 65 years. Psychotic depressions are more common in late life than at other stages of the life cycle (Meyers 1992). Medical illness, such as hypothyroidism, frequently leads to an organic mood disorder. An adjustment disorder with depressed mood secondary to physical disability and/or chronic illness is among the most frequent causes of depressed mood among older individuals.

Diagnostic Workup

As with the diagnosis of other geriatric psychiatry syndromes, the patient's history and a collateral history from a family member are the keys to making the diagnosis of depression in late life. Although older persons may exhibit some tendency to "mask" their depressive symptoms, a careful interview almost invariably reveals significant depression if it is present. The history should be complemented by a thorough mental status examination with attention to disturbances of motor behavior and perception, presence or absence of hallucinations, disturbances of thinking, and thorough cognitive testing. Psychological testing may be implemented to distinguish depression from dementia but should not be performed in the midst of a severe depressive episode. Some tests, such as the blood count and measurement of vitamin B_{12} and folate levels, are useful in screening for medical illnesses that may present with depressive symptoms. The thyroid panel is essential in the diagnosis of the depressed older patient, given that subclinical hypothyroid disorders are frequently uncovered in the workup.

Although the abnormalities in sleep associated with depression frequently parallel those associated with normal aging, experienced polysomnographers can distinguish them. MRI is optional despite the association of subcortical white matter hyperintensities with late-life depression. The physician ordering laboratory tests for a depressed older patient also must consider the potential adverse health consequences for an older adult experiencing a severe or chronic mood disorder. For example, major depression is associated with decreased bone mineral density, placing older women with depression at greater risk for osteoporosis (Michelson et al. 1996).

Treatment

Clinical management involves pharmacotherapy, electroconvulsive therapy (ECT), psychotherapy, and work with the family. The pharmacological treatment of choice at pres-

Table 20–13. Antidepressant therapy for seniors with typical starting doses

Selective serotonin reuptake inhibitors
  Fluoxetine (Prozac) 10 mg/day
  Sertraline (Zoloft) 50 mg/day in divided doses
  Paroxetine (Paxil) 10 mg/day
  Citalopram (Celexa) 10 mg/day
  Trazodone (Desyrel) 50 mg at night

Serotonin–norepinephrine reuptake inhibitors
  Venlafaxine (Effexor) 37.5 mg/day
  Duloxetine (Cymbalta) 20 mg qd or bid

Tricyclic antidepressants
  Nortriptyline 50–75 mg at night

Note. qd=once daily; bid=twice daily.

ent is one of the new-generation antidepressant medications (Table 20–13). Despite the advent of these newer agents, some geriatric psychiatrists still prefer to first administer one of the secondary amines, such as nortriptyline, in healthy older adults. The SSRIs fluoxetine, sertraline, paroxetine, and citalopram can be used at somewhat lower dosages than are prescribed at earlier stages of the life cycle (e.g., 10 mg/day for paroxetine). The most common adverse effects that limit the use of SSRIs are agitation and persistent weight loss. Paroxetine has been shown to significantly (but not dramatically) improve the symptoms of minor depression and dysthymia at dosages between 10 and 40 mg/day (Williams et al. 2000). If treatment with an SSRI is not successful, then the second-choice medications are usually the serotonin–norepinephrine reuptake inhibitors (SNRIs), such as venlafaxine (beginning at around 37.5 mg/day) or duloxetine (beginning with 20 mg/day) (Alexopoulos et al. 2001).

The older person who does not respond to antidepressant medications or who experiences significant side effects from the medications may be a candidate for ECT. Depressed older persons who are experiencing a severe depressive episode are candidates for ECT; they are especially likely to respond if they are experiencing psychotic symptoms. With proper medical support, ECT is a safe and effective treatment for older adults. Despite a higher level of physical illness and cognitive impairment, even the oldest patient with severe major depression may tolerate ECT as well as younger patients do and may demonstrate similar or better acute response. Unilateral nondominant ECT is preferred. If the treatment is successful, then maintenance ECT at progressively extended intervals is a method of preventing relapse.

Several studies have demonstrated the effectiveness of cognitive and behavioral therapies (including interpersonal psychotherapy) in outpatient treatment of older persons who have major depression without melancholia (Lynch and Aspnes 2004). Cognitive therapy also may be an adjunct for severe melancholic depressions that are treated concomitantly with medications. Cognitive-behavioral therapy is well tolerated by older people because of its limited duration and educational orientation, as well as the active interchange between the therapist and the patient.

Any effective therapy for depression in older persons must include work with the family. Families are often the most important allies of the clinician working with depressed older patients. Families should be informed as to the danger signs, such as potential for suicide, in a severely depressed older family member. In addition, the family can provide structure for reengaging a withdrawn and depressed older person into social activities.

Hypochondriasis

Hypochondriasis among older persons is one of the more common and frustrating of the somatoform disorders encountered by health care professionals. An essential feature of hypochondriasis in older persons is their belief that they have one of several serious illnesses (Table 20–14). This belief derives from an exaggerated interpretation of physical signs

Table 20–14. Characteristics of hypochondriasis in the elderly

Belief of suffering from one or more serious illnesses

Exaggerated interpretation of physical signs

Chronic course

Symptoms frequently focused in the abdominal and genitourinary areas

Concerns not relieved by reassurance from the physician

Exaggerated side effects from medications

and sensations. The medical workup often will reveal some physical abnormality but does not support a medical diagnosis that can account for the severity and breadth of symptoms experienced. However, hypochondriacal symptoms do not reach the level of somatic delusions.

Frequency and Origins

In community surveys, exaggerated concern about health was found among 10% of older persons (Blazer and Houpt 1979). Most older persons assessed their health accurately, with no trend for older individuals inaccurately perceiving their health as being worse than it actually is. Hypochondriacal older persons overuse health care services, and therefore one or two hypochondriacal older patients in a primary care physician's practice may occupy an appreciable amount of time, leading the physician to believe that hypochondriasis is a common condition.

The etiology of hypochondriasis is, by definition, not biological. This does not mean, however, that hypochondriacal older persons do not experience physical illness or that the symptoms reported by some older individuals are not, to some degree, the expression of actual physical problems. Exaggeration of symptoms (as opposed to the invention of symptoms) is the manifestation of hypochondriasis.

Contributing Factors

Several mechanisms may contribute to hypochondriasis in older persons. First, the symptoms may be used to shift anxiety from specific psychological conflicts to more concrete problems with body functioning. An older person may fear the loss of his or her mind, the loss of a spouse, the loss of personal capabilities, or the loss of a social role. Fear of these losses is then replaced by a preoccupation with physical health in hypochondriasis.

Social factors are probably the major reason that aging persons are at risk for developing hypochondriasis. Older persons often have difficulty meeting personal and/or social expectations. Family members may wish the older family member to participate in activities that are beyond his or her capability, such as taking a long walk, lifting luggage, or preparing a meal. Failure to meet these family expectations, or perhaps anger at the family for insisting that these expectations be met, can lead the older person to focus on his or her physical problems to the exclusion of facing the issue directly. Older persons also use hypochondriasis as a means of adapting to the real problem of isolation. Preoccupation with physical problems and help-seeking for those physical problems in some cases become the center of the older person's life. Frequent visits to the physician require assistance with transportation from family or friends and provide social contact with persons in the health care professional's office.

Diagnostic Workup

The diagnostic workup of the hypochondriacal older patient consists of a thorough history and a routine physical examination. Routine laboratory studies should be performed, but once the clinician is assured that the patient does not have a severe or undetected physical problem that contributes to the symptoms, then he or she should limit further laboratory studies. The differential diagnosis includes major depression and dysthymia, anxiety disorders (both generalized anxiety and panic), schizophrenic disorder (if the exaggerated physical concern expressed by the patient borders on delusional thinking), and dementing disorders. The diagnosis of hypochondriasis does not exclude the diagnosis of other psychiatric disorders. Many older persons with hypochondriasis meet criteria for a somatoform disorder and, for example, a dementing disorder.

Treatment

Working with the hypochondriacal older patient requires both tact and patience. The development of a management strategy should be based on management goals (Table 20–15). Older patients with hypochondriasis are best managed by a primary care physician as opposed to a psychiatrist. After the initial evaluation, the hypochondriacal older patient should be seen for relatively brief but regularly scheduled visits, in general lasting no more than 10–20 minutes each. Emphasis during the follow-up visits initially should be on a brief review of interval historical information coupled with a brief physical examination (including checking pulse and blood pressure). The remainder of the visit should be relatively unstructured and should focus on events in the patient's life. The clinician should refrain from interpretations connecting the physical problems with specific life events, instead encouraging the patient to

Table 20–15. Goals for managing hypochondriasis in the older adult

Control excessive use of health care services.

Decrease concern and anxiety in the patient.

Provide assurance of professional commitment to managing the patient's condition.

Decrease family stress and facilitate capability of family to provide social support.

Decrease the anxiety, anger, and frustration of the health care professional treating the patient.

Prescribe medications with caution.

discuss concerns about family, friends, perceived isolation, and so forth. The clinician may prescribe medications but must recognize that older patients with hypochondriasis are at increased risk for becoming dependent on psychotropic medications. Placebos are generally not appropriate, because discovery that a placebo has been prescribed undoubtedly will destroy the relationship between patient and doctor.

Medications that can be used for treating the hypochondriacal older patient include those that have relatively few side effects and those that have been demonstrated to be at least minimally effective in alleviating the symptoms expressed by the patient. For example, L-tryptophan can be prescribed for problems with sleeping (2 grams of this drug at night would be an appropriate dose). Another mildly sedating drug is trazodone, given at a dose of 25–50 mg (taken at night). Neither of these drugs will lead to habituation.

Conclusion

The seven geriatric syndromes discussed in this chapter account for most of the psychopathology that both psychiatrists and geriatricians encounter while working with older adults. The syndromal approach permits the clinician to focus on the functional impairment that results from psychopathology and on the day-to-day management of the older person in both the hospital and the outpatient clinic. A syndromal approach also provides a more realistic conceptualization of late-life psychopathology, which often is comorbid across psychiatric diagnoses and comorbid with physical illnesses.

Key Points

- Acute confusion is much more common in hospitalized older adults than usually recognized. Careful screening is necessary to identify these patients.

- Working with the family of the patient with memory loss is key to easing the suffering of the patient and preventing institutionalization prior to when absolutely necessary.

- Good sleep hygiene is more important than pharmacological management of insomnia in older adults.

- Generalized anxiety is usually comorbid with other conditions, such as depression or physical illness. Diagnosing comorbid conditions is the first step to managing anxiety in older adults.

- Suspiciousness and agitation are the most disruptive symptoms of dementing disorders.

- Uncomplicated depression in late life is as responsive to treatment as in midlife. Depression comorbid with physical illness or memory loss is much more difficult to treat.

- Implementing a structured approach to each patient contact with a hypochondriacal patient can reduce the overuse of health care services significantly.

Suggested Readings

Alexopoulos GS, Katz IR, Reynolds CF 3rd, et al: The Expert Consensus Guideline Series. Pharmacotherapy of depressive disorders in older patients. Postgrad Med (Special Issue: Pharmacotherapy):1–86, 2001

Blazer DG: Generalized anxiety disorder. Harv Rev Psychiatry 5:18–27, 1997

Blazer DG: Psychiatry and the oldest old. Am J Psychiatry 157:1915–1924, 2000

Blazer DG: Depression in late life: review and commentary. J Gerontol A Biol Sci Med Sci 58:249–265, 2003

Blazer DG, Hybels CF: Origins of depression in later life. Psychol Med 35:1241–1252, 2005

Blazer DG, Steffens D (eds): The American Psychiatric Publishing Textbook of Geriatric Psychiatry, 4th Edition. Washington, DC, American Psychiatric Publishing, 2009

Inouye S: Delirium in older persons. N Engl J Med 354:1157–1165, 2006

Jeste D, Wetherell J, Dolder C: Schizophrenia and paranoid disorders, in The American Psychiatric Publishing Textbook of Geriatric Psychiatry, 3rd Edition. Edited by Blazer DG, Steffens D, Busse E. Washington, DC, American Psychiatric Publishing, 2004, pp 269–281

Roses A: Genetic testing for Alzheimer disease: practical and ethical issues. Arch Neurol 54:1226–1229, 1997

References

Alexopoulos GS, Meyers BS, Young RC, et al: Executive dysfunction increases the risk for relapse and recurrence of geriatric depression. Arch Gen Psychiatry 57:285–290, 2000

Alexopoulos GS, Katz IR, Reynolds CF 3rd, et al: The Expert Consensus Guideline Series. Pharmacotherapy of depressive disorders in older patients. Postgrad Med (Special Issue: Pharmacotherapy):1–86, 2001

American Psychiatric Association: Diagnostic and Statistical Manual of Mental Disorders, 3rd Edition. Washington, DC, American Psychiatric Association, 1980

American Psychiatric Association: Diagnostic and Statistical Manual of Mental Disorders,

4th Edition, Text Revision. Washington, DC, American Psychiatric Association, 2000

Ancoli-Israel S: Insomnia in the elderly: a review for the primary care practitioner. Sleep 23 (suppl 1):S23–S30, 2000

Ancoli-Israel S, Ayalon L: Diagnosis and treatment of sleep disorders in older adults. Am J Geriatr Psychiatry 14:95–103, 2006

Blazer DG: Generalized anxiety disorder. Harv Rev Psychiatry 5:18–27, 1997

Blazer DG: Psychiatry and the oldest old. Am J Psychiatry 157:1915–1924, 2000

Blazer DG: Depression in Late Life, 3rd Edition. New York, Springer, 2002

Blazer DG: Depression in late life: review and commentary. J Gerontol A Biol Sci Med Sci 58:249–265, 2003

Blazer DG, Houpt J: Perception of poor health in the healthy older adult. J Am Geriatr Soc 27:330–334, 1979

Blazer DG, George L, Landerman R, et al: Psychiatric disorders: a rural/urban comparison. Arch Gen Psychiatry 42:651–656, 1985

Blazer DG, Hughes D, George L: The epidemiology of depression in an elderly community population. Gerontologist 27:281–287, 1987

Blazer DG, Hughes D, George L: Generalized anxiety disorder, in Psychiatric Disorders in America. Edited by Robins L, Regier D. New York, Free Press, 1991, pp 180–203

Breitner J, Zandi P: Do nonsteroidal antiinflammatory drugs reduce the risk of Alzheimer's disease? N Engl J Med 345:1567–1568, 2001

Christenson R, Blazer D: Epidemiology of persecutory ideation in an elderly population in the community. Am J Psychiatry 141:1088–1091, 1984

Foley D, Monjan A, Brown S, et al: Sleep complaints among elderly persons: an epidemiological study of three communities. Sleep 18:425–432, 1995

Folstein M, Folstein S, McHugh P: Mini-Mental State: a practical method for grading the cognitive state of patients for the clinician. J Psychiatr Res 12:189–198, 1975

Inouye S: Prevention of delirium in hospitalized older patients: risk factors and targeted interventions. Ann Intern Med 32:257–263, 2000

Inouye S: Delirium in older persons. N Engl J Med 354:1157–1165, 2006

Inouye SK, Bogardus ST Jr, Charpentier PA, et al: A multicomponent intervention to prevent delirium in hospitalized older patients [see comments]. N Engl J Med 340:669–676, 1999

Jeste D: Tardive dyskinesia in older patients. J Clin Psychiatry 61 (suppl 4):27–32, 2000

Jeste D, Wetherell J, Dolder C: Schizophrenia and paranoid disorders, in The American Psychiatric Publishing Textbook of Geriatric Psychiatry, 3rd Edition. Edited by Blazer D, Steffens D, Busse E. Washington, DC, American Psychiatric Publishing, 2004, pp 269–281

Katz I, Jeste D, Mintzer J, et al: Comparison of risperidone and placebo for psychoses and behavioral disturbances with dementia: a randomized double-blind trial. Risperidone Study Group. J Clin Psychiatry 60:107–115, 1999

Koenig H, Meador K, Cohen H, et al: Depression in elderly hospitalized patients with medical illness. Arch Intern Med 148:1929–1936, 1988

Lowenthal M: Lives in Distress. New York, Basic Books, 1964

Lynch T, Aspnes A: Individual and group psychotherapy, in The American Psychiatric Publishing Textbook of Geriatric Psychiatry, 3rd Edition. Edited by Blazer D, Steffens D, Busse E. Washington, DC, American Psychiatric Publishing, 2004, pp 443–458

Martin N, Stones M, Young J: Development of delirium: a prospective cohort study in a community hospital. Int Psychogeriatr 12:117–127, 2000

Meyers B: Geriatric delusional depression. Clin Geriatr Med 8:299–308, 1992

Michelson D, Stratakis C, Hill L: Bone mineral density in women with depression. N Engl J Med 335:1176–1181, 1996

Reifler B, Teri L, Raskind M, et al: Double-blind trial of imipramine in Alzheimer's disease patients with and without depression. Am J Psychiatry 146:45–49, 1989

Roses A: Apolipoprotein E affects the rate of Alzheimer disease expression: beta-amyloid burden is a secondary consequence dependent on APOE genotype and duration of disease. J Neuropathol Exp Neurol 53:429–437, 1994

Roses A: Genetic testing for Alzheimer disease: practical and ethical issues. Arch Neurol 54:1226–1229, 1997

Williams J, Barrett J, Oxman T, et al: Treatment of dysthymia and minor depression in primary care: a randomized controlled trial in older adults. JAMA 284:1519–1526, 2000

21

PSYCHIATRY AND THE LAW

Robert I. Simon, M.D.
Daniel W. Shuman, J.D.

Psychiatrist–Patient Relationships and the Law

General Contours of the Relationship

Informed Consent

The decision to initiate a treatment or diagnostic procedure belongs to the patient, who has the right to determine what will be done to his or her body (Schloendorff v. Society of New York Hospital 1914). Concomitantly, a physician occupies a fiduciary role to assist in the patient's decision. The law seeks to make that decision meaningful by requiring a physician to inform the patient about the available choices, known as an *informed consent*. Included among factors to be disclosed are the potential benefits, risks, alternatives, and consequences of the diagnostic or treatment procedure. The failure to satisfy this requirement of informed consent is a breach of the duty that the physician owes a patient and is actionable as a tort (Appelbaum et al. 1987).

The courts typically require that a decision be knowing, intelligent, and voluntary to satisfy the requirements of informed consent (Long v. Jaszczak 2004). We use "competency" instead of "intelligence" and "information" instead of "knowing," believing them to be more practical psychiatric considerations for clinical psychiatrists. We do not, however, intend to change the substantive requirements:

- Competency (intelligence)
- Information (knowing)
- Voluntariness

Usually, clinicians provide the first level of screening in identifying patient competency and in deciding whether to accept a patient's treatment decision. The patient or a bona fide representative must be given an adequate description of the treatment. If the patient who refuses treatment appears to lack health care decision-making capacity, it does not mean that the patient cannot be treated. An appropriate substitute decision maker can provide (or withhold) consent. To be able to provide informed consent, the patient or substitute decision maker should be told about the risks, benefits, and prognosis both with and without treatment, as well as alternative treatments and their risks and benefits. In addition, the competent patient must voluntarily consent to or refuse the proposed treatment or procedure.

The legal doctrine of informed consent is consistent with the provision of good clinical care. The informed consent doctrine allows patients to become partners in making treatment determinations that accord with their own needs and values. In the past, physicians operated under the "do no harm" principle. Today, psychiatrists are increasingly required to practice within the model of informed consent and patient autonomy. Most psychiatrists find increased patient autonomy desirable in fostering development of the therapeutic alliance that is so essential to treatment. Furthermore, patient autonomy is the goal of most psychiatric treatments (Beahrs and Gutheil 2001).

Competency (intelligence). It is clinically useful to distinguish the terms *incompetence* and *incapacity. Incompetence* refers to a court adjudication, whereas *incapacity* indicates a functional inability as determined by a clinician (Mishkin 1989). Legally, only competent persons may give informed consent. An adult patient is presumed competent unless adjudicated incompetent or temporarily incapacitated because of a medical emergency. Incapacity does not prevent treatment; it merely requires the clinician to obtain substitute consent or an exception to the requirement of informed consent. Absent an emergency, treating an incompetent patient without substituted consent is not permitted.

Legal competence is typically thought to refer to cognitive capacity. The conception derives largely from the laws governing transactions. Important clinical concepts such as

affective incompetence are not usually recognized by the law as dispositive. For example, a severely depressed but cognitively intact patient may be regarded as competent to refuse antidepressant medication. Manic patients tend to emphasize the risks of medications while downplaying their benefits. Schizophrenic patients tend to be fearful that medication will cause them serious harm. These patients may be unable to make a balanced assessment that considers both the risks and the benefits of a proposed drug. One study, in which three instruments were used to assess competency for treatment decisions, found that the schizophrenia and depression groups demonstrated poorer understanding of treatment disclosures, poorer reasoning in decision making regarding treatment, and a greater likelihood of failing to appreciate their illness or the potential treatment benefits (Grisso and Appelbaum 1995a). Denial of illness often interferes with insight and the ability to appreciate the significance of information provided to the patient. In *In the Guardianship of John Roe* (1992), the Massachusetts Supreme Judicial Court recognized that denial of illness can render a patient incompetent to make treatment decisions.

Competency is not a scientifically determinable state and is situation specific. The issue of competency arises in a number of civil, criminal, and family law contexts. Although there are no hard-and-fast definitions, the patient's ability to do the following is legally germane to determining competency:

- Understand the particular treatment choice being proposed
- Make a treatment choice
- Communicate that choice verbally or nonverbally

A review of case law and scholarly literature reveals four standards for determining incompetency in decision making (Appelbaum et al. 1987). In order of increasing levels of mental capacity required, these standards are as follows:

1. Communication of choice
2. Understanding of relevant information provided
3. Appreciation of available options and consequences
4. Rational decision making

Patients with severe mental disorders frequently deny their illness. Although they may communicate a choice and understand the information provided, these patients may lack the insight or ability to appreciate the information provided (Grisso and Appelbaum 1995b). Rational decision making is impaired as well. For example, patients with schizophrenia tend to fear some idiosyncratic harm from the treatment while ignoring the actual risk of medication side effects.

Most psychiatrists prefer a rational decision-making standard in determining incompetency. Most courts prefer the first two standards mentioned earlier but often combine competency standards. A truly informed consent that considers the patient's autonomy, personal needs, and values occurs when rational decision making is applied by the patient to the risks and benefits of appropriate treatment options provided by the clinician.

Grisso and Appelbaum (1995a) found that the choice of standards determining competence affected the type and proportion of patients classified as impaired. When compound standards were used, the proportion of patients identified as impaired increased. These authors advised that clinicians be aware of the applicable standards in their jurisdictions.

A valid consent can be either *expressed* (oral or in writing) or *implied* from the patient's actions. The competency issue is particularly sensitive when dealing with minors or mentally disabled persons who lack the requisite cognitive capacity for health care decision making. In both cases, it is generally recognized in the law that an authorized representative or guardian may consent for the patient.

Information (knowing).   The standard for exercising a legally sufficient disclosure var-

ies from state to state. Traditionally, the duty to disclose was measured by a professional standard: either what a reasonable physician would disclose under the circumstances or what the customary disclosure practices of physicians are in a particular community. In the landmark case *Canterbury v. Spence* (1972), a patient-oriented standard was applied. This standard focused on the "material" information that a *reasonable* person in the patient's position would want to know to make an informed decision. An increasing number of courts have applied this standard, and some have expanded "material risks" to include information regarding the consequences of not consenting to the treatment or procedure (Truman v. Thomas 1980). Even in patient-oriented jurisdictions, there is no duty to disclose every possible risk. A material risk is defined as one in which a physician knows or should know what would be considered significant by a reasonable person in the patient's position.

Voluntariness.   For consent to be considered legally voluntary, it must be given freely by the patient and without coercion, fraud, or duress. In evaluating whether consent is truly voluntary, the courts typically examine all the relevant circumstances, including the psychiatrist's manner, the environmental conditions, and the patient's mental state.

Malcolm (1992) noted subtle differences in the concepts of persuasion and coercion. *Persuasion* is defined as the physician's aim "to utilize the patient's reasoning ability to arrive at a desired result" (p. 241). *Coercion* occurs "when the doctor aims to manipulate the patient by introducing extraneous elements which have the effect of undermining the patient's ability to reason" (p. 241).

Exceptions and liability.   There are two basic exceptions to the requirement of obtaining informed consent. When immediate treatment is necessary to save a life or prevent serious harm, and it is not possible to obtain either the patient's consent or that of someone authorized to provide consent for the patient, the law typically presumes that the consent would have been granted. Two considerations are relevant when applying this exception. First, the emergency must be serious and "imminent"; second, the patient's condition, and not the surrounding circumstances (e.g., adverse environmental conditions), determines the existence of an emergency.

The second exception, *therapeutic privilege,* excepts informed consent if a psychiatrist determines that a complete disclosure of possible risks and alternatives might have a deleterious impact on the patient's health and welfare. Jurisdictions vary in their application of this exception. Absent specific case law or statutes outlining the factors relevant to such a decision, a doctor must substantiate a patient's inability psychologically to withstand being informed of the proposed treatment. Some courts have held that therapeutic privilege may be invoked only if informing the patient will worsen his or her condition or will so frighten the patient that rational decision making will be precluded (Canterbury v. Spence 1972; Natanson v. Kline 1960). Therapeutic privilege cannot be used as a means of circumventing the legal requirement for obtaining informed consent from the patient before initiating treatment.

Waivers. A physician need not disclose risks of treatment when the patient has competently, knowingly, and voluntarily waived his or her right to be informed (e.g., when the patient does not want to be informed of drug risks). This is not an exception to the requirement of informed consent but rather a patient choice to decide with limited information.

Absent a waiver or an exception, treatment without an adequate informed consent opens the door to a damage claim for an intentional tort if the treatment is initiated without consent or a negligence tort if treatment is initiated without an adequate consent.

Confidentiality and Privilege

Confidentiality refers to the right of a patient, and the correlative duty of a professional, of nondisclosure of relational communications to outside parties without implied or expressed authorization. The duty of confidentiality limits the actions of the professional but does not limit the power of a judge to compel disclosure of relevant relational confidences. *Privilege,* or more accurately *relational privilege,* is a limitation on the power of the judge to compel disclosure of relational confidences. A psychiatrist–, psychotherapist–, or physician–patient privilege may be recognized by case law (Jaffee v. Redmond 1996) but is more typically a statute or rule of evidence that permits the holder of the privilege (e.g., the patient) to prevent the person to whom confidential information was given (e.g., the psychiatrist) from being compelled by a judge to disclose it in a judicial proceeding.

Confidentiality. Although the law relating to confidentiality of health information has been state law, the Health Insurance Portability and Accountability Act of 1996 (HIPAA) adds a layer of federal law to protect patient health care information. If state and federal laws conflict, the more protective rule prevails. HIPAA limits disclosure of patient health information without patient authorization except as necessary for treatment, payment, and health care operations; however, the limitation is not absolute. For example, HIPAA permits disclosure in a judicial or administrative (e.g., workers' compensation or Social Security) proceeding when there is 1) the patient's written consent, 2) a subpoena, or 3) a court order signed by a judge. A separate consent is required to permit the disclosure of psychotherapy notes.

Clinical–legal foundation. Relational privileges require courts to compromise their search for truth by not availing themselves of relevant evidence. Thus courts have typically been reluctant to recognize a privilege and quick to find an exception applicable (Shuman and Weiner 1987). Indeed, the common law did not recognize physician–patient or psychotherapist–patient privilege. When courts have done so, it has been because they have been convinced of its necessity to further a relationship of great utility to society. For example, in 1996 the U.S. Supreme Court ruled that confidential communications between psychotherapist and patient are privileged and, unless an exception applies, may not be compelled in federal trials (Jaffee v. Redmond 1996). In the majority of cases where a privilege is recognized by statute or rule of evidence, there is typically an acknowledgment of similar reasoning.

Breaching of confidentiality. Once the doctor–patient relationship has been created, the professional assumes a duty to safeguard a patient's disclosures. This duty is not absolute, and there are circumstances in which breaching confidentiality is both ethical and legal.

Patients also waive confidentiality in a variety of situations, especially in managed care settings. Medical records may be sent to potential employers or to insurance companies when benefits are requested. A limited waiver of confidentiality ordinarily exists when a patient participates in group therapy. Whether one group member can be compelled in court to disclose information shared by another group member during group therapy is still unsettled legally (Slovenko 1998). Many state confidentiality statutes provide statutory exceptions to confidentiality between the psychiatrist and the patient in one or more situations (Brakel et al. 1985) (Table 21–1).

If a patient gives the psychiatrist good reason to believe that a warning should be issued to an endangered third party, the duty of confidentiality of the communication that gave rise to the warning may be limited. Psychiatrists who have issued warnings have been compelled to testify in criminal cases (Leong et al. 1992), although the obligation to breach confidentiality may not resolve the privilege issue at trial.

Privilege. The patient, not the psychiatrist, is the holder of the physician–, psychiatrist–, or psychotherapist–patient privilege and is entitled to determine whether to assert it. Re-

Table 21–1. Common limitations of testimonial privilege

Valid patient consent
Civil commitment proceedings
Criminal proceedings
Child custody disputes
Court-ordered report
Patient-litigant exception
Child abuse proceedings

Source. Reprinted with permission from Simon RI: *A Concise Guide to Psychiatry and the Law for Clinicians,* 3rd Edition. Washington, DC, American Psychiatric Publishing, 2001, p. 54.

lational privileges govern disclosures in the judicial setting (e.g., deposition, trial); the duty of confidentiality governs disclosures in extrajudicial settings (e.g., cocktail parties, memoirs, visits by the police). Privilege statutes or case law recognition represents recognition by the state of the importance of protecting information provided by a patient to a psychotherapist. This recognition moves away from the essential purpose of the American system of justice (e.g., "truth finding") by insulating certain information from disclosure in court. This protection is justified on the basis that the special need for privacy in the psychotherapist–patient relationship outweighs the unbridled quest for an accurate outcome in court.

Privilege statutes usually are drafted with reference to one of the following four relationships, depending on the type of practitioner:

1. Physician–patient (general)
2. Psychiatrist–patient
3. Psychologist–patient
4. Psychotherapist–patient

Privilege statutes also specify exceptions to testimonial privilege. Although exceptions vary, the most common are summarized in Table 21–1.

The *patient-litigant exception* commonly occurs in the insanity defense, will contests, workers' compensation cases, child custody disputes, personal injury actions, and medical malpractice actions.

Liability. An unauthorized or unwarranted breach of the duty of confidentiality can cause a patient emotional harm and result in a claim based on at least four theories:

1. Malpractice (breach of professional duty of confidentiality)
2. Breach of statutory duty of confidentiality
3. Invasion of privacy
4. Breach of (implied) contract

Competency

The ability to effectively exercise rights recognized by the law demands a minimal mental capacity or competence. One articulation of the meaning of *competency* is "having sufficient capacity, ability…[or] possessing the requisite physical, mental, natural, or legal qualifications" (Black 1990, p. 285). This conceptualization is deliberately vague because *competency* is a broad concept encompassing many different legal issues and contexts. As a result, its requirements can vary widely depending on the circumstances in which it is being measured (e.g., making health care decisions, executing a will, or confessing to a crime).

Competency refers to a *minimal* mental, cognitive, or behavioral ability, trait, or capability required to perform a particular act (e.g., waive counsel) or to assume a particular role (e.g., practice dentistry). A determination of incompetency is ultimately a judicial determination. The term *incapacity*, which is often interchanged with *incompetency*, refers to an individual's functional inability to understand or to form an intention with regard to some act as determined by health care providers (Mishkin 1989).

The legal designation of "incompetent" is applied to an individual who fails one of the mental tests of capacity and is therefore considered *by law* to be not mentally capable of performing a particular act or assuming a particular role. The adjudication of incompetence by a court is now, more commonly, subject or issue specific. For example, the fact that a psychiatric patient is adjudicated incompetent to drive does not automatically render that patient incompetent to do other things, such as consent to treatment, testify as a witness, marry, or enter into a contract.

Generally, the law only gives effect to decisions by a competent individual and seeks to protect incompetent individuals from the harmful effects of their acts. Adults (age 18 years or older; U.S. Department of Health and Human Services 1981) are presumed to be competent (Meek v. City of Loveland 1929). This presumption, however, may be rebutted by evidence of incapacity (Scaria v. St. Paul Fire and Marine Ins. Co. 1975). For the psychiatric patient, perception, short- and long-term memory, judgment, language comprehension, verbal fluency, and reality orientation are mental functions that a court will scrutinize when the issues of "capacity" and "competency" have been raised.

As a matter of law, incompetency may not be presumed from either treatment for mental illness (Wilson v. Lehman 1964) or institutionalization (Rennie v. Klein 1978). Mental disability or illness does not necessarily render a person incompetent in any or in all areas of functioning. Instead, scrutiny is given to determine whether specific functional incapacities exist that render a person incapable of making a particular kind of decision or performing a particular type of task.

Respect for individual autonomy (Schloendorff v. Society of New York Hospital 1914) demands that individuals be allowed to make decisions of which they are capable, even if they are seriously mentally ill, developmentally arrested, or organically impaired. A judicial determination of incompetence must precede an abridgement of that decision-making authority. Physical and mental illness is but one factor to be weighed in determining competency.

Guardianship

Guardianship is a method of substitute decision making for individuals who have been judicially determined to be unable to act for themselves (Drakel et al. 1985). Historically, the state or sovereign possessed the power and authority to safeguard the estate of incompetent persons (Regan 1972). This traditional role still reflects the purpose of guardianship today. In some states, there are separate provisions for the appointment of a "guardian of one's person" (e.g., health care decision making) and for a "guardian of one's estate" (e.g., authority to make contracts to sell one's property; Sales et al. 1982). The latter type of guardian is frequently referred to as a *conservator,* although this designation is not uniformly used throughout the United States. A further distinction, also found in some jurisdictions, is between *general (plenary)* and *specific* guardianship (Sales et al. 1982). As the name implies, the specific guardian is restricted to exercising decisions about a particular subject area. For instance, he or she may be authorized to make decisions about major or emergency medical procedures, with the disabled person retaining the freedom to make decisions about all other medical matters. General guardians, in contrast, have total control over the disabled individual's person, estate, or both (Sales et al. 1982).

Guardianship arrangements are increasingly used with patients who have dementia, particularly AIDS-related dementia and Alzheimer's disease (Overman and Stoudemire 1988). Under the Anglo-American system of law, an individual is presumed to be competent unless adjudicated incompetent. Incompetence is a legal determination made by a court of law on the basis of evidence provided by health care providers and others that the individual's functional mental capacity is significantly impaired. The Uniform Guardianship and Protective Proceedings Act (UGPPA) or the Uniform Probate Code (UPC) is used as a basis for laws governing competency in many states (Mishkin 1989). Drafted by legal scholars and practic-

ing attorneys, the uniform acts serve as models for the purpose of achieving consistency among the state laws by enactment of model laws (UGPPA § 5–101). *General incompetency* is defined by the UGPPA as meaning "impaired by reason of mental illness, mental deficiency, physical illness or disability, advanced age, chronic use of drugs, chronic intoxication, or other cause (except minority) to the extent of lacking sufficient understanding or capacity to make or communicate reasonable decisions."

Some patients with psychiatric disorders may meet the preceding definition. Generally, the appointment of a guardian is limited to situations in which the individual's decision-making capacity is so impaired that he or she is unable to care for personal safety or provide such necessities as food, shelter, clothing, and medical care, with the likely result of physical injury or illness (In re Boyer 1981). The standard of proof required for a judicial determination of incompetency is *clear and convincing evidence.* Although the law does not assign percentages to proof, if it did, clear and convincing evidence would likely be in the range of 75% certainty (Simon 1992a).

States vary on the extent of their reliance on psychiatric assessments. Nonmedical personnel such as social workers, psychologists, family members, friends, colleagues, and even the individual who is the subject of the proceeding may testify.

Health Care Decision Making

Because psychiatric patients frequently have impaired mental capacity, the difficulty associated with obtaining a valid informed consent to proposed diagnostic procedures and treatments can be both challenging and frustrating. The need to obtain competent informed consent is not negated simply because it "appears" that the patient is in need of medical intervention or would likely benefit from it. Instead, clinicians must assure themselves that the patient or an appropriate substitute decision maker has given a competent consent before proceeding with treatment. An increasing number of states require a judicial determination of incompetence and the court's substituted consent prior to the administration of antipsychotic medications to a patient who is deemed by a health care provider to lack the functional mental capacity to consent (Simon 1992a).

Only a *competent* person is legally able to give informed consent. Competent patients must not be treated against their objections. Health care providers work with patients who sometimes are of questionable competence because of mental illness, narcotic abuse, or alcoholism. When psychiatrists treat patients with neuropsychiatric deficits, the responsibility to obtain a valid informed consent can be clinically daunting because of the vacillating and unpredictable mental states associated with many central nervous system disorders.

Psychiatric patients who have been determined to lack the requisite functional mental capacity to make a treatment decision (Frasier v. Department of Health and Human Resources 1986) should have an authorized representative or guardian appointed to make health care decisions on their behalf (Aponte v. United States 1984). A number of consent options may be available for such patients, depending on the jurisdiction.

Right to Die

Legal decisions addressing the issue of a patient's "right to die" can be divided into two categories: decisions dealing with individuals who were incompetent at the time removal of life support systems was sought (In re Conroy 1985; In re Quinlan 1976) and decisions dealing with competent patients.

Incompetent patients. The U.S. Supreme Court ruled, in *Cruzan v. Director, Missouri Department of Health* (1990), that the state of Missouri may refuse to remove a food and water tube surgically implanted in the stomach of Nancy Cruzan without clear and convincing evidence of her wishes. Ms. Cruzan was in a persistent vegetative state for 7 years. Without clear and convincing evidence of a pa-

tient's decision to have life-sustaining measures withheld in a particular circumstance, the state has the right to maintain that individual's life, even to the exclusion of the family's wishes.

The importance of the *Cruzan* decision for physicians treating severely or terminally impaired patients is that physicians must seek clear and competent instructions regarding foreseeable treatment decisions. For example, a psychiatrist treating a patient with progressive degenerative diseases should attempt to ascertain the patient's wishes regarding the use of life-sustaining measures *while that patient can still competently articulate those wishes.* This information is best provided in the form of a living will, durable power-of-attorney agreement, or health care proxy. Although physicians may fear civil or criminal liability for stopping life-sustaining treatment, liability may also arise from overtreating critically or terminally ill patients (Weir and Gostin 1990). Legal liability may occur for providing unwanted treatment to an autonomous patient or treatment that is against the best interests of a nonautonomous patient.

Competent patients. A growing body of cases has emerged involving *competent* patients—with excruciating pain and terminal diseases—who seek the termination of further medical treatment. Beginning with the fundamental tenet that "no right is held more sacred...than the right of every individual to the possession and control of his own person" (Schloendorff v. Society of New York Hospital 1914; Union Pacific Realty Co. v. Botsford 1891), courts have taken this principle of autonomy seen in informed consent cases and applied it to right-to-die cases.

The right to decline life-sustaining medical intervention, even for a competent person, is not absolute. As noted in *In re Conroy* (1985), four countervailing state interests generally exist that may limit the exercise of that right: 1) preservation of life, 2) prevention of suicide, 3) safeguarding of the integrity of the medical profession, and 4) protection of innocent third parties. Balancing autonomy and these countervailing state interests, the trend has been to support a competent patient's right to have artificial life-support systems discontinued (Bartling v. Superior Court 1984; Bouvia v. Superior Court 1986; In re Farrell 1987; In re Jobes 1987; In re M.B. 2006; In re Peter 1987; Tune v. Walter Reed Army Medical Hospital 1985).

As a result of the *Cruzan* decision, courts now focus on the reliability of the evidence proffered in establishing the patient's competence, specifically the clarity and certainty with which a decision to withhold medical treatment is made. When a fully informed, competent terminally ill patient has chosen to forgo any further medical intervention, courts are less likely to overrule the patient's decision.

Advance Directives

The use of advance directives such as a living will, health care proxy, or durable medical power of attorney is recommended to avoid ethical and legal complications associated with requests to withhold life-sustaining treatment measures (Simon 1992a; Solnick 1985). The Patient Self-Determination Act, which took effect on December 1, 1991, requires hospitals, nursing homes, hospices, managed care organizations (MCOs), and home health care agencies to advise patients or family members of their right to accept or refuse medical care and to execute an advance directive (LaPuma et al. 1991). These advance directives provide a method for individuals, while competent, to choose proxy health care decision makers in the event of future incompetency. A living will can be contained as a subsection of a durable power of attorney agreement. In the ordinary power of attorney created for the management of business and financial matters, the power of attorney generally becomes null and void if the person creating it becomes incompetent.

The right to formulate an advance directive is determined by state law. All 50 states and the District of Columbia permit individuals to create a *durable* power of attorney (i.e.,

one that endures even if the competence of the creator does not) (Cruzan v. Director, Missouri Department of Health 1990). Several states and the District of Columbia have durable power of attorney statutes that expressly authorize the appointment of proxies for making health care decisions (Cruzan v. Director, Missouri Department of Health 1990).

Generally, a durable power of attorney has been construed to empower an agent to make health care decisions. Such a document is much broader and more flexible than a living will, which covers only the period of a diagnosed terminal illness, specifying only that no "extraordinary treatments" be used that would prolong the act of dying (Mishkin 1985). To rectify the sometimes uncertain status of the durable power of attorney as applied to health care decisions, a number of states have passed or are considering passing health care proxy laws. The health care proxy is a legal instrument akin to the durable power of attorney but specifically created for health care decision making. Despite the growing use of advance directives, there is increasing evidence that physician values rather than patient values are more decisive in end of life decisions (Orentlicher 1992).

In a durable power of attorney or health care proxy, general or specific directions are set forth about how future decisions should be made in the event a person becomes unable to make these decisions. The determination of a patient's competence is not specified in most durable power of attorney and health care proxy statutes. Because this is a medical or psychiatric question, the examination by two physicians to determine the patient's ability to understand the nature and consequences of the proposed treatment or procedure, ability to make a choice, and ability to communicate that choice is usually minimally sufficient. This information, like all significant medical observations, should be clearly documented in the patient's file.

Several states have enacted laws that authorize a person to designate in writing a health care surrogate to make health care decisions reflecting that person's values, which comes into effect when the person authorizing the surrogate is determined to be incapacitated. Some states authorize separate surrogates for mental health care decisions. Unless time limited on its face, the authorization continues until revoked. If the person who executed the designation attempts to revoke it when a psychiatric disorder exists and it is not clear whether he or she is incapacitated, it may be appropriate to obtain a judicial determination of the capacity to revoke.

Substituted Judgment

Psychiatrists often find that the time required to obtain an adjudication of incompetence is unduly burdensome and that the process frequently interferes with the provision of quality treatment. Moreover, families are often reluctant to face the formal court proceedings necessary to declare their family member incompetent, particularly when sensitive family matters are disclosed. A common solution to both of these problems is to seek the legally authorized proxy consent of a spouse or relative serving as guardian when the refusing patient is believed to be incompetent. Proxy consent, however, is becoming less available as a consent option (Simon 1992a). Many states exclude surrogate authorizations for the treatment of mental disorders.

There are clear advantages associated with having the family serve as decision makers (Perr 1984). First, use of responsible family members as surrogate decision makers maintains the integrity of the family unit and relies on the sources who are most likely to know the patient's wishes. Second, it is more efficient and less costly than an attempt to prove incompetency. There are some disadvantages, however. Proxy decision making requires synthesizing the diverse values, beliefs, practices, and prior statements of the patient for a given specific circumstance (Emanuel and Emanuel 1992). As one judge characterized the problem, any proxy decision making in the absence of specific directions is "at best only an optimistic approxima-

tion" (In re Jobes 1987). Ambivalent feelings, conflicts within the family and with the patient, and conflicting economic interests may make certain family members suspect as guardians (Gutheil and Appelbaum 1980). Also, relatives may not be available or may not want to get involved. Moreover, next of kin may possess dubious competence or even less competence than the patient.

The President's Commission for the Study of Ethical Problems in Medicine and Biomedical and Behavioral Research (1982) recommended that the relatives of incompetent patients be selected as proxy decision makers for the following reasons:

1. The family is generally most concerned about the good of the patient.
2. The family is usually most knowledgeable about the patient's goals, preferences, and values.
3. The family deserves recognition as an important social unit to be treated, within limits, as a single decision maker in matters that intimately affect its members.

Several states permit proxy decision making by statute, mainly through informed consent statutes (Solnick 1985). Some state statutes specify that another person may authorize consent on behalf of the incompetent patient, whereas others mention specific relatives.

Unless proxy consent by a relative is provided by statute or by case law authority in the state where the psychiatrist practices, it is not recommended that the good-faith consent by next of kin be relied on in treating a psychiatric patient believed to lack health care decision-making capacity (Klein et al. 1983). The legally appropriate procedure to follow is to seek judicial recognition of the family member as the substitute decision maker.

A debate continues about the theory of substitute decision making. Should the substitute decision maker (i.e., guardian, designated surrogate) act in the patient's best interest (the "objective test"), or should he or she rely on what the patient would have decided if competent (the "subjective" or "substituted judgment" approach)? The increasingly used subjective test is difficult to implement for patients who have never been competent, who have made improvident or less than competent decisions in the past, or who have never openly stated choices to be implemented by others. Also, the values of substitute decision makers can be easily substituted for the patient regardless of which test is used (Roth 1985). Both the best interests and the substituted judgment standards lead to predictable biases by those who implement them. Use of the best interests standard leads to treatment of patients and sustaining life. Application of the substituted judgment standard favors treatment refusal and the upholding of civil liberties (E.D. Robertson 1989).

The substituted judgment standard has found considerable judicial favor. It is based on the incompetent person's "right to privacy" translated into the medical context as the right to refuse treatment. The right to privacy is the constitutional expression of the autonomy Americans claim as free persons living in a free society. On this point, courts find authority and inspiration from John Stuart Mill:

> The only purpose for which power can be rightfully exercised over any member of a civilized community against his will, is to prevent harm to others. His own good, either physical or moral, is not a sufficient warrant. He cannot rightfully be compelled to do or forebear because it will be better for him to do so, because it will make him happier, because in the opinion of others, to do so would be wise, or even right. (Mill 1859/1951)

High-Risk Relationships

Psychiatric Malpractice

Medical malpractice is a tort (i.e., a civil wrong not grounded in criminal or contract law). Most medical malpractice claims are based in negligence rather than intentional

torts (e.g., battery, false imprisonment), if for no other reason than to avoid the exclusionary language in most professional liability policies for intentional acts. *Negligence*, the fundamental concept underlying most malpractice claims, is the failure to act reasonably under the circumstances. In the case of medical malpractice, negligence involves either doing something that a physician should not have done with a patient under the circumstances or failing to do something that a physician should have done with a patient under the circumstances. However, acting unreasonably is not alone sufficient to support a negligence claim.

For a psychiatrist to be found *liable* to a patient for malpractice, four fundamental elements must be established by a preponderance of the evidence (i.e., more likely than not): 1) there was a duty of care owed by the defendant, 2) the duty of care was breached, 3) the plaintiff (i.e., the patient) suffered actual damages, and 4) the defendant's deviation was the direct cause of the damages. Each of these four elements must be met for the claim to prevail. A psychiatrist may have rendered substandard care, but if the jury finds that this caused no legally recognized harm or that any harm was caused by another actor or condition, the claim fails.

In most states, whether the psychiatrist's duty to his or her patient has been breached turns on whether the fact finder decides that the defendant acted with the degree of skill and care of the average physician in that specialty under the circumstances (Stepakoff v. Kantar 1985). The use of a somatic therapy, including electroconvulsive therapy (ECT), is evaluated no differently from the use of any other medical treatment or procedure with respect to potential liability. The same standard of the degree of skill and care of the average physician practicing that specialty governs the assessment of whether a psychiatrist's use of or failure to use a somatic intervention is negligent.

It is generally acknowledged within the psychiatric profession that there is no *absolute standard* protocol for the administration of psychotropic medication or ECT. Nevertheless, the existence of professional treatment guidelines and procedures that are generally accepted or used by a significant number of psychiatrists should alert clinicians to consider such guidelines as practice reference sources. For example, the American Psychiatric Association (APA) has published comprehensive findings and guidelines such as the task force reports concerning ECT (American Psychiatric Association 2001a), tardive dyskinesia (American Psychiatric Association 1992), and the treatment of psychiatric disorders (American Psychiatric Association 2004). Official guidelines are relevant evidence in setting the standard but neither bind the fact finder at trial nor preempt sound professional judgment in attending to the specific clinical needs of patients.

Guidelines and procedures publications of private nongovernmental organizations cannot bind the courts and thus do not establish the standard of care by which a psychiatrist's actions must be measured in malpractice litigation. Along with expert testimony, they are sources of relevant information for the fact finder to consider in setting the standard of care (Shuman 2001). Therefore, a reasonable psychiatrist should be familiar with and should have considered the APA's and other similar guidelines (Stone v. Proctor 1963).

There is less professional autonomy and flexibility associated with the use of ECT. Usually, the reasonable care standard applied to psychiatric treatment is construed in a fairly broad manner. Some psychiatric treatments such as ECT, however, are more rigidly regulated than others. For instance, the Joint Commission considers ECT to be a *special treatment* procedure to be regulated by written policies. Whenever ECT is used, the procedure must be adequately justified and documented in the patient's medical chart (Joint Commission on Accreditation of Healthcare Organizations 2006). The ECT policies of treatment facilities as well as judicial decisions and statutory regulation of ECT can also serve as establishing the basis for liability, if violated.

The standard for judging the use and administration of medication, on the other hand, appears to be consistent with the more flexible and general reasonable care requirement. Another reference source is the *Physicians' Desk Reference* (PDR), which may be used to establish or dispute the reasonableness of a psychiatrist's pharmacotherapy procedures. The PDR is a commercially distributed and privately published reference of medication products used in the United States. The U.S. Food and Drug Administration (FDA) requires that drug manufacturers have their official package inserts reported in the PDR (Simon 1992a). Accordingly, psychiatrists consult publications such as the PDR as needed to keep abreast of current and accurate medication information. Although numerous courts have cited the PDR as a credible source of medication-related information in the medical profession, the PDR does not by itself establish the standard of care (Gowan v. United States 1985; Witherell v. Weimer 1986). Instead, it is simply relevant evidence to establish the standard of care in a particular situation (Callan v. Norland 1983; Doerr v. Hurley Medical Center 1984). Courts generally follow the reasoning in *Ramon v. Farr* (1989), holding that drug inserts alone do not set the standard of care. They are only one element to be considered, along with previous clinical experience, the scientific literature, approvals in other countries, expert testimony, and other pertinent factors. The presence of a substantial scientific literature that justifies the clinician's treatment is more persuasive than FDA approval. The PDR or any other reference cannot serve as a substitute for the psychiatrist's sound clinical judgment.

Courts recognize the importance of professional judgment and give psychiatrists, like other medical specialists, latitude in explaining special diagnostic or treatment considerations that guide their decision making.

For instance, the clinical data regarding pharmacological treatment of rapid-cycling bipolar disorder indicate that a variety of potentially useful drug therapies exist, some of which are considered experimental or on the cutting edge (Simon 1997). Various drugs and hormones are useful as mood stabilizers, such as carbamazepine, clozapine, thyroid and estrogen replacement, calcium channel blockers, antihypertensives, neuroleptics, atypical antipsychotics, and other anticonvulsants (lamotrigine, valproate, gabapentin).

The courts do not demand professional orthodoxy. Evidence that a treatment procedure is accepted by at least a respectable minority of professionals in the field can establish that a particular treatment is a reasonable professional practice (Simon 1993). The standard of care associated with the use of a somatic therapy to treat a psychiatric patient, *at a minimum,* is summarized in Table 21–2.

Theories of liability. The potential for negligence by a psychiatrist is greatest in clinical situations involving the use of psychotropic medication. Unlike talk therapies, in which the causation of harm is more diffuse (i.e., whether a different talk therapy likely would have produced a different result), medication errors tend to be more stark and their consequences easier to trace. Although no reliable compilation of malpractice claims data has been published, anecdotal information suggests that medication-related lawsuits constitute a significant share of claims filed against psychiatrists. Claims data from the APA Professional Liability Insurance Program showed that medication error and drug reaction constituted 7% of malpractice allegations (Benefacts 1996). Allegations of drug mismanagement are a significant contributor to "incorrect treatment," the most common malpractice category.

A review of the relevant case law indicates that various mistakes, omissions, and poor medication treatment practices commonly result in malpractice actions brought against psychiatrists. The following discussion, al-

Table 21–2. Required minimum standard of care for a somatic treatment of a psychiatric patient

Pretreatment

Complete clinical history (medical, psychiatric)

Complete physical examination as clinically indicated (performed by another physician or, if necessary, by the psychiatrist)

Administration of necessary laboratory tests and review of past test results

Disclosure of sufficient information to the patient to obtain informed consent, including information about the risks and benefits both of treatment and of no treatment

Thorough documentation of all treatment decisions, informed consent information, pertinent patient responses, and other relevant treatment data

Posttreatment

Careful monitoring of the patient's response to treatment, including adequate follow-up evaluations and appropriate laboratory testing

Prompt adjustments in treatment, as clinically indicated

Arrangement for additional informed consent when treatment is altered appreciably or new treatment initiated

though not intended to be exhaustive, provides a framework for identifying problem areas associated with medication treatment.

Failure to adequately evaluate. Sound clinical practice requires that before any form of treatment is initiated, the patient should be adequately evaluated. The nature and extent of an evaluation are largely dictated by the type of treatment being contemplated and the medical and psychiatric condition of the patient. A physical examination should be conducted or obtained, if clinically indicated. A recently performed physical examination may suffice, or patients may be referred elsewhere if the psychiatrist does not perform physical examinations. The duty to ensure that proper informed consent is obtained can be fulfilled at this time.

Failure to monitor.   Probably the most common act of negligence associated with pharmacotherapy is the failure to monitor the patient while he or she is taking medication, including carefully following the patient for adverse side effects. Once psychotropic medication is prescribed, it is the psychiatrist's duty to monitor the patient. Consultation or referral may be necessary according to the clinical needs of the patient. Monitoring may require the use of laboratory testing. Serum drug levels are obtainable for a number of psychotropic medications. The primary indications for these laboratory tests include assessment of therapeutic and toxic levels of medication and patient compliance with treatment. The use of carbamazepine, valproate, and clozapine requires periodic monitoring of the hematopoietic system and the liver. Failure to supervise patients to ensure that they are taking medications properly can delay or prevent the detection of harmful side effects or the necessity to change to more effective treatment. If a patient is harmed, a malpractice action might result (Chaires v. St. John's Episcopal Hospital 1984; Clifford v. United States 1985; Kilgore v. County of Santa Clara 1982; Muldrow v. Re-Direct, Inc. 2005).

Split treatment.   Split-treatment situations require that the psychiatrist stay fully informed of the patient's clinical status as well as of the nature and quality of treatment the patient is receiving from the nonmedical therapist (Sederer et al. 1998). In a collaborative relationship, responsibility for the patient's care is shared according to the qualifications and limitations of each clinician. The responsibilities of each discipline do not diminish those of the other disciplines. Patients should be informed of the separate responsibilities of each discipline. Periodic evaluation by the psychiatrist and the nonmedical therapist of the patient's clinical condition and needs is necessary to determine whether the collaboration should continue. On termi-

nation of the collaborative relationship, the patient should be informed by the clinicians either separately or jointly. In split treatments, if negligence is claimed on the part of the nonmedical therapist, it is likely that the collaborating psychiatrist will be sued, and vice versa (Woodward et al. 1993).

In managed care or similar treatment settings, the mere prescribing of medication without an informed, working doctor–patient relationship does not meet generally accepted standards of good clinical care. Fragmented care, in which the psychiatrist functions only as a prescriber of medication while remaining uninformed about the patient's overall clinical status, constitutes substandard treatment. Such a practice may diminish the efficacy of the drug treatment itself or even lead to the patient's failure to take the prescribed medication.

Psychiatrists who prescribe medications in split-treatment arrangements should be able to hospitalize patients if necessary. If the psychiatrist does not have admitting privileges, prearrangements should exist with other psychiatrists who can hospitalize patients if emergencies arise.

In managed care settings, psychiatrists may be required to prescribe medications from a restrictive or closed formulary. Psychiatrists, in their professional discretion, should determine which medications will be prescribed according to the special clinical needs of the patient. Split treatment is increasingly used by MCOs and is a potential malpractice minefield (Meyer and Simon 1999).

Negligent prescription practices.   The selection of a medication, determination of initial dosage and form of administration, and other related procedures are all decisions left to the professional discretion of the treating psychiatrist. In managed care settings, psychiatrists should vigorously resist attempts to limit their choice of drugs. The prescribing of specific medications should be determined by the psychiatrist and the clinical needs of the patient. An appeal should be filed if a drug that is not formulary approved

Table 21–3. Common negligent prescription practices

Exceeding recommended dosages without clinical indications

Prescribing multiple drugs inappropriately

Prescribing medication for unapproved uses without a documented rationale

Prescribing unapproved medications

Failing to disclose medication risks

is denied. The law recognizes that the physician is in the best position to "know the patient" and to determine what course of treatment is best under the circumstances. The standard by which a psychiatrist's prescription practices will be evaluated is reasonableness. In administering psychotropic medication, psychiatrists need only conform their procedures and decision making to those that are *ordinarily* practiced by other psychiatrists under similar circumstances.

A review of cases involving allegations of negligent prescription procedures reveals several common practices representing potential deviations from generally accepted treatment practice (Table 21–3).

As stated earlier, any physician who prescribes medication has a duty to first obtain the informed consent of the patient (Table 21–4). Obtaining competent informed consent may be complicated by the fact that some psychiatric patients have compromised mental capacity for health care decision making. Patients lacking such decision-making capacity require consent for treatment by substitute decision makers (Table 21–5).

Each time a medication is changed and a new drug is introduced, informed consent should be obtained. Failure to inform a patient properly of the risks and benefits of a prescribed medication is a ground for a malpractice action if the patient is injured as a result (Karasik v. Bird 1984; Moran v. Botsford General Hospital 1984; Wright v. State 1986).

Other medication-related issues that have resulted in legal action include 1) failure to treat side effects after they have been recog-

Table 21–4. Informed consent: reasonable information to be disclosed

Although there exists no consistently accepted set of information to be disclosed for any given medical or psychiatric situation, five areas of information are generally provided:

1. Diagnosis: Description of the condition or problem
2. Treatment: Nature and purpose of proposed treatment
3. Consequences: Risks and benefits of the proposed treatment
4. Alternatives: Viable alternatives to the proposed treatment, including risks and benefits
5. Prognosis: Projected outcome with and without treatment

Source. Reprinted with permission from Simon RI: *Clinical Psychiatry and the Law,* 2nd Edition. Washington, DC, American Psychiatric Press, 1992, p. 128.

nized or should have been recognized, 2) failure to monitor a patient's compliance with prescription limits, 3) failure to prescribe medication or appropriate levels of medication according to the treatment needs of the patient, 4) failure to refer a patient for consultation or treatment by a specialist when indicated, and 5) negligent withdrawal from medication and unclear or illegible prescriptions.

Table 21–5. Common consent options for patients lacking the mental capacity for health care decisions

Proxy consent of next of kin, as permitted by state law[a]

Adjudication of incompetence and appointment of a guardian

Substituted consent of the court

Advance directives (living will, durable power of attorney, health care proxy)

[a]May be excluded for treatment of mental disorders.
Source. Adapted with permission from Simon RI: *Clinical Psychiatry and the Law,* 2nd Edition. Washington, DC, American Psychiatric Press, 1992, p. 109.

National Practitioner Data Bank

On September 1, 1990, the National Practitioner Data Bank established by the Health Care Quality Improvement Act of 1986 went into effect. The data bank tracks disciplinary actions, malpractice judgments, and settlements against physicians, dentists, and other health care professionals (Johnson 1991).

Hospitals, health maintenance organizations, MCOs, professional societies, state medical boards, and other health care organizations are required to report any disciplinary action taken against providers lasting more than 30 days. Disciplinary actions include limitation, suspension, or revocation of privileges or professional society membership. MCOs are not required to report physicians to the data bank if they do not follow treatment protocols. However, when a physician is deselected by an MCO for a quality-of-care issue, the MCO must report it ("The National Practitioner Data Bank and MCOs" 1999). Medical malpractice payments account for approximately three-quarters of reports made to the data bank. Under the Health Care Quality Improvement Act, immunity from liability is granted for health care entities and providers making peer review reports in good faith (Walzer 1990).

Hospitals are required to request information from the data bank concerning all physicians applying for staff privileges. Every 2 years, a query of the data bank is required concerning each physician or other practitioner on the hospital staff. Hospitals that do not comply face loss of immunity for professional peer review activities.

The public does not have access to the data bank. Plaintiffs' attorneys can have access to the data bank only if they can prove that the hospital failed to query the data bank about the physician in question. The information obtained can be used only to sue the hospital for negligent credentialing. Physicians can request information from the data bank about their own file. A study found that hospital reporting of actions taken regarding clinical privileges from 1991 to 1995 declined, raising concerns about underreporting (Baldwin et al. 1999).

The Suicidal Patient

The most common malpractice claim arising from psychiatric care is the failure to provide reasonable protection to patients from harming themselves. There are categories of negligent failings that are frequently asserted: diagnostic failures (i.e., failure to assess the potential for suicide), treatment failures (i.e., failure to use reasonable treatment interventions and precautions), and implementation failures (i.e., failure to carry out treatment properly and not negligently).

These categorical failings, each of which applies to inpatient and outpatient settings, are simply different ways in which the practitioner's duty of care may have been breached by unreasonable conduct. Claims for conduct resulting in the death of a patient are governed by the same tort principles that apply when a living patient brings a malpractice claim. However, because tort claims in common law did not survive the death of a patient, most states have legislation permitting the survival of such actions by the former patient's estate under the banner of wrongful death. Although they apply traditional tort principles, most wrongful-death actions brought for patient suicides turn on the legal concepts of *foreseeability, reasonableness,* and *causation.* As a general rule, a psychiatrist who exercises reasonable care in compliance with accepted medical practice will not be held liable for any resulting injury. Thus, if the fact finder concludes that a patient's suicide was not reasonably foreseeable, that the precautions taken by the psychiatrist were reasonable, or even if they were not that the suicide was caused by an unforeseeable intervening factor, the claim will fail.

Foreseeable suicide. The evaluation of suicide risk is one of the most complex, difficult, and challenging clinical tasks in psychiatry (Simon 2004). Suicide is a rare event. A systematic assessment of a patient's suicide risk forms the basis of a sound clinical management plan. Using reasonable care in assessing suicide risk can preempt the problem of predicting the actual occurrence of suicide, for which professional standards do not exist. Standard approaches to the assessments of suicide risk are described in the psychiatric literature (Simon and Hales 2006). Time attenuates suicide risk assessments, requiring that assessment be a process, not an event.

As an accepted standard of care, an evaluation of suicide risk should be done with all patients, regardless of whether they present with overt suicidal complaints. A review of case law shows that reasonable care requires that a patient who is either suspected of being or confirmed to be suicidal must be the subject of certain affirmative precautions. A failure either to reasonably assess a patient's suicide risk or to implement an appropriate precautionary plan after the suicide potential becomes foreseeable is likely to render a practitioner liable if the patient is harmed because of a suicide attempt. The law permits the fact finder to conclude that suicide is preventable if it is foreseeable. Foreseeability, however, should not be confused with preventability. In hindsight, many suicides seem preventable that were clearly not foreseeable.

When suicide risk assessments are competently performed and recorded, the psychiatrist demonstrates careful and thorough management of the suicidal patient. Moreover, evidence of a reasonable suicide risk assessment also demonstrates that the psychiatrist adhered to the prevailing standard of care. Although psychiatrists cannot ensure favorable outcomes with suicidal patients, they can ensure that the process of suicide risk assessment was competently performed (Simon 2002).

Inpatients.   Intervention in an inpatient setting usually requires the following:

- Screening evaluations
- Development of an appropriate treatment plan
- Implementation of that plan
- Ongoing case review by clinical staff

Careful documentation of assessments and management interventions with changes responsive to the patient's clinical situation are evidence of clinically and legally sufficient psychiatric care. Assessing suicide risk and protective factors is only half of the equation. Documenting the benefits of a psychiatric intervention (e.g., ward change, pass, discharge) against the risk of suicide permits an evenhanded approach to the clinical management of the patient.

Psychiatrists are more likely to be sued successfully when a psychiatric inpatient commits suicide. The law permits the fact finder to conclude that the opportunities to foresee (i.e., anticipate) and control (i.e., treat and manage) suicidal patients are greater in the hospital (Hofflander v. St. Catherine's Hospital 2003).

Outpatients.   Psychiatrists are expected to reasonably assess the severity and imminence of a foreseeable suicidal act. The result of the assessment dictates the treatment and safety management options. Psychiatrists are not strictly liable whenever an outpatient commits suicide (Speer v. United States 1981). Instead, the reasonableness of the psychiatrist's efforts is determinative.

Suicide prevention pacts.   Suicide prevention contracts created between the clinician and the patient attempt to develop an expressed understanding that the patient will call for help rather than act out suicidal thoughts or impulses. These contracts have no legal authority; although they may be helpful in solidifying the therapeutic alliance, they may falsely reassure the psychiatrist. Suicide prevention agreements between psychiatrists and patients must not be used in place of adequate suicide assessment (Simon 1999).

Legal defenses.   A psychiatrist's Answer to a malpractice claim arising out of a patient suicide may consist of a denial of allegations in the plaintiff's Complaint, from which the fact finder might reject the allegation that the psychiatrist breached a duty that proximately caused the patient's suicide. In addition, the defendant's Answer to the Complaint might include affirmative defenses that have the legal effect of defeating the claim even if the defendant's negligence proximately caused the patient's suicide.

One approach to denying a crucial allegation of the plaintiff's case is to prove that the care and supervision provided were reasonable. One example of that denial of negligence is the best-judgment defense asserting that the patient was properly assessed and treated for suicide risk but committed suicide anyway (J.D. Robertson 1991). In some cases the treatment may appear to contribute to the risk. This has proved to be controversial in the use of the "open door" policy in which patients are allowed freedom of movement for therapeutic purposes. In these cases, the individual facts and reasonableness of the staff's application of the "open door" policy appear to be paramount. Nevertheless, courts have difficulty with abstract treatment notions such as personal growth when faced with a dead patient.

The plaintiff must persuade the fact finder that the psychiatrist's negligence more likely than not caused the patient's suicide. Thus proof that the suicide was caused by an unforeseeable intervening cause negates a critical element of the claim. For example, a fact finder may find a psychiatrist not liable for the suicidal act of a borderline patient who experienced a traumatic loss of a romantic relationship between therapy sessions and then impulsively attempted suicide without trying to contact the psychiatrist.

Affirmative defenses, like the statute of limitations, bar untimely claims regardless of their merits. Governmental or sovereign immunity, where it exists, bars claims regardless of the strength of the plaintiff's claim.

The Violent Patient

As a general rule, absent a special relationship, one person has no duty to control the conduct of a second person to prevent that person from harming a third person (Restatement [Second] of Torts 1965). Applying this rule to psychiatric care, psychiatrists traditionally have had only a limited duty owed to third persons to control their patients. Included in this limited class of duty to third persons for the acts of their patients is negligent discharge of a dangerous patient who harms a third person or the failure to warn a patient about the risks of driving while taking certain medications, resulting in injury to others (Felthous 1990). After *Tarasoff* (Tarasoff v. Regents of the University of California 1976), the therapist's legal duty and potential liability significantly expanded in the outpatient setting in many, but not all, states (Thapar v. Zezulka 1999). In *Tarasoff*, the California Supreme Court reasoned that a duty to protect third parties was imposed when a special relationship existed between the individual whose conduct created the danger and the defendant. Finding this special relationship requirement met in this setting, the court concluded that "the single relationship of a doctor to his patient is sufficient to support the duty to exercise reasonable care to protect others [from the violent acts of patients]." Critical to recognizing a duty in this situation was the court's assumption about mental health professionals and the foreseeability of violence.

Psychiatrists do not have the ability to predict violence with any accuracy. Violent behaviors are the result of the complex interplay among social, clinical, and personality factors that vary significantly across situations and time (Widiger and Trull 1994). Nonetheless, clinical methods for assessing the risk of violence exist that reflect the current standard of care (Baxter and Beck 1998; Monahan and Steadman 1994; Simon 1992a; Tardiff 2002).

Assessment of risk of violence is essentially a clinical judgment. Because the validity of violence risk assessments is only modestly greater than chance, the MacArthur Violence Risk Assessment Study was established. The purpose of the study was to improve clinical risk assessment validity, enhance effective clinical risk management, and provide data on mental disorders and violence for informing mental health law and policy (Monahan et al. 2001). In this study, violence risk assessments were found to have a validity that was modestly better than chance. Until more studies are available, sound clinical practice requires that thorough violence risk assessments be routinely performed with potentially violent patients on the basis of current knowledge of violence risk factors. Although violence risk assessments need to be made at such critical points as the initiation of ward status changes, passes, and discharge, violence risk assessment is more of a continuing process rather than a solitary event. All such assessments should be duly recorded.

The index of suspicion for potential violence should be high in patients with a past history of violence who are currently making serious threats of harm toward specific individuals. The potential for violence is further heightened if the patient is acutely psychotic, substance abusing, angry, or fearful of being harmed or is experiencing delusions of being controlled or influenced (Link and Stueve 1994).

Following *Tarasoff,* courts in other jurisdictions have interpreted the case variously. Some states have adopted the *Tarasoff* holding, whereas others have limited or extended its scope and reach. In most states, psychotherapists have a duty, established by case law or statute, to act affirmatively to protect an endangered third party from a patient's violent or dangerous acts. A few courts have declined to find a *Tarasoff* duty in a specific case, whereas some courts have simply rejected the *Tarasoff* duty (Evans v. United States 1995; Green v. Ross 1997). In *Thapar v. Zezulka* (1999), the Texas Supreme Court ruled that the state statute on confidentiality *permits* but does not *require* disclosures by therapists of threats of harm to endangered third parties by their patients.

When courts have found a duty to protect, they have required an "imminent" threat of serious harm to a foreseeable victim. The

term *imminent,* however, is a problematic construct for assessing violence (Simon 2006). Just as the decisions have sought to narrow the time frame within which the violence that triggers the duty might arise, so they have sought to limit the persons who are at risk. Only a small minority of courts have held that a duty to protect exists for the population at large; most require an identifiable victim to be at risk. In some jurisdictions, courts have held that the need to safeguard the public well-being overrides all other considerations, including confidentiality. Despite the fact that the *Tarasoff* duty is still not law in some jurisdictions and is subject to different interpretations by individual courts, the duty to protect is, in effect, a national standard of practice.

Several states have enacted statutes that immunize the psychiatrist from legal liability arising from a patient's violent acts toward others when the psychiatrist facing this predicament takes certain action such as warning the endangered third party and/or notifying the authorities (Appelbaum et al. 1989). The duty-to-protect language stated in some statutes allows for a greater variety of clinical interventions.

Evolving trends. An important evolving trend is the application of the *Tarasoff* duty to sexual abuse cases by an alleged pedophile. A psychiatrist was denied dismissal of a claim against him by a child patient who was abused by his psychiatric resident/patient for not reporting to the medical school that his student/patient was a pedophile (Garamella v. New York Medical College 1998). The resident/patient molested the child at a hospital crisis center. The court reasoned that the defendant psychiatrist's control over the psychiatric resident was far greater than in the typical psychiatrist–patient relationship, leaving for trial whether the plaintiff "was within a foreseeable class of victims to whom Dr. Ingram [the residency supervisor] might owe a duty of care arising from DeMasi's [the resident] disclosure. The issue of foreseeability is a disputed one, properly reserved for the trier of fact" (pp. 174–175).

A *Tarasoff* duty was also found where a spouse had knowledge of her husband's sexually abusive behavior against children in the neighborhood (J.S. v. R.T. 1998; Touchette v. Ganal 1996). In another case, the court found that a *Tarasoff* duty could exist but declined to find the parents of a babysitter liable for his dangerous sexual behavior (People v. Rose 1998). The court determined that no evidence existed that the parents knew of their son's proclivity to commit a sexual assault.

Release of potentially violent patients. Under managed care, discharging violent or potentially violent inpatients presents unique challenges for treating psychiatrists (Simon 1998). The treatment of psychiatric inpatients has changed dramatically in the managed care era (Lazarus and Sharfstein 1994). Most psychiatric units, particularly in general hospitals, have become short-stay, acute-care psychiatric facilities. Generally, only suicidal, homicidal, or gravely disabled patients with major psychiatric disorders pass strict precertification review for hospitalization (Tischler 1990). Close scrutiny by utilization reviewers permits only short hospitalization for these patients (Wickizer et al. 1996). The purpose of hospitalization is crisis intervention and management to stabilize patients and to ensure their safety, and the treatment of patients is provided by a variety of mental health professionals. Nonetheless, the psychiatrist often must bear the ultimate burden of liability for treatments gone awry ("Why Are Liability Premiums Rising?" 1996). Limited opportunity usually exists during the hospital stay to develop a therapeutic alliance with patients. The ability to communicate with patients—the psychiatrist's stock-in-trade—is often severely curtailed. All of these factors contribute to a greatly increased risk of malpractice suits against psychiatrists that allege premature or negligent discharge of patients due to cost containment policies.

There is more control over the patient in the hospital than is available in an outpatient setting. Courts closely evaluate decisions made by psychiatrists treating inpatients that adversely affect the patients or a third party. Liability imposed on psychiatric facilities that had custody of patients who injured others outside the institution after escape or release is clearly distinguishable from the factual situation of *Tarasoff*. Duty-to-warn cases generally involve patients in outpatient treatment. Liability arises from the inaction of the therapist who fails to take affirmative measures to warn or protect endangered third parties. In negligent-release cases, liability may arise from the allegation that the institution's affirmative act in releasing the patient caused injury to the third party. Moreover, allegations may be made that a psychiatrist or hospital personnel failed, prior to the patient's discharge, to warn individuals known to be at risk of harm from that patient. Lawsuits stemming from the release of foreseeably dangerous patients who subsequently injure or kill others are roughly five to six times more common than outpatient duty-to-warn lawsuits (Simon 1992b).

The psychiatrist's liability is determined by reference to professional standards. Consultation with other psychiatrists may provide additional protection when the discharge of a potentially violent patient appears problematic. Consulting with an attorney may help clarify legal obligations, but clinicians ultimately must exercise their professional judgment.

The patient's willingness to cooperate with the psychiatrist is critical to maintaining follow-up treatment. The psychiatrist's obligation focuses on structuring the follow-up visits in such a manner as to encourage compliance. A study of Department of Veterans Affairs (VA) inpatient referrals to a VA mental health outpatient clinic showed that of the 24% of inpatients who were referred, approximately one-half failed to keep their first appointments (Zeldow and Taub 1981). Nevertheless, limitations do exist on the extent of the psychiatrist's ability to ensure follow-up care. Most patients retain the right to refuse treatment. These limitations must be acknowledged by both the psychiatric and legal communities (Simon 1992a). The American Medical Association Council on Scientific Affairs has developed evidence-based discharge criteria for safe discharge from the hospital (American Medical Association 1996).

In either the outpatient or inpatient situation, psychiatrists are in compliance with the responsibility to warn and protect others from potentially violent patients if they reasonably assess the patients' *risk* for violence and make clinically appropriate interventions based on their findings. Professional standards do exist for assessment of the risk factors for violence (Simon 2001), but no standard of care exists for the prediction of violent behavior. The clinician should assess the risk of violence frequently, updating the risk assessment at significant clinical junctures (e.g., room and ward changes, passes, discharge). A risk–benefit assessment should be conducted and recorded before a pass or discharge is issued. Assessing the risk of violence is a "here and now" determination performed at the time of discharge. After the patient is discharged, the potential for violence against self or others depends on the nature and course of the mental illness, adequacy of future treatment, adherence to treatment recommendations, and exposure to unforeseeable stressful life events.

Involuntary Hospitalization

Involuntary hospitalization of persons with mental disorders is limited to statutorily defined criteria in all states. Based on the state's decision to exercise its constitutional authority, all states have authorized civil commitment of individuals who are mentally ill and dangerous to self or others, and some states also permit commitment of individuals who are mentally ill and unable to provide for their basic needs. Generally, each state spells out which criteria are required and what each means. Terms such as *mentally ill* are of-

ten loosely described, thus placing the responsibility for appropriate diagnosis on the clinical judgment of the petitioner.

Some states have enacted legislation that permits involuntary hospitalization of three other distinct groups in addition to individuals with mental illness: developmentally disabled persons, substance-addicted persons, and mentally disabled minors. Special commitment provisions may exist governing requirements for the admission and discharge of mentally disabled minors as well as numerous due process rights afforded these individuals (Parham v. J.R. 1979).

Involuntary hospitalization of psychiatric patients usually arises when violent behavior threatens to erupt toward self or others and when patients become unable to care for themselves. These patients frequently manifest mental disorders and conditions that meet the substantive criteria for involuntary hospitalization.

Courts, not clinicians, have the authority to commit patients. The psychiatrist initiates the process that brings the patient before the court, usually after a brief period of hospitalization for evaluation or after an evaluation of a prospective patient at the request of the court. The psychiatrist must be guided by the treatment needs of the patient in seeking involuntary hospitalization, within the constraints of commitment standards.

Commitment statutes do not require involuntary hospitalization but are permissive (Appelbaum et al. 1989). The statutes enable mental health professionals and others to seek involuntary hospitalization for persons who meet certain substantive criteria. The duty to seek involuntary hospitalization is a standard-of-care issue. Patients who are mentally ill and pose a serious threat to themselves or others may require involuntary hospitalization as a primary psychiatric intervention.

Liability. Because psychiatrists are often granted conditional immunity for their good-faith participation in involuntary hospitalization proceedings, it is not surprising that most malpractice claims involving involuntary hospitalization allege an absence of good faith in the psychiatrists' behavior. Often these lawsuits are brought under the theory of false imprisonment. Other areas of liability that may arise from wrongful commitment include assault and battery, malicious prosecution, abuse of authority, and intentional infliction of emotional distress (Simon 1992a).

The use of reasonable professional judgment is perhaps the best evidence that the psychiatrist's actions were taken in good faith (Mishkin 1989). Performing a careful examination of the patient, abiding by the requirements of the law, and ensuring that sound reasoning motivates the certification of the patient are good clinical practice and only secondarily good risk management. Evidence of willful, blatant, or gross failure to adhere to statutorily defined commitment procedures may expose a psychiatrist to a lawsuit.

Rights of involuntarily hospitalized patients. Most states recognize the right of inpatients to refuse treatment. Even though the patient is involuntarily hospitalized, the order for hospitalization, without a more specific finding, does not negate a presumption of competence. In most states, patients involuntarily hospitalized who refuse medication are entitled to a separate court hearing for an adjudication of incompetence and the provision of substituted consent by the court. In a civil rights action by a state prisoner challenging involuntary treatment with antipsychotic drugs without a prior judicial hearing (Washington v. Harper 1990), the U.S. Supreme Court ruled involuntary treatment of a prisoner was constitutionally permissible when the prisoner was found to be a serious danger to himself or others as the result of a mental illness and the treatment was in the prisoner's medical interest. The Court found that, in lieu of a judicial hearing, administrative procedures that included review by an administrative panel satisfied procedural due process requirements.

Hospitalized patients possess other rights. Patients possess rights of visitation, although these rights can be temporarily suspended for proper cause relating to a patient's care and treatment. Free communications of hospitalized patients through mail, telephone, or visitors are considered a right, unless protection of the patients or others requires supervision of communications. The right to privacy includes allowing patients to have secure locker space, private toilet and shower facilities, and a minimum square footage of floor space. Protection of confidentiality is also included. Economic rights include the right to have and spend money and to handle one's own financial affairs responsibly. In most jurisdictions, involuntarily hospitalized patients do not lose their civil rights, such as the right to manage their own money. Hospitalized patients must be paid for their work unless it is truly therapeutic labor (i.e., intended to benefit the patient, not the hospital). "Patients' rights" are not absolute and often must be tempered by the clinical judgment of the mental health professional. Inevitably, disputes over perceived or real violations of patients' rights arise. In some jurisdictions, a civil rights officer or ombudsman is mandated by statute to mediate these disputes.

Seclusion and Restraint

The psychiatric legal issues surrounding seclusion and restraint are complex. Seclusion and restraint have both indications and contraindications as clinical management tools (American Psychiatric Association 1985; see Tables 21–6 and 21–7). The legal regulation of seclusion and restraint has become increasingly more stringent over the past decade.

Legal challenges to the use of seclusion and restraints have been made on behalf of the institutionalized mentally ill and the mentally retarded. Frequently, these lawsuits do not stand alone but are part of a challenge to a wide range of alleged abuses within a hospital.

Generally, the courts have held that seclusion and restraints are an intrusion on a pa-

Table 21–6. Indications for seclusion and restraint

1. Prevent harm to the patient or others.
2. Prevent disruption to treatment program or physical surroundings.
3. Assist in treatment as part of ongoing behavior therapy.
4. Decrease sensory overstimulation (seclusion only).
5. Respond to patient's reasonable voluntary request.[a]

[a]First seclusion; then, if necessary, restraints.
Source. Adapted with permission from Simon RI: *Concise Guide to Psychiatry and Law for Clinicians,* 3rd Edition. Washington, DC, American Psychiatric Publishing, 2001, p. 114.

Table 21–7. Contraindications to seclusion and restraint

1. Unstable medical and psychiatric conditions[a]
2. Delirious patients or patients with dementia who are unable to tolerate decreased stimulation[a]
3. High-risk suicidal patients[a]
4. Patients with severe drug reactions or overdoses or patients requiring close monitoring of drug dosages[a]
5. For punishment of the patient or for convenience of staff

[a]Unless close supervision and direct observation are provided.
Source. Adapted with permission from Simon RI: *Concise Guide to Psychiatry and Law for Clinicians,* 3rd Edition. Washington, DC, American Psychiatric Publishing, 2001, p. 117.

tient's constitutionally protected interests and may be implemented only when a patient presents a risk of harm to self or others and no less restrictive alternative is available. Some courts have also required the following:

1. Restraint and seclusion may be implemented only by a written order from an appropriate medical official.
2. Orders must be confined to specific, time-limited periods.
3. A patient's condition must be regularly reviewed and documented.
4. Any extension of an original order must be reviewed and reauthorized.

Sexual Misconduct

Therapist–patient sex is usually preceded by progressive boundary violations in treatment (Simon 1989). As a consequence, patients are often psychologically damaged by the precursor boundary violations as well as the eventual sexual misconduct of the therapist (Simon 1991). An excellent account of the gradual erosion of treatment boundaries leading to near loss of control with a client is given by Rutter (1989).

General boundary guidelines exist for conducting psychiatric treatment (Simon 1992c). Awareness of these guidelines and of

their transgression may help alert the therapist to progressive boundary violations (Simon 1994). Sexual misconduct does not occur in isolation but usually involves a variety of negligent acts of omission and commission.

Three types of legal responses to sexual misconduct have been enacted: reporting, civil liability, and criminal prosecution. *Reporting statutes* require a therapist who learns of any past or current therapist–patient sex to disclose this information. Some states have enacted *civil statutes* that make it explicit that sexual misconduct is a violation of the standard of care and authorize a damage claim (Bisbing et al. 1995). *Criminal statutes* addressing sexual misconduct have also been enacted. They may be appropriate given the therapist's behavior and may be the only remedy for exploitative therapists who do not have malpractice insurance, therapists who are unlicensed, or therapists who do not belong to professional organizations.

Civil liability. Psychiatrists who sexually exploit their patients are subject to civil and criminal sanctions as well as ethical and professional licensure disciplinary proceedings. *The Principles of Medical Ethics With Annota-*

tions Especially Applicable to Psychiatry (American Psychiatric Association 2001b) states that sex with a current or former patient is unethical (Section 2, Annotation 1). However, a malpractice claim is probably the most common legal response.

In a medical malpractice claim for sexual misconduct, in order to prevail the plaintiff has the burden of proving, by a preponderance of the evidence (i.e., "more likely than not"), among other things, that the exploitation took place. This burden can be met by corroborating evidence such as letters, pictures, hotel receipts, and identification of incriminating body markings of the exploited, as well as the testimony of other abused (former) patients. The plaintiff is also required to demonstrate that the misconduct caused harm such as a worsened psychiatric condition, suicide attempts, or the necessity for hospitalization. Expert psychiatric testimony is usually required to establish the type and extent of psychological damages as well as to establish whether a breach of the standard of care occurred.

A few states have enacted civil statutes proscribing sexual misconduct (Simon 1992a). Several states make therapist sexual misconduct a crime (Bisbing et al. 1995). Some states prosecute sexual exploitation suits under their sexual assault statutes. A number of states have enacted statutes that provide civil and criminal remedies to patients who were sexually abused by their therapists (Appelbaum 1990; Strasburger et al. 1991). For instance, Minnesota enacted legislation that states the following:

> A cause of action against a psychotherapist for sexual exploitation exists for a patient or former patient for injury caused by sexual contact with the psychotherapist if the sexual contact occurred: 1) during the period the patient was receiving psychotherapy…or 2) after the period the patient received psychotherapy…if a) the former patient was emotionally dependent on the psychotherapist; or b) the sexual contact occurred by means of thera-

peutic deception. (Minn. Stat. Ann. § 148A.02 2005)

A person who engages in sexual penetration with another person is guilty of criminal sexual conduct in the third degree if any of the following circumstances exists:

> (h) the actor is a psychotherapist and the complainant is a patient of the psychotherapist and the sexual penetration occurred: (i) during the psychotherapy session; or (ii) outside the psychotherapy session if an ongoing psychotherapist–patient relationship exists. Consent by the complainant is not a defense. (Minn. Stat. Ann. § 609.344 2005)

It is not a recognized defense to these common-law or statutory remedies that the patient was aware that sex was not a part of treatment, that the sex occurred outside the treatment setting, that treatment ended before the sexual relationship began, or that the patient consented to the sexual contact. Patients cannot consent to malpractice. In sexual misconduct cases, the issue is never patient consent but always breach of fiduciary trust by the therapist and the harm it caused.

There is no "respected minority" in the profession that claims sexual relations with patients is therapeutic. This position had a few adherents at one time but is no longer publicly advocated by credible mental health professionals.

Criminal sanctions. Sexual exploitation of a patient may be classified as rape or sexual assault (Hoge et al. 1995). Many of the new wave of statutes criminalizing therapist–patient sexual misconduct assume, as a matter of law, that a current patient is incapable of giving consent to sexual relations with his or her therapist and treat all sexual relations between therapist and patient as a criminal act committed by the therapist (Minn. Stat. Ann. § 609.344 2005). In states without such a provision, sex with a current patient may be criminally actionable under sexual assault statutes if the state can prove that the patient was coerced into engaging in the sexual act. Typically, this type of evidence is limited to the use of some form of substance (e.g., medication) either to induce compliance or to reduce resistance. Anesthesia, ECT, hypnosis, drugs, force, and threat of harm have been used to coerce patients into sexual submission (Schoener et al. 1989). To date, claims of psychological coercion through the manipulation of transference phenomena have not been successful in establishing the coercion necessary for a criminal case. In cases involving a minor patient, the issue of consent or coercion is irrelevant because minors and adult incompetent persons are considered unable to provide valid consent. Therefore, sex with a child or an incompetent person is automatically considered a criminal act.

Professional disciplinary action. For the purposes of adjudicating allegations of professional misconduct, licensing boards are typically granted certain regulatory and disciplinary authority by state statutes. As a result, state licensing organizations, unlike professional associations, may discipline an offending professional by suspending or revoking his or her license to practice. There is no cost to a patient to seek redress through this means, nor are licensure boards constrained by statutes of limitations. A review of published reports of sexual misconduct cases adjudicated before licensing boards revealed that in the vast majority of cases, the evidence was reasonably sufficient to substantiate a claim of exploitation, leading to revocation of the professional's license or suspension from practice for varying lengths of time, including permanent suspension.

Patients can bring ethical charges against psychiatrists before the district branches of the APA at any time. Ethical violators who are members may be reprimanded, suspended, or expelled from the APA. All national organizations of mental health professionals have ethically proscribed sexual relations between therapist and patient.

Psychiatry in the Courtroom

Psychiatry and Criminal Law: Criminal Proceedings

Individuals charged with committing crimes may display significant psychiatric and neurological impairment that played a causal role in the commission of the crimes or was precipitated by the charges against them. The causal connection between brain damage and violence, however, remains frustratingly obscure. Violent behavior spans a wide spectrum from a normal response to a threatening situation to violence emanating directly from an organic brain disorder. Moreover, violent behavior is often the result of the interaction between an individual and a specific situation. Brain damage and mental illness may or may not play a significant role in this equation.

Criminal Intent (Mens Rea)

Under the common law, criminal culpability for most serious crimes requires 1) the mental state or level of intent to commit the act (known as the *mens rea*, or guilty mind), 2) the act itself or conduct associated with committing the crime (known as *actus reus*, or guilty act), and 3) a concurrence in time between the guilty act and the guilty mental state (Bethea v. United States 1976). To convict a person of a particular crime, the state must prove beyond a reasonable doubt that the defendant committed the criminal act with the requisite intent. All three elements are necessary to satisfy the threshold requirements for the imposition of criminal sanctions.

The defendant's intent determines not only the culpability for an offense but also the gravity of the offense. For instance, a person who deliberately plans to commit a crime is subject to more serious prosecution and punishment than one who does so impulsively. The difficulty, of course, is in assessing intent retrospectively (Simon and Shuman 2002).

Traditionally, legislative definitions of offenses required proof of general intent for some crimes and proof of specific intent to meet the *mens rea* requirement for others. *Specific intent* refers to the *mens rea* in crimes in which a *further intention* exists beyond the presence of a general criminal intent. For instance, the intent necessary for first-degree murder typically includes a "specific intent to kill" (Rogers and Shuman 2005). Unlike general intent, specific criminal intent may not be presumed from the unlawful criminal act alone. Because of the difficulties inherent in these categories, modern statutory codes have created more precise criteria for defining mental states that distinguish intentional, knowing, reckless, and negligent behavior (Rogers and Shuman 2005).

Mental handicaps or impairments present a host of problems across the criminal justice system. From assessing appropriateness of diversion to the specialized mental health courts or the mental health system, the risks posed by release on bail, or competence to stand trial to face criminal charges (Dusky v. United States 1960); to addressing *mens rea* or an affirmative defense of insanity and the disposition of an insanity aquittee (M'Naughten's Case 1843; United States v. Brawner 1972); to sentencing of convicted offenders and determination of eligibility for a sentence of death (Penry v. Lynaugh 1989; Tennard v. Dretke 2004), as well as competence to be executed (Ford v. Wainwright 1986), the impact of mental impairment pervades the criminal justice system. The first and most common context in which mental impairment arises is competence to stand trial. We do not require every defendant to be assessed and found competent before a trial begins; competence is presumed. However, when as the result of the defendant's conduct a question arises, the defense counsel, prosecutor, or judge may raise the issue, thus requiring the court to decide whether the defendant understands the charges brought against him or her and is capable of rationally assisting counsel with the defense.

Competency to Stand Trial

The legal standard for assessing pretrial competency was established by the U.S. Supreme Court in *Dusky v. United States* (1960). To be competent to make decisions during the pretrial process, at trial, and during an appeal, the court succinctly and without embellishment required that the defendant have "sufficient present ability to consult with his lawyer with a reasonable degree of rational understanding" and "a rational as well as factual understanding of the proceedings against him" (Dusky v. United States 1960). Subsequent decisions have clarified that the level of understanding required need not be sophisticated.

Although the *Dusky* test does not require the absence of understanding resulting from the presence of a mental disease or defect, that is typically the case. However, a defendant may be found incompetent to stand trial even if he or she does not have a mental disease or defect as defined by the latest version of DSM, as in the case of a physical illness that affects cognition.

Although most impairments implicated in competency examinations are functional rather than organic (Reich and Wells 1985), various forms of neuropsychiatric impairments typically raise questions about a defendant's competency to stand trial. In *Wilson v. United States* (1968), the defendant had no memory of the time of an alleged robbery because he had permanent retrograde amnesia. This impairment was caused by injuries he sustained in an automobile accident that occurred as he was being pursued by the police after the offense. Of the various criteria that the court established in determining the defendant's competency to stand trial, the following are directly relevant to the issue of neuropsychiatric impairment (Wilson v. United States 1968):

1. The extent to which the amnesia affected the defendant's ability to consult with and assist his lawyer

2. The extent to which the amnesia affected the defendant's ability to testify in his own behalf

Any disorder, whether functional or organic, that significantly impairs a defendant's cognitive and communicative abilities is likely to have an impact on competency. Nevertheless, it is the actual *functional* mental capability to meet the minimal standard of trial competency, and not the severity of the deficits, that determines whether an individual is cognitively capable to be tried. For example, Slovenko (1995) questioned whether psychiatric diagnosis is relevant to competency to stand trial. The presence or absence of a mental illness is irrelevant if the defendant is capable of meeting competency requirements. It is legal criteria, not medical or psychiatric diagnosis, that govern competency. Diagnosis is relevant only to the question of restoring the defendant's competency to stand trial with treatment.

Checklists and structured interviews have been developed to assess specific psychological factors applicable to the competency standards established in *Dusky*. The Interdisciplinary Fitness Interview, designed for use by lawyers and mental health professionals (Schreiber et al. 1987), provides for a detailed examination of psychopathology and legal knowledge using explicit scales for rating each response to the competency evaluation. *Evaluating Competencies: Forensic Assessments and Instruments,* by Thomas Grisso (1986), is a standard reference in the field.

A defendant's impairment in one particular function, however, does not automatically render him or her incompetent. For example, the fact that the defendant is manifesting certain deficits because of damage to the parietal lobe does not necessarily mean that he or she lacks the requisite cognitive ability to aid in his or her own defense at trial (Tranel 1992). The ultimate determination of incompetency is for the court to decide (United States v. David 1975). Moreover, the impairment must be considered in the context of the particular case or proceeding. Mental impairment that may render an individual incompetent to stand trial in a complicated tax fraud case might not for a misdemeanor trial.

Psychiatrists and psychologists who testify as expert witnesses regarding the effect of psychiatric problems on a defendant's competency to stand trial are most effective if their findings are framed according to the degree to which the defendant is cognitively capable of meeting the standards enunciated in *Dusky*.

Insanity Defense

One of the most controversial issues in American criminal jurisprudence is the insanity defense. Defendants with functional or organic mental disabilities who are found competent to stand trial may seek acquittal claiming that they were not criminally responsible for their actions because of insanity at the time the offense was committed. The retrospective assessment of the offender's mental state at the time of the crime in insanity defense cases is one of the most challenging evaluations that the forensic psychiatrist performs (Simon and Shuman 2002).

Criminals may commit crimes for many reasons, but the law presumes that they do so of their own free will and that it is therefore just to impose punishment. Some offenders, however, are so mentally disturbed in their thinking and behavior that they are thought to be incapable of making a choice that could have been deterred by the criminal law and for which retribution is justified. Historically, albeit controversially, the common law has long recognized some form of limitation on the punishment of a "crazy" or insane person (Blackstone 1769; Coke 1680). Larger in legend than in life, the insanity defense is rarely used and even more rarely successful. Approximately 1% of criminal defendants plead not guilty by reason of insanity; of these, only 10%–25% are successful. The chance of exculpation is greatest when the criminal defendant was found to be psychotic at the time of the crime by the pretrial assessment (Brakel et al. 1985).

A universally accepted definition of legal insanity does not exist. Over the years, tests of insanity have been subject to much controversy, modification, and refinement (Brakel et al. 1985). Thus, there is variability in the insanity defense standard in the United States, depending on which state's or jurisdiction's law applies.

Following the acquittal by reason of insanity of John Hinckley Jr. on charges of attempting to assassinate President Reagan and murder others, an outraged public demanded changes in the insanity defense. Federal and state legislation to accomplish that result ensued. Between 1978 and 1985, approximately 75% of all states made some sort of substantive change in their insanity defense (Perlin 1989). Nevertheless, a number of states continued to adhere to the American Law Institute (ALI) insanity defense standard or some version of it. The ALI test provides that a person is not responsible for criminal conduct if at the time of such conduct, as a result of mental disease or defect, he or she lacks substantial capacity either to appreciate the criminality (wrongfulness) of his or her conduct or to conform that conduct to the requirements of law. As used in this article, the terms *mental disease* or *defect* do not include an abnormality manifested only by repeated criminal or otherwise antisocial conduct (Model Penal Code § 4.01 [1962]).

This standard contains both a cognitive and a volitional prong. The *cognitive prong* derives from the 1843 M'Naughten rule exculpating the defendant who does not know the nature and quality of the alleged act or does not know the act was wrong. The *volitional prong* is a vestige of the irresistible impulse test, which states that the defendant who is overcome by an irresistible impulse that leads to an alleged act is not responsible for that act.

By contrast, defendants tried in a federal court and most state courts are governed by a cognitive, pre-ALI standard. The federal standard is contained in the Comprehensive Crime Control Act of 1984 (P.L. 98–473 1984), which provides that it is an affirmative de-

fense to all federal crimes that, at the time of the offense, "the defendant, as a result of a severe mental disease or defect, was unable to appreciate the nature and quality or the wrongfulness of his acts. Mental disease or defect does not otherwise constitute a defense." This codification eliminates the volitional or irresistible impulse portion of the insanity defense—that is, it does not allow an insanity defense based on a defendant's inability to conform his or her conduct to the requirements of the law. The defense is limited to defendants who are unable to appreciate the wrongfulness of their acts (i.e., the *cognitive portion* of the defense). The rule applicable in the federal courts requires the defendant to prove insanity by clear and convincing evidence. The standard of persuasion varies among the states. In a minority of states, the prosecution has the burden of proving beyond a reasonable doubt that the defendant was sane. In most states, the defendant must bear the burden of proving by a preponderance of the evidence that she or he was insane (Melton et al. 1997). A few states have abolished the affirmative defense of insanity, leaving defendants who claim that their mental state at the time of the crime should render them not responsible to attempt to negate *mens rea* with a more formidable burden.

Depending on the definitions contained in the criminal code or case law, the lack of capacity due to mental defects other than mental illness may be sufficient. For instance, mental retardation may represent an adequate basis for the insanity defense under certain circumstances. However, the impulse disorders—intermittent explosive disorder, kleptomania, pathological gambling, and pyromania—have not fared well under an insanity defense both because some of these disorders are specifically excluded in some states and because in jurisdictions with only a cognitive test, these disorders do not satisfy the cognitive impairment requirement. Absent class-wide exclusions of these disorders and with a volitional prong applicable, case-by-case scrutiny is appropriate. Pathological gambling has had little success as a basis for an insanity defense (Rosenthal and Lorenz 1992). McGarry (1983) pointed out that the lack of volitional control over the isolated act of gambling does not assume a lack of control concerning criminal acts committed in the service of the impulse to gamble. Compulsive gambling, however, has been raised as a mitigating factor at sentencing (Rosenthal and Lorenz 1992).

Depending on the severity of the functional or organic mental disorder and its effect on an offender's cognitive and affective processes, a defense of insanity might be warranted. At the least, the presence of a psychiatric disorder should be investigated as a *mitigating* factor that may have caused the offender to have diminished capacity.

Diminished Capacity

Because the insanity defense is an affirmative defense, it is only presented in a case after the prosecution has presented sufficient evidence to persuade a reasonable juror that the state has met its burden of proof on *mens rea* and *actus reus*. There are, however, degrees of mental impairment that are relevant to *mens rea* but do not negate it. In recognition of this, the concept of *diminished capacity* was developed (Melton et al. 1997).

Diminished capacity, where it is recognized, permits the accused to introduce medical and psychological evidence relating directly to the *mens rea* for the crime charged without having to assert a defense of insanity (Melton et al. 1997). Typically, when this is available, it applies to specific intent crimes. When a defendant's *mens rea* for the crime charged is nullified by psychiatric evidence, the defendant is acquitted only of that charge but is likely held responsible for an offense requiring a lesser *mens rea*, such as manslaughter (Melton et al. 1997). Patients with psychiatric disorders who commit criminal acts may be eligible for a diminished capacity defense.

Guilty But Mentally Ill

In a number of states, an alternative verdict of *guilty but mentally ill* has been established.

Under these statutes, if the defendant pleads not guilty by reason of insanity, this alternative verdict is available to the jury. Under an insanity plea, the verdict may be

- Not guilty
- Not guilty by reason of insanity
- Guilty but mentally ill
- Guilty

Guilty but mentally ill is an alternative verdict that is not different in its legal effect from finding the defendant guilty. The court must still impose a sentence on the convicted person, and the length of sentence and terms of confinement are not altered. Although the verdict directs that the convicted person receive necessary treatment, treatment should also be available to any prisoner with a mental disorder. The frequent unavailability of appropriate psychiatric treatment for prisoners adds to the spuriousness of this verdict.

Psychiatry and Civil Law: Expert Testimony

Civil litigation in psychic injury and head trauma cases may require the evaluation and testimony of psychiatrists, often working in conjunction with neurologists, other physicians, psychologists, neuropsychologists, and allied mental health professionals. Psychiatrists become involved in litigation as witnesses in one of two ways: as treaters (fact witnesses) or as forensic experts.

The Treating Clinician

The treating psychiatrist and the forensic psychiatric expert have different roles in litigation. Treatment and expert roles do not mix (Greenberg and Shuman 1997; Strasburger et al. 1997). The treating psychiatrist must rely heavily on the subjective reporting of the patient. In the treatment context, psychiatrists are interested primarily in the patient's perception of his or her difficulties, not necessarily the objective reality. As a consequence, treating psychiatrists usually do not speak to third parties or check pertinent records to gain additional information about a patient or to corroborate the patient's statements. The law, however, is interested in truth as scrutinized by the crucible of the adversary system. Uncorroborated patient reports relied on by a treating psychiatrist are vulnerable to attack as unreliable.

Credibility issues also abound. The treating psychiatrist is, and must be, an ally of the patient. This bias *in favor of* the patient is a proper treatment stance that fosters the therapeutic alliance. The psychiatrist looks for mental disorders to treat. A treatment rather than a litigation agenda is the appropriate stance for the treating psychiatrist.

In court, credibility is critical. Opposing counsel may attempt to portray the treating psychiatrist as an advocate for the patient-litigant, which may or may not be true. Also, court testimony by the treating psychiatrist may compel the disclosure of information that is not *legally* privileged but nonetheless is viewed as intimate and confidential by the patient. This disclosure by a trusted therapist is bound to cause psychological damage to the therapeutic relationship (Strasburger 1987). In addition, psychiatrists must be careful to inform patients about the consequences of releasing treatment information, especially in legal matters. Section 4, Annotation 2, of *The Principles of Medical Ethics With Annotations Especially Applicable to Psychiatry* (American Psychiatric Association 2001b) states, "The continuing duty of the psychiatrist to protect the patient includes fully apprising him/her of the connotations of waiving the privilege of privacy. This may become an issue when the patient is being investigated by a government agency, is applying for a position, or is involved in legal action."

Finally, when the treating psychiatrist testifies concerning the need for further treatment, a conflict of interest is readily apparent. In making such treatment prognostications, the psychiatrist stands to benefit economically from the recommendation of further treatment. Although this may not be the intention of the psychiatrist, opposing counsel will be sure to point out that the psychiatrist has a financial interest in the case.

The American Academy of Psychiatry and the Law (1989/1991), in its ethics statement, advises that "a treating psychiatrist should generally avoid agreeing to be an expert witness or to perform an evaluation of his patient for legal purposes because a forensic evaluation usually requires that other people be interviewed and testimony may adversely affect the therapeutic relationship" (p. xii). The treating psychiatrist should attempt to remain solely in a treatment role. If it becomes necessary to testify on behalf of the patient, the treating psychiatrist should testify only as a fact witness rather than as an expert witness. As a fact witness, the psychiatrist will be asked to describe the number and length of visits, the diagnosis, the treatment, and the prognosis. The treatment relationship does not provide an adequate basis for going beyond these issues. Psychiatrists must remain ever mindful of the many double-agent roles that can develop when mixing psychiatry and litigation (Simon 1987, 1992a).

The Forensic Expert

The forensic expert is usually free from the encumbrances of the treating psychiatrist in litigation. No doctor–patient relationship, with its treatment biases toward the patient, is created during forensic evaluation. The forensic expert typically reviews various records and looks to multiple sources of information to verify the factual assumptions that underlie any opinions drawn (Shuman and Greenberg 2003). Furthermore, the forensic expert considers the possibility of exaggeration or malingering because of a clear appreciation of the litigation context and the absence of treatment bias. Finally, the forensic psychiatrist does not face a conflict of interest for recommending treatment from which he or she would personally (i.e., financially) benefit. However, this same absence of a traditional doctor–patient relationship may subject the expert to being labeled as a "hired gun."

Conclusion

The legal issues surrounding the treatment and management of psychiatric patients are challenging and complex. The forensically informed psychiatrist is in a stronger position to provide good clinical care to the patient within the regulation of psychiatry by the courts and through governmental legislation. Moreover, psychiatrists will be increasingly required to testify in court concerning psychiatric patients. Familiarity and comfort with the role of a fact or expert witness will facilitate competent psychiatric testimony.

Key Points

- While the risk of being sued is inherent in the practice of psychiatry, spending time and talking with patients reduces the chances of being sued when things go bad.

- Except in an emergency, a psychiatrist must obtain informed consent—intelligent, knowing, and voluntary—from a competent patient before providing treatment. If the patient is not competent, an alternative method of consent (e.g., advance directive, guardianship) must be used.

- Patient confidences are sacrosanct and may be disclosed only when authorized in writing by the patient, ordered by the court, or excepted by law (e.g., elder or child abuse).

- Although psychiatrists may be competent in many roles, they should avoid conflicting roles such as forensic expert and therapist for the same patient-litigant.

- The psychiatrist who remains informed about the legal regulation of psychiatry can more effectively manage complex clinical-legal issues that inevitably arise with patients.

Suggested Readings

American Psychiatric Association: The Principles of Medical Ethics With Annotations Especially Applicable to Psychiatry. Washington, DC, American Psychiatric Association, 2001

Appelbaum PS, Gutheil TG: Clinical Handbook of Psychiatry and the Law, 3rd Edition. Baltimore, MD, Williams & Wilkins, 2000

Lifson LE, Simon RI (eds): The Mental Health Professional and the Law: A Comprehensive Handbook. Cambridge, MA, Harvard University Press, 1998

Melton GB, Petrila J, Poythress NG, et al: Psychological Evaluations for the Courts: A Handbook for Mental Health Professionals and Lawyers, 2nd Edition. New York, Guilford, 1997

Monahan J, Steadman HJ, Silver E, et al: Rethinking Risk Assessment: The MacArthur Study of Mental Disorder and Violence. New York, Oxford University Press, 2001

Morris R, Sales BD, Shuman DW: Doing Legal Research: A Guide for Social Scientists and Mental Health Professionals. Thousand Oaks, CA, Sage, 1996

Rogers R, Shuman DW: Fundamentals of Forensic Practice: Mental Health and Criminal Law. New York, Springer, 2005

Sales BD, Shuman DW: Experts in Court: Accommodating Law, Science and Expert Knowledge. Washington, DC, American Psychological Association, 2005

Schoener GR, Milgrom JH, Gonsiorek JC, et al: Psychotherapists' Sexual Involvement With Clients. Minneapolis, MN, Walk-In Counseling Center, 1989

Shuman DW: Psychiatric and Psychological Evidence, 3rd Edition. Rochester, NY, Thomson West, 2005

Simon RI: Assessing and Managing Suicide Risk: Guidelines for Clinically Based Risk Management. Washington, DC, American Psychiatric Publishing, 2004

Simon RI, Gold LH (eds): American Psychiatric Publishing Textbook of Forensic Psychiatry. Washington, DC, American Psychiatric Publishing, 2004

Simon RI, Hales RE (eds): American Psychiatric Publishing Textbook of Suicide Assessment and Management. Washington, DC, American Psychiatric Publishing, 2006

Simon RI, Shuman DW (eds): Predicting the Past: The Retrospective Psychiatric Assessment of Mental States in Litigation. Washington, DC, American Psychiatric Publishing, 2002

Slovenko R: Psychotherapy and Confidentiality: Testimonial Privileged Communication, Breach of Confidentiality, and Reporting Duties. Springfield, IL, Charles C Thomas, 1998

Slovenko R: Psychiatry in Law, Law In Psychiatry. New York, Brunner-Routledge, 2002

References

American Academy of Psychiatry and the Law: Ethical Guidelines for the Practice of Forensic Psychiatry. Adopted May 1987. Revised October 1989, 1991

American Medical Association: Report of the Council on Scientific Affairs: Evidence-Based Principles of Discharge and Discharge Criteria (CSA Report 4-A-96). Chicago, IL, American Medical Association, 1996

American Psychiatric Association: The Psychiatric Uses of Seclusion and Restraint (APA Task Force Report No 22). Washington, DC, American Psychiatric Association, 1985

American Psychiatric Association: Tardive Dyskinesia: A Task Force Report of the American Psychiatric Association. Washington, DC, American Psychiatric Association, 1992

American Psychiatric Association: The Practice of Electroconvulsive Therapy: Recommendations for Treatment, Training, and Privileging. A Task Force Report of the American Psychiatric Association, 2nd Edition. Edited by Weiner RD. Washington, DC, American Psychiatric Association, 2001a

American Psychiatric Association: The Principles of Medical Ethics With Annotations Especially Applicable to Psychiatry. Washington, DC, American Psychiatric Association, 2001b

American Psychiatric Association: Practice Guidelines for the Treatment of Psychiatric Disorders. Arlington, VA, American Psychiatric Association, 2004

Appelbaum PS: Statutes regulating patient–therapist sex. Hosp Community Psychiatry 41:15–16, 1990

Appelbaum PS, Lidz CW, Meisel A: Informed Consent: Legal Theory and Clinical Practice. New York, Oxford University Press, 1987, pp 84–87

Appelbaum PS, Zonana H, Bonnie R, et al: Statutory approaches to limiting psychiatrists' liability for their patients' violent acts. Am J Psychiatry 146:821–828, 1989

Baldwin LM, Hart LG, Oshel RG, et al: Hospital peer review and the National Practitioner Data Bank. JAMA 282:349–355, 1999

Baxter P, Beck JC: The violent patient: minimize your risk, in Practicing Psychiatry Without Fear: Guidelines of Liability Prevention. Edited by Lifson LE, Simon RI. Cambridge, MA, Harvard University Press, 1998

Beahrs JO, Gutheil TG: Informed consent in psychotherapy. Am J Psychiatry 158:4–10, 2001

Benefacts. A Message from the APA-sponsored Professional Liability Insurance Program. Psychiatric News, April 19, 1996, pp 1, 26

Bisbing SB, Jorgenson LM, Sutherland PK: Sexual Abuse by Professionals: A Legal Guide. Charlottesville, VA, Michie, 1995

Black HC: Black's Law Dictionary, 6th Edition. St Paul, MN, West Publishing, 1990

Blackstone W: Commentaries, Vol 4, 1769, pp 24–25

Brakel SJ, Parry J, Weiner BA: The Mentally Disabled and the Law, 3rd Edition. Chicago, IL, American Bar Foundation, 1985

Coke E: Third Institute 6, 6th Edition, 1680

Emanuel EJ, Emanuel LL: Proxy decision making for incompetent patients: an ethical and empirical analysis. JAMA 267:2067–2071, 1992

Felthous AR: The duty to warn or protect to prevent automobile accidents, in American Psychiatric Press Review of Clinical Psychiatry and the Law, Vol 1. Edited by Simon RI. Washington, DC, American Psychiatric Press, 1990, pp 221–238

Greenberg SA, Shuman DW: Irreconcilable conflict between therapeutic and forensic roles. Journal of Professional Psychology: Research and Practice 28:50–56, 1997

Grisso T: Evaluating Competencies: Forensic Assessments and Instruments. New York, Plenum, 1986

Grisso T, Appelbaum PS: Comparison of standards for assessing patients' capacities to make treatment decisions. Am J Psychiatry 152:1033–1037, 1995a

Grisso T, Appelbaum PS: The MacArthur treatment competence study, III: abilities of patients to consent to psychiatric and medical treatments. Law Hum Behav 19:149–174, 1995b

Gutheil TG, Appelbaum PS: Substituted judgement and the physician's ethical dilemma: with special reference to the problem of the psychiatric patient. J Clin Psychiatry 41:303–305, 1980

Hoge SK, Jorgenson L, Goldstein N, et al: APA resource document: legal sanctions for mental health professional–patient sexual misconduct. Bull Am Acad Psychiatry Law 23:433–448, 1995

Johnson ID: Reports to the National Practitioner Data Bank. JAMA 265:407–411, 1991

Joint Commission on Accreditation of Healthcare Organizations: Comprehensive Accreditation Manual for Behavioral Healthcare Hospital Accreditation Standards PC 13.50. Oak Brook Terrace, IL, Joint Commission on Accreditation of Healthcare Organizations, 2006

Klein J, Onek J, Macbeth J: Seminar on Law in the Practice of Psychiatry. Washington, DC, Onek, Klein and Farr, 1983

LaPuma J, Orentlicher D, Moss RJ: Advance directives on admission: clinical implications and analysis of the Patient Self-Determination Act of 1990. JAMA 266:402–405, 1991

Lazarus JA, Sharfstein SS: Changes in the economics and ethics of health and mental health care, in American Psychiatric Press Review of Psychiatry, Vol 13. Edited by Oldham JM, Riba MB. Washington, DC, American Psychiatric Press, 1994, pp 389–413

Leong GB, Eth S, Silva JA: The psychotherapist as witness for the prosecution: the criminalization of *Tarasoff*. Am J Psychiatry 149:1011–1015, 1992

Link BG, Stueve A: Psychotic symptoms and the violent/illegal behavior of mental patients compared to community controls, in Violence and Mental Disorder: Developments in Risk Assessment. Edited by Monahan J, Steadman H. Chicago, IL, University of Chicago Press, 1994, pp 137–159

Malcolm JG: Informed consent in the practice of psychiatry, in American Psychiatric Press Review of Clinical Psychiatry and the Law, Vol 3. Edited by Simon RI. Washington, DC, American Psychiatric Press, 1992, pp 223–281

McGarry AL: Pathological gambling: a new insanity defense. Bull Am Acad Psychiatry Law 11:301–308, 1983

Melton GB, Petrila J, Poythress NG, et al: Psychological Evaluations for the Courts: A Handbook for Mental Health Professionals and Lawyers, 2nd Edition. New York, Guilford, 1997

Meyer DJ, Simon RI: Split treatment: clarity between psychiatrists and psychotherapists. Psychiatr Ann 29:241–245, 327–332, 1999

Mill JS: On liberty (1859), in The World in Literature. Atlanta, GA, Scott, Foresman, 1951, pp 316–333

Mishkin B: Decisions in Hospice. Arlington, VA, National Hospice Organization, 1985

Mishkin B: Determining the capacity for making health care decisions, in Issues in Geriatric Psychiatry (Advances in Psychosomatic Medicine, Vol 19). Edited by Billig N, Rabins PV. Basel, Switzerland, S Karger, 1989, pp 151–166

Monahan J, Steadman H (eds): Violence and Mental Disorder: Developments in Risk Assessment. Chicago, IL, University of Chicago Press, 1994

Monahan J, Steadman HJ, Silver E, et al: Rethinking Risk Assessment: The MacArthur

Study of Mental Disorder and Violence. New York, Oxford University Press, 2001

The National Practitioner Data Bank and MCOs, in Psychiatric Practice and Managed Care, Vol 5, No 5. Washington, DC, American Psychiatric Association, 1999, pp 1, 9–10

Orentlicher D: The illusion of patient choice in end-of-life decisions. JAMA 267:2101–2104, 1992

Overman W Jr, Stoudemire A: Guidelines for legal and financial counseling of Alzheimer's disease patients and their families. Am J Psychiatry 145:1495–1500, 1988

Perlin ML: Mental Disability Law: Civil and Criminal, Vol 3. Charlottesville, VA, Michie, 1989

Perr IN: The clinical considerations of medication refusal. Legal Aspects of Psychiatric Practice 1:5–8, 1984

President's Commission for the Study of Ethical Problems in Medicine and Biomedical and Behavioral Research: Making Health Care Decisions, Vol 1: A Report on the Ethical and Legal Implications of Informed Consent in the Patient–Practitioner Relationship. Washington, DC, U.S. Government Printing Office, October 1982

Regan M: Protective services for the elderly: commitment, guardianship, and alternatives. William Mary Law Rev 13:569–573, 1972

Reich J, Wells J: Psychiatric diagnosis and competency to stand trial. Compr Psychiatry 26:421–432, 1985

Robertson ED: Is "substituted judgment" a valid legal concept? Issues Law Med 5:197–214, 1989

Robertson JD: The trial of a suicide case, in American Psychiatric Press Review of Clinical Psychiatry and the Law, Vol 2. Edited by Simon RI. Washington, DC, American Psychiatric Press, 1991, pp 423–441

Rogers R, Shuman DW: Fundamentals of Forensic Practice: Mental Health and Criminal Law. New York, Springer, 2005

Rosenthal RJ, Lorenz VC: The pathological gambler as criminal offender: comments on the evaluation and treatment. Psychiatr Clin North Am 15:647–660, 1992

Roth LH: Informed consent and its applicability for psychiatry, in Psychiatry, Vol 3. Edited by

Cavenar JO. Philadelphia, PA, JB Lippincott, 1985, pp 1–17

Rutter P: Sex in the Forbidden Zone: When Therapists, Doctors, Clergy, Teachers and Other Men in Power Betray Women's Trust. Los Angeles, CA, JP Tarcher, 1989

Sales B, Powell DM, Van Duizend R: Disabled Persons and the Law: State Legislative Issues. New York, Plenum, 1982, p 461

Schoener GR, Milgrom JH, Gonsiorek JC, et al: Psychotherapists' Sexual Involvement With Clients. Minneapolis, MN, Walk-In Counseling Center, 1989

Schreiber J, Roesch R, Golding S: An evaluation of procedures for assessing competency to stand trial. Bull Am Acad Psychiatry Law 155:187–203, 1987

Sederer LI, Ellison J, Keyes C: Guidelines for prescribing psychiatrists in consultative, collaborative, and supervisory relationships. Psychiatr Serv 49:1197–1202, 1998

Shuman DW: Expertise in law, medicine, and health care. J Health Polit Policy Law 26:267–290, 2001

Shuman DW, Greenberg SA: Expert witnesses, the adversary system, and the voice of reason: reconciling impartiality and advocacy. Professional Psychology: Research and Practice. 34:219–224, 2003

Shuman DW, Weiner MF: The psychotherapist-patient privilege: a critical examination. Springfield, IL, Charles C Thomas, 1987

Simon RI: The psychiatrist as a fiduciary: avoiding the double agent role. Psychiatr Ann 17:622–626, 1987

Simon RI: Sexual exploitation of patients: how it begins before it happens. Psychiatr Ann 19:104–112, 1989

Simon RI: Psychological injury caused by boundary violation precursors to therapist-patient sex. Psychiatr Ann 21:614–619, 1991

Simon RI: Clinical Psychiatry and the Law, 2nd Edition. Washington, DC, American Psychiatric Press, 1992a

Simon RI: Clinical risk management of suicidal patients: assessing the unpredictable, in American Psychiatric Press Review of Clinical Psychiatry and the Law, Vol 3. Edited by Simon RI. Washington, DC, American Psychiatric Press, 1992b, pp 3–63

Simon RI: Treatment boundary violations: clinical, ethical, and legal considerations. Bull Am Acad Psychiatry Law 20:269–288, 1992c

Simon RI: Innovative psychiatric therapies and legal uncertainty: a survival guide for clinicians. Psychiatr Ann 23:473–479, 1993

Simon RI: Treatment boundaries in psychiatric practice, in Forensic Psychiatry: A Comprehensive Textbook. Edited by Rosner R. New York, Van Nostrand Reinhold, 1994

Simon RI: Clinical risk management of the rapid cycling bipolar patient. Harv Rev Psychiatry 4:245–254, 1997

Simon RI: Psychiatrists' duties in discharging sicker and potentially violent patients in the managed care era. Psychiatr Serv 49:62–67, 1998

Simon RI: The suicide prevention contract: clinical, legal and risk management issues. J Am Acad Psychiatry Law 27:445–450, 1999

Simon RI: Concise Guide to Psychiatry and the Law for Clinicians, 3rd Edition. Washington, DC, American Psychiatric Publishing, 2001

Simon RI: Suicide risk assessment: what is the standard of care? J Am Acad Psychiatry Law 30:340 344, 2002

Simon RI: Assessing and Managing Suicide Risk: Guidelines for Clinically Based Risk Management. Washington, DC, American Psychiatric Publishing, 2004

Simon RJ: The myth of "imminent" violence in psychiatry and the law. University of Cincinnati Law Review 75:631–644, 2006

Simon RI, Hales RE (eds): American Psychiatric Publishing Textbook of Suicide Assessment and Management. Washington, DC, American Psychiatric Publishing, 2006

Simon RI, Shuman DW (eds): Predicting the Past: The Retrospective Psychiatric Assessment of Mental States in Litigation. Washington, DC, American Psychiatric Publishing, 2002

Slovenko R: Assessing competency to stand trial. Psychiatr Ann 26:392–393, 397, 1995

Slovenko R: Psychotherapy and Confidentiality: Testimonial Privileged Communication, Breach of Confidentiality, and Reporting Duties. Springfield, IL, Charles C Thomas, 1998

Solnick PB: Proxy consent for incompetent nonterminally ill adult patients. J Leg Med 6:1–49, 1985

Strasburger LH: "Crudely, without any finesse": the defendant hears his psychiatric evaluation. Bull Am Acad Psychiatry Law 15:229–233, 1987

Strasburger LH, Jorgenson L, Randles R: Criminalization of psychotherapist–patient sex. Am J Psychiatry 148:859–863, 1991

Strasburger LH, Gutheil TG, Brodsky A: On wearing two hats: role conflict in serving as both psychotherapist and expert witness. Am J Psychiatry 154:448–456, 1997

Tardiff K: The past as prologue: assessment of future violence in individuals with a history of past violence, in Retrospective Assessment of Mental States in Litigation: Predicting the Past. Edited by Simon RI, Shuman DW. Washington, DC, American Psychiatric Publishing, 2002

Tischler GL: Utilization management of mental health services by private third parties. Am J Psychiatry 147:967–973, 1990

Tranel D: Functional neuroanatomy: neuropsychological correlates of cortical and subcortical damage, in The American Psychiatric Press Textbook of Neuropsychiatry, 2nd Edition. Edited by Yudofsky SC, Hales RE. Washington, DC, American Psychiatric Press, 1992, pp 70–75

U.S. Department of Health and Human Services: The Legal Status of Adolescents 1980. Washington, DC, U.S. Department of Health and Human Services, 1981

Walzer RS: Impaired physicians: an overview and update of legal issues. J Leg Med 11:131–198, 1990

Weir RF, Gostin L: Decisions to abate life-sustaining treatment for nonautonomous patients: ethical standards and legal liability for physicians after Cruzan. JAMA 264:1846–1853, 1990

Why are liability premiums rising? Psychiatric News, June 21, 1996, pp 1, 24–25

Wickizer TM, Lessler D, Travis KM: Controlling inpatient psychiatric utilization through managed care. Am J Psychiatry 153:339–345, 1996

Widiger TA, Trull TJ: Personality disorders and violence, in Violence and Mental Disorder: Developments in Risk Assessment. Edited by Monahan J, Steadman H. Chicago, IL, University of Chicago Press, 1994, pp 203–226

Woodward B, Duckworth K, Gutheil TG: The pharmacotherapist-psychotherapist collaboration, in Annual Review of Psychiatry, Vol 12. Edited by Oldham J. Washington, DC, American Psychiatric Press, 1993

Zeldow PB, Taub HA: Evaluating psychiatric discharge and aftercare in a VA medical center. Hosp Community Psychiatry 32:57–58, 1981

Legal Citations

Aponte v. United States, 582 F.Supp 65 (D PR 1984)

Bartling v. Superior Court, 163 Cal.App.3d 186, 209 Cal.Rptr. 220 (1984)

Bethea v. United States, 365 A.2d 64 (D.C. App. 1976), cert. denied, 433 U.S. 911 (1977)

Bouvia v. Superior Court, 179 Cal.App. 3d 1127, 225 Cal.Rptr. 297 (1986)

Callan v. Norland, 114 Ill.App.3d 196, 448 N.E.2d 651 (1983)

Canterbury v. Spence, 464 F.2d 772 (D.C. Cir. 1972), cert denied, Spence v. Canterbury, 409 U.S. 1064 (1972)

Chaires v. St. John's Episcopal Hospital, No. 808/75 N.Y. Cty.Sup.Ct (N.Y. Feb 21, 1984)

Clifford v. United States, No 82-5002 USDC (SD 1985)

Comprehensive Crime Control Act (CCCA), P.L. 98–473, 1984

Cruzan v. Director, Missouri Department of Health, 497 U.S. 261 (1990)

Doerr v. Hurley Medical Center, No 82–674–39 NM Mich Aug (1984)

Dusky v. United States, 362 U.S. 402 (1960)

Evans v. United States, 883 F.Supp. 124 (SD Miss 1995)

Ford v. Wainwright, 477 US 399 (1986)

Frasier v. Department of Health and Human Resources, 500 So.2d 858, 864 (La. Ct. App. 1986)

Garamella v. New York Medical College, 23 F.Supp. 2d 167 (D Conn 1998)

Gowan v. United States, 601 F.Supp. 1297 (D. Or. 1985)

Green v. Ross, 691 So.2d 542 (Fla. 2d DCA 1997)

Hofflander v. St. Catherine's Hospital, 664 N.W.2d 545 (WI 2003)

In re Boyer, 636 P.2d 1085, 1089 (Utah 1981)

In re Conroy, 98 N.J. 321, 486 A.2d 1209, 1222–23 (1985)

In re Farrell, 108 N.J. 335, 529 A.2d 404 (1987)

In re Jobes, 108 N.J. 394, 529 A.2d 434 (1987)

In re M.B., 2006 WL 721511, Court of Appeals N.Y., Mar 23, 2006

In re Peter, 108 N.J. 365, 529 A.2d 419 (1987)

In re Quinlan, 70 N.J. 10, 355 A.2d 647, cert denied, 429 U.S. 922 (1976)

In the Guardianship of John Roe, 411 Mass. 666 (1992)

Jaffee v. Redmond, 518 U.S. 1 (1996)

J.S. v. R.T., 714 A.2d 924 (N.J. 1998)

Karasik v. Bird, 98 A.D.2d 359, 470 N.Y.S.2d 605 (1984)

Kilgore v. County of Santa Clara, No. 397–525 (Santa Clara Cty. Super. Ct. Cal. 1982)

Long v. Jaszczak, 688 N.W.2d 173 (N.D. 2004)

Meek v. City of Loveland, 85 Colo. 346, 276 P. 30 (1929)

Minn. Stat. Ann. § 148A.02 (West 2005)

Minn. Stat. Ann. § 609.344 (West 2005)

M'Naughten's case. 10 Cl. & Fin. 200, 8 Eng. Rep 718 (HL 1843)

Model Penal Code (1962)

Moran v. Botsford General Hospital, No. l 81–225–533, Wayne Cty. Cir. Ct. (MI Oct. 1, 1984)

Muldrow v. Re-Direct, Inc., 397 F.Supp.2d 1 (D.D.C. 2005)

Natanson v. Kline, 186 Kan. 393, 350 P.2d. 1093 (1960)

Parham v. J.R., 442 U.S. 584 (1979)

Penry v. Lynaugh, 492 U.S. 302 (1989)

People v. Rose, 573 N.W.2d 765 (Neb 1998)

Ramon v. Farr, 770 P.2d 131 (Utah 1989)

Rennie v. Klein, 462 F.Supp. 1131 (D. N.J. 1978), remanded, 476 F.Supp. 1294 (D. N.J. 1979), aff'd in part, modified in part and remanded, 653 F.2d 836 (3d. Cir. 1980), vacated and remanded, 458 U.S. 1119 (1982), 720 F.2d 266 (3rd Cir. 1983)

Restatement [Second] of Torts 315(a) (1965)

Scaria v. St. Paul Fire and Marine Ins. Co., 68 Wis.2d 1, 227 N.W.2d 647 (1975)

Schloendorff v. Society of New York Hospital, 211 N.Y. 125, 105 N.E. 92 (1914), overruled, Bing v. Thunig, 2 N.Y.2d 656, 143 N.E.2d 3, 163 N.Y.S.2d 3 (1957)

Speer v. United States, 512 F.Supp. 670 (N.D. Tex. 1981), aff'd, Speer v. United States, 675 F.2d 100 (5th Cir. 1982)

Stepakoff v. Kantar, 473 N.E.2d 1131 (Mass. 1985)

Stone v. Proctor, 259 N.C. 633, 131 S.E.2d 297 (1963)

Tarasoff v. Regents of the University of California, 17 Cal.3d 425, 551 P.2d 334; 131 Cal. Rptr. 14 (1976)

Tennard v. Dretke, 542 U.S. 274 (2004)

Thapar v. Zezulka, 944 S.W.2d 635 (Tex. 1999)

Touchette v. Ganal, 922 P.2d 347 (Haw. 1996)

Truman v. Thomas, 27 Cal.3d 285, 611 P.2d 902, 165 Cal. Rptr. 308 (1980)

Tune v. Walter Reed Army Medical Hospital, 602 F.Supp. 1452 (D.D.C. 1985)

Uniform Guardianship and Protective Proceedings Act (1997)

Union Pacific Realty Co. v. Botsford, 141 U.S. 250, 251 (1891)

United States v. Brawner, 471 F.2d 969 (D.C. Cir. 1972), superseded by statute, see Shannon v. United States, 512 U.S. 573 (1994)

United States v. David, 511 F.2d 355 (D.C. Cir. 1975)

Washington v. Harper, 494 U.S. 210 (1990)

Wilson v. Lehman, 379 S.W.2d 478, 479 (Ky. 1964)

Wilson v. United States, 391 F.2d 460, 463 (D.C. Cir. 1968)

Witherell v. Weimer, 148 Ill. App.3d 32, 499 N.E.2d 46 (1986), rev'd on other grounds, 118 Ill. 2d 515 N.E.2d 68 (1987)

Wright v. State, No. 83-5035 Orleans Parish Civ. Dist. Ct. (LA April 1986)

22

SUICIDE

Robert I. Simon, M.D.

There are two kinds of clinical psychiatrists: those who have had patient suicides, and those who will have patient suicides. Every patient suicide is also a tragedy for the clinician and for the suicide survivors. Patient suicide is an occupational hazard of psychiatric practice, accompanied by increased malpractice liability exposure. The only way to avoid patient suicide attempts or patient suicides is to not treat patients.

Suicide Risk Assessment

Suicide risk assessment is a core competency that psychiatrists are expected to acquire during their residency training (Scheiber et al. 2003). The purpose of suicide risk assessment is to identify modifiable, treatable risk and protective factors that inform the patient's treatment and safety management needs.

A standard of care does not exist for the prediction of suicide (Pokorny 1983, 1993). Attempting to predict who will commit suicide creates false-positive and false-negative predictions (R.I. Simon 2004). The standard of care for suicide risk assessment is an elusive concept (R.I. Simon and Shuman 2006). An examination of what constitutes the standard of care for suicide risk assessment reveals differences of opinion among competent clinicians, academics, and researchers who testify as experts in suicide cases. Clinicians are expected to perform reasonable suicide risk assessments (R.I. Simon 2002). The bedeviling question is—what is reasonable?

A number of suicide risk assessment methods have been proposed (Beck et al. 1998; Clark and Fawcett 1999; Jacobs et al. 1999; Linehan 1993; Mays 2004; Rudd et al. 2001; Shea 2004; R.I. Simon 2004). No suicide risk assessment method has been empirically tested for reliability and validity (Busch et al. 1993). Clinicians can create their own systematic suicide risk assessment methodology reflecting their training, clinical experience, and knowledge of the evidence-based psychiatric literature. A systematic suicide risk assessment, whichever method is used, should more than meet the standard of care.

Systematic suicide risk assessment encourages the clinician to gather sufficient information to perform a competent assessment. Risk and protective factors are assessed dimensionally as low, moderate, or high according to the clinical presentation of the patient. An overall assessment of the level of suicide risk is determined. The assessment of suicide risk and protective factors creates an individualized mosaic of the patient's overall suicide risk. The clinician assesses the acute high-risk suicide factors, especially the response to treatment, over the patient's clinical course. Protective factors are also monitored. *Acute* is defined as the magnitude and intensity of the symptom, for example, early-morning waking versus debilitating global insomnia. A high-risk factor is supported by an evidence-based strong association with suicide.

The suicide risk assessment method in Table 22–1 is one way of conceptualizing risk assessment. It is *not* intended to be used as a suicide risk assessment form or protocol. Obviously, suicidal patients may present with only a few risk factors or with risk factors not identified on a form or protocol. No form or

Table 22–1. Systematic suicide risk assessment: conceptual model

Assessment factors[a]	Risk	Protective
Individual		
Unique clinical features		
Clinical		
Current attempt (lethality)		
Panic attacks[b]		
Psychic anxiety[b]		
Loss of pleasure and interest[b]		
Alcohol abuse[b]		
Depressive turmoil (mixed states)[b]		
Diminished concentration[b]		
Global insomnia[b]		
Suicide plan		
Suicidal ideation (command hallucinations)[c]		
Suicide intent[c]		
Hopelessness[c]		
Prior attempts (lethality)[c]		
Therapeutic alliance		
Psychiatric diagnoses (Axis I and Axis II)		
Symptom severity		
Comorbidity		
Recent discharge from psychiatric hospital		
Drug abuse		
Impulsivity		
Agitation		
Physical illness		
Family history of mental illness (suicide)		
Mental competency		

Table 22–1. Systematic suicide risk assessment: conceptual model *(continued)*

Assessment factors[a]	Risk	Protective
Interpersonal relations		
Work or school		
Family		
Spouse or partner		
Children		
Situational		
Living circumstances		
Employment or school status		
Financial status		
Availability of guns		
Managed care setting		
Statistical		
Age		
Gender		
Marital status		
Race		
Overall risk ratings[d]		

[a]Rate risk and protective factors present as low (L), moderate (M), high (H), nonfactor (0), or range (e.g., L–M, M–H).
[b]Risk factors statistically significant within 1 year of assessment (Fawcett et al. 1990).
[c]Associated with suicide 2–10 years following assessment (Fawcett et al. 1990).
[d]Judge overall suicide risk as low, moderate, high, or a range of risk.

protocol can encompass all possible risk factors. Using stand-alone risk assessment forms may lead to robotic assessments that fail to capture the highly individual risk and protective factors presented by every patient at risk for suicide. Invariably, crucial risk factors are omitted.

Standardized suicide risk prediction scales do not identify which patient will attempt or commit suicide (Busch et al. 1993). Single scores on suicide risk assessment scales and inventories should not be the sole basis for clinical decision making. Structured or semistructured suicide scales may complement but are not a substitute for systematic suicide risk assessment (American Psychiatric Association 2003). Malone et al. (1995b), however, found that semistructured screening instruments improved routine clinical assessments in the documentation and detec-

tion of lifetime suicidal behaviors. Oquendo et al. (2003) discussed the advantages and limitations of research instruments in assessing suicide risk. The standard of care does not require that specific psychological tests or checklists be used as part of systematic suicide risk assessment (Bongar et al. 1992).

The standard of care requires psychiatrists and other mental health professionals to reasonably assess patients at risk for suicide. It is foreseeable that failing to perform a reasonable suicide risk assessment can harm the patient. Suicide risk assessment is an integral part of the psychiatric examination. Systematic suicide risk assessment that evaluates both risk and protective factors should exceed any reasonable definition of "adequate" (G.E. Simon et al. 2006). Systematic suicide assessment is an inductive process, reasoning from specific patient data to arrive at a clinical judgment that informs treatment and safety management.

A certain analogy exists between suicide risk assessment and weather forecasting (Monahan and Steadman 1996; R.I. Simon 1992). Suicide risk assessments are "here and now" determinations made for the purpose of treatment and management; they are not predictions. Moreover, there are no suicide risk factors for "imminent" suicide. *Imminence* is another word for a short-term prediction that is not supported by evidence-based research (R.I. Simon 2006). Like weather forecasts, suicide risk assessments require frequent updating. The analogy, however, is imperfect. Weather forecasters can predict the weather with reasonable accuracy, but they cannot change it. Psychiatrists cannot predict who will commit suicide, but they can reduce or even eliminate the threat of suicide through treatment and safety management.

Professional organizations have developed practice guidelines for the assessment and management of individuals at risk for suicide. The American Academy of Child and Adolescent Psychiatry (2001) has published practice parameters for children and adolescents with suicidal behaviors. The American Psychiatric Association (2003) has also developed practice guidelines for the treatment and management of patients at suicide risk.

Suicide Risk and Protective Factors

Risk Factors

Suicide is the result of multifaceted determinants, including diagnostic (psychiatric and medical), psychodynamic, genetic, familial, occupational, environmental, social, cultural, and contextual factors. No pathognomonic risk factors exist. A single risk factor does not have the statistical power upon which to base a suicide risk assessment. General risk assessment factors have been identi-

fied through retrospective community-based psychological autopsies and studies of completed suicides (Fawcett et al. 1993). To be useful, general risk factors must be adapted to the clinical presentation of the individual patient. Evidence-based research finds that high-risk factors associated with attempted suicide in adults include depression, prior suicide attempts, hopelessness, suicidal ideation, alcohol abuse, cocaine abuse, and recent loss of an important relationship (Murphy et al. 1992).

Short-term suicide risk factors derived from a 10-year prospective study of patients with affective disorders were statistically significant within 1 year of assessment (Fawcett et al. 1990). The short-term risk factors were panic attacks, psychic anxiety, loss of pleasure and interest, moderate alcohol abuse, depressive turmoil, diminished concentration, and global insomnia. Short-term risk factors were predominantly severe, anxiety driven, and treatable by a variety of drugs (Fawcett 2001). Acute suicide risk factors are usually treatable or modifiable. For example, treating anxiety or severe insomnia in a depressed patient can rapidly lower suicide risk. Modifying just a few acute risk factors can significantly reduce a patient's risk for suicide (Table 22–2).

Long-term suicide risk factors in patients with major affective disorders were associated with suicides completed 2–10 years after assessment (Fawcett et al. 1990). Long-term risk factors include suicidal ideation, suicidal intent, severe hopelessness, and prior suicide attempts.

Clarity of diagnosis is essential in suicide risk assessment. All mental disorders except mental retardation are associated with an increased risk of suicide. Harris and Barraclough (1997) abstracted 249 reports from the medical literature on the mortality of mental disorders. They compared the observed number of suicides with the expected rate. A standardized mortality ratio (SMR) was calculated for each disorder. The SMR determines the relative risk of suicide for a partic-

Table 22–2. Examples of modifiable and treatable suicide risk factors

Depression	Impulsivity
Anxiety	Agitation
Panic attacks	Physical illness
Psychosis	Difficult situations
Sleep disorders	(e.g., family, work)
Substance abuse	Lethal means
Command hallucinations	(e.g., guns, drugs)

Source. Reprinted from Simon RI: *Assessing and Managing Suicide Risk: Guidelines for Clinically Based Risk Management.* Washington, DC, American Psychiatric Publishing, 2004, p. 26.

ular disorder compared with the expected rate in the general population. It is calculated by dividing the observed mortality by the expected mortality (Table 22–3).

Patients with Axis I psychiatric disorders such as schizophrenia, anxiety disorders, major affective disorders, and substance abuse disorders (especially alcohol) often present with acute (state) suicide risk factors. Sareen et al. (2005) demonstrated that a preexisting anxiety disorder is an independent risk factor for the onset of suicidal ideation and attempts. Patients with Axis II disorders often display chronic (trait) suicide risk factors. Exacerbation of a personality disorder or comorbidity with an Axis I disorder (including substance abuse) can transform a chronic suicide risk factor into an acute factor. Suicide risk increases with the total number of risk factors, providing a quasi-quantitative dimension to suicide risk assessment (Murphy et al. 1992).

Personality disorder, recent negative life events, and Axis I comorbidity were found in a large sample of suicides (Heikkinen et al. 1997). Recent stressful life events, including workplace problems, family strife, unemployment, and financial trouble, were highly represented among patients with personality disorder. Personality disorders associated with depressive symptoms and substance abuse disorders are highly represented among patients who complete suicide (Isometsa et al. 1996).

Table 22–3. Suicide risk associated with various mental and physical disorders

Disorder	Standardized mortality ratio[a]
Eating disorders	23.14
Major depression	20.35
Sedative abuse	20.34
Mixed drug abuse	19.23
Bipolar disorder	15.05
Opioid abuse	14.00
Dysthymia	12.12
Obsessive-compulsive disorder	11.54
Panic disorder	10.00
Schizophrenia	8.45
Personality disorders	7.08
AIDS	6.58
Alcohol abuse	5.86
Epilepsy	5.11
Child and adolescent psychiatric	4.73
Cannabis abuse	3.85
Spinal cord injury	3.82
Neuroses	3.72
Brain injury	3.50
Huntington's chorea	2.90
Multiple sclerosis	2.36
Malignant neoplasms	1.80
Mental retardation	0.88

[a]Standardized mortality ratio is calculated by dividing observed mortality by expected mortality.

Source. Adapted from Harris and Barraclough 1997.

Patients with personality disorders have a sevenfold increased risk of suicide compared with the general population (Harris and Barraclough 1997). Cluster B personality disorders, especially borderline and antisocial personality disorders, place patients at increased risk for suicide (Duberstein and Conwell 1997). In borderline patients, impulsivity was associated with a high number of suicide attempts, after controlling for substance abuse and a lifetime diagnosis of depressive disorder (Brodsky et al. 1997). Impulsivity can be assessed clinically by asking patients about violent rages, assaultive behaviors, arrests, destruction of property, spending sprees, speeding tickets, sexual indiscretions, and other indicia of poor impulse control.

The lifetime suicide rate for schizophrenia is between 9% and 13%. The lifetime rate for suicide attempts is between 20% and 40%. The estimated number of suicides annually in the United States among schizophrenic patients is 3,600, or 12% of total suicides. Suicide is the leading cause of death among persons with schizophrenia who are younger than 35 years (Meltzer 2001). Suicide tends to occur in the early stages of a schizophrenic illness and during acute exacerbations (Meltzer 2001). Suicide remains a risk throughout the individual's life cycle. Palmer et al. (2005), in a reexamination of the psychiatric literature, estimated that 4.9% of schizophrenic patients will complete suicide, usually near the onset of illness. Recent studies have found an increased rate of suicide among patients with psychotic disorders (Radomsky et al. 1999; Warman et al. 2004). No differences exist in rates of suicide between depressed patients with and without melancholic features (Kessing 2003).

Prior suicide attempts by any method had the highest SMR of 38.36. Suicide risk was highest in the 2 years after the first attempt (Harris and Barraclough 1997). Between 7% and 12% of patients who make suicide attempts complete suicide within 10 years. Thus, a suicide attempt is a significant risk factor for suicide. Most suicides, however, occur in patients with no prior history of attempts (Malone et al. 1995a).

Suicidal ideation is an important risk factor. Suicidal *ideation* should be differentiated from suicide *intent. Suicidal ideation* can be passive, fleeting, intermittent, active, and intense, with or without the intent to die. *Suicide intent* is the subjective expectation and desire to die by a self-destructive act. *Lethality* refers to the danger to life posed by a suicide method or act. An individual who takes 10 aspirins in the mistaken belief that he or she will die forms the intent to complete suicide even though the method is not lethal. A person who accidentally dies by hanging, as in autoerotic asphyxia, does not intend to die.

In the National Comorbidity Survey, the transition from suicide ideation to suicide plan was 34% and from plan to attempt was 72% (Kessler et al. 1999). The transition from suicide ideation to an unplanned attempt was 26%. Approximately 90% of unplanned and 60% of planned first attempts occurred within 1 year of the onset of suicide ideation. Mann et al. (1999) found that the severity of suicidal ideation is an indicator of risk for attempting suicide. Beck et al. (1990) discovered that when patients were asked about suicidal ideation at its worst point, patients with higher scores were 14 times more likely to complete suicide than patients with lower scores.

Approximately 25% of patients who are at risk for suicide do not admit having suicidal ideation to clinicians but do tell their families (Robins 1981). When patients withhold permission to speak with families, the psychiatrist can listen to families without violating confidentiality. Hall et al. (1999) found that 69 of 100 patients had only fleeting or no suicidal thoughts before they made a suicide attempt. No patient reported a specific plan before making an impulsive suicide attempt. A prior suicide attempt had not occurred in 67% of the patients. Patients who are determined to commit suicide regard the psychiatrist and other mental health professionals as the enemy (Resnick 2002). Thus, a patient's denial of suicidal ideation requires additional assessment for the presence of other suicide risk factors.

A family history of mental illness, especially of suicide, is a significant suicide risk factor. The offspring of patients with mood disorders who attempt suicide are at a markedly increased risk for suicide (Brent et al. 2002). Genetic and familial transmission of suicide risk is independent of the transmission of psychiatric illnesses (Brent et al. 1996). The Copenhagen Adoption Study showed that adoptees who completed suicide had a sixfold increased rate of suicide among their biological relatives compared with matched adoptees who did not commit suicide (Schulsinger et al. 1979). Trémeau et al. (2005) found that a family history of suicide was associated with an increased risk for suicide attempt, with lethality of method, with repeated attempts, and with the number of attempts. Mann et al. (1999) proposed a stress–diathesis model of suicide behavior. For suicide to occur, a trigger (stress)—usually a psychiatric disorder—and a preexisting vulnerability to suicidal behaviors (diathesis) must both be present. The neurobiology and genetics of suicide were reviewed by Mann et al. (2001).

Protective Factors

A competent suicide risk assessment evaluates both risk and protective factors (R.I. Simon 2004). The self-report Reasons for Living Inventory measures beliefs that may act as preventive factors against suicide (Linehan et al. 1983). The preventive factors include survival and coping skills, responsibility to family, child-related concerns, fear of suicide, fear of social disapproval, and moral/religious values. Other protective factors may include availability and community access to effective clinical care for mental, physical, and substance abuse disorders; adherence with recommended treatments; family and community support; life-affirming cultural values that discourage suicide; skills in problem solving and nonviolent conflict resolution; children at home; and pregnancy (Goldsmith et al. 2001). The inventory can be

used to monitor patients at chronic high suicide risk and to assess the effectiveness of treatment. Dervic et al. (2004) found that religious affiliation was associated with less suicide behavior in depressed patients. Severely depressed patients, however, may feel angry and abandoned by God or that "God will understand," increasing their risk of suicide.

The presence of a therapeutic alliance can be an important protective factor against suicide (R.I. Simon 1998). The therapeutic alliance is influenced by a number of factors, especially the nature and severity of the patient's mental disorder. It can change from session to session. It cannot be assumed, therefore, that a therapeutic alliance will remain a protective factor between sessions. Clinicians are shocked and bewildered when a patient with whom they believed they had a sustaining therapeutic alliance attempts or completes suicide between sessions. The absence of a therapeutic alliance with a patient at risk for suicide is a significant risk factor (R.I. Simon 2004).

Protective factors, like risk factors, vary with the clinical presentation of the individual patient at suicide risk. An ebb and flow exists between risk and protective factors. Protective factors are easier for patients to talk about and thus tend to be overvalued by the patient and the clinician. Protective factors can be overcome, however, by the acuteness and severity of the patient's illness. Identification and marshaling of protective factors are important aspects of patient discharge planning.

Using Patterns to Assess Risk

Patients display distinctive suicide risk and protective factors. Suicide patterns can be identified by obtaining a detailed history of the patient's past suicide crises or attempts. Understanding a patient's psychodynamic responses to past and current life stressors is also important. Identifying a patient's recurrent prodromal symptomatology provides the clinician with insight in treating and managing the patient's current clinical condition.

A suicide attempt, especially if recent, may be a rehearsal for completed suicide. Although a patient may repeat the method of prior attempts, there is no assurance that a subsequent attempt will use the same methods. Isometsa and Lonnqvist (1998) found that 82% of suicide attempters used at least two different methods in subsequent suicide attempts and completions. Sixty-two percent of males and 38% of females died in their first attempt. The risk of suicide is highest during the first year after a suicide attempt.

Treatment

Treatment of the patient at risk for suicide requires a full commitment of time and effort by the clinician. A realistic self-appraisal should help the clinician decide whether such a commitment can be made. The treatment of patients at risk for suicide can be emotionally taxing and professionally threatening. Some clinicians decline to treat suicidal patients, if at all possible. Countertransference reactions often occur during the treatment of suicidal patients; these reactions need to be identified and constructively managed so as not to interfere with treatment. Anger, despair, frustration, hopelessness, hate, and a threat to one's competence are some of the feelings evoked in clinicians (Gabbard and Allison 2006). Acting as a savior and attempting to reparent the patient are countertransference traps. Clinicians must be able to effectively manage the inevitable anxieties and vicissitudes that arise in the treatment of suicidal patients.

Psychotherapies

Psychotherapies have an essential role in the treatment and management of patients at risk for suicide. Evidence-based research has identified psychotherapeutic treatments that reduce the risk of suicide attempts or completions in psychiatric patients. In a randomized, controlled trial, cognitive therapy was found effective in preventing suicide attempts for adults who had recently attempted suicide (Brown et al. 2005).

Linehan et al. (2006) demonstrated, in a 2-year randomized, controlled trial, that dialectical behavior therapy (DBT) was uniquely effective in reducing suicide attempts. In comparison with therapy by experts for suicidal behaviors and borderline personality disorder, DBT was associated with better outcomes during a 2-year treatment and follow-up period.

Guthrie et al. (2001, 2003) randomly assigned 119 patients who were seen in the emergency department after deliberate self-poisoning to either psychodynamic interpersonal therapy or treatment as usual (outpatient follow-up by a general practitioner). The patients who received therapy experienced a significantly greater reduction in suicidal ideation at a 6-month follow-up as compared with the control subjects. Also, they were less likely to report repeat self-harm attempts.

Treatment of borderline personality disorder using a randomized, controlled trial of psychodynamically based partial hospitalization demonstrated dramatic reductions in suicide behavior (Bateman and Fonagy 2000, 2004). Ninety-five percent of the sample of 39 borderline patients attempted suicide in the 6 months before the beginning of the study. Only 5.3% made attempts in the 6 months after treatment.

There is, however, limited evidence-based research for treatments that effectively prevent recurrent suicide attempts (Hawton et al. 2005). Nonetheless, psychosocial interventions are critically important in the treatment and management of suicidal patients.

Somatic Therapies

Lithium significantly decreases suicide risk in patients with bipolar disorder (Baldessarini et al. 2001). The risk of suicide attempts in bipolar patients taking lithium is more than eight times lower than among patients not taking the medication. Even with lithium, however, the completed suicide rate among bipolar patients is still 10 times higher than the suicide rate in the general population (Baldessarini 2003). The potential for lethal overdose should guide the quantity of lithium prescribed for a patient at risk for suicide. In some responders, antidepressant medication can have a significant therapeutic benefit within several weeks. Most responders require 8–12 weeks for maximum benefit following the initiation of antidepressant treatment (Gelenberg and Chesen 2000). Patients should be informed that an antidepressant requires time to become effective, and educating patients about the "ups and downs" in depressive symptoms that commonly occur in the course of improvement helps combat hopelessness. According to some researchers, other than prior suicide attempts, hopelessness is the best indication of suicide risk (Beck et al. 1985; Malone et al. 1995b). During this "down time," the patient must be carefully monitored.

Clozapine reduces the suicide attempt and completion rates in schizophrenia and schizoaffective disorder (Meltzer 2001; Meltzer et al. 2003). The U.S. Food and Drug Administration (FDA) has approved clozapine for the treatment of recurrent suicidal behaviors in patients with schizophrenia or schizoaffective disorder.

Suicidal ideation, intent, and plan in selected patients with mood and psychotic disorders are indications for electroconvulsive therapy (ECT), especially when alternative treatments are not appropriate or have not been effective (American Psychiatric Association 2001). ECT should be the treatment of choice when rapid results are needed for the patient at high risk for suicide for whom a delay would be life threatening. A rapid clinical response with reduction or resolution of suicidal behaviors often occurs with ECT, presumably by treating the underlying psychiatric disorder (Prudic and Sackheim 1999). A study by Kellner et al. (2005) showed that suicidal intent in depressed patients was rapidly relieved by ECT. The authors recommended that ECT be given earlier consideration rather than thought of as a last option.

There is little evidence that ECT imparts long-term beneficial effects on suicidal behaviors or completed suicide (Sharma 1999). Administration of inpatient ECT may be followed by outpatient maintenance ECT. The effectiveness ascribed to ECT can be difficult to distinguish from the coadministration of pharmacotherapy. As with any treatment, there is a certain percentage of patient nonresponders.

In 2004, the FDA began requiring black box warnings of increased suicide risk for children and adolescents with major depressive disorders and other psychiatric disorders during the first few months of treatment with selective serotonin reuptake inhibitors (SSRIs). In 2005, the FDA issued similar warnings for adults treated with antidepressants. Hammad et al. (2006) reviewed all placebo-controlled trials submitted to the FDA, consisting of 4,582 patients in 24 trials. The trial periods ranged from 4 to 16 weeks. They found that the use of antidepressant medications is associated with a "modestly" increased risk of suicide.

The FDA has told manufacturers of antidepressants to issue stronger warnings on their labels regarding the monitoring of both pediatric and adult patients for the emergence of suicidal ideation and the worsening of depression. Precursors to worsening depression and suicidal ideation include symptoms of activation syndrome such as anxiety, agitation, panic attacks, insomnia, irritability, hostility, impulsivity, akathisia, hypomania, and mania. Psychiatrists should document the rationale, including risk–benefit assessments, for prescribing an antidepressant drug to a child or adolescent. At a minimum, FDA monitoring requirements should be followed. Hopelessness and suicide may be averted by informing all patients and the parents of children and adolescents that activation symptoms can be a drug reaction, a worsening of the psychiatric disorder, or some combination of both. Close follow-up by the clinician is indicated according to the clinical needs of the patient. The practitioner's clinical experience, the consensus experience of colleagues, and case reports in the psychiatric literature are important guides to prescribing drugs for children and adolescents. For further discussion of antidepressant use in children and adolescents, see Ash (2006) and Kim et al. (2006).

A study by Gibbons et al. (2007) demonstrated an association between decreased SSRI prescriptions for children and adolescents and increased suicide cases in this population in the United States and Finland. SSRIs continue to be considered the first-line treatment for depression with associated suicidal behaviors. While psychiatrists wait for further studies to definitively settle the question, the risks and benefits of SSRIs should be thoroughly explained (with documentation) to patients and their families, according to the current state of scientific knowledge.

The psychiatrist's clinical focus must necessarily be on treating the patient's current condition. Treatment of the patient's current episode of psychiatric illness is frequently successful in decreasing or eliminating the associated acute risk of suicide. Factors unrelated to the efficacy of psychiatric treatment also affect suicide mortality rates in the long run. For example, Ostamo and Lonnqvist (2001), in a 5-year follow-up study of patients treated in hospitals after suicide attempts, found an increase in mortality from suicide, homicide, and other causes. The nature of the patient, the efficacy of treatments, and the adherence and access to or availability of mental health resources are central to determining treatment outcomes.

Collaborative or Split Treatment

Assessment and management of patients at risk for suicide are especially challenging in collaborative or split-treatment arrangements. The hospital length of stay is brief for most psychiatric patients. Patients referred to partial hospitalization are discharged rapidly to outpatient split treatment.

The medication management of patients at risk for suicide who are in split treatment requires close monitoring. Psychiatrists owe a duty of care to their patients for the duration of their drug prescriptions. The patient may be given a 90-day prescription that can be mailed to a pharmacy. Such "mail-away" bulk prescriptions lower the cost of medication. In addition, the patient's copayment is reduced from once a month to once every 90 days. However, the prescription of large quantities of medications for patients at risk for suicide can be lethal. For example, a patient is prescribed 1,000 mg/day of an anticonvulsant mood stabilizer; 1,500 mg/day of lithium; 15 mg/day of an atypical antipsychotic; and 900 mg/day of sleep medication. A 90-day prescription or a 30-day prescription renewable three times gives the patient 90,000 mg of anticonvulsant mood stabilizer, 135,000 mg of lithium; 1,350 mg of an atypical antipsychotic, and 81,000 mg of sleep medication. Even a 30-day supply of these medications would be lethal. The potential lethality of the medications prescribed for the patient should be conveyed to the psychotherapist (Silk 2001).

Patients at risk for suicide commonly have more than one psychiatric diagnosis and often are taking several medications. If the patient is scheduled for a 15-minute medication check once every 30, 60, or 90 days, the risk for suicide may increase over this period. The psychiatrist must rely on the psychotherapist's assessment and management of suicide risk during the 90-day period. The "we are in this together" part of split treatment is negated unless frequent communication between psychiatrist and therapist is maintained according to the clinical needs of the patient. Close monitoring of patients at risk for suicide who are taking potentially lethal amounts of medication should be standard psychiatric practice (R.I. Simon 2004).

Safety Management

In the safety management of suicidal patients, the tension between providing safety and allowing freedom of movement creates uncertainty (R.I. Simon 2006). Clinicians also experience dissonance between the need to provide adequate supervision for patients at suicidal risk and the denial of insurance coverage by third-party payers for these services. As noted earlier, the only certainty is that effective treatment and safety management of the suicidal patient require the clinician's full commitment of time and effort.

Systematic suicide risk assessment informs the safety management of patients at risk for suicide. Patients who are determined to commit suicide will find a way (Fawcett et al. 2003). Fawcett et al. (2003), in a review of 76 inpatient suicides, found that 42 of these patients were on 15-minute checks. Nine percent of patients were on one-to-one observation or with a staff member at the time of suicide. Deception and lack of patient cooperation complicate safety assessments.

Gun safety management may be necessary. The psychiatrist usually asks a responsible family member to remove and secure guns and ammunition outside the home. Guns may also be kept by the suicidal patient in his or her car or office or at another location. The psychiatrist must receive a timely call-back from the responsible person confirming that the guns and ammunition have been removed and separately secured according to plan. A call-back is essential. The complex subject of gun safety management is discussed in detail elsewhere (R.I. Simon 2007).

Outpatients

The ability to exercise control over outpatients at suicide risk, including those attending partial hospitalization programs, is limited. In outpatient settings, patient safety is usually managed by clinical intervention such as increasing the frequency of visits, strengthening the therapeutic alliance, providing or adjusting medications, and involving family or other concerned persons in the treatment, if the patient permits. Voluntary or, if necessary, involuntary hospitalization remains an option for suicidal patients at high suicide risk who can no longer be safely treated as outpatients. In the managed care era, most suicidal patients at moderate suicide risk and even some patients at high risk are treated in outpatient settings.

Whether to hospitalize a patient can be a trying decision for the clinician. The decision is considerably more complicated when the need for hospitalization is clear but the patient refuses. The action that the clinician takes at this point is critical for the patient's treatment and for risk management.

The clinician, after systematic suicide risk assessment, may determine that the suicidal patient requires hospitalization. The risks and benefits of continuing outpatient treatment are weighed against the risks and benefits of hospitalization, and these are shared with the patient. If the patient agrees, arrangements for immediate hospitalization are made. The patient must go *directly* to the hospital, accompanied by a responsible person. The patient should not stop to do errands, get clothing, or make last-minute arrangements. A detour can provide the patient with the opportunity to attempt or to complete suicide. If the patient is driven to the hospital, an additional passenger may be needed to prevent the patient from jumping out of the car. In some cases, clinicians have accompanied the patient to the hospital. The clinician, however, has no legal duty to assume physical custody of the patient (Farwell v. Un 1990).

Involuntary Hospitalization

If the patient rejects the clinician's recommendation for hospitalization, the matter is immediately addressed as a treatment issue. Because the need for hospitalization is acute, a prolonged inquiry into the patient's reasons for rejecting the recommendation for hospitalization is not feasible. Furthermore, the therapeutic alliance may be strained. Consultation and referral are options for the clinician to consider, if time and the patient's condition permit. It is this situation that tries the professional and personal mettle of the clinician.

The uncompensated time required, the inconvenience, the disruption of the clinician's schedule, the possibility of a court appearance, and the fear of a lawsuit by the patient may dissuade the clinician from initiating involuntary hospitalization. However, failure to involuntarily hospitalize a patient judged to be at high risk for suicide who subsequently attempts or completes suicide may result in a malpractice suit against the clinician. State commitment statutes grant clinicians immunity from liability when they use reasonable judgment, follow statutory commitment procedures, and act in good faith.

Documenting suicide risk assessment and the rationale for involuntary hospitalization represents good clinical care and provides sound risk management. When involuntary hospitalization is sought on reasonable clinical grounds, it must be left to the courts to resolve uncertainty about commitment. The clinician's proper focus is the patient's treatment and safety.

Inpatients

There must be a rational nexus between patient autonomy in the hospital setting and the patient's diagnosis, treatment, and safety needs. With patients at risk for suicide, standard safety precautions must be observed where indicated, such as removal of shoelaces, belts, sharp objects, glass products, and even pillowcases that can be used for suffocation and other potentially lethal instruments. A thorough search for contraband is standard procedure on admission. Psychiatric units are usually fitted, at a minimum, with non-weight-bearing fixtures and shower curtain rods, very short cords for electrical beds (properly insulated), cordless telephones or telephones with safety cords, jump-proof windows, barricade-proof doors, and closed-circuit video cameras. The most common and available method of committing suicide by inpatients is strangulation, usually accomplished by a belt, articles of clothing, shoelaces, or a bedsheet hooked up to the patient's bed, door, or bathroom fix-

tures. Safe installation of plumbing pipes for toilets and use of solid ceilings are necessary to diminish the risk of hanging. The most dangerous place on the psychiatric unit is the patient's room, especially the bathroom. Seclusion rooms should have windows or audiovisual surveillance capability (Lieberman et al. 2004).

Determining safety precautions is complicated by court directives that require highly disturbed patients to be treated by the least restrictive means (R. I. Simon 2000). In *Johnson v. United States* (1976), the Court noted that an "open door" policy creates a higher potential for danger. The Court went on to say:

> Modern psychiatry has recognized the importance of making every effort to return a patient to an active and productive life. Thus, the patient is encouraged to develop his self-confidence by adjusting to the demands of everyday existence. Particularly because the prediction of danger is difficult, undue reliance on hospitalization might lead to prolonged incarceration of potentially useful members of society.

The tension between promoting individual freedom and preventing self-injury introduces an inherent uncertainty in the safety management of suicidal patients (Amchin et al. 1990). In malpractice suits, the individual facts of the case and the reasonableness of the staff's application of the open door policy are determinative.

Suicide Prevention Contracts

The suicide prevention contract has achieved wide acceptance, although no studies demonstrate that it is effective in preventing suicide (Stanford et al. 1994). The suicide prevention contract can increase patients' risk of suicide when used in place of adequate suicide risk assessments. Suicide risk assessment is a *process*, whereas contracts tend to be *events*. The suicide prevention contract goes by a variety of names, such as the "no-harm contract," the "no-suicide contract," or the "contract for safety." It is frequently used by mental health professionals in outpatient and inpatient settings and in hospital emergency departments. In managed care settings, a criterion for admission to an inpatient unit may be based on a patient's refusal to sign a suicide prevention contract. If the patient is willing to sign a no-harm contract, third-party payers may not authorize admission. Suicide prevention contracts are frequently used in nursing assessments (Egan 1997).

A suicide prevention contract is a clinical, not a legal, contract. It is a mutual understanding reached between the clinician and the patient regarding collaboration to prevent suicide. The trustworthiness of the arrangement is contingent upon many variables. The contract establishes that the patient is at risk of suicide but does not establish that suicide risk has been assessed.

Suicide prevention measures work best when a therapeutic alliance exists between the psychiatrist and patient. The therapeutic alliance is a dynamic, changeable interaction between the clinician and the patient that is influenced by the course of the patient's illness as well as situational and other factors. The therapeutic alliance that supports a patient's safety during one session may dissipate before a next scheduled session due to an acute exacerbation of the illness. The status of the therapeutic alliance should be assessed regularly and documented. The presence or absence of a therapeutic alliance can be a key preventive or suicide risk factor.

Suicide Aftermath

Suicide aftermath presents the clinician with conflicting tensions between maintaining patient confidentiality, providing support to the suicide survivors, and implementing risk management principles that limit liability exposure. After a patient's death, the duty to maintain confidentiality of the patient's record continues unless a court decision or statute provides otherwise. Careful documentation and maintenance of confidentiality of the patient's records provide a sound

defense in malpractice litigation, in administrative hearings, and in ethics proceedings.

Gutheil recommends family outreach by the clinician as crucial for devastated family members following a patient's suicide (T.G. Gutheil, personal communication, October 1989). This recommendation, which is based primarily on humanitarian concerns for survivors, has important risk management implications. Gutheil pointed out that "bad feelings" combined with a bad outcome often lead to litigation. The persons who lived with the patient before the suicide not only experience intense emotional pain currently but also shared it with the patient before death. Some lawsuits are filed because of the clinician's refusal to express, in some way, feelings of condolence, sympathy, and regret for the patient's death.

In Massachusetts, an "apology statute" exists that renders various benevolent human expressions such as condolences, regrets, and apologies "inadmissible as evidence of an admission of liability in a civil action" (Mass. Gen. Laws 1986). Slovenko (2002) noted that Texas and California enacted legislation similar to that in Massachusetts. The highest courts of Georgia and Vermont provided apology protection by judicial opinions in 1992. Despite the enactment of legislation regarding apologies, Regehr and Gutheil (2002) stated that "the current empirical evidence is insufficiently solid to support the proposition that apology by oppressors, perpetrators, and a defendant is a panacea leading to healing of trauma under all circumstances" (pp. 429–430).

Risk Management

Risk management is a reality of psychiatric practice, especially in the assessment and management of patients at risk for suicide. Many risk management guidelines are derived from malpractice cases, often recommending *ideal* or *best* liability prevention practices. The actual standard of care required of a psychiatrist is the skill and care

Table 22–4. Basic elements of therapeutic risk management

Patient centered

Supports treatment and the therapeutic alliance

Working knowledge of legal regulation of psychiatry

Clinical management of psychiatric–legal issues

Wellness, not legal agenda

"First do no harm" ethic

Consultation, "never worry alone"

Source. Adapted from Simon RI: *Assessing and Managing Suicide Risk: Guidelines for Clinically Based Risk Management.* Washington, DC, American Psychiatric Publishing, 2004, p. 19.

Table 22–5. Sample suicide risk assessment note: contents

Suicide risk factors assessed and weighed (low, moderate, high)

Protective factors assessed and weighed (low, moderate, high)

Overall assessment rating (low, moderate, high, or range)

Treatment and management intervention informed by the assessment

Effectiveness of interventions evaluated

Source. Reprinted from Simon RI: "Suicide Risk: Assessing the Unpredictable," in *The American Psychiatric Publishing Textbook of Suicide Assessment and Management.* Edited by Simon RI, Hales RE. Washington, DC, American Psychiatric Publishing, 2006, p. 25.

"ordinarily provided" or reasonable, prudent care. These standards can be confused by expert witnesses who testify in malpractice cases (R.I. Simon 2005). Moreover, suicide cases are fact specific, challenging, multifaceted, and nuanced, making it difficult to provide precise assessment and management guidelines. Although most risk management guidelines commonly set forth best practices, therapeutic risk management is embedded in the provision of sound clinical care and the use of common sense.

Therapeutic risk management is patient centered. It supports the treatment process and the therapeutic alliance (Table 22–4). At a minimum, it follows the fundamental ethical principle in medicine of "first do no harm." A working knowledge of the legal regulation of psychiatry enables the psychiatrist to manage clinical-legal issues more effectively. Therapeutic risk management provides the psychiatrist with a significant measure of practice comfort that permits continued maintenance of the treatment role with patients at risk for suicide.

Performing systematic suicide risk assessments that inform treatment and management interventions is good clinical care and, secondarily, sound therapeutic risk management. Documentation of the risk assessments supports good patient care and substantiates

clinical judgment (American Psychiatric Association 2003). The argument can be made in court by plaintiff's counsel that a suicide risk assessment that was not documented was not performed. Documentation of suicide risk assessments can be done efficiently (Table 22–5). Important clinical assessments require documentation. It is worth repeating that good care of patients at suicidal risk requires the clinician's full commitment to the patient's evaluation, treatment, and management. The clinical imperative holds true as well in collaborative treatment relationships with other mental health professionals.

Conclusion

Suicide risk assessment is a core competency. Systematic suicide risk assessment identifies risk and protective factors that inform the patient's treatment and management. Suicide risk factors must be aggressively treated and protective factors rapidly mobilized. The treatment and management of the suicidal patient require the clinician's full commitment of time and effort.

Patient suicides are an occupational hazard of clinical practice. The psychiatrist should carry comprehensive malpractice insurance from an established professional liability insurer.

Key Points

- Systematic suicide risk assessment informs treatment and management for patients at risk for suicide. It is secondarily a risk management technique.

- Treatable and modifiable acute suicide risk factors should be identified early and treated aggressively.

- Systematic suicide assessment identifies and weights the clinical importance of both risk and protective factors.

- Suicide risk assessment is a process, not an event. Psychiatric inpatients should have suicide risk assessments conducted at admission and discharge and at other important clinical junctures during treatment.

- Suicide prevention contracts must not take the place of conducting systematic suicide risk assessments.

- Contemporaneous documentation of suicide risk assessments is good clinical care and standard practice.

- Systematic suicide risk assessment performed at the time of discharge informs the patient's postdischarge plan.

- During the treatment of patients at significant risk for suicide, it may be necessary to contact family members or others to facilitate hospitalization, to mobilize support, and to acquire information of clinical importance to the clinician. Whenever possible, this should be done with the patient's permission.

- Suicide risk assessment is the responsibility of the psychiatrist. It should not be delegated to others.

- The treatment and management of the patient at risk for suicide require the clinician's full commitment of time and effort, despite denial of services and cost-containment policies of third-party payers.

Suggested Readings

American Academy of Child and Adolescent Psychiatry: Summary of the practice parameters for the assessment and treatment of children and adolescents with suicidal behaviors. J Am Acad Child Adolesc Psychiatry 40:495–499, 2001

American Psychiatric Association: Practice guidelines for the assessment and treatment of patients with suicidal behaviors. Am J Psychiatry 160 (suppl):1–60, 2003

Berman AL, Jobes DA, Silverman M: Adolescent Suicide: Assessment and Intervention, 2nd Edition. Washington, DC, American Psychological Association, 2006

Chiles JA, Strosahl KD: Clinical Manual for Assessment and Treatment of Suicidal Patients. Washington, DC, American Psychiatric Publishing, 2006

Goldsmith SK, Pellman TC, Kleinman AM, et al. (eds): Reducing Suicide: A National Imperative. Washington, DC, National Academies Press, 2001

Rudd MD, Joiner T, Rajab MH: Treating Suicidal Behavior: An Effective, Time-Limited Approach. New York, Guilford, 2001

Shea SC: The delicate art of eliciting suicidal ideation. Psychiatr Ann 34:385–400, 2004

Simon RI: Assessing and Managing Suicide Risk: Guidelines for Clinically Based Risk Management. Washington, DC, American Psychiatric Publishing, 2004

Simon RI, Hales RE (eds): The American Psychiatric Publishing Textbook of Suicide Assessment and Management. Washington, DC, American Psychiatric Publishing, 2006

References

Amchin J, Wettstein RM, Roth LH: Suicide, ethics, and the law, in Suicide Over the Life Cycle. Edited by Blumenthal SJ, Kupfer DJ. Washington, DC, American Psychiatric Press, 1990, pp 637–663

American Academy of Child and Adolescent Psychiatry: Summary of the practice parameters for the assessment and treatment of children and adolescents with suicidal behaviors. J Am Acad Child Adolesc Psychiatry 40:495–499, 2001

American Psychiatric Association: The Practice of Electroconvulsive Therapy: Recommendations for Treatment, Training, and Privileging. A Task Force Report of the American Psychiatric Association, 2nd Edition. Edited by Weiner RD. Washington, DC, American Psychiatric Association, 2001

American Psychiatric Association: Practice guidelines for the assessment and treatment of patients with suicidal behaviors. Am J Psychiatry 160 (suppl):1–60, 2003

Ash P: Children and adolescents, in The American Psychiatric Publishing Textbook of Suicide Assessment and Management. Edited by Simon RI, Hales RE. Washington, DC, American Psychiatric Publishing, 2006, pp 35–56

Baldessarini RJ: Lithium effects on depression and suicide. J Clin Psychiatry (visuals), January 2003

Baldessarini RJ, Tondo L, Henner J: Treating the suicidal patient with bipolar disorder: reducing suicide risk with lithium. Ann NY Acad Sci 932:24–38, 2001

Bateman AW, Fonagy P: Psychotherapy for Borderline Personality Disorder: Mentalization-Based Treatment. Oxford, England, Oxford University Press, 2000

Bateman AW, Fonagy P: Mentalization-based treatment of BPD. J Personal Disord 18:36–51, 2004

Beck AT, Steer RA, Kovacs M, et al: Hopelessness and eventual suicide: a 10-year prospective study of patients hospitalized with suicidal ideation. Am J Psychiatry 142:559–562, 1985

Beck AT, Brown G, Berchick RJ, et al: Relationship between hopelessness and ultimate suicide: a replication with psychiatric outpatients. Am J Psychiatry 147:190–195, 1990

Beck AT, Steer RA, Ranieri WF: Scale for suicidal ideation: psychometric properties of a self-report version. J Clin Psychol 44:499–505, 1998

Bongar B, Maris RW, Bertram AL, et al: Outpatient standards of care and the suicidal patient. Suicide Life Threat Behav 22:453–478, 1992

Brent DA, Bridge J, Johnson BA, et al: Suicidal behavior runs in families. Arch Gen Psychiatry 53:1145–1152, 1996

Brent DA, Oquendo M, Birmaher B, et al: Familial pathways to early onset suicide attempt. Arch Gen Psychiatry 59:801–807, 2002

Brodsky BS, Malone KM, Ellis SP, et al: Characteristics of borderline personality disorder associated with suicidal behavior. Am J Psychiatry 154:1715–1719, 1997

Brown GK, Ten Have T, Henriques GR, et al: Cognitive therapy for the prevention of suicide attempts. JAMA 294:536–570, 2005

Busch KA, Clark DC, Fawcett J, et al: Clinical features of inpatient suicide. Psychiatr Ann 23:256–262, 1993

Clark DC, Fawcett J: An empirically based model of suicide risk assessment of patients with affective disorders, in Suicide and Clinical Practice. Edited by Jacobs DJ. Washington, DC, American Psychiatric Association, 1999, pp 55–73

Dervic K, Oquendo MA, Grunebaum MF, et al: Religious affiliation and suicide attempt. Am J Psychiatry 161:2303–2308, 2004

Duberstein P, Conwell Y: Personality disorders and completed suicide: a methodological and conceptual review. Clinical Psychology: Science and Practice 4:359–376, 1997

Egan MP: Contracting for safety: a concept analysis. Crisis 18:23, 1997

Farwell v. Un, 902 F.2d 282 (4th Cir. 1990)

Fawcett J: Treating impulsivity and anxiety in the suicidal patient. Ann NY Acad Sci 932:94–105, 2001

Fawcett J, Scheftner WA, Fogg L, et al: Time-related predictors of suicide in major affective disorder. Am J Psychiatry 147:1189–1194, 1990

Fawcett J, Clark DC, Busch KA: Assessing and treating the patient at suicide risk. Psychiatr Ann 23:244 255, 1993

Fawcett J, Busch KA, Jacobs DG: Clinical correlates of inpatient suicide. J Clin Psychiatry 64:14–19, 2003

Gabbard GO, Allison SE: Psychodynamic treatment, in The American Psychiatric Publishing Textbook of Suicide Assessment and Management. Edited by Simon RI, Hales RE. Washington, DC, American Psychiatric Publishing, 2006, pp 221–234

Gelenberg AJ, Chesen CL: How fast are antidepressants? J Clin Psychiatry 61:712–721, 2000

Gibbons RD, Brown CH, Hur K, et al: Early evidence on the effects of regulators' suicidality warnings on SSRI prescriptions and suicide in children and adolescents. Am J Psychiatry 164:1356–1363, 2007

Goldsmith SK, Pellman TC, Kleinman AM, et al (eds): Reducing Suicide: A National Imperative. Washington, DC, National Academies Press, 2001

Guthrie E, Kapur N, Mackway-Jones K, et al: Randomized controlled trial of brief psychological intervention after deliberate self-poisoning. BMJ 323:135–138, 2001

Guthrie E, Kapur N, Mackway-Jones K, et al: Predictors of outcome following brief psychodynamic-interpersonal therapy deliberate self-poisoning. Aust N Z J Psychiatry 37:532–536, 2003

Hall RC, Platt DE, Hall RC: Suicide risk assessment: a review of risk factors for suicide in 100 patients who made severe suicide attempts: evaluation of suicide risk in a time of managed care. Psychosomatics 40:18–27, 1999

Hammad TA, Laughren T, Raloosin J: Suicidality in pediatric patients treated with antidepressant drugs. Arch Gen Psychiatry 63:332–339, 2006

Harris CE, Barraclough B: Suicide as an outcome for mental disorders. Br J Psychiatry 170:205–228, 1997

Hawton K, Townsend E, Arensman E, et al: Psychosocial and pharmacological treatments for deliberate self-harm. Cochrane Database Syst Rev (2):CD001764, 2005

Heikkinen ME, Henriksson MM, Erkki T, et al: Recent life events and suicide in personality disorders. J Nerv Ment Dis 185:373–381, 1997

Isometsa ET, Lonnqvist JK: Suicide attempts preceding completed suicide. Br J Psychiatry 173:531–535, 1998

Isometsa ET, Henriksson ME, Heikkinen ME, et al: Suicide among subjects with personality disorders. Am J Psychiatry 153:667–673, 1996

Jacobs DG, Brewer M, Klein-Benheim M: Suicide assessment: an overview and recommended protocol, in Guide to Suicide Assessment and Intervention. Edited by Jacobs DJ. San Francisco, CA, Jossey-Bass, 1999, pp 3–39

Johnson v. United States, 409 F.Supp. 1283 (M.D. Fla. 1976); revised, 576 F.2d 606 (5th Cir. 1978); cert denied, 451 U.S. 1019 (1981)

Kellner CH, Fink M, Knapp R, et al: Relief of expressed suicidal intent by ECT: a consortium of research in ECT study. Am J Psychiatry 162:977–982, 2005

Kessing LV: Subtypes of depressive episodes according to ICD-10: prediction of risk of relapse and suicide. Psychopathology 36:285–291, 2003

Kessler RC, Borges G, Walters EE: Prevalence of and risk factors for lifetime suicide attempts in the National Comorbidity Survey. Arch Gen Psychiatry 55:617–626, 1999

Kim HF, Marangell LB, Yudofsky SC: Pharmacological treatment and electroconvulsive therapy, in The American Psychiatric Publishing Textbook of Suicide Assessment and Management. Edited by Simon RI, Hales RE. Washington, DC, American Psychiatric Publishing, 2006, pp 199–220

Lieberman DZ, Resnik HLP, Holder-Perkins V: Environmental risk factors in hospital suicide. Suicide Life Threat Behav 34:448–453, 2004

Linehan MM: Cognitive Behavioral Treatment of Borderline Personality Disorder. New York, Guilford, 1993

Linehan MM, Goodstein JL, Nielsen SL, et al: Reasons for staying alive when you are thinking of killing yourself: the Reasons for Living Inventory. J Consult Clin Psychol 51:276–286, 1983

Linehan MM, Comtois KA, Murray AM, et al: Two-year randomized controlled trial and follow-up of dialectical behavior therapy vs therapy by experts for suicidal behaviors and borderline personality disorder. Arch Gen Psychiatry 63:757–766, 2006

Malone KM, Haas GL, Sweeney JA, et al: Major depression and the risk of attempted suicide. J Affect Disord 34:173–185–1995a

Malone KM, Szanto K, Corbitt EM, et al: Clinical assessment versus research methods in the assessment of suicidal behavior. Am J Psychiatry 152:1601–1607, 1995b

Mann JJ, Waternaux C, Haas GL, et al: Toward a clinical model of suicidal behavior in psychiatric patients. Am J Psychiatry 156:181–189, 1999

Mann JJ, Brent DA, Arango V: The neurobiology and genetics of suicide and suicide attempts: a focus on the serotonergic system. Neuropsychopharmacology 24:467–477, 2001

Mass. Gen. Laws, Ch. 233, Sec 23D (1986)

Mays D: Structured assessment methods may improve suicide prevention. Psychiatr Ann 34:367–372, 2004

Meltzer HY: Treatment of suicidality in schizophrenia. Ann NY Acad Sci 932:44–58, 2001

Meltzer HY, Alphs L, Green AI, et al: Clozapine treatment for suicidality in schizophrenia. Arch Gen Psychiatry 60:82–91, 2003

Monahan J, Steadman HJ: Violent storms and violent people: how meteorology can inform risk communication in mental health law. Am J Psychol 51:931–938, 1996

Murphy GE, Wetzel RD, Robins E, et al: Multiple risk factors predict suicide in alcoholism. Arch Gen Psychiatry 49:459–462, 1992

Oquendo MA, Halberstam, Mann JJ: Risk factors for suicidal behavior: the utility and limitation of research instruments, in Standardized Evaluation in Clinical Practice. Edited by First MB (Review of Psychiatry Series, Vol 22; Oldham JM and Riba MB, series eds). Washington, DC, American Psychiatric Publishing, 2003, pp 103–130

Ostamo A, Lonnqvist J: Excess mortality of suicide attempters. Soc Psychiatry Psychiatr Epidemiol 36:29–35, 2001

Palmer BA, Pankratz S, Bostwick JM: The lifetime risk of suicide in schizophrenia. Arch Gen Psychiatry 62:247–253, 2005

Pokorny AD: Predictions of suicide in psychiatric patients: report of a prospective study. Arch Gen Psychiatry 40:249–257, 1983

Pokorny AD: Suicide prediction revisited. Suicide Life Threat Behav 23:1–10, 1993

Prudic J, Sackheim H: Electroconvulsive therapy and suicide risk. J Clin Psychiatry 60 (suppl):104–110, 1999

Radomsky ED, Haas GL, Mann JJ, et al: Suicidal behavior in patients with schizophrenia and other psychotic disorders. Am J Psychiatry 156:1590–1595, 1999

Regehr C, Gutheil TG: Apology, justice and trauma recovery. J Am Acad Psychiatry Law 30:425–430, 2002

Resnick PJ: Recognizing that the suicidal patient views you as an adversary. Curr Psychiatr 1:8, 2002

Robins E: The Final Months: Study of the Lives of 134 Persons Who Committed Suicide. New York, Oxford University Press, 1981

Rudd MD, Joiner T, Rajab MH: Treating Suicidal Behavior: An Effective, Time-Limited Approach. New York, Guilford, 2001

Sareen J, Cox BJ, Afifi TO, et al: Anxiety disorders and risk for suicidal ideation and suicide attempts: a population-based longitudinal study of adults. Arch Gen Psychiatry 62:1249–1257, 2005

Scheiber SC, Kramer TSM, Adamowski SE: Core Competence for Psychiatric Practice: What Clinicians Need to Know. Washington, DC, American Psychiatric Publishing, 2003

Schulsinger F, Kety SS, Rosenthal D, et al: A family study of suicide, in Origins, Prevention and Treatment of Affective Disorders. Edited by Schou M, Stromgen F. London, Academic Press, 1979, pp 277–287

Sharma V: Retrospective controlled study of inpatient ECT: does it prevent suicide? J Affect Disord 56:183–187, 1999

Shea SC: The delicate art of eliciting suicidal ideation. Psychiatr Ann 34:385–400, 2004

Silk K: Split (collaborative) treatment for patients with personality disorders. Psychiatr Ann 31:615–622, 2001

Simon GE, Savarino J, Opersklaski B, et al: Suicide risk during antidepressant treatment. Am J Psychiatry 163:41–47, 2006

Simon RI: Clinical Psychiatry and the Law, 2nd Edition. Washington, DC, American Psychiatric Press, 1992

Simon RI: The suicidal patient, in The Mental Health Practitioner and the Law: A Comprehensive Handbook. Edited by Lifson LE, Simon RI. Cambridge, MA, Harvard University Press, 1998, pp 329–343

Simon RI: Taking the "sue" out of suicide: a forensic psychiatrist's perspective. Psychiatr Ann 30:399–4071, 2000

Simon RI: Suicide risk assessment: what is the standard of care? J Am Acad Psychiatry Law 30:340–344, 2002

Simon RI: Assessing and Managing Suicide Risk: Guidelines for Clinically Based Risk Management. Washington, DC, American Psychiatric Publishing, 2004

Simon RI: Best practices or reasonable care? J Am Acad Psychiatry Law 33:8–11, 2005

Simon RI: Patient safety versus freedom of movement: coping with uncertainty, in The American Psychiatric Publishing Textbook of Suicide Assessment and Management. Edited by Simon RI, Hales RE. Washington, DC, American Psychiatric Publishing, 2006, pp 423–439

Simon RI: Gun safety management with patients at risk for suicide. Suicide Life Threat Behav 37:518–526, 2007

Simon RI, Shuman DW: The standard of care in suicide risk assessment: an elusive concept. CNS Spectr 11:442–445, 2006

Slovenko R: Psychiatry in Law/Law in Psychiatry. New York, Brunner-Routledge, 2002

Stanford EJ, Goetz RR, Bloom JD: The no harm contract in the emergency assessment of suicidal risk. J Clin Psychiatry 55:344–348, 1994

Trémeau F, Staner L, Duval F, et al: Suicide attempts and family history of suicide in three psychiatric populations. Suicide Life Threat Behav 35:702–713, 2005

Warman DM, Forman E, Henriques GR, et al: Suicidality and psychosis: beyond depression and hopelessness. Suicide Life Threat Behav 34:77–86, 2004

INDEX

*Page numbers printed in **boldface** type refer to tables or figures.*